William M. Wells
Alan Colchester   Scott Delp   (Eds.)

Medical Image Computing and Computer-Assisted Intervention – MICCAI'98

First International Conference
Cambridge, MA, USA, October 11-13, 1998
Proceedings

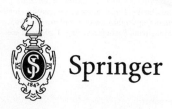

Springer

Series Editors

Gerhard Goos, Karlsruhe University, Germany
Juris Hartmanis, Cornell University, NY, USA
Jan van Leeuwen, Utrecht University, The Netherlands

Volume Editors

William M. Wells
Harvard Medical School and
Brigham and Women's Hospital, Department of Radiology
75 Francis Street, Boston, MA 02115, USA
E-mail: sw@ai.mit.edu

Alan Colchester
University of Kent
Canterbury, Kent CT2 7NT, UK
E-mail: a.colchester@ukc.ac.uk

Scott Delp
Northwestern University
Departments of Biomedical Engineering
and Physical Medicine and Rehabilitation
345 East Superior Street, Chicago, IL 60611, USA
E-mail: delp@nwu.edu

Cataloging-in-Publication data applied for

Die Deutsche Bibliothek - CIP-Einheitsaufnahme

Medical image computing and computer assisted intervention : first international conference ; proceedings / MICCAI '98, Cambridge, MA, USA, Ocober 11 - 13, 1998. William M. Wells ... (ed.). - Berlin ; Heidelberg ; New York ; Barcelona ; Budapest ; Hong Kong ; London ; Milan ; Paris ; Singapore ; Tokyo : Springer, 1998
  (Lecture notes in computer science ; Vol. 1496)
  ISBN 3-540-65136-5

CR Subject Classification (1991): I.5, I.3.5-8. I.2.9-10, I.4, J.3

ISSN 0302-9743
ISBN 3-540-65136-5 Springer-Verlag Berlin Heidelberg New York

This work is subject to copyright. All rights are reserved, whether the whole or part of the material is concerned, specifically the rights of translation, reprinting, re-use of illustrations, recitation, broadcasting, reproduction on microfilms or in any other way, and storage in data banks. Duplication of this publication or parts thereof is permitted only under the provisions of the German Copyright Law of September 9, 1965, in its current version, and permission for use must always be obtained from Springer-Verlag. Violations are liable for prosecution under the German Copyright Law.

© Springer-Verlag Berlin Heidelberg 1998
Printed in Germany

Typesetting: Camera-ready by author
SPIN 10639055   06/3142 – 5 4 3 2 1 0   Printed on acid-free paper

Preface

MICCAI was formed by the joining of the vigorous strands of research in the fields of medical image analysis, computer assisted interventions, medical robotics, and visualization. In the past, these activities were highlighted in three parallel conferences: Visualization in Biomedical Computing (VBC), Medical Robotics and Computer Assisted Surgery (MRCAS), and Computer Vision, Virtual Reality, and Robotics in Medicine (CVRMED). All of these conferences originated in the early 1990's, with VBC having the longest tradition.

The substantial overlap of the research and the communities represented by these meetings led to the idea of forming a single international flagship meeting, to be held annually. A series of discussions quickly led to a unanimous agreement on the form of the conference: a representation of the highest possible quality of research in the combined community, to be selected by peer review from full papers and to be presented in a single track of oral and poster sessions. Slightly more time was needed to name the conference, and the community finally settled on MICCAI.

Due to the interdisciplinary nature of our emerging field, interested scientists are burdened with the need to train in additional areas – the computer scientists have to learn about medicine, while the medical doctors have to learn about computer science. Beyond the challenges of their own research, they have to address the issue of how to communicate their science to those in other fields. We hope that MICCAI will serve as a forum to encourage this cross-disciplinary discussion, and enable each sub-community to appreciate the issues of most concern to their counterparts.

We are delighted with the response from the community for this inaugural meeting, which is reflected by the high quality of the papers in these proceedings. The program chairs relied on our highly qualified program committee for the reviews. Each paper was reviewed independently by 2–4 reviewers, matched as well as possible in their background to the topic of the paper. For the final process, we assembled a group of senior members of the executive and program committees in Boston in order to decide on the papers. Of the 243 papers submitted for review, 134 were accepted for presentation. With such strong interest we can already plan for next year's meeting in England.

It is our distinct pleasure to welcome you to Boston and Cambridge. We look forward to an exciting conference.

October 1998　　　　　Takeyoshi Dohi, W. Eric L. Grimson and Ron Kikinis
General Co-Chairs
MICCAI98

Organization

First International Conference on
Medical Image Computing and Computer-Assisted Intervention
Massachusetts Institute of Technology, Cambridge, MA, USA
October 11–13, 1998

A unified conference formed by the merger of CVRMed, MRCAS, and VBC
Computer Vision, Virtual Reality and Robotics in Medicine, Medical Robotics
and Computer Assisted Surgery, Visualization in Biomedical Computing

Executive Committee

Nicholas Ayache   INRIA Sophia Antipolis, France
Anthony DiGioia   Shadyside Hospital – USA
James Duncan   Yale University, USA
Karl-Heinz Höhne   University of Hamburg, Germany
Stephane Lavallée   Laboratoire TIMC/IMAG, FR
Stephen Pizer   University of North Carolina, USA
Richard Robb   Mayo Clinic, USA
Russell Taylor   Johns Hopkins University, USA

General Co-Chairs

Takeyoshi Dohi   University of Tokyo, JP
Ron Kikinis   Harvard Medical School, USA
W. Eric L. Grimson   MIT, USA

Program Committee Co-Chairs

Alan Colchester   University of Kent, UK
Scott Delp   Northwestern University, Chicago, USA
William Wells   Harvard Medical School, USA

Program Committee

James Anderson	Johns Hopkins University, USA
Takehide Asano	Chiba University, JP
Nicholas Ayache	INRIA Sophia Antipolis, FR
Ruzena Bajcsy	University of Pennsylvania, USA
Andre Bauer	Berufsgenossenschaftliche Unfallklinik, DE
Isabelle Bloch	Ecole Nationale Superieure de Telecom, FR
Michel Bolla	Grenoble Hospital, FR
Fred Bookstein	University of Michigan, USA
Michael Brady	Oxford University, UK
Peter Brett	University of Bristol, UK
Richard Bucholz	St. Louis University Medical Center, USA
Grigore Burdea	Rutgers University, USA
Colin Caro	Imperial College, UK
Steven Charles	University of Tennessee, USA
Phillipe Cinquin	Laboratoire TIMC/IMAG, FR
Jean-Louis Coatrieux	Rennes University, FR
Ela Clarigde	University of Birmingham, UK
Court Cutting	New York University, USA
Jacques Darcourt	Nice University, FR
Paolo Dario	ARTS Lab, IT
Brian Davies	Imperial College, UK
Anthony DiGioia	Shadyside Hospital, USA
Takeyoshi Dohi	University of Tokyo, JP
James Drake	Hospital for Sick Children, USA
James Duncan	Yale University, USA
Alan C. Evans	Montreal Neurological Institute, CAN
Norberto Ezquerra	Georgia Tech, USA
Elliot Fishman	Johns Hopkins University, USA
J. Michael Fitzpatrick	Vanderbilt University, USA
Thomas Fortin	Grenoble University, FR
Henry Fuchs	University of North Carolina, USA
Toshi Fukuda	Nagoya University, USA
Guido Gerig	Communications Tech. Lab, CH
Sarah Gibson	Mitsubishi Electric Research Lab, USA
Michael Goris	Stanford University Medical Center, USA
Frank Gosse	Hanover Medical School, USA
Erik Granum	Aalborg University
W. Eric L. Grimson	MIT, USA
Blake Hannaford	University of Washington, USA
David Hawkes	Guy's Hospital, UK
William Heinrichs	Stanford University, USA
Derek Hill	Guy's Hospital, UK
Karl-Heinz Höhne	University of Hamburg, DE
Robert Howe	Harvard University, USA
Koji Ikuta	Nagoya University, JP
Branislav Jaramaz	Shadyside Hospital, USA
Chris Johnson	University of Utah, USA

Program Committee

Ferenc Jolesz	Harvard Medical School, USA
Leo Joskowicz	Hebrew University of Jerusalem, ISR
Takeo Kanade	Carnegie Mellon University, USA
Arie Kaufman	State Univ. of New York, Stony Brook, USA
Louis Kavoussi	Johns Hopkins University, USA
Peter Kazanzides	Integrated Surgical Systems, USA
Ron Kikinis	Harvard Medical School, USA
Yong Min Kim	University of Washington, USA
Andres Kriete	University of Giessen, DE
Heinz Lemke	Tech. University, DE
Stephane Lavallée	Laboratoire TIMC/IMAG, FR
Bill Lorensen	General Electric, USA
Robert Maciunas	Vanderbilt University, USA
Grégoire Malandain	INRIA Sophia, FR
Majrilio Marcacci	Istituti Ortopedici Rizzoli, IT
Tim McInerney	MIT USA, University of Toronto, CAN
Dwight Meglan	Mitsubishi Electric Research Lab, USA
Philippe Merloz	Grenoble Hospital, FR
Dimitris Metaxas	University of Pennsylvania, USA
Chuck Meyer	University of Michigan, USA
Brent Mittlestadt	Integrated Surgical Systems, USA
Heinrich Muller	University of Dortmund, DE
Alison Noble	Oxford University, UK
Lutz Nolte	M.E. Muller Institute, CH
Wieslaw Nowinski	Kent Ridge Digital Labs, Singapore
Charles Pelizzari	University of Chicago, USA
Michael Peshkin	Northwestern University, USA
Stephen Pizer	University of North Carolina, USA
Rob Playter	Cambridge Dynamics, USA
Glenn Preminger	Duke University Medical Center, USA
Jerry Prince	Johns Hopkins University, USA
Klaus Radermacher	Helmholtz Inst of Aachen, DE
Hans Reinhardt	Neurosurgical University Clinic, CH
Richard Robb	Mayo Clinic, USA
Jean-Marie Rocchisani	Hopital Avicenne, FR
Joseph Rosen	Dartmouth-Hitchcock Medical Center, USA
Jonathan Sackier	UCSD Medical Center, USA
Ichiro Sakuma	Tokyo Denki University, JP
Tim Salcudean	University of British Columbia, CAN
Kenneth Salisbury	MIT, USA
Richard Satava	Yale University, USA
Paul Schenker	Jet Propulsion Laboratory, USA
Achim Schweikard	TU Muenchen, DE
H. Siegfried Stiehl	University of Hamburg, DE
David Stulberg	Northwestern University, USA
Paul Suetens	KU Leuven, BEL

Program Committee

Naoki Suzuki   Tokyo Jikei University, JP
Gabor Szekèly   Communications Tech. Lab, CH
Mark Talamini   Johns Hopkins University, USA
Chris Taylor   University of Manchester, UK
Russ Taylor   Johns Hopkins University, USA
Frank Tendick   University of California San Francisco, USA
Demetri Terzopoulos   University of Toronto, CAN
Jean-Philippe Thirion   INRIA Sophia, FR
David Thomas   National Hospital, UK
Andrew Todd-Pokropek   University College London, UK
Jocelyne Troccaz   Laboratoire TIMC/IMAG, FR
Jay Udupa   University of Pennsylvania, USA
Dirk Vandermeulen   University of Leuven, BEL
Marcel Van Herk   The Netherlands Cancer Institute, NETH
Michael Vannier   University of Iowa Hospitals and Clinics, USA
Baba Vemuri   University of Florida, USA
Max A. Viergever   Utrecht University, NETH
Simon Warfield   Harvard Medical School, USA
Eiju Watanabe   Tokyo Metropolitan Police Hospital, JP
Lee Weiss   Carnegie Mellon University, USA
James Zinreich   Johns Hopkins University, USA

Sponsoring Institutions

Harvard Medical School, Boston, MA, USA
Massachusetts Institute of Technology, MA, USA

Table of Contents

Surgical Planning

Planning and Evaluation of Reorienting Osteotomies of the Proximal Femur in Cases of SCFE Using Virtual Three-Dimensional Models 1
    J.A. Richolt, M. Teschner, P. Everett, B. Girod, M.B. Millis and R. Kikinis

Computer-Aided Planning of Patellofemoral Joint OA Surgery: Developing Physical Models from Patient MRI 9
    Z.A. Cohen, D.M. McCarthy, H. Roglic, J.H. Henry, W.G. Rodkey, J.R. Steadman, V.C. Mow and G.A. Ateshian

Computer Assisted Orthognathic Surgery 21
    B. Mollard, S. Lavallée and G. Bettega

Computer-Aided Image-Guided Bone Fracture Surgery: Modeling, Visualization, and Preoperative Planning 29
    L. Tockus, L. Joskowicz, A. Simkin and C. Milgrom

Surgical Navigation and Measurements

A Surgical Planning and Guidance System for High Tibial Osteotomies ... 39
    C.Y. Tso, R.E. Ellis, J. Rudan and M.M. Harrison

Measurement of Intraoperative Brain Surface Deformation Under a Craniotomy 51
    C.R. Maurer, Jr., D.L.G. Hill, R.J. Maciunas, J.A. Barwise, J.M. Fitzpatrick and M.Y. Wang

Clinical Experience with a High Precision Image-Guided Neurosurgery System 63
    W.E.L. Grimson, M.E. Leventon, G. Ettinger, A. Chabrerie, F. Ozlen, S. Nakajima, H. Atsumi, R. Kikinis and P. Black

Three-Dimensional Reconstruction and Surgical Navigation in Pediatric Epilepsy Surgery... 74
    A. Chabrerie, F. Ozlen, S. Nakajima, M.E. Leventon, H. Atsumi, W.E.L. Grimson, E. Keeve, S. Helmers, J. Riviello Jr., G. Holmes, F. Duffy, F. Jolesz, R. Kikinis and P. Black

Treatment of Pelvic Ring Fractures: Percutaneous Computer Assisted Iliosacral Screwing 84
    L. Carrat, J. Tonetti, S. Lavallée, P. Merloz, L. Pittet and J.-P. Chirossel

Cardiac Image Analysis

Model Tags: Direct 3D Tracking of Heart Wall Motion from Tagged
Magnetic Resonance Images 92
    A.A. Young

Quantitative Three Dimensional Echocardiograpy: Methodology,
Validation, and Clinical Applications 102
    F.H. Sheehan, E.L. Bolson, R.W. Martin, G. Bashein and J. McDonald

Measurement of 3D Motion of Myocardial Material Points from Explicit
B-Surface Reconstruction of Tagged MRI Data 110
    A.A. Amini, P. Radeva, M. Elayyadi and D. Li

Cardiac Image Analysis II

Multiscale Vessel Enhancement Filtering 130
    A.F. Frangi, W.J. Niessen, K.L. Vincken and M.A. Viergever

Fast Quantification of Abdominal Aortic Aneurysms from CTA Volumes .. 138
    O. Wink, W.J. Niessen and M.A. Viergever

3-D Fusion of Biplane Angiography and Intravascular Ultrasound for
Accurate Visualization and Volumetry 146
    A. Wahle, G.P.M. Prause, S.C. DeJong and M. Sonka

Patient-Specific Analysis of Left Ventricular Blood Flow 156
    T.N. Jones and D.N. Metaxas

Dense 2d Displacement Reconstruction from SPAMM-MRI with
Constrained Elastic Splines: Implementation and Validation 167
    A.A. Amini, Y. Chen, J. Sun and V. Mani

Motion Analysis of the Right Ventricle from MRI Images 177
    E. Haber, D.N. Metaxas and L. Axel

Magnetic Resonance Guided Radiofrequency Ablation: Creation and
Visualization of Cardiac Lesions 189
    A.C. Lardo, H. Halperin, C. Yeung, P. Jumrussirikul, E. Atalar and E. McVeigh

Medical Robotic Systems

Human Versus Robotic Organ Retraction During Laparoscopic Nissen
Fundoplication 197
    B. Poulouse, M. Kutka, M. Mendoza-Sagaon, A. Barnes, C. Yang,
R.H. Taylor and M. Talamini

A New Laparoscope Manipulator with an Optical Zoom 207
    E. Kobayashi, K. Masamune, T. Dohi and D. Hashimoto

A Newly Developed Stereotactic Robot with Detachable Drive for
Neurosurgery 215
    K. Masamune, L.H. Ji, M. Suzuki, T. Dohi, H. Iseki and K. Takakura

Calibration of Video Cameras to the Coordinate System of a Radiation
Therapy Treatment Machine 223
    S.W. Hadley, L.S. Johnson and C.A. Pelizzari

An Image Overlay System for Medical Data Visualization 232
    M. Blackwell, C. Nikou, A.M. DiGioia and T. Kanade

Surgical Systems and Simulators

Volumetric Image Guidance via a Stereotactic Endoscope 241
    R. Shahidi, B. Wang, M. Epitaux, R. Grzeszczuk and J. Adler

The Application Accuracy of the Frameless Implantable Marker System
and Analysis of Related Affecting Factors 253
    Q. Li, L. Zamorano, Z. Jiang, F. Vinas and F. Diaz

Multi-level Strategy for Computer-Assisted Transbronchial Biopsy 261
    I. Bricault, G. Ferretti and P. Cinquin

A Fast, Accurate and Easy Method to Position Oral Implant Using
Computed Tomography. Clinical Validations 269
    G. Champleboux, T. Fortin, H. Buatois, J.L. Coudert and E. Blanchet

Experimental Protocol for Accuracy Evaluation of 6-d Localizers for
Computer-Integrated Surgery: Application to Four Optical Localizers 277
    F. Chassat, S. Lavallée

Visualization and Evaluation of Prostate Needle Biopsy 285
    J. Zeng, C. Kaplan, J. Bauer, I.A. Sesterhenn, J.W. Moul and S.K. Mun

Virtual Endoscope System with Force Sensation 293
    K. Ikuta, M. Takeichi and T. Namiki

Using Region-of-Interest Based Finite Element Modeling for Brain-Surgery
Simulation 305
    K.V. Hansen, O.V. Larsen

An Image Processing Environment for Guiding Vascular MR Interventions 317
  R. van der Weide, K.J. Zuiderveld, C.J.G. Bakker, C. Bos, H.F.M. Smits, T. Hoogenboom, J.J. van Vaals and M.A. Viergever

Fluroscopic Image Processing for Computer-Aided Orthopaedic Surgery .. 325
  Z. Yaniv, L. Joskowicz, A. Simkin, M. Garza-Jinich and C. Milgrom

Probe Design to Robustly Locate Anatomical Features 335
  K.B. Inkpen, R.J Emrich and A.J. Hodgson

Concepts and Results in the Development of a Hybrid Tracking System
for Computer Aided Surgery 343
  W. Birkfellner, F. Watzinger, F. Wanschitz, G. Enislidis, M. Truppe, R. Ewers and H. Bergmann

Computer-Assisted Interstitial Brachytherapy 352
  W. Freysinger, E. Hensler, A.R. Gunkel, R.J. Bale, M. Vogele, A. Martin, T. Auer, P. Eichberger, A. Szankay, T. Auberger, K.H. Künzel, O. Gaber, W.F. Thumfart and P.H. Lukas

3-D Model Supported Prostate Biopsy Simulation and Evaluation 358
  J. Xuan, Y. Wang, I.A. Sesterhenn, J.W. Moul and S.K. Mun

Human Factors in Tele-inspection and Tele-surgery: Cooperative
Manipulation under Asynchronous Video and Control Feedback 368
  J.M. Thompson, M.P. Ottensmeyer and T.B. Sheridan

Computer Assisted Coronary Intervention by Use of On-line
3d Reconstruction and Optimal View Strategy........................ 377
  S.-Y. J. Chen and J.D. Carroll

Medical Robotic Systems II

A Robotic Approach to HIFU Based Neurosurgery 386
  B.L. Davies, S. Chauhan and M.J.S Lowe

Virtual Surgery System Using Deformable Organ Models and Force
Feedback System with Three Fingers 397
  N. Suzuki, A. Hattori, A. Takatsu, T. Kumano, A. Ikemoto and Y. Adachi

A Modular Surgical Robotic System for Image Guided Percutaneous
Procedures 404
  D. Stoianovici, L.L. Whitcomb, J.H. Anderson, R.H. Taylor and L.R. Kavoussi

Optimum Designed Micro Active Forceps with Built-in Fiberscope for
Retinal Microsurgery 411
  K. Ikuta, T. Kato and S. Nagata

Gauging Clinical Practice: Surgical Navigation for Total Hip Replacement . 421
  J.E. Moody Jr., A.M. DiGioia, B. Jaramaz, M. Blackwell, B. Colgan and C. Nikou

Segmentation

Adaptive Template Moderated Spatially Varying Statistical Classification . 431
  S.K. Warfield, M. Kaus, F.A. Jolesz and R. Kikinis

Automatic Quantification of MS Lesions in 3D MRI Brain Data Sets: Validation of INSECT 439
  A. Zijdenbos, R. Forghani and A.C. Evans

Computer-Aided Diagnostic System for Pulmonary Nodules Using Helical CT Images 449
  K. Kanazawa, Y. Kawata, N. Niki, H. Satoh, H. Ohmatsu, R. Kakinuma, M. Kaneko, K. Eguchi and N. Moriyama

Enhanced Spatial Priors for Segmentation of Magnetic Resonance Imagery 457
  T. Kapur, W.E.L. Grimson, R. Kikinis and W.M. Wells

Exploring the Discrimination Power of the Time Domain for Segmentation and Characterization of Lesions in Serial MR Data 469
  G. Gerig, D. Welti, C.R.G. Guttmann, A.C.F Colchester and G. Székely

Computational Neuroanatomy

Reconstruction of the Central Layer of the Human Cerebral Cortex from MR Images 481
  C. Xu, D.L. Pham, J.L. Prince, M.E. Etemad and D.N. Yu

Regularization of MR Diffusion Tensor Maps for Tracking Brain White Matter Bundles 489
  C. Poupon, J.-F. Mangin, V. Frouin, J. Régis, F. Poupon, M. Pachot-Clouard, D. Le Bihan and I. Bloch

Measurement of Brain Structures Based on Statistical and Geometrical 3D Segmentation 499
  M. Á. González Ballester, A. Zisserman and M. Brady

Automatic Identification of Cortical Sulci Using a 3D Probabilistic Atlas .. 509
  G. Le Goualher, D.L. Collins, C. Barillot and A.C. Evans

Segmentation and Measurement of the Cortex from 3D MR Images 519
  X. Zeng, L. H. Staib, R.T. Schultz and J.S. Duncan

Biomechanics

A Biomechanical Model of Soft Tissue Deformation, with Applications to
Non-rigid Registration of Brain Images with Tumor Pathology 531
    S. K. Kyriacou and C. Davatzikos

Building Biomechanical Models Based on Medical Image Data:
An Assessment of Model Accuracy 539
    W.M. Murray, A.S. Arnold, S. Salinas, M.M. Durbhakula, T.S. Buchanan and S.L. Delp

Modeling of Soft Tissue Deformation for Laparoscopic Surgery Simulation. 550
    G. Székely, C. Brechbuehler, R. Hutter, A. Rhomberg and P. Schmid

Detection in Medical Images

A Colour Image Processing Method for Melanoma Detection 562
    O. Colot, R. Devinoy, A. Sombo and D. de Brucq

Abnormal Masses in Mammograms: Detection Using Scale-Orientation
Signatures 570
    R. Zwiggelaar and C.J. Taylor

Detecting and Inferring Brain Activation from Functional MRI by
Hypothesis-Testing Based on the Likelihood Ratio 578
    D. Ekatodramis, G. Székely and G. Gerig

Data Acquisition and Processing

A Fast Technique for Motion Correction in DSA Using a Feature-Based,
Irregular Grid 590
    E.H.W. Meijering, K.J. Zuiderveld and M.A. Viergever

Autofocusing of Clinical Shoulder MR Images for Correction of Motion
Artifacts 598
    A. Manduca, K.P. McGee, E.B. Welch, J.P. Felmlee and R.L. Ehman

Reconstruction of Elasticity and Attenuation Maps in Shear Wave
Imaging: An Inverse Approach 606
    A. Manduca, V. Dutt, D.T. Borup, R. Muthupillai, R.L. Ehman and J.F. Greenleaf

Understanding Intensity Non-uniformity in MRI 614
    J.J. Sled and G.B. Pike

Neurosurgery and Neuroscience

3D Reconstruction from Projection Matrices in a C-Arm Based 3D-Angiography System 119
    N. Navab, A. Bani-Hashemi, M. S. Nadar, K. Wiesent, P. Durlak, T. Brunner, K. Barth and R. Graumann

An Automatic Threshold-Based Scaling Method for Enhancing the Usefulness of Tc-HMPAO SPECT in the Diagnosis of Alzheimer's Disease 623
    P. Saxena, D.G. Pavel, J.C. Quintana and B. Horwitz

Automatic Computation of Average Brain Models...................... 631
    A. Guimond, J. Meunier and J.-P. Thirion

Brain Shift Modeling for Use in Neurosurgery 641
    O. Škrinjar, D. Spencer and J.S. Duncan

Proximity Constraints in Deformable Models for Cortical Surface Identification 650
    D. MacDonald, D. Avis and A.C. Evans

Fast Analysis of Intracranial Aneurysms Based on Interactive Direct Volume Rendering and CTA.. 660
    P. Hastreiter, Ch. Rezk-Salama, B. Tomandl, K.E.W. Eberhardt and T. Ertl

Visualizing Spatial Resolution of Linear Estimation Techniques of Electromagnetic Brain Activity Localization 670
    A.K. Liu, J.W. Belliveau and A.M. Dale

Biomechanics and Kinematics

Biomechanical Simulation of the Vitreous Humor in the Eye Using an Enhanced ChainMail Algorithm 679
    M.A. Schill, S.F.F. Gibson, H.-J. Bender and R. Männer

A Biomechanical Model of the Human Tongue and Its Clinical Implications... 688
    Y. Payan, G. Bettega and B. Raphaël

Three-Dimensional Joint Kinematics Using Bone Surface Registration: A Computer Assisted Approach with an Application to the Wrist Joint in Vivo 696
    J.J. Crisco, R.D. McGovern and S.W. Wolfe

Range of Motion after Total Hip Arthroplasty: Simulation of Non-axisymmetric Implants 700
    C. Nikou, B. Jaramaz and A.M. DiGioia

Shape Analysis and Models

4D Shape-Preserving Modeling of Bone Growth 710
    P.R. Andresen, M. Nielsen and S. Kreiborg

AnatomyBrowser: A Framework for Integration of Medical Information ... 720
    P. Golland, R. Kikinis, C. Umans, M. Halle, M.E. Shenton and J.A. Richolt

Automatic, Accurate Surface Model Inference for Dental CAD/CAM 732
    C.-K. Tang, G. Medioni and F. Duret

Initial In-Vivo Analysis of 3d Heterogeneous Brain Computations for Model-Updated Image-Guided Neurosurgery 743
    M. Miga, K. Paulsen, F. Kennedy, J. Hoopes, A. Hartov and D. Roberts

A New Dynamic FEM-based Subdivision Surface Model for Shape Recovery and Tracking in Medical Images 753
    C. Mandal, B.C. Vemuri and H. Qin

Automatic Quantification of Changes in the Volume of Brain Structures .. 761
    G. Calmon, N. Roberts, P. Eldridge and J.-P. Thirion

Automatic Analysis of Normal Brain Dissymmetry of Males and Females in MR Images 770
    S. Prima, J.-P. Thirion, G. Subsol and N. Roberts

Marching Optimal-Parameter Ridges: An Algorithm to Extract Shape Loci in 3D Images 780
    J.D. Furst and S.M. Pizer

Singularities as Features of Deformation Grids 788
    F.L. Bookstein

Morphological Analysis of Terminal Air Spaces by Means of Micro-CT and Confocal Microscopy and Simulation within a Functional Model of Lung .. 798
    A. Kriete, H. Watz, W. Rau and H.-R. Duncker

Feature Extraction and Image-Based Measurements

2D+T Acoustic Boundary Detection in Echocardiography 806
    M. Mulet-Parada and J.A. Noble

Automatically Finding Optimal Working Projections for the Endovascular Coiling of Intracranial Aneurysms 814
    D.L. Wilson, J. A. Noble, D. Royston and J. Byrne

Computer Assisted Quantitative Analysis of Deformities of the Human Spine 822
    B. Verdonck, P. Nijlunsing, F.A. Gerritsen, J. Cheung, D.J. Wever, A. Veldhuizen, S. Devillers and S. Makram-Ebeid

Motion Measurements in Low-Contrast X-ray Imagery 832
  M. Berger and G. Gerig

Pitfalls in Comparing Functional Magnetic Resonance Imaging and
Invasive Electrophysiology Recordings 842
  D.L.G. Hill, A. Simmons, A.D. Castellano Smith, C.R. Maurer Jr.,
T.C.S. Cox, R. Elwes, M.F. Brammer, D.J. Hawkes and C.E. Polkey

Medical Image-Based Modeling

Specification, Modeling and Visualization of Arbitrarily Shaped Cut
Surfaces in the Volume Model 853
  B. Pflesser, U. Tiede and K.-H. Höhne

An Object-Based Volumetric Deformable Atlas for the Improved
Localization of Neuroanatomy in MR Images 861
  T. McInerney and R. Kikinis

Automated Labeling of Bronchial Branches in Virtual Bronchoscopy
System 870
  K. Mori, J.-i. Hasegawa, Y. Suenaga, J.-i. Toriwaki, H. Anno and K. Katada

Building a Complete Surface Model from Sparse Data Using Statistical
Shape Models: Application to Computer Assisted Knee Surgery
System 879
  M. Fleute and S. Lavallée

Constrained Elastic Surface Nets: Generating Smooth Surfaces from
Binary Segmented Data.. 888
  S.F.F. Gibson

Medical Simulation

Assessing Skill and Learning in Surgeons and Medical Students Using a
Force Feedback Surgical Simulator 899
  R. O'Toole, R. Playter, T. Krummel, W. Blank, N. Cornelius, W. Roberts,
W. Bell and M. Raibert

Virtual Reality Vitrectomy Simulator................................ 910
  P.F. Neumann, L.L. Sadler and J. Gieser

An Experimental Image Guided Surgery Simulator for
Hemicriolaryngectomy and Reconstruction by Tracheal Autotransplantation 918
  F. Schutyser, J. Van Cleynenbreugel, V.V. Poorten, P. Delaere, G. Marchal
and P. Suetens

Virtual Endoscopy of Mucin-Producing Pancreas Tumors 926
    T. Nakagohri, F.A. Jolesz, S. Okuda, T. Asano, T. Kenmochi, O. Kainuma, Y. Tokoro, H. Aoyama, W.E. Lorensen and R. Kikinis

Augmented Reality Visualization for Laparoscopic Surgery 934
    H. Fuchs, M.A. Livingston, R. Raskar, D. Colucci, K. Keller, A. State, J.R. Crawford, P. Rademacher, S.H. Drake and A.A. Meyer

Registration

Evaluation of Control Point Selection in Automatic, Mutual Information Driven, 3D Warping... 944
    C. Meyer, J. Boes, B. Kim and P. Bland

3D/2D Registration via Skeletal Near Projective Invariance in Tubular Objects.. 952
    A. Liu, E. Bullitt and S.M. Pizer

Measuring Global and Local Spatial Correspondence Using Information Theory 964
    F. Bello and A.C.F. Colchester

Non-linear Cerebral Registration with Sulcal Constraints................ 974
    D.L. Collins, G. Le Goualher and A.C. Evans

Surgical Planning II

A Double Scanning Procedure for Visualisation of Radiolucent Objects in Soft Tissues: Application to Oral Implant Surgery Planning 985
    K. Verstreken, J. Van Cleynenbreugel, G. Marchal, D. van Steenberghe and P. Suetens

Interactive Pre-operative Selection of Cutting Constraints, and Interactive Force Controlled Knee Surgery by a Surgical Robot 996
    S.J. Harris, M. Jakopec, R.D. Hibberd, J. Cobb and B.L. Davies

Multimodal Volume-Based Tumor Neurosurgery Planning in the Virtual Workbench.. 1007
    L. Serra, R.A. Kockro, C.G. Guan, N. Hern, E.C.K. Lee, Y.H. Lee, W.L. Nowinski and C. Chan

Ultrasound

Real-Time Tools for Freehand 3D Ultrasound......................... 1016
    R. Prager, A. Gee and L. Berman

Computer-Based Determination of the Newborn's Femoral Head Coverage using Three-Dimensional Ultrasound Scans............................ 1024
    H.M. Overhoff, P. Heinze, D. Lazovic and U. von Jan

Ultrasound Imaging Simulation: Application to the Diagnosis of Deep
Venous Thromboses of Lower Limbs 1032
    D. Henry, J. Troccaz, J.L. Bosson and O. Pichot

Isolating Moving Anatomy in Ultrasound Without Anatomical Knowledge:
Application to Computer-Assisted Pericardial Punctures 1041
    A. Bzostek, G. Ionescu, L. Carrat, C. Barbe, O. Chavanon and J. Troccaz

A New Branching Model: Application to Carotid Ultrasonic Data 1049
    A. Moreau-Gaudry, P. Cinquin and J.-P. Baguet

Registration II

Multi-modal Volume Registration Using Joint Intensity Distributions 1057
    M.E. Leventon and W.E.L. Grimson

Multimodality Deformable Registration of Pre- and Intraoperative Images
for MRI-guided Brain Surgery 1067
    N. Hata, T. Dohi, S.K. Warfield, W.M. Wells, R. Kikinis and F.A. Jolesz

A Novel Approach for the Registration of 2D Portal and 3D CT Images
for Treatment Setup Verification in Radiotherapy 1075
    R. Bansal, L.H. Staib, Z. Chen, A. Rangarajan, J. Knisely, R. Nath and
J.S. Duncan

Multimodality Imaging for Epilepsy Diagnosis and Surgical Focus
Localization: Three-Dimensional Image Correlation and Dual Isotope
SPECT 1087
    B.H. Brinkmann, R.A. Robb, T.J. O'Brien, M.K. O'Connor and
B.P. Mullan

Non-rigid Multimodal Image Registration Using Mutual Information 1099
    T. Gaens, F. Maes, D. Vandermeulen and P. Suetens

Feature-Based Registration of Medical Images: Estimation and Validation
of the Pose Accuracy 1107
    X. Pennec, C.R.G. Guttmann and J.-P. Thirion

The Correlation Ratio as a New Similarity Measure for Multimodal
Image Registration 1115
    A. Roche, G. Malandain, X. Pennec and N. Ayache

Real-Time Registration of 3D Cerebral Vessels to X-ray Angiograms..... 1125
    Y. Kita, D.L. Wilson and J.A. Noble

Multi-object Deformable Templates Dedicated to the Segmentation of Brain
Deep Structures 1134
    F. Poupon, J.-F. Mangin, D. Hasboun, C. Poupon, I.E. Magnin and V.
Frouin

Non-rigid Registration of Breast MR Images Using Mutual Information ... 1144
    D. Rueckert, C. Hayes, C. Studholme, P. Summers, M. Leach and D.J. Hawkes

A Comparison of Similarity Measures for use In 2D-3D Medical Image Registration 1153
    G.P. Penney, J. Weese, J.A. Little, P. Desmedt, D.L.G. Hill and D.J. Hawkes

Elastic Model Based Non-rigid Registration Incorporating Statistical Shape Information 1162
    Y. Wang and L.H. Staib

Image Registration Based on Thin-Plate Splines and Local Estimates of Anisotropic Landmark Localization Uncertainties 1174
    K. Rohr

Segmentation II

Segmentation of Carpal Bones from 3d CT Images Using Skeletally Coupled Deformable Models 1184
    T.B. Sebastian, H. Tek, J.J. Crisco, S.W. Wolfe and B.B. Kimia

Segmentation of Bone in Clinical Knee MRI Using Texture-Based Geodesic Active Contours 1195
    L.M. Lorigo, O. Faugeras, W.E.L. Grimson, R. Keriven and R. Kikinis

Tensor Controlled Local Structure Enhancement of CT Images for Bone Segmentation 1205
    C.-F. Westin, S.K. Warfield, A. Bhalerao, L. Mui, J.A. Richolt and R. Kikinis

Segmentation of Magnetic Resonance Images Using 3D Deformable Models 1213
    J. Lötjönen, I.E. Magnin, P.-J. Reissman, J. Nenonen and T. Katila

Automatic Segmentation of Brain Tissues and MR Bias Field Correction Using a Digital Brain Atlas 1222
    K. Van Leemput, F. Maes, D. Vandermeulen and P. Suetens

Robust Brain Segmentation Using Histogram Scale-Space Analysis and Mathematical Morphology 1230
    J.-F. Mangin, O. Coulon and V. Frouin

Vascular Shape Segmentation and Structure Extraction Using a Shape-Based Region-Growing Model 1242
    Y. Masutani, T. Schiemann and K.-H. Höhne

Author Index 1251

Planning and Evaluation of Reorienting Osteotomies of the Proximal Femur in Cases of SCFE Using Virtual Three-Dimensional Models

Jens A. Richolt[1], Matthias Teschner[2], Peter Everett[1], Bernd Girod[2], Michael B. Millis[3], and Ron Kikinis[1]

[1]Surgical Planning Laboratory, Brigham and Women's Hospital, Harvard Medical School,
75, Francis Street, Boston, MA, 02115, USA
{jens, peverett, kikinis}@bwh.harvard.edu
http://splweb.bwh.harvard.edu:8000/pages/index.html
[2]Telecommunications Institute, University Erlangen-Nuremberg,
Cauer Strasse 7, D-91058 Erlangen, Germany
[3]Children's Hospital, Orthopaedic Surgery, Harvard Medical School,
300, Longwood Avenue, Boston, MA, 02115, USA

Abstract. Slipped Capital Femoral Epiphysis (SCFE) is a disease affecting the geometry of adolescent hips. Evaluation of the slippage as well planning of correction surgeries is a major three-dimensional problem. Therefore, the current clinical approach, which is based on biplanar plain radiographs, is not satisfying.

We have developed a software environment for planning and evaluation of reorienting osteotomies in severe cases of SCFE. In our system CT-based virtual surface models fitted by oriented bounding boxes (OBB) are manipulated. The hip motion as well as a correction surgery can be simulated. Both are controlled by collision detection. Therefore, the motion is based on the surface geometry of the joint partners rather than on a predefined, fixed rotation center. The pre- and simulated postoperative evaluation uses the range of motion as the essential parameter. The surgeon can obtain valuable information about the geometric correlation of the physiologic joint faces along hip motion.

1 Introduction

Slipped Capital Femoral Epiphysis (SCFE) is a condition affecting the proximal femur of adolescents. The SCFE is defined as the slippage of the femoral head on the proximal growth plate against the femoral neck. Usually this displacement occurs in a posterior and inferior direction (Fig. 1). In severe cases these events can determine a significant loss of hip function. Initially the loss of motion may be well tolerated, but eventually pain and stiffness of the joint will result from arthritic degeneration [2].

The standard procedure (so called in-situ-pinning) in SCFE aims towards the prevention of further slippage, which does not affect the post slippage geometry. In severe cases an additional correction osteotomy might be considered to improve the range of motion and the containment of femoral head and acetabulum [6,13]. The central part of this surgery consists of a cut through the proximal femur and a reorientation of the proximal part. The most common approach is the intertrochanteric osteotomy, which is performed as a horizontal cut between the lesser and major trochanter. Cuts closer to the deformity (i.e. in the femoral neck) are a more direct approach concerning the correction, but it is recognized that these have a much higher incidence of postoperative femoral head necrosis.

Since Imhäuser and Southwick described the guidelines for intertrochanteric osteotomies, little has changed in the planning of these surgeries [6,13]. In general the deformity is diagnosed and the amount of the displacement is measured on biplanar plain radiographs. The measurements give the values for the amount and direction of the reorientation of the proximal part.

The major uncertainties of this method are the poor reproducibility of the positioning for radiographs and the projectional errors [3]. In addition, the reorientation consists of a combination of rotations along different axes. A surgical plan based on biplanar radiographs doesn't address this complex procedure adequately.

The ability to acquire volumetric image data instead of projectional images and digital image post-processing could improve surgical planning. So far the planning of reorienting osteotomies in SCFE does not benefit from those technologies on a routine basis. Some earlier proposed systems and algorithms could be applied to this problem [1,4,9,10,14], but all of them are either missing interactivity or lack the ability to functionally evaluate the simulated procedure.

It was therefore our goal to develop an environment for the simulation of reorienting osteotomies. Such a system should be:
• fast enough for routine clinical use,
• able to simulate an osteotomy,
• able to realign anatomical objects separately and
• able to allow a functional evaluation.

2 Methods

We developed a surgical planning environment for reorienting osteotomies in cases of SCFE. Three-dimensional surface models represent the relevant anatomical structures in our approach.

In the first step, the preoperative range of motion based on the bony constraints can be determined by simulating the hip motion. Collision detection is used to control the motion in the hip joint. Our model does not use a fixed and predetermined rotation center.

The next step is the simulation of the osteotomy and the reorientation. Then the surface models are saved in the new position and finally reevaluated by the motion simulation.

In the following paragraphs, the underlying techniques are described in detail.

2.1 Visualization

In this study CT volume scans are used to reconstruct three-dimensional surface models. Segmentation of femur and pelvis is done with commonly used intensity thresholding techniques. Operator interaction is needed ensure proper separation of pelvis and femur and to determine the border between femoral head and neck. The latter is equivalent to the growth plate, which appears much darker than calcified bone in CT images.

The segmented files are reconstructed using "The Visualization Toolkit" (VTK) [11] implementation of the marching cubes algorithms [7] to the following objects: pelvis, femoral head and femoral neck with proximal femur (Fig. 1). In addition, the position of the knee condyles is represented to check for ante-/retroversion and the rotation of the femur. The surface models typically consist of about 50,000 triangles, after application of a triangle reduction algorithm [12].

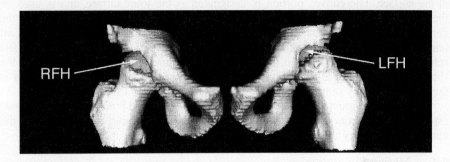

Fig. 1. Frontal view of the surface models of both hips in neutral position. The left hip is affected by SCFE. The left femoral head (LFH) is displaced posterior and slightly inferior. The right femoral head (RFH) shows a normal geometry.

The discrimination between femoral heads and the rest of the femur distinguishes between objects with and without articular cartilage.

The rendering uses the VTK libraries as well [11].

2.2 Collision Detection

For collision detection, we used the VCollide library of the University of North Carolina at Chapel Hill [5]. This library checks for interference between triangles of different geometric objects. The objects have to be represented as so-called polygon soups. The objects do not have to be convex and they are not considered to have any special properties. In our case we have convex and concave objects as well.

In a first step, VCollide computes a hierarchical tree-structure of oriented bounding boxes (OBB). Following certain rules, a generated OBB is separated in two areas with nearly the same number of triangles. For each of these areas, a new OBB is generated and so on. This leads to a hierarchical OBB-tree-representation.

OBB's are especially useful in interference tests (aka. collision detection). Only the OBB's are transformed – not the whole object. Only if two OBB's are not disjoint is the next layer of OBB's tested. If leaf nodes are reached in both structures, then all the triangles, which are represented by these nodes, are transformed and tested for interference. This method reduces the amount of transformations as well as the amount of interference tests, and is largely responsible for the interactive performance of our system.

2.3 Determination of an arbitrary rotation center

We model flexion and abduction as rotations of the femur. Therefore, we need to estimate an arbitrary center of these rotations for both femora. The positions of these centers relative to the acetabulum will change during motion simulation, as each femur is repositioned to mate its joint surface with the corresponding surface of the acetabulum.

The femoral head can be approximated as part of a sphere of which we can compute the center. We designated the triangle in the segmented femoral head with the most superior centroid as belonging to the convex surface of the joint.

With these assumptions we can easily classify the convex and concave portions of the surface. The convex portion is designated as the joint surface, and is used for the fully automatic determination of the rotation center. For several points of the convex portion we estimate the normals. On a perfect sphere, these normals would all intersect at the center of rotation. Because our segmentation result is not a perfect sphere, the normals usually do not intersect each other. Therefore, we determine the shortest connection of all these normals; the center of gravity of these connections is then called arbitrary center of rotation.

It is not important for the rotation center to be computed precisely. An inaccurate estimation only reduces the performance of the simulation process by increasing the number of iterations needed to reposition the femora in order to mate joint surfaces.

2.4 Motion Simulation

Motion simulation consists of reorienting the femur by small increments while maintaining contact between paired joint surfaces, and checking that no other pairs come into contact. Motion stops when further rotation of the femur under these constraints is impossible.

Since contacts of parts not covered with cartilage are non-physiologic, only our femoral head model is allowed to collide with the pelvis object.

To hold the femur in the acetabulum, we simulate a force to the femur towards the acetabulum. For each step of the simulation process, the femur is forced in this direction as far as possible. If a collision is detected, small steps perpendicular to the direction of the force are performed. For each of these steps, it is checked whether the femur can move further towards the acetabulum. With this iterative scheme, we find the optimal position of the femur.

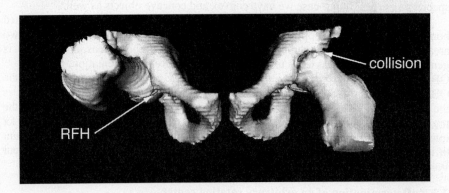

Fig. 2. Frontal view of the surface models of both hips, maximal simulated flexion. The left femur is flexed 29°, the right femur 105°. The location of the bony motion-limiting collision is indicated for the left femur.

After the optimal position is found, the program tries to rotate the femur along a user-defined axis (i.e. for flexion or abduction). This process is performed stepwise as well and alternates with the formerly described femur position adjustment. This alternating scheme allows a motion adapted to the individual surface geometry of the joint partners without being committed to an arbitrary rotation center.

For each simulation step, the collision detection algorithm is applied. The simulation process stops as soon as femoral parts other than the head collide with any part of the pelvis (Fig. 2 and 4).

Remark. In order to bias these findings, we have to put the femora in a neutral position before simulation. Most important in this aspect seems to be the femoral rotation. Due to the slippage of the epiphysis the patient keeps the leg in external rotation. The virtual models of the knee condyles enable us to correct for this problem.

2.5   Osteotomy Simulation

The osteotomy simulation tool permits the operator to read, view, cut, and reorient segmented surface models. The visualization functions are based on the VTK libraries [11], but it adds the ability to perform boolean operations between different surface models. In the case of osteotomy simulation, it is the boolean subtraction of the cutter model (i.e. virtual saw) from the bone model with interactive performance. At the core of the operation is the calculation of intersections between the edges of one model and the triangles of the other model [8].

The same OBB hierarchy mentioned earlier is used to rapidly identify regions of potential interaction between cutter surface and bone surface [5]. Therefore, topology and transformations are only computed for those sets of triangles that are identified in the OBB hierarchy for potential interaction.

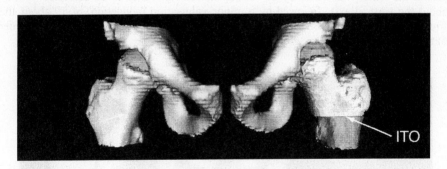

Fig. 3. Frontal view of the surface models of both hips after simulated cutting and repositioning. ITO indicates the location of the intertrochanteral osteotomy. The portion of the femur that is distal to the intertrochanteral cut is shown in a darker shade. The proximal femur was repositioned by 20° of flexion, 25° of derotation and 5° of adduction. Note the increased appearance of symmetry in the placement of the left femoral head towards the acetabula.

The cutter model has mouse-driven interface, which can be used to position and orient the tool with respect to the bone. Once positioned, a button press signals the subtraction of the tool volume from the bone volume. For a simple cut, a single subtraction may be sufficient, but multiple cuts can be made. After the osteotomy, the bone model consists of two or more topologically disjoint segments (Fig.3). Each segment is identified and written out as an independently orientable model.

The mouse-driven interface can also be used to reposition one segment with respect to the others. During a surgical simulation, the surgeon can reorient the proximal part interactively. While comparing the relative position of femoral head and acetabulum to the position on the healthy side, he can simulate an arbitrary reorientation (Fig. 3).

The same OBB-tree based collision detection that is used for range of motion analysis is also used to prevent positioning with overlapping volumes. At this point, the user may wish to use some of the measuring tools provided for measuring the angles and distances between features of the model.

Once the desired repositioning is achieved, the segments are reunited into a single model, which can be input to the post-surgical range of motion analysis. If the result of the 'postoperative' finding is not satisfying another reorientation can be simulated.

3 Results

3.1 Illustrative Case

Figures 1-6 are based on the datasets from a 13-year-old boy with SCFE of his left hip (Fig. 1). By simulating the bone determined range of motion we could assess a maximal flexion of 105° on the healthy side and 29° on the affected side (Fig. 2). The measurements for abduction were 76° and 49° respectively (Fig. 3).

In the next step, an intertrochanteric osteotomy was simulated. The proximal part of the femur was flexed by 20° about the left-right axis, then derotated by 25° about the vertical axis, followed by a minor valgisation (adduction) of 5° about the front-back axis. It is important to realize that the final orientation depends on the order of these rotations.

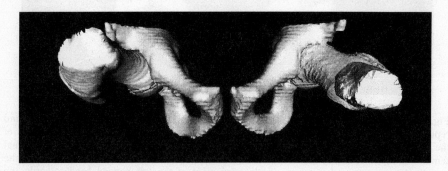

Fig. 4. Frontal view of the surface models of both femora in maximal simulated post-surgical flexion. The left femur is flexed 69°, an improvement of 40° from the pre-surgical simulation. The right femur is unchanged at 105°.

3.2 Performance

We tested our implementation on a SUN ULTRA 30, 300MHz, 128MB RAM, with Creator3D graphics acceleration and on a SGI O$_2$, R10000, 180Mhz, 128MB RAM, with standard 3D triangle acceleration. Our scenes usually consist of 8 objects with approximately 50,000 triangles. In general, the data size for those models is about one MByte.

Table 1. Performance of our collision detection system on different computer systems.

Computer System	Preparing OBB-structure	Collision detection
SUN	3.20 sec	0.05 sec or 16 fps
SGI	4.77 sec	0.07 sec or 14 fps

For these measurements, the collision detection is performed in real time using a standard UNIX workstation. A full motion to maximal flexion / abduction for both sides takes usually between 10 and 30 seconds.

The osteotomy simulation is performed in real time as well.

4 Discussion

We present a system for the preoperative evaluation, simulation of reorienting osteotomies and the 'postoperative' reevaluation in cases of SCFE.

Previously described systems generally applicable to this topic lack some important features. Simple and fast simulation systems are mostly based on surface models. These systems are able to perform osteotomies, but due to their lack of collision detection, they are neither able to simulate the improvement in the range of motion nor to simulate a hip motion without a fixed center of rotation [1,9].

Gerber's approach uses volume rendering to display the motion of the hip joint [4]. This procedure comes at the cost of time. The vast amount of necessary computations makes real time interaction impossible.

Pflesser et al. used a method of ray composition and rendering [10]. This method can display interpenetrating volumes. However, the motion of the hip joint requires a predefined and fixed center of rotation. In addition, this system does not detect and avoid the collision automatically. It needs the evaluation of a user.

For the known problems in surgical simulation systems, we developed a system based on surface models, which we fitted by oriented bounding boxes (OBB). The combination of OBB's and surface models is the basis for the high performance of our system. In contrast to axis-aligned bounding boxes (AABB), OBB's fit the object better [5]. Although the computation of OBB's is more time-consuming than that of AABB's, OBB's do not have to be recomputed if the object is transformed.

Anatomically, our system currently lacks the interaction of ligaments and muscles. Therefore, in some cases, non-physiological degrees of motion could be observed. The addition of ligament modeling to the existing environment is currently in progress. This will make the current system applicable to many other joints and surgical planning problems.

Using the current system, a surgeon can already obtain valuable information for the planning of reorienting osteotomies in cases of SCFE. Instead of estimating the impact of his planned osteotomy to the improvement of range of motion, he can visualize and quantify that impact in a three dimensional environment.

Due to the performance of the system, even on standard workstations, the practicality of the system has a major advantage over earlier programs. In addition, the data preparation can be done in a reasonable amount of time.

On the whole, the presented system can be used for the planning of reorienting osteotomies in cases of SCFE on a routine clinical basis.

5 References

1. Altobelli D, Kikinis R, Mulliken J, Cline H, Lorensen W, and Jolesz F, 1993
   Computer-assisted three-dimensional planning in cranofacial surgery.
   Plast Reconst Surg, 92: 576-585.
2. Boyer DW, Mickelson MR, and Ponseti IV, 1981
   Slipped capital femoral epiphysis. Long-term follow-up study of one hundred and twenty-one patients.
   J Bone Joint Surg [Am], 63: 85-95.
3. Cohen MS, Gelberman RH, Griffin PP, Kasser JR, Emans JB, and Millis MB
   Slipped capital femoral epiphysis: assessment of epiphyseal displacement and angulation.
   J Pediatr Orthop, 6: 259-264.
4. Gerber JD, Ney DR, Magid D, and Fishman EK, 1991
   Simulated Femoral Repositioning with Three-Dimensional CT.
   J Comput Assist Tomogr, 15: 121-125.
5. Gottschalk S, Lin M, and Manocha D, 1996
   OBB-Tree: A Hierarchical Structure for Rapid Interference Detection.
   Proc. ACM Siggraph '96, 171-180.
6. Imhäuser G, 1957
   Zur Pathogenese und Therapie der jugendlichen Hüftkopflösung.
   Z Orthop, 88: 3-41.
7. Lorensen W and Cline H, 1987
   Marching cubes: A high resolution 3D surface construction algorithm.
   Computer Graphics, 21: 163-169.
8. Mantyla M, 1988
   An Introduction to Solid Modelling.
   Computer Science Press, Rockville, MD.
9. Murphy SB, Kijewski PK, Millis MB, and Harless A, 1989
   Simulation of Osteotomy Surgery about the Hip Joint.
   Computer Assisted Radiology, Proc. CAR '91, Lemke, H. U. et al. (eds.), Springer-Verlag, Berlin.
10. Pflesser B, Tiede U, and Höhne KH, 1994
    Simulating Motion of Anatomical Object with Volume-Based 3D-Visualisation.
    Visualization in Biomedical Computing, Proc., R. A. Robb (ed.), SPIE 2359, Rochester, MN, 291-300.
11. Schroeder W, Martin K, and Lorensen W, 1997
    The Visualization Toolkit.
    2nd ed., Prentice-Hall, New Jersey.
12. Schroeder, W., J. Zarge, and W. Lorensen. 1992.
    Decimation of Triangle Meshes.
    Computer Graphics 26(2):65-70.
13. Southwick WO, 1967
    Osteotomy through the Lesser Trochanter for Slipped Capital Femoral Epiphysis.
    J Bone Joint Surg, 49-A: 807-835.
14. Vannier M and Marsh J, 1996
    Three-dimensional imaging, surgical planning and image-guided therapy.
    Rad Clin North Am, 34: 545-563.

Computer-Aided Planning of Patellofemoral Joint OA Surgery: Developing Physical Models from Patient MRI

Zohara A. Cohen[1,2], Denise M. McCarthy[3], Hrvoje Roglic[1,2], Jack H. Henry[2], William G. Rodkey[4], J. Richard Steadman[4], Van C. Mow[1,2], and Gerard A. Ateshian[1,2]

[1] Department of Mechanical Engineering, Columbia University, 500 W 120th St, MC4703, New York, NY 10027

[2] Orthopaedic Research Laboratory, Department of Orthopaedic Surgery, Columbia-Presbyterian Medical Center, 630 West 168th St, BB1412, New York, NY 10032

[3] Department of Radiology, Columbia-Presbyterian Medical Center, Milstein Hospital Building, 3-248, New York, NY 10032

[4] Steadman-Hawkin Sports Medicine Foundation, 181 W. Meadow Drive, Suite 1000, Vail, CO 81657

Abstract. Generally, the surgical procedures employed in the treatment of patellofemoral joint (PFJ) osteoarthritis (OA) aim, either explicitly or implicitly, to alter the biomechanics of the osteoarthritic joint (i.e., improve motion and load transmission characteristics). Because of the mechanical nature of some of these surgical objectives, they can be evaluated prior to and subsequent to surgery by using an appropriate patient-specific physical model of the patient's PFJ, derived from 3D MRI data. This study describes the process by which such patient-specific physical models can be created using standard clinical imaging modalities.

Introduction

Currently, the clinical consensus is that the success of surgery for PFJ OA is highly variable and often unpredictable. Much of the data used in the decision making process derive from clinical examinations, supported by standard radiographic images that provide only indirect evidence of the severity of osteoarthritic damage in the diseased joint. The results of various procedures for the treatment of PFJ OA as well as patellar instability have been described in the literature for decades. The estimated success rate of patellofemoral PFJ surgery for osteoarthritis OA is 60%, excluding replacement arthroplasty. The long-term aim of this project is to improve this success rate by providing a new set of tools to help orthopaedic surgeons in planning their surgical treatment of PFJ OA.

One of the leading hypotheses for the initiation and progression of PFJ OA is that excessive stresses in the articular layers lead to degeneration by promoting a rate of tissue degradation that exceeds its rate of repair. From a clinical perspective, it is also believed that excessive articular contact stresses may contribute to the pain experienced by OA patients. Therefore, the premise of the current study is that successful planning of the outcome of PFJ OA surgery is dependent on a reliable prediction of changes in the articular contact area and stresses which would result from surgery. Because of the complexity of the articular topography of the PFJ, an accurate representation of the surfaces is required, which can be obtained from magnetic resonance imaging (MRI). Furthermore, such surgical planning is dependent on the ability to predict the forces which develop within the various structures of the joint, including articular contact forces, ligament forces, and other soft tissue interactions, that are dependent on the muscle forces acting across the joint. In this study, we describe our current progress on the development of physical models of patient knee joints from MRI, which can be used for the calculation of such parameters as contact areas, stresses and forces across the PFJ under various configurations of loading, as well as changes in these parameters following surgical simulations.

Computer-Aided Orthopaedic Surgery

Several investigators have used computer models to evaluate orthopaedic surgical procedures. Delp and co-workers developed a computer model [14,18] which they applied to investigate surgical treatments on the ankle [15,16], hip, and knee [17] joints, as well as gait [19]. Chao and co-workers applied a 2-D rigid-body-spring-model to evaluate wrist [3,27,31] and knee joint mechanics [9,32]. Furthermore, Chao and co-workers proposed methods to plan various surgeries for individual patients using their model [9] and created a computer software program to analyze knee osteotomy [8]. Other authors have also investigated the use of computer models to plan surgeries, mostly for the hip joint [7,37,38,39,40,51], but for the wrist [33] and tibia [48] as well. Finally, some investigators have reported use of guidance tools and robots in the operating room to aid the surgeons [35, 9,41]. However, these studies generally have not focused on OA nor have they relied on such parameters as articular contact forces, areas and stresses. As a result, they have not attempted to reproduce the articular surfaces accurately. In this study, accurate topographic models of the patient's PFJ are developed from MRI data.

MRI of Articular Cartilage

Magnetic resonance imaging of articular cartilage has been the subject of intense research in recent years. Until recently, identification of cartilage defects could be made only by arthroscopy or surgery. Accurate, early, MR diagnosis can potentially tailor arthroscopy and surgery. The use of MR imaging has also been considered to show promise as a potential outcome measure for therapeutic studies by a task force of the Osteoarthritis Research Society [2]. The appearance of cartilage has been described on many MR sequences. T1- and T2-weighted spin echo images, which have both been advocated, are limited by a minimum practical slice thickness of 2-3 mm. Newer techniques include magnetization transfer and gradient echo imaging. Magnetization transfer techniques have been used to increase the contrast between cartilage and bone [50], however, magnetization transfer is not widely available and the subtraction method required introduces error.

Gradient echo imaging allows acquisition of thin contiguous slices in a volume which can be reformatted in multiple planes. Furthermore, gradient echo imaging has greater signal-to-noise in each slice than spin echo images [45]. In 1993, a study which compared T1-weighted, proton density, T2-weighted, spoiled GRASS, GRASS, and fat suppressed spoiled GRASS concluded spoiled GRASS best for cartilage [44]. Fat suppressed spoiled GRASS images were also more accurate than magnetization transfer in cartilage thickness determination of cadaver ankle articular cartilage [52]. High resolution volume spoiled GRASS cartilage sequences have been used in cadavers with 1-2 mm slice thickness to determine cartilage thickness in cadaver knees with precision [11-13,23]. In our own prior studies, we compared cadaver knee joint MRI measurements of cartilage topography and thickness against stereophotogrammetric measurements, and demonstrated sub-pixel accuracies (0.16 mm on average for topographic measurements, 0.32 mm on average for thickness measurements, on the patella and femur) [13].

Currently, for patient MRIs, we acquire two sets of images for each patient visit. The first set employs the cartilage-specific sequence proposed by Disler et al. and Peterfy et al. [20,21,42,43], which we have successfully implemented in our own studies [12,13]. This sequence consists of a 3-D volume spoiled GRASS with fat suppression, sagittal acquisition, TR=52 ms, TE=5 ms, flip angle=40°, field of view (FOV) = 12 to 16 cm (to enclose the entire articular layers of the knee), matrix = 256x160, 1 NEX, 60 contiguous 1.5 mm slices, with a duration of 8:56 minutes, and with the knee in full extension inside a linear extremity coil (Fig. 1a). The second set (Fig. 1b) consists of a sagittal acquisition, TR=550 ms, TE=15 ms, FOV = 16 cm, matrix = 256x192, slice thickness = 4 mm, acquisition time = 3:35 minutes, acquired in the body coil (50 cm diameter) at the maximum knee flexion angle permitted within the space constraints (typically, 50°-70° of flexion, 60° on average). The first set of images is used to get accurate anatomic measurements of the articular layers while the second set of images is used to determine the position of the patella relative to the femur, at a flexion angle where the PFJ contact force, contact area and contact stresses are close to their highest values.

Segmentation of MR images is performed using a custom-written semi-automated cubic B-spline snake procedure to extract the contours of the articular and subchondral bone surfaces (Fig. 2). This technique has been shown to achieve equal accuracy as manual segmentation in our previous cadaver study [13] while decreasing the time required for segmentation of all 60 slices by more than tenfold, down to approximately 2 hours.

Using the femoral and patellar bone contours from the two MRI sequences, a surface registration procedure is applied to realign the highly accurate cartilage surfaces acquired near full knee extension in the first sequence into the flexed position assumed by the patient in the second sequence. A surface proximity algorithm [5,47,49] is employed to determine the articular contact areas in the patient PFJ for the given flexed position (Fig. 3a). This articular contact area represents the baseline contact configuration which may serve for analyzing subsequent changes, either from post-surgical MRI or from surgical simulations performed on the physical model constructed from MRI data. Other information of significant value which can be obtained from the first MRI sequence is the thickness of the articular layer over the entire joint surface. Thickness maps can be used to track the changes in a patient's cartilage layer over time. A repeatability study performed on the knee of one volunteer over two sets of measurements showed a root-mean-square difference in thickness of 0.40mm, 0.27mm and 0.60 mm for the patella, femur and tibia respectively, precisions which compare favorably with the thickness measurement accuracy determined in the cadaver study [13]. Correlations may be found in some patients between regions of cartilage degeneration, as assessed from the thickness maps, and the location of the articular contact areas (Fig 5 a,c).

3D Multibody Modeling of the Patellofemoral Joint

Building on the work of previous investigators [6,24,25,28,29,30], we have recently developed a general interactive mathematical 3D model, capable of simulating different joints [34]. The model employs a quasi-static equilibrium analysis that predicts the equilibrium pose, contact areas, contact forces, and ligament forces of multiple bodies (bones and soft tissues) interacting together. Complex bone and articular surfaces are accurately represented by mathematical surfaces, and the contact stress between surfaces is approximated by various functions of the surface proximities. Ligaments are modeled as line segments whose forces are linearly or nonlinearly dependent on their length, stretch, or strain. Constant loads are applied through tendons to simulate muscle forces, and the tendons may loop through tendon pulleys connected to various bones. The model permits wrapping of the tendons and ligaments around bone and articular surfaces (e.g. the quadriceps tendon wrapping around the femoral trochlea) by imbedding particles in the ligaments and tendons, and letting these particle bodies interact with the surfaces. External forces and moments can be applied to any of the bodies, either in a body-fixed coordinate system or in a global coordinate system (e.g., to simulate gravitational forces). Finally, any of the translational or rotational degrees-of-freedom of a moving body may be optionally constrained (e.g., the knee flexion angle).

The Newton-Raphson iterative procedure was used to solve efficiently for the equilibrium condition; to expedite the calculations all components of the Jacobian matrix are evaluated analytically. The model was validated by reproducing results of actual cadaver knee joint experiments [34]. By using an analytical Jacobian formulation, the model converges very rapidly (2 to 10 seconds for most analyses). It provides graphical display of the results, and it allows the user to interactively change any of the input parameters.

In patient studies, a physical (multibody) model is constructed for the patient PFJ using the articular surface data, tendon and ligament insertions and bone contour data acquired from the first MRI sequence (Fig. 4,b and 5a ,b). The lines of action of the various quadriceps muscle components (vastus medialis obliqus, vastus lateralis, rectus femoris+vastus intermedius+vastus medialis longus can be inferred from manual segmentation of the muscle contours, and current work is in progress to assess the accuracy of this process. The muscle force magnitudes are adjusted so that the contact map generated from MRI is reproduced by the model. The properties of the soft tissue structures incorporated into the patient PFJ multibody model (articular cartilage, quadriceps tendon and patellar ligament stiffnesses) are currently obtained from the literature, since these properties cannot as yet be determined from MRI using current techniques.

Surgical Simulations

Many operations are available for the treatment of PFJ OA. These treatments may be divided into four categories:
1. Arthroscopic Procedures: lateral retinacular release, patellar shaving, lysis of adhesions, combinations.
2. Open Procedures: tibial tuberosity transfer (Hughston, Maquet, Elmslie-Trillat, Fulkerson), advancement of the VMO, lateral retinacular release, combinations.
3. Osteotomy: high tibial, distal femoral.
4. Resection: facetectomy, patellectomy.

However, not all patients respond to a given operation [1,26] and most of the surgical procedures relieve pain to a disappointingly variable degree. Therefore, in view of the numerous surgical procedures that have been used with variable success for the treatment of PFJ OA, there exists a significant need for aiding the orthopaedic surgeon in the planning of surgery by providing estimates of the potential outcome for each of these procedures, alone or in combinations. Such a mechanism ideally should provide a quantitative measure to allow proper assessment of each procedure. In this study, we propose to use such measures as PFJ articular contact areas, forces and stresses.

For the purpose of surgical simulations, many of the procedures described above require relatively minimal modifications to the physical multibody model of the joint, relative to the baseline patient-specific data. For example, tibial tuberosity transfer operations can be simulated by relocating the insertion points of the patellar ligament bundles on the tibia and adjusting the applied quadriceps forces to maintain the same flexion moment on the tibia (Fig. 4a,b). The patient shown in Fig 4 previously had a tibial tuberosity transfer, but complains of persistent knee pain. Reverse surgical simulation shows that the transfer procedure did in fact decrease the stress in the patient's knee. However, looking at the contact map of the current configuration, the contact is still positioned laterally on the patella, perhaps a source of her current pain. Lateral retinacular release may be performed by decreasing the force in the vastus lateralis (VL) component of the quadriceps force, while, similarly, adjusting other muscle forces to maintain a fixed moment about the knee (Fig. 5). On the femur of the patient represented by Fig 5 there is a focal lesion that coincides with the location of maximum contact stress for that knee. A simulated VL release shows that this patient may receive only limited benefit from such surgery, due to the limited amount of medial shift in contact area and the small decrease in contact stress (0.46 MPa to 0.43 MPa). Likewise, advancement of the vastus medialis obliquus can be simulated by relocating the insertion of this muscle component onto the patella. Osteotomies would require re-orienting the lines of action of the muscles and/or relocating the patellar ligament insertion. Other procedures involve more elaborate modifications such as changes to the solid model representation of the patella for resection procedures or patella shaving (Fig. 6) which can be performed with a solid modeler, or incorporation of additional soft-tissue structures for the simulation of adhesions [47].

The sophistication of the patient-specific multibody model of the PFJ can be increased by modeling more of the soft-tissue structures surrounding the joint, such as capsular tissues or the fat pad. The need for incorporating more details into the model should be based on experimental verification of the model's predictive ability in the simulation of various surgeries. Such experimental verifications are currently under way in a clinical setting involving the efforts of orthopedic surgeons, radiologists and engineers at four institutions across the United States.

Conclusion

Generally, the aims of surgical procedures employed in the treatment of PFJ OA are to alter the biomechanics of the osteoarthritic joint (i.e., improve motion and load transmission characteristics). For example, the explicitly stated goals of the Maquet or Fulkerson procedures have been to reduce the joint contact forces or stresses, to increase the size or to shift the location of the contact areas, to increase the moment arm of various tendons, or a combination thereof. Within the clinical setting, it is generally believed that reduction of PFJ contact forces and stresses, as well as re-establishment of normal joint kinematics, will decrease joint pain and improve the patient outcome. However, a direct correlation between such biomechanical variables and patient outcome has never been investigated. Because of the mechanical nature of some of these surgical objectives, they can be evaluated prior to and subsequent to surgery by using an appropriate patient-specific physical model of the patient's PFJ, derived from 3D MRI data. This paper has summarized some of the technical aspects of our current progress toward this objective.

Acknowlegement: This study was supported in part by the Steadman-Hawkins Sports Medicine Foundation.

References

1. Aglietti P, Buzzi R, De Biase P, Giro n F: Surgical treatment of recurrent dislocation of the patella. Clin Orthop 308 (1994) 8-17
2. Altman R, Brandt K, Hochberg M, Moskowitz R: Design and conduct of clinical trials in patients with osteoarthritis: recommendations from a task force of the Osteoarthritis Research Society. Osteoarthritis Cartilage 4 (1996) 217-243
3. An KN, Himeno S, Tsumura H, Kawai T, Caho E YS: Pressure distribution on articular surfaces: application to joint stability evaluation. J Biomech 23 (1990) 1013-1020
4. Ateshian GA, Soslowsky LJ, and Mow VC : Quantitation of articular surface topography and cartilage thickness in knee joints using stereophotogrammetry. J Biomech 24 (1991) 761-776
5. Ateshian GA, Kwak SD, Soslowsky LJ, M ow VC: A stereophotogrammetric method for determining in situ contact areas in diarthrodial joints, and a comparison with other methods. J Biomech 27 (1994) 111-124
6. Blankevoort L, Kuiper JH, Huiskes R, Grootenboer HJ: Articular contact in a three-dimensional model of the knee. J Biomech 24 (1991) 1019-1031
7. Burk DL Jr, Mears DC, Cooperstein LA, Herman GT, Udupa JK: Acetabular fractures: three-dimensional computed tomographic imaging and interactive surgical planning. J Comput Tomogr 10 (1986) 1-10
8. Chao EYS, Lynch JD, Vanderploeg MJ: Simulation and animation of musculoskeletal joint system. J Biomech Eng 115 (1993) 562-568
9. Chao EYS, Sim FH: Computer-aided preoperative planning in knee osteotomy. Iowa Orthop J 15 (1995) 4-18
10. Cohen ZA, Kwak SD, Ateshian GA, Blankevoort L, Henry JH, Grelsamer RP, Mow VC: The effect of tibial tuberosity transfer on the patellofemoral joint: A 3-D simulation. Adv Bioeng, ASME, BED 33 (1996) 387-388
11. Cohen ZA, McCarthy DM, Ateshian GA, Kwak SD, Peterfy CG, Alderson P, Grelsamer RP, Henry JH, Mow VC: In vivo and in vitro knee joint cartilage topography, thickness, and contact areas from MRI. Trans Orthop Res Soc 22 (1997) 625
12. Cohen ZA, McCarthy DM, Ateshian GA, Kwak SD, Peterfy CG, Alderson P, Grelsamer RP, Henry JH, Mow VC: Knee joint topography and contact areas: validation of measurements from MRI. Proc Bioeng, ASME, BED 35 (1997) 45-46
13. Cohen ZA, McCarthy DM, Kwak SD, Legrand P, Fogarasi F, Ciaccio EJ, Ateshian GA: Knee cartilage topography, thickness, and contact areas from MRI: In vitro calibration and in vivo measurements. Osteoarthritis Cart (in press)
14. Delp SL, Loan JP, Hoy MG, Zajac FE, Topp EL, Rosen JM: An interactive, graphics-based model of the lower extremity to study orthopaedic surgical procedures. IEEE Trans Biomed Eng 37 (1990) 757-767
15. Delp SL, Statler K, Carroll NC: Preserving plantar flexion strength after surgical treatment for contracture of the triceps surae: a computer simulation study. J Orthop Res 13 (1994) 96-104
16. Delp SL, Komattu AV, Wixson RL: Superior displacement of the hip in total joint replacement: effects of prosthetic neck length, neck-stem angle, and anteversion angle on the moment-generating capacity of the muscles. J Orthop Res 12 (1994) 860-870
17. Delp SL, Ringwelski DA, Carroll NC: Transfer of the rectus femoris: effects of transfer site on moment arms about the knee and hip. J Biomech 27 (1994) 1201-1211
18. Delp SL, Loan JP: A graphics-based software system to develop and analyze models of musculoskeletal structures. Comput Biol Med 25 (1995) 21-34

19. Delp SL, Arnold AS, Speers RA, Moore CA: Hamstrings and psoas lengths during normal and crouch gait: implications for muscle-tendon surgery. J Orthop Surg 14 (1996) 144-151
20. Disler DG, Peters TL, Muscoreil SJ, Rat ner LM, Wagle WA, Cousins JP, Rifkin MD: Fat-suppressed imaging of knee hyaline cartilage: technique optimization and comparison with conventional MR imaging. Am J Radiol 163 (1994) 887-892
21. Disler DG, McCauley TR, Wirth CR, Fuchs MD: Detection of knee hyaline cartilage defects using fat-suppressed three-dimensional spoiled gradient-echo MR imaging: comparison with standard MR imaging and correlation with arthroscopy. Am J Radiol 165 (1995) 377-382
22. Eckstein F, Sittek H, Milz S, Putz R, Reiser M: The morphology of articular cartilage assessed by magnetic resonance imaging (MRI): reproducibility and anatomical correlation. Surg Radiol Anat 16 (1994) 429-38
23. Eckstein F, Gavazzeni A, Sittek H, Ha ubner M, Losch A, Milz S, Englmeier KH, Schulte E, Putz R, Reiser M: Determination of knee joint cartilage thickness using three-dimensional magnetic resonance chondro-crassometry (3D MR-CCM). Magn Reson Med 36 (1996) 256-65
24. van Eijden, TMGJ, Kouwenhoven E, Verbur g J, Weijs WA: A mathematical model of the patellofemoral joint. J Biomech 19 (1986) 219-229
25. Essinger JR, Leyvraz PF, Heegard JH, Robertson DD: A mathematical model for the evaluation of the behaviour during flexion of condylar-type knee prostheses. J Biomech 22 (1989) 1229-1241
26. Fulkerson JP, Schutzer, SF: After failure of conservative treatment for painful patellofemoral malalignment: lateral release or realignment? Orthop Clin North Am 17 (1986) 283-288
27. Garcia-Elias M, An KN, Cooney WP, Linsc heid RL, Chao EY: Transverse stability of the carpus: an analytic study. J Orthop Res 7 (1989) 738-743
28. Garg A, Walker PS: Prediction of total kn ee motion using a three-dimensional computer-graphics model. J Biomech 23 (1990) 45-58
29. Heegaard J, Leyvraz PF, Curnier A, Ra kotomanana L, Huiskes R: The biomechanics of the human patella during passive knee flexion. J Biomech 28 (1995) 1265-1279
30. Hirokawa S: Three-dimensional mathema tical model analysis of the patellofemoral joint. J Biomech 24 (1991) 659-671
31. Horii E, Garcia-Elias M, An KN, Bishop A T, Cooney WP, Linscheid RL, Caho EYS: Effect on force transmission across the carpus in procedures used to treat Kienböck's disease. J Hand Surg 15A (1990) 393-400
32. Hsu RWW, Himeno S, Coventry MB, Chao EYS: Normal axial alignment of the lower extremity and load-bearing distribution at the knee. Clin Orthop 255 (1990) 215-227
33. Jupiter JB, Ruder J, Roth DA: Computer -generated bone models in the planning of osteotomy of multidirectional distal radius malunions. J Hand Surg 17A (1992) 406-415
34. Kwak SD, Ateshian GA, Blankevoort L, Ahm ad, CS, Gardner TR, Grelsamer RP, Henry JH, Mow VC: A general mathematical multibody model for diarthrodial joints: application and validation using the patellofemoral joint. Adv Bioeng, ASME, BED 33 (1996) 239-240
35. Matsen FA 3rd, Garbini JL, Sidles JA, P ratt B, Baumgarten D, Kaiura R: Robotic assistance in orthopaedic surgery. Clin Orthop 296 (1993) 178-186
36. Millis MB, Murphy SB: The use of comput ed tomographic reconstruction in planning osteotomies of the hip. Clin Orthop 274 (1992) 154-159

37. Murphy SB, Kijewski PK, Simon SR, Chand ler HP, Griffin PP, Reilly DT, Penenberg BL, Landy MM: Computer-aided simulation, analysis, and design in orthopedic surgery. Orthop Clin North Am 17 (1986) 637-649
38. Murphy SB, Kijewski PK, Millis MB, Hall JE, Simon SR, Chandler HP: The planning of orthopaedic reconstructive surgery using computer-aided simulation and design. Comput Med Imaging & Graph 12(1988) 33-45
39. Nolte LP, Zamorano LJ, Jiang Z, Wang Q, Langlotz F, Berlemann U: Image-guided insertion of transpedicular screws: a laboratory set-up. Spine 20:497-500 (1995)
40. O'Toole RV, Jaramaz B, DiGioia AM 3rd, Visnic CD, Reid RH: Biomechanics for preoperative planning and surgical simulations in orthopaedics. Comput Biol Med 25 (1995) 183-191
41. Paul H, Bargar WL, Mittlestadt B, Musits B, Taylor RH, Kanzanzides P, Zuhars J, Williamson B, Hanson W: Development of a surgical robot for cementless total hip arthroplasty. Clin Orthop 285 (1992) 57-66
42. Peterfy CG, van Dijke CF, Janzen DL, Gluer CG, Namba R, Majumdar S, Lang P, Genant HK: Quantification of articular articular cartilage in the knee with pulsed saturation transfer subtraction and fat-suppressed MR imaging: optimization and validation. Radiology 192 (1994) 485-491
43. Peterfy CG, Majumdar S, Lang P, van D ijke CF, Sack K, Genant HK: MR Imaging of the arthritic knee: improved discrimination of cartilage, synovium, and effusion with pulsed saturation transfer and fat-supressed T1-weighted sequences. Radiology 191 (1994) 413-419
44. Recht MP, Kramer J, Marcelis S, Pathria MN, Trudell D, Haghighi P, Sartoris DJ, Resnick D: Abnormalities of articular cartilage in the knee: analysis of available MR techniques. *Radiology* 187 (1993) 473-478
45. Recht MP, Resnick D: MR imaging of artic ular cartilage: current status and future directions. Am J Radiol 163 (1994) 283-290
46. Roglic H, Kwak SD, Henry JH, Ateshian G A, Rodkey W, Steadman JR, Mow VC: Adhesions of the patellar and quadriceps tendons: mathematical model simulation. Adv Bioeng, ASME, BED 36 (1997) 261-262
47. Ronsky J, van den Bogert A, Nigg B: In vivo quantification of human patellofemoral joint contact. Proc Can Soc Biomech 8 (1994) 82
48. Sangeorzan BJ, Sangeorzan BP, Hansen ST, Judd RP: Mathematically directed single-cut osteotomy for correction of tibial malunion. J Orthop Trauma 3 (1989) 267-275
49. Scherrer PK, Hillberry BM, Van Sickle DC: Determining the in vivo areas of contact in the canine shoulder. J Biomech Eng 101 (1979) 271-278
50. Seo GS, Aoki J, Moriya H, Karakida O, Sine S, Hikada H, Katsuyama T: Hyaline cartilage: in vivo and in vitro assessment with magnetization transfer imaging. Radiology 201 (1996) 525-530
51. Sutherland CJ, Bresina SJ, Gayou DE : Use of general purpose mechanical computer assisted engineering software in orthopaedic surgical planning: advantages and limitations. Comput Med Imaging Graph 18 (1994) 435-442
52. Tan TCF, Wilcox DM, Frank L, Shih C, Trude ll DJ, Sartoris DJ, Resnick D: MR imaging of articular cartilage in the ankle: comparison of available imaging sequences and methods of measurement in cadavers. Skeletal Radiol 25 (1996) 749-755

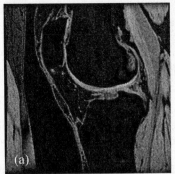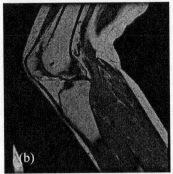

Fig. 1. Two image sequences are acquired for each patient: (a) a 9 minute cartilage sequence at full extension in a linear extremity coil and (b) a 4 minute sequence at 50°-70° of flexion in the full-body coil of the MRI scanner. This patient's patella exhibits arthritic lesions which can be visualized from the cartilage-specific sequence.

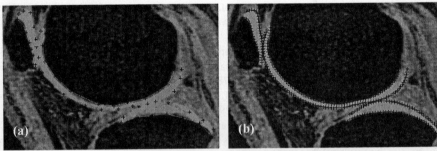

Fig. 2. Semi-automated segmentation of the cartilage layers from MRI: (a) A piecewise linear curve is first provided along the desired edge by manual digitizing (shown here for the cartilage and subchondral bone surfaces of the patella, femur and tibia). (b) A snake algorithm finds a best-fit cubic B-spline curve along the desired edges. The number of B-spline control points and knot spacing is determined from the initial curve [13].

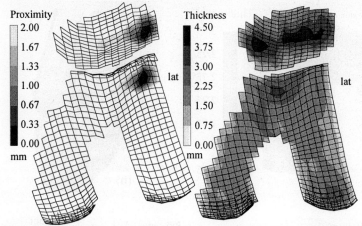

Fig. 3. Segmentation of patellar and femoral cartilage layers from patient MRI: (a) Contact map for patient with lateral subluxation at 70° flexion. (b) Cartilage thickness maps for same patient, showing a normal thickness distribution.

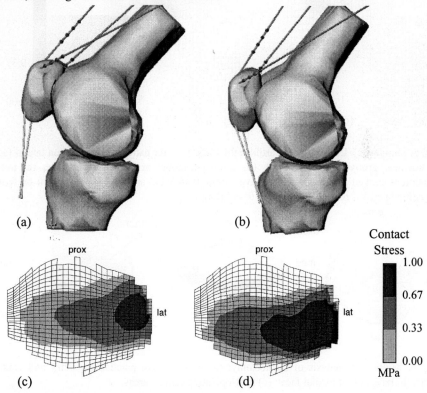

Fig. 4. Multibody model of the knee joint of a patient with previous tibial tuberosity elevation surgery. (a) Current configuration, (b) probable configuration before surgery (tuberosity shifted 15 mm posteriorly), (c) map of current stress distribution on the patella (avg. stress: 0.44 MPa) and (d) map of probable stress distribution before surgery (avg. stress: 0.57 MPa)

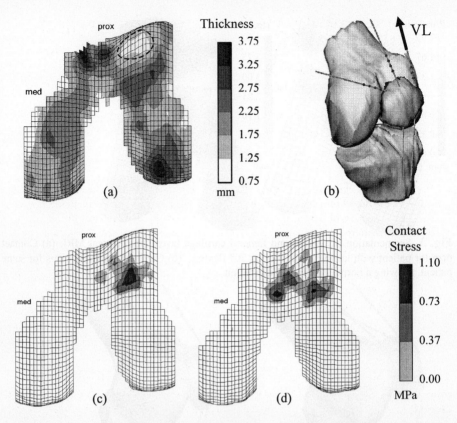

Fig. 5. Simulated VL release. (a) Cartilage thickness map for patient with lesion on lateral facet of trochlear groove (dashed curve), (b) computer model of same patient knee, (c) initial location of contact area on the femur (avg. stress: 0.46 MPa) and (d) contact pattern on femur after simulated VL release (avg. stress: 0.43 MPa)

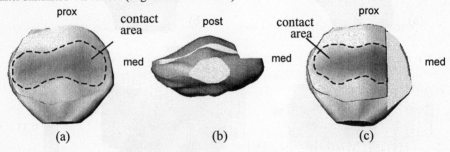

Fig. 6. Multibody analysis of facetectomy: (a) Pre-operative patellar geometry and contact areas; (b) resection of medial facet; (c) post-operative contact areas.

Computer Assisted Orthognathic Surgery

B. Mollard*, S. Lavallée* and G. Bettega+
*TIMC Laboratory - IAB, Faculté de Médecine de Grenoble
38706 LA TRONCHE, FRANCE
+Plastic and Maxillo-facial Surgery department
CHU A. Michallon - B.P. 217 38043 GRENOBLE CEDEX, FRANCE
Benoit.Mollard@imag.fr

Abstract. This paper presents a surgical simulator for orthognathic surgery based on the integration of dental models and 3D cephalometry. The objective of dental models integration is to make coherent informations gathered from different sources (occlusal analysis and CT scan), and for that purpose, a system using a 3D optical localizer is used. The 3D Cephalometry analysis is used for the detection of dysmorphosis and surgical planning. This cephalometry integrates the Inferrence process for improving the surgical system. Both elements of our simulator have been implemented and technically validated with success.

1 Introduction

Planning cranio-facial surgical procedures, particularly orthognathic surgery, requires integration of multiple and complex data gathered from different sources: clinical examination (anthropometry), orthodontic (dental models), radiological (cephalometry) and intra-operative data (constraints and position information). This heterogeneity makes the therapeutic decision difficult, particularly in asymmetrical dysmorphosys. This is the reason why several three-dimensional (3D) surgical analysis and simulation softwares and methods have been developed [2, 8, 6, 11, 7].
This paper introduces a 3D cephalometric analysis system and a surgical simulator for orthognatic surgery developed by Bettega et al. [2]. Our simulator is based on the integration of dental models (section 2) and 3D cephalometry (section 3). We discuss the notion of *Inferrence* and its benefit in terms of improvement of the surgical system (section 4). Those concepts are illustrated on concrete and quantified data.

2 Dental Models Integration

The goal of dental model integration is to transpose the results of the occlusal analysis carried out on teeth plaster cast by the prosthesist into the 3D CT scan models visualized and manipulated by the surgeon. The objective is to make both informations coherent, for better accuracy and efficiency. For that purpose, we use a three-dimensional optical localizer (Optotrak, NorthernDigital, Toronto). First, two intercuspidation splints are constructed. These resine splints

are modeled with the plaster casts, according to the usual procedure followed by
the orthodontist and the prosthesist. The initial intercuspidation splint (ICS_i) is
used to materialize the mandible position in preoperative occlusion and to allow
the ulterior fusion of the data given by the localizer and those extracted from
the CT slices (Figure 1). During the acquisition of the patient CT-scan, ICS_i
will guaranty that the preoperative occlusion is respected. This plate is also used
to support a rigid body (infra-red emitting system) localized by Optotrak . The
final intercuspidation splint (ICS_f) corresponds to the occlusal correction. It
is used to mobilise the plaster casts, which are manually displaced in order to
engage the teeth in the desired position after the intervention. The final splint is
built by the prosthesist using an articulation jaw and plaster casts, following a
long-term orthodontic treatment which has displaced the teeth towards a desired
position.

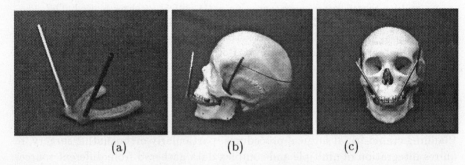

(a) (b) (c)

Fig. 1. Lateral(b) and facial(c) views of a dry skull equipped with ICS_i (a).
This splint is equipped with external landmarks made up of two aluminium
tubes (implanted on the splint with a guide plate) easily identifiable in CT scan
slices (without causing radiological artefacts) and constituting a 3D referential
visible by Optotrak. These landmarks tubes allow matching the CT scan and
the dental data with accuracy.

The change from the initial splint to the final one is represented by a displacement matrix T_1 (Figure 2 (a)). In other words, T_1 defines the relative position
of maxilla in relation to the mandible after the intercuspidation splint has been
changed. The scheme for accurate determination of T_1 consists of digitizing the
position of infra-red emitting systems firmly fixed to plaster cast, first with **ICS_i**,
then with **ICS_f**. The relative displacement given by $T1$ has to be transferred into
the tridimensional reconstruction of the CT-scan referential. This is done by the
application of a registration algorithm between landmarks tubes digitized with
Optotrak, and those tubes pointed on CT-scan slices (Figure 2 (b)). In order to
evaluate the accuracy of the landmarks tube-based registration method, we have
compared it with a 3D-3D rigid registration algorithm using octree-splines [9]
(Figure 3). We have compared the rotation and translation components of both
transformations:

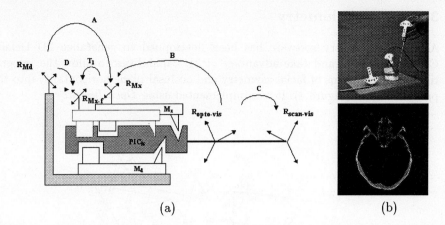

Fig. 2. (a) Identification of the different matrices - (b) Digitization of Landmarks Tubes: it consists of making a sensor equipped with a rigid body sliding and rotating into the tube. About one hundred points are digitized in this way and for each tube - Calculation of the line which goes through the longitudinal axis of each tube after manual localisation on each CT-scan slice of the center of both tube slices

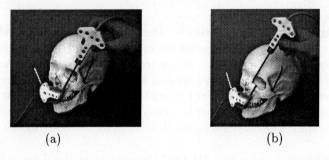

Fig. 3. (a) Evaluation of matrix C using the tubes (b) Evaluation of matrix C using the 3D-3D non-rigid registration algorithm: on the bone surface of a dry skull equipped with ICS_i, 200 points are digitized in $R_{opto-vis}$ referential. A 3D CT scan reconstruction of the bone surface is performed in $R_{scan-vis}$ referential. Therefore, the optical data (cloud of points) are matched with the CT scan data (points extracted from the 3D reconstruction of the bone surface).

The rotation error is $0.93 dg$. The translation error is $0.43 mm$.
Both transforms are obtained using very different data. Results show that they are probably both equally accurate. Those results are quite acceptable and validate our approach. With our system, it is possible to integrate the dental models in the 3D cephalometry and so, in the surgical simulator.

3 3D Cephalometry

A 3D cephalometry software has been developped to generalize 2D Delaire Cephalometry [4] and take advantage of 3D capabilities to allow the integration of the problems of facial asymetry and occlusal plane horizontality into the profile analysis (Figure 4). It was implemented using *Open-Inventor*.

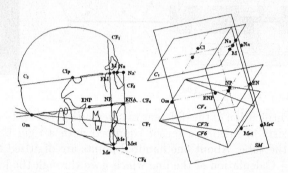

Fig. 4. 2D Representation of simplified Delaire analysis and 3D Representation of cephalometric points and planes

3D Reconstruction Modalities - The *Marching Cubes* method is used to reconstruct the skull from computer tomography [10]. The rendering quality is excellent but the number of triangles generated to reconstruct the bone surfaces is too huge to allow an interactive surgical simulation. We don't use compression algorithms to reduce the number of facets because the operator must have a sufficiently precise model to identify correctly the cephalometrical points without losing any detail. The chosen solution is to build an "hybrid" model of the skull (Figure 5).

3D Cephalometry - The 3D Cephalometrical analysis procedure is then divided in 3 steps: definition of sagittal median plane (Figure 6 (a)), determination of 10 cephalometrical anatomical landmarks (Figure 6 (b)) and the analysis itself, which is automatically calculated (Figure 6 (c)). Each step of the analysis is validated and if necessary manually corrected.

Virtual Osteotomies - The goal is to isolate on the 3D model a part of the maxilla and of the mandible from the rest of the skull. In the same way, one must dissociate the maxilla above the intercuspidation splint and the mandible (below the splint). The osteotomies are performed using a parallelepiped cutting pattern (Figure 6 (d)). It is interactively placed on the skull model and dimensioned with the manipulation tools provided by *Open-Inventor*. Those tools are sufficient to obtain a realistic model of surgical cutting off.

Dental Models Integration - The orthognatic diagnosis is subsenquently established (3D position of maxilla, mandible, chin compared to normal) and the surgical simulation is carried out. The $T1$ matrix is applied to the dissociated dental portions to correct the occlusion on the CT representation. This corrected

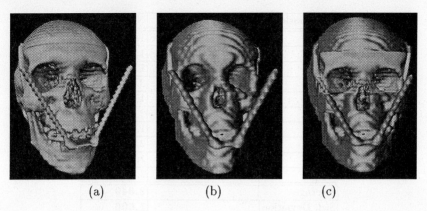

Fig. 5. (a) High Resolution Model (b) Low Resolution Model (c) Hybrid model. Hybrid model consists of building two models: a high resolution model and a low resolution model reconstructed from averaged CT scan slices. Then, both models are divided into blocks that have the same size. The hybrid model is a combination of these two models divided in blocks. For each cephalometrical point, a default configuration has been defined, but it can also be personnalized by the operator. The low resolution blocks can also be dismissed in order to improve the interactivity and focus on the region of interest.

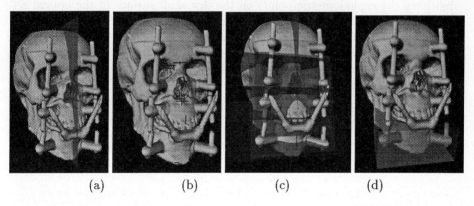

Fig. 6. 3D Cephalometrical analysis

maxillo-mandibular set is then positionned into the remaining skull respecting the previous orthognathic diagnosis. At this point, the necessity of a genioplasty is evaluated and performed if needed.

Validation of the 3D Cephalometry - The 3D cephalometry used in our simulator has to be validated at two levels. The first level consists of verifying that it is possible to define on the 3D model reconstructed from CT scan slices the anatomical landmarks (cephalometrical elements). The second level concerns the validation of the 3D cephalometrical analysis itself and its protocol. The pro-

Landmark	Error	Norm (mm)
M_d	-0.853 -0.0339 -1.508	1.733
M_g	-0.448 1.184 -0.148	1.275
NA	-0.292 -0.450 -1.299	1.406
Me	-1.607 -2.259 1.769	3.289
ENA	1.801 0.027 0.007	1.802
II_s	0.205 0.418 -2.417	2.461
Clp_d	1.168 -0.527 -0.902	1.567
Clp_g	1.840 -1.976 -0.763	2.806
Np_d	-1.549 1.596 -1.384	1.533
Np_g	-0.691 -0.417 -1.303	2.620
Average		**2.049**
Std. Deviation		**1.606**
Minimum		**1.275**
Maximum		**3.289**

Table 1. Results

cedure of validation is realised on a dry skull equipped with its landmarks (tubes) and examinated by computerized tomography. It consists, on the one hand, of digitizing the cephalometric points on the dry skull surface in the optical reference system, and on the other hand, of locating the same points on the 3D surface model in the CT scan reference system. The C transformation matrix between both referentials is then calculated, either by using the tube-based registration method that has been previously validated, or by using the rigid 3D surface registration algorithm. Therefore, both sets of points are compared and the precision that can be achieved by the operator using the simulator is evaluated.

The results for the 10 chosen anatomical landmarks are shown in Table 1. Those results are rather satisfactory, since the largest errors (3.3 mm) correspond to points that are difficult to determine accurately in the real space.

4 Inferrence

In order to have a very effective cephalometrical analysis, the determination of the cephalometrical points must be done with accuracy. But this task is very repetitive; it requires all the attention of the operator during a long time. For this reason, we have integrated in the simulator a procedure which defines automatically an initial position for each landmark and their viewpoints. This is done by *Inferrence*, the process by which the properties of a model are mapped in the patient space using the 3D Octree-splines Transformation. We can use the result of Inferrence between a model and the patient data to display the initial position of the landmarks and to associate viewpoints to each landmark

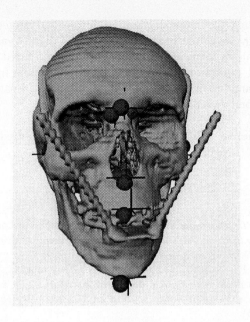

Fig. 7. Illustration of the Inferrence principle. The spheres are landmarks of another model which have been inferred to this model and constitute the initial position for the landmark definition. One can appreciate their relative proximity in comparaison with the final position of the landmarks (crosses).

by inferrence of the model viewpoint. This application is illustrated in Fig. 7. Initial registration is obtained by alignment of CT coordinate systems (without additional translation or rotation). In this position, the mean distance between landmarks is 21.8mm (min/max = 14.2 mm / 29.5 mm). After elastic registration and inferrence, the mean distance between landmarks is 5.7 mm (min/max = 4.3 mm /8.2 mm).

5 Conclusion

In this paper, we have presented the concepts of the elements necessary for integrated cephalometry analysis, with particular emphasis on the integration of orthodontic information, for optimal and coherent surgical planning. All those elements have been implemented and technically validated with success.

The complete integration and test of the system is now necessary. It will be based on two kinds of experiments. In the first experiment, standard osteotomies and bone displacements can be performed on a dry skull in order to simulate a dysmorphosis. The 3D cephalometry analysis should be able to detect and correct the dysmorphosis. In the second experiment, we will apply the simulation system on the skull of a normal subject. The 3D cephalometry analysis shouldn't detect any dysmorphosis.

Finally, reproducing the surgical planning during real surgery will be possible by using two elements of the puzzle that we have already validated. First, registration is possible by using the intercuspidation plate fitted with a rigid body, exactly described in section 2. Second, alignment of bone fragments to a predefined position and orientation has been validated on 14 patients, using a passive system for condyle repositionning [5, 3, 1].

Acknowledgements: this research is financially supported by the european project IGOS HC1026HC.

References

1. G. BETTEGA, *La Chirurgie orthognathique assistée par ordinateur: de la planification à la réalisation*, PhD thesis, Université Joseph Fourier - Grenoble 1, 23 Novembre 1997.
2. G. BETTEGA, P. CINQUIN, S. LAVALLEE, AND B. RAPHAEL, *Dispositif de détermination d'un déplacement entre des positions relatives de 2 moulages dentaires et système de simulation d'intervention en chirurgie orthognatique*, patent FR 9616066, (1996).
3. G. BETTEGA, V. DESSENNE, B. RAPHAEL, AND P. CINQUIN, *Computer assisted mandibular condyle positioning in orthognatic surgery*, J. Oral Maxillo Facial Surgery, (1996), pp. 553–558.
4. J. DELAIRE, *L'analyse architecturale et structurale cranio-faciale (de profil). Principes theoriques. Quelques exemples d'emploi en chirurgie maxillo-faciale.*, Revue de Stomatologie et de chirurgie Maxillo-faciale, 79 (1978), pp. 1–33.
5. V. DESSENNE, G. BETTEGA, S. LAVALLEE, P. CINQUIN, AND B. RAPHAEL, *Computer-assisted mandibular condyle positioning in orthognatic surgery*, in Second Symposium on Medical Robotics and Computer Assisted Surgery Proc. (MRCAS'95), Baltimore, 1995, Wiley, pp. 215–221.
6. J. M. ET AL., *Applications of computer graphics in craniofacial surgery*, Clin. Past. Surg., (1986), pp. 441–8.
7. M. V. ET AL., *Three-dimensional computer graphics for craniofacial surgical planning and evaluation*, in Computer Graphics, vol. 17, 1983, pp. 263–74.
8. E. KEEVE, S. GIROD, AND B. GIROD, *Computer-Aided Craniofacial Surgery*, in Computer Assisted Radiology, H. Lemke and al., eds., P.O. Box 211 - 1000 AE Amsterdam - The Nederlands, 1996, Elsevier Science B.V., pp. 757–763.
9. S. LAVALLEE, R. SZELISKI, AND L. BRUNIE, *Anatomy-based registration of 3-D medical images, range images, X-ray projections, 3-D models using Octree-Splines*, in Computer Integrated Surgery, R. Taylor, S. Lavallee, G. Burdea, and R. Mosges, eds., MIT Press, Cambridge, MA, 1996, pp. 115–143.
10. LORENSEN, *Marching cube: a High Resolution 3D Surface Construction Algorithm*, Computer Graphics, SIGGRAPH'87, 21 (1987), pp. 163–169.
11. R. ROBB AND D. HANSON, *The ANALYZE software system for visualization and analysis in surgery simulation*, in Computer-integrated surgery, R. e. a. Taylor, ed., MIT Press, Cambridge, MA, 1996, ch. 10.

Computer-Aided Image-Guided Bone Fracture Surgery: Modeling, Visualization, and Preoperative Planning

L. Tockus[1,4], L. Joskowicz[1], A. Simkin[2], and C. Milgrom[3] MD

[1] Institute of Computer Science, The Hebrew Univ., Jerusalem 91904 Israel.
[2] Lab. of Experimental Surgery, Hadassah Univ. Hospital, Jerusalem 91120 Israel.
[3] Dept. of Orthopaedic Surgery, Hadassah Univ. Hospital, Jerusalem 91120 Israel.
[4] Biomedicom, Technology Park, Malha, Mail Stop IIL 376 Jerusalem 91487, Israel
lana@biomedicom.co.il, josko@cs.huji.ac.il
ruskin@vms.huji.ac.il,milgrom@md2.huji.ac.il

Abstract. This paper describes the FRACAS computer-integrated orthopaedic system for assisting surgeons in closed long bone fracture reduction. FRACAS' goals are to reduce the surgeon's cumulative exposure to radiation and improve the positioning accuracy by replacing uncorrelated static fluoroscopic images with a virtual reality display of 3D bone models created from preoperative CT and tracked intraoperatively in real-time. Fluoroscopic images are used to register the bone models to the intraoperative situation and to verify that the registration is maintained. This paper describes the system concept, and the software prototypes of the modeling, preoperative planning, and visualization modules.

1 Introduction

Fluoroscopy-based orthopaedic procedures crucially depend on the ability of the surgeon to mentally recreate the spatio-temporal intraoperative situation from uncorrelated, two-dimensional fluoroscopic X-ray images. Significant skill, time, and frequent use of the fluoroscope are required, leading to positioning errors and complications in a non-negligible number of cases, and to significant cumulative radiation exposure of the surgeon [12]. Recent research shows that computer-aided systems can significantly improve the accuracy of orthopaedic procedures by replacing fluoroscopic guidance with interactive display of 3D bone models created from preoperative CT studies and tracked in real time. Examples include systems for acetabular cup placement [13], for total knee replacement, and for pedicle screw insertion [5, 8].

We are currently developing a computer-integrated orthopaedic system, called FRACAS, for closed medullary nailing of long bone fractures. Medullary nailing is a very frequent routine procedure that restores the integrity of the fractured bone by means of a nail inserted in the medullary canal [1]. The nail is placed without surgically exposing the fracture through an opening close to the piriformus fossa in the proximal femoral bone. The surgeon manually aligns the bone

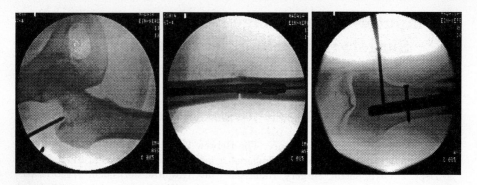

Fig. 1. Fluoroscopic images showing the steps of closed medulary nailing (from left to right): opening of the medulary canal; alignement of the bone fragments and nail insertion; and distal locking.

fragments, inserts a guide wire, reams the canal if necessary, and drives the nail in with a hammer. Lateral proximal and distal interlocking screws are inserted to prevent fragment rotation and bone shortening. All these steps are performed under fluoroscopic guidance (Fig. 1).

The most common errors and complications in closed medullary fixation come from limited viewing capabilities. Because all alignment, reaming, and positioning must be done under fluoroscopy, the surgeon must mentally reconstruct the location of the parts in space and time, manipulate the tools and the bone without visual feedback, and confirm the position with a new set of fluoroscopic images. This often imprecise, slow, and tedious procedure can cause improper positioning and alignment, inadequate fixation, malrotation, bone cracking, cortical wall penetration, bone weakening with multiple or enlarged screw holes in the worst case. The surgeon's direct exposure to radiation in each procedure is between 3 to 30 min with 31-51% spent on distal locking [12] depending on the patient and the surgeon's skill. When the bone fragments are difficult to align, the surgeon reverts to open techniques. The surgeon's radiation exposure and the reported number of complications of this kind motivates the search for improved solutions.

FRACAS' goals are to reduce the surgeon's cumulative exposure to radiation and improve the positioning and navigation accuracy by replacing uncorrelated static fluoroscopic images with a virtual reality display of 3D bone models created from preoperative CT and tracked intraoperatively in real-time (Figure 2). Fluoroscopic images are used for registration – to establish a common reference frame – between the bone models and the intraoperative situation, and to verify that the registration is maintained. This paper describes the system concept and the software prototypes of the modeling, preoperative planning, and visualization, modules. A companion paper describes fluoroscopic image processing.

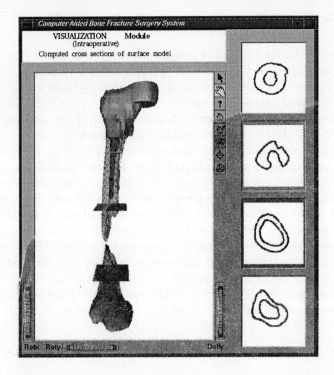

Fig. 2. Intraoperative three-dimensional distal and proximal bone fragment models that replace the fluoroscopic images, as displayed by the Visualization module. Their location is tracked and updated in real time during surgery. The four windows on the right show the inner and outer bone contours at the selected cross sections corresponding to planes on the left.

2 Previous work

Two computer-based systems for long bone fracture reduction [10, 15] and [3] focus on distal screw locking. Both use intraoperative fluoroscopy and optical tracking without preoperative CT images. [10, 15] uses a passive mechanical arm with optical encoders to guide the surgeon to the right drilling position. It automatically identifies the distal holes in the fluoroscopic images, plans the drilling trajectory, and constraints passive arm motions. The advantage of the system is that it eliminates trial-and-error drill positioning. The disadvantage is that it requires additional mechanical hardware. [3] continuously displays the projection of the surgical tools as they move on preselected fluoroscopic images, thus approximating continuous fluoroscopy. Since the images are correlated, the surgeon can simultaneously view the tool's progression from several viewpoints. This is similar to the conventional procedure and reduces the number of images needed. However, it does not provide preoperative planning support, does not display 3D views, and does not update the bone fragment positions in real time

3 Goals and rationale

Our goal in developing FRACAS is to assist the surgeon in all the steps of fracture reduction, not just in distal locking. It provides 3D bone modeling, preoperative planning, fluoroscopic image processing, and anatomy-based registration of the 3D model with the fluoroscopic images.

We believe that the additional cost and time of the preoperative CT study is outweighed by the potential reduction in more expensive intraoperative time, in minimizing mistakes and repetitive attempts at fracture reduction, and in reducing the surgeon's exposure to radiation. In many centers, including ours, CT is readily available for trauma patients, adding little preoperative time, risk, and morbidity. Cases of fracture femur may be divided into those in which the sole injury is the fractured femur, and those which there is multiple trauma. Multiple trauma patients are likely to have other CT studies done anyhow, e.g., abdomen and pelvis. In both cases, the patient's leg is immobilized on a Thomas splint which makes transport on the emergency room stretcher and transfer to the CT table easy and relatively pain free, with minimal fracture movement. Any fracture movement that does occur would not be associated with an increased risk for pulmonary emobilism.

4 FRACAS: system description

The FRACAS system [4] comprises three units: a standard fluoroscopic C-arm, a real-time position tracking optical system, and a computer workstation with data processing and visualization software. The fluoroscopic unit is used to capture images that are used to establish a common reference frame (registration) between the intraoperative bone position and preoperative bone fragment models. The tracking unit is used to provide accurate, real-time spatial object positions with optical cameras following infrared light-emitting diodes (LEDs) rigidly mounted on the surgical instruments or attached to the bones via bone screws [5, 9]. The computer workstation is used preoperatively for modeling and planing, and intraoperatively for data fusion and display.

The envisaged sequence of the procedure is as follows: preoperatively, a CT of the healthy and fractured bones is acquired. Surface and canal bone models are constructed by the modeling module. Using the planning modules, the surgeon interactively selects the distal and proximal bone fragments and nail type, length, and diameter. Shortly before the surgery, the fluoroscopic and tracking units are calibrated by a technician. The patient is then brought into the operating room and the surgeon prepares and exposes the femur canal following the usual procedure.

To track the position of the bone fragments, the surgeon rigidly implants two specially prepared bone screws with LEDs attached to them. Fluoroscopic images are then captured by a technician (without the nearby presence of the surgeon) to perform an anatomy-based registration with the preoperative bone fragment models. With the LEDs in place, the technician activates the optical tracking

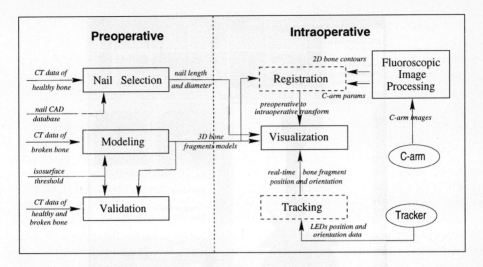

Fig. 3. Flow diagram of FRACAS's main software modules. Solid rectangles are implemented modules, dashed ones are under construction.

system to capture the location of the bone fragments and surgical instruments. The images are imported into the workstation via a video frame grabber, and the tracking data via a serial port. The visualization module constructs the virtual reality image showing the bone fragments and surgical instrument models and presents it to the surgeon on a high-definition monitor. The surgeon manipulates the bone fragments and surgical tools, following their relative positions and orientations on the monitor. Once the desired positioning is achieved, a new set of fluoroscopic images is captured and registered to confirm the intraoperative situation with the displayed model. This process is repeated for the different steps of the procedure.

Figure 3 shows the main FRACAS software modules and the data flow between them. We describe the modeling and validation, nail selection, and visualization modules in detail next. The fluoroscopic image processing module is presented in [16]. The registration and tracking modules are under development.

5 Modeling

The modeling module inputs the CT data and a user-defined bone density threshold value. It outputs the inner and outer surface models of the selected proximal and distal bone fragments. The models are produced in two steps. First, polygonal surface models of the bone external and internal fragment surfaces are created. Then, the surgeon interactively defines the extent of the proximal and distal fragments of interest with cutting planes. Figure 4 shows the modeling module window with a segmental comminuted fracture.

The bone fragment surface models are meshes of connected triangles. They are extracted from the CT data using an extended Marching Cubes algorithm

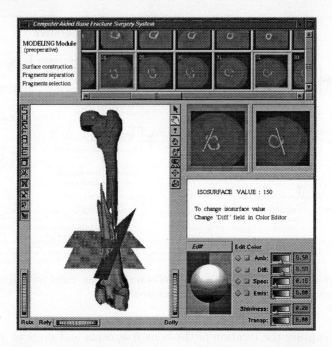

Fig. 4. The Modeling module display. The top window shows the original CT slices. The left bottom window shows the surface model of the fractured bone (the canal surface is hidden). The horizontal planes indicate the position of the selected CT slices shown in detail on the two windows on the right. The slanted plane is the user-defined cutting plane that separates the bone fragments. The bottom right window shows the bone density threshold and the material and viewing parameters.

[7] which classifies surface triangles as proximal, distal, canal, or outer surface. The size of the triangular meshes depends on the CT data, typically consisting of several tens of thousands of triangles. For example, the CT set in Figure 4 consists of 44 slices at 10mm intervals, image size 160x160, pixel size 1mm^2; it yields a model of about 75,000 triangles.

Since the bone fragments are usually in contact due to the action of the muscles, bone and canal surface models are frequently lumped together (a single connected piece for linear fractures, several pieces for segmental and comminuted fractures). An additional step is necessary to separate the fragment models because threshold information alone is not sufficient to determine when a new fragment begins and when one ends when they are in contact.

The fragment models are separated into different pieces by means of user-defined cutting planes whose intersection defines regions of interest. Cutting planes can be positioned in one of two ways. One is by defining the plane in a default configuration and bringing it to the desired location using manipulation dials (on the left and bottom part of the window in Figure 4). The drawback is that the cutting plane is initially in an arbitrary position and might require a series of non-intuitive dial manipulations to bring it to the desired position.

A more suitable method is to interpolate a cutting rectangle from two line segments defined in two CT slices close to the area of the desired separation (the white line segments in the two detailed CT windows on the right in Figure 4). To avoid separating model parts that are far from the cutting area, the plane is automatically clipped to a rectangle. The position of the resulting cutting plane can be interactively fine-tuned by changing the position of the segment endpoints or by using the manipulation dials. This procedure is repeated until one or more planes are in the desired position. The fragments are then separated according to their point membership classification relative to each plane. Undesired bone fragments and bone particles are eliminated by clicking on them with the mouse. To differentiate between them, the selected bone fragments are displayed in different colors (dark upper fragment in Figure 4).

To verify that the computed surface model closely matches the CT data, we developed a visual validation module. For each CT slice, the module computes the cross section of the geometric model at the CT slice location and shows it superimposed with the original CT data. The discrepancy between the two can be determined by visual inspection by moving up and down the CT slices. Quantitative measures could be computed if necessary. To improve the fit, the bone density threshold value can be adjusted accordingly.

6   Nail selection

The nail selection module assists the surgeon to select the optimal nail size and length when a CT of the healthy bone is available. It inputs the CT data of the healthy bone and a predefined CAD library of nail models available on site. Its output is the universal nail type, its length, and its diameter. The module constructs a bone and canal surface model and allows the surgeon to perform spatial measurements on it. Figure 5 shows the nail selection window.

To select a nail, the surgeon performs a series of canal diameter and height measurements. Canal diameter measurements are performed on the CT slices (four right windows in Figure 5) by moving the endpoints of a measuring segment (shown in white). Its length is interactively updated and appears in the top left corner of the window. Height measurements are performed on the 3D window (left window) by moving the endpoints of the measuring segment (black segment). Its length is interactively updated and appears in the top left corner of the window. Having determined the closest standard diameter and nail length, the surgeon enters the nail size, and the system retrieves the corresponding CAD model from the nail library. Nail diameters typically come in intervals of 1mm, lengths in intervals of 20mm. The nail model is then interactively positioned with the manipulator dials inside the bone to ensure that the diameter is adequate and that there is no impingement with the knee or hip joint. Although the actual nail deforms when it is inserted into the canal, the displayed nail position is close enough for the preoperative evaluation and selection.

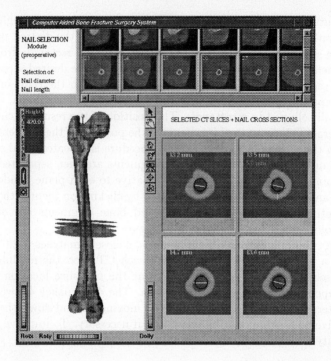

Fig. 5. The Nail Selection module display. The top window shows the original CT slices. The left bottom window shows the healthy bone surface model, the selected nail model, and the planes of the four selected CT slices shown in detail on the four windows to the right of it. The detailed CT slices windows on the right show the nail cross section (dark circle) superimposed on the original CT image.

7 Visualization

The visualization module provides the surgeon with a virtual reality view of the intraoperative position and orientation of the proximal and distal fragments, the nail, and the surgical instruments. The positions are updated with real-time data from the tracking unit, after the preoperative model and the intraoperative situation have been registered (Figure 2). The inputs are the proximal and distal fragment models, the nail model, the registration transformation, and the on-line tracking position information. The output is a display of the updated virtual reality model, which can be seen from any desired perspective, as illustrated in Figure 2 (the nail is omitted; models of locking screws and other surgical instruments can be readily incorporated).

Since the main task is to align the proximal and distal canal, FRACAS displays the central part of the exterior bone fragments translucid and highlights the canal surface inside. The femoral head and the condyles are displayed opaque to provide a reference frame for the joint and bone axes. Note that because of the fracture, the canal can vanish altogether before the end of the fragment. The virtual reality window provides standard viewing capabilities, e.g., zooming, viewpoint and perspective modification. It also includes four windows for cross section visualization, which can be interactively moved up and down the bone (note that the original CT image cannot be displayed, as the bone fragment position has changed).

8 Conclusion

We have described the design and implementation of the modeling, nail selection, and visualization modules of the FRACAS computer-integrated system for closed medullary nailing. The goal of system is to overcome most of the planning, viewing and spatial positioning difficulties associated with orthopaedic image-guided surgery. FRACAS constructs a 3D model of the exterior and canal surface bone fragments and displays an updated view of their position and orientation. It assists surgeons in selecting the optimal nail length and diameter by interactively positioning a CAD nail model inside the healthy bone model. Its main advantages are spatial display and real-time image update, akin to continuous fluoroscopy. To date, we have conducted evaluation trials on five patient data sets to test the user interface and validate the prototype.

Current work on the FRACAS system includes fluoroscopic image processing (image dewarping, C-arm calibration, and contour extraction) [16] and anatomic 2D/3D registration. Near term plans include real-time tracking, system integration and in-vitro prototype testing.

Acknowledgments

Leo Joskowicz is supported by a Guastalla Faculty Fellowship. Lana Tockus was supported by a Silicon Graphics Biomedical (now Biomedicom) grant.

References

1. Brumback R.J., "Regular and Special Features - The Rationales of Interlocking Nailing of the Femur, Tibia, and Humerus" *Clinical Orthopaedics and Related Research*, **324**, Lippincott-Raven, 1996.
2. Fadda M. Bertelli, D., Martelli S. Marcacci, M., Dario P., Carmella D. and Trippi D., "Computer Assisted Planning for Total Knee Arthroplasty" *CVRMed-MRCAS'97*, Lecture Notes in Computer Science 1205, Troccaz et al. eds., Springer 1997.
3. Hofstetter, R., Slomczykowski, M. Bourquin, I, Nolte, L.P, "Fluoroscopy Based Surgical Nagivation – Concept and Clinical Applications", *Proc. 11th Int. Symp. on Computer Assisted Radiology and Surgery*, H.U. Lemke, et al. eds, Springer 1997.
4. Joskowicz, L., Tockus, L., Yaniv, Z, Simkin, A., Milgrom, C. "Computer-Aided Image-Guided Bone Fracture Surgery – Concept and Implementation", *Proc. 12th Int. Symp. on Computer Assisted Radiology and Surgery*, H.U. Lemke et. al. eds, 1998.
5. Lavallée, S., Sautot, P., Troccaz, J., Cinquin, P., Merloz, P. "Computer Assisted Spine Surgery: a Technique for Accurate Transpedicular Screw Fixation Using CT Data and a 3D Optical Localizer", *J. of Image-Guided Surgery* 1(1), 1995.

6. Leitner F., Picard F., Minfelde R., Schultz H.J., Cinquin P. and Saragaglia D., "Computer-assisted knee surgical total replacement" *CVRMed-MRCAS'97*, Lecture Notes in Computer Science 1205, Troccaz et al. eds., Springer 1997
7. Lorensen W.E. and Cline H.E., "Marching Cubes: A High Resolution 3D Surface Construction Algorithm", *SIGGRAPH'87*, Vol. 21(4), July 1987.
8. Li Q.H., Holdener H.J., Zamorano L., *et. al.* Nolte L.P., Visarius H., and Diaz F., "Computer-assisted transpedicular screw insertion" *Lecture Notes in Computer Science*, Springer, 1996.
9. Nolte, L.P., Zamorano L., et. al. "A Novel Approach to Computer Assisted Spine Surgery", *Proc. 1st Int. Symp. on Medical Robotics and Computer Assisted Surgery*, Pittsburgh, 1994.
10. Phillips R., Viant W.J., Mohsen A.M.M.A., Griffits J.G., Bell M.A., Cain T.J., Sherman K.P. and Karpinski M.R.K., "Image Guided Orthopaedic Surgery - Design and Analysis" *IEEE Transactions on Robotics and Control*, March 1996.
11. Russel T.A., "Fractures of Lower Extremity" *Campbell's Orthopaedic Encyclopedia*, 1995.
12. Sanders R., "Exposure of the Orthopaedic Surgeon to Radiation", *J. of Bone Joint Surgery* 75 A(3), 1993.
13. Simon, D.A, Jaramaz, B, Blackwell, *et al.* "Development and Validation of a Navigational Guidance System for Acetabular Implant Placement", *Proc. of CVRMed-MRCAS'97*, Lecture Notes in Computer Science 1205, Springer 1997.
14. Tockus, L. "A System for Computer-Aided Image-Guided Bone Fracture Surgery: Modeling, Visualization, and Preoperative Planning", Msc Thesis, Hebrew U., Jerusalem, July 1997.
15. Viant, W.J., Phillips, R., Griffiths, et al. "A Computer Assisted Orthopaedic System for Distal Locking of Intramedullary Nails", *Proc. of MediMEC'95*, 1995.
16. Yaniv, Z., Joskowicz, L., Simkin, A. Garza-Jinich, M, Milgrom C. "Fluoroscopic Image Processing for Computer-Aided Orthopaedic Surgery" *1st Int. Conf. on Medical Computing and Computer-Assisted Intervention*, Boston, 1998.

A Surgical Planning and Guidance System for High Tibial Osteotomies

C. Y. Tso*   R. E. Ellis*   J. Rudan[†]   M. M. Harrison[†]

* Department of Computing and Information Science
[†] Department of Surgery

Queen's University at Kingston, Ontario, Canada

Abstract

A three-dimensional pre-surgical planner and image-guided surgery system for high tibial osteotomy has been developed. The planning software permits a surgeon to establish the tibial axes, plan the corrective osteotomy, and visualize both the preoperative state and the predicted postoperative state in three dimensions. The parameters that describe the placement and orientation of the osteotomy resection planes can be transmitted to an accompanying guidance system that allows the surgeon to accurately perform the planned procedure. Tests were performed *in vitro* to compare the accuracy of the computer-enhanced technique to the traditional technique, and an *in vivo* pilot study has been initiated. The computer-enhanced technique produced a significant reduction in the error of correction and is simple to use while performing the surgical procedure. The work indicates that three-dimensional planning and surgical performance of high tibial osteotomy is essential to the accuracy of the procedure.

1 Rationale and Objectives

An osteotomy is a surgical procedure to realign a bone in order to change the biomechanics of a joint, especially to change the force transmission through a joint. Theses procedures must be performed accurately, not only to create the desired geometries but also to provide biological environments for rapid and effective healing. In particular, the high tibial osteotomy (HTO) is a corrective surgical procedure in which the upper part of the tibia is resected so that the lower limb can be realigned. The most common form of HTO is the closing wedge osteotomy, in which the realignment is achieved by removing a lateral wedge of bone from the proximal tibia.

High tibial osteotomies are indicated for the relatively young and active patient who has painful unicompartmental knee arthrosis, especially an arthrosis due to an early stage of osteoarthritis. The most common surgical alternative to the procedure is a total knee arthroplasty (TKA) or unicompartmental arthroplasty. TKA has a typical survival rate of 90% at 15 years after the procedure, but the polyethylene articulating surfaces generate wear particles that lead to loosening or failure and subsequent revision. By contrast, HTO preserves the joint's original cartilaginous surfaces and corrects the fundamental mechanical problem of the knee. This advantage of HTO is especially important to the young active patient, for whom an arthroplasty has a greater probability of earlier failure than is likely for an older inactive patient. Economically, the cost of an osteotomy is approximately 1/3 that of an arthroplasty.

The major difficulty with HTO is that the outcome is not predictable, and the major suspected reason for the unpredictability is that it is difficult to attain the desired correction angle. Numerous long-term clinical studies have shown that osteotomy results are improved if the femoral-tibial alignment angle is between 7° and 13° of varus alignment [19, 13]. Immediate postoperative results show a large variability – by averaging the variances of reported results, calculation shows that the overall standard deviation of angular correction is 2.5° for HTO performed with jig systems and 5.6° for those without the use of jigs[7, 16, 15, 17, 10, 14]. Significant changes in the angle of correction after operation can be observed, which can be attributed to fragment mobility. Recent results have suggested that proper patient selection, more careful planning, and more precise execution of the osteotomy can produce a longer-lasting HTO[12, 18]. For example, an extensive clinical review[20] reports on 128 knees that were studied for up to 15 years, finding a revision rate was only 10.9%.

1.1 The Traditional Technique for High Tibial Osteotomy

The most common form of HTO is the closing wedge osteotomy, popularized by Coventry in 1973 [3]. The wedge is first planned on a frontal-plane standing X-ray by drawing a wedge of the desired correction angle, where the wedge's upper plane is parallel to the tibial plateau and the lower plane is above the tibial tubercle. Ideally, the wedge will produce a hinge of cortical bone approximately 2–5 mm in thickness.

Upon surgical exposure of the proximal tibia, the correction is mapped to the bones of the patient via a ruler or a jig system. The surgery is then performed either freehand or with assistance of Kirschner wires (K-wires) as cutting guides. Intraoperative fluoroscopic X-ray is often employed for verification before and during the procedure. Technical difficulties often arise from the use of fluoroscopy, such as image-intensifier nonlinearities and distortions that compromise accuracy, and parallax errors that can provide misleading angular and positional guidance.

1.2 A Computer Technique for High Tibial Osteotomy

The major contribution of computer assisted surgery to HTO has so far been in preoperative planning, whereby the surgeon is provided with a prediction of postoperative alignment or loading. One such system, developed by the Tsumura group[23], used a two-dimensional static biomechanical model originally proposed by Coventry and Insall[4, 11]. The other preoperative planner, developed by Chao et al., used a two-dimensional rigid-body spring model to simulate the forces across the articular surfaces[1, 2, 9]. It also attempted to account for ligamentous effects, and simulated two-dimensional dynamic loading.

A drawback of these approaches is that planning and simulation of the three-dimensional osteotomy are carried out in only two dimensions. There are many inherent problems in executing a two-dimensional plan in three-dimension space. For example, tilting of the saw blade in the anterior/posterior direction is not controlled by the traditional technique. Further, if the axis for closing the osteotomy is not perpendicular to the frontal plane, an unintended internal/external rotation of the foot is induced.

We submit that the premature failures and large variability in HTO are due to: (1) the inability of current planning methods to address the fact that HTO is a three-dimensional procedure; and (2) the incapability of manual surgeries to produce the planned amount of axis shift accurately. It is insufficient to plan a three-dimensional surgery using the traditional two-dimensional X-ray information. Also, substantial spatial reasoning and surgical experience are required to accurately cut a three-dimensional wedge through the limited surgical exposure.

Our approach to solving these problems is to use computer assistance to achieve accurate three-dimensional corrections. A surgical enhancement system has been developed that facilitates preoperative planning in three-dimensional space. This three-dimensional plan can then be executed in an image-guided surgery system. The inherent precision in the image-guided surgery system is expected to lead to better reliability, consistency and speed in HTO than can be achieved by the traditional techniques.

The goal was to reduce the incidence of the common postoperative problems. With a three-dimensional guidance and planning system it should be possible to eliminate, or greatly reduce the probability of (a) incorrect valgus alignment, (b) incorrect proximal/distal location of the osteotomy, and (c) inadvertent internal/external foot rotation. If proximal-fragment fracture is due to proximity of the osteotomy to the joint, especially because of inadvertent anterior/posterior sloping of the proximal resection, then the probability of fracture should be reduced. Finally, if the post-osteotomy fixation is also planned and guided, the danger of fixation into the joint articulation should also be reduced.

2 Computer-Assisted Planning and Guidance

The computer-assisted high tibial osteotomy was performed in nine steps:

1. Three or more radio-opaque markers were inserted into the tibia under local anesthesia, placed slightly distal to the tibial tubercle.
2. CT images of the knee were acquired from the femoral condyles to below the tibial tubercle, using axial mode slices of 3mm width spaced 2mm apart.
3. A three-dimensional surface model of the tibia was reconstructed from the CT images by isosurface extraction.
4. With the isosurface model, and data from standardized weight-bearing radiographs, the surgeon used preoperative planning software to plan the procedure. Given the desired correction in the sagittal and frontal planes, the planner simulated a closing-wedge osteotomy. The surgeon could visually inspect the three-dimensional position of the resection planes and adjust the planes as desired.
5. Intraoperatively, the pre-implanted fiducial markers were located in three dimensions with a precision mechanical arm.

6. The coordinate system common to the CT scan, the computerized tibia model, and the planned osteotomy were mapped onto the coordinate system of the patient by means of a fiducial registration algorithm [5].
7. The accuracy-critical step of the surgical procedure was performed by attaching a drill to the locating device. A full-screen computer animation displayed the relative positions of surgical instruments superimposed on the planned resection planes, with several screen updates per second. Referring to the online computer graphics, the surgeon then inserted two K-wires into the proximal tibia for each resection plane.
8. The wires were then used as saw guides to perform the osteotomy in a manner similar to the traditional Coventry technique [3]. Osteoclasis was used to complete the formation of a medial hinge.
9. After the bone wedge was removed and the tibia adjusted to the new angulation, standard step staples were used to immobilize the fragments and the surgical field was closed.

2.1 A Preoperative Planning System

The closing-wedge osteotomy is rotation about a cortical bone hinge, which when modeled as rotation about an axis in space makes the procedure particularly suited to computer-assisted planning. The planning process is linear and well structured, so the planner was implemented as a *wizard-based* system in which each window had text describing the step and a graphical interface for effecting that step. The preoperative planning system was implemented in X/Motif, and its major function was to allow the surgeon to specify two resection planes on a graphical model of a tibia.

The triangulated isosurface model of the tibia was first loaded and displayed. The user selected the tibial anatomical axis and the transverse axis, from which the system computed the frontal axis. The second step was selection of the tibial plateau, which was rendered as a plane that could obscure or be obscured by the proximal tibial surface. The user had control over the varus/valgus tilt, the anterior/posterior tilt, and the proximal/distal placement of where the plateau plane intersected the anatomical axis. Typically the surgeons viewed the superimposed axes and plateau carefully to ensure that they fully understood the anatomy of the individual patient.

The third and final step was selection of the resection planes. The user moved the proximal plane down to an appropriate level (usually 10–14 mm) and then specified the correction angle of the wedge. The angle could be measured from a pre-operative plain X-ray film or could be found as an adjustment to the tibial-plateau/tibial-shaft angle automatically calculated by the system. The user could translate the hinge axis in proximal/distal and medial/lateral directions, and could rotate it about the internal/external axis.

The most powerful computation performed in the planning system was a simulation of the result of the osteotomy in the third step. The two resection planes intersected the model to produce four components: the proximal fragment, the distal fragment, the lateral wedge, and the medial hinge. The system discarded the wedge, rotated the distal fragment to contact the proximal fragment, and "stretched" the hinge component with an affine transformation to provide a smooth rendering of the medial cortex. This stretching was completed by retriangulation of the faces that had been split by intersection with the resection planes.

The original tibia with superimposed resection planes was displayed on one side of the monitor, and on the other side was the predicted result including pre-operative and predicted post-operative axes. The images could be visualized from any viewpoint, to facilitate understanding of the full three-dimensional consequences of the osteotomy. Because the tibial cortex was modeled as a triangular mesh, which allowed a desktop UNIX workstation running OpenGL to render each virtual surgery within one or two seconds. Figure 1 shows a sample completed plan for a plastic tibial model used in a laboratory study.

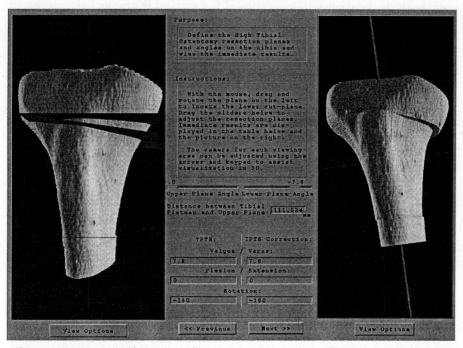

Fig. 1. A preoperative planning system for high tibial osteotomy. The system displays the preoperative and postoperative models of the tibia at real time, as well as the three anatomical angles as changed by the simulated surgery.

The software program guided the user through the steps of preoperative planning. Control of objects in all three dimensions was primarily by means of a mouse, with transformations smoothly rendered by interpolating rotations as quaternions [8, 21, 22]. The osteotomy's geometry was rendered visually and the rotational parameters were displayed as the Grood-Suntay parameters of valgus/varus, internal/external rotation, and flexion/extension [6]. The user could adjust the osteotomy's correction via a mouse, or enter values via a keyboard, to achieve the desired correction.

2.2 An Image-Based Guidance System

The image guidance system was composed of software running on a desktop UNIX workstation (SUN Microsystems, Sunnyvale CA) and a mechanical localizer (FARO Technologies, Lake Mary, FL). Registration was accomplished by touching three or more pre-implanted fiducial markers with the localizer, then calculating the least-squares rigid transformation between localizer coordinates and CT coordinates [5]. With registration accomplished, it was possible to transform any model or action represented in one coordinate system to the other coordinate system. The surgeons found that the most helpful information was (a) rendering transverse, frontal, and sagittal planes from CT volumetric data, with the location and orientation of the surgical instrument superimposed in color on the gray-scale images, and (b) using solid modeling to render the three-dimensional surface model of the tibia, models of the resection planes, and a three-dimensional model of a virtual surgical instrument. Additional guidance information was available digitally, as required by the surgeon, by means of simple queries to the software. Figure 2 shows the screen layout of the guidance system.

3 Laboratory Tests

The laboratory tests were mock surgeries performed on plastic bone models (Pacific Research Laboratories, WA). Prior to testing, the bone models were prepared for registration and scanned with CT. Four registration markers were inserted into accurately milled holes on the antero-lateral surface of each model. The positions were selected such that the markers would be within a realistic surgical exposure and would also be located only on the distal fragment of the tibia after osteotomy.

To facilitate resection each bone model was fixed in a special jig that held the tibia model at a 45° angle from the horizontal. Black closed-cell foam masked the proximal part of the bone model, to simulate the visual obstructions created by soft tissue that appear clinically. After the wedge was removed, the distal and proximal fragments of the tibia were held together by strong adhesive (Shoe Goo) and with woodworking staples delivered from a staple gun.

Thirty mock surgeries were performed, with intended corrections of 9°, 14°, and 19°. The tasks were to (a) perform the osteotomy with fluoroscopic guidance of the saw blade followed by conventional cutting and osteoclasis, and (b) perform the osteotomy by computer-enhanced planning and guidance of pin placement followed by conventional cutting and osteoclasis. For each task each angular correction was performed five times in a randomized sequence, alternating tasks (a) and (b).

Subsequently, the wedge angles were measured. These measurements took advantage of the presence in the models of a transverse hole approximately 15mm inferior to the tibial plateau; this hole is parallel to the Cartesian **X** axis

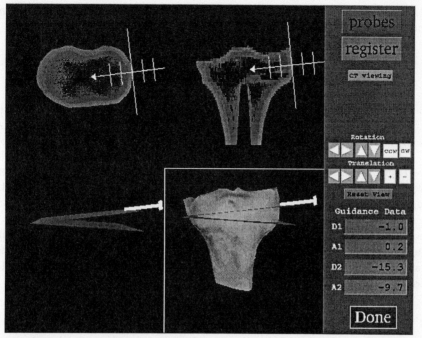

Fig. 2. An image-based guidance system for orthopedic surgery. The surgery software displays the position of the surgical instrument in several reconstructed CT planes, and also shows the tibial model, the planned resection planes, and a virtual surgical instrument.

of the Grood-Suntay coordinate system [6]. The wedges were placed in a jig that fixed the wedges via the transverse hole, and surface points were collected from the superior wedge surface using a precision mechanical arm (Faro Technologies, FL). Varus/valgus angulations were calculated as the total rotation about the Cartesian **Y** axis of the Grood-Suntay coordinate system of the tibia.

3.1 Laboratory Results

The surgeons found that the two major pieces of software – the 3–D preoperative planner and image-based guidance system – provided an appropriately user-friendly interface. The modeling of preoperative and postoperative alignment gave them an unprecedented control and preview of the surgical procedure. The information provided by the image-based guidance system was very useful, in that they easily installed the guide wires by looking solely at the screen (as they do when performing an arthroscopic procedure).

The test osteotomies were analysed by examining the wedge angles. For traditional and computer-enhanced techniques, the mean and standard deviations of the differences between the intended varus/valgus angle and the achieved varus/valgus angle were computed. Results are shown in Table 1. According to the classic F-test, the reduction in standard deviations are significant to a 95%

confidence level. Differences in the mean errors are not statistically significant, and in both sets are very low.

Table 1. Summary of Laboratory Test Results
Errors are the difference between the measured varus/valgus angle and the intended angle. The range is the difference between the largest and smallest error.

Wedge Errors, Traditional			Wedge Errors, Computer-Enhanced		
Mean	Std. Dev.	Range	Mean	Std. Dev.	Range
$-0.4°$	$2.3°$	$8.4°$	$0.1°$	$1.4°$	$3.7°$

There were no training effects observed in the trials, i.e. the errors were evenly distributed through time. The errors were larger for larger correction angles, which is not a surprising result.

A particularly interesting observation was the accurate formation of the osteotomy hinge when operating with computer assistance. In every trial the hinge was between 1 mm and 3 mm in thickness. When operating in the traditional way, with fluoroscopic guidance of the saw blade, the hinge could be non-existent (totally mobile fragments) or up to 5 mm in thickness.

4 Clinical Trials

Clinical tests involved five patients, all having arthrosis confined to the medial compartment. Each patient was preoperatively instrumented with titanium-alloy markers 1.9 mm diameter, 3.5 mm length; the markers were the screws of soft-tissue anchors (Wright Medical) and were inserted percutaneously into the anterolateral aspect of the proximal tibia under local anesthesia. Each patient was then imaged with Roentgen stereogrammetric analysis (to validate the absolute accuracy of the intraoperative registration), with Questor Precision Radiographs (to establish clinical axes in weight-bearing stance), and with axial-mode computed tomography (to provide accurate three-dimensional images of the anatomy and the markers). Instrumentation and imaging were approximately one week prior to surgery. No infection arose from the marker implantation and the patients reported only minor discomfort.

Image preparation and preoperative planning were conducted in a manner identical to the methods used in the laboratory trials. During surgery the patient's lower affected leg was held in a specially constructed holder that could rigidly hold the leg in angles from full extension to over 90° flexion. Marker identification was simple, and little preparation of the bone surface or surrounding soft tissues was required to expose the tiny markers. Intraoperative registration and drilling of the two guide wires required a maximum of 6 minutes, compared to a minimum of 12 minutes for typical fluoroscopically guided wire insertion. Resection, reduction, and fixation with step-staples were conducted in the traditional manner. Postoperative plain X-ray films were taken to assess the osteotomy and to ensure that the staples did not intrude into joint.

For each patient, the intraoperative evaluation of the procedure was that the medial hinge was correctly placed and of the correct thickness. The resected bone surfaces were visually smooth and flat. Technically each osteotomy was not only acceptable but was judged to be between very good to excellent. The postoperative radiographic examination in each case showed very good to excellent bone-surface contact and no fixation problems. Figure 3 shows a representative fluoroscopic image of a reduced and stapled osteotomy, which has excellent mating of the cut surfaces.

Traditional radiographic analysis was conducted for the four patients whose pre-operative and post-operative X-ray films were available. The pre-operative and post-operative tibial-plateau/tibial-shaft angles were calculated, and their differences were compared to the intended corrections that had been established using the pre-operative planning system. Table 2 summarizes these results.

5 Discussion

The major contribution of this work has been the development of software that supports preoperative planning of a closing-wedge high tibial osteotomy in three dimensions, and accompanying software that guides the surgeon to achieve the desired result. Work by other investigators, even with the use of computers, planned in only two dimensions. It is possible that the inability of two-dimensional planning to control for all of the angulation variables has contributed to the reputation of high tibial osteotomy as unpredictable.

Table 2. Pre-operative, post-operative, and intended tibial-plateau/tibial-shaft correction angles, and the resulting error, measured from frontal X-ray films. Complete films were unavailable for the first patient.

Patient	\multicolumn{2}{c}{Tibial-plateau/tibial-shaft angles, in degrees}			
	Pre-op	Post-op	Correction	Goal	Error
2	4.0 varus	6.5 valgus	10.5	9.0	+1.5
3	5.5 varus	7.0 valgus	12.5	11.0	-1.5
4	4.0 varus	5.5 valgus	9.5	11.0	-1.5
5	1.0 varus	5.5 valgus	6.5	8.0	-1.5

The fundamental problem with planning in only the frontal plane is the implicit assumption that the hinge axis is always perpendicular to the frontal plane. The intended kinematics of this plan will be reproduced in the patient only if this edge of closure is exactly as dictated. When the hinge axis deviates from being perpendicular to the frontal plane, extension/flexion and internal/external rotations are inevitably introduced. Elementary 3D geometry can be used to show that that a small deviation in the location of the hinge axis can easily lead to $10°$ or more unintended internal-external rotation of the foot, which in turn can produce abduction or adduction moments on the knee during normal daily activities. Such unintended effects may contribute to a poor biomechanical environment that does not adequately treat the arthrosis from which the patient suffers.

An important clinical advantage of the computer-assisted technique is the accurate placement of the medial hinge. With simple measurements it is relatively easy to control the thickness of the lateral portion of the wedge, but it is much more difficult to place the apex of the wedge with a millimeter or two

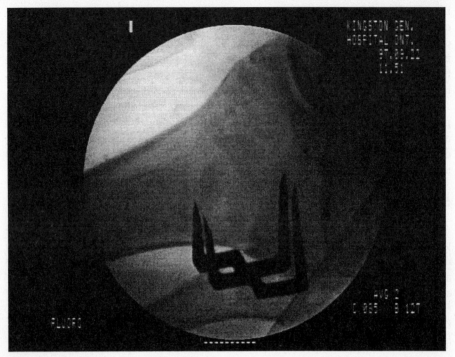

Fig. 3. Fluoroscopic image of a completed computer-enhanced osteotomy.

of the medial tibial cortex. Jig systems can control the wedge angle, but again the placement of the apex is difficult to ensure even with fluoroscopic imaging. Apex placement is important because small lateral misplacement of the position of the wedge apex can produce a relatively large overcorrection – the small medial changes are propagated across the width of the tibia. If the wedge apex is placed too far medially then medial soft tissues can be disrupted, decreasing the stability of the osteotomy during healing.

The laboratory results show that the angle of the removed lateral wedge can be controlled to an accuracy at least as good as the best jig system. Because the location of the medial cortical hinge can also be controlled, it is expected that computer-enhanced osteotomy will provide superior outcomes than the current course of treatment offers. Use of the computer-assisted HTO system has clarified the importance of incorporating all three dimensions in the planning and execution of this type of osteotomy. In particular, the laboratory tests have revealed some pitfalls that arose from neglecting three-dimensional aspects of osteotomy techniques, and shown that the standard deviation of angular error can be half that of the traditional technique.

The clinical results are in a pilot-study stage but are promising. To date the maximum radiologically measured error is smaller than the standard deviation of the best jig systems. We will continue to recruit patients into our study, and also will follow the progress of the cohort to determine the quality of bone union and retainment of alignment that result from the computer-enhanced technique.

A shortcoming of the traditional and our computer-enhanced techniques is that neither accurately controls the flexion/extension correction or the internal/external rotation. Flexion/extension can be controlled by use of additional wires, or by determining an additional control point on each resection plane for the initial phase of the saw cut. The computer-assisted technique can also be modified to provide the surgeon with real-time feedback of the foot rotation, so that a desired overall limb alignment can be achieved. This is not trivial to do with a single mechanical arm for location sensing, but is relatively straightforward if optoelectronic position sensors are employed. It may also be possible to track the saw and/or an osteotome so that the surgeon can gain greater control of the osteotomy in the posterior aspect of the tibia, which is not readily seen from an anterolateral surgical approach.

This initial attempt at three-dimensional osteotomy planning concentrated on the development of a three-dimensional environment with geometric simulations. Future work could include biomechanical simulation accounting for the ligaments and for predicted medial/lateral displacement of the joint by normal walking forces. The high tibial osteotomy is a particular use of the closing-wedge osteotomy and the current system could be adapted for application in other anatomical regions. The closing-wedge osteotomy is only one of many corrective orthopedic procedures that could benefit from computer-assisted planning and image-guided surgical techniques.

Acknowledgments

This research was supported in part by the Natural Sciences and Engineering Research Council of Canada and by Communications and Information Technology Ontario (an Ontario Centre of Excellence). We are grateful to Gordon Goodchild for his careful programming of the guidance system and his assistance in performing the studies. Patricia McAllister and Cameron McLeod coordinated the clinical studies and assisted in marker implantation.

References

1. E. Y. S. Chao and F. H. Sim. "Computer-aided preoperative planning in knee osteotomy". *Iowa Orthopaedic Journal*, 15:4–18, 1995.
2. E. Y. S. Chao, J. D. Lynch, and M. J. Vanderploeg. "Simulation and animation of musculoskeletal joint system". *Journal of Biomechanical Engineering*, 115(4B):562–568, November 1993.
3. M. B. Coventry. "Osteotomy about the knee for degenerative and rheumatoid arthritis". *Journal of Bone and Joint Surgery [Am]*, 55(1):23–48, January 1973.
4. M. B. Coventry. "Upper tibial osteotomy for osteoarthritis". *Journal of Bone and Joint Surgery [Am]*, 67(7):1136–1140, 1985.
5. R. E. Ellis, S. Toksvig-Larsen, and M. Marcacci. "Use of a biocompatible fiducial marker in evaluating the accuracy of computed tomography image registration". *Investigative Radiology*, 31(10):658–667, October 1996.
6. E. S. Grood and W. J. Suntay. "A joint coordinate system for the clinical description of three-dimensional motions: application to the knee". *ASME Journal of Biomechanical Engineering*, 105:136–144, May 1983.

7. B. Hagstedt, O. Norman, T. H. Olsson, and B. Tjornstrand. "Technical accuracy in high tibial osteotomy for gonarthrosis". *Acta Orthopaedica Scandinavica*, 51(6):963–970, December 1980.
8. J. C. Hart, G. K. Francis, and L. H. Kauffman. "Visualizing quaternion rotation". *ACM Transactions on Graphics*, 13(3):256–276, 1994.
9. A. D. Hassen and E. Y. S. Chao. *High Tibial Osteotomy*, volume 2 of *Knee Surgery*, pages 1121–1134. Williams and Wilkins, Baltimore, 1994.
10. A. A. Hofmann, R. W. B. Wyatt, and S. W. Beck. "High tibial osteotomy. Use of an osteotomy jig, rigid fixation, and early motion versus conventional surgical technique and cast immobilization". *Clinical Orthopaedics and Related Research*, 271:212–217, October 1991.
11. J. N. Insall, M. D. Joseph, and C. Msika. "High tibial osteotomy for varus gonarthrosis: A long term follow-up study". *Journal of Bone and Joint Surgery [Am]*, 66(7):1040–1048, 1984.
12. R. B. Jakob and S. B. Murphy. "Tibial osteotomy for varus gonarthrisis: Indication, planning and operative technique". *Instructional Course Lectures*, 41:87–93, 1992.
13. J. S. Keene, D. K. Monson, J. M. Roberts, and J. R. Dyreby Jr. "Evaluation of patients for high tibial osteotomy". *Clinical Orthopaedics and Related Research*, 243:157–165, June 1989.
14. J. L. Knight. "A precision guide-pin technique for wedge and rotatory osteotomy of the femur and tibia". *Clinical Orthopaedics and Related Research*, 262:248–255, January 1991.
15. T. Koshino, T. Morii, J. Wada, H. Saito, N. Ozawa, and K. Noyori. "High tibial osteotomy with fixation by a blade plate for medial compartment osteoarthritis of the knee". *Orthopedic Clinics of North America*, 20(2):227–243, April 1989.
16. R. Myrnerts. "Clinical results with the SAAB jig in high tibial osteotomy for medial gonarthrosis". *Acta Orthopaedica Scandinavica*, 51(3):565–567, June 1980.
17. S. Odenbring, N. Egund, and A. Lindstrand. "A guide instrument for high tibial osteotomy". *Acta Orthopaedica Scandinavica*, 60(4):449–451, 1989.
18. D. Paley and J. E. Herzenberg. "New concepts in high tibial osteotomy for medial compartment osteoarthritis". *Orthopedic Clinics of North America*, 25(3):483–498, July 1994.
19. J. F. Rudan and M. A. Simurda. "High tibial osteotomy - A Prospective Clinical and Roentgenographic Review". *Clinical Orthopaedics and Related Research*, 255:251–256, June 1990.
20. J. F. Rudan and M. A. Simurda. "Valgus high tibial osteotomy - a long-term follow-up study". *Clinical Orthopaedics and Related Research*, 268:157–160, July 1991.
21. K. Shoemake. "Animating rotation with quaternion curves". *Computer Graphics*, 19(3):245–254, 1985.
22. K. Shoemake. "Arcball: A user interface for specifying three-dimensional orientation using a mouse". In *Proceedings of Graphics Interface*, pages 151–156, May 1992.
23. H. Tsumura, S. Himeno, and T. Kawai. "The computer simulation on the correcting osteotomy of osteoarthritis of the knee". *Journal of Japanese Orthopaedic Association*, 58:565–566, 1984.

Measurement of Intraoperative Brain Surface Deformation Under a Craniotomy

Calvin R. Maurer, Jr.[1], Derek L. G. Hill[1], Robert J. Maciunas[2], John A. Barwise[2], J. Michael Fitzpatrick[2], and Matthew Y. Wang[2]

[1] Division of Radiological Sciences and Medical Engineering, King's College London, UK
{c.maurer, d.hill}@umds.ac.uk
[2] Departments of Neurological Surgery (rjm), Anesthesiology (jab), and Computer Science (jmf, myw), Vanderbilt University, Nashville, Tennessee

Abstract. We measured the deformation of the dura and brain surfaces between the time of imaging and the start of surgical resection for 21 patients. All patients underwent intraoperative functional mapping, allowing us to measure brain surface motion at two times that were separated by nearly an hour after opening the dura but before resection. The positions of the dura and brain surfaces were recorded and transformed to the coordinate space of a preoperative MR image using the Acustar neurosurgical navigation system. The mean displacements of the dura and the first and second brain surfaces were 1.2, 4.4, and 5.6 mm, respectively, with corresponding mean volume reductions under the craniotomy of 6, 22, and 29 ml. The maximum displacement was greater than 10 mm in approximately one-third of the patients for the first brain surface measurement and one-half of the patients for the second. In all cases the direction of brain shift corresponds to a "sinking" of the brain intraoperatively, compared with its preoperative position. We observed two patterns of the brain surface deformation field depending on the inclination of the craniotomy with respect to gravity. Separate measurements of brain deformation within the closed cranium caused by changes in patient head orientation with respect to gravity suggested that less than 1 mm of the brain shift recorded intraoperatively could have resulted from the change in patient orientation between the time of imaging and the time of surgery. These results suggest that intraoperative brain deformation is an important source of error that needs to be considered when using neurosurgical navigation systems.

1 Introduction

It is becoming increasingly common for neurosurgical procedures to be performed with the assistance of a localizer and computer system that enables the surgeon to relate the position of a surgical instrument to structures of interest visible in preoperative images. Procedures performed using such systems are often described as image-guided surgery. The most established image-guided surgery systems use a stereotactic frame. More recently, a variety of frameless systems have been developed. Methods of physical space localization include articulated mechanical arms, ultrasonic range-finding systems, electromagnetic systems, and active and passive optical techniques. All current neurosurgical navigation systems assume that the head and its contents behave as a rigid body and use extrinsic features (skin-affixed or bone-implanted markers) or anatomical structures (point landmarks or surfaces) to determine the rigid-body registration transformation.

Errors in image-guided surgery caused by errors in identifying the external features used for registration, geometrical distortion in the preoperative images, and errors in the tracking of surgical instruments have been well documented for several systems [3, 7]. Another potentially important source of errors is brain deformation between the time of imaging and the time of surgery or during surgery. Such deformations will invalidate the rigid-body assumption and consequently introduce inaccuracies into the system that will not be detected by the standard measures of registration or tracking error.

Surprisingly, little quantitative measurement of brain deformation has been published. A number of investigators have reported motion of brain structures while resection is underway. As far as we are aware, preliminary quantitative measurements were first reported by a number of groups, including us, at several recent conferences [1, 2, 5, 9].

In this study, which follows a pilot study of five patients [5], we measured the deformation of the dura and brain surfaces between the time of imaging and the start of surgical resection for 21 patients. All patients underwent intraoperative functional mapping prior to resection, providing us with the opportunity to measure brain surface shift at two times that were separated by nearly an hour after opening the dura but before performing surgical resection of the lesion. The positions of the dura and brain surfaces were recorded and transformed to the coordinate space of a preoperative MR image using the Acustar neurosurgical navigation system [7].

2 Methods

2.1 Clinical Material

We evaluated intraoperative brain surface movement by analyzing data obtained from 21 patients that underwent craniotomies for the resection of cerebral lesions at Vanderbilt University Medical Center between September 1996 and May 1997. Patients undergoing a second operation were excluded from consideration in this study. The cases included tumors that were located primarily in the left hemisphere (18 left, 3 right). The types of tumors were as follows: 13 low-grade gliomas, 5 anaplastic astrocytomas, 2 glioblastomas multiforme, and 1 teratoma. The tumor locations were as follows: 2 frontal, 5 temporal, 1 parietal, 6 fronto-temporal, 1 fronto-parietal, 4 temporo-parietal, 1 temporo-occipital, and 1 parieto-occipital. The patients ranged in age from 19 to 68 years (mean $\pm$ SD = 39 $\pm$ 15 yr). The patients were operated on in the supine position with the head oriented 90° right or left (for the left and right tumors, respectively). Functional mapping of sensory, motor, and/or language areas was performed using intraoperative cortical stimulation for all patients in this study. This provided an opportunity to measure brain surface movement at two times that were separated by nearly an hour after opening the dura but before performing surgical resection of the lesion.

The anesthesia was as standardized as possible. All patients received 20 mg of dexamethasone every 3 hours beginning just before surgery. Mannitol (1 g/kg) was administered at the start of the creation of the craniotomy burr holes. Serum osmolality was generally in the 280–290 osmol range before mannitol administration and increased to 300–310 osmol after 30 minutes, at which point it remained fairly constant during the surface measurements. No patient was given narcotics or benzodiazepines. All patients received 60 ml of 0.5% lidocaine with 0.125% bupivacaine applied to their scalp incisions and Mayfield clamp sites for local analgesia. Patients initially received propofol (50–200 μg/kg/min total anesthesia administered intravenously). The infusion was reduced to 25–75 μg/kg/min at the start of the creation of the burr holes and was stopped when the section of cranium was elevated. Breathing resumed spontaneously after this through a laryngeal mask airway, which was removed when the patient responded to commands. The patients were aroused and awake by the time the section of cranium was elevated and for all surface measurements. Pulse and blood pressure were maintained within 20% of their preoperative values.

2.2 Preoperative Image Acquisition

The surgeries were performed using the Acustar neurosurgical navigation system (manufactured by Johnson & Johnson Professional, Inc., Randolph, MA; the Acustar trademark is now owned by Picker International, Highland Heights, OH) for intraoperative guidance [7]. Before the patient was imaged, the surgeon implanted four plastic posts into the outer table of the cranium of the patient, with one end remaining outside the skin. The specific locations of the posts were determined by individual clinical circumstances, but generally the posts were widely separated and placed on both sides of the head, with two of the markers inferior and two superior to the region of surgical interest. Image markers that contain contrast fluid and generate high intensity in both CT and MR images were attached to the posts just before image acquisition.

Both CT and MR images were acquired preoperatively for all patients (except that no CT image was acquired for one patient). Imaging studies were performed the day before or the morning of the surgical procedure. The CT images were acquired using a Siemens Somatom Plus scanner. Each image volume contained between 39 and 47 transverse slices with 512 × 512 pixels. The voxel dimensions were 0.4 × 0.4 × 3.0 mm. All CT image volumes in this study were stacks of image slices with no interslice gap or slice overlap. The gantry tilt angle was zero. Three-dimensional (3-D) MP-RAGE MR image volumes were acquired using the head coil in a Siemens Magnetom SP4000 1.5 T scanner. Each image volume contained 128 coronal slices with 256 × 256 pixels. The voxel dimensions were typically 1.0 × 1.0 × 1.6 mm. The readout gradient was oriented in the cranio-caudal direction with a magnitude of 4.7 mT/m.

The centroid of each image marker was determined using the marker localization algorithm described in [11].

2.3 Intraoperative Measurements

Intraoperatively, the head was fixed in a Mayfield clamp, physical-space markers were attached to the marker posts, a localization probe was calibrated, and the markers were localized. The localization probe is equipped with an array of infrared emitting diodes (IREDs). Physical space tracking of the probe was accomplished with optical triangulation using an Optotrak 3020 (Northern Digital, Ontario, Canada). The physical-space markers are manufactured with a hemispherical divot, the center of which corresponds to the centroid of the image markers. The tip of the probe is a spherical ball. Intraoperative localization of each marker was performed by placing the ball-point tip into the divot and pressing a button on the probe handle.

The standard Acustar system registers images to each other and to the intraoperative physical coordinate system. When the localizer tip is placed near or within the patient, triplanar reformatted images intersecting at the corresponding position in image coordinates are generated. The Acustar system used for the work presented here was enhanced so that it could also record probe tip positions after registration was performed. To collect a dura or brain surface point, the surgeon placed the probe tip on the surface and recorded its 3-D coordinates by pressing a button. It took two or three seconds to acquire each point. The number of points collected in each acquisition ranged from 39 to 69 (mean $\pm$ SD = 56 $\pm$ 7). We attempted to collect surface points as uniformly distributed over the craniotomy as possible. We attempted to collect brain surface points on the gyral "envelope." Specifically, we avoided recording tip positions inside the sulci.

Dura surface points were collected soon after elevating the craniotomy. Points on the brain surface were collected twice, once after opening the dura but before functional mapping, and once after mapping but before performing surgical resection of the tumor. Immediately before every surface data acquisition, we recorded the position of a marker visible in the surgical field and collected approximately eight skull surface points around the edge of the craniotomy. To test the reproducibility of the surface data points, for four patients, we had two surgeons each collect a set of brain surface points, one immediately after the other.

2.4 Data Analysis

The distance between a dura, brain, or cranial surface point collected intraoperatively and the corresponding surface in the preoperative images was found by first transforming the physical space point to the image coordinate system using the rigid-body transformation provided by the Acustar system and then calculating the closest point on a triangle set representation of the image surface [6]. The image-to-physical rigid-body transformation was determined by fitting the image and physical space marker positions in a least-squares sense [7]. The dura and brain surfaces were manually delineated in the preoperative MR images using an interactive segmentation tool. The brain contours were drawn around the gyral envelope and did not invaginate into the sulci. Each resulting stack of polygonal surface contours was converted into a triangle set as described in [6]. A triangle set representation of the cranial surface was automatically extracted from each CT image using the tetrahedral decomposition method of Gueziec & Hummel [4]. Because the localization probe tip is a spherical ball, the recorded position was systematically displaced from the true surface position by a distance equal to the radius of the spherical tip, which was 1.5 mm for all of the measurements made in this study. The calculated point-to-surface distances were positive if the intraoperatively recorded points were outside the brain image surface and negative if the points were inside the surface. The systematic displacement introduced by the finite diameter of the probe tip was corrected for by subtracting the tip's radius from these point-to-surface distances before further analysis. To test the reproducibility of dura and brain surface segmentation, we had two people each draw contours for four of the patients.

The craniotomy area was estimated from the skull surface points collected around the edge of the craniotomy as follows. The plane that best fit the skull points in a least-squares sense was determined, the points were projected onto this plane, and the area of the polygon formed by these projected points was computed. For three patients, the craniotomy inclination was estimated by computing the angle between the normal to the plane fit through the skull points and the gravity field direction. The direction of gravity was estimated as the normal to a plane fit through approximately eight points collected on the surface of a pan of water placed within the optical field of view.

With the Acustar system, a "reference emitter" containing an array of IREDs is rigidly attached to the Mayfield head clamp via a multijointed arm. The reference emitter defines the intraoperative coordinate system and thus allows movement of the operating table and repositioning of the Optotrak 3020 when necessary, e.g., to maintain an optical line of sight. This technique does not compensate for patient movement relative to the Mayfield clamp. We estimated the magnitude of gross head motion relative to the Mayfield clamp between registration and the collection of a set of surface points in two ways: 1) by computing the distance between the position of a marker visible in the surgical field at the time of surface point collection and its position at the time of registration, and 2) by computing the distance between skull points collected around the edge of the craniotomy immediately before the dura or brain surface points were collected and a triangle set representation of the skull surface derived from the CT scans.

2.5 Effect of Orientation

Patients are normally operated on in a different position from that in which they are imaged. For example, all the patients studied here were imaged supine but operated on with their heads in a lateral position. To assess what proportion of the intraoperative brain shift we measured might be due to the change in brain orientation relative to gravity, we acquired MR images for two patients in both a conventional supine position and a prone position. We chose these two patient orientations because we were unable to get the patients positioned comfortably in the MR scanner in the operative position (head orientation 90° left or right), and also because we believe that imaging a patient both prone and supine is likely to give an upper bound on the motion of the brain with respect to the cranium resulting from change in patient orientation.

We used three techniques to estimate the brain shift resulting from the change in patient orientation. The first technique is analogous to the method used to assess intraoperative shift. We manually delineated the brain surface from both scans using the Analyze software package (Biomedical Imaging Resource, Mayo Foundation, Rochester, MN), and transformed the prone brain surface contours to the supine image coordinate space using the registration transformation calculated from the bone-implanted markers. Triangle set representations of each surface were created as described in Section 2.4, and the difference in brain surface position was calculated for the portion of the cerebrum superior to the orbital-meatal line. The second technique is a comparison of the bone-implanted marker registration transformation ("cranial transformation") and a voxel-similarity registration transformation computed using the segmented brains ("brain transformation"). The voxel-similarity registration algorithm automatically finds the rigid-body transformation between the two segmented brains that maximizes the normalized mutual information of the joint probability distribution of the two images [10]. The discrepancy between these two transformations provides an estimate of the motion of the brain with respect to the skull caused by the change in patient orientation. We calculated the mean and maximum discrepancy in position of the brain voxels resulting from the difference in these transformations. Finally, we visually assessed brain deformation by computing thresholded boundaries in the prone images and overlaying them on the supine images, using both the cranial and brain transformations.

3 Results

3.1 Intraoperative Brain Deformation

The distance between the position of each dura and brain surface point collected intraoperatively with a localization probe and the nearest point on the same surface manually segmented from the preoperative MR images was calculated. Positive distances represented physical points outside the image surface and negative distances points inside the surface. Thus, negative distance values represented a "sinking" of surface points relative to the cranium, compared with their preoperative position. Similarly, positive values represented "bulging" or "protruding" points.

Because of the possibility that the patient may move with respect to the coordinate system defined by the reference emitter, e.g., within the Mayfield clamp, we verified that the registration was still accurate at the time of surface point collection. The two measures we used to assess the validity of the registration at the time of surface point collection were the distance between a marker visible in the surgical field and its position at the time of registration, and the distance of skull surface points from the skull surface segmented from a CT image. For two patients, both the marker displacement and mean skull point distance were greater than 1.5 mm. For the remaining 19 patients, the mean marker displacement was 0.3–0.4 mm, and the maximum displacement for all measurements was 0.8 mm. The mean cranial point distance was 0.7–0.8 mm, and the maximum distance was 1.2 mm. These small numbers suggested that for these 19 patients, the image-to-physical transformation determined at the beginning of surgery was still accurate at the time of surface point collection.

Table 1 lists summary statistics of dura and brain surface displacement for these 19 patients. Dura surface points were collected soon after elevating the craniotomy. Brain surface points were collected after opening the dura but before performing cortical stimulation (Brain 1) and after stimulation but before performing surgical resection of the tumor (Brain 2). The first and second sets of brain points were collected 53 ± 27 (mean $\pm$ SD) and 98 ± 31 minutes, respectively, after the dura points were collected. The 10 and 90% distance values were determined by sorting the distances in descending order and taking the $(0.10n)$th and $(0.90n)$th elements in the sorted list, where n is the number of values (one for each point). The 10 and 90% distance values approximated the range of brain movement. We used them rather than the minimum and maximum values to eliminate the possibility that the extreme values represented erroneous outliers. The three displacements (dura and two brain surfaces) were significantly different from

Table 1. Intraoperative Dura and Brain Surface Displacement (mm)

	Surface	Mean	10%	90%
Mean ± SD	Dura	−1.2 ± 2.0	0.5 ± 1.6	−3.0 ± 2.5
	Brain 1	−4.4 ± 1.9	−1.0 ± 1.1	−7.9 ± 3.2
	Brain 2	−5.6 ± 1.9	−1.2 ± 1.1	−10.3 ± 3.2
Min to Max	Dura	2.0 to −4.8	3.4 to −1.9	0.9 to −8.1
	Brain 1	−1.3 to −7.1	2.8 to −2.5	−2.3 to −13.2
	Brain 2	−3.1 to −8.5	2.4 to −3.0	−6.2 to −15.0

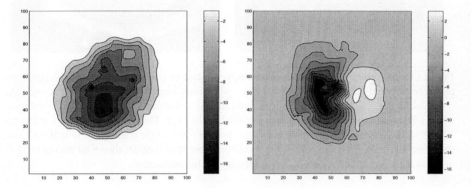

Fig. 1. Plots showing the spatial distribution of brain surface movement.

each other (two-tailed paired t test, $P < 0.01$). This is true for both the mean and 90% displacement values. The 90% displacement was greater than 10 mm in approximately one-third of the patients (7 of 19 patients) for the first brain surface and approximately one-half of the patients (10 of 19 patients) for the second.

Figure 1 shows contour plots of brain surface displacement. The left plot was created from data regarding a patient whose craniotomy inclination was 6 degrees, and is typical of most of the patients in this study. The brain was sinking under the craniotomy relative to its preoperative position. The displacement field was shaped somewhat like a bowl, with the largest displacement near the center of the craniotomy. The right plot was created from data regarding a patient whose craniotomy inclination was 34 degrees. Again the brain was sinking over much of the area of the craniotomy, but there was a region that was bulging or protruding (positive displacement values). This protruding region was at the lowest edge of the craniotomy. A similar pattern of bulging at the gravitationally dependent edge was observed in two other patients. Figure 2 shows the intraoperatively recorded brain surface overlayed as a white line on coronal slices from the preoperative MR image volumes for the same two patients shown in Fig. 1.

To test the reproducibility of dura and brain surface segmentation, for four patients, we had two people each draw contours. The mean distance between the surfaces obtained by each person ranged from −0.6 to 0.5 mm for dura and −0.4 to 0.5 mm for brain. The overall means were 0.1 and 0.2 mm for dura and brain, respectively. To test

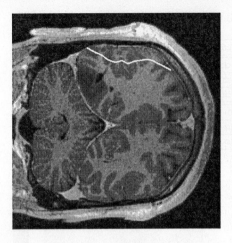
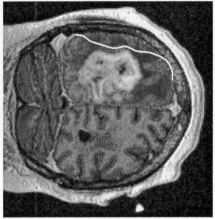

Fig. 2. Coronal image slices from the MR image volumes of two patients, showing the intraoperatively recorded brain surface overlayed as a white line. These images correspond to the data presented in Fig. 1. The image slices have been rotated to indicate the intraoperative orientation of the patient, with the direction of gravity vertical on the page. The patient's left side is at the top in each image. The ends of the white lines represent the edges of the craniotomy. In both patients, the brain was sinking under much of the craniotomy, but in the patient shown on the right, there was a slightly protruding region at the lowest edge of the craniotomy.

the reproducibility of the measurement of intraoperative brain surface movement, we had two surgeons each collect a set of brain surface points, one immediately after the other. Brain surface displacement was calculated for each set of measurements. The difference in mean brain surface displacement obtained by each surgeon ranged from −0.4 to 0.3 mm. The difference in overall means was 0.1 mm.

Patient age, craniotomy size, mannitol dose, time since mannitol infusion, net fluid volume change, and partial pressure of arterial carbon dioxide might all contribute to the amount of dura and brain surface shift. We examined plots of and calculated linear regressions of surface point displacement as compared with these variables. There were no visually obvious trends and no statistically significant correlations.

3.2 Effect of Orientation

The effect of orientation on the deformation of the brain within the closed cranium was assessed for two patients who were imaged prone and supine. Brain deformation between these imaging studies was quantified using the three techniques described in Section 2.5. The mean and SD of the brain surface displacement calculated using the first technique were less than 1 mm for both patients. Using the second technique, we determined that the mean discrepancy between the cranial and brain transformations for the two patients was less than 0.5 mm and that the maximum discrepancy was less than 1 mm. Both sets of measurements suggested that motion of the brain relative to the cranium resulting from a change in patient orientation only (i.e., without a craniotomy) is less than 1 mm. The mean discrepancies we obtained were only slightly larger than

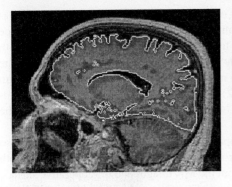 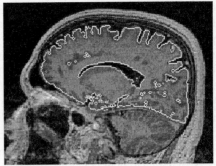

Fig. 3. Visual assessment of the effect of head orientation on brain shift. Threshold boundaries were computed in the prone images and overlayed on the supine images. In the left and right columns, boundaries were mapped using the cranial and brain transformations, respectively. There was no visually apparent brain shift using either transformation.

the expected error of the bone-implanted marker system, so the actual brain shift may have been smaller than these upper-bound figures suggest. Figure 3 shows the threshold boundary overlays for one of the two patients. There is no visually apparent brain shift using either the cranial or brain transformation.

4 Discussion

4.1 Sources of Error

There are several sources of error in a surgical navigation system: error inherent in the registration process, geometrical distortion in the images, movement of the patient with respect to the system during surgery, and movement of the brain relative to the cranium between scanning and the time of surgery. Because the purpose of this paper is to measure the latter, we need to examine the magnitude of the former.

The accuracy of the Acustar system was determined, in an earlier clinical trial, to be 1.0 ± 0.5 mm (mean $\pm$ SD) for CT-physical registration and 1.3 ± 0.6 mm for MR-physical registration [7]. These values include error in localizing the marker positions, error in tracking (i.e., finding the position of) the localization probe, and geometrical distortion in the image. The image-to-physical registrations using MP-RAGE MR images in the current study are likely to have been more accurate than the registrations obtained using the spin-echo MR images that were used in our previous studies [7].

The mean degradation in accuracy of the Acustar system during surgery was determined, in an earlier study, to be approximately 0.5 mm, with a change greater than 1.5 mm observed in 3 of 24 patients [7]. We believe that such head movement, some of which may occur during elevation of the craniotomy, is the principal cause of the degradation in accuracy. If the measured displacement of the brain were caused by head motion relative to the Mayfield clamp, then the bone surface and brain surface would be displaced in the same way. Thus, in this study, at the time of surface point collection, we measured the displacement of a marker visible in the surgical field relative to its position at the time of registration and calculated the distance of skull surface points from the skull surface segmented from a CT image. In 2 of 21 patients, both marker displacement and mean skull point distance were greater than 1.5 mm. In the remaining patients, the mean (maximum) marker displacement was 0.3–0.4 (0.8) mm and skull point distance was 0.7–0.8 (1.2) mm. For these 19 patients, the image-to-physical transformation determined at the beginning of surgery was still accurate at the time of surface point collection.

Surface segmentation error and intraoperative surface point localization error also contribute to brain shift measurement error. We assessed the reproducibility of both manual delineation of the brain surface from the MR images and intraoperative surface point collection and determined that different observers produced results that differed by less than 0.5 mm for both measurements. There is also the possibility of bias in our surface measurements resulting from the finite size of the spherical probe tip and the depression of the brain surface when recording measurements with the probe. The small values of the skull surface point distances after correcting for the size of the probe tip and the very small brain shifts measured at the edge of the craniotomies (see Figs. 1 and 2) suggested that our surface measurements are substantially free of bias.

It is important to note that we calculated the distance between a surface point collected intraoperatively and the nearest point on the same surface manually segmented from the preoperative MR image. The nearest point on the segmented surface was not necessarily the corresponding point, and thus, our displacement values are clearly lower bound estimates. In summary, the cortical surface shifts we calculated were substantially higher than our measurement error. The actual shifts are probably higher than our calculated shifts because we were using nearest image surface points rather than corresponding points.

4.2 Possible Causes of Brain Shift

We were surprised by the magnitude of the brain surface shift that we recorded. Exploring the reasons for the shift might make it possible to develop enhancements to surgical navigation systems to enable them to compensate for it.

High speed MR imaging techniques have previously been used to measure brain motion during imaging [8]. Pulsatile motion with the same period as the cardiac cycle and an amplitude of up to 0.5 mm was reported. The intraoperative brain shift we measured in our study was an order of magnitude larger than the reported pulsatile motion. The intraoperative brain surface deformation was also substantially larger than shift caused by a change in the orientation of the patient's head between the time of imaging and the time of surgery.

It is standard surgical practice to reduce intracranial pressure (ICP) before performing neurosurgical procedures. Steroids are often administered preoperatively to reduce inflammation. Intraoperatively, cerebral blood volume can be controlled by manipulating ventilation to alter carbon dioxide concentration in the blood and by tilting the bed to increase or reduce venous drainage. Cerebrospinal fluid (CSF) volume can be altered by reducing CSF production or by draining CSF. The water content of the brain can be reduced by administering an osmotically active drug, e.g., the sugar alcohol mannitol.

The effect these parameters have on ICP is well documented, but little is known about the resulting volume changes and brain deformation they cause in humans.

We approximated the volume between the brain surface in the image and the brain surface recorded intraoperatively by integrating the volume under surface displacement plots such as those shown in Figs. 1. This provides a reasonable approximation to the volume change under the craniotomy because the craniotomies are relatively flat and because the displacements are approximately normal to the plane of the craniotomy. This estimate does not include any volume change associated with brain shift outside the craniotomy. The mean ± SD volume changes under the craniotomy were -6 ± 11, -22 ± 10, and -29 ± 11 ml for the dura, first, and second brain surfaces, respectively. The mean change for the dura surface was less than 1% of typical brain volume. The mean changes for the brain surfaces were approximately 1–2%.

4.3 Consequences for Image-Guided Surgery

Motion of the brain surface relative to the cranium may not be an important factor in some types of neurosurgery. For example, if a lesion of interest is at the base of the cranium, surrounded by cranial nerves and blood vessels, it may move much less relative to the skull than the brain surface immediately underneath a craniotomy. Our measurements are unlikely to have much applicability for assessing errors at such deep structures. Furthermore, we measured brain motion only in the direction perpendicular to the brain surface. This type of motion has only a minor influence on the accuracy of image-guided surgery for planning the position of a craniotomy.

The motion that we measured in this study will directly affect the accuracy with which a surgeon can judge his or her depth into the brain in the vicinity of the surface. For example, if the surgical navigation system is being used to assist the surgeon in identifying the distal edge of a superficial lesion, then brain motion in the direction perpendicular to the brain surface directly degrades the accuracy of the system.

The goal of this study was to accurately quantify intraoperative deformation of the brain cortical surface. Clearly the ultimate goal of this field of research is to quantify 3-D brain deformation. Bucholz [1] recently reported some preliminary studies of subsurface structure displacement using intraoperative ultrasonography. The brain cortical surface is a good starting point for measuring subsurface deformation because the surface is visible and it is possible to obtain very accurate measurements of the surface. Intraoperative ultrasound images typically have a low signal-to-noise ratio, and segmentation of subsurface structures is often difficult. It might be possible to quantify 3-D brain motion using elastic deformation models. Measurements of surface displacement similar to those we have reported in this study can potentially be used as boundary conditions for such models. Further work is necessary to quantify the deformation of subsurface structures and to determine how deformation is influenced by the resection process. It is possible that further studies will find that for some types of neurosurgical procedures requiring high accuracy, brain deformation is substantial and too variable to be corrected using computational algorithms. If this turns out to be the case, then accurate imaging guidance for these procedures could be provided only by high-quality intraoperative imaging, such as interventional MR imaging.

Any evidence of brain motion derived from this study, especially in the context of otherwise satisfactory deep brain target localization, must not be used to justify inaccurate systems or pessimism about system accuracy in general. Instead, it should prompt renewed efforts to develop techniques to minimize this motion or correct for it dynamically in order to achieve better registration.

References

1. Bucholz RD, Yeh DD, Trobaugh J, et al: The correction of stereotactic inaccuracy caused by brain shift using an intraoperative ultrasound device. In: Troccaz J, Grimson E, Mösges R (eds): *CVRMed-MRCAS '97*, Berlin, Springer-Verlag, 1997, pp 459–466.
2. Dorward NL, Alberti O, Velani B, et al: Early clinical experience with the EasyGuide neuronavigation system and measurement of intraoperative brain distortion. In: Hellwig D, Bauer BL (eds): *Minimally Invasive Techniques for Neurosurgery*, Heidelberg, Springer-Verlag, 1997, pp 193–196.
3. Golfinos JG, Fitzpatrick BC, Smith LR, Spetzler RF: Clinical use of a frameless stereotactic arm: Results of 325 cases. *J Neurosurg* 83:197–205, 1995.
4. Gueziec A, Hummel R: Exploiting triangulated surface extraction using tetrahedral decomposition. *IEEE Trans Visualization Comput Graph* 1:328–342, 1995.
5. Hill DLG, Maurer CR Jr, Wang MY, et al: Estimation of intraoperative brain surface movement, In: Troccaz J, Grimson E, Mösges R (eds): *CVRMed-MRCAS '97*, Berlin, Springer-Verlag, 1997, pp 449–458.
6. Maurer CR Jr, Aboutanos GB, Dawant BM, et al: Registration of 3-D images using weighted geometrical features. *IEEE Trans Med Imaging* 15:836–849, 1996.
7. Maurer CR Jr, Fitzpatrick JM, Wang MY, et al: Registration of head volume images using implantable fiducial markers. *IEEE Trans Med Imaging* 16:447–462, 1997.
8. Poncelet BP, Wedeen VJ, Weisskoff RM, Cohen MS: Brain parenchyma motion: Measurement with cine echoplanar MR imaging. *Radiology* 185:645–651, 1992.
9. Reinges MHT, Krombach G, Nguyen H, et al: Assessment of intraoperative brain tissue movements by frameless neuronavigation. *Comput Aided Surg* 2:218, 1997 (abstract).
10. Studholme C, Hill DLG, Hawkes DJ: Automated 3D registration of MR and PET brain images by multi-resolution optimisation of voxel similarity measures. *Med Phys* 24:25–35, 1997.
11. Wang MY, Maurer CR Jr, Fitzpatrick JM, Maciunas RJ: An automatic technique for finding and localizing externally attached markers in CT and MR volume images of the head. *IEEE Trans Biomed Eng* 43:627–637, 1996.

Clinical Experience with a High Precision Image-Guided Neurosurgery System[*]

E. Grimson[1], M. Leventon[1], G. Ettinger[4], A. Chabrerie[2], F. Ozlen[3], S. Nakajima[2], H. Atsumi[3], R. Kikinis[2], and P. Black[3]

[1] MIT AI Laboratory, Cambridge MA, USA
welg@ai.mit.edu
[2] Radiology, Brigham & Womens Hospital, Harvard Medical School, Boston USA
[3] Neurosurgery, Brigham & Womens Hospital, Harvard Medical School, Boston USA
[4] Alphatech, Burlington MA USA

Abstract. We describe an image-guided neurosurgery system which we have successfully used on 70 cases in the operating room. The system is designed to achieve high positional accuracy with a simple and efficient interface that interferes little with the operating room's usual procedures, but is general enough to use on a wide range of cases. It uses data from a laser scanner or a trackable probe to register segmented MR imagery to the patient's position in the operating room, and an optical tracking system to track head motion and localize medical instruments. Output visualizations for the surgeon consist of an "enhanced reality display," showing location of hidden internal structures, and an instrument tracking display, showing the location of instruments in the context of the MR imagery. Initial assessment of the system in the operating room indicates a high degree of robustness and accuracy.

1 Introduction

Many surgical procedures require highly precise localization, often of deeply buried structures, in order for the surgeon to extract targeted tissue with minimal damage to nearby structures. While methods such as MRI and CT are valuable for imaging and displaying the internal 3D structure of the body, the surgeon must still relate what he sees on the 3D display with the actual patient.

Traditional clinical practice often only utilizes 2D slices of MR or CT imagery, requiring the surgeon to mentally transform that information to the actual patient, thus there is a need for techniques to register 3D reconstructions of internal anatomy with the surgical field. Such image-guided surgical tools allow the surgeon to directly visualize important structures, and plan and act accordingly. Visualization methods include "enhanced reality visualization" [11], in which rendered internal structures are overlaid on the surgeon's field-of-view, and instrument tracking, in which medical instruments acting on the patient are localized and visualized in the 3D MR or CT imagery.

---

[*] This report describes research supported in part by DARPA under ONR contract N00014-94-01-0994.

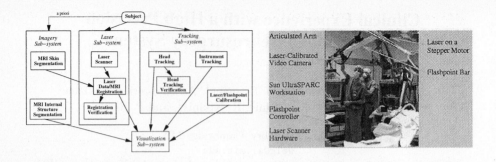

Fig. 1. (left) Image-guided surgery system architecture. (right) Setup of system in operating room.

The key components of an accurate, reliable, image-guided surgery system are: creating accurate, detailed, patient-specific models of relevant anatomy for the surgical procedure; registering the models, and the corresponding imagery, to the patient; maintaining the registration throughout the surgical procedure; and tracking medical instruments in the surgical field in order to visualize them in the context of the MR/CT imagery and the reconstructed models.

We have developed a system which addresses these issues, primarily in neurosurgery. We had earlier reported our registration algorithms [11], and algorithmic testing of the system [10]. The important developments we report here are integration of tracking techniques, engineering of the system into an effective surgery tool, evaluation of the system's performance under control conditions, and initial experience of using the system on 70 cases in the operating room.

2 Image-Guided Neurosurgery System

Neurosurgery is an ideal application for image-guided techniques, by virtue of the high precision it requires, the need to visualize nearby tissue, the need for planning of optimal trajectories to target tissue, and the need to localize visually indistinguishable, but functional different, tissue types. Early attempts to achieve image-guided neurosurgery consisted of stereotactic frames which directly provided the fiducials for registering the MRI or CT data to the patient [8]. More recently, frameless stereotaxy systems have been pursued by many groups [1, 2, 5, 15, 18, 23], and usually consist of two components: registration and tracking. We have added a third, initial, component to our system – reconstructed models of the patient's anatomy. The system's components are described below.

The architecture of our image-guided surgery system (Figure 1) supports frameless, non-fiducial, registration of medical imagery by matching surface data, and supports optical tracking of patient and instrument locations. The system (Figure 1) consists of a portable cart containing a Sun UltraSPARC workstation and the hardware to drive the laser scanner and Flashpoint tracking system. On top of the cart is mounted an articulated extendable arm to which we attach a bar housing the laser scanner and Flashpoint cameras. The three linear Flashpoint cameras are inside the bar. The laser is attached to one end of the bar, and a video camera to the other. The joint between the arm and scanning bar has three degrees-of-freedom to allow easy placement of the bar in desired configurations.

2.1 Imagery Sub-system

MRI is the prime imaging modality for the neurosurgery cases we support. The images are acquired prior to surgery without a need for special landmarking strategies. To process the imagery, a wide range of methods (e.g., [25, 21, 16, 19, 22]) have been applied to the segmentation problem, i.e. identifying different tissue types in medical imagery. Our current approach to segmentation uses an automated method to initially segment into major tissue classes while removing gain artifacts from the imager [25, 13], then uses operator driven interactive tools to refine this segmentation. This latter step primarily relies on 3D visualization and data manipulation techniques to correct and refine the initial automated segmentation. The segmented tissue types include skin, used for registration, and internal structures such as brain, tumor, vessels, and ventricles. These segmented structures are processed by the Marching Cube algorithm [14] to construct isosurfaces and support surface rendering for visualization.

The structural models of patients constructed using such methods can be augmented with functional information. For example, functional MRI methods or transcranial magnetic stimulation methods [7] can be used to identify motor or sensory cortex. This data can then be fused with the structural models [26] to augment such models. In each case, segmentation produces information in a local coordinate frame, which must be merged together. We currently use a registration method based on Mutual Information [26] to do this. The result is an augmented, patient-specific, geometric model of relevant structural and functional information.

2.2 Registration Sub-system

Registration is the process by which the MRI or CT data is transformed to the coordinate frame of the patient. The most common form of registration uses fiducials [1, 15, 20, 23]: either markers attached to the skin or bone prior to imaging or anatomically salient features on the head. The fiducials are manually localized in both the MR or CT imagery and on the patient and the resulting correspondences are used to solve for the registration. Fiducial systems may not be as accurate as frame-based methods–Peters [17] reports fiducial accuracy about an order of magnitude worse than frame-based methods, but Maciunas [15] reports high accuracy achieved with novel implantable fiducials.

Another registration approach is surface alignment in which the MRI skin surface is aligned with the patient's scalp surface in the operating room. Ryan [18] generates the patient's scalp surface by probing about 150 points with a trackable medical instrument. Colchester [5] uses an active stereo system to

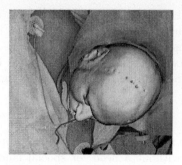 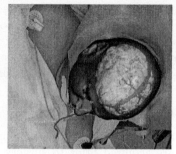

Fig. 2. (left) Initial alignment of laser and MRI data, showing overlay of MRI skin data on laser scanner's video image. (right) Enhanced reality visualization of the patient showing hidden internal structures overlaid on the surgeon's view of the patient.

construct the scalp surface. We also perform the registration using surface alignment[9], benefiting from its dense data representation, but use either a laser scanner to construct the patient's scalp surface or a trackable probe to obtain data points from the patient's skin surface for registration.

We have used two related methods to register the reconstructed model to the actual patient position. In the first method, we use a laser scanner to collect 3D data of the patient's scalp surface as positioned on the operating table. The scanner is a laser striping triangulation system consisting of a laser unit (low power laser source and cylindrical lens mounted on a stepper motor) and a video camera. The laser is calibrated a priori by using a calibration gauge of known dimensions to calculate the camera parameters and the sweeping angles of the laser. In the operating room the laser scanner is placed to maximize coverage of the salient bony features of the head, such as nose and eye orbits. To ensure accurate registration we can supplement the laser data with points probed with a Flashpoint pointer, similar to [18], to include skin points that are not visible to the laser in the registration. The acquired laser data is overlaid on the laser scanner's video image of the patient for specification of the region of interest. This process uses a simple mouse interface to outline the region of the head on which we want to base the registration. This process need not be perfect—the registration is designed to deal robustly with outliers. The laser scan takes about 30 seconds once the sensor is appropriately placed above the patient.

An alternative method is to simply use a trackable probe to acquire data. In this case, we trace paths on the skin of the patient with the trackable probe, recording positional information at points along each path. These points are not landmarks, but simply replace the lines of laser data. The registration process is the same, whether matching laser data or trackable probe data to the skin surface of the MRI model.

One of the keys to our system is the integration of a reliable and accurate data-to-MRI registration algorithm. Our registration process is described in detail in [11]. It is a three step process performing an optimization on a six parameter rigid transformation, which aligns the data surface points with the MRI skin surface. The steps consist of: (1) A manual initial alignment in which we roughly align the two surfaces. Accurate manual alignment can be very difficult, but we aim only to be within 20° of the correct transformation which subsequent steps solve for. This process is performed using two displays and takes about 60 seconds. In one display, the rendered MRI skin is overlaid on the laser scanner's video view of the patient, and the MRI data is rotated and translated in 3D to achieve a qualitatively close alignment. In the second display, the laser data is projected onto three orthogonal projections of the MRI data. The projected MRI data is colored such that intensity is inversely proportional to distance from the viewer. In each overlay view, the laser data may be rotated and translated in 2D to align the projections. An alternative to manual initial alignment is to record three known points using the trackable probe (e.g. tip of the nose, tip of the ear), then identify roughly the same point in the MRI model. This process determines a rough initial alignment of the data to the MR reconstruction, and typically takes less then 5 seconds. (2) Automated interpolated alignment which performs optimization over a large region of convergence [9–11]. This process runs in about 10 seconds on a Sun UltraSPARC workstation. The method basically solves for the transform that optimizes a Gaussian weighted least-squares fit of the two data sets. (3) Automated detailed alignment which performs optimization to accurately localize the best surface data to MRI transformation[9–11]. This process runs in about 10 seconds on a Sun UltraSPARC workstation. The method basically solves a truncated least-squares fit of the two data sets, refining the transformation obtained in the previous step.

Three verification tools are used to inspect the registration results as the objective functions optimized by the registration algorithm may not be sufficient to guarantee the correct solution. One verification tool overlays the MRI skin on the video image of the patient, (Figure 2), except that we animate the visualization by varying the blending of the MRI skin and video image. A second verification tool overlays the sensed data on the MRI skin by color-coding the sensed data by distance between the data points and the nearest MRI skin points. Such a residual error display identifies possible biases remaining in the registration solution. A third verification tool compares locations of landmarks. Throughout the surgery, the surgeon uses the optically tracked probe to point to distinctive anatomical structures. The offset of the probe position from the actual point in the MR volume is then observed in the display.

2.3 Tracking Sub-system

Tracking is the process by which objects are dynamically localized in the patient's coordinate system. Of particular interest to us is the tracking of medical instruments and the patient's head. Optical trackers use multiple cameras to triangulate the 3D location of flashing LEDs that may be mounted on any object to be tracked. Such devices are generally perceived as the most accurate, efficient, and reliable localization system [2, 4]. Other methods, such as acoustic or magnetic field sensing are being explored as well, but tend to be more sensitive

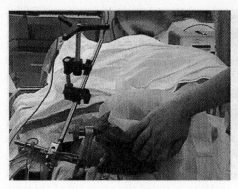
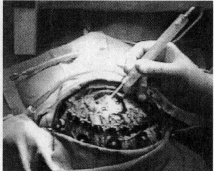

Fig. 3. Trackable configuration of LEDs attached to head clamp, or to the skin flap.

to environmental effects. We use optical tracking, the Flashpoint system by IGT Inc., Boulder, CO, USA, due to its accuracy and ease-of-use benefits.

Tracking patient head motion is often necessary since the head is not always clamped to the operating table, the head may move relative to the clamp, the operating table may be moved, or the hardware performing the tracking may be moved to rearrange lights or other equipment in the operating room. Although not all image-guided surgery systems account for patient motion, [1, 2, 5, 15, 18] solve this problem by attaching trackable markers to the head or clamp. We also currently utilize an optically trackable configuration of markers attached to a Mayfield clamp (Figure 3). We have also experimented with directly attaching trackable LEDs to the skin surface of the patient. Our experience is that while in most cases this worked well, it required that the surgeon carefully plan the location of the LEDs to ensure that they did not move between initial placement and opening of the skin flap.

We require direct line-of-sight from the Flashpoint cameras to the LEDs at times when the surgeon requires image-guidance. In order to maintain such line-of-sight we can re-locate the scanning bar such that it is both out of the way of the surgeon but maintains visibility of the LEDs. Such dynamic reconfiguration of the scanning bar is a benefit of the head tracking process.

Instrument tracking is performed by attaching two LEDs to a sterile pointer. The two LEDs allow us to track the 3D position of the tip of the pointer as well as its orientation, up to the twist angle which is not needed for this application. Figure 3 shows the surgeon using the trackable pointer in the opened craniotomy.

2.4 Visualization Sub-system

Two types of visualizations are provided to the surgeon on the workstation monitor. One is an enhanced reality visualization in which internal structures are overlaid on the video image of the patient. The video image is set up to duplicate the surgeon's view of the patient. Any segmented MR structures may be displayed at varying colors and opacities (see Figure 2).

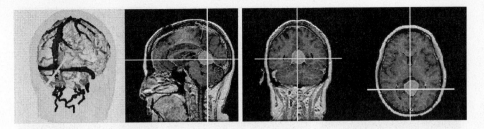

Fig. 4. Pointer tracking in 3D MRI rendering and three orthogonal MRI slices.

A second visualization shows the location of the pointer tip in a 3D rendering of selected MRI structures and in three orthogonal MRI slices (see Figure 4). These visualizations are updated twice per second as the pointer is moved.

3 Operating Room Procedure

Using our system, as seen from the surgeon's perspective, involves: (1) Prepare patient for surgery as per usual procedure including clamping the head. Head is still visible. (2) Attach a configuration of LEDs to the head clamp, and record the positions of the LEDs in the Flashpoint system. (3) Register MRI to patient by placing our scanner bar over patient's head. The bar is generally about $1.5m$ away from head. Scan patient's head by swabbing a trackable probe across the skin. Typically several swabs are used, designed to cover a wide range of positions on the patient. It is often convenient to include swabs along known paths such as across the cheeks or down the nose, as these paths will aid in inspecting the resulting registration. (4) The Flashpoint/laser bar may be re-positioned at any point to avoid interference with equipment and to maintain visibility of LEDs. (5) Sterilize and drape patient. Any motion of the patient during this process will be recorded by movements of the LED configuration attached to the head clamp. (6) Proceed with craniotomy and surgical procedure. (7) At any point, use sterile Flashpoint pointer to explore structures in the MR imagery.

4 Performance Analysis

To evaluate the performance of our registration and tracking subsystems, we have performed an extensive set of controlled perturbation studies [6]. In these studies, we have taken existing data sets, simulated data acquisition from the surface of the data, added noise to the simulated surface data, then perturbed the position of data and solved for the optimal registration. Since we know the starting point of the data, we can measure the accuracy with which the two data sets are re-registered.

While extensive details of the testing are reported in [6], the main conclusions of the analysis are:

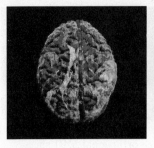 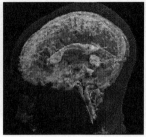 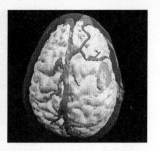

Fig. 5. Examples of neurosurgical cases. The last example includes a fusion of fMR data overlaid on top of the structural model.

- accurate and stable registration is achieved for up to 45 degree rotational offsets of the data sets, with other perturbations;
- accurate and stable registration is achieved for up to 75 degree rotational offsets of the data sets, with no other perturbations;
- robust registration is obtained when the surface data spans at least 40% of the full range of the surface, and is generally obtained with as little as 25% coverage;
- small numbers of outliers do not affect the registration process.

5 Operating Room Results

We have used the described image-guided neurosurgery system on 70 patients. These cases included: 44 Supratentorial - 22 high grade, 22 low grade; 6 Meningiomas; 3 Metastases; 2 Posterior Fossa; 1 Meningioangiomatosis; 7 Intractable Epilepsy; 4 Vascular; 2 Biopsies; and 1 Demyelinating lesion.

In all cases the system effectively supported the surgery:

- by providing guidance in planning bone cap removal – this was done through the augmented reality visualization in which the surgeon could visualize paths to the critical tissue and plan an appropriate entry point.
- identifying margins of tumor – this was done by tracing the boundaries of tissue with the trackable probe.
- localizing key blood vessels.
- and orienting the surgeon's frame of reference.

Selected examples are shown in Figure 5.

To qualitatively validate the system's performance, the surgeon placed the pointer on several known landmarks: skull marks from previous surgeries, ventricle tip, inner skull bones such as eye orbits, sagittal sinus, and small cysts or necrotic tissues. He then estimated their position in the MRI scan, and we compared the distance between the expected position and the system's tracked

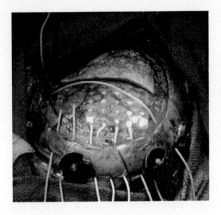 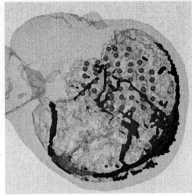

Fig. 6. Grid of electrodes placed on cortical surface. Location of grid points overlaid onto MR reconstruction, with focal area highlighted.

position. In all cases, this error was less than two voxels (MRI resolution was $0.9375mm \times 0.9375mm \times 1.5mm$).

One example of the effectiveness of the system is illustrated by the following study. Twenty patients with low-grade gliomas underwent surgery with the system. The pathologies included 10 low grade astrocytomas (grades I, II out of IV), 7 oligoastrocytomas (without anaplastic features) and 3 oligodendrogliomas. Thirteen patients underwent cortical mapping including 7 who underwent speech and motor mapping, 2 motor alone, 1 speech alone and 3 motor and sensory. 31% had a subtotal resection, the remainder had total resection. One patient exhibited temporary left-sided weakness. Cortical mapping had represented the sensory cortex diffusely behind this patient's gross tumor. The post-operative weakness was temporary and was thought to be due to swelling. One patient showed a mild, left upper extremity proprioreceptive deficit which was due to a vascular accident on post-operative day one. The remaining patients were neurological intact following the procedure.

In addition to the tumor resection cases, we have also used the system in 10 pediatric epilepsy cases [3]. In the first stage of this two stage surgery, the patient's cortex is exposed and a grid of electrical pickups is placed on the cortical surface. A lead from each pickup is threaded out through the skin for future monitoring. In addition to registering the MRI model of the patient to his/her position, the location of each electrical contact is recorded and transformed to MRI coordinates. The patient is then closed up and monitored for several days. During any seizure event, the activity from each cortical probe is monitored, and transformed to the MRI model. This enables the surgeon to isolate potential foci in MRI coordinates. During a second surgical procedure, the augmented MRI model is reregistered to the patient and the locations of the hypothesized foci are presented to the surgeon for navigational guidance. An example of this is shown in Figure 6.

To see the range of cases handled by our system, we encourage readers to visit the web site:

http://splweb.bwh.harvard.edu:8000/pages/comonth.html

which shows selected cases with descriptions of the use and impact of the navigation system on the case.

6 Summary

We have described an image-guided neurosurgery system, now in use in the operating room. The system achieves high positional accuracy with a simple, efficient interface that interferes little with normal operating room procedures, while supporting a wide range of cases. Qualitative assessment of the system in the operating room indicates strong potential. In addition to performing quantitative testing on the system, we are also extending its capabilities by integrating a screw-based head tracking system and improved visualization capabilities.

References

1. L. Adams, et al., "An Optical Navigator for Brain Surgery". *IEEE Computer*, **29**(1):48–54, Jan. 1996.
2. D.R. Bucholtz, K.R. Smith. "A Comparison of Sonic Digitizers Versus Light Emitting Diode-Based Localization". R.J. Maciunas, ed., *Interactive Image-Guided Neurosurgery*, Amer. Assoc. Neur. Surg., 1993.
3. A. Chabrerie, F. Ozlen, S. Nakajima, M. Leventon, H. Atsumi, E. Grimson, E. Keeve, S. Helmers, J. Riviello, G. Holmes, F. Duffy, F. Jolesz, R. Kikinis, P. Black, "Three-Dimensional Reconstruction and Surgical Navigation in Pediatric Epilepsy Surgery", Medical Image Computation and Computer Assisted Interventions, Boston, October 1998.
4. P. Cinquin et al., "Computer Assisted Medical Interventions". *IEEE EMB*, 254–263, May/June 1995.
5. A.C.F. Colchester et al., "Development and Preliminary Evaluation of VISLAN, a Surgical Planning and Guidance System Using Intra-Operative Video Imaging". *Medical Image Analysis*, **1**(1):73–90, March 1996.
6. G. Ettinger, "Hierarchical three-dimensional medical image registration", Ph.D. Thesis, MIT, 1997.
7. G. Ettinger, et al., "Experimentation with a Transcranial Magnetic Stimulation System for Functional Brain Mapping", *Medical Image Analysis*, **2**(2):133–142, 1998.
8. R. Galloway. "Stereotactic Frame Systems and Intraoperative Localization Devices". R. Maciunas, ed., *Interactive Image-Guided Neurosurgery*, Amer. Assoc. Neur. Surg., 1993.
9. W.E.L. Grimson, et al., "An Automatic Registration Method for Frameless Stereotaxy, Image Guided Surgery, and Enhanced Reality Visualization", Comp. Vis. and Pattern Recognition Conference, Seattle, June 1994.

10. W.E.L. Grimson, et al., "Evaluating and Validating an Automated Registration System for Enhanced Reality Visualization in Surgery". *First CVRMED*, Nice France, April 1995, pp. 3–12.
11. W.E.L. Grimson, et al., "An Automatic Registration Method for Frameless Stereotaxy, Image Guided Surgery, and Enhanced Reality Visualization". *IEEE TMI*, **15**(2):129–140, April 1996.
12. B. Horn. "Closed-form Solution of Absolute Orientation Using Unit Quaternions". *JOSA A*, **4**:629–642, April 1987.
13. T. Kapur, W.E.L. Grimson, R. Kikinis. "Segmentation of Brain Tissue from MR Images". *First CVRMED*, Nice France, April 1995, pp. 429–433.
14. W.E. Lorensen, H.E. Cline. "Marching Cube: A High Resolution 3-D Surface Construction Algorithm". *Computer Graphics*, **21**(3):163–169, 1987.
15. R. Maciunas, et al., "Beyond Stereotaxy: Extreme Levels of Application Accuracy Are Provided by Implantable Fiducial Markers for Interactive Image-Guided Neurosurgery". R.J. Maciunas, ed., *Interactive Image-Guided Neurosurgery*, Amer. Assoc. Neur. Surg., 1993.
16. T. McInerney, D. Terzopoulos. "Medical image segmentation using topologically adaptable snakes". *CVRMed* 1995.
17. T. Peters, et al., "Three-Dimensional Multimodal Image-Guidance for Neurosurgery". *IEEE TMI*, **15**(2):121–128, April 1996.
18. M.J. Ryan, et al., "Frameless Stereotaxy with Real-Time Tracking of Patient Head Movement and Retrospective Patient-Image Registration". *J. Neurosurgery*, **85**:287–292, August 1996.
19. G. Szekely, et al. "Segmentation of 3d objects from MRI volume data using constrained elastic deformations of flexible fourier surface models". *CVRMed* 1995.
20. S. Tebo, et al., "An Optical 3D Digitizer for Frameless Stereotactic Surgery". *IEEE Comp. Graph. Appl.*, **16**(1):55–64, Jan. 1996.
21. K.L. Vincken, A.S.E. Koster, M.A. Viergever. "Probabilisitc hyperstack segmentation of MR Brain Data", *CVRMed*, 1995.
22. S. Warfield, et al., "Automatic identification of grey matter structures from MRI to improve the segmentation of white matter lesions". *Journal of Image Guided Surgery* **1**(6):326–338, June 1996.
23. E. Watanabe, "The Neuronavigator: A Potentiometer-Based Localizing Arm System". R. Maciunas, ed., *Interactive Image-Guided Neurosurgery*, Amer. Assoc. Neur. Surg., 1993.
24. W.M. Wells. "Adaptive Segmentation of MRI Data". *First CVRMED*, Nice France, April 1995, pp. 59–69.
25. W.M. Wells, III, W.E.L. Grimson, R. Kikinis, F.A. Jolesz, "Adaptive Segmentation of MRI data", *IEEE Trans. Medical Imaging*, **15**(4):429–442, August 1996.
26. W.M. Wells, et al. "Multi-modal volume registration by maximization of mutual information" *Medical Image Analysis*, **1**(1): 35–51, 1996.

Three-Dimensional Reconstruction and Surgical Navigation in Padiatric Epilepsy Surgery

Alexandra Chabrerie[1,3], Fatma Ozlen[1,3], Shin Nakajima[1,3],
Michael Leventon[2], Hideki Atsumi[1], Eric Grimson[2], Erwin Keeve[1],
Sandra Helmers[4], James Riviello Jr.[4], Gregory Holmes[4], Frank Duffy[4],
Ferenc Jolesz[1], Ron Kikinis[1], and Peter Black[3]

[1] Surgical Planning Laboratory, Brigham and Women's Hospital,
Harvard Medical School, Boston, MA
[2] Artificial Intelligence Laboratory,
Massachusetts Institute of Technology, Cambridge, MA
[3] Division of Neurosurgery, Brigham and Women's Hospital, Children's Hospital,
Harvard Medical School, Boston, MA
[4] Department of Neurology, Children's Hospital,
Harvard Medical School, Boston, MA

Abstract. We have used MRI-based three-dimensional (3D) reconstruction and a real-time, frameless, stereotactic navigation device to facilitate the removal of seizure foci in children suffering from intractable epilepsy. Using this system, the location of subdural grid and strip electrodes is recorded on the 3D model to facilitate focus localization and resection. Ten operations were performed – two girls and eight boys ranging in age from 3-17 – during which 3D reconstruction and surgical instrument tracking navigation was used. In all cases, the patients tolerated the procedure well and showed no post-operative neurological deficits.

1 Introduction

Although most children suffering from epilepsy have a good prognosis for remission, a small percentage of cases are resistant to conventional Anti-Epileptic Drugs. For these patients, surgical intervention for seizure focus removal to stop the seizures and to prevent further brain injury provides great hope [1]. Subdural grid and strip electrodes in chronic monitoring of the Electroencephalogram (EEG) have become more widely used as a means of accurately obtaining the necessary localization of the focus with a minimum morbidity [2]. Implanting subdural electrodes directly on the brain surface allows the epilepsy investigator to record a series of ictal and interictal recordings, with ample time for a complete and precise mapping [3]. In addition, cortical stimulation for localizing an epileptic focus also determines its relation to eloquent areas and surrounding cortical function [4].

Magnetic Resonance Imaging (MRI) is a highly reliable neuroimaging procedure in patients with partial or localized epilepsy [4]. For several years, we have been making computerized, 3D reconstructions of pre-operative MRI scan

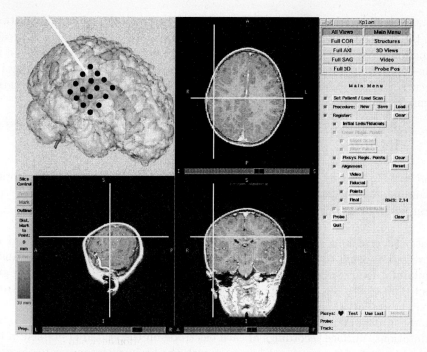

Fig. 1. The interface displayed on the computer monitor during surgery. The position of the LED probe is simultaneously displayed on the 3D model (white arrow). The position on the corresponding MRI splices is displayed in the axial, sagittal and coronal planes. The subdural electrodes are shown as black spheres.

data for surgical planning [5] and intraoperative navigation. We have recently developed a novel neurosurgical navigator in which medical image registration and instrument tracking automatically establishes correspondence between the medical images from MRI scans, the three-dimensional model and the actual patient environment [6]. Using this intraoperative guidance, medical instruments acting on the patient are localized in the 3D coordinate frame of the MRI imagery. Consequently, the surgeon is allowed to view a patient and at the same time display, in exact alignment, that view and all other surrounding internal structures on both the reconstructed model and three views on the original MRI scans. Most importantly, any point may be recorded and displayed on the 3D model as an arrow or simple dot (see Figure 1).

We have combined functional diagnostic tools including EEG results and subdural strip and grid electrodes results, with real-time, intra-operative imaging and 3D reconstruction to increase the precision of localization and subsequent resection of seizure foci. The 3D models constructed from pre-operative MRI scans allow pre-operative surgical planning as well as intraoperative navigation. The latter is used as guidance for the surgeon to the correct location of the abnormality and to establish its boundaries for safe resection without affecting neighboring areas and decreasing the invasion of eloquent cortex. Most importantly, it allows the recording of the subdural grid and strip electrode positions on the 3D model and as a result, provides an accurate, 3D visualization. A precise functional and structural map of the patient's brain is thus created and used for pre-operative planning and intraoperative navigation, ultimately increasing the accuracy localization of the focus and decreasing the likelihood of post-operative neurological deficits.

2 Methods

Patients: 3D reconstructions using MR images were created and used for surgical planning in 10 pediatric patients (ages 3 -18 yrs; 2 girls and 8 boys), all suffering from intractable seizures.

Subdural grid and strip placement: Criteria for surgical intervention and investigation using cortical surface electrodes included intractable seizures and a unilateral focus believed to be cortical, temporal or extra-temporal. The grid and strip electrodes most often used initially are either a 4x8 or 8x8 electrode contact grid array (AdTech Medical Instruments; Racine, Wisc., USA) and were modified depending on the result of the pre-operative assessment or operative limitations. Surface recordings of each electrode on the grid are obtained in the operating room to ensure good contact with the brain surface prior to closure.

MR data acquisition and transfer: The MR data were obtained by a 1.5 Tesla MR unit (Signa; GE Medical Systems, Milwaukee, WI). A series of 124 images of post-contrast, 3D SPGR (SPoiled Gradient Recalled acquisition in the steady-state, 1.5 mm thickness, 256x256 matrix of 220-240 mm FOV) were obtained. An MR angiogram in either the axial or the sagittal plane for 3D reconstruction of the vasculature was used. The velocity encoding (VENC) was chosen according to the specific pathology. For cortical/subcortical tumors, we chose 20 cm/sec VENC to visualize small cortical vessels. For arterial information, we used 60 cm/sec. The data were digitally transferred to the workstation (SPARC 20; Sun Microsystems, Inc., Mountain View, CA) via a computer network.

Image processing: Each image was pre-processed to reduce noise using anisotropic diffusion filtering [7]. A segmentation based on signal intensities and voxel connectivity [8, 9] was then performed using one of the MR series (SPGR and MR angiogram). Imperfections in the 3D objects were corrected by manual editing. From these images, 3D models of the skin, brain, vessels, focal lesion and ventricles were reconstructed using the marching cubes algorithm and a surface rendering method [8–10]. These objects were then integrated and displayed on a computer workstation (Ultra-1; Sun Microsystems, Inc.) with a graphic accelerator (Creator 3D; Sun Microsystems Inc.) and 3D display software (LAVA; Sun Microsystems, Inc.). Each object thus may be rendered partially or completely transparent and oriented according to the viewer's choice. T2-weighted images and MR angiogram images can be registered to the base series (SPGR) using a

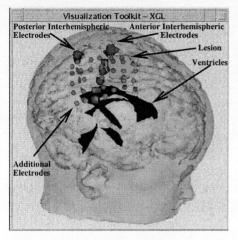 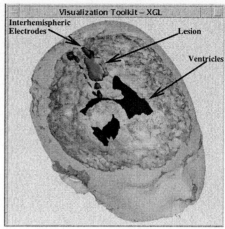

Fig. 2. 3D reconstruction showing the position of the subdural electrodes. 96 electrodes were applied directly to the cortical surface, including a posterior and an anterior interhemispheric strip. The parietal and frontal electrodes were localized using the trackable probe. The interhemispheric electrodes were segmented from an internal scan.

multi-modal volume registration method by maximization of mutual information [36]. Each object may be individually colored to facilitate visualization.

Surgical navigation: For intra-operative navigation, a real-time, Light Emitting Diode-based (LED), frameless, stereotactic device developed in the laboratory was used. Prior to surgery, a dynamic reference frame carrying three LED's (Image Guided Technologies, Inc.) is fixed next to the patient's head. A series of points from the patient's skin are recorded using an LED probe (Image Guided Technologies, Inc.). The information is tracked using an optical digitizer (Flashpoint 5000; Image Guided Technologies, Inc.). The points recorded in real space are then matched to the 3D model in two stages. An initial alignment is obtained by recording the real-space location of three points, then manually matching those points on the MRI model. This initial registration is refined by finding the optimal transformation that aligns all of the points onto the skin surface of the model [6, 14]. After registration the surgeon points to a known area on the patient using the LED probe, to confirm correspondence between the patient and the 3D model and MRI slices. During surgery, the surgeon uses a sterile LED probe to select any point on or inside the patient's brain. Any point may be recorded and displayed on the 3D model using an arrow or simple dot (see Figure 2).

3 Results and Illustrative Cases

Ten patients were pre-operatively evaluated in the Surgical Planning Laboratory at Brigham and Women's Hospital, Boston, MA. Their ages ranged from

Case	Diagnosis	Sex	Age	Outcome
1	Epilepsy	M	7	No new seizures
2	Left frontal focus	M	10	No new seizures
3	Left frontoparietal focus	M	3	No new seizures
4	Hypothalamic Hamartoma	M	18	No new seizures
5	Right parietal focus	M	12	No new seizures
6	Temporal epilepsy	M	15	No new seizures
7	Left temporal lobectomy	M	8	No new seizures
8	Left temporal lobectomy	F	5	Severe seizures remaining
9	Tuberous sclerosis	M	10	Seizure-free for approx two months post-operatively
10	Tuberous sclerosis	F	3	Seizures remaining but different in pattern than during pre-operative evaluation

Table 1. Summary of cases.

3 to 18, including two females and eight males. The females included one left temporal lobectomy and one right frontal tuber removal. The males included one left subcortical tuber removal and callosotomy, one left temporal lobectomy and hippocampectomy, one right parietal lobe mass removal, one left frontoparietal focus removal, one temporal epilepsy, one hypothalamic hamartoma with gelastic seizures, one right frontal interhemispheric focus removal (Table 1). The pre-operative and post-operative diagnosis was identical in all patients. Seven remained seizure free post-operatively. One girl suffering from tuberous sclerosis still experienced seizures but different in pattern from those recorded pre-operatively. The young boy suffering from the same congenital disorder remained seizure free for two months. The girl suffering from temporal lobe epilepsy showed atypical EEG readings during the initial evaluation and still had severe seizures post-operatively. No patient exhibited new post-operative neurological deficits.

For all the cases, the 3D imaging allowed the accurate evaluation of the lesions' anatomic location and relationship with neighboring cortical functionally relevant areas. The following cases illustrate the applications of our system.

Case 1: A seven year old boy with a one-year history of focal seizures and a lesion in the parasagittal posterior frontal lobe which on the MRI seemed consistent with hamartoma or dysplasia was admitted for subdural grid and strip placement and long-term monitoring. During the initial operation, 96 electrodes were applied directly to the cortical surface, including one posterior interhemispheric strip placed directly vertically down within the interhemispheric fissure posterior to the central sulcus and another placed anteriorly (Figure 2). One frontal and one parietal grid were placed subdurally on the lateral surface of the posterior frontal and the parietal lobes respectively. The location of the electrodes was recorded on the 3D model using the LED probe (black dots). Electrographic monitoring detected that all episodes were identical and consisted of abrupt and simultaneous onset of low amplitude fast activity in electrodes F32 of the frontal grid and AI11 and AI12 of the anterior interhemispheric strip. Using these results and intra-operative navigation the lesion was removed with careful motor and sensory monitoring. The patient tolerated the procedure well and has remained seizure free since then.

Case 2: An 8 year old boy suffering from intractable seizures was examined. The MRI showed no apparent lesions. Previous EEG results suggested a left temporal origin for seizure which prompted the decision to insert subdural grids and strips on that area to refine the seizure focus area. The location of the grids and strips was recorded and used as a map during bedside stimulation. Cortical stimulation was performed through the indwelling grids and strip electrodes. A mild interference with language in the superior portion of the posterior portion of the left latero-temporal grid in a region corresponding to Broca's area. As a result, it was decided to conducted a left temporal lobectomy as well as hippocampectomy. The hippocampus was reconstructed, displayed on the 3D model and used for guidance during surgery (Figure 1). The patient tolerated the procedure well and remained seizure free post-operatively.

Case 3: A two and a half year old girl with a history of tuberous sclerosis and cardiac disrrhythmia was admitted for seizure focus removal using subdural grids and strips and 3D reconstruction and navigation. A 32-contact grid was placed over the right lateral frontal region and an 8 contact strip was placed interhemispherically on the right frontal region. During the intracranial monitoring, it was noted that the seizure onset was localized to several contacts on the grid which were in the immediate region of the cortical tuber. Using 3D reconstruction and navigation, the tuber which was lying directly beneath the electrodes and which had been identified as the zone of epileptogenicity was removed (Figure 3). Following the operation, the patient remained free of post-operative neurological deficits with an MRI which showed a nice resection cavity.

4 Discussion

The system described above provides a novel application for surgical navigation systems for epilepsy assessment and surgery. EEG investigation results are merged with MRI imaging, and 3D reconstruction, to offer a functional as well as structural map for guidance during epileptic focus resection.

For the evaluation of epilepsy cases, EEG remains the cornerstone for the localization of seizure foci [11]. Interictal as well as ictal epileptiform activity which include such abnormalities as sharp waves, spikes, focal slowing and asymmetries of beta activity are used for the localization [1]. However, it is common that the EEG results, clinical neuroimaging results and clinical findings are not congruent, in which case the procedure of subdural grid and strip evaluation become quite useful. These electrodes are used for the planning of a safe resection, especially if the source of epileptic activity is located near eloquent cortex. In such a case, functional mapping of the area surrounding the lesion using successive electrical stimulation of the electrodes is also conducted. This procedure

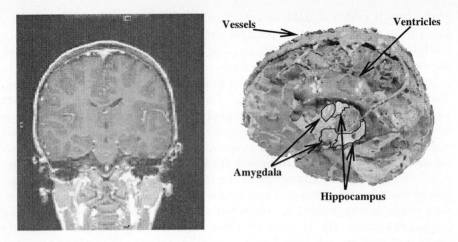

Fig. 3. LEFT: Coronal MRI showing no anatomically evident seizure foci. RIGHT: Three-dimensional reconstruction based on the patient's MRI scan used for pre-operative planning and surgical guidance.

has been conducted routinely [12] and although it is associated with risks (e.g., bleeding and infection), it is tolerated remarkably well by children [13].

Because of the limitations of the surgeons' views of the brain prior to and during the surgery, they have had to create a mental picture of the lesion(s) and their spatial arrangement to neighboring structures using pre-operative EEG results and MRI scan data. By integrating the above, a physical map of the child's brain can be created, both for surgical planning and intraoperative navigation. The 3D models that are created pre-operatively in which each structure can be phased in and out, rotated in any direction and enlarged according to the view that is desired, essentially provide a means for the neurosurgical team to "look inside the brain". Moreover, the application of these models for intraoperative use, contributes to a higher definition of a lesion's location and margins. In addition, the possibility of recording the location of each electrode on the subdural grids and strips, on a model in which the brain is made more transparent and in which the lesion is labeled in a separate color, represents a great leap from the conventional two dimensional X-ray visualization.

The increased use of 3D-reconstruction [6, 15-24] and surgical navigation [25-30,33-36] have substantially influenced neurosurgery. Although numerous navigation systems have been widely used for epilepsy surgery, the ability to establish a correspondence between the subdural electrodes that are placed on the brain surface and on the 3D model has not yet been described. Conventional methods of viewing these grids and strips include X-ray films [1] which in turn do not allow proper assessment of the underlying soft tissue.

We have developed the routine use of 3D reconstructions in surgical navigation for seizure focus removal in epilepsy surgery. Pre-operatively, the 3D model is used for surgical planning [30, 16, 17], facilitating the evaluation of the surgical approach. Intraoperatively, this system enables recording of the subdural grid and strip electrodes directly on the 3D model, providing an intuitive way to visualize the electrodes which can easily be translated into the surgical field.

The fusion of several techniques routinely used in the operating room for neurological evaluation with imaging algorithms provides an optimal array of resources available for seizure focus evaluation and resection. The registration process, for instance, in which multiple MRI modalities including T1 and T2-weighted, pre and post-gadolinium injection and MR angiogram scans, can be fused together to generate the final 3D model [36], substantially increases the precision of the 3D model and positioning of the focus with neighboring structures. The visualization of blood vessels surrounding the focus provides a useful reference point for localization. Furthermore, areas which cannot be seen on T1-weighted images but which are seen on T2-weighted slices, may be combined on the same model for a more accurate map for navigation and resection.

During pediatric epilepsy surgery, the selectivity of resection is crucial, especially in foci near eloquent cortex. The ability to visualize the brain anatomy, seizure focus location and grid and strip electrodes in 3D provides an additional tool for focus localization and margin determination both pre- and intraoperatively. The fusion of modalities including EEG evaluation results, MRI scans, subdural electrode stimulation results and 3D reconstruction increases the selectivity of abnormal versus normal brain tissue and as a result, increases the likelihood of a favorable surgical outcome.

5 Acknowledgments

The authors thank Marianna Jacob, Mark Anderson, Caryn Sefton and Sheila Harney. This research was supported by NIH grants RO1 CA 46627-08, PO1 CA67165-01A1, PO1 AG04953-14, NSF grants BES 9631710 and DARPA grant F41624-96-2-0001. It was also supported by the Boston Neurosurgical Foundation.

References

1. Holmes GL: Intractable epilepsy in children. *Epilepsia* 37:14-27, 1996
2. Rosenbaum TJ, Laxer KD, Vessely M, Smith WD: Subdural electrodes for seizure focus localization. *Neurosurgery* 19:73-81, 1986
3. Luders H, Lesser RP, Dinner DS, Morris HH, Hahn J, Freidman L, Skipper G, Wyllie G, Friedman D: Localization of Cortical Function: New information from extraoperative monitoring of patients with epilepsy. *Epilepsia* 28: S56-S65, 1988.
4. Cascino GD. Structural neuroimaging in partial epilepsy. *Neurosurg Clin North Am* 6:455-464, 1995.
5. Kikinis R, Gleason PL, Moriarty TM, Moore MR, Alexander E III, Stieg PE, Matsumae M, Lorensen WE, Cline HE, Black PM, Jolesz FA. Computer-assisted interactive three-dimensional planning for neurosurgical procedures. *Neurosurgery* 38:640-651, 1996

6. Leventon ME: A registration, tracking and visualization system for image-guided surgery. MIT Master's Thesis, May 1997
7. Gerig G, Kubler O, Kikinis R, Jolesz FA: Nonlinear anisotropic filtering of MRI data. *IEEE Trans Med Imaging* 11/2: 221-232, 1992
8. Cline HE, Dumoulin CL, Lorensen WE, Hart HR, Ludke S: 3D reconstruction of the brain from magnetic resonance images using a connectivity algorithm. *Magn Reson Imaging* 5:345-352, 1989
9. Cline HE, Lorensen WE, Kikinis R, Jolesz FA: Three-dimensional segmentation of MR images of the head using probability and connectivity. *J Comput Assist Tomogr* 14: 1037-1045, 1990
10. Cline HE, Lorensen WE, Souza SP, Jolesz FA, Kikinis R, Gerig G, Kennedy TE : 3D surface rendered MR images of the brain and its vasculature. Technical note *J Comput Assist Tomogr* 14: 344-351, 1991
11. Engel J Jr: A practical guide for routine EEG studies in epilepsy: *J Clin Neurophysiol* 1:109-42, 1984
12. Adelson PD, Black PMcL, Madsen JR, Kramer, U, Rockoff, MA, Riviello, JJ, Helmer, SL, Mikati, M, Holmes, GL: Use of subdural grids and strip electrodes to identify a seizure focus in children. *Pediatr Neurosurg* 22:174-180, 1995
13. Riviello JJ Jr, Kramer U, Holmes G, . Safety of invasive electroencephalic monitoring: a comparison of adults and children. *Neurology* 43(suppl):A288, 1993
14. Grimson WEL, Ettinger, GJ, White SJ, Lozano-Perez T, Wells WM, Kikinis R. A automatic registration method for frameless stereotaxy, image guided surgery, and enhanced reality visualization. *IEEE Trans Med Imaging* 15:129-140, 1996
15. Gleason PL, Kikinis R, Altobelli D, Wells WM, Alexander E III, Black PMcL, Jolesz FA :Video registration virtual reality for nonlikage stereotactic surgery. *Stereotact Funct Neurosurg* 63:139-43, 1994
16. Nakajima S, Atsumi H, Kikinis R, Moriarty TM, Metcalf DC, Jolesz FA, Black PMcL: Use of cortical surface vessel registration for image-guided neurosurgery. *Neurosurgery* 41: 1209, 1997.
17. Nakajima S, Atsumi H, Bhalerao AH, Computer assisted surgical planning for cerebrovascular neurosurgery. *Neurosurgery* 41:403-409, 1997
18. Kettenbach J, Richolt JA, Hata N, et al (1997) Surgical planning Laboratory: a new challenge for radiology *Computer Assisted Radiology*, Elsevier, Amsterdam (in press)
19. Hu X, Tan KK, Levin DN, Galhatra S, Mullan JF, Hekmatpanah J, Spire JP: Three- dimensional magnetic resonance images of the brain: application to neurosurgical planning. *J Neurosurg* 72: 433-440, 1990
20. Aoki S, Sasaki Y, Machida Y, Ohkubo T, Minami M, Sasaki Y: Cerebral aneurysms: detection and delineation suing 3D CT angiography. *AJNR* 13: 1115-1120, 1992
21. Schwartz RB, Jones KM, Chernoff DM, Mukheyi SK, Khorasani T, Tice HM, Kikinis R, Hooton SM, Stieg PE, Polak JF: Common carotid artery bifurcation: evaluation with spiral CT work in progress. *Radiology* 185: 513-519, 1992
22. Castillo M, Wilson JD. CT angiography of the common carotid artery bifurcation: Comparison between two techniques and conventional angiography. *Neuroradiology* 36: 602-604, 1994
23. Schwartz, RB. Neuroradiology applications of spinal CT. *Semin Ultrasound*, CT, MR 15: 139-147, 1994
24. Watanabe E, Watanabe T, Manaka S, Mayanagi Y, Takakura K. Three-dimensional digitizer (neuro-navigator): New equipment of CT-guided stereotaxic surgery. *Surg Neurol* 27: 543-547, 1987

25. Watanabe E, Mayanagl Y, Kosugi Y, et al, Open surgery assisted by neuronavigator, a stereotactic, articulated, sensitive arm. *Neurosurg* 28: 792-800, 1991
26. Kato A, Yoshimine T, Hayakawa T, et al. A frameless, armless navigational system for computer assisted neurosurgery. Technical note. *J Neurosurg* 74: 845- 849, 1991
27. Barnett GH, Kormos DW, Steiner CP, et al. Intraoperative localization using an armless, frameless stereotatic wand. *J Neurosurg* 78:510-514, 1993
28. Tan KK, Grzeszczuk R, Levin DN, et al. A frameless stereotactic approach to surgical planning based on retrospective patient-image registration. Technical note. *J Neurosurg* 79:296-303, 1993
29. Reinhardt HF, Hortsmann GA, Gratzl O. Sonic stereometry in microsurgical procedures for deep-seated brain tumors and vascular malformations. *Neurosurg* 32:51-57, 1993
30. Barnett GH, Kormos DW, Steiner CP, et al Use of a frameless, armless, stereotactic wand for brain tumor localization and three-dimensional neuroimaging. *Neurosurg* 33:674-678, 1993
31. Golfinos JG, Fitzpatrick BC, Smith LR, et al. Clinical use of a frameless stereotactic arm: results of 325 cases. *J Neurosurg* 83:197-205, 1995
32. Friets EM, Strohbehn JW, Hatch JF, et al. A frameless stereotaxic operating microscope for neurosurgery. *IEEE Trans Biomed Eng* 36:608-617, 1989
33. Koivukangas J, Louhisalmi Y, Alakuijala J, et al. Ultrasound-controlled neuronavigator-guided brain surgery. *J Neurosurg* 79:36-42, 1993
34. Laborde G, Gilsbach J, Harders A, et al. Computer-assisted localizer for planning of surgery and intra-operative orientation. *Acta Neurochi* (Wien)119:166-170, 1992
35. Robert DW, Strobehn JW, Hatch JF, et al. A frameless stereotaxic integration of computerized tomographic imaging and the operating microscope. *J Neurosurg* 65:545-549, 1986
36. Wells WM III, Viola P, Atsumi H, Nakajima S, Kikinis R: Multi-modal volume registration by maximization of mutual information. *Medical Image Analysis* 1:35-51, 1996.

Treatment of Pelvic Ring Fractures: Percutaneous Computer Assisted Iliosacral Screwing

Lionel CARRAT[a], Jerome TONETTI[b], M.D., Stephane LAVALLEE[a], Ph.D.
Philippe MERLOZ[c], M.D., Laurence PITTET[d], M.D. and Jean-Paul CHIROSSEL[b], M.D.

[a] TIMC Laboratory, Faculté de Médecine, I.A.B., 38706 La Tronche (France)
[b] Anatomy Laboratory, Pr Chirossel, University Joseph Fourier 38043 Grenoble
[c] Orthopaedic Department, CHU A. Michallon - BP 217 - 38043 Grenoble
[d] Radiology Department, CHU A. Michallon - BP 217 - 38043 Grenoble
e-mail : Lionel.Carrat@imag.fr

Abstract. This paper describes the development and preliminary testing of an image-guided system for the placement of iliosacral screws to stabilize pelvic ring fractures percutaneously, with the aim of decreasing the incidence of surgical complications and increasing the accuracy of screw placement. Pre-operative planning of screw trajectories is performed on a 3D model of the pelvis constructed from CT scans. During surgery, a 6D optical localizer is used to track the positions and orientations of an ultrasound probe, a surgical drill and a reference frame fixed to the posterior iliac crest. Registration of the pre-operative model with curves segmented from the ultrasound scans is performed using a surface-based algorithm. The drill tip and axis are displayed relative to the desired screw trajectories in real time. The accuracy of the system has been verified in four cadaver specimens by comparing actual screw trajectories to the desired trajectories and by measuring the distance from each screw to important anatomical landmarks on post-operative CT scans. All screws were considered to be in correct position.

1 Introduction

Unstable pelvic ring fractures with complete posterior ring disruption (Fig. 1) justify a surgical fixation as described in [1]. The non-operative treatment is not adequate to stabilize the closed reduction in order to prevent hemipelvic ascension or pseudarthrosis of the fracture.
The current technique is open reduction with internal fixation, described in [2, 3, 4], which consists in introducing 2 screws through the iliosacral joint into the sacral ala and the body of the first sacral vertebra (Fig. 2). The trajectory of the drill must respect the close anatomic elements [5] which are the first sacral nerve root in the S1-S2 foramen, lumbosacral nerve trunc, roots of the cauda equina, iliac vessels and the peritonial cavity. In order to secure the procedure, empirical reference marks must be taken. As a consequence, a large surgical exposure of the sacrum and the posterior part of the fossa iliaca lateral must be done. Complications like blood loss, hematoma and wound infection are not rare

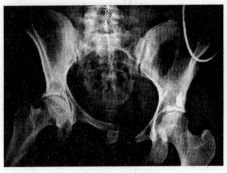 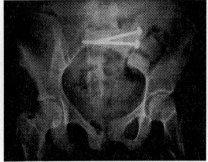

Fig. 1. Unstable pelvic ring fracture with complete disruption of the posterior arch. **Fig. 2.** The screwing technique

after such exposure because of the perineum's proximity. Percutaneous technique using fluoroscopy or computer tomography, described in [6, 3, 7], minimize the rate of wound complications. But these techniques require a great experience of the surgeon [5]. Furthermore, digestive gases make the vision difficult.

This article presents a technique using computer assisted guiding method in order to increase accuracy and to decrease the rate of wound complications. Our approach is based on standard computer assisted surgery using pre-operative CT-scan model registered with ultrasound data of the anatomical subject during surgery.

2 Material and methods

Our protocol is divided into three steps.
Surgical planning.
A CT-scan acquisition of nearly 50 images with a 3mm slice thickness is performed with a spiral CT GE Hispeed Advantage. The examination field include all the pelvic bone from the top of the iliac crest to the ischiatic process. A semi-automatic segmentation of the bone is performed in order to have a 3D model of the pelvis. The surgeon defines the optimal placement of the screws described by the entry point, direction, length and diameter. An interactive interface allows the surgeon to compute planes of arbitrary orientation in the volume of CT-scan images. For each pelvis 3 optimal screw positions have been defined on one side of the pelvis (one from supraforaminal S1-S2 superior into the S1 vertebra's body, one from supraforaminal S1-S2 inferior into the S1 body and one from infraforaminal S1-S2 into the S2 body). The screw tips are defined on the mid-sagittal line of the sacrum.
Intra-operative registration and tracking.
During surgery, a 6D optical localizer Optotrak (Northern Digital, Toronto, Canada) (Fig. 3A) locates the position and orientation of infra-red LED's fixed on customized rigid-bodies (TIMC, laboratory) and on a standard ultrasound

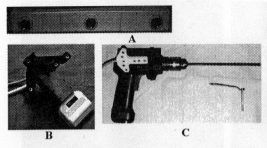
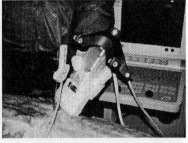

Fig. 3. During surgery, an optical localizer (A) locates in 3D the position and orientation of LED's fixed on rigid-bodies. A standard ultrasound probe (B) and a standard power drill (C) are equipped with such rigid-bodies.

Fig. 4. The surgeon makes the ultrasound acquisition. Thanks to the localizer, images are located in 3D in the intra-operative coordinate system.

probe (Fig. 3B) of 7.5 MHz (EUB-405 Hitachi inc, Tokyo, Japan). A rigid-body is also fixed on a standard surgical power drill (Fig. 3C) which will be used for the drilling step. The accuracy of the localizer is better than 0.6 mm inside a $1m^3$ volume. A reference rigid-body is firmly fixed, thanks to a pin, in the posterior iliac crest. It defines the intra-operative reference coordinate system which is used during the whole surgery, whatever the displacements of the bone are. As described in [8, 9], we use a standard ultrasound probe to image the bone and soft tissue interface of the iliac ala ipsilateral to the screwing (iliac crest, fossa iliaca lateral, ischiatic processus and posterior side of the sacrum). Nearly 60 ultrasound images are acquired (Fig. 4). Then, a segmentation procedure enables us to build curves of 2D points that belong to the bone surface on each image. In most cases, nearly 40 of them are segmented which requires 20 minutes. Several images are not segmented because of their poor quality but acquisition should be better on living humans than on cadavers. Using the 6D location and the calibration of ultrasound image planes, those curves are converted in clouds of 3D points referenced in the intra-operative coordinate system. Those clouds of points are registered with the 3D CT-scan model of the pelvis using surface based registration algorithms of the Stealth software (Sofamor-Danek inc, Memphis, USA)(Fig. 5), thereby avoiding the need to insert fiducial markers into the bones when constructing the pre-operative model. Results of the registration indicate an average rms (root mean squares) error of 0.6 mm measured on the four pelvis. As a result, the optimal screw positions defined on the CT-scan are known in the intra-operative coordinate system.

Passive drilling guidance.
The passive guidance process can then be started (Fig. 6). The standard power drill, equipped with a rigid-body, is calibrated. The tip and axis positions can thus be localized and reported in real-time on the computer screen. For each screwing, the optimal trajectory and the real position of the drill are displayed on the screen. The position of the drill is shown on each anatomical view of the

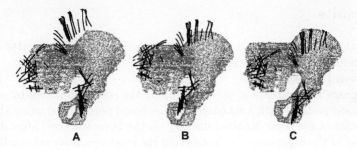

Fig. 5. Registration between the CT model (in grey) and the points segmented on ultrasound images of the pelvic (in black). The initial position (A) is the result of a pre-registration made on few data. After a couple of surface-based algoritms iterations, set of data looks like in (B) and the final position is shown in (C).

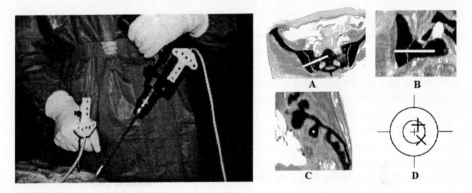

Fig. 6. Passive drilling guidance.   **Fig. 7.** Real-time monitoring.

pelvic. (Fig. 7A) is the axial view, (Fig. 7B) is the axe view and (Fig. 7C) is the coronal view. On (Fig. 7D) the optimal trajectory is represented by a central cross-hair. The drill tip and axis are projected on a view orthogonal to this trajectory and are represented by two different cross-hairs. The surgeon must superimpose the drill cross-hairs with the central cross-hair. In order to increase the legibility of the visual comparison two circles are displayed. The smaller represents a difference of 2.5mm, the other represents 5mm. During the drilling process, the depth penetration of the drill is also displayed and compared with the maximum depth penetration allowed by the CT-scan planning. At the end of the drilling process, the guidance's results are stored. These values are used in order to evaluate the surgeon's accuracy and the drilling process feasibility. We store the distance between real and optimal entry points, target points and depth penetration. Thanks to this assisted guidance, 6.5mm diameter screws for cancellous bones (Synthes inc, Etupe, France) are easily inserted in the drilled guide holes.

3 Results

This method has been tested on four cadaver pelvis. We have inserted 3 screws with various trajectories in each.

Ultrasound registration.

With regards to registration, we can compare the results obtained by our ultrasound based method with a standard surface-based registration using 3D points. These points have been digitized directly on the bone surfaces, after dissection at the end of the experiment, by preserving the intra-operative referential. Then, we performed a very stable and accurate registration in order to obtain a gold standard for ultrasound-based registration evaluation. The post-experiment comparison between registration matrix obtained with ultrasound images and with digitized 3D points are measured in terms of rotation and translation. The average errors are $1.47°$ in rotation and 2.57mm in translation. Those values can be considered as the absolute errors of ultrasound based registration.

Drilling guidance.

Regarding drilling guidance, the user interface was found to be very practical. However, a minor problem was encountered concerning the mechanical deflection of the drill. As a consequence, the localisation of the tip was inaccurate and errors can be larger than 5 mm. It has been notified for a few specific trajectories. This problem has been solved by using a different mechanical system for guidance (Fig. 8). LED's used for the power drill axis localisation are placed on the drill guide in order to avoid errors introduced by the deflection during the drilling process. Furthermore, we can use the guidance during the screwing process which was not possible before. The depth penetration is still measured thanks to the rigid-body fixed on the power drill and the calibration of the drill tip. At the end of the process, we have saved values which show the accuracy of the guidance. We have measured the distance between optimal and real position

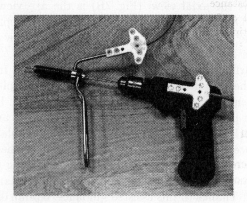

Fig. 8. New materiel used for drilling process.

of the drill for the entry point, target point and the depth of the tip point for each pelvis. The average errors are 1.9 mm for entry point, 1.7 mm for target point and 0.81 mm for the depth.

Screw positions.
Screw positions have been checked thanks to a post-operative CT-scan acquisition (Fig. 9). For supraforaminal S1-S2 screws, we have measured the distance from the screw to the anterior cortex of the sacrum, the distance from the screw to the spinal canal or the foramen and the distance from the tip of the screw to the mid-sagittal line of the sacrum (Fig. 9). For infraforaminal screws, we have measured the distance from the screw to the anterior cortex of the sacrum, the distance from the screw to the S2-S3 foramen and the distance from the tip of the screw to the mid-sagittal line of the sacrum. Those values are reported in (Fig. 10). All screws were considered to be in correct position and preserves the close anatomic elements.

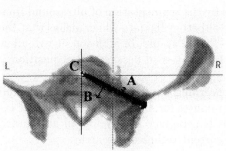

Fig. 9. Exemple of an image taken for CT-verification with method of measurement for screws'position. A is the distance from the screw to the anterior cortex of the sacrum. B is the distance from the screw to the spinal canal or foramen. C is the distance from the tip of the screw to the mid-sagittal line of the sacrum.

	Screws	A	B	C
Pelvis 1	Suprafor. S1-S2 sup.	0.5	5	3
	Suprafor. S1-S2 inf.	2	2	1
	Infrafor. S1-S2	8	0.5	1
Pelvis 2	Suprafor. S1-S2 sup.	4	15	1
	Suprafor. S1-S2 inf.	2	14	5
	Infrafor. S1-S2	9.5	4	5
Pelvis 3	Suprafor. S1-S2 sup.	10	1	2
	Suprafor. S1-S2 inf.	3	8	1
	Infrafor. S1-S2	3	3	2
Pelvis 4	Suprafor. S1-S2 sup.	7	9	1
	Suprafor. S1-S2 inf.	2	6	2.5
	Infrafor. S1-S2	4	2	0
Average		4.6	5.8	2

Fig. 10. Measurement of screws placement. A, B and C are in millimeters. A and B values are never equal to 0. The more the C value is close to 0, the better the depth guidance is. (Max. value is 5 mm).

4 Discussion

Final position of screws depends on the planning, the accuracy of the registration and the drilling process. During the surgical planning, the trajectory is chosen as natural as possible, means into the bony corridor created by the cortical walls of the sacral ala and the sacral vertebra. Guidance process is easier when the tip of the drill is introduced into the bone exactly at the optimal entry point. If so, the drill go deep naturally into the cancellous bone without running against the cortical bone. As a consequence, a great accuracy is required at the beginning of the guidance process.

Values measured on CT-scan images for verification were difficult to take, because of artefacts due to the steel of the screws. We have thus measured the narrowest distance between the screw's image and the cortical bone.

Actually, the ultrasound acquisition is performed on the iliac crest, fossa ilaca lateral, ischiatic process and posterior side of the sacrum. The intra-operative reference coordinate system is fixed in the posterior iliac crest. Our current research consists in performing the registration only on the sacrum because accuracy needs to be more important on this part of the pelvis with respect to anatomic elements. Furthermore, it will also avoid the problem of motion at fracture sites relative to pre-operative CT-scan. The intra-operative coordinate system is firmly fixed on the spinal process of the first sacral vertebral of the sacrum. Our approach is to acquire ultrasound images on the sacrum with a smaller probe and to digitize points directly with a pointer. These points are digitized by using short incision used for the fixation of the rigid-body. These data are mixed with 3D curves obtained by the segmentation of ultrasound images. This method should take advantage of better 3D data which means that the registration should be more accurate and more stable. In addition, it will allow to reduce the reconstruction diameter of the CT-scan because the acquisition is performed only on the sacrum.

The major drawback of our method is concerning the segmentation of ultrasound images. This step takes time (nearly 20 minutes for 40 images) and required experience from the surgeon. Therefore, it is necessary to develop an automated and accurate segmentation. This is our current technical research.

Computer assisted methods have been proposed to perform pelvic surgery [10]. Some authors have already described a material-based registration method in order to insert iliosacral screws [11]. They use a carrier fixed with pins which are implanted in the posterior part of the scarum before the CT-scan examination. With our approach no pelvic instrumentation is performed before the CT-scan. It makes the medical intervention non invasive, pinless and frameless.

5 Conclusion

In the framework of computer assisted surgery applied to orthopaedics, this article has presented a percutaneous fixation method for pelvic ring fractures using ultrasound based registration. Our percutaneous technique takes advantage of some previously developed method for spine surgery [12, 13, 14] because of the decreasing of wound complications. It has been validated successfully on 4 cadaver specimens, which encourages us to start clinical validation. This technique could be applied to fractures with possible closed reduction [7]. But it could also be applied to any other applications of percutaneous orthopaedic surgery.

Acknowledgements: This research is financially supported by the European project CRIGOS BMH4-CT97-2427.

References

1. Waddel J.P. Pennal G.F., Tile M. and Garside H. Pelvic disruption : Assessment and classification. *Clinical Orthopaedic*, (151):12–21, 1980.
2. E. Letournel. Pelvic fractures. *Rev. Chir. Orthop.*, (10):145–148, 1978.
3. JM. Matta and T. Saucedo. Internal fixation of pelvic fracture. *Clin. Orthop.*, (242):83–97, 1989.
4. M. Tile and GF. Pennal. Pelvic disruption : Principe of management. *Clin. Orthop.*, (151):56–64, 1980.
5. Freese J. Templeman D., Schmidt A. and Weisman I. Proximity of iliosacral screws to neurovascular structures after internal fixation. *Clinical Orthopaedic*, (329):194–198, 1996.
6. Coombs R.J. Jackson W.T. Ebraheim N.A., Russin J.J. and Holiday B. Percutaneous computer-tomography stabilization of pelvic fractures. *Prelimnary report*. *J. Orthop. Trauma.*, (1):197–204, 1987.
7. M.L. Routt and P.T. Simonian. Closed reduction and percutaneous skeletal fixation of sacral fractures. *Clinical Orthopaedic*, (329):121–128, 1996.
8. C. Barbe, J. Troccaz, B. Mazier, and S. Lavallee. Using 2.5D echography in computer assisted spine surgery. In *IEEE Engineering in Medicine and Biology Society Proceedings*, pages 160–161. IEEE, 1993.
9. R. Mosges and S. Lavallee. Multimodal information for computer-integrated surgery. In R. Taylor, S. Lavallee, G. Burdea, and R. Mosges, editors, *Computer-integrated surgery: technology and clinical applications*, pages 5–20. MIT Press, Cambridge, MA, 1996.
10. A.L. Jacob. Computer assistance in pelvic and acetabular fractures. In L. Nolte, editor, *CAOS'96 (Computer Assisted Orthopaedic Surgery)*, Bern (CH), 1996. Muller Institute.
11. R. Hu, N. Glossop, D. Steven, and J. Randle. Accuracy of image guided placement of iliosacral lag screws. In J. Troccaz and al., editors, *CVRMed-MRCAS'97 Proc., LNCS Series 1205*, pages 593–596. Springer, 1997.
12. S. Lavallee, P. Sautot, J. Troccaz, P. Cinquin, and P. Merloz. Computer Assisted Spine Surgery : a technique for accurate transpedicular screw fixation using CT data and a 3D optical localizer. *Journal of Image Guided Surgery*, 1(1):65–73, 1995.
13. S. Lavallee, R. Szeliski, and L. Brunie. Anatomy-based registration of 3-D medical images, range images, X-ray projections, 3-D models using Octree-Splines. In R. Taylor, S. Lavallee, G. Burdea, and R. Mosges, editors, *Computer Integrated Surgery*, pages 115–143. MIT Press, Cambridge, MA, 1996.
14. P. Merloz, J. Tonetti, A. Eid, C. Faure, S. Lavallee, J. Troccaz, P. Sautot, A. Hamadeh, and P. Cinquin. Computer Assisted Spine Surgery. *Clinical Orthopaedics and related Research*, (337):86–96, 1997.

Model Tags: Direct 3D Tracking of Heart Wall Motion from Tagged MR Images

Alistair A. Young

Department of Anatomy with Radiology,
University of Auckland, Private Bag 92019, Auckland, New Zealand.
a.young@auckland.ac.nz, http://www.auckland.ac.nz/anat/ayoung/

Abstract. A method is presented for the reconstruction of 3D heart wall motion directly from tagged magnetic resonance (MR) images, without prior identification of ventricular boundaries or tag stripe locations. Model tags were created as material surfaces which defined the location of the magnetic tags within the model. Image-derived forces acted on the model tags, while the model could also be manipulated by a small number of user-controlled guide points. The method was applied to simulated images in which the true motion was specified, as well as to clinical images of a normal volunteer. The RMS errors in displacement and strain calculated from the simulated images were similar to those obtained using previous stripe tracking and model fitting methods. A significant improvement in analysis time was obtained for the normal volunteer, making the method more clinically viable.

1 Introduction

Magnetic resonance (MR) tissue tagging is a useful clinical tool for the non-invasive measurement of heart wall motion [1], [2]. Typically, multiple parallel tagging planes of magnetic saturation are created orthogonal to the image plane in a short time interval (5-12 msec) on detection of the R wave of the ECG. Often a grid of tag planes is created, whose intersection with the image plane give rise to dark bands ("image stripes"), 1-2 mm in width and spaced 5-10 mm apart, which deform with the tissue and fade according to the time constant T1 (700 msec in myocardium). Techniques for stripe tracking and strain estimation have been developed and validated in both 2D [3] and 3D [4]. Recently, a number of clinical studies have used MR tagging to characterize regional left ventricular wall motion and deformation in normal and diseased hearts [5], [6]. The clinical utility of this technique is currently limited by the prohibitively long time required for image analysis. Most analysis methods require the prior extraction of the inner and outer boundaries of the left ventricle in each image together with the localization of the image tag stripes in each frame [4], [7], [8], [9], [10], [11], [12]. Several semi-automatic methods have been developed for tracking the tags and identifying the boundaries [4], [13], [14]. However, the image intensity information is insufficient to completely characterize the boundary and tag locations, due to limited spatial and temporal resolution, lack of contrast between muscle and blood, and respiration and gating artifacts. User interaction with the tracking and segmentation processes is therefore essential. As 3D studies typically comprise more than 200 images (5-12 short axis slices and 5-8 long axis slices, each with 5-20 frames), the time required for user interaction can be substantial. This paper describes a method for reconstructing regional left ventricular (LV) motion and deformation directly and simultaneously from a set of long and short axis tagged MR images, without the need for separate boundary and image stripe tracking.

2 Methods

2.1 Finite Element Model

As done previously, a 16 element finite element (FE) model was constructed to describe the geometry and motion of the left ventricle [4],[6]. Each element employed bicubic Hermite interpolation in the circumferential and longitudinal directions, with linear interpolation transmurally. Nodes shared position and derivative information between elements, giving C^1 continuity. Within each element, the geometric field $\mathbf{x}$ was given as a function of element (material) coordinates ξ as a weighted average of nodal values:

$$\mathbf{x}(\xi_1, \xi_2, \xi_3) = \sum_n \Psi_n(\xi_1, \xi_2, \xi_3) \mathbf{x}^n \qquad (1)$$

where $\mathbf{x}^n$ are the nodal values and Ψ_n are the element basis functions. Note that the element coordinates ξ of material points do not change (by definition) as the model deforms.

As a first step in the motion reconstruction problem, the approximate geometry of the LV at end-diastole (ED) must be determined. This was done interactively by fitting a small number of guide points by linear least squares. A smoothing term constrained the model to smoothly approximate the guide points. In practice, the geometry of a subsequent time frame (eg. the second or third frame) was constructed first, then deformed to ED using the relative motion of the tag stripes to indicate the displacement of the guide points.

2.2 Model Tags

Image stripes provide information about the underlying deformation of the heart but do not represent the motion of material points. Due to the tomographic nature of the imaging process, material points move through the fixed image slice planes during the deformation. This can result in the appearance and disappearance of image stripes due to the elliptical shape of the left ventricle. In order to apply the correct image motion constraints to the model, a set of "model tags" was created within the FE model. Model tags represent the material surfaces within the heart tissue which are tagged with magnetic saturation and which deform with the heart.

The location and orientation of the tag planes at the time of their creation (ED) are determined by the tagging pulse sequence parameters. Each tag plane P_t was described by a point on the plane $\mathbf{p}_t$ and a normal $\mathbf{n}_t$ to the plane. Similarly each image slice plane P_i was described by a point $\mathbf{p}_i$ and normal $\mathbf{n}_i$. Each tag plane was associated with one or more image slice planes; let T_i denote the set of tag planes associated with each image plane P_i. Model tags were found using a subdivision algorithm [15],[17]. Each element was subdivided into N subelements with subelement nodes equally spaced in ξ space. The tag planes were then intersected with the subelement mesh assuming linear variation between subelement nodes. The result was a set of triangles whose vertices were given in element (material) coordinates. Fig. 1a shows a schematic of this procedure.

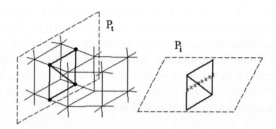

Fig. 1. Calculation of model tags (a, left) and model tag-image intersections (b, right). a) thin lines: model subelement boundaries; dashed lines: tag plane P_t; thick lines: model tag triangles. b) thick lines: model tag triangles; dashed lines: image plane P_i; x: MTI points.

2.3 Model Deformation

At any stage in the model fitting process, a collection of model tag - image intersection (MTI) points could be found by intersecting the model tags with the image planes. For each intersecting model tag triangle, the intersecting edges were interpolated to result in a set of MTI points spaced approximately 1-2 mm apart (Fig. 1b). Let $M(i,t)$ denote the set of MTI points associated with each $P_t \in T_i$. The model was deformed from frame to frame to minimize the following objective function:

$$E(\mathbf{x}) = S(\mathbf{x}) + \sum_{P_i} \sum_{P_t \in T_i} \sum_{n \in M(i,t)} w_n \left[\mathbf{n}_t \cdot (\mathbf{x}(\xi_n) - \mathbf{x}_n) \right]^2 \qquad (2)$$

where S is a smoothing term, $\mathbf{x}(\xi_n)$ are MTI points associated with tag plane P_t intersecting image P_i, and $\mathbf{x}_n$ are image stripe points associated with $\mathbf{x}(\xi_n)$. The w_n are weights derived from the image intensity function and $\mathbf{n}_t$ are the normals to the original tagging plane P_t. The smoothing term measured the variation of the deformation from a prior geometry, as described previously [4]:

$$S(\mathbf{x}) = \int_\Omega \sum_k \left\| \frac{\partial \mathbf{F}}{\partial \xi_k} \right\|_F^2 \partial \Omega \qquad (3)$$

where F is the deformation gradient tensor defined with respect to the rectangular Cartesian coordinate system. The smoothing weights were set small enough to have negligible effects in regions containing sufficient data points. In regions with few or no data points, the effect of this smoothing term is to reduce the variation of deformation across the model.

The error function eqn. (2) was minimized using an iterative nonlinear least squares procedure (see Appendix and [15]). In summary, each iteration consisted of the solution of eqn. (2) by linear least squares (keeping the ξ_n constant). After each iteration, the MTI points $\mathbf{x}(\xi_n)$ were recalculated, along with their associated image stripe points $\mathbf{x}_n$. The dot product employed in eqn. (2) is a statement of the aperture problem: The image stripes provide information about where the material point is in the direction normal to the tag, whereas the position of the material point along the tag is unknown. This constraint is similar to that used previously in optical flow problems [18].

2.4 Image Stripe Points

Image stripe points were associated with each MTI point by searching the image in a small neighborhood for the most likely point on the image to which the MTI point should move. The likelihood function measured the probability that each pixel was located on the center of an image stripe. This was given by the output of stripe detection filters (one for each stripe orientation) convolved with the image. The filters had a Gaussian shape in the direction parallel to the stripe and a second derivative of a Gaussian in the direction normal to the stripe. The scale of the filter was tuned to the width of the tag stripes (in this paper all filters had $\sigma = 1.5$ pixels). The search was carried out in a small neighborhood centered about each MTI point consisting of those pixels in the direction orthogonal to the image stripe and less than half a stripe spacing away from the MTI point. Rather than take the image point with the maximum filtered image value, the centroid of the neighbourhood (the average of all the points in the neighborhood weighted by their filtered image values) was used as the most likely stripe point. This was a more robust measure of the position of the stripe center than the maximum filtered value, and allowed the calculation of the image stripe center to subpixel resolution. Center-of-mass image constraints have previously been employed for active contour models and are more stable than gradient-based image constraints [19]. Finally, the weight w_n for each neighbourhood was calculated as the maximum value of the filtered image in the neighborhood. Myocardial pixels with low weight are located between stripes (where the search neighborhood did not include a stripe center) and on stripes running in the other direction.

Previous studies have shown that image stripe orientations do not change substantially during the cardiac cycle (typically less than 20°). The search direction was therefore kept constant throughout the tracking process (orthogonal to the original stripes). This enabled the result of the search to be precalculated before the stripe tracking process. For each image, a displacement image was generated which stored the displacement in pixels from each pixel to the centroid of the filtered image in the search neighbourhood. To maintain subpixel resolution, the displacement was multiplied by a scaling factor before being stored as a 1 byte/pixel image. The weight for each pixel was similarly precalculated as an image. Fig. 2 shows an example of a short axis image at end-systole (ES), showing raw, filtered, displacement and weighting images.

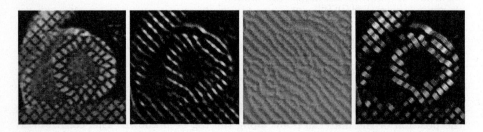

Fig. 2. Precalculation of image forces as images. From left: raw image; result of the stripe detection filter in one orientation; displacement image (lighter greylevels indicate displacement towards the top right, darker greylevels indicate displacement in the opposite direction); weight image (lighter greylevels indicate higher weighting)

2.5 User Interaction

It is not uncommon for model tags to move more than one stripe spacing between frames. In order to bring the model into approximate correspondence with the image stripes a fit to guide points was performed. This involved the minimization of eqn. (2) above with small number of guide points in place of the image stripe points. The smoothing term ensured a smooth interpolation between guide point displacements. To define a guide displacement the user clicked on a MTI point on the image and then clicked on a point to which the MTI point should move. The normal in the dot product of eqn. (2) was the tag normal associated with the MTI point. After these "guide iterations" the MTI points should be within range of the image stripe forces and the fit could proceed with "image iterations" as above. The user was also able to interact with the image iteration by selecting a group of MTI points and redefining their associated image stripe points.

2.6 Image Acquisition

In vivo clinical images of a normal volunteer were acquired with a Siemens Vision MR scanner using breath-hold segmented k-space imaging sequences. Eight parallel short axis slices were obtained orthogonal to the central axis of the LV spaced 11.5 mm apart, together with six long axis slices oriented 30° apart about the LV central axis. Each slice was 8 mm thick and comprised 19 frames through the cardiac cycle. The image resolution ranged from 1.17 to 1.37 mm per pixel, depending on the field of view.

2.7 Simulated Deformation

Simulated images were also generated of a prescribed deformation, in order to determine whether errors are introduced in the calculation of model tags and MTI points or in the search for image stripe centroids. An initial regular ED geometry was constructed in prolate spheroidal coordinates (focal length of 42 mm), with inner surface at $\lambda = 0.60$ and outer surface at $\lambda = 0.85$. The final ES geometry had an inner surface at $\lambda = 0.40$ and outer surface at $\lambda = 0.82$, with a longitudinal contraction of 15% in μ and uniform twist in θ from 24° and 21° at the endocardial and epicardial apex respectively to $-8°$ and $-7°$ at the endocardial and epicardial base respectively. The prolate model was converted to rectangular Cartesian coordinates and model tags (8mm apart) were calculated for 8 short axis images spaced 10 mm apart and 6 long axis images spaced 30° apart about the central axis. The images were then simulated by assigning each pixel within the inner and outer boundaries to a representative myocardial greylevel and each pixel within 1 mm of a MTI point to a representative stripe greylevel.

The simulated images were also analyzed using previously described stripe tracking and model fitting procedures [4]. Briefly, the stripes were tracked in each slice using an active contour model of the 2D tagging grid. The finite element model was then used to reconstruct the 3D displacements of material points by fitting the motion from ES to ED. Then the ED model was deformed to ES by fitting the reconstructed 3D displacements of the stripe data.

3 Results

3.1 Initial Geometry

In total 103 guide points were required for the ED geometry of the normal volunteer (53 for the endocardial surface and 50 for the epicardial surface). As there were 14 image slices this represents 3-4 points per surface per slice. The geometry in the third frame was determined first, then the guide points were moved to match the motion of the stripes back to the ED frame. The entire process required less than 10 minutes to complete, compared with approximately 30 minutes to manually define each boundary on each slice individually.

3.2 Model Deformation

Using the ideal tag plane positions and orientations derived from the imaging parameters, 182 model tags were found within the ED geometry. The model was then deformed to each frame by fitting the location of the MTI points to the image stripes. A small motion occurred between the tag creation and the time of the ED image, so this frame was also fitted in the same manner. The deformed ED geometry was then used as the prior (undeformed state) in the smoothing term for all subsequent frames. Fig. 3 shows three of the model tags (two from the short axis images and one from a long axis image) at tag creation and ES. Fig. 3

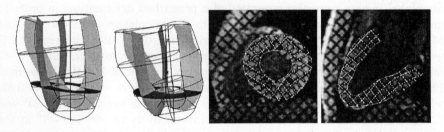

Fig. 3. a (left): Model tags at the time of creation (left) and at ES (right). The two lighter tags are from the short axis images, while the dark tag is from a long axis image. b (right): Short (left) and long (right) axis images at ES with MTI points overlayed.

shows short and long axis images at ES with MTI points overlayed. Typically, one guide iteration (∼30 guide points) and two image iterations (∼4900 points) were sufficient to achieve good correspondence between image stripes and MTI points.

The 3D tracking procedure took ∼5 min per frame, representing a considerable time saving over the previous method [4] which required definition of the inner and outer boundaries and image stripe tracking for each frame followed by 3D model fitting (∼45 min per frame). Each iteration (least squares fit) took ∼30 sec to compute on a 180 Mhz R5000 workstation, however the code has not been optimized for execution speed.

3.3 Simulated Deformation

The simulated ED geometry was deformed to fit the simulated image stripes in the same manner as above. Typically, 2 guide points per frame were required to bring the model into approximate correspondence. The root mean squared (RMS) errors in the displacement were 0.38 mm in x, 0.34 mm in y and 0.34 mm in z (the image pixel size was 1.17 mm). RMS errors in strain were 0.022 in circumferential strain (true range -0.357 to 0.088), 0.021 in longitudinal strain (true range -0.350 to -0.117) and 0.187 for radial strain (true range 0.446 to 0.930).

These images were also analyzed using a previously described 2D stripe tracking algorithm and 3D finite element model fitting technique. The RMS errors of the resulting displacement were 0.29 mm in x, 0.38 mm in y and 0.38 mm in z. Strain estimates had RMS errors of 0.023 in circumferential strain, 0.020 in longitudinal strain and 0.186 in radial strain. Thus the direct 3D tracking method resulted in similar errors to the 2D tracking/3D fitting method. The error was greatest in the radial (transmural) direction and was mainly due to the lack of tag resolution in this direction, especially at the apex where there was only one stripe orthogonal to the radial direction.

4 Discussion

This paper describes a method for directly reconstructing the shape and motion of the LV. Use of a 3D model to track the stripes implicitly constrains the motion in each slice to be compatible with its 3D neighbours. Thus, all stripes in all images contribute to the tracking process in a coherent 3D manner. User interaction is also constrained to act on the 3D model, thereby maintaining compatibility between displacements and reducing the amount of interaction to a minimum. Features of the method were: a) the use of very sparse guide points in combination with model smoothing to estimate the approximate geometry at ED and gross motion of the LV, b) the calculation of model tags and MTI points for use in the objective function eqn. (2) and c) precalculation of the image displacements, reducing the search for corresponding image stripe points to a simple look-up operation.

Park et al. [8],[9] developed a class of deformable model with parametric global deformations which varied locally to capture the heart motion. Rather than model the tag surfaces, tag planes were assumed to translate without bending in the through-plane direction from frame to frame. O'Donnell et al. [10],[11] described a deformable model with both global and local components of motion. Deformation parameters were fitted to a priori contour and stripe data. The 3D displacements of the stripe data were reconstructed by estimating the motion from each deformed frame back to the first frame (ED), as in [4]. Denney [14] described a stripe tracking procedure which did not require prior knowledge of the inner and outer contours of the heart. An active contour model was used to track stripes across an entire region of interest and a maximum a posteriori hypothesis test was used to segment myocardial tag stripes from background. Such contour-free stripe data could be used as input to model- free motion reconstruction methods such as the method developed by Denney and McVeigh [12], or that of Kerwin and Prince [20]. These methods do not require the prior formation of a geometric model; however regional analysis of material strains requires further processing.

References

1. Axel, L. and L. Dougherty. Heart Wall motion: Improved method of spatial modulation of magnetization for MR imaging. Radiology. 172: 349-350, 1989.
2. Zerhouni, E.A., D.M. Parish, W.J. Rogers, A. Yang and E.P. Shapiro. Human heart: Tagging with MR imaging - A method for noninvasive assessment of myocardial motion. Radiology. 169: 59-63, 1988.

3. Young, A.A., L. Axel, L. Dougherty, D.K. Bogen and C.S. Parenteau. Validation of tagging with MRI to estimate material deformation. Radiology. 188: 101-108, 1993.
4. Young, A.A., D.L. Kraitchman, L. Dougherty and L. Axel. Tracking and finite element analysis of stripe deformation in magnetic resonance tagging. IEEE Trans Medical Imaging. 14: 413-421, 1995.
5. Palmon L.C., N. Reichek, S.B. Yeon, N.R. Clark, D. Brownson, E. Hoffman, and L. Axel. Intramural myocardial shortening in hypertensive left ventricular hypertrophy with normal pump function. Circulation, 89(1):122-131, 1994.
6. Young, A.A., C.M. Kramer, V.A. Ferrari, L. Axel and N. Reichek. Three-dimensional left ventricular deformation in hypertrophic cardiomyopathy. Circulation. 90: 854-867, 1994.
7. O'Dell, W.G., C.C. Moore, W.C. Hunter, E.A. Zerhouni, and E.R. McVeigh. Three-dimensional myocardial deformations: Calculation with displacement field fitting to tagged MR images. Radiology, 195(3):829-835, 1995.
8. Park, J., D. Metaxas, A.A. Young, and L. Axel. Deformable models with parameter functions for cardiac motion analysis from tagged MRI data. IEEE Trans. Medical Imaging, 15(3):278-289, 1996.
9. Park, J., D. Metaxas, and L. Axel. Analysis of left ventricular wall motion based on volumetric deformable models and MRI-SPAMM. Medical Image Analysis, 1(1):53-71, 1996.
10. O'Donnell, T., A. Gupta and T. Boult. The hybrid volumetric ventriculoid: New model for MR-SPAMM 3-D analysis. Proceedings of Computers in Cardiology, pp 5-8, Vienna, September 1995.
11. O'Donnell, T., T. Boult and A. Gupta. Global models with parametric offsets as applied to cardiac motion recovery. Proceedings of Computer Vision and Pattern Recognition, pp 293-299, San Francisco, June 1996.
12. Denney T.S. Jr. and E.R. McVeigh. Model-free reconstruction of three-dimensional myocardial strain from planar tagged MR images. J. Magnetic Resonance Imaging, 7:799-810. 1997.
13. Guttman, M.A., J.L. Prince and E.R. McVeigh. Tag and contour detection in tagged MR images of the left ventricle. IEEE Trans. Medical Imaging, 13(1): 74-88, 1994.
14. Denney, T.S. Jr., Identification of myocardial tags in tagged MR images without prior knowledge of myocardial contours. XVth International Conference on Information Processing in Medical Imaging, pp 327-340, Poultney, Vermont, June 1997.
15. Young A.A., F.A. Fayad and L. Axel. Right ventricular midwall surface motion and deformation using magnetic resonance tagging. American Journal of Physiology: Heart and Circulatory Physiology. 271:H2677-H2688, 1996.
16. Terzopoulos, D. The computation of visible-surface representations. IEEE Trans. Pattern Analysis and Machine Intelligence. 10: 417-438, 1988.
17. Lorensen, W.E. and H.E. Cline. Marching cubes: A high resolution 3D surface construction algorithm. Computer Graphics. 21: 163-169, 1987.
18. Hildreth, E.C. Computations underlying the measurement of visual motion. Artificial Intelligence 23:309-354, 1984.
19. Davatzikos, C.A. and J.L. Prince. Convexity Analysis of Active Contour Problems. Proceedings of Computer Vision and Pattern Recognition, San Francisco, June 1996.
20. Kerwin, W.S. and J.L. Prince, J.L. Generating 3D cardiac material markers using tagged MRI. XVth International Conference on Information Processing in Medical Imaging. pp 313-326. Poultney, June 1997.

21. Marquardt, D.W. An algorithm for least squares estimation of nonlinear parameters. J Soc Indust Appl Math. 11: 431-441, 1963.

Appendix: Minimization Algorithm

A Levenburg-Marquardt algorithm [21] was used to minimize eqn. (2), as done previously for RV surface models [15]. The objective function eqn. (2) can be written:

$$E = \|Sq\|^2 + \|Jq - p\|^2 \qquad (4)$$

where S is a matrix derived from the smoothing term, J is a matrix containing model basis functions evaluated at ξ_n and weighted by the tag normals, p is a vector containing components of x_n weighted by the tag normals and q is a vector of model parameters. Note that J varies with q, but S does not.

The Newton method minimizes E by neglecting terms higher than second order in the Taylor series expansion, giving the following iteration:

$$H_k(q_{k+1} - q_k) = -\left.\frac{\partial E}{\partial q}\right|_k \qquad (5)$$

where H is the Hessian matrix of second derivatives of E. The right hand side of eqn. (5) has a component due to the fact that ξ_n can change with q. However, the error function eqn. (2) measures the squared distance from each data point to the model position ξ_n in the direction approximately perpendicular to the model tag surface. Since ξ_n can only change within the model tag surface, the contribution to the first derivative of the error function due to changes in model position will be small. We therefore use the linear approximation:

$$\frac{\partial E}{\partial q} = S^T S q + J^T J q - J^T p \qquad (6)$$

Replacing the Hessian H with the linear approximation $S^T S + J^T J$, and adding a term $\Lambda I (\Lambda > 0)$ to avoid non-positive definite H, gives the iteration:

$$(S^T S + J_k^T J_k + \Lambda I) q_k + 1 = \Lambda I + J_k^T p \qquad (7)$$

If λ is large the step becomes small and in the direction of steepest descent; if λ is small the update becomes a full Gauss-Newton step. In practice, all the iterations were performed with $\lambda = 0$, equivalent to solving the linear problem that arises if the ξ_n are assumed to be constant over the step.

Quantitative Three Dimensional Echocardiography: Methodology, Validation, and Clinical Applications

Florence H. Sheehan M.D.[1], Edward L. Bolson M.S.[1], Roy W. Martin, Ph.D.*, Gerard Bashein M.D. Ph. D.*, and John McDonald Ph.D.+

ABSTRACT

Three dimensional (3D) ultrasound imaging provides the most accurate measurement of the volume of the heart's left ventricle. We have developed methods for acquiring and quantitatively analyzing 3D echocardiograms to measure the size, shape, and function not only of the left ventricle but also the mitral annulus and other structures in the mitral apparatus. These methods provide a powerful tool to investigate structure-function relationships, evaluate surgical procedures, and assess patient prognosis.

1 INTRODUCTION

Although multiple modalities are available clinically to image the heart, the elegant but complex structure of this organ is only now being revealed with the recent advent of 3D imaging techniques. Much of the research in 3D echocardiography to date has been devoted to volume rendering for visualization, e.g. of congenital heart defects. However quantitative analysis has the potential for much wider applications in adult cardiology.

Our research team has devoted 11 years to the development and validation of hardware and software for quantitative 3D echo. Acquiring a 3D echo study of a patient is performed using a magnetic field system to track the spatial location and orientation of each image. Our software allows us to display the images, trace the borders of heart structures, review the border tracings, reconstruct the left ventricle (LV), mitral valve, and associated structures in 3D, and measure their dimensions, shape, and function.

This report presents the results of studies validating the accuracy of these techniques in phantoms and in heart specimens, and discusses applications of these techniques to clinical investigation.

2 METHODS

Image Acquisition (Fig. 1) Imaging is performed using commercial ultrasound equipment. The 3D image set is acquired over four to six 6-10 sec periods of held end-expiration, depending on each patient's breath holding ability and image quality. The first two scans cover the parasternal long axis view and angulated short axis views of the LV. At the apical window, two or three separate scans are used to acquire the

---

[1] From the Depts. of Medicine/Cardiology (Box 356422, phone (206) 543-4535, fax (206) 685-9394), Anesthesiology*, and Statistics+, University of Washington, Seattle, WA 98195

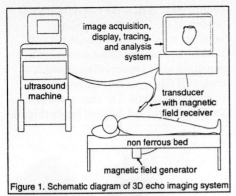

Figure 1. Schematic diagram of 3D echo imaging system

long axis images and complete a 180° rotation. The sixth scan is performed if and where additional coverage is needed.

A magnetic field system (Flock of Birds™ model 6D-FOB, Ascension Technology Corp., Burlington, VT) is used to track the ultrasound scanhead (1). The system consists of a magnetic field transmitter, a receiver, and electronic circuitry which interfaces with a computer. During imaging the transmitter is placed under the mattress and the receiver is attached to the ultrasound scanhead. Images are digitized using a framegrabber and registered with position data, hemodynamic parameters, and scanning parameters such as image depth.

Quantitative Analysis Techniques: The images are reviewed and those corresponding to end diastole and end systole are manually selected as the frames of maximum and minimum cavity area, respectively. The borders of the LV and of anatomic features are then manually traced in the selected images (Fig. 2). The border points are converted to x,y,z coordinates using probe position and orientation data. The traced borders are reviewed immediately in 3D using a software interface (Advanced Visual Systems, Waltham MA). All images are traced using

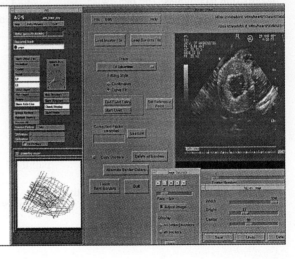

Figure 2. User interface for image display and border tracing program. The 2D image is displayed at right and can be reviewed in cine loop format. The traced borders are converted into x,y,z coordinates and presented in a 3D window, lower left, for comparison with other traced borders of the same or other structures. This facilitates confirmation of image registration and border editing.

the leading-edge technique with the border passing through the middle of the bright part of the lateral echoes.

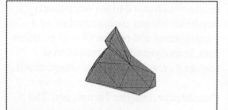

Figure 3. Control Mesh for LV Endocardium.

3D Reconstruction of the LV endocardium and epicardium: A piecewise smooth subdivision surface is fit to 3D points sampled from the traced borders. This method was developed to avoid the inherent limitations of other methods which restricted their anatomical accuracy or application to different 3D image acquisition techniques. The piecewise smooth subdivision has been shown to accurately measure volume, and is the only method shown to reproduce LV shape with anatomical accuracy (1). This is essential for analysis of regional LV function and geometry. Triangulated control meshes are designed as models for the LV endocardium and epicardium (Fig. 3).

The control mesh is recursively subdivided to produce a mesh of 576 faces. Parts of the control mesh can be marked as sharp to allow for creases at the mitral annulus and outflow track and a sharp point at the apex in the final piecewise smooth subdivision surface. The control mesh is fit to the manually traced borders of the LV, valves, papillary muscles, apex, and other anatomic landmarks in a process that minimizes a penalized least-squares criterion which trades off fidelity to the borders against surface smoothness. The same mesh is used for both normal and diseased hearts (Fig.4).

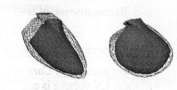

Figure 4. Reconstructions of the LV endocardium at end diastole (mesh) and end systole (solid) in a patient with cardiomyopathy (right) and a normal subject (left).

The piecewise smooth subdivision method is also used to reconstruct the surfaces of the papillary muscles (Fig. 5)

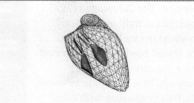

Figure 5. 3D reconstruction of the LV, papillary muscles, and chordae tendineae.

and of the mitral valve leaflets (Fig. 6).

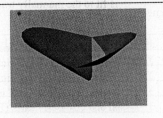

Figure 6. Reconstruction of mitral valve leaflets.

Quantitative Analysis of Cardiac Parameters: LV volume is computed by summing the volumes of the tetrahedra formed by connecting a point inside the LV cavity with the vertices of each triangular face on the reconstructed 3D surface. The LV volumes determined at end diastole and end systole are used to calculate stroke volume, ejection fraction, and cardiac output, as well as the respective volume indices. LV mass is calculated as the difference between the volumes of the LV endocardial and epicardial surface reconstructions, multiplied by the specific gravity of cardiac muscle.

To measure regional wall thickness, a medial surface (CenterSurface™) is constructed midway between the epicardial and endocardial surface reconstructions (2) (Fig. 7). Chords are drawn perpendicular to the CenterSurface™ and extended to their intersection with the endocardium and epicardium. The length of each chord is a measure of the local orthogonal wall thickness. Comparison of the wall thickness at end diastole and end systole at each triangular face of the LV surface provides a measure of wall thickening, a parameter of regional LV function.

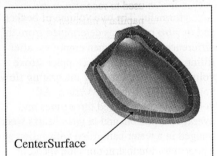

Figure 7. Cutaway view of reconstructions of the LV endocardium and epicardium and the CenterSurface™.

To reconstruct the mitral valve annulus the traced points are ordered and then connected to form a polygon. A smooth curve is constructed using Fourier series approximations in x,y, and z relative to path length along the polygon (3). The mitral annulus orifice area is determined from the least squares plane fitted to the annular data. Other dimensions such as annular height, circumference, eccentricity, as well as the distance from the LV apex to the annulus, the distance between high points on the annulus, the distance between low points on the annulus, and the magnitude of annular motion are analyzed from the reconstructed annulus.

Table 1. *In vitro* Validation of Volume Measurement by 3D Echo

Standard	Range, ml	N	Regression	r	SEE, ml
beaker phantom	48-151	9	y=1.05x-0.59	0.995	3.5
balloon phantoms	40.6-182.5	12	y=1.00x-0.6	1.000	1.3
in vitro hearts	30.2-104.1	5	y=1.02x-1.3	1.000	0.4
Doppler stroke volume	67.2-117.8	5	y=1.18x-17.9	0.990	2.8

Table 2. *In vitro* Validation of Mass Measurement by 3D Echo

Standard	Range, gm	N	Regression	r	SEE, gm
in vitro hearts	116.5-191.8	5	y=0.98x+1.4	0.998	2.5

Table 3. *In Vitro* Validation of Measurements of Mitral Annulus Size and Shape

Parameter	N	r squared	SEE
Annulus area, cm^2	10	0.99	0.9
Annulus circumference, cm	10	0.99	0.3
Anterior leaflet area, cm^2	9	0.990	1.0
Posterior leaflet area, cm^2	9	0.933	1.1
Annulus height (maximum deviation from least squares fitted plane), cm	40		0.1

3 RESULTS OF VALIDATION STUDIES

The accuracy of volume determination has been evaluated using phantoms, *in vitro* hearts, and *in vivo* by comparison with Doppler stroke volume (1, 4). Beaker phantoms consisted of plastic beakers whose rims were cut in a saddle shape to mimic the mitral annulus and covered with parafilm "leaflets". Balloon phantoms were imaged both in their natural ellipsoid shape and after shape distortion with an equatorial constriction. *In vitro* porcine and calf hearts were obtained from the slaughterhouse, stuffed, and fixed in formalin. The true volume of beaker and *in vitro* hearts was determined from the difference in weight when empty vs. after filling with water. *In vivo* Doppler stroke volume was determined by integrating flow velocity at the LV outflow track. All volumes were measured three times and averaged. Phantom and *in vitro* hearts were imaged in a water bath filled with saline at a concentration that mimics the speed of ultrasound in tissue at room temperature. The results indicate that our 3D echo methods are highly accurate (Table 1). Note that in the regression equation y=volume calculated by 3D echo and x=true volume.

N=number; r=correlation coefficient; SEE=standard error of the regression. However *in vivo* validation has only been performed on a small patient population to date, and additional data are needed to establish the validity of this methodology.

The accuracy of mass determination was evaluated using *in vitro* hearts. The porcine and calf hearts described above were trimmed, fixed, weighed in triplicate, and imaged in a saline bath (4).

The accuracy of mitral annulus and leaflet reconstruction was validated using the beaker phantoms used to validate volume measurement (3).

4 CLINICAL APPLICATIONS

We feel that 3D echo offers unparalleled opportunity to explore the complex relationship between the left ventricle and mitral valve apparatus. Accordingly, we applied our 3D echo techniques to investigate the etiology of functional mitral regurgitation. This condition is characterized by a structurally normal but dysfunctional valve. It has been attributed by various investigators to distortion of the size, shape, position, or motion of the LV, left atrium, mitral valve annulus, and/or papillary muscles.

We analyzed the size, shape, and motion of the mitral annulus in patients with normal hearts undergoing noncardiac surgery and in patients with functional mitral regurgitation secondary to coronary artery disease undergoing bypass graft surgery and/or mitral valve repair. 3D echo was performed using a transesophageal echo probe following induction of anesthesia. Images were acquired at 30 frames/sec every 5-8° over a 180° rotation. The annulus was traced manually in every frame through a normal cardiac cycle. The traced points were converted to x,y,z coordinates and used to reconstruct the annulus with a Fourier technique (3). The analysis showed that in functional mitral regurgitation the annulus is larger, rounder, and flatter and its deformational changes during systole are reduced in magnitude, compared to normal (Fig.8) (5).

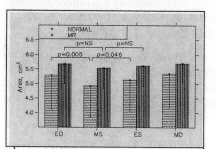

Figure 8. Fluctuation in mitral annulus area over the cardiac cycle in normal subjects and patients with functional mitral regurgitation.

Further studies are in progress using the quantitative 3D echocardiographic techniques that we have developed to measure the size and shape of the LV and all of the elements of the mitral valve apparatus in patients with functional mitral regurgitation. This will make it possible for the first time to compare the contribution of abnormalities in each structure's shape to the severity of valvular dysfunction. Other applications of quantitative 3D echocardiography include diagnosis of ischemic heart disease by stress echocardiography (comparing regional wall thickening at baseline and after dobutamine), endpoint measurements for clinical trials (due to the method's accuracy and reproducibility), and investigation of ventricular remodeling following acute myocardial infarction or partial left ventriculectomy.

5 Discussion

Earlier studies have already established the superior accuracy and reproducibility of 3D echocardiography for the measurement of LV volume, mass, and infarct size (6, 7).

Our methodology for 3D echocardiography is the first to provide comprehensive quantitative analysis of not only the LV but also the mitral annulus, leaflets, chordae tendineae, and papillary muscles. Other structures such as the right ventricle can also be analyzed using the same approach. The accuracy of this methodology is comparable to that of other 3D echocardiographic systems. However the advantage of our approach is flexibility, and this is the reason why it can be applied to so many more analyses than simply volume and mass measurement.

The first source of flexibility is the magnetic field system, which allows us to acquire a 3D scan using freehand scanning in the same manner as a 2D study. Images can be acquired from any combination of intersecting, parallel, or oblique imaging planes and from multiple acoustic windows, an important feature for enlarged or aneurysmal LV's and for acquiring data about other structures of interest. Because the magnetic field receiver is tiny, unlike sound emitters, it does not impinge on the mattress or interfere with apical scanning. The methods can be applied to transesophageal as well as transthoracic scanning.

The second source of flexibility is in image analysis. Borders and partial borders of any number of anatomical structures can be traced and stored. This makes it easy, for example, to measure the distance and angle between any pair of structures, or between points within the same structure.

Third, the piecewise smooth subdivision method of 3D surface reconstruction allows tremendous flexibility. Independent of geometric assumptions, it can accept borders from different combinations of views and acoustic windows. It can reconstruct any structure once the model is defined in the form of a control mesh. Mesh design is facilitated by a 3D editor allowing immediate refitting to show the effect of a design change.

Finally, we have designed the analysis software to be independent of imaging modality. That is, the same measurements can be made from magnetic resonance or computed tomography images.

In summary, our methodology allows a wider range of parameters and inter structure relationships to be analyzed than previously possible. Our plan is to apply these techniques to clinical research while at the same time researching methods for automating image analysis, in order to convert this into a clinical tool.

REFERENCES

1. Legget ME, Leotta DF, Bolson EL, et al. System for quantitative three dimensional echocardiography of the left ventricle based on a magnetic field position and orientation sensing system. IEEE Trans Biomed Eng 1998;(in press).

2. Bolson EL, Sheehan FH, Legget ME, et al. Applying the centersurface model to 3-D reconstructions of the left ventricle for regional function analysis. In: Computers in Cardiology. Long Beach, CA: IEEE Computer Society, pp. 63-66 1995.

3. Legget ME, Bashein G, McDonald JA, et al. Three dimensional measurement of the mitral annulus using multiplane transesophageal echocardiography: In vitro validation and in vivo demonstration. J Am Soc Echo 1998;(in press).

4. Leotta DF, Munt B, Bolson EL, et al. Quantitative three-dimensional echocardiography by rapid imaging from multiple transthoracic windows: In vitro validation and initial in vivo studies. J Am Soc Echo (in press) 1997.

5. Kaplan S, Sheehan FH, Bashein G, et al. Three-dimensional echocardiographic assessment of annular dimensions, shape, and dynamics in the normal and regurgitant mitral valve (abstr.). J Am Coll Cardiol 1998;31(Suppl. A):284A.

6. Jiang L, de Prada JAV, Handschumacher MD, et al. Quantitative three-dimensional reconstruction of aneurysmal left ventricles: In vitro and in vivo validation. Circulation 91: 222-230 1995.

7. Gopal AS, Keller AM, Shen Z, et al. Three-dimensional echocardiography: In vitro and in vivo validation of left ventricular mass and comparison with conventional echocardiographic methods. J Am Coll Cardiol 24: 504-513 1994.

Measurement of 3D Motion of Myocardial Material Points from Explicit B-Surface Reconstruction of Tagged MRI Data

Amir A. Amini, Petia Radeva, Mohamed Elayyadi, and Debiao Li

CVIA Lab, Box 8086, 660 S. Euclid,
Washington University Medical Center,
St. Louis, MO 63110-1093,
email: amini@mobius.wustl.edu
home page: http://www-cv.wustl.edu

Abstract. MRI is unique in its ability to non-invasively and selectively alter tissue magnetization, and create tag planes intersecting image slices. The resulting grid of signal voids allows for tracking deformations of tissues in otherwise homogeneous-signal myocardial regions. In this paper, we propose a specific Spatial Modulation of Magnetization (SPAMM) imaging protocol together with efficient techniques for measurement of 3D motion of material points of the human heart from images collected with the SPAMM method. The techniques make use of tagged images in orthogonal views by explicitly reconstructing 3D B-spline surface representation of each tag plane (two intersecting the short-axis (SA) image slices and one intersecting the long-axis (LA) image slices). The developed methods allow for viewing deformations of 3D tag surfaces, spatial correspondence of long-axis and short-axis image slice and tag positions, as well as non-rigid movement of myocardial material points as a function of time.

1 Introduction

Non-invasive techniques for assessing the dynamic behavior of the human heart are invaluable in the diagnosis of heart disease, as abnormalities in the myocardial motion sensitively reflect deficits in blood perfusion [12]. MRI is a non-invasive imaging technique that provides superb anatomic information with excellent spatial resolution and soft tissue contrast. Conventional MR studies of the heart provide accurate measures of global myocardial function, chamber volumes and ejection fractions, and regional wall motions and thickening. In MR tagging, the magnetization property of selective material points in the myocardium are altered in order to create tagged patterns within a deforming body such as the heart muscle. The resulting pattern defines a time-varying curvilinear coordinate system on the tissue. During tissue contractions, the grid patterns move, allowing for visual tracking of the grid intersections over time. The intrinsic high spatial and temporal resolutions of such myocardial analysis schemes provide unsurpassed information about local contraction and deformation in the heart wall which can be used to derive local strain and deformation indices from different myocardial regions.

Previous work for analysis of tagged images includes work by Young, Kraitchman, Dougherty, and Axel [11] who adopted an analysis system for tagged images based on snakes. Once the tag positions on the myocardium are found, coordinates of these points in deformed images are determined within a volumetric finite element model fitted to endocardial and epicardial contours. The work of Park, Metaxas, and Axel [9] considers geometric primitives which are generalization of volumetric ellipsoids, through use of parameter functions which allow for spatial variations of aspect ratios of the model along the long axis of the LV. This model is specially useful for computing the twisting motion of the heart. Prince and McVeigh and Gupta and Prince developed an optical flow based approach to the analysis of tagged MR images [4]. The approach of Guttman, Prince, and McVeigh [5] for analysis of radial tagged images is to use a graph-search technique that determines the optimal inner and outer boundaries of the myocardium as well as tag lines by finding points one after the other in a sequence, using initial search starting points on the determined LV boundaries. In Amini, Curwen, and Gore [1, 2], tag lines are tracked with Dynamic Programming B-snakes and coupled B-snake grids. Spline warps then warp an area in the plane such that snake grids obtained from two SPAMM frames are brought into registration, interpolating a dense displacement vector field. A volumetric B-solid model was proposed in Radeva, Amini, and Huang [10] to concurrently analyze and track tag lines in different image slices by implicitly defined B-surfaces which align themselves with tagged data. The solid is a 3D tensor product B-spline whose isoparametric curves deform under image forces from tag lines in different image slices. In [6], tag surfaces were constructed using thin-plate splines, and subsequently intersection of the thin-plate spline surfaces were computed based on an alternating projection algorithm to yield displacements of material points.

Although the latter 2 articles provide novel techniques for computation of tag surfaces from discrete image slices, the former paper ([10]) can not reconstruct tag surfaces independent of a B-solid. The latter article ([6]) leads to a somewhat compute intensive algorithm for tag surface reconstruction; in particular requiring inversion of the thin-plate spline matrix [3] of order $O(n \times n)$ (n being the total number of tag points on all image slices.) It is not difficult to see that n can approach upwards of 200. Furthermore, intersecting thin-plate spline surfaces has to be performed in the Euclidean space since the surfaces are not of parametric form. The present article provides machinery for very fast computation of tag surfaces using B-snakes on individual slices, does not require *a priori* computation of a solid, and furthermore since by design the surfaces are parametric, it leads to a naturally easy to implement algorithm for computing 3D material points.

2 Reconstruction of Tag Planes from Coupled B-Snake Grids

B-splines are suitable for representing a variety of industrial and anatomical shapes [1,7,8]. The advantages of B-spline representations are: (1) They are smooth, continuous parametric curves which can represent open or closed curves. For our application, due to parametric continuity, B-splines will allow for sub-pixel localization of tags, (2) B-splines are completely specified by few control points, and (3) Individual movement of control points will only affect their shape locally. In medical imaging, local tissue deformations can easily be captured by movement of individual control points without affecting static portions of the curve.

A B-spline curve is expressed as

$$\alpha(u) = \sum_{i=0}^{N-1} p_i B_i(u) \qquad (1)$$

where $B_i(u)$ are the B-spline basis functions having polynomial form, and local support, and p_i are the sequence of control point of the B-spline curve. Two remarks should be made regarding the sequence of control points: a) The number of control points is much fewer in number than a sampling of the curve $\alpha(u)$ on a pixel grid, and b) p_i rarely reside on the actual curve. To localize a tag line based on B-snakes, an external energy can be defined and optimized in order to locate feature points on individual image slices [1,10]. Given a spatial stack of m curves on m image slices, each represented by n control points, a matrix of control points is constructed as follows:

$$\begin{bmatrix} V_{11} & \cdots & V_{1n} \\ & \cdots & \\ V_{m1} & \cdots & V_{mn} \end{bmatrix} \qquad (2)$$

where the second index may denote ordering along the x axis, and the first index may denote ordering along the z axis (image slices). The matrix immediately gives rise to the surface

$$S(u,v) = \sum_{ij} V_{ij} B_{i,k}(u) B_{j,k}(v) \qquad (3)$$

where we have used non-periodic blending functions as defined in [8]. We have applied cubic splines (i.e., of order $k = 4$) to ensure that there is the necessary flexibility in parametrized shapes (it should be noted that $B_{j,k}$ takes on an identical form to $B_{i,k}$). Furthermore, given that tag lines and images are of approximately equal distance, uniform B-splines are considered so that the knots are spaced at consecutive integer values of parametric variables.

Figures 1 and 2 illustrate the construction of intersecting cubic B-spline tag surfaces from a spatial stack of coupled B-snake grids.

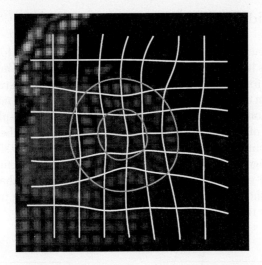

Fig. 1. A grid of B-spline snakes on short-axis image slices in mid-systole. Note that for better illustration, in this figure as well as all analysis to follow every second tag line is utilized. The analysis area of interest is the region within the myocardial borders of the LV.

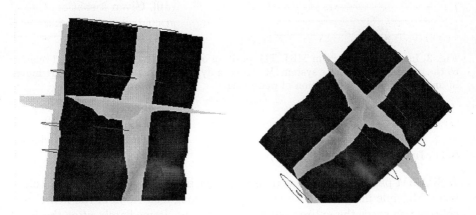

Fig. 2. Figure illustrates the reconstruction of two orthogonal tag surfaces from a sequence of coupled B-spline curves in short-axis image slices (as in figure 1). Two views of the same tag planes are shown. The dark surface corresponds to the second vertical grid line from the right in figure 1. The bright vertical surface orthogonal to this surface corresponds to the fourth horizontal grid line from the top. Finally, the bright horizontal surface is the long-axis tag plane corresponding to the short-axis image slice.

3 Non-Rigid Tracking

The procedure outlined in section 2 provides a mechanism for tracking points within short-axis image slices. However, as shown in figure 3, in MRI, position of image slices are fixed relative to the magnet's coordinate system, and therefore this approach can only yield within short-axis-slice motion of material points. To obtain information about movement of points in the "out-of-plane" direction, a second sequence of images is acquired with slices parallel to the heart's long-axis and with the requirement that tag planes intersecting the new slices be in parallel to short axis images. This requirement however is not sufficient for 3D tracking, and there should yet be an additional requirement, namely that the same set of material points should be imaged in both views. The imaging protocol in section 3.1 accomplishes this goal.

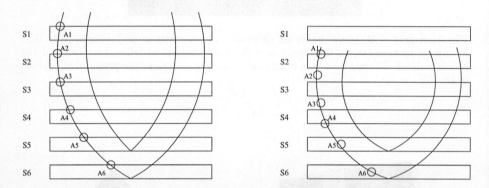

Fig. 3. Imaging geometry in MRI. The position of slices $(S1, \cdots, S6)$ are fixed relative to the magnet's coordinate system. However, a dynamic organ such as the heart moves in-and-out of the slices. Motion of points $A1, \cdots, A6$ illustrates this.

3.1 Imaging Protocol

A SPAMM pulse sequence was used to collect images of normal healthy volunteers. Multiple images in both short-axis and long axis views of the heart were collected to cover the entire volume without gaps. Immediately after the ECG trigger, rf tagging pulses were applied in two orthogonal directions. The repetition time (TR) of the imaging sequence was approximately 7.1 msec, the echo time (TE) was 2.9 msec, the rf pulse flip angle was 15 degrees, and the time extent of rf tag pulses was 22 msec. Echo sharing was used in collecting each time-varying image sequence for given slice position (called a Cine sequence). Five data lines were collected for any time frame during each heart cycle, but two data lines were overlapped between two consecutive cardiac frames, resulting in an effective temporal resolution of approximately 22 $msec$. Other imaging parameters were: field of view = $330mm$, data acquisition matrix size = 160×256

(phase encoding by readout), in-plane resolution = $2.1 \times 1.3 mm^2$, slice thickness = $7mm$, and tag spacing = $7mm$. The total imaging time was therefore 32 heart beats for each Cine sequence, and the subject was instructed to breath only following each Cine acquisition. Since there were 19 volumetric temporal frames and 17 spatial slices in each image volume, all of the images were acquired in 544 heartbeats. In the long-axis view, there were also 19 temporal frames. However, 13 slices covered the entire heart in this case resulting in 416 heart beats of total imaging time.

The image orientations for the short-axis and long-axis views of the heart were first determined by collecting multiple oblique angle scout images. For the short-axis images, one of the tagging planes was placed parallel to the long-axis imaging planes of the heart by manually setting the angles of the tagging plane in the coordinate system of the magnet to be the same as those of the long-axis view as determined from scout images. The coordinates of the center of the central tagging plane in the reference coordinates system (relative to the center of the magnet) were set to be the same as those of the center of one of the long-axis image planes to be acquired, again determined by the scout images. As a result, one set of tagging planes intersecting short-axis image slices coincided with long-axis images since both tag spacing and slice thickness were 7 mm center-to-center. The other short-axis tagging plane was placed orthogonal to the first tagging plane. Similarly, long-axis images were acquired with their tag planes coinciding with short-axis slice positions. Figure 4 displays position of the short-axis image slices on one long-axis image at end-diastole.

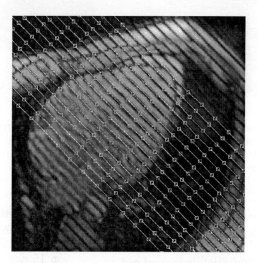

Fig. 4. Position of short-axis image slices at the time of tag placement is drawn on a long-axis image acquired at the same time point in the heart cycle.

As a result of the imaging protocol outlined in this section, the tag intersections from short-axis images are the material points corresponding precisely to the intersection of three tag planes, and revealing for all time points in the cardiac cycle, 3D motion of these special points.

3.2 Computing Time-Dependent Coordinates of Material Points

As we did in the case of coupled B-snakes of short-axis images, once again we measure deformations of tag planes in the long-axis orientation by creating B-spline surfaces from stacks of B-snakes. The difference between short-axis and long-axis image acquisitions is however that there is only one set of parallel tag planes intersecting long-axis images. Figure 5 illustrates a tag surface constructed from a spatial sequence of long-axis images.

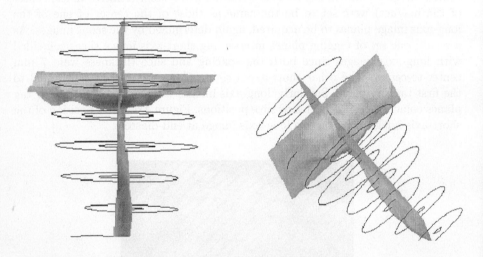

Fig. 5. B-spline surface representation of a long-axis tag plane reconstructed from a spatial stack of B-snakes. Two views of a reconstructed long-axis tag surface is displayed horizontally. "Out-of-plane" movement of the heart is visualized by deviation from flatness of the long-axis B-surface.

Coordinates of material points may be obtained by computing intersections of three intersecting B-spline surfaces representing three intersecting tag surfaces. For each triplet of intersecting B-spline surfaces, $(S_1(u_1,v_1), S_2(u_2,v_2), S_3(u_3,v_3))$, the following computation is carried out

$$\min_{P_1,P_2,P_3} d^2(S_1,S_2) + d^2(S_1,S_3) + d^2(S_2,S_3) \quad (4)$$

where point P_i belongs to surface S_i and d is the Euclidean distance metric. The minimization is carried out using the method of Conjugate Gradient Descent which insures fast convergence of the method. Note that the overall distance function above can be written as

$$||S_1(u_1,v_1) - S_2(u_2,v_2)||^2 +$$
$$||S_2(u_2,v_2) - S_3(u_3,v_3)||^2 +$$
$$||S_1(u_1,v_1) - S_3(u_3,v_3)||^2 \qquad (5)$$

with the goal of finding the parameters (u_i, v_i) for the triplet of surfaces. The computed parameters will in fact be surface parameters of the intersection point. For the iterative optimization process, a good initial set of parameters has been found to be parameters of the intersection point assuming linear B-spline bases. The algorithm was tested on an image sequence which included 17 slices and 19 frames (17 × 19 images) yielding temporal position of around 250 material points over the heart cycle. In a movie of these material points, the 3D motion of individual SPAMM points of the myocardium is clearly apparent.

Figure 6 displays results of the intersection computation for few of the material points.

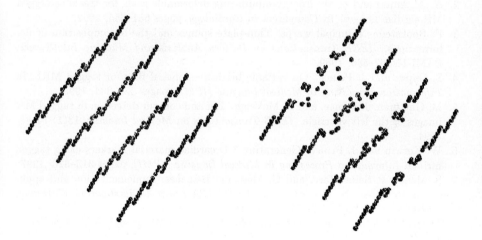

Fig. 6. Location of the material points for every fourth slice of the MRI data is displayed on the left. New computed location of material points one-third through systole is shown on the right. Non-rigid motion of material points of the heart can be appreciated: points further up in slices (around the base) move downwards, whereas points near the heart's apex are relatively stationary.

4 Conclusions

In conclusion, we have described efficient methods for visualization and tracking of 3D material points of the heart from 2 sets of orthogonal tagged MR views.

We have argued that in comparison to other forms of tag representation, use of B-splines has several advantages, including immediate generation of tag surfaces, subpixel accuracy for tag plane localization and parametric continuity, as well as the need to only assign the location of few control points in order to determine the location of a complete tag plane. Currently, the system is being used in actual clinical situations as part of a large clinical study.

Acknowledgements

This work is supported in part by a grant from Whitaker Biomedical Engineering Foundation, and grant 1R29HL57628 from the National Institutes of Health.

References

1. A. A. Amini, R. W. Curwen, and John C. Gore. Snakes and splines for tracking non-rigid heart motion. In *European Conference on Computer Vision*, pages 251–261, University of Cambridge, UK, April 1996.
2. A. A. Amini and et al. Energy-minimizing deformable grids for tracking tagged MR cardiac images. In *Computers in Cardiology*, pages 651–654, 1992.
3. F. Bookstein. Principal warps: Thin-plate splines and the decomposition of deformations. *IEEE Transactions on Pattern Analysis and Machine Intelligence*, PAMI-11:567–585, 1989.
4. S. Gupta and J. Prince. On variable brightness optical flow for tagged MRI. In *Information Processing in Medical Imaging (IPMI)*, pages 323–334, 1995.
5. M. Guttman, J. Prince, and E. McVeigh. Tag and contour detection in tagged MR images of the left ventricle. *IEEE Transactions on Medical Imaging*, 13(1):74–88, 1994.
6. W. Kerwin and J. Prince. Generating 3-D cardiac material markers using tagged mri. In *Information Processing in Medical Imaging (IPMI)*, pages 313–326, 1997.
7. S. Menet, P. Saint-Marc, and G. Medioni. B-snakes: Implementation and application to stereo. In *Proceedings of the DARPA Image Understanding Workshop, Pittsburgh, PA*, pages 720–726, Sept. 1990.
8. Michael E. Mortenson. *Geometric Modeling*. John Wiley and Sons, New York, 1985.
9. J. Park, D. Metaxas, and L. Axel. Volumetric deformable models with parameter functions: A new approach to the 3d motion analysis of the LV from MRI-SPAMM. In *International Conference on Computer Vision*, pages 700–705, 1995.
10. P. Radeva, A. Amini, and J. Huang. Deformable B-Solids and implicit snakes for 3D localization and tracking of SPAMM MRI data. *Computer Vision and Image Understanding*, 66(2):163–178, May 1997.
11. A. Young, D. Kraitchman, L. Dougherty, and L. Axel. Tracking and finite element analysis of stripe deformation in magnetic resonance tagging. *IEEE Transactions on Medical Imaging*, 14(3):413–421, September 1995.
12. E. Zerhouni, D. Parish, W. Rogers, A. Yang, and E. Shapiro. Human heart: Tagging with MR imaging – a method for noninvasive assessment of myocardial motion. *Radiology*, 169:59–63, 1988.

3D Reconstruction from Projection Matrices in a C-Arm Based 3D-Angiography System

N. Navab[1], A. Bani-Hashemi[1], M. S. Nadar[1]
K. Wiesent[2], P. Durlak[2], T. Brunner[2], K. Barth[2] and R. Graumann[2]

[1] Siemens Corporate Research, Inc.
755 College Road East
Princeton, NJ 08540
navab@scr.siemens.com

[2] Siemens AG, Medical Engineering Group
Erlangen, Germany

Abstract. 3D reconstruction of arterial vessels from planar radiographs obtained at several angles around the object has gained increasing interest. The motivating application has been interventional angiography. In order to obtain a three-dimensional reconstruction from a C-arm mounted X-Ray Image Intensifier (XRII) traditionally the trajectory of the source and the detector system is characterized and the pixel size is estimated. The main use of the imaging geometry characterization is to provide a correct 3D-2D mapping between the 3D voxels to be reconstructed and the 2D pixels on the radiographic images.
We propose using projection matrices directly in a voxel driven backprojection for the reconstruction as opposed to that of computing all the geometrical parameters, including the imaging parameters. We discuss the simplicity of the entire calibration-reconstruction process, and the fact that it makes the computation of the pixel size, source to detector distance, and other explicit imaging parameters unnecessary.
A usual step in the reconstruction is sinogram weighting, in which the projections containing corresponding data from opposing directions have to be weighted before they are filtered and backprojected into the object space. The rotation angle of the C-arm is used in the sinogram weighting. This means that the C-arm motion parameters must be computed from projection matrices. The numerical instability associated with the decomposition of the projection matrices into intrinsic and extrinsic parameters is discussed in the context. The paper then describes our method of computing motion parameters without matrix decomposition. Examples of the calibration results and the associated volume reconstruction are also shown.

1 Background and Justification

Interventional angiography has motivated many research and development work on 3D reconstruction of arterial vessels from planar radiographs obtained at several angles around the subject. The endovascular therapy of subarachnoid aneurysms using detachable Guglielmi coils is an application where an imaging system with 3D-capabilities is very useful, [4]. The success of this intravascular procedure critically depends on the packing of the aneurysm. Coils projecting into parent vessels may cause thrombosis, while incomplete filling may lead to regrowth of the aneurysm. Other applications that would benefit from the 3D capabilities are the treatment of carotid stenoses and high resolution bone imaging.

In order to obtain a three-dimensional reconstruction from a C-arm mounted XRII traditionally the trajectory of the source and detector system is characterized and the pixel size is computed. Variety of methods have been proposed in the literature to compute different sets of characterization parameters [15], [2], [4], [3]. Rouge et al. [15] use a non-linear minimization method to compute the position and orientation of the X-ray system relative to the world coordinate system, as well as the image center and scale, using a spiral phantom. Koppe et al. [2] use two consecutive calibration steps to compute 15 parameters explicitly. These parameters are the source position, iso-center, focus parameters, position and orientation. The main use of the imaging geometry characterization is however to provide a correct 3D-2D mapping between the 3D voxels to be reconstructed and the 2D pixels on the radiographic images. We suggest a simple calibration procedure that results in the 3D-2D mapping, as well as, the backprojection algorithm that uses this mapping. As a result we avoid explicit computation of quantities such as pixel size, source to detector distance, and the scale factors due to image digitization. This makes the whole calibration-reconstruction process simple and accurate. An X-ray calibration phantom can be positioned around the head of the patient. This will only occupy a small portion of the X-ray image. The projection matrices are then easily computed. These matrices are then directly used for the back-projection. There is then no need for decomposing these matrices into different geometry and imaging parameters.

If we use the projection matrices computed using an X-ray calibration phantom for 3D reconstruction, the result will be in the coordinate system attached to the calibration phantom. It is however important to present the reconstructed volume in a coordinate frame that is intuitive and natural for the clinicians. During the interventional procedures the C-arm is often moved in the cranial to caudal and LAO to RAO directions to find an optimum view of the lesion. One of the main advantages of this 3D reconstruction is the off-line examination of the vessel tree in order to define an optimum view. This will minimize the radiation exposure to the patient, as well as, the injection of contrast material. Another factor in interventional neuroradiology is the proper placement of the patient to target an organ or a lesion for imaging. An intuitive reference frame is needed for proper placement of patient prior to data collection.

The iso-center of the C-arm is a natural choice, and the effective (average) rotation axis of the gantry is also a natural way to describe a principle axis in the equipment coordinate frame. Therefore, the 3D reconstruction must be presented in this coordinate frame. The matrices mapping 3D voxels to 2D projections must now map the voxels from the C-arm coordinate frame to the projection plane. This makes it necessary to compute the motion of the C-arm. Due to numerical instabilities of matrix decomposition, it is desired to compute this motion directly without matrix decomposition. This is done quite accurately, and new mathematical formulation for the use of Quaternion representation is introduced [12].

We show that parameters such as X-ray source position and intra-frame motion of the imaging system can be computed without the decomposition of the projection matrix. A series of X-ray source positions result in a mean iso-center and a mean axis of rotation. This helps define an intuitive coordinate system at the iso-center of the C-arm. The mean axis of rotation defines one of the principle axes.

The only assumption made is that the intrinsic parameters do not vary between two consecutive frames. Due to small angular motion of the C-arm and the normalization done through distortion correction process[10, 5], this assumption is in practice always satisfied.

We suppose that the image intensifier is free of distortion effect. This is in our application done through an off-line distortion characterization and an on-line distortion correction. The coming generation of X-ray angiography systems use solid state detectors. These detectors are free of geometric distortion, so in the future the distortion correction step will be unnecessary.

2 Definition of Projection Geometry

The 3D-2D mapping is represented by $\mathbf{P}$ a 3×4 homogeneous matrix of projection. This matrix can be computed by imaging a known phantom and establishing correspondences between feature points on the phantom and their radiographic image. The projection matrix $\mathbf{P}$ is defined up to a scale factor. This matrix represents all the imaging geometry parameters. These parameters can be divided into two sets. The first set is called the extrinsic parameters. These parameters define the position and orientation of the imaging system in a world coordinate system, e. g. the coordinate system associated with the calibration phantom. The second set of parameters is called the intrinsic parameters. These parameters only depend on internal parameters of our radiographic imaging system such as pixel size, image center, and source to detector distance.

The imaging system is modeled after a simple pinhole camera. This model proves to be sufficiently accurate for this application. A C-arm coordinate system is defined with its origin at the X-ray source. We define the z-axis parallel to the normal dropping from X-ray source onto the image plane. The x-axis and y-axis are parallel to the row and column vectors of the 2D detector plane.

The homogeneous matrix $\mathbf{P}$ maps voxels from the C-arm coordinate frame to the image plane. We have:

$$\mathbf{P} \cong [\mathbf{AR} \quad \mathbf{AT}] \quad (1)$$

where $\mathbf{A} \begin{bmatrix} \alpha_u & 0 & u_0 \\ 0 & \alpha_v & v_0 \\ 0 & 0 & 1 \end{bmatrix}$.

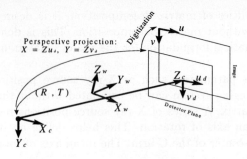

Fig. 1. Mapping between different coordinate systems

The symbol ≅ is used to emphasize that the equality is in homogeneous coordinates and therefore up to scale. The parameters defining **R**, and **T** are called the extrinsic parameters. The matrix **A** incorporates scaling along the horizontal and vertical directions. It also incorporates shifting of the coordinate center from the image center (intersection of optical axis with the image plane) to any arbitrary point on the image. The parameters α_u and α_v also incorporate in them any horizontal and vertical scale changes due to the digitization process. They also include the changes due to the increase or decrease of the relative distance between source and detector. It is important to note that the matrix **P** relates every 3D point in the world coordinate frame to a pixel in the image. Figure 1 illustrates the imaging process including: (a) going from a point in the world coordinate system (X_w, Y_w, Z_w) to a C-arm coordinate system (X_c, Y_c, Z_c), (b) perspective projection onto the detector plane, and (c) the digitization process and change of the coordinate center to an arbitrary point (upper left corner).

In the traditional computed tomography reconstruction, the motion of the C-arm, the relation between the X-ray source and the image intensifier, and the pixel size are computed in different steps. These quantities are later used in the mathematical formulation of the back-projection geometry, from image coordinates in pixels to 3D coordinates in voxels (for example, in millimeters). Here we directly compute the projection matrix **P**. This can be done simply by solving the homogeneous linear system of equations:

$$\bar{\mathbf{x}}_i \cong \mathbf{P}\bar{\mathbf{X}}_i \tag{2}$$

where $\bar{\mathbf{x}}_i = [u_i, v_i, 1]$ and $\bar{\mathbf{X}}_i = [x_i, y_i, z_i, 1]$ are the homogeneous coordinates of the image pixel and 3D voxel in the canonical homogeneous coordinate system.

3 Direct Computation of C-Arm Motion

We first show that during the motion of the C-arm, the consecutive positions of the X-ray source $\mathbf{C} = -\mathbf{R}^t\mathbf{T}$, in the world coordinate system can be computed without decomposing the projection matrix **P**.

Let us define the 3 × 3 matrix $\mathbf{p}_{13}$ and the 3-D vector $\mathbf{p}_4$ such that $\mathbf{P} = [\mathbf{p}_{13}\ \mathbf{p}_4]$. Using Eq. 1, we have $\mathbf{p}_{13} = \mathbf{AR}$ and $\mathbf{p}_4 = \mathbf{AT}$. We have therefore: $\mathbf{p}_{13}^{-1}\mathbf{p}_4 = \mathbf{R}^{-1}\mathbf{T}$. Matrix $\mathbf{R}$ is a rotation matrix and therefore $\mathbf{R}^t = \mathbf{R}^{-1}$.

We can then compute the position of the X-ray source $\mathbf{C}$ without decomposing the matrix $\mathbf{P}$. We have:

$$\mathbf{C} = -\mathbf{p}_{13}^{-1}\mathbf{p}_4 \qquad (3)$$

In order to estimate the motion of the C-arm from projection matrices $\mathbf{P}_i$, the classical method [9, 7, 6] is to decompose each projection matrix into intrinsic and extrinsic parameters. If $\mathbf{P}^i$ and $\mathbf{P}^j$ are the projection matrices obtained at two arbitrary positions of the C-arm, the inter-frame motion is then computed:

$$\mathbf{P}^i \cong [\mathbf{A}_i\mathbf{R}_i \quad \mathbf{A}_i\mathbf{T}_i]$$
$$\mathbf{P}^j \cong [\mathbf{A}_j\mathbf{R}_j \quad \mathbf{A}_j\mathbf{T}_j]$$
$$\mathbf{R}_{(i,j)} = \mathbf{R}_i^T\mathbf{R}_j$$
$$\mathbf{T}_{(i,j)} = \mathbf{R}_i^T(\mathbf{T}_j - \mathbf{T}_i)$$

If the imaging parameters stay constant during the C-arm motion, we show that the motion of the C-arm can also be computed without the decomposition of the projection matrices. The motion of the C-arm ($\mathbf{R}_{(i,j)}, \mathbf{T}_{(i,j)}$), and the two projection matrices, $\mathbf{P}^i$ and $\mathbf{P}^j$, satisfy the following equation:

$$\mathbf{P}^j \cong \mathbf{P}^i \begin{bmatrix} \mathbf{R}_{(i,j)} & \mathbf{T}_{(i,j)} \\ \mathbf{0}^T & 1 \end{bmatrix} \qquad (4)$$

The C-arm motion is therefore directly computable, [3]:

$$\mathbf{R}_{(i,j)} = \kappa \mathbf{p}_{13}^{i}{}^{-1}\mathbf{p}_{13}^{j} \text{ and } \mathbf{T}_{(i,j)} = \mathbf{p}_{13}^{i}{}^{-1}(\kappa \mathbf{p}_4^j - \mathbf{p}_4^i) \qquad (5)$$

We may solve this system of equations by first solving for the scale factor κ. The orthogonality of the rotation matrix can be used to write:

$$\mathbf{p}_{13}^{i}\mathbf{p}_{13}^{i}{}^T = \kappa^2 \mathbf{p}_{13}^{j}\mathbf{p}_{13}^{j}{}^T \qquad (6)$$

This results in a least square estimation of κ. A first estimation of the rotation matrix $\tilde{\mathbf{R}}_{ij}$ can be then computed from equation 5. This may not, however, be an orthogonal matrix. A method for finding the corresponding orthogonal matrix is proposed in the literature. This method finds the orthogonal matrix $\mathbf{R}$ as a result of the following minimization [6], [11]:

$$Min_{\mathbf{R}} \sum_{i=1..3} \|\mathbf{R}\mathbf{v}_i - \mathbf{e}_i\| \qquad (7)$$

where $\mathbf{e}_i$ is the ith column of the identity matrix, and $\mathbf{v}_i$ is the ith column of the matrix $\tilde{\mathbf{R}}_{ij}^T$.

This minimization is usually done using the Quaternion representation of the rotation [16], [11]. Once the scale factor κ and then the rotation matrix $\mathbf{R}_{ij}$ are computed, the translation $\mathbf{T}_{ij}$ can be estimated from Eq.5.

We, however, propose a new method for computing the motion and the scale parameter from Eq.5. This method gives more accurate results compared to the two previous methods. The basic idea is to first compute the rotation matrix $\mathbf{R}_{(i,j)}$, followed by the computation of the translation $\mathbf{T}_{(i,j)}$ and the scale factor κ.

We also use the Quaternion representation of the rotation matrices in order to reduce the number of unknowns and get accurate results. The Quaternion has been used in the past to solve problems of the form $\mathbf{Ru} = \mathbf{u}'$, where $\mathbf{u}$ and $\mathbf{u}'$ are unit vectors. Here the problem is that the unknown scalar κ makes our equations of the form: $\mathbf{Rv} = \kappa\mathbf{v}'$. One possible solution is to normalize the vectors and write these equations in the standard form. We, however, propose a method to use the Quaternion representation to accurately compute the rotation matrix $\mathbf{R}$, by directly solving equations of the form $\mathbf{Rv} = \kappa\mathbf{v}'$. The results are more accurate than the standard minimization after normalization. This is based on a new finding on the Quaternion formulation presented in [12].

Our method of computing the rotation, followed by scale and translation is compared with computing scale first, followed by rotation and translation. Simulations and experiments with real data show that more accuracy is obtained using our method. Figure 2 shows the error in estimating the rotational angle. A number of 3D points from our calibration phantom are projected onto two images using two projection matrices taken from a real experiment. Gaussian noise is then added to the coordinates of each projected point. At each noise level one thousand pairs of images have been automatically generated. The projection matrices and the motion parameters are then computed. Figure 2 shows the behavior of error for the following three methods: (a) decomposition of the projection matrix, (b) direct computation of scale, followed by rotation and translation, and (c) our direct estimation of rotation first, followed by scale and translation. The decomposition of the projection matrices results in the worst estimation of the angular motion. The direct method proposed in [12] results in higher accuracy, particularly when increasing the noise level.

3.1 Computation of C-Arm Coordinate Frame

It is very important to establish an intuitive and natural coordinate frame within which the reconstructed volume can be presented. It was mentioned earlier that the C-arm gantry is a good frame of reference. Therefore, it is necessary to compute the X-ray source position position for each projection. This source position is assumed to move in a quasi-circular orbit. In this section we define an effective iso-center and axis of rotation for this orbit. That would be sufficient to establish the desired coordinate frame.

Once the rotations between all consecutive frames are estimated, we can compute the axis $\mathbf{r}_i$ and the angle θ_i of each rotational motion. These angles are later used in sinogram weighting[13]. Sinogram weighting means that the

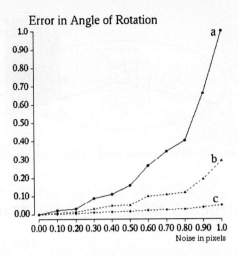

Fig. 2. The error in the estimation of angle of rotational motion from projection matrices: a) by decomposing the projection matrix, b) direct computation of scale, followed by rotation and translation, c) our direct estimation of rotation, followed by scale and translation.

projections containing corresponding data from opposing directions have to be weighted before they are filtered and backprojected into the object space.

We also need to compute the average axis of rotation. If there are n frames, the average axis of rotation is:

$$\mathbf{r} = \frac{1}{n-1} \sum_{i=1}^{n-1} \mathbf{r}_i \qquad (8)$$

where $\mathbf{r}_i$ is the axis of rotational motion between two consecutive frames i and $i+1$.

The approximate motion of the system is then a sequence of pure rotational motion around the axis of rotation $\mathbf{r}$. In order to find the best candidate for an iso-center, we fit a cylinder, parallel to the axis of rotation, to all X-ray source positions $\mathbf{C}_i$, $i = 1..n$. Next, we fit a plane orthogonal to the axis of rotation $\mathbf{r}$ to all the X-ray source positions $\mathbf{C}_i$, $i = 1..n$. The intersection of this plane with the cylinder axis is the estimated iso-center.

We now represent the projection matrices, computed in the unintuitive coordinate system of the calibration phantom, in an intuitive coordinate system with its origin at the effective iso-center and one of its coordinate axis along the average axis of rotation. Note, that this is purely a change of coordinate systems and introduces no additional errors.

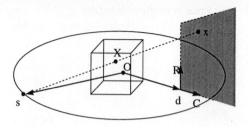

Fig. 3. Physical parameters traditionally used in the backprojection step of 3D cone beam reconstruction.

4 3D Reconstruction Using Projection Matrices for Back-Projection

CT reconstruction using two dimensional detectors are commonly referred to as cone-beam reconstruction techniques. In 1984 Feldkamp *et. al.* , [8], proposed an *approximate* 3D reconstruction algorithm which has been widely accepted. For an overview of *exact* cone beam reconstruction, refer to the work of Clack and Defrise, [1], and the work of Smith, [14]. Feldkamp reconstruction technique could be considered as a generalization of the 2D fan beam reconstruction extended to the third dimension. This method is based on filtered-backprojection. Stated very concisely, in this method, all the 2D projection images are filtered, backprojected into the volume and combined to form the volume data. Filtered-backprojection-type techniques including Feldkamp reconstruction have been developed in the community of CT specialists, therefore different implementations have been greatly influenced by the existing tradition. In this tradition physical parameters of the system are used in the backprojection. For the cone beam reconstruction these parameters are illustrated in Figure 3. s is the X-ray source that is moving on an orbit around the center of rotation O. d is a vector connecting the center of rotation to the origin of the two dimensional detector. r and c are two unit vectors signifying the orientation of the orthogonal axes on the detector plane. A principle step of Filtered-backprojection-type cone beam reconstruction algorithms is backprojection. This consists of tracing a ray from each pixel on the image intensifier back to the X-ray source in order to mark all the 3D voxels which have contributed to this projection.

In this paper we are interested in a voxel oriented approach to backprojection. This approach involves tracing a ray from the X-ray source to a voxel and continued until it intersects the image intensifier at point, marking the point by which the voxel is affected during the backprojection step. The computed tomography community is accustomed to using individual parameters of the geometry for backprojection. These parameters are computed at different calibration steps. We have designed a calibration apparatus and software that provides a transformation matrix relating each voxel in the world coordinate system to a point in the image. This matrix incorporates all the physical parameters involved in the 3-D to 2-D projection. These are the parameters that have been traditionally used in the backprojection step. We have successfully used the transformation matrix in the backprojection step directly, without the need to know the individual physical parameters. This approach is helpful in the following ways:

1. Eliminating the need for running separate calibration steps to compute different physical parameters.
2. Finding a mapping between the voxels to the pixels in the image plane, thereby, eliminating the effect of scale and shift caused by the image digitization process.
3. Providing a more accurate backprojection by computing all the parameters at once, keeping the overall projection error at a minimum (in a least squared sense).
4. Formulating a voxel driven backprojection method based on homogeneous transformation matrices results in an elegant and efficient algorithm.

5 Results

The 3D calibration and reconstruction results presented here have been obtained from prototype installations at four medical and university sites. The prototype system encompasses additional components not discussed in this paper. The geometry of the rotational angiography imaging system, a Siemens NEUROSTAR T.O.P, has been found to be reproducible. The calibration results have remained stable for over a period of more than four months. In an off-line process a calibration phantom has been positioned on the operating table, and a set radiographic images has been taken. The Pose Determination Software (PDS) has automatically made the 3D-2D correspondences between the makers on the calibration ring and their radiographic images. The PDS has then computed the projection matrices, the iso-center, and the inter-frame motions as described in the previous sections. The projection matrices are then transformed into the intuitive coordinate system with its origin at the estimated iso-center as described in the paper.

During the reconstruction of the patient data, only these projection matrices have been used for the back-projection process. The pixel size, image center and source to detector distances have neither been computed nor used during the calibration and reconstruction process.

Typical parameters for the prototype runs are as follows: The exposure was performed over a total angle of 200 degrees in 5 seconds, LAO to RAO; the injection rate of the contrast agent was 2.5 cc/s, for a total of about 14 cc, with contrast agent being iodine (80 to 100%); the XRII format was either 22 or 33 cm (9 or 13"), the dosage at the XRII entrance was one of two settings, 0.48 or 1.2 μGy (55 or 140 μR). The dosage is about ten times lower than that for CT. However, the primary limitation of the system is not from the noise but from the low number of projections which limits the image quality. The contrast is good since the Hounsfield units are markedly above those of bone, (from 2000 to 6000 HU) due to the arterial injection of contrast agent. However, for the case of

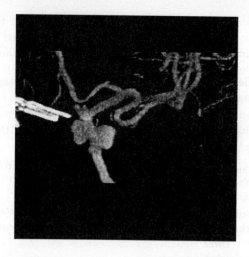

Fig. 4. Shaded-surface display image of a reconstructed volume of a human patient.

CT-Angio with venous injection, the Hounsfield units are between 200 and 300 HU only. The spatial resolution is approximately 0.2 mm "isotropic". A typical reconstruction volume is $256 \times 256 \times 256$, sometimes $512 \times 512 \times 256$ with voxel resolution being somewhere in between 0.1 to 0.3 mm.

Figure 4 shows a portion of the shaded-surface display image of a 3D reconstructed volume from patient data.

6 Conclusions

A simple calibration and back-projection algorithm was described using projection matrices directly in a voxel driven backprojection for the reconstruction as opposed to that of computing all the geometrical parameters, including the imaging parameters. We discussed the simplicity of the entire calibration-reconstruction process, and the fact that it makes the computation of the pixel size, source to detector distance, and other explicit imaging parameters unnecessary. A robust motion estimation scheme was proposed in order to compute the motion of the C-arm and recover the average iso-center and axis of rotation, without decomposing the projection matrices into different geometric and imaging parameters. The whole process becomes therefore quite simple. For a reproducible system, such as the NEUROSTAR T.O.P, the calibration phantom is placed and the projection matrices are computed for an exposure over a total angle of 200 degrees. This is done once every few months. For a non reproducible system the projection matrices can be computed using the patient run. The calibration ring designed to only cover a small portion of the image in this case, and does not interfere with the region of interest. This projection matrices are then directly used during the back-projection process. This calibration and reconstruction process was tested on the results obtained from prototype installation on medical sites, and the results are quite satisfactory.

References

1. R. Clack and Michel Defrise. Overview of reconstruction algorithms for exact cone-beam tomography. pages 230–241. Proc. SPIE 2299, 1994.
2. R. Koppe E. Klotz J. Op de Beek and H. Aerts. 3D vessel reconstruction based on rotational angiography. In *Computer Assitsted Radiology*, pages 101–107. Springer, June 1995.
3. N. Navab et. al. Dynamic geometrical calibration for 3D cerebral angiography. pages 361–370. Proc. SPIE 2708, 1996.
4. R. Fahrig, A. J. Fox, and D. W. Holdsworth. Characterization of a C-arm mounted XRII for 3D image reconstruction during interventional neuroradiology. pages 351–360. Proc. SPIE 2708, 1996.
5. R. Fahrig, M. Moreau, and D. W. Holdsworth. Three-dimensional computer tomographic reconstruction using a C-arm mounted XRII: Correction of image intensifier distortion. *Medical Physics*, 24:1097–1106, 1997.
6. O.D. Faugeras. *Three-Dimensional Computer Vision: A Geometric Viewpoint*. MIT Press, Cambridge, MA, 1993.
7. O.D. Faugeras and G. Toscani. The calibration problem for stereo. In *Proc. IEEE Conf. Comput. Vision Pattern Recog.*, pages 15–20, Miami, FL, June 1986. IEEE.
8. L. A. Feldkamp, L. C. Davis, and J. W. Kress. Practical cone-beam algorithm. *J. Opt. Soc. Am. A, Opt. Image Sci.*, 1(6):612–619, June 1984.
9. S. Ganapathy. Decomposition of trnasformation matrices for robot vision. In *Proc. International Conference on Robotics and Automation*, pages 130–139, 1984.
10. E. Gronenschild. The accuracy and reproducibility of a global method to correct for geometric image distortion in the X-ray imaging chain. *Medical Physics*, 24:1875–1888, 1997.
11. R. Horaud, F. Dornaika, B. Lamiroy, and S. Christy. Object pose: The link between weak perspective, paraperspective and full perspective. *Int'l J. Comput. Vision*, 22(2):173–189, March 1997.
12. N. Navab. Direct estimation of rotation: A new quaternion formulation. Technical Report SCR-98-TR-631, Siemens Corporate Research, 755 College Road East, Princeton, NJ 08540, July 1998.
13. D. L. Parker. Optimal short scan convolution reconstruction for fanbeam CT. *Medical Physics*, 9(2):254–257, March/April 1982.
14. B. D. Smith. Cone-beam tomography: Recent advances and tutorial review. *Optical Engineering*, 29(5):524–534, May 1990.
15. A. Rougée A. C. Picard Y. Trousset and C. Ponchut. Geometrical calibration for 3D X-ray imaging. In *Image Capture, Formatting, and Display*, volume 1897, pages 161–168. SPIE, February 1993.
16. Z. Zhang and O. Faugeras. *3D Dynamic Scene Analysis: A Stereo Based Approach*. Springer, Berlin, Heidelberg, 1992.

Multiscale Vessel Enhancement Filtering*

Alejandro F. Frangi, Wiro J. Niessen, Koen L. Vincken, Max A. Viergever

Image Sciences Institute, Utrecht University Hospital
Room E.01.334, Heidelberglaan 100, 3584 CX Utrecht, the Netherlands
{alex,wiro,koen,max}@isi.uu.nl

Abstract. The multiscale second order local structure of an image (*Hessian*) is examined with the purpose of developing a vessel enhancement filter. A vesselness measure is obtained on the basis of all eigenvalues of the Hessian. This measure is tested on two dimensional DSA and three dimensional aortoiliac and cerebral MRA data. Its clinical utility is shown by the simultaneous noise and background suppression and vessel enhancement in maximum intensity projections and volumetric displays.

1 Introduction

Accurate visualization and quantification of the human vasculature is an important prerequisite for a number of clinical procedures. Grading of stenoses is important in the diagnosis of the severity of vascular disease since it determines the treatment therapy. Interventional procedures such as the placement of a prosthesis in order to prevent aneurysm rupture or a bypass operation require an accurate insight into the three dimensional vessel architecture.

Both two-dimensional projection techniques, such as DSA, and three-dimensional modalities as X-ray rotational angiography, CTA and MRA are employed in clinical practice. Although CTA and MRA provide volumetric data, the common way of interpreting these images is by using a maximum intensity projection.

The main drawbacks of maximum intensity projections are the overlap of non-vascular structures and the fact that small vessels with low contrast are hardly visible. This has been a main limitation in time-of-flight MRA [4]. In contrast enhanced MRA [12] the delineation of these vessels is considerably improved, but other organs can be still projected over the arteries.

The purpose of this paper is to enhance vessel structures with the eventual goal of vessel segmentation. A vessel enhancement procedure as a preprocessing step for maximum intensity projection display will improve small vessel delineation and reduce organ over-projection. Segmentation of the vascular tree will facilitate volumetric display and will enable quantitative measurements of vascular morphology.

There are several approaches to vessel enhancement. Some of them work at a fixed scale and use (nonlinear) combinations of finite difference operators applied in a set of orientations [2–4]. Orkisz *et al.* [11] presents a method that applies a median filter in the direction of the vessel. All these methods have shown problems to detect vessels over a large size range since they perform a fixed scale analysis. Moreover, to handle voxel anisotropy, these methods usually need to resample the dataset or to resource to $2\frac{1}{2}D$ processing (cf. [11]). Multi-scale approaches to vessel enhancement include "cores" [1], steerable filters [7, 8], and assessment of local orientation via eigenvalue analysis of the Hessian matrix [10, 13].

---

* This research was sponsored by the Netherlands Ministry of Economic Affairs (Program IOP Beeldverwerking). We are indebted to our colleagues Dr. Theo van Walsum, Onno Wink and Joes Staal for fruitful discussions and various contributions to the paper.

The multiscale approach we discuss in this paper is inspired by the work of Sato *et al.* [13] and Lorenz *et al.* [10] who use the eigenvalues of the Hessian to determine locally the likelihood that a vessel is present. We modify their approach by considering all eigenvalues and giving the vesselness measure an intuitive, geometric interpretation. Examples on medical image data are included.

2 Method

In our approach we conceive vessel enhancement as a filtering process that searches for geometrical structures which can be regarded as tubular. Since vessels appear in different sizes it is important to introduce a measurement scale which varies within a certain range.

A common approach to analyze the local behavior of an image, L, is to consider its Taylor expansion in the neighborhood of a point $\mathbf{x}_o$,

$$L(\mathbf{x}_o + \delta\mathbf{x}_o, s) \approx L(\mathbf{x}_o, s) + \delta\mathbf{x}_o^T \nabla_{o,s} + \delta\mathbf{x}_o^T \mathcal{H}_{o,s} \delta\mathbf{x}_o \qquad (1)$$

This expansion approximates the structure of the image up to second order. $\nabla_{o,s}$ and $\mathcal{H}_{o,s}$ are the gradient vector and Hessian matrix of the image computed in $\mathbf{x}_o$ at scale s. To calculate these differential operators of L in a well-posed fashion we use concepts of linear scale space theory [5,6]. In this framework differentiation is defined as a convolution with derivatives of Gaussians:

$$\frac{\partial}{\partial x} L(\mathbf{x}, s) = s^\gamma L(\mathbf{x}) * \frac{\partial}{\partial x} G(\mathbf{x}, s) \qquad (2)$$

where the D-dimensional Gaussian is defined as:

$$G(\mathbf{x}, s) = \frac{1}{\sqrt{(2\pi s^2)}^D} e^{-\frac{\|\mathbf{x}\|^2}{2s^2}} \qquad (3)$$

The parameter γ was introduced by Lindeberg [9] to define a family of normalized derivatives. This normalization is particularly important for a fair comparison of the response of differential operators at multiple scales. When no scale is preferred γ should be set to unity.

Analyzing the second order information (Hessian) has an intuitive justification in the context of vessel detection. The second derivative of a Gaussian kernel at scale s generates a probe kernel that measures the contrast between the regions inside and outside the range $(-s,s)$ in the direction of the derivative (figure 1). This approach is the one followed in this work.

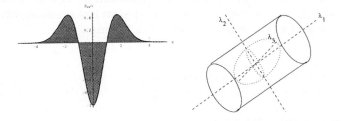

Fig. 1. *Left*: The second order derivative of a Gaussian kernel probes inside/outside contrast of the range $(-s,s)$. In this example $s = 1$. *Right*: The second order ellipsoid describes the local principal directions of curvature.

The third term in Equation (1) gives the second order directional derivative,

$$\delta \mathbf{x}_o^T \mathcal{H}_{o,s} \delta \mathbf{x}_o = (\frac{\partial}{\partial \delta \mathbf{x}_o})(\frac{\partial}{\partial \delta \mathbf{x}_o}) L(\mathbf{x}_o, s) \tag{4}$$

The idea behind eigenvalue analysis of the Hessian is to extract the principal directions in which the local second order structure of the image can be decomposed. Since this directly gives the direction of smallest curvature (along the vessel) application of several filters in multiple orientations is avoided. This latter approach is computationally more expensive and requires a discretization of the orientation space.

Let $\lambda_{s,k}$ denote the eigenvalue corresponding to the k-*th* normalized eigenvector $\hat{\mathbf{u}}_{s,k}$ of the Hessian $\mathcal{H}_{o,s}$, all computed at scale s. From the definition of eigenvalues:

$$\mathcal{H}_{o,s} \hat{\mathbf{u}}_{s,k} = \lambda_{s,k} \hat{\mathbf{u}}_{s,k} \tag{5}$$

and it follows that

$$\hat{\mathbf{u}}_{s,k}^T \mathcal{H}_{o,s} \hat{\mathbf{u}}_{s,k} = \lambda_{s,k} \tag{6}$$

By analyzing Equations (4)-(6) a nice geometric interpretation arises. The eigenvalue decomposition extracts three orthonormal directions which are invariant up to a scaling factor when mapped by the Hessian matrix. In particular, a spherical neighborhood centered at $\mathbf{x}_o$ with radius 1, $\mathcal{N}_{\mathbf{x}_o}$, will be mapped by $\mathcal{H}_o$ onto an ellipsoid whose axes are along the directions given by the eigenvectors of the Hessian and the corresponding axis' semi-lengths are the magnitudes of the respective eigenvalues.

This ellipsoid locally describes the second order structure of the image (thus we coin it *second order ellipsoid* -figure 1-) and can be used as an intuitive tool for the design of geometric similarity measures.

In the remainder of the paper λ_k will be the eigenvalue with the k-*th* smallest magnitude ($|\lambda_1| \leq |\lambda_2| \leq |\lambda_3|$). Under this assumption Table 1 summarizes the relations that must hold between the eigenvalues of the Hessian for the detection of different structures. In particular, a pixel belonging to a vessel region will be signaled by λ_1 being small (ideally zero), and λ_2 and λ_3 of a large magnitude and equal sign (the sign is an indicator of brightness/darkness). The respective eigenvectors point out singular directions: $\hat{\mathbf{u}}_1$ indicates the direction along the vessel (minimum intensity variation) and $\hat{\mathbf{u}}_2$ and $\hat{\mathbf{u}}_3$ form a base for the orthogonal plane. We are interested in "vesselness" measures suited for medical images. In MRA and CTA, vessels emerge as bright tubular structures in a darker environment. This *prior* information related to the imaging modality can be used as a consistency check to discard structures present in the dataset with a polarity different than the one sought. Accordingly, we shall look for structures whose λ_2 and λ_3 are both simultaneously negative.

To summarize, for an ideal tubular structure in a $3D$ image:

$$|\lambda_1| \approx 0 \tag{7}$$
$$|\lambda_1| \ll |\lambda_2| \tag{8}$$
$$\lambda_2 \approx \lambda_3 \tag{9}$$

and the sign of λ_2 and λ_3 indicate its polarity.

We emphasize that all three eigenvalues play an important role in the discrimination of the local orientation pattern. This will yield expressions that differ from the similarity measures proposed by Sato *et al.* [13] and Lorenz *et al.* [10] who only make use of two eigenvalues in their respective $3D$ line filters. In particular, Sato's approach [13] uses a different eigenvalue ordering scheme: they are sorted in increasing *value* (not absolute value), and only the two largest are considered in the line filter. This implies that dark and bright lines are not treated in a similar manner.

Our dissimilarity measure takes into account two geometric ratios based on the second order ellipsoid. The first ratio accounts for the deviation from a blob-like structure but cannot distinguish between a line- and a plate-like pattern:

$$\mathcal{R}_\mathcal{B} = \frac{\text{Volume}/(4\pi/3)}{(\text{Largest Cross Section Area}/\pi)^{3/2}} = \frac{|\lambda_1|}{\sqrt{|\lambda_2 \lambda_3|}} \qquad (10)$$

This ratio attains its maximum for a blob-like structure and is zero whenever $\lambda_1 \approx 0$, or λ_1 and λ_2 tend to vanish (notice that λ_1/λ_2 remains bounded even when the second eigenvalue is very small since its magnitude is always larger than the first).

The second ratio refers to the largest area cross section of the ellipsoid (in the plane orthogonal to $\hat{u}_1$) and accounts for the aspect ratio of the two largest second order derivatives. This ratio is essential for distinguishing between plate-like and line-like structures since only in the latter case it will be zero,

$$\mathcal{R}_\mathcal{A} = \frac{(\text{Largest Cross Section Area})/\pi}{(\text{Largest Axis Semi-length})^2} = \frac{|\lambda_2|}{|\lambda_3|} \qquad (11)$$

The two geometric ratios we introduced so far are grey-level invariant (i.e., they remain constant under intensity re-scalings). This ensures that our measures only capture the geometric information of the image. However, in MRA and CTA images there is additional knowledge available: vessel structures are brighter than the background and occupy a (relatively) small volume of the whole dataset. If this information is not incorporated background pixels would produce an unpredictable filter response due to random noise fluctuations. However, a distinguishing property of background pixels is that the magnitude of the derivatives (and thus the eigenvalues) is small, at least for typical signal-to-noise ratios present in acquired datasets. To quantify this we propose the use of the norm of the Hessian. We use the Frobenius matrix norm since it has a simple expression in terms of the eigenvalues when the matrix is real and symmetric. Hence we define the following measure

2D		3D			orientation pattern
λ_1	λ_2	λ_1	λ_2	λ_3	
N	N	N	N	N	noisy, no preferred direction
		L	L	H-	plate-like structure (bright)
		L	L	H+	plate-like structure (dark)
L	H-	L	H-	H-	tubular structure (bright)
L	H+	L	H+	H+	tubular structure (dark)
H-	H-	H-	H-	H-	blob-like structure (bright)
H+	H+	H+	H+	H+	blob-like structure (dark)

Table 1. Possible patterns in $2D$ and $3D$, depending on the value of the eigenvalues λ_k (H=high, L=low, N=noisy, usually small, +/- indicate the sign of the eigenvalue). The eigenvalues are ordered: $|\lambda_1| \leq |\lambda_2| \leq |\lambda_3|$.

of "second order structureness",

$$S = \|\mathcal{H}\|_F = \sqrt{\sum_{j \leq D} \lambda_j^2} \tag{12}$$

where D is the dimension of the image.

This measure will be low in the background where no structure is present and the eigenvalues are small for the lack of contrast. In regions with high contrast compared to the background, the norm will become larger since at least one of the eigenvalues will be large. We therefore propose the following combination of the components to define a vesselness function,

$$\mathcal{V}_o(s) = \begin{cases} 0 & \text{if } \lambda_2 > 0 \text{ or } \lambda_3 > 0, \\ (1 - \exp\left(-\frac{\mathcal{R}_A^2}{2\alpha^2}\right)) \exp\left(-\frac{\mathcal{R}_B^2}{2\beta^2}\right)(1 - \exp\left(-\frac{\mathcal{S}^2}{2c^2}\right)) \end{cases} \tag{13}$$

where α, β and c are thresholds which control the sensitivity of the line filter to the measures $\mathcal{R}_A$, $\mathcal{R}_B$ and $\mathcal{S}$. The idea behind this expression is to map the features in Equations (10)-(12) into probability-like estimates of vesselness according to different criteria. We combine the different criteria using their product to ensure that the response of the filter is maximal only if all three criteria are fulfilled. In all the results presented in this work α and β were fixed to 0.5. The value of the threshold c depends on the grey-scale range of the image and half the value of the maximum Hessian norm has proven to work in most cases. However, future research will be directed towards automating this threshold selection. We expect that this threshold can be fixed for a given application where images are routinely acquired according to a standard protocol.

The vesselness measure in Equation (13) is analyzed at different scales, s. The response of the line filter will be maximum at a scale that approximately matches the size of the vessel to detect. We integrate the vesselness measure provided by the filter response at different scales to obtain a final estimate of vesselness:

$$\mathcal{V}_o(\gamma) = \max_{s_{min} \leq s \leq s_{max}} \mathcal{V}_o(s, \gamma) \tag{14}$$

where s_{min} and s_{max} are the maximum and minimum scales at which relevant structures are expected to be found. They can be chosen so that they will cover the range of vessel widths.

For $2D$ images we propose the following vesselness measure which follows from the same reasoning as in $3D$,

$$\mathcal{V}_o(s) = \begin{cases} 0 & \text{if } \lambda_2 > 0, \\ \exp\left(-\frac{\mathcal{R}_B^2}{2\beta^2}\right)(1 - \exp\left(-\frac{\mathcal{S}^2}{2c^2}\right)) \end{cases} \tag{15}$$

Here, $\mathcal{R}_B = \lambda_1/\lambda_2$ is the blobness measure in $2D$ and accounts for the eccentricity of the second order ellipse.

Equations (13) and (15) are given for bright curvilinear structures (MRA and CTA). For dark objects (as in DSA) the conditions (or the images) should be reversed.

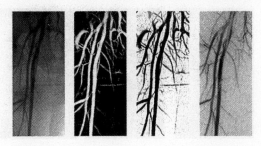

Fig. 2. *Left*: Part of a contrast X-ray image of the peripheral vasculature. *Middle-left*: Calculated vesselness of the left image. *Middle-right*: Calculated vesselness after inversion of the grey-scale map. *Right*: Image obtained by subtracting reference (without contrast) image from left image; shown here to facilitate visual inspection of the results of the filtering procedure.

3 Results

3.1 2D DSA images

In this section we show some results of vessel enhancement filtering in $2D$ DSA images. These images are obtained by acquiring an X-ray projection when intra-arterial contrast material is injected. A reference image is first acquired without contrast, which is subtracted from the image with contrast for background suppression. If no motion artifacts are present the subtracted images are of such good quality, that further processing is not desirable. We therefore only apply our enhancement filter to the contrast images directly, and use the subtracted images to be able to judge the performance of the vessel enhancement filter.

In figure 2, a part of an image of the peripheral vasculature is shown, where performance of subtraction is usually quite good. Although contrast is not very high in the contrast images, the method detects most vessels, over a large size range. Notice however that some artifacts where introduced in regions where background fluctuations have line patterns.

3.2 3D MRA images

We have applied our method to three-dimensional aortoiliac MRA datasets, to show the potential of enhancement filtering to improve visualization of the vasculature. In figure 3 (left) we show a maximum intensity projection which is applied directly to the grey-scale data of an MRA dataset of the aortoiliac arteries. By determining the vesselness of the MRA image at multiple scales we obtain separate images depicting vessels of various widths. This is shown in figure 4. Here we plotted maximum intensity projections of the vesselness at four scales. The rightmost image shows how we can combine these multiscale measurements by using a scale selection procedure (recall that we work with normalized derivatives), eventually yielding a display of both the small and large vessels. The figure also shows that small and large vessels can be distinguished, which can for example be used in artery/vein segmentation. Since the enhancement filtering does not give a high output at other structures, additional information can more easily be visualized. In the middle frame of figure 3 we show the maximum intensity projection which is obtained after vessel enhancement filtering. In the right frame a closest vessel projection is shown. In this case, it is possible to determine the order in depth of various vascular structures. The excellent noise and background suppression provided by the vesselness measure greatly facilitates the use

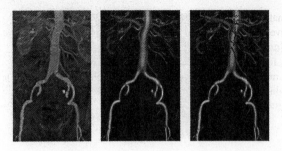

Fig. 3. *Left*: Original maximum intensity projection of a contrast (Gd-DTPA) MRA image. *Middle*: Maximum intensity projection of vessel enhanced image. We obtain quite good background suppression. *Right*: Closest vessel projection, facilitated by the filter's excellent background suppression.

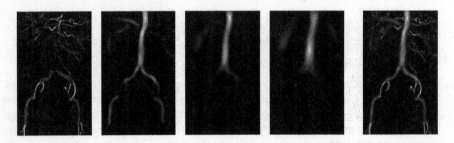

Fig. 4. The first four images show the vesselness obtained at increasing scales. The last image is the result after the scale selection procedure.

of a closest vessel projection. In order to compare the results of the vessel enhancement procedure with renderings obtained using a threshold on the original image, we show both renderings in figure 5. We see that the original image has more background disturbance. However, the vessels tend to be narrower in the vessel enhancement image compared to the original dataset. This is due to the fact that at the boundaries of vessels the vesselness is not very high. The vessel enhancement filtering should be used in a subsequent segmentation procedure for obtaining quantitative measurements on the vasculature.

4 Discussion

We have presented a method for vessel enhancement filtering which is based on local structure. To this end we examined the local second order ellipsoid. Since we use information about all axes of the second order ellipsoid (all eigenvalues), the approach is a generalization of other existing approaches on the use of second order information for line detection. Recently, Sato *et al.* [13] and Lorenz *et al.* [10] used eigenvalue analysis of the Hessian for vessel enhancement, but they did not use all eigenvalues simultaneously. We have shown the excellent noise and background suppression in a two clinical image modalities, underlying the potential of the approach.

It is important to realize that we do not obtain a segmentation of the vasculature. Only if an accurate model of the typical luminance in the perpendicular direction of the vessel is known, an estimate of the size of the vessel can be made based on the response of the filter over scales. However this is often not the case. For example, in MRI it is common to reduce the reconstruction time by restricting the number of lines in k-space (scan percentage) which accounts for a reduction of the effective Fourier spectrum of the measured signal. This technique can lead to ringing artifacts (overshoot) in high transition steps (for example, in vessels boundaries) thus violating simplified profile models (Gaussian/bar-like [7, 10]). The vesselness measure can serve as a preprocessing step for segmentation of this type of images.

References

1. S. Aylward, *et al.*. Intensity ridge and widths for tubular object segmentation and description. In A. A. Amini, F. L. Bookstein, and D. C. Wilson, eds., *Math. Meth. in Biomed. Imag. Anal.*, pages 131–138, 1995.
2. H. Chen and J. Hale. An algorithm for MR angiography image enhancement. *MRM*, 33(4):534–40, April 1995.
3. Y. P. Du and D. L. Parker. Vessel enhancement filtering in three-dimensional MR angiography. *JMRI*, 5(3):353–359, 1995.
4. Y. P. Du and D. L. Parker. Vessel enhancement filtering in three-dimensional MR angiograms using long range signal correlation. *JMRI*, 7(2):447–450, 1997.
5. L. M. J. Florack, *et al.*. Scale and the differential structure of images. *Imag. and Vis. Comp.*, 10(6):376–388, July/August 1992.
6. J. J. Koenderink. The structure of images. *Biol. Cybern.*, 50:363–370, 1984.
7. T. M. Koller, *et al.*. Multiscale detection of curvilinear structures in 2-D and 3-D image data. In E. Grimson, S. Shafer, A. Blake, and K. Sugihara, editors, *Proc. Fifth Int. Conf. on Comp. Vis.*, pages 864–869, 1995.
8. T. M. Koller. *From Data to Information: Segmentation, Description and Analysis of the Cerebral Vascularity*. Diss. ETH no. 11367, Swiss Federal Institute of Technology ETHZ, 1995.
9. T. Lindeberg. Edge detection and ridge detection with automatic scale selection. In *Proc. Conf. on Comp. Vis. and Pat. Recog.*, pages 465–470, San Francisco, CA, June 1996.
10. C. Lorenz, *et al.*. Multi-scale line segmentation with automatic estimation of width, contrast and tangential direction in 2D and 3D medical images. In J. Troccaz, E. Grimson, and R. Mösges, eds., *Proc. CVRMed-MRCAS'97*, LNCS, pages 233–242, 1997.
11. M. M. Orkisz, *et al.*. Improved vessel visualization in MR angiography by nonlinear anisotropic filtering. *MRM*, 37(6):914–9, June 1997.
12. M. R. Prince. Gadolinium-enhanced MR aortography. *Radiol.*, 191:155–164, 1994.
13. Y. Sato, *et al.*. 3D multi-scale line filter for segmentation and visualization of curvilinear structures in medical images. In J. Troccaz, E. Grimson, and R. Mösges, eds., *Proc. CVRMed-MRCAS'97*, LNCS, pages 213–222, 1997.

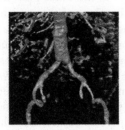
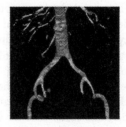

Fig. 5. *Left*: Volume rendering based on threshold of the original dataset. *Right*: Volume rendering based on threshold of the vesselness image.

Fast Quantification of Abdominal Aortic Aneurysms from CTA Volumes

O. Wink, W.J. Niessen, M.A. Viergever

Image Sciences Institute, Room E 01.334,
University Hospital Utrecht, Heidelberglaan 100,
3584 CX Utrecht, the Netherlands
{onno,wiro,max}@isi.uu.nl
http://www.isi.uu.nl

Abstract. A method is presented which aids the clinician in obtaining quantitative measurements of an abdominal aortic aneurysm from a CTA volume. These measurements are needed in the preoperative evaluation of candidates for minimally invasive aneurysmal repair. The user initializes starting points in the iliac artery. Subsequently, an iterative tracking procedure outlines the central lumen line in the aorta and the iliac arteries. Quantitative measurements on vessel morphology are performed in the planes perpendicular to the vessel axis. The entire process is performed in less than one minute on a standard workstation. In addition to the presentation of the calculated measures, a 3D view of the vessels is generated. This allows for interactive inspection of the vasculature and the tortuosity of the vessels.

1 Introduction

An abdominal aortic aneurysm (AAA) is a life threatening dilation of the main artery, occurring mainly in men at older age. Standard treatment of an AAA involves the replacement of the dilated part of the aneurysm by a prosthesis. This invasive procedure has a postoperative mortality rate of about 7%. Recently a less invasive, alternative treatment with potentially lower risk has emerged, which implies the introduction of a folded aortic graft through the femoral artery, using a groin incision. The dimensioning of grafts for this endovascular intervention is a key issue in the effort to minimize peri- and postoperative complications. The most common complications of inaccurate graft sizing are persistent endoleak and thrombosis of the graft body or limbs. In order to minimize inaccuracy in graft sizing, diameter measurements should be performed in planes perpendicular to the central vessel axis [1]. This central lumen line, the very basis for the dimensioning of the grafts, is currently drawn by the clinician, using three orthogonal views. The entire dimensioning process is very labor intensive, user dependent, and takes roughly one hour per patient.

The purpose of this study is to develop a fast objective method for the detection of the central lumen line, and to subsequently determine different quantitative measures along this line, in order to facilitate the preoperative evaluation of candidates scheduled for endovascular repair.

2 Related work

Most methods of 3D line detection [2-4], are based on a two phase process. First a feature image is constructed that yields high responses in the center of the lumen. Second, a search process is started that tries to connect the different maxima from the preceding stage into a connected structure. These methods are computationally intensive, and exhibit varying results, especially in highly curved regions, and at the bifurcations.

In contrast, the homing cursor [5] directly explores the 3D volume, but assumes smoothly varying contours, and a Gaussian cross section. Because of the large variations in width of the vessels, and the presence of calcifications, this method is not suited for our application.

Other 3D applications [6-8] that are able to cope with the varying width of the vessel structure either use different preprocessing steps, like segmentation and/or manual delineation of the central lumen, before the actual quantification process takes place. Fiebich et al. [9] report successful automated segmentation of the aorta and its branching vessels, based on two different thresholds. However, the more difficult problem of segmenting the iliac and femoral arteries is not solved by this procedure. The variation in contrast of the iliac and femoral arteries is too large for a single threshold to yield a successful segmentation.

The method presented here, directly explores the 3D data. As a result, no segmentation is needed before the method can be applied. User interaction is minimal, only two starting points have to be indicated. Furthermore, the method can be used interactively.

3 Current practice

In current clinical practice at our hospital, the operator manually determines the central lumen line on a Philips EasyVision workstation, using three orthogonal views. Based on this line, and its perpendicular planes, it is determined whether the patient is suited for endovascular repair. If the iliac trajectory for example has a diameter less than 5 mm, the graft may not be able to pass. The different measurements result in the dimensions of the graft and the preferred entry side (left or right), through which the graft will be introduced. In order to get an overview of the vasculature and the tortuosity of the iliac trajectory, the aorta is segmented manually. The segmentation is performed in the 2D slices, using basic thresholding and region growing techniques.

4 Description of the method

We propose a near automatic method for the detection of the central lumen line of the aorta and the iliac and femoral arteries. After the initial points have been determined by the operator, the tracking process is started. In every iteration the central lumen line is extended by one point. At this new position, a plane perpendicular to the central lumen line is constructed. This plane is subsequently searched for the center of the lumen, which results in an update of the central lumen line. During the process, the central lumen line and a corresponding confidence level are presented. This enables the user to monitor the process, and take over control if needed. In the next sections the different phases will be described in detail. First, the most important step, determining the lumen center, is discussed.

4.1 Determination of the lumen center

Given a plane, perpendicular to the central lumen line, we aim to compute the center of the lumen. Figure 1 gives three examples of such a cutplane. These

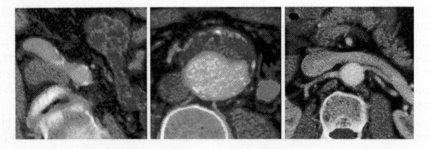

Fig. 1. Three examples of a perpendicular plane, in which the center of the lumen must be determined. In the left image, two iliac arteries, just below the bifurcation are visible. In the middle image the aneurysm itself is displayed. The right image shows the neck of the aneurysm and two renal arteries.

examples illustrate some specific problems that may be encountered in determining the center of the lumen. First, the calcifications appear as very dense spots, yielding a high response to any gradient integration based method. Second, both shape and size of the contour of the lumen are very unpredictable. This hampers template based or model based methods, and methods based on a fixed scale. Third, it may occur that the cutplane is almost parallel to one of the joining arteries, or is positioned at a bifurcation. Fourth, the intensity of the pixels in the contrast filled lumen may vary considerably.

We propose a method which is capable of coping with the problems described above. A schematic example of the method is given in figure 2. From the point

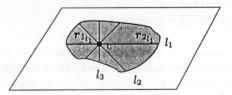

Fig. 2. Determination of the lumen center. From the point c, a number of rays is cast. For line l_1 there exists a pair of rays $(r_{1_{l_1}}, r_{2_{l_1}})$.

c in the perpendicular plane, a number of 'rays' is cast. Every ray r stops at the first gradient maximum above a threshold t. The gradient ∇L at scale σ is computed using a convolution of the original image with a Gaussian derivative in the direction of the ray:

$$\frac{\partial L}{\partial r} = \frac{|r.\nabla L|}{|r|} \qquad (1)$$

For every pair of rays $(r_{1_{l_i}}, r_{2_{l_i}})$ along every line i, the length is determined. The confidence level CL of a point is determined using:

$$CL = \frac{1}{N} \sum_{i=1}^{N} \frac{\min(|r_{1_{l_i}}|, |r_{2_{l_i}}|)}{\max(|r_{1_{l_i}}|, |r_{2_{l_i}}|)} \qquad (2)$$

where N is the number of lines. When the confidence level is computed for every point in a 30x30 grid around the center of the leftmost cutplane in figure 1, we get the surface as shown in figure 3. The point with the highest confidence

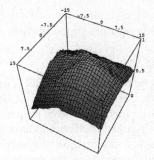 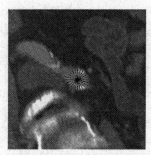

Fig. 3. Confidence level surface, and the rays used in computing the maximum confidence level, $\sigma = 3, t = 4, N = 12$.

level is assumed to be the center of the lumen. The rays used to compute this maximum, are displayed in the right image of figure 3.

The confidence level has several interesting properties, Some of these will now be discussed.

Calcifications: because the gradient is computed in the direction of the ray, the calcification is treated as being part of the lumen (see the right image in figure 3). If only the gradient magnitude would be used, the ray would have stopped at the first boundary of the calcification it detects, thus giving an underestimate of the lumen width, and a possible error in the determined lumen center.

If a significant amount of calcium is present in one of the perpendicular planes, the method might find the center of a calcification instead of the center of the lumen. Therefore, we put a constraint on the minimum length of the lines. If the length of a line is below this threshold, the contribution to the confidence level will be zero.

Bifurcations: if the cutplane is positioned at a bifurcation, the confidence level is still able to find the center. In figure 4 an example of a bifurcation is given. In

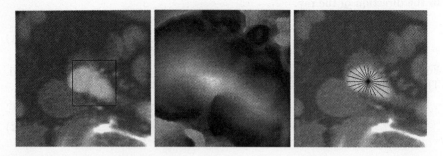

Fig. 4. An example of a bifurcation (left), and its confidence level image (middle), showing the largest peak in the middle. The right image displays the rays used, $\sigma = 3, t = 4, N = 12$.

the middle image of figure 4, the confidence level corresponding to the square in the left figure, is shown. This figure shows three definite peaks, with the largest in the middle. In the right image, the different rays are superimposed over the original image.

Intensity, scale and rotational invariance: the confidence level is invariant to the absolute value of the intensities in the lumen and to its size. However, several criteria have to be met, in order for the method to give proper results. Because of the thresholding of the gradient, the lumen itself should have a rather continuous grey level, and have higher intensity values than the surrounding tissue. The rotational invariance of the method depends on the number of lines that are used in computing the confidence level. The larger the number of lines, the better it approximates rotational invariant behaviour.

Outliers: if one of the rays 'misses' the border of the lumen, and stops at the edge of another more remote structure the contribution to the confidence level is almost zero. This is also the case if one of the rays accidentally enters one of the joining vessels, like the renal arteries as shown in the rightmost image from figure 1.

Interactivity: because of the normalization, the confidence level CL is always within the range $[0, 1]$. The confidence level can therefore be used to determine whether the tracking process went outside the artery, by inspecting its value or change in value during the tracking process.

Indication of the lumen borders: the confidence level is supposed to give a high value in the vicinity of the lumen center. Furthermore, the positions where the casting of the ray is terminated, give an indication of the lumen border. This information can be used as an initialization for more sophisticated segmentation methods, like active contour models [10]. In the quantification process, the minimum length of the lines (d_{min}) used in determining the lumen center, is stored. This measure is not very robust to noise and irregularities in the image, but is used to give a quick overview of the vessel morphology.

4.2 Presentation of the results

When the method is applied to a CTA dataset, the results are presented in several ways. The central lumen line is displayed on the EasyVision workstation during the tracking process. The quantitative results are presented in a 'click able' graph, displaying the minimum diameter d_{min} and the confidence level CL at every cut plane, as shown in figure 5. The graph can be used to interactively

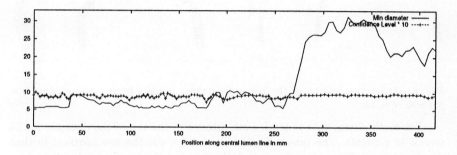

Fig. 5. Minimimum diameter in mm. and confidence level, $\sigma = 3, t = 4, N = 24$.

inspect the lumen cross sections. Pressing a position in the graph generates the corresponding cut plane along the computed central lumen line. Possible problem areas can thus be inspected.

During the tracking process, the end positions of the rays in every perpendicular plane are stored. Connecting these points to polygons yields a 3D representation of the computed lumen borders as shown in figure 6. This 3D representation can be interactively manipulated to get an overview of the tortuosity of the iliac trajectory, and the neck of the aneurysm.

5 Experiments and results

The method was applied to 15 patients. For every patient, a starting position was manually determined in both left and right iliac arteries. The CTA acquired for the evaluation of candidates for the endovascular procedure, typically consist of 183 slices of 512 x 512 pixels, with a pixel size of 0.49 mm, and an effective slice thickness of 2.0 mm. A total of 140 cc of contrast fluid is given intravenously with an injection rate of 3 cc/sec. Scanning is performed at 140 KV/225 mA., starting 30 seconds after onset of injection.

Based on experimental evidence, we selected default values for the free parameters t, σ and N, which remained fixed for all clinical studies.

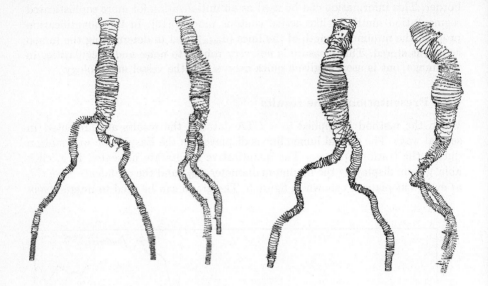

Fig. 6. 3D representations of the computed lumen borders from two patients, $\sigma = 3, t = 4, N = 24$.

The method was able to track both arteries to the top of the datasets for 14 out of 15 patients. The reason for the one failure was the low contrast in that specific dataset. The method accidentally detected the border of the thrombus, instead of the border of the lumen. The iliac arteries were correctly tracked in all the patients.

The average time for performing 150 iterations, including the computation of the d_{min} and the storage of the endpoints of the rays was less than one minute, on a SUN Sparc 5, 170 MHz.

6 Conclusions and future work

A method has been presented that is able to delineate an abdominal aorta aneurysm in less than one minute. The method is robust to typical problems occurring in 3D CTA data such as branching vessels, calcifications and shape variations. User initialization is minimal, and the clinician is able to supervise the tracking procedure interactively. The results are displayed in order to access problem areas quickly.

Initial experiments showed that in 14 out of 15 datasets, both vessels were completely tracked. Even in the highly curved iliac arteries the method was able to generate a central lumen line.

Currently, the results with respect to the minimum diameter are being validated with manually determined measurements. Also the method will be compared with manually determined central lumen lines.

The computed central lumen line and the estimated lumen borders will be used as an initialization for more advanced segmentation procedures.

Acknowledgments

We thank Dr Ivo Broeders from the Department of Vascular Surgery of our hospital for providing us the CTA datasets. Paul Desmedt from Philips Medical Systems Best is acknowledged for his help in building the prototype within the EasyScil reformat facility. This research is done within the context of the EASI project "European Applications for Surgical Interventions", subsidized by the European Commission under contract HC1012 in their "4th Framework Telematics Applications for Health" RTD programme.

References

1. I. A. J. M. Broeders, J. D. Blankensteijn, M. Olree, W. P. Th. M. Mali, and B. C. Eikelboom. Preoperative sizing of grafts for transfemoral endovascular aneurysm management: a prospective comparative study of spiral CT angiography, arteriography, and conventional CT imaging. *Journal of Endovascular Surgery*, 4:252–261, 1997.
2. C. Lorenz, I. C Carlsen, T. M. Buzug, C. Fassnacht, and J. Weese. Multi-scale line segmentation with automatic estimation of width, contrast and tangential direction in 2D and 3D medical images. In *Proc. CVRMed and MRCAS 1997*, number 1205 in Lecture notes in Computer Science, pages 233–242. Springer Verlag, Berlin, 1997.
3. V. Prinet and O. Monga. Vessel representation in 2D and 3D angiograms. In H. U. Lemke, M. W. Vannier, and K. Inamura, editors, *Computer Assisted Radiology and Surgery*, pages 240–245. Elsevier Publishers, Amsterdam, 1997.
4. Th. M. Koller, G. Gerig, G. Székely, and D. Dettwiler. Multiscale detection of curvilinear structures in 2D and 3D image data. In *Fifth International Conference on Computer Vision*, pages 864–869, 1995.
5. A. B. Houtsmuller, A. W. M. Smeulders, H. T. M. van der Voort, J. L. Oud, and N. Nanninga. The homing cursor: A tool for three-dimensional chromosome analysis. *Cytometry*, 14:501–509, 1993.
6. T. O'Donnel, A. Gupta, and T. Boult. A new model for the recovery of cylindrical structures from medical image data. In *Proc. CVRMed and MRCAS 1997*, number 1205 in Lecture notes in Computer Science, pages 223–232. Springer Verlag, Berlin, 1997.
7. V. Juhan, B. Nazarian, K. Malkani, R. Bulot, J. M. Bartoli, and J. Sequeira. Geometrical modelling of abdominal aortic aneurysms. In *Proc. CVRMed and MRCAS 1997*, number 1205 in Lecture notes in Computer Science, pages 243–252. Springer Verlag, Berlin, 1997.
8. J. Beier, R. Siekmann, F. Müller, J. Tröger, H. Schedel, G. Biamino, E. Fleck, and R. Felix. Planning and control of aortic stent implantations using 3D reconstructions based on computer tomography. In H. U. Lemke, M. W. Vannier, and K. Inamura, editors, *Computer Assisted Radiology*, pages 716–720. Elsevier Publishers, Amsterdam, 1996.
9. M. Fiebich, M. Tomiak Mitchell, R. M. Engelmann, and K. R. Hoffmann. Automatic segmentation in CT angiography of the abdominal aorta. In H. U. Lemke, M. W. Vannier, and K. Inamura, editors, *Computer Assisted Radiology and Surgery*, pages 277–282. Elsevier Publishers, Amsterdam, 1997.
10. M. Kass, A. P. Witkin, and D. Terzopoulos. Snakes: Active contour models. *International Journal of Computer Vision*, 1:321–331, 1988.

3-D Fusion of Biplane Angiography and Intravascular Ultrasound for Accurate Visualization and Volumetry

Andreas Wahle[1], Guido P. M. Prause[1,3], Steven C. DeJong[2], and Milan Sonka[1]

[1] The University of Iowa, Department of Electrical and Computer Engineering
Iowa City, IA 52242, USA
{andreas-wahle,milan-sonka}@uiowa.edu
[2] The University of Iowa, Department of Internal Medicine
Iowa City, IA 52242, USA
[3] MeVis Institute at the University of Bremen
D-28359 Bremen, Germany

Abstract. Coronary angiography delivers accurate information about the vessel topology and shape, but only limited data concerning the vessel cross-section. Intravascular ultrasound provides detailed information about the cross-sectional shape as well as the composition of vessel wall and plaque, but fails to consider the geometric relationships between adjacent images. In this paper, we present a new approach for combination of both methods to allow accurate assessment of coronary arteries regarding both longitudinal and cross-sectional dimensions.

1 Introduction

During the last decades, quantitative analyses from selective coronary contrast angiographic images have been established as de-facto standard for the diagnosis of coronary artery disease. Well-established systems for single-plane analysis of local stenoses [1–3] have been complemented by accurate spatial reconstructions from biplane angiograms, allowing assessment of complex diffuse disease affecting the entire coronary artery system [4–6]. However, the major limitation of X-ray angiography is its restriction to the inner lumen. The cross-sectional shape is mostly approximated by elliptical contours, and the wall thickness as well as the plaque composition cannot be determined at all.

Recently, intravascular ultrasound (IVUS) of the coronary arteries evolved as an additional method in cardiovascular diagnosis. A catheter with an ultrasonic transducer in its tip is placed at the distal end of the desired vessel segment and pulled back with an approximately constant speed during imaging. The luminal cross-sections can be determined as well as the wall thickness, and even the composition of the plaque [7–9]. On the other hand, IVUS is not able to consider vessel curvature and torsion when assigning the detected plaque to specific locations. Spatial reconstructions as performed up to now by straight stacking of the images are geometrically incorrect and thus do not allow proper volumetric analyses. For a correct reconstruction, the following effects have to be dealt with [10–12]:

- Due to vessel *curvature*, the IVUS slices are not parallel. Thus, volume fragments at the inner side of the vessel related to its curvature will be overestimated and fragments on the outer side underestimated during volumetric analysis.
- Due to vessel *torsion* as defined by differential geometry, the axial orientation of an ideal IVUS catheter within the vessel is no longer constant. The torsion of the catheter path is zero only if the vessel lies within a plane. Whenever the vessel moves outside of this plane, the catheter twists axially, and this rotation must be considered in the 3-D reconstruction as well.

Our solution for these problems is derived using the combination of the data obtained from coronary angiography and intravascular ultrasound to provide an exact assignment of the cross-sectional data to the vessel segment in both location and orientation. The 3-D vessel shape and topology are determined by accurate reconstruction from biplane angiograms of approximately known imaging geometry. The vessel cross-sections are extracted from IVUS data acquired in the same session as the angiographic images. For both tasks, our previously developed and validated systems are utilized.

2 Methods

2.1 Image Acquisition and Preprocessing

Placement and pullback of the IVUS catheter is usually supervised by fluoroscopy, thus all required data can be obtained in a single step. Both angiograms and IVUS images have to be digitized since they are usually acquired on conventional media like cine film and S-VHS tapes. It is desirable to avoid this step by direct digital access to the imaging devices in standardized formats in the near future.

While the IVUS sequence reflects the entire pullback, angiograms are taken only at the start of the pullback, eventually an additional pair at the end. A low amount of radio-opaque contrast dye may be injected to allow an identification of the vessel lumen without covering the IVUS catheter itself. A constant supervision of the catheter tip movement by angiography as proposed by Evans et al. [11] is not acceptable in clinical applications, due to physical limitations of the imaging device and the additional X-ray exposure of the patient.

The angiograms are corrected for geometric distortions like the pincushion and sigmoidal effects [13]. Further visual manipulations, e.g. edge enhancement by unsharp masking, adaptive histogram equalization, zooming, etc., can be performed to allow a better identification of the catheter (Fig. 1).

2.2 Generation of Spatial IVUS Frames

In this section, the basis for the geometrically correct reconstruction of the IVUS images is described. For each of the 2-D images, a 3-D *frame* is calculated, which

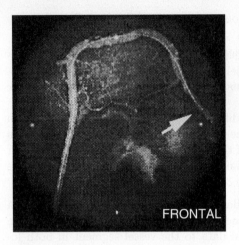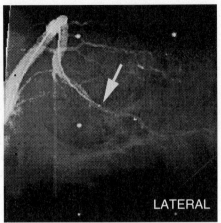

Fig. 1. Preprocessed biplane angiograms in a right coronary artery of an extracted cadaveric pig heart with inserted IVUS catheter; the arrows mark the location of the IVUS transducer at pullback start, i.e. at the most distal location.

represents a mapping function of the planar images into spatial dimensions. Once these frames are calculated, they may be filled with the plain pixel data as well as the high-level results from the segmentation. The frames are determined from the information contained in the angiograms, by extracting the path of the catheter, mapping the IVUS images to locations, and calculating their orientations.

Catheter Extraction. From the rectified angiograms, the catheter may be extracted by conventional methods for vessel detection [2, 3]. Furthermore, we developed a new dynamic programming approach to find the correct path of the catheter even in vessels filled with contrast dye. The starting point of the pullback has to be marked in both projections, and then some proximal guide points, at least up to the end of the pullback. The catheter is detected within an adaptable region of interest (ROI) along the guide points. A recent approach combines catheter extraction and 3-D reconstruction in a single step using active contour models (3-D *snakes* [14]).

3-D Reconstruction of the Trajectory. The IVUS catheter is reconstructed as a single line in 3-D without cross-sectional information from the angiographic projections. A single point, identified in both projections, can be reconstructed by calculating its projection rays in 3-D from the known imaging geometry. The reconstruction algorithm as initially reported in [13] has meanwhile been replaced by the comprehensive approach as developed at the German Heart Institute of Berlin [6, 15] to achieve higher accuracy. For each object point P visible in both projections p, its projection rays can be calculated from the known locations of the X-ray sources A_p and the points B_p, resulting from the transformation of the respective image points to image intensifier level. Theoretically, these rays should intersect in the original 3-D location P at imaging time, provided that the assumed imaging geometry is correct and both projection points have been identified accurately. Since this is hard to ensure, an approximation has to be performed to find the location of the point to be reconstructed. This is done by using the weighted mean of those points Q_p on both rays (A_p, B_p) that mark the nearest distance between them (Fig. 2).

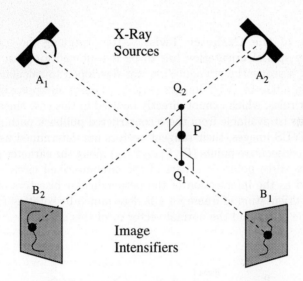

Fig. 2. Principle of point reconstruction from two projections.

After estimating the initial geometry from the parameters given by the gantry, the assumed imaging geometry is refined using n unique reference points in the angiograms by an approximation method minimizing the reconstruction error $|\mathbf{Q}_1(i) - \mathbf{Q}_2(i)|$ over all points $0 \leq i < n$.

Furthermore, the ray bundles resulting from the catheter extraction have to be matched, i.e. those pairs of elements have to be found that correspond in both projections. The initial discrete mapping algorithm as introduced by Parker et al. [16], which assigns pairs of 2-D elements within a cost matrix to yield the optimum combinations, has been extended to interpolate intermediate elements for determination of a more accurate correspondence. Further enhancements were done to stabilize the cost matrix approach when applied to larger vessel segments by smoothing in the correspondence domain, mainly to eliminate distortions from local roughness.

Mapping of the Image Locations. In the following step, the frame of each IVUS image has to be assigned to a specific location along the pullback path. Due to the fact that a continuous supervision of the catheter pullback is not available, its speed is assumed to be constant, which is approximately true if a mechanical pullback device is used [10]. Since the length from pullback start to any location on the path can be determined accurately [6, 15], the location of each frame can be determined from its timestamp. If — in addition to the start image — another biplane angiographic pair exists for the end of the pullback, this information can be used to calculate the real mean pullback speed for a better assignment.

Calculation of the Catheter Twist. After assigning the frames to their locations, the spatial orientation has to be determined for each of them. For this purpose, a sequential triangulation was developed to calculate the relative twist between adjacent IVUS images (Fig. 3). This is an approximation to the Frenet-Serret rules, which cannot directly be used in this case since only a set of discrete points ist available from the reconstructed pullback path. For each pair of adjacent IVUS images, their tangent vectors are determined using the three surrounding consecutive points (P_i, P_{i+1}, P_{i+2}) along the catheter path. The arc through these three points is a part of the circumscribed circle, whose center is determined as the intersection of the perpendicular bisectors of the tangent vectors. The orientation of frame $i+1$ is determined by rotating frame i by the enclosed angle α_i around the normal vector n_i of this triangle.

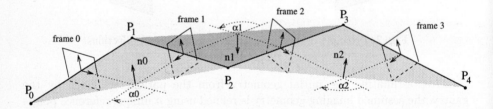

Fig. 3. Calculation of the relative twist by sequential triangulation.

Although the relative twist can be calculated, the absolute orientation remains ambiguous. One way to achieve a correct overall match of the IVUS and angiography data is to use anatomic landmarks like branching vessels. Unfortunately, the locations and orientations of branches frequently cannot be determined accurately enough both in angiographic and IVUS images [13]. Algorithms to solve this problem automatically by using additional information and physical constraints are under development. Currently, the absolute orientation is determined by user interaction.

Fig. 4 shows the reconstructed frames from the angiograms of Fig. 1. The longitudinally resampled slice of the geometrically correct reconstructed IVUS cube corresponds to the orientation of the frontal angiogram.

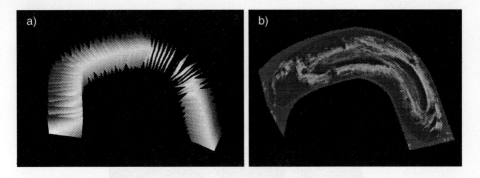

Fig. 4. Spatially correct IVUS reconstruction: a) Calculated IVUS frames with color-coded corners; b) after mapping the pixel data into the frames, a longitudinal slice of the descending arc has been extracted.

2.3 IVUS Segmentation

Our method as earlier described in [7] automatically identifies the plaque/media interface (internal lamina, internal wall border), the media/adventitia interface (external lamina, external wall border), and the plaque/lumen interface (plaque border). Due to the use of a-priori information about 2-D and 3-D anatomy of coronary vessels and ultrasound imaging physics, the method can automatically determine vessel wall morphology and plaque volumes. The two key aspects of the approach are as follows:

1. Graph searching is utilized to identify globally optimal borders.
2. A-priori information is incorporated into the border detection process through the computation of local cost values.

In particular, to identify the position of the internal and external wall borders, the method searches for edge triplets representing the leading and trailing edges of the laminae echoes. The interactively defined elliptical shape of the ROI serves as a model of the preferred vessel shape. Knowledge of the vessel wall thickness is also used to constrain the search for the external and internal wall borders.

To facilitate a fully automated 3-D analysis of IVUS pullback image sequences, the region of interest in which the borders are determined must be automatically identified when the 3-D border detection is performed. The 3-D border detection algorithm was designed to use contextual information for the estimation of the ROI size and position changes in the successive frames. The general steps of the 3-D IVUS segmentation algorithm are as follows: A single elliptic region of interest is interactively identified in the first image of the pullback sequence. Inside the ROI, internal and external wall, and plaque borders are automatically identified using the graph-search based segmentation approach. In subsequent images, current ROIs are automatically determined from the computer-detected borders in the preceding images.

Fig. 5 shows an example of automated inner and outer vessel wall detection in an IVUS image of the sequence for the angiograms in Fig. 1 with our algorithm.

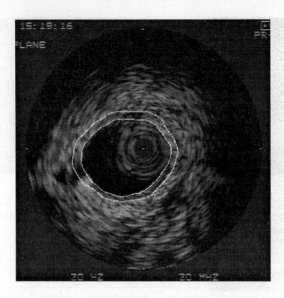

Fig. 5. Segmented IVUS image with inner and outer borders of the vessel wall.

2.4 3-D Visualization

After mapping of the pixel data into 3-D space, the volume cube may be analyzed with the conventional methods for volume rendering (Fig. 4b). A detailed surface model of the inner and outer borders of the vessel wall, as well as the plaque, can be generated after segmentation. This model is represented together with the spatially correct locations of the angiograms and the X-ray sources in a VRML-2.0 world, thus allowing visualizations platform-independently by any appropriate viewer (Fig. 6).

3 Results

3.1 Frame Mapping

For validation of the frame generation, studies in both phantoms and cadaveric pig hearts were performed. Analyses in helical phantoms have shown a good match of the measured and the analytically determined twist [12]. The predicted axial rotation of the IVUS images in helices of different displacements per revolution showed high correlations of $r=0.99$, but also some overestimation of the real twist by 0.87–1.0% per centimeter of pullback.

For the in-vitro studies in right coronary arteries, with a typical pullback length of 100–120 mm, the overall twisting range along individual pullbacks was 41.8° in the least tortuous up to 118.1° in the most tortuous vessel. Two of the hearts which we evaluated were supplied with metal markers (Fig. 7). Three pullbacks per heart were performed by a highly experienced person, instructed

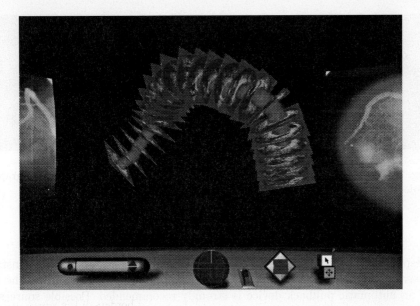

Fig. 6. VRML-2.0 model after triangulation of the segmented contours: internal and external laminae along with some IVUS images inserted according to their calculated spatial frames; X-ray sources (behind the viewpoint) and angiograms are included as well; the lower part of the scene shows the control panel of the VRML viewer.

to maintain a constant pullback speed of 1 mm/s. However, using the clips as landmarks, a pullback speed of 1.14±0.34 mm/s resulted, which indicates that the manual pullback is significantly non-uniform. The RMS error of the predicted frame orientations over all six pullbacks was 21.96° with a standard deviation of 4.87°. The highest deviations from mean were measured for the clips located in areas of high local twisting, where the slight mismatches in their locations are quite significant. Other important influences include intraobserver variability due to manual pullback with an RMS error of 5.01° (max. 27.5°), as well as additional twisting of the mechanically driven catheter system due to friction and non-uniform rotation distortions. In phantom experiments, the twisting showed errors up to 57° in areas of bending (curvature of 50° over a segment of 15 mm in length). During saline flush, we could measure a twisting of up to 70°, presumptively due to the increased pressure.

3.2 IVUS Segmentation

The automated method for the detection of borders in IVUS images was validated in cadaveric hearts as well as in-vivo in single images and image pullback sequences [7]. Lumen and plaque area measurements correlated well with those determined manually by expert observers (r=0.98, y=1.01x+1.51; r=0.94, y=1.06x−0.09; respectively). Root-mean-square wall and plaque border positioning errors were under 0.15 mm.

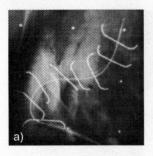 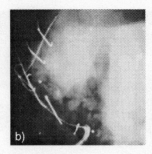 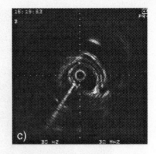

Fig. 7. Cadaveric pig heart with metal clips: a) frontal and b) lateral angiographic projections; c) IVUS image with peak caused by a clip.

4 Conclusion

Despite the fact that the manual pullback cannot be assumed to be of constant speed, the matching algorithms showed a very good accuracy. However, the use of an automatic pullback device is strongly recommended. Possible sources of the errors in the frame orientations, aside the manual pullback, were found in systematic torsions within the catheter system. These effects may be avoided or at least reduced by using solid-state catheter systems with no rotating parts.

In conclusion, our system provides high accuracy in 3-D reconstruction of the vessel topology, and a spatially correct assignment of plaque and wall data as delivered by the IVUS segmentation.

Acknowledgments

This work has been supported in part by grants Pr 507/1-2 and Wa 1280/1-1 of the *Deutsche Forschungsgemeinschaft*, Germany, and by grants IA-94-GS-65 and IA-96-GS-42 of the *American Heart Association*, Iowa Affiliate.

References

1. Kirkeeide R. L., Fung P., Smalling R. W., and Gould K. L., Automated evaluation of vessel diameter from arteriograms, in: Proc. Computers in Cardiology 1982, Seattle WA. IEEE-CS Press, Los Alamitos CA (1982) 215–218.
2. Beier J., Oswald H., Sauer H. U., and Fleck E., Accuracy of measurement in quantitative coronary angiography (QCA), in: Lemke H. U., Rhodes M. L., Jaffe C. C., and Felix R. (eds.), Computer Assisted Radiology (CAR '91). Springer, Berlin/New York (1991) 721–726.
3. Sonka M., Winniford M. D., and Collins S. M., Robust simultaneous detection of coronary borders in complex images. IEEE Transactions on Medical Imaging **14** (1995) 151–161.
4. Guggenheim N., Doriot P. A., Dorsaz P. A., Descouts P., and Rutishauser W., Spatial reconstruction of coronary arteries from angiographic images. Physics in Medicine and Biology **36** (1991) 99–110.

5. Seiler C., Kirkeeide R. L., and Gould K. L., Basic structure-function relations of the epicardial coronary vascular tree; basis of quantitative coronary arteriography for diffuse coronary artery disease. Circulation **85** (1992) 1987–2003.
6. Wahle A., Wellnhofer E., Mugaragu I., Sauer H. U., Oswald H., and Fleck E., Assessment of diffuse coronary artery disease by quantitative analysis of coronary morphology based upon 3-D reconstruction from biplane angiograms. IEEE Transactions on Medical Imaging **14** (1995) 230–241.
7. Sonka M., Zhang X., Siebes M., Bissing M. S., DeJong S. C., Collins S. M., and McKay C. R., Segmentation of intravascular ultrasound images: A knowledge-based approach. IEEE Transactions on Medical Imaging **14** (1995) 719–732.
8. Dijkstra J., Wahle A., Koning G., Reiber J. H. C., and Sonka M., Quantitative coronary ultrasound: State of the art, in: Reiber J. H. C. and van der Wall E. E. (eds.), What's New in Cardiovascular Imaging? Vol. 204 of Developments in Cardiovascular Medicine, Kluwer, Dordrecht (1998) 79–94.
9. Sonka M. and Zhang X., Assessment of plaque composition using intravascular ultrasound, in: Reiber J. H. C. and van der Wall E. E. (eds.), What's New in Cardiovascular Imaging? Vol. 204 of Developments in Cardiovascular Medicine, Kluwer, Dordrecht (1998) 183–196.
10. Laban M., Oomen J. A., Slager C. J., Wentzel J. J., Krams R., Schuurbiers J. C. H., den Boer A., von Birgelen C., Serruys P. W., and de Feyter P. J., ANGUS: A new approach to three-dimensional reconstruction of coronary vessels by combined use of angiography and intravascular ultrasound, in: Proc. Computers in Cardiology 1995, Vienna AT. IEEE Press, Piscataway NJ (1995) 325–328.
11. Evans J. L., Ng K. H., Wiet S. G., Vonesh M. J., Burns W. B., Radvany M. G., Kane B. J., Davidson C. J., Roth S. I., Kramer B. L., Meyers S. N., and McPherson D. D., Accurate three-dimensional reconstruction of intravascular ultrasound data; spatially correct three-dimensional reconstructions. Circulation **93** (1996) 567–576.
12. Prause G. P. M., DeJong S. C., McKay C. R., and Sonka M., Towards a geometrically correct 3-D reconstruction of tortuous coronary arteries based on biplane angiography and intravascular ultrasound. International Journal of Cardiac Imaging **13** (1997) 451–462.
13. Prause G. P. M., DeJong S. C., McKay C. R., and Sonka M., Semi-automated segmentation and 3-D reconstruction of coronary trees: Biplane angiography and intravascular ultrasound data fusion, in: Proc. Medical Imaging 1996: Physiology and Function from Multidimensional Images, Newport Beach CA. Vol. 2709, SPIE, Bellingham WA (1996) 82–92.
14. Molina C., Prause G. P. M., Radeva P., and Sonka M., 3-D catheter path reconstruction from biplane angiograms, in: Proc. Medical Imaging 1998: Image Processing, San Diego CA. Vol. 3338, SPIE, Bellingham WA (1998) 504–512.
15. Wahle A., Präzise dreidimensionale Rekonstruktion von Gefäßsystemen aus biplanen angiographischen Projektionen und deren klinische Anwendung. No. 152 in Fortschritt-Berichte, Reihe Biotechnik (17), VDI Verlag, Düsseldorf (1997).
16. Parker D. L., Pope D. L., van Bree R. E., and Marshall H. W., Three-dimensional reconstruction of moving arterial beds from digital subtraction angiography. Computers and Biomedical Research **20** (1987) 166–185.

Patient-Specific Analysis of Left Ventricular Blood Flow

Timothy N. Jones and Dimitris N. Metaxas

VAST Lab, Department of Computer and Information Science
University of Pennsylvania, Philadelphia, PA 19104-6389, USA
tnj@graphics.cis.upenn.edu, dnm@central.cis.upenn.edu
http://www.cis.upenn.edu/~tnj/

Abstract. We use a computational fluid dynamics (CFD) solver to simulate the flow of blood through the left ventricle (LV). Boundary conditions for the solver are derived from actual heart wall motion as measured by MRI-SPAMM. This novel approach allows for the first time a patient-specific LV blood flow simulation using exact boundary conditions.

1 Introduction

The development of a patient specific LV blood flow simulator is an open and challenging research problem. There are imaging techniques such as phase velocity MR which can indirectly measure velocity, but the resulting data must be reconstructed and tends to be very noisy and requires significant post-processing to be of any use. A detailed description of these methods is beyond the scope of this paper. There has been a large body of work in the mechanical engineering literature over the past few decades related to the computational simulation of fluid dynamics (CFD). Some of the more approachable texts are those of Ferziger and Perić [3], Fletcher [4], Patankar [7], and Roache [11]. There have been many varieties of numerical methods developed for simulating different types of fluids (liquids and gases) with various physical properties (density and viscosity) undergoing varying types of flows (laminar, turbulent, supersonic) in different types of physical environments (those with external temperature and chemical influences). While the general problem of CFD is one of the more challenging in computational science, good results have been obtained using techniques designed for specific problems.

Several researchers have developed CFD techniques to simulate blood flow through the heart with varying degrees of realism. Peskin and McQueen [9][5] developed the immersed fiber method, in which the heart wall is modeled by a woven stand of fibers immersed in a viscous, incompressible fluid. The fibers are arranged in a shape which approximates that of the heart, and exert forces in the tangential direction. These forces are applied to the Navier-Stokes equations to induce motion in the fluid. The result is an effect similar to that caused by the contracting heart wall. While the results are convincing from a computational point of view, the fibers have no physical connection to the actual heart. Yoganathan et al. [15] later addressed the anatomical issue by constructing the fibers to represent the shape of the LV. Pelle et al. [8] used the Laplace equation to simulate velocity in a cylindrical model of the LV, neglecting viscous effects and assuming irrotational flow. The Bernoulli equation computes pressure from velocity in a linked model. The velocity equations were augmented with terms to more closely approximate the local structure of the heart wall. Thomas and Weyman [14] used a Navier-Stokes solver to simulate ventricular filling in a simplified geometrical model. Dubini et al. [2] used a Navier-Stokes solver to simulate the installation of a by-pass device in a simplified model of the right ventricle. Taylor et al. [13] used the shape of a digitized canine LV in a Navier-Stokes simulation. The motion of the wall was described by having it moved toward the center of the aortic outlet.

While these contributions and others have allowed important quantitative analysis of simplified models of hearts, none of them have used realistic data from actual patients. The goal of our work has been to address this shortcoming. In this paper, we adapt a computational fluid dynamics (CFD) solver to develop for the first time a patient specific blood flow simulator for the left ventricle (LV). Boundary conditions for the solver are derived from actual heart wall motion as measured by MRI-SPAMM. Visualization of preliminary results is presented.

2 Boundary Data Extraction

The model of blood flow described in the next section uses as input boundary data extracted from the LV's endocardium motion. The volumetric analysis of the LV from MRI-SPAMM data was developed by Park et al.[6]. The method uses as input boundary and tagged data to fit a volumetric deformable model with parameter functions that can capture the motion of the LV. These parameters capture the contraction and twist of the LV which are essential for modeling correctly the blood flow within the LV. In this paper we use the 3D time-varying position of points on the LV endocardium that are sampled from the volumetric LV model. These data are used as boundary conditions in the blood flow simulation described next.

3 Modeling Blood Flow

In this section we describe the equations that govern the dynamics of our blood flow model.

We use an Eulerian approach for the description of the flow field, in which the variables (pressure and velocity) of the fluid are solved for across the domain of interest. The Lagrangian formulation, in which variables of the fluid are tracked at the position of an object (such as a blood molecule) as it moves through the domain, or mixed Eulerian-Lagrangian formulation, are useful in other situations such as solid body dynamics or mixed media interfaces and will not be used here.

The fundamental laws to be considered in the description of fluid flow are the conservation of mass (continuity) and momentum, repectively:

$$\frac{dm}{dt} = 0 \quad \text{and} \quad \frac{d(m\mathbf{v})}{dt} = \sum \mathbf{f}, \tag{1}$$

where m is mass, t is time, $\mathbf{v}$ is velocity, and $\mathbf{f}$ are forces.

Our Eulerian approach deals not with parcels of matter, but rather with parcels of space known as control volumes. We therefore need to convert the control mass-oriented conservation equations above into control volume-oriented forms. The amount of mass in a control mass CM can be defined as:

$$m = \int_{\Omega_{CM}} \rho d\Omega, \qquad (2)$$

where Ω_{CM} is the volume of the control mass and ρ is the density of the matter. Inserting this definition into Eq. 1 and applying Green's theorem yields the control volume equation for mass conservation (for control volumes fixed in space):

$$\frac{\partial}{\partial t}\int_{\Omega_{CM}} \rho d\Omega = \frac{\partial}{\partial t}\int_{\Omega_{CV}} \rho d\Omega + \int_{S_{CV}} \rho \mathbf{v} \cdot \mathbf{n} dS = 0, \qquad (3)$$

where Ω_{CV} is the volume of the control volume CV, S_{CV} is the surface of the control volume, and $\mathbf{n}$ is the outward-facing normal to the surface. This equation states that the rate of change of the amount of mass of a control volume is the rate of change within the volume plus the next flux of mass through the boundaries of the volume due to fluid motion (convection). For incompressible fluids (liquids) such as blood, density is constant and the first term in Eq. 3 disappears, leaving:

$$\int_S \rho \mathbf{v} \cdot \mathbf{n} dS = 0. \qquad (4)$$

Applying a similar technique to the momentum equation yields the control volume form:

$$\frac{\partial}{\partial t}\int_{\Omega_{CV}} \rho \mathbf{v} d\Omega + \int_{S_{CV}} \rho \mathbf{v}\mathbf{v} \cdot \mathbf{n} dS = \sum \mathbf{f}. \qquad (5)$$

The forces $\mathbf{f}$ in the momentum equation are surface forces such as pressure and stress and body forces such as buoyancy and gravity. The blood is treated as a Newtonian fluid, that is, one in which stress is linearly dependent on velocity. The stress tensor, which represents the rate of transport of momentum, with constant viscosity is then:

$$\mathsf{T} = -p\mathsf{I} + \mu(\mathrm{grad}\mathbf{v}), \qquad (6)$$

where μ is the dynamic viscosity, I is the unit tensor, and p is the static pressure. Ignoring body forces and utilizing Eq. 6 in Eq. 5 the momentum conservation equation becomes:

$$\frac{\partial}{\partial t}\int_{\Omega_{CV}} \rho \mathbf{v} d\Omega + \int_{S_{CV}} \rho \mathbf{v}\mathbf{v} \cdot \mathbf{n} dS = \int_{S_{CV}} \mathsf{T} \cdot \mathbf{n} dS. \qquad (7)$$

The continuity and momentum equations are collectively referred to as the Navier-Stokes equations.

4 Numerical Methods

We describe the technique we use to approximate the continuous equations of our mathematical model with discrete versions suitable for solution on a computer.

4.1 Discretization

Any system of partial differential/integral equations such as those in our mathematical model derived above must be approximated by algebraic equations for solution on a computer. This is done by defining a numerical grid, which samples points in space with nodes. The original equations are approximated by a system of linear algebraic equations in which the values of the variables at the grid nodes are the unknowns. Each node provides one algebraic equation which relates variable values at that node with the values at neighboring nodes on the grid. This is assembled into a system of the form:

$$a_P \phi_P + \sum_k a_k \phi_k = q_P, \tag{8}$$

where ϕ represents the unknown, P denotes the node at which the equation is being solved, k spans the neighboring nodes involved in the approximations, the a are coefficients involving geometrical and fluid properties, and q contains the terms in which all variable values are known (source terms). The system can be written in matrix form as:

$$\mathbf{A}\phi = \mathbf{q}, \tag{9}$$

where $\mathbf{A}$ is the coefficient matrix, ϕ is the vector containing the variables at the grid nods, and $\mathbf{q}$ is the vector containing the source terms. The solution of this system will be addressed below. For now we are only interested in its construction.

There are several methods for discretizing partial differential equations. The finite difference method is the oldest and simplest to implement. The partial derivatives in the differential form of the conservation equations are replaced by approximations in terms of nodal values of the variables. A structured grid is used. In the finite element method, the domain of interest is divided into a set of discrete volumes, or elements, that may be unstructured. The equations in the mathematical model are multiplied by a weight function before being integrated over the domain. The weight function describes how the variable varies over an element. While this method provides the most accuracy in irregular geometric domains, the formulation of the element equations does not have an easy physical interpretation.

The finite volume method, which we employ, divides the domain of interest into a finite number of small control volumes (cells), and places the numerical grid nodes at the center of the cells[3][7]. The grid is constructed such that adjacent cells share a face. The sum of the integral equations derived in the previous section for the individual cells is then equal to the global equation since surface integrals for adjacent cells cancel out. To obtain algebraic equations for each cell, the integrals must be approximated by quadrature formulae. A diagram of a 2D finite volume is shown in Fig. 1.

In Cartesian coordinates, 3D cells have six faces, denoted e, w, n, s, t, and b. Net boundary flux through a cell is the sum of integrals over the faces:

$$\int_S f \mathrm{d}S = \sum_k \int_{S_k} f \mathrm{d}S, \tag{10}$$

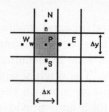

Fig. 1. 2D finite volume around node P, neighbors E, W, N, S, faces e, w, n, s

where k spans the six faces and f is the component of the convective or diffusive vector in the direction normal to the face k. The surface integral in the right side of Eq. 10 is approximated in terms of variable values at a finite number of locations on the face. The values on the face are approximated in terms of nodal values at the two cells which share the face. We use the midpoint rule, a second-order accurate method in which the integral is approximated as the product of the variable value at the face center and the area of the face. For the face 'e' we have:

$$F_e = \int_{S_e} f dS \approx f_e S_e. \qquad (11)$$

Since variables are solved for at nodes which lie in the center of cells, the value at the face centers must be interpolated. These values must be obtained with at least second-order accuracy to maintain that of the midpoint rule. Central differencing, described above, is a suitable approach.

Approximation of volume integrals is performed similarly to that of surface integrals; the volume integral is replaced by the product of the variable value at the center of the cell and the volume of the cell.

4.2 Matrix System Construction

For the unsteady term of Eq. 7, we use a second order three time level scheme. This leads to the approximation:

$$(\frac{\partial}{\partial t} \int_\Omega \rho u_i d\Omega)_P \approx \frac{\rho \Delta \Omega}{2 \Delta t}(3u_i^{n+1} - 4u_i^n + u_i^{n-1}) = A_P^t u_{i,P}^{n+1} - Q_{u_i}^t, \qquad (12)$$

where:

$$A_P^t = \frac{3\rho \Delta \Omega}{2 \Delta t} \quad \text{and} \quad Q_{u_i}^t = \frac{\rho \Delta \Omega}{2 \Delta t}(4u_i^n - u_i^{n-1}). \qquad (13)$$

The index n refers to the time iteration step.

We split the surface integrals in the convective, viscous, and pressure terms into six faces as described above. The nonlinear terms are approximated by the product of an old value (from the preceding iteration) and a new value. The mass flux across the 'e' face is:

$$\dot{m}_e^m = \int_{S_e} \rho \mathbf{v} \cdot \mathbf{n} dS \approx (\rho u)_e^{m-1} S_e, \qquad (14)$$

where m refers to the implicit solver iteration step. The convective flux of u_i momentum is then:

$$F_{i,e}^c = \int_S \rho u_i \mathbf{v} \cdot \mathbf{n} dS \approx \dot{m}_e u_{i,e}. \tag{15}$$

The diffusive flux requires the stresses τ_{xx}, τ_{yx}, and τ_{zx} at the face 'e'. Central difference approximations give:

$$(\tau_{xx})_e = \mu \left(\frac{\partial u}{\partial x}\right)_e \approx \mu \frac{u_E - u_P}{x_E - x_P}, \tag{16}$$

and similarly for $(\tau_{yx})_e$ and $(\tau_{zx})_e$.

The pressure term is approximated by:

$$Q_u^P = -\int_S p\mathbf{i} \cdot \mathbf{n} dS \approx -(p_e S_e - p_w S_w)^{m-1}, \tag{17}$$

which leads to the complete approximation for the momentum equation:

$$A_P^t u_{i,P} + F_i^c - F_i^d = Q_i^t + Q_i^P, \tag{18}$$

where:

$$F^c = F_e^c + F_w^c + F_n^c + F_s^c + F_t^c + F_b^c, \tag{19}$$
$$F^d = F_e^d + F_w^d + F_n^d + F_s^d + F_t^d + F_b^d. \tag{20}$$

The complete algebraic system for the u momentum has the form:

$$A_P^u u_P + \sum_k A_k^u u_k = Q_P^u \tag{21}$$

The coefficient A_E in the A matrix is:

$$A_E^u = \min(\dot{m}_e^u, 0) - \frac{\mu S_e}{x_E - x_P}, \tag{22}$$

and the coefficients for the other faces are analogous. The A_P coefficient is:

$$A_P^u = A_P^t - \sum_k A_k^u, \tag{23}$$

and the Q vector is:

$$Q_P^u = Q_u^t + Q_u^p. \tag{24}$$

The construction of the system for the v and w equations are analogous.

Pressure Correction Because the solution for the momentum equations uses old values of pressure for the calculation of the pressure term (Eq. 17), the result does not in general satisfy the continuity equation. To resolve this problem, we use the SIMPLE algorithm first developed by Caretto et al. [1]. We first solve the momentum equations as described above, and then gradually "correct" the pressure, and hence the velocity by way of the pressure term, until the continuity equation is satisfied to within some small numerical tolerance.

For the continuity equation to be satisfied, the net mass flux through a cell must be zero. After solving the momentum equations above, the net mass flux is:

$$\Delta \dot{m}_P = \dot{m}_e + \dot{m}_w + \dot{m}_n + \dot{m}_s + \dot{m}_t + \dot{m}_b. \tag{25}$$

The velocity corrections u', v', and w' will cause this term to become zero.

The pressure correction p' is related to the velocity correction u' by:

$$u'_e = -\frac{\sum_k A_k^u u'_k}{A_P} - \frac{S_e}{A_P^u}(p'_E - p'_P). \tag{26}$$

Substituting this into the continuity equation leads to the pressure-correction equation:

$$A_P^p p'_P + \sum_k A_k^p p'_k = -\Delta \dot{m}_P, \tag{27}$$

where the A coefficients are:

$$A_P^p = -\sum_k A_k^p \quad \text{and} \quad A_E^p = -\left(\frac{\rho S^2}{A_P^u}\right)_e, \tag{28}$$

and similarly for the other faces.

4.3 Matrix System Solution

The construction of our discrete approximation to the Navier-Stokes equations results in a matrix system in the form of Eq. 9. Many techniques have been devised to solve such systems, but they vary greatly in their utility (see Press et al. [10] for an excellent overview). Direct methods are applicable to any type of matrix, but their poor performance prevents their use in most interesting engineering problems. Gauss elimination, the most basic method, reduces a matrix to an upper triangular form through a series of linear operations on rows or columns. A back substitution phase then computes the unknowns from the upper triangular matrix. LU decomposition improves on the Gauss technique by constructing the triangular matrix in a way that does not require the source vector, resulting in considerable speedup for systems that use the same coefficient matrix repeatedly. Structured matrices, in which non-zero coefficients occur in small, structured areas of the matrix such as along the diagonal, reduce the computational and storage complexity of solvers for them substantially, but direct solvers are frequently still too slow for practical application.

Iterative solvers start out with an approximate solution to the system (for example, the solution at the previous time iteration), and add a residual to the solution until the unknown reaches zero (to within a small tolerance). Using large residuals allows the solver to complete faster, but too large a residual induces divergence, in which the solution error increases. Our numerical method uses the algorithm of Stone's "strongly implicit solver" [12], an iterative solver specifically designed for approximations to partial differential equations. The matrices resulting from these approximations are highly structured, with non-zero coefficients occuring only along the main diagonal and a few nearby neighboring diagonals (depending on the neighborhood used in the approximation of derivatives). An approximate LU decomposition is performed in which the resulting triangular matrices have a similar sparsity to the original matrix. Stone's method takes advantage of the smoothness of the PDEs being solved to greatly improve convergence.

5 Boundary Conditions

In this section we describe the boundary condition requirements of our mathematical model and numerical implementation, and how we derive them from MRI-SPAMM LV wall motion data.

The Navier-Stokes equations require boundary conditions at all points on the boundary of the solution domain for uniqueness. These are either Dirichlet conditions, in which the velocity at a boundary point is specified, or Neumann conditions, in which the derivative of velocity at a boundary point is specified. In the latter case, velocity values at interior points adjacent to the boundary are extrapolated to satisfy the derivative condition.

For our finite volume discretization, this means that the solution domain must be surrounded by boundary cells. We utilize three types of boundary cells: inlet (Dirichlet), outlet (Neumann), and wall (zero normal velocity). At walls, the convective flux in the normal direction and normal viscous stress are zero. At inlet boundaries, the velocity normal to the boundary (mass flux) is usually specified. This specification of velocity at wall and inlet boundaries means that the pressure correction across these boundaries should be zero. This is implemented by extrapolating pressure at the exterior cells along the boundary so that the pressure gradient across the interior boundary cells is zero. Outlet cells generally have a zero velocity gradient in the normal direction. These boundaries are ignored in the momentum equations, and their values copied from the adjacent interior cells. Their mass flux is allowed to adjust during the pressure correction step to ensure continuity.

We approximate sloped or curved boundaries by blocking off cells in our regular grid which lie outside the true boundary. While this introduces a discretization error, good results can be obtained by using a sufficiently fine grid resolution. Alternative coordinate representations such as cylindrical can also reduce this error for appropriate shapes such as the LV.

5.1 Heart Wall Boundary Conditions

Our goal in this work has been to simulate the flow through the LV of specific patients. The availability of MRI-SPAMM imaging tools provides us with a motion model of the walls of the LV. We use the motion data computed for the inner wall as boundary conditions as we now describe.

The output of the MRI-SPAMM tracking algorithm is a 4D time-series of the positions of fixed points on the LV wall throughout the cardiac cycle. Dividing the displacement of point positions by the time period computed from the pulse rate gives us the velocity at a finite number of positions on the wall. Unfortunately, these points are irregularly sampled, so we must interpolate them at regular intervals corresponding to our numerical grid. We do this by connecting the points on the wall to form a surface using splines or line segments. This wall surface is then intersected with planes which cut through the numerical grid at regular intervals along a specified axis. This intersection gives us a 2D cross section of the wall surface. The intersection plane is then divided into cells corresponding to the spacing of our numerical grid along the other two axes. A series of point-in-polygon tests is used to compute the grid cells which the wall surface intersects. The union of the intersection cells across all cut planes through the dataset provides us with the boundary cells required to solve the mathematical model. Because the boundary cells correspond to points on the wall surface, and the MRI-SPAMM data provides us with the velocity of these points, the boundary cells are of the inlet type. Recalling that "inlet" refers to the Dirichlet condition, the fact that the wall may be expanding at these points does not present a problem - the term inlet merely indicates a specified velocity and not the direction of fluid flow. Because the velocities at the boundary cells are interpolated from the irregularly sampled MRI-SPAMM data points, the velocities on the numerical grid boundaries are scaled to yield the same total flux across the wall.

The "outlet" (Neumann) boundaries are more complex. Because the MRI-SPAMM method does not track the base of the LV containing the valve, our input model is "open-ended." The results presented here treated the entire open area as an outlet area, but any valve model is straightforward to implement. Different valve configurations can be simulated by reconfiguring the boundary cells at the base, or improved MRI techniques in the future which image the base will be handled automatically by our method.

6 Results

We show the results of our method on a sample MRI-SPAMM dataset from a normal subject of a half cardiac cycle from end diastole to end systole.

Figure 2 shows a visualization of the blood flow in three frames of a half cardiac cycle. A small number of points was seeded across a plane perpendicular to the long axis and integrated in both time directions with the velocity field. The lines indicate the paths of the points, and the cones indicate the direction of motion. Speed is indicated by color. A 40x20x20 numerical grid was used with 40 slices perpendicular to the long axis of the LV. Approximately 1500 boundary points (depending on the frame) were interpolated from 91 MRI-SPAMM data points. Figure 2(a) is at end diastole, as the LV starts to contract. We see that the velocity shows a strong outflow pattern to the center of the base. Flow along the walls is toward the apex, which is consistent with the contraction of the walls. Figure 2(b) is a bottom view (from the apex) of the flow at end diastole. Here we can clearly see the rotational pattern induced in the blood flow by the twisting motion of the endocardium. The flat side of the cones indicates the outward (toward the base) motion of the flow in the interior region, while

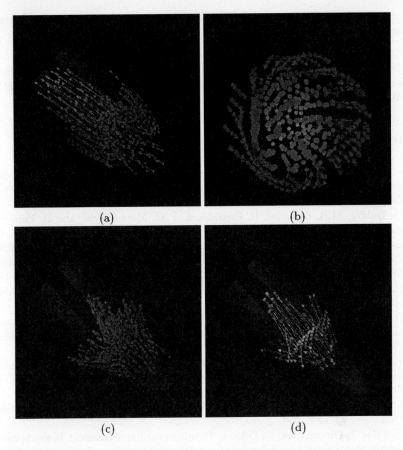

Fig. 2. Visualization of blood flow: (a) end diastole, (b) end diastole from apex, (c) mid systole, (d) end systole

the motion along the walls is in the opposite direction. Figure 2(c) is midway through systole, and we see the outflow pattern beginning to diminish as the LV approaches full contraction. The shorter lines indicate reduced speed as the flow begins to change direction. Figure 2(d) is at end systole, as the LV is beginning to expand again. Here we see the flow pattern from the base reversed, as blood begins to rush in again. Flow along the walls is directed away from the apex, consistent with the wall motion as the LV begins to expand.

7 Conclusions

In this paper we have described a novel approach to the patient-specific simulation of blood flow within the left ventricle. By utilizing MRI-SPAMM data as boundary conditions to a Navier-Stokes based CFD solver, we are able to produce convincing results which capture the full 3D contraction and twist of endocardial motion. Results from a sample dataset qualitatively consistent with clinical experience are presented. Ongoing work focuses on the application of our method to various types of cardiac disease and the extraction of relevant quantitative information.

8 Acknowledgements

This research has been funded by grants from the NSF (Career Award 96-24604), the Whitaker Foundation, and the NIH/NLM (LM06638-01).

References

1. L.S. Caretto, A.D. Gosman, S.V. Patankar, and D.B. Spalding. Two calculation procedures for steady, three-dimensional flows with recirculation. In *Proc. 3rd Int. Conf. Num. Methods Fluid Dyn.*, 1972.
2. G. Dubini, M.R. de Leval, R. Pietrabissa, F.M. Montevecchi, and R. Fumero. A numerical fluid mechanical study of repaired congenital heart defects. application to the total cavopulmonary connection. *J. Biomechanics*, 29(1):111–121, 1996.
3. J.H. Ferziger and M. Perić. *Computational Methods for Fluid Dynamics*. Springer-Verlag, 1996.
4. C.A.J. Fletcher. *Computational Techniques for Fluid Dynamics*. Springer-Verlag, 1991.
5. D.M. McQueen and C.S. Peskin. A three-dimensional computational method for blood flow in the heart: Ii. contractile fibers. *J. Computational Physics*, 82:289–297, 1989.
6. J. Park, D. Metaxas, and L. Axel. Analysis of left ventricular wall motion based on volumetric deformable models and mri-spamm. *Medical Image Analysis*, 1(1):53–71, 1996.
7. S.V. Patankar. *Numerical Heat Transfer and Fluid Flow*. Hemisphere Publishing, 1980.
8. G. Pelle, J. Ohayon, and C. Oddou. Trends in cardiac dynamics: Towards coupled models of intracavity fluid dynamics and deformable wall mechanics. *J. de Physique III*, 4(6):1121–1127, 1994.
9. C.S. Peskin and D.M. McQueen. A three-dimensional computational method for blood flow in the heart: I. immersed elastic fibers in a viscous incompressible fluid. *J. Computational Physics*, 81:372–405, 1989.
10. W.H. Press, S.A. Teukolsky, W.T. Vetterling, and B.P. Flannery. *Numerical Recipes in C*. Cambridge, 2nd ed. edition, 1992.
11. P.J. Roache. *Computational Fluid Dynamics*. Hermosa Publishers, 1972.
12. S.H. Stone. Iterative solution of implicit approximations of multidimensional partial differential equations. *SIAM J. Numerical Analysis*, 5:530–558, 1968.
13. T.W. Taylor, H. Suga, Y. Goto, H. Okino, and T. Yamaguchi. The effects of cardiac infarction on realistic three-dimensional left ventricular blood ejection. *Trans. ASME*, 118:106–110, 1996.
14. J.D. Thomas and A.E. Weyman. Numerical modeling of ventricular filling. *Annals Biomedical Engineering*, 20(1):19–39, 1992.
15. A.P. Yoganathan, Jr. J.D. Lemmon, Y.H. Kim, P.G. Walker, R.A. Levine, and C.C. Vesier. A computational study of a thin-walled three-dimensional left ventricle during early systole. *J. Biomechanical Engineering*, 116:307–314, 1994.

Dense 2D Displacement Reconstruction from SPAMM-MRI with Constrained Elastic Splines: Implementation and Validation[1]

Amir A. Amini[1], Yasheng Chen[1], Jean Sun[1], and Vaidy Mani[2]

[1] CVIA Lab, Box 8086, 660 S. Euclid,
Washington University Medical Center, St. Louis, MO 63110
email: amini@mobius.wustl.edu
home page: http://www-cv.wustl.edu
[2] Iterated Systems, Inc., Atlanta, Georgia

Abstract. Efficient constrained thin-plate spline warps are proposed in this paper which can warp an area in the plane such that two embedded snake grids obtained from two SPAMM frames are brought into registration, interpolating a dense displacement vector field. The reconstructed vector field adheres to the known displacement information at the intersections, forces corresponding snakes to be warped into one another, and for all other points in the myocardium, where no information is available, a C^1 continuous vector field is interpolated. The formalism proposed in this paper improves on our previous variational-based implementation and generalizes warp methods to include biologically relevant contiguous open curves, in addition to standard landmark points. The method has been extensively validated with a cardiac motion simulator, in addition to *in-vivo* tagging data sets.

1 Introduction

MR tagging is an imaging method which offers an excellent technique for measuring non-rigid motion of the myocardium. With this method, the magnetization property of selective material points are altered in order to create dark stripe patterns within a deforming body such as the heart muscle. The resulting pattern defines a time-varying curvilinear coordinate system on the tissue [5, 15], which deforms with the contracting tissue. Tagged MRI, however, is limited in that it can only mark a sparse set of lines and points in the myocardial tissue for tracking of deformations. The problem which we address in this paper is that of reconstruction of dense motion fields from sparse noisy data, not very different from the surface reconstruction problem encountered in stereo vision [8, 12]. An original solution to the motion reconstruction problem was proposed in [1, 3].

---
[1] Supported in part by a grant from Whitaker Biomedical Engineering Foundation, and grant IRI-9796207 from the National Science Foundation

However, in this formulation only information at tag crossings were utilized as part of the reconstruction algorithm. In [2], the method was further extended to that of constrained thin-plate reconstruction of the displacement field from points and lines based on a variational solution (for related work, also please see [11].) In this paper, we improve on the reconstruction paradigm in [2] and present extensive validation of the methodologies. One advantage of this line of work is that it allows for reconstruction of dense deformations between 2 arbitrary frames in a sequence of tagged images, as dense motion reconstruction methods generally produce displacement vector fields relative to undeformed tags in the initial frame. (For related work by other researchers please see [7, 9, 14].)

2 Constrained Thin-Plate Splines

Tracking tissue deformations with SPAMM using snake grids provides 2D displacement information at tag intersections and 1D displacement information along other 1D snake points [2]. The displacement measurement from tag lines however are sparse; interpolation is required to reconstruct a dense displacement field from which strain, torsion, and other mechanical indices of function can be computed at all myocardial points. In this section, we describe an efficient solution to the formulation in [2] (this improves on methods in computation time and order of convergence) for reconstructing a dense displacement vector field using localized coordinates of tag positions. In this development, we assume only 2D motion (as is roughly the case towards the apical end of the heart). Although thin-plate warps have been investigated by Bookstein [6], they have been used to interpolate a warp given specified landmarks.

To proceed more formally, the vector field continuity constraint is the bending energy of a thin-plate which is applied to the x and y component of the displacement field $(u(x,y), v(x,y))$:

$$\Phi_1 = \int\int u_{xx}^2 + 2u_{xy}^2 + u_{yy}^2 \, dxdy + \\ \int\int v_{xx}^2 + 2v_{xy}^2 + v_{yy}^2 \, dxdy \qquad (1)$$

This serves as the smoothness constraint on the reconstructed vector field, characterizing approximating thin-plate splines.

With intersection "springs" in place, the intersections of two grids are "pulled" towards one another by minimizing

$$\Phi_2 = \sum (u - u_{int})^2 + (v - v_{int})^2 \qquad (2)$$

In (2), u_{int} and v_{int} are the x and y components of displacement at tag intersections as well as at intersections of myocardial contours with tag lines. The form of the intersection spring constraints is similar to depth constraints in surface reconstruction from stereo, and has also been used in a similar spirit in [14].

Assuming 2D tissue motion, a further physical constraint is necessary: any point on a snake in one frame must be displaced to lie on its corresponding snake in all subsequent frames. This constraint is enforced by introducing a sliding spring. One endpoint of the spring is fixed on a grid line in the first frame, and its other endpoint is allowed to slide along the corresponding snake in the second frame, as a function of iterations. We minimize

$$\Phi_3 = \sum \left\{ (x + u - \bar{x})^2 + (y + v - \bar{y})^2 \right\} \quad (3)$$

along 1D snake points. In the above equation, (x, y) are the coordinates of a point on the snake in the current frame, and $(\bar{x}, \bar{y})$ is the closest point to $(x + u, y + v)$ on the corresponding snake in the second frame.

2.1 Conjugate gradient and quasi-Newton algorithms

Let $(u(x,y), v(x,y))$ be the displacement field as before. The objective function $\Phi(u,v)$ which needs to be minimized is the linear combination

$$\Phi = \lambda_1 \Phi_1 + \lambda_2 \Phi_2 + \lambda_3 \Phi_3. \quad (4)$$

Note that $\bar{x}$ and $\bar{y}$ are dependent on u and v respectively which makes the function $\Phi_3(u,v)$ non-quadratic. We can derive the Euler-Lagrange equations for the variational problem in (4) and solve the resulting system of equations [2]. In this paper, we develop a more efficient approach. We follow [8] and straightaway discretize the function Φ in (4). Assuming the distance between two adjacent grid points to be

$$u_{i+1,j} - u_{ij} = u_{i,j+1} - u_{ij} = h, \quad (5)$$

the second order partial derivatives $(u_{xx})_{ij}$, $(u_{xy})_{ij}$ and $(u_{yy})_{ij}$ at the point (i,j) can be approximated by

$$(u_{xx})_{ij} = \frac{u_{i+1,j} - 2u_{i,j} + u_{i-1,j}}{h^2}$$

$$(u_{xy})_{ij} = \frac{u_{i+1,j+1} - u_{i+1,j} - u_{i,j+1} + u_{i,j}}{h^2}$$

$$(u_{yy})_{ij} = \frac{u_{i,j+1} - 2u_{i,j} + u_{i,j-1}}{h^2} \quad (6)$$

The discrete form of the function Φ_1 can be obtained by substituting the discrete derivatives into the first equation in (1). The partial derivatives of Φ_1 can be calculated using the computational molecule approach discussed in [12] though special attention should be paid in computing the molecules near the endocardial and epicardial boundaries where the smoothness constraint should break in order not to smooth over the motion discontinuity. The endocardial and epicardial boundaries were each manually segmented through-out a slice sequence using a 6 control point cubic B-spline contour. The discretization of the function Φ_2 and calculation of its partial derivatives is almost trivial. Let us consider the function Φ_3 which is non-quadratic. The partial derivatives

$$(\Phi_3)_u = (u + x - \bar{x})(1 - \bar{x}_u) + (v + y - \bar{y})(-\bar{y}_u)$$
$$(\Phi_3)_v = (v + y - \bar{y})(1 - \bar{y}_v) + (u + x - \bar{x})(-\bar{x}_v) \quad (7)$$

For simplification, we now make two approximations. For vertical grids, the x-coordinates of curves only vary slightly, and as the grid lines are spatially continuous, $\bar{x}_u$ is expected to be small. Furthermore, for vertical grids $\bar{y}$ changes minutely as a function of u, so that $\bar{y}_u \approx 0$. For horizontal grids, the y coordinates of curves also vary slightly along the length of grid lines, and since these are spatially continuous curves, $\bar{y}_u$ is expected to be small. Note that these approximations will hold under smooth local deformations, as is expected in the myocardial tissue. Only $\bar{x}_u$ for horizontal grids, and $\bar{y}_v$ for vertical grids is expected to vary more significantly. The approximate derivates are now given by:

$$(\Phi_3)_u = (u + x - \bar{x})(1 - T_{hor}\bar{x}_u)$$
$$(\Phi_3)_v = (v + y - \bar{y})(1 - T_{ver}\bar{y}_v) \quad (8)$$

The variables T_{hor} and T_{ver} are predicates equal to one if the snake point of interest lies on a horizontal, or a vertical grid line. Needless to say, the above functions can be discretized by replacing the continuous values by the corresponding values at the grid points.

After discretization, a typical quadratic optimization problem takes the following form:

$$f(\mathbf{x}) = c - \mathbf{b}^T\mathbf{x} + \frac{1}{2}\mathbf{x}^T\mathbf{A}\mathbf{x} \quad (9)$$

where $\mathbf{x}$ is the vector of variables, $\mathbf{A}$ is the constant Hessian matrix of second order partial derivatives and $\mathbf{b}$ and $\mathbf{c}$ are constant vectors. In the present problem, the terms Φ_1 and Φ_2 can be cast in the above form. Unfortunately, in the term Φ_3, the values $\bar{x}$ and $\bar{y}$ are dependent on x and y respectively which makes Φ_3 non-quadratic. The discrete optimization function form of Φ is given by:

$$\Phi(\mathbf{x}) = c - \mathbf{b}^T\mathbf{x} + \frac{1}{2}\mathbf{x}^T\mathbf{A}\mathbf{x} + \lambda_3\Phi_3(\mathbf{x}) \quad (10)$$

where $\mathbf{A}$, $\mathbf{b}$ and $\mathbf{c}$ are constants and include the contributions from $\lambda_1\Phi_1$ and $\lambda_2\Phi_2$. we are now ready to look at specific minimization algorithms.

The first algorithm we investigate is the conjugate gradient (CG) algorithm. For an order N quadratic problem, the CG algorithm is guaranteed to converge in N iterations. Moreover, it does not store the Hessian matrix and requires $o(N)$ storage for an order N optimization problem. Note that the CG algorithm does not explicitly calculate or store the Hessian matrix $\mathbf{A}$ and can be adapted to the function Φ in (10). We do not know the Hessian matrix for Φ. However, we do know how to calculate the derivative $\nabla\Phi(\mathbf{p})$ using the derivatives for the functions Φ_1, Φ_2 and Φ_3. We use this knowledge of the gradient of Φ in the implementation of the CG algorithm. As a final point, since Φ is non-quadratic, the algorithm may not converge in N iterations. For a description of the CG algorithm please refer to [10].

Quasi-Newton algorithm is a different optimization method that we have investigated. It differs from CG in that it has higher memory requirements but better convergence properties for non-quadratic functions. By quasi-Newton method we mean techniques which use an approximation to the inverse Hessian matrix in each iteration as opposed to Newton methods which use the exact inverse. A generic quasi-Newton algorithm calculates and stores an approximation to the inverse Hessian matrix in each iteration. Hence for an order N optimization problem, this method needs $o(N^2)$ storage. The advantage of a quasi-Newton algorithm lies in that it has quadratic convergence properties for general smooth functions (not necessarily quadratic). A specific quasi-Newton algorithm is characterized by the approximation it uses for the Hessian matrix. The quasi-Newton method used in this paper is called the Davidon-Fletcher-Powell (DFP) algorithm. An overview of which is given in the [10].

2.2 Validations

Cardiac Simulator

To test and validate the algorithm an environment based on a 13 parameter kinematic model of Arts et al. [4] has been implemented as described in [13] for simulating a time sequence of tagged MR images.

The motion model involves application of a cascade of linear transformations describing rigid (rotations and translations) as well as non-rigid transformations (radial compression, torsion, ellipticalization in SA and LA, as well as shear along x, y, and z axes). Once a chosen discretization step is assumed and a mesh for tessellating the 3D space is generated, the linear matrix transformations are applied in a sequence to all the mesh points so as to deform the reference model. The parameters of the motion model, referred to as k-parameters, and the transformations to which they correspond are as follows: 1) k_1: Radially dependent compression, 2) k_2: Left ventricular torsion 3) k_3: Ellipticalization in long-axis (LA) planes 4) k_4: Ellipticalization in short-axis (SA) planes 5) k_5: Shear in x direction 6) k_6: Shear in y direction 7) k_7: Shear in z direction 8) k_8: Rotation about x-axis 9) k_9: Rotation about y-axis 10) k_{10}: Rotation about z-axis 11) k_{11}: Translation in x direction 12) k_{12}: Translation in y direction 13) k_{13}: Translation in z direction In order to simulate MR images, a plane intersecting the geometric model is selected, and tagged spin-echo imaging equations are applied for simulating the imaging process.

For the purposes of validating 2D displacement field reconstructions, we have used the parameters k_2, k_4, k_5, and k_{10} for generating 2D deformations of the geometric model, based on which images and in addition 2D displacement vector fields of *actual* material points are produced. The error norms used in comparing the ground truth vector field (V_g) with the vector field measured by our warp algorithm (V_m) are:

$$\varepsilon_L = \frac{1}{N} \sum ||V_m| - |V_g||, \tag{11}$$

$$\varepsilon_\theta = \frac{1}{\sum |V_g|} \sum |V_g| \cdot \arccos \frac{V_g \cdot V_m}{|V_g||V_m|} \tag{12}$$

where ε_L measures the average difference in length between V_g and V_m, and ε_θ measures the deviation in angle between V_g and V_m. ε_θ requires further explanation. As can be seen from (12), we weigh individual angle deviations by the magnitude of the material point displacement vector; normalized by the sum of magnitude of all ground truth vectors. The reason for this is to emphasize angle deviation of points which have large displacements, and similarly to de-emphasize the angle deviation of points which have a smaller displacement.

TS	IP	D_0	TE	TR	T1	T2
0.9 cm	0.5 cm	300	0.03 sec	10 sec	0.6 sec	0.1 sec
k_x	k_y	θ	R_i	R_o	δ	ss
7 rad/cm	7 rad/cm	45 deg.	0.25	0.6	4 cm	0.05 cm/pixel

Table 1. Imaging parameters and dimensions of geometric model. Please note that TS is tag separation, IP is the image plane position, R_i and R_o are the inner and outer radii of the 2 prolate spheroids, and ss is the sample size.

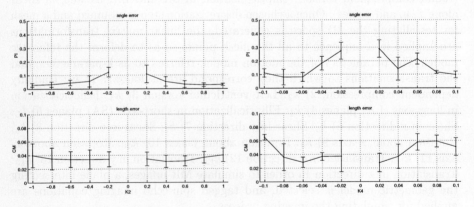

Fig. 1. The error plots for angle and length error for k_2 and k_4. Please see text for details.

Figures 1 and 2 show the angle and length errors by comparing V_m and V_g as a function of a range of values of k_2, k_4, k_5, and k_{10}, keeping the rest of the

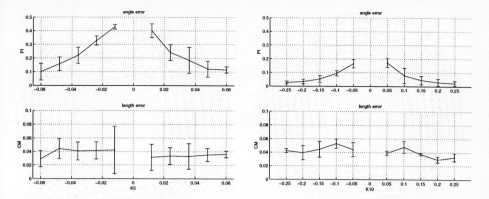

Fig. 2. The error plots for angle and length error for k_5 and k_{10}. Please see text for details.

k parameters constant. The imaging and geometric parameters of the model for these experiments is shown in table 1. Additionally, as part of the validations and in order to test the sensitivity of the algorithms to different values of λ_1, λ_2, and λ_3, we varied each of these coefficients individually between the integers: 0 and 10, keeping the other 2 at the constant value of 1 (excluding $\lambda_1 = 0$). The error bars in these plots show the 3σ range on either side of the error mean for particular values of each k parameter. As can be seen from the figures, to a large degree the algorithm is insensitive to the exact values of λ_i's. An additional remarkable point regarding the error plots is the fact that for smaller motions, the value of ε_θ is larger than that for bigger motions. The reason for this unintuitive result can only be attributed to the larger percent inaccuracies in reconstruction of smaller displacements by the warping algorithm. Also, it should be noted that error plots in figures 1 and 2 subsume the errors incurred in localization of tags and myocardial contours (in this paper, tag and contour localization is performed through manual placement of control points of B-spline curves [2].) Although the magnitude of errors are bound to be smaller if accurate location of contour and tag lines in the simulated images were to be used, our complete system for tracking and reconstruction of tag lines would not be tested, and furthermore since the exact location of tags and contours are not known in real images, results may not be a good model of realistic situations.

Finally, Figure 3 displays true and reconstructed vector fields corresponding to torsion of the computational phantom.

In-Vivo Validations

Since "out-of-plane" movement of the LV occurs in slices close to the valve-plane; i.e., at the top of the LV, for the purposes of extraction of 2D deformations, here we only consider SPAMM image slices acquired near the ventricular apex. Results of application of techniques to *in vivo* data of a normal human volunteer is shown in figure 4. Note that in this case, the computed dense motion

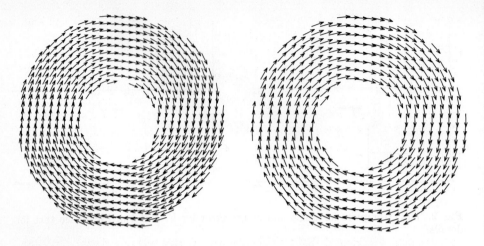

Fig. 3. Comparison of computed (left) and true (right) displacement vector fields corresponding to torsion ($k_2 = -1.0$).

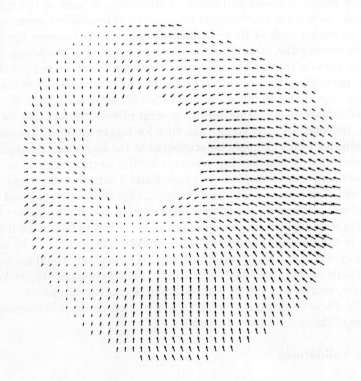

Fig. 4. The reconstructed vector field by CG computed from deforming a 7×7 B-spline grid for an apical slice acquired at 90 and 180 msec after the ECG trigger. The vector field is displayed on the myocardial region in the 90 msec image.

is computed from two *deformed* grids. The endocardial and epicardial contours were each manually segmented through-out the sequence using a 6 control point B-spline representation, as we have found automatic determination of myocardial contours in a SPAMM image sequence to be a formidable task due to the presence of tag lines. In order to assess the sensitivity of the vector field to different λ_i coefficient values, the following study was undertaken. The vector field for the uniform weight factors $\lambda_1 = 1$, $\lambda_2 = 1$, and $\lambda_3 = 1$ was chosen as the ground-truth. Vector fields corresponding to different coefficient values were subsequently compared with this vector field. Results are illustrated in table 2.

3 Conclusions

We have described new methods for efficient reconstruction of dense displacement vector fields from SPAMM grids. The constrained thin-plate spline methods warp an area in the plane such that two embedded grids of curves are non-rigidly registered, thereby interpolating a dense displacement vector field. The new warp method treats intersection points of SPAMM grids as standard landmarks and forces these to come together. Furthermore, it corresponds complete tag curves and brings these into alignment. Finally, where no information is available, it interpolates a C^1 continuous vector field.

In addition to the developed machinery in this paper, methods were evaluated using a cardiac motion simulator. The methods have been tested for accuracy in length as well as angle of the reconstructed displacement vectors from the known ground-truth, and the results indicate that constrained thin-plate spline reconstructions of myocardial deformations is sufficiently accurate for measurement of in-plane tissue deformations within a reasonable time and between any two frames in a sequence of tagged images.

λ_1	λ_2	λ_3	Angle Error	Length Error
1	1	1	0	0
5	1	1	0.006	0.019
10	1	1	0.008	0.029
1	5	1	0.005	0.012
1	10	1	0.006	0.015
1	1	5	0.005	0.015
1	1	10	0.008	0.021
1	1	0	0.007	0.018
1	0	1	0.011	0.043

Table 2. The values for angle (fraction of π) and length errors (in cm) as a function of λ_1, λ_2, and λ_3. The "ground-truth" in this case was chosen to be the reconstructed displacement field with $\lambda_i = 1$.

References

1. A. A. Amini. Automated methods for cardiac motion analysis from MR tagging. Proposal funded by The Whitaker Foundation, 1992.
2. A. A. Amini, R. W. Curwen, and John C. Gore. Snakes and splines for tracking non-rigid heart motion. In *European Conference on Computer Vision*, pages 251–261, University of Cambridge, UK, April 1996.
3. A. A. Amini and et al. MR physics-based snake tracking and dense deformations from tagged MR cardiac images (oral presentation). In *AAAI Symposium on Applications of Computer Vision to Medical Image Processing*, Stanford University, Stanford, California, March 1994.
4. T. Arts, W. Hunter, A. Douglas, A. Muijtjens, and R. Reneman. Description of the deformation of the left ventricle by a kinematic model. *J. Biomechanics*, 25(10):1119–1127, 1992.
5. L. Axel and L. Dougherty. MR imaging of motion with spatial modulation of magnetization. *Radiology*, 171(3):841–845, 1989.
6. F. Bookstein. Principal warps: Thin-plate splines and the decomposition of deformations. *IEEE Transactions on Pattern Analysis and Machine Intelligence*, PAMI-11:567–585, 1989.
7. T. Denney and J. Prince. Reconstruction of 3-d left ventricular motion from planar tagged cardiac MR images: An estimation-theoretic approach. *IEEE Transactions on Medical Imaging*, 14(4):625–635, December 1995.
8. W. Grimson. An implementation of a computational theory of visual surface interpolation. *Computer Vision, Graphics, and Image Processing*, 22:39–69, 1983.
9. J. Park, D. Metaxas, and L. Axel. Volumetric deformable models with parameter functions: A new approach to the 3d motion analysis of the LV from MRI-SPAMM. In *International Conference on Computer Vision*, pages 700–705, 1995.
10. W. Press, B. Flannery, S. Teukolsky, and W. Vetterling. *Numerical recipes in C*. Cambridge University Press, Cambridge, 1988.
11. P. Radeva, A. Amini, and J. Huang. Deformable B-Solids and implicit snakes for 3d localization and tracking of SPAMM MRI data. *Computer Vision and Image Understanding*, 66(2):163–178, May 1997.
12. D. Terzopoulos. *Multiresolution Computation of Visible Representation*. PhD thesis, MIT, 1984.
13. E. Waks, J. Prince, and A. Douglas. Cardiac motion simulator for tagged MRI. In *Proc. of Mathematical Methods in Biomedical Image Analysis*, pages 182–191, 1996.
14. A. Young, D. Kraitchman, L. Dougherty, and L. Axel. Tracking and finite element analysis of stripe deformation in magnetic resonance tagging. *IEEE Transactions on Medical Imaging*, 14(3):413–421, September 1995.
15. E. Zerhouni, D. Parish, W. Rogers, A. Yang, and E. Shapiro. Human heart: Tagging with MR imaging – a method for noninvasive assessment of myocardial motion. *Radiology*, 169:59–63, 1988.

Motion Analysis of the Right Ventricle From MRI Images

Edith Haber[1], Dimitris N. Metaxas[2], and Leon Axel[3]

[1] Department of Bioengineering
[2] VAST Lab, Department of Computer and Information Science
[3] Department of Radiology
University of Pennsylvania, Philadelphia, PA 19104-6389, USA
edith@seas.upenn.edu
http://www.cis.upenn.edu/~edith/

Abstract. Both normal and abnormal right ventricular (RV) wall motion is not well understood. In this paper, we use data from *tagged* MRI images to perform the first 3D motion study of the entire right ventricle to date. Our technique is an adaptation of a physics-based deformable modeling methodology that was successfully used on the left ventricle(LV). As opposed to the previous approach, currently we use segmented contours to generate the geometry, 1D tags for our input data (due to the thinner RV), and localized degrees of freedom (DOFs) with finite elements. Although we build a biventricular model, our results focus on method validation and visualizing clinically useful parameters that describe RV wall motion.

1 Introduction

Abnormal motion of the RV serves as an indicator of several types of heart disease, such as RV ischemia and hypertrophy [3]. However, there is no in-depth knowledge of the RV motion and its correlation to the various diseases. One reason that researchers do not agree about the exact pumping mechanism of the normal RV may be regional variations in contraction patterns occuring at different phases of systole. Since studies have found that RV contraction varies with increases in pressure and volume, and ischemia [3], a method for accurately assessing RV wall motion can both answer questions into its normal function and can be used as an indicator of various diseases.

The RV receives blood from the right atrium and pumps it into the pulmonary artery. It appears crescent-like in a cross-sectional view and, unlike the LV, is difficult to define with any parameterized 3D shape. The RV shares a septum with the LV, while its outer free wall is in mechanical contact with the pericardium and the lungs. The RV cavity can be conceptually separated into an inflow tract, a highly-trabeculated apical portion, and a relatively smooth outflow tract [6] (Fig. 1). The $3mm$-thick free wall is thin relative to the $7mm$-thick LV free wall. This relative thinness and complex geometry make it difficult to capture RV wall motion using regular imaging modalities.

This paper presents a new methodology for modeling and analyzing the RV shape and motion from MRI-tagged data. We make significant modifications to

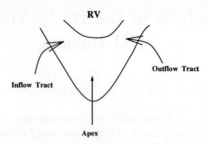

Fig. 1. Schematic of right ventricular compartments

the physics-based deformable modeling framework of [8, 12], which was applied to MRI tag intersections for LV wall motion reconstruction. At the currently available image resolution, a small number of tag point intersections fall within the normally thin-walled RV. In order to capture the full 3D motion, the new method uses different constraints to incorporate input data consisting of the entire lengths of 1D tags extracted from multi-view MRI-SPAMM images. Also, due to the complex shape of the RV, we cannot construct our initial model by fitting a deformable geometric primitive to the initial contour data. Instead, we build a deformable model of the biventricular geometry directly from the initial contours. Although this model includes both the right and left ventricles, we focus on the analysis of the RV in this paper.

The initial geometric model is a volumetric finite element model (FEM) mesh that we fit to subsequent contour and tag data. Due to the complex RV geometry and motion, the analysis consists of using the maximum possible DOFs. Instead of lumping them into parameter functions as in [12], we use stiffness from finite elements to smooth the sparse input data which result from imaging the thin RV wall. However, in order to make our analysis clinically useful we convert the model's DOFs into equivalent lumped parameters such as scaling and twisting.

In addition to the quantitative analysis, we use computer graphics techniques to visualize the reconstructed RV shape and motion by color mapping the distribution of derived parameters onto our model. Our preliminary results quantify previously documented knowledge of the RV motion and provide a more detailed motion analysis of the RV compared to previous methods. In addition, having a biventricular model opens the way for the quantitative study of inter-ventricular dependence and relative motion.

2 Related Work

Right ventricular wall motion has been studied invasively by implanting markers into small portions of the RV wall and using an imaging modality to track the motion of the markers [16, 4, 18, 14]. While results from these techniques showed regional variations in contraction, questions remain about whether the invasive nature of these techniques affect contraction patterns [4]. Although, the MRI tagging method has provided a non-invasive method for studying heart wall motion, most of these studies have centered on the LV. Since the two-dimensional

(2D) images do not capture important through-plane motion, data from multiple views must be integrated by fitting a 3D model to the data [12, 19, 9]. To the best of our knowledge, the only work that has used entire tag lines (as opposed to tag intersections) is that of O'Dell,et al. [11]. These researchers developed a displacement field fitting technique which was used to fit an ellipsoidal finite element model to LV data.

Up to now the only MRI tagging study of the RV free wall was performed by Young, et al. [20], who fit a *surface* model to intersections of mid-wall contours with the tags. In the past, RV *geometry* has been reconstructed from both CT and MR images as these technologies developed [10]. Integrated models for the RV-LV geometry have also been developed using tools from constructive solid geometry [13]. In addition, the right ventricular free wall was modeled as a thin shell by fitting biquadratic surface patches [15].

3 Image Acquisition and Data Extraction

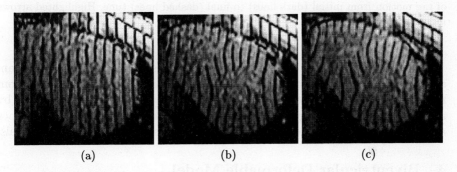

(a) (b) (c)

Fig. 2. Mid-wall short-axis 1D tagged MR images at (a) beginning systole (b) mid-systole (c) end-systole.

In order to capture the motion in the ventricular walls using MRI images, we use a 1D SPAMM (SPAtial Modulation of Magnetization) tagging technique [2]. This non-invasive technique produces a family of parallel tagging planes by using a sequence of non-selective radio frequency excitation separated by intervals of magnetic field gradient in the direction perpendicular to these planes prior to imaging. The intersection of these tagging planes with the imaging plane produces dark stripes (Fig. 2) which represent actual tissue. Therefore, the initially straight lines deform as the heart contracts. Due to through-plane motion, the portion of the tag plane seen in an initial image may move out of the imaging plane and be replaced by the intersection of a different portion of the same tag plane with the imaging plane. Thus, the stripes only provide information about motion in the direction perpendicular to the initial tag plane and we need 3 different views to capture the full 3D motion, e.g., 2 short axis views (one with horizontal and one with vertical stripes), and a long-axis view (Fig. 3). The figure depicts how each tag plane/image plane combination provides information about motion in mutually perpendicular directions.

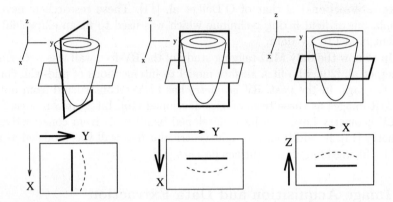

Fig. 3. 1st row: Image and tag (dark) planes. 2nd row: 2D image planes with example of tag motion from initial (dark lines) to final (dashed lines) time. Highlighted arrows indicate for which direction we get motion information.

We extract tags and contours from the images using SPAMMVU, a program developed in the Department of Radiology at our institution [1]. Tags from multiple time phases (between end-diastole and end-systole) were tracked by adapting the deformable mesh scheme of [21] for 1D stripes. The extracted stripes are approximated as a series of points by sampling the tag lines at $2mm$ intervals.

4 Biventricular Deformable Model
4.1 Model Geometry

Although the RV cannot be defined by any simple parameterized geometric primitive, an accurate geometric model is important for a model-based fitting technique. Since the septum plays a role in the function of both ventricles, our approach is to create a biventricular geometric model. Due to the complex geometries involved, we build a discretized mesh of volumetric finite elements directly from contours extracted from end-diastolic images [5]. The short-axis contours were used to generate the finite element mesh, with the insertion points of the RV free wall into the septum as guide points. Points sampled for the contours then became the nodes of the finite elements. This geometric model could also be used for volume measurement, and, given cardiac material properties, for stress analysis.

Our deformable model fitting technique results in the displacement of over 500 nodes through time. In order to make these results clinically meaningful we convert nodal displacements into scaling and twisting parameters. Since it would be less relevant to describe the twisting of the RV with respect to the long axis of the LV (or vice versa), we define a local coordinate system for

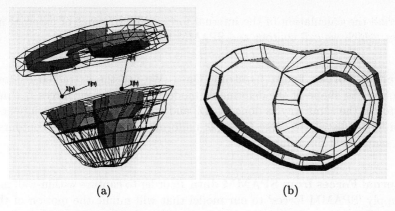

Fig. 4. Initial finite element mesh. (a) Anterior view of with sections cut away to show local coordinate systems. Note that the RV apex is above that of the LV apex. (b) Cross sectional view of a layer elements which connects contours from two image planes

each ventricle. The axes of the coordinate systems are the eigenvectors of the matrix of central moments [8], with the eigenvector corresponding to the smallest eigenvalue is the one with the most inertia being labeled the z-axis (see Fig. 4). The transformation of position **x** with respect to the global, non-inertial frame to the local position **s**, is

$$\mathbf{x} = \mathbf{c} + \mathbf{R}\mathbf{s} \qquad (1)$$

where **c** is the origin of the local frame and **R** is the rotation matrix which takes a point from the global to the local coordinate system. The RV free wall is in the RV coordinate system, while the LV free wall and septum are both in the LV coordinate system. Some of the finite elements connect nodes across the model so that two systems remain connected. The finite element mesh, with a shaded RV and LV endocardium, is also shown in Fig. 4.

4.2 Model Dynamics

Our basic approach is to fit the model to the data with physics-based deformations as in [12]. Unlike the previous work, our model deforms with different kinds of DOFs, i.e., the position, $\mathbf{q}_i$, of each node i of the finite element mesh. We use a non-inertial model and integrate the following equation of motion to solve for $\mathbf{q}_i$:

$$\dot{\mathbf{q}}_i = \mathbf{f}_{i,internal} + \mathbf{f}_{i,external} \qquad (2)$$

where $\mathbf{f}_{i,internal}$ is the finite element stiffness force, and $\mathbf{f}_{i,external}$ is the force derived from the image data. The forces are only used to deform our model and are not meant to replicate the actual forces in the heart wall muscle. The large number of DOFs requires we have internal stiffness forces in order to maintain continuity in the motion. As mentioned earlier, we later lump those DOFs to parameters which are more recognizable to physicians. In the following, we describe the calculation of the internal force and two types of external images forces, which we call contour and SPAMM forces.

External Forces From Contour Data We use the extracted contours to maintain the shape of the deformable model. These contour forces $\mathbf{f}_{i,c}$, are calculated in the same way as done by [12] and applied to the appropriate node(s). In order to distribute these forces as uniformly as possible, the contours were first sampled at $5mm$ intervals.

External Forces from SPAMM data In order to capture within-wall motion, we apply 'SPAMM forces' to our model that will mimic the motion of the tag stripes. We can accomplish this because we have a time correspondence between stripes and the finite elements allow us to register the initial stripes locations to the model. We register each point on the stripe to the non-deforming, stationary local coordinate system of the appropriate finite element. The transformation from the local position, (e, n, s), to the global position of a point, (x, y, z), is written in terms of the finite element shape functions:

$$x = \sum_{j=1}^{n} N_j(e,n,s)x_j, \ y = \sum_{j=1}^{n} N_j(e,n,s)y_j, \ z = \sum_{j=1}^{n} N_j(e,n,s)z_j \quad (3)$$

where x_j, y_j, z_j is the position of the jth node in the element numbering system. The shape functions, N_j, can be seen as weighting the global coordinate of a node according to where a point lies in the (e, n, s) system. In this paper, we use six-noded wedge and eight-noded parallelepiped elements, whose linear shape functions are given in [22]. Since we only know the positions of the nodes (x_j, y_j, z_j) and the position of a tag point on the stripe (x, y, z), we solve the set of three equations (Eq. 3) for the local coordinates (e, n, s) using Newton-Raphson. Since each finite element is defined to be a 2 by 2 cube centered at the origin of its local coordinate system, the point falls within a particular element if: $-1 <= e, n, s <= 1$.

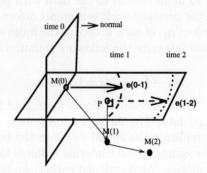

Fig. 5. Application of SPAMM forces

For each material point from an extracted tag, we define the spring-like SPAMM force, $\mathbf{f}_S$, to be a scalar multiple of the distance vector, $\mathbf{e}$: $\mathbf{f}_S = \kappa \mathbf{e}$, where κ is the strength. $\mathbf{e}$ is a vector in the direction of the tag plane normal which extends from a material point to its corresponding tag stripe at the next time phase (see Fig. 5). After time 0, the material point will move out of the plane due to forces applied on other points in other directions. For these cases, i.e. time 1, the projected point (P) of the material point (M(1)) onto the original image plane, rather than the material point itself, is used to calculate $\mathbf{e}$.

The SPAMM force, $\mathbf{f}_S$, is applied within the element and must be distributed to the nodes of that element. The force on each node is weighted by the shape functions:

$$\mathbf{f}_{j,S} = N_j \mathbf{f}_S \tag{4}$$

where the subscript j refers to the node number within an element. This is the manner in which concentrated loads are distributed to the nodes in finite element theory, so that the collection of material points registered to the model have a 'line of forces' applied to them. If the same node receives forces from different material points, the final force is the average of all $f_{j,S}$.

The total external force on each global node, i, is the sum of the contour and the SPAMM forces, i.e., $\mathbf{f}_{i,external} = \mathbf{f}_{i,c} + \mathbf{f}_{i,S}$.

Internal forces due to stiffness In our formulation, we model stiffness as an internal force, $\mathbf{f}_{i,internal}$. We use stiffness to impose a continuity and smoothing constraint on our many DOFs, and not to model the actual cardiac material properties (a topic of future research). As a result, we consider each element to consist of an isotropic, linear, incompressible material. The stiffness force, $\mathbf{f}_{i,internal}$, on a node from a particular element can be computed from

$$\mathbf{f}_{i,internal} = \mathbf{Kd} \tag{5}$$

where $\mathbf{d}$ are the nodal displacements. The stiffness matrix, $\mathbf{K}$, incorporates the geometry and material properties of the element and is computed from

$$\mathbf{K} = \int\int\int \mathbf{B}^T \mathbf{D} \mathbf{B} \, dV \tag{6}$$

where $\mathbf{D}$ is the stress-strain matrix and $\mathbf{B}$ is the strain-displacement matrix, whose formulations are given in [22].

4.3 Model Parameters: Twisting

We convert the reconstructed displacement results into a twisting parameter, θ, of a point (s_x, s_y, s_z) about the z-axis of the local coordinate system. The equations which define twisting are $s_x = s_X \cos\theta - s_Y \sin\theta$ and $s_y = s_X \sin\theta + s_Y \cos\theta$, where an uppercase subscript denotes the point at its initial position. Since simply subtracting the angles will give erroneous results when a point moves across the $\theta = 0$ line, we solve the two equations for $\sin\theta$ and $\cos\theta$, and solve for θ:

$$\theta = \arctan \frac{s_X s_y - s_Y s_x}{s_Y s_y + s_X s_x} \tag{7}$$

5 Results

5.1 Validation

In order to validate the fitting method, we built a computational phantom in the shape of a thick-walled, annular cylinder. We deform the model using equations in cylindrical coordinates [19, 7]:

$$z = \lambda Z + \phi R \tag{8}$$

$$\theta = \Theta + \Omega(R - R_i) + \gamma(Z - Z_{min}) + \Theta_{min} \tag{9}$$

$$r = f(R) = \sqrt{\frac{\alpha}{\lambda}(R^2 - R_i^2) + r_i^2} \tag{10}$$

where (R, Θ, Z) = initial position, (r, θ, z) = deformed position, R_i = internal radius, and Z_{min} = minimum height. Twisting within the cylinder is the superposition of a minimum twist (Θ_{min}), twisting between short-axis layers (controlled by Ω), and twisting between the inner and outer walls (controlled by γ). Axial deformation is varied in the axial and radial directions with the use of the λ and ϕ parameters, respectively. Finally, an incompressibility constraint leads to radial deformation being a function of the initial radius.

We generate parallel tag planes with a $7mm$ separation with tag points sampled every $2mm$ along a stripe. Simulated short-axis image plane (5 total) were separated at $7.2mm$ intervals, and simulated rotating long-axis image planes (as in our actual imaging protocol) were separated at 20 degree intervals. As done in [19] , we use Eq. (8 -10) to solve for unknown r, θ, Z tag and contour positions from known R, Θ, z for the short axis, and to solve for unknown r, Θ, z tag and contour positions from known R, θ, Z for the long axis. Geometric and deformation parameters are shown in Table 1.

Phantom Parameters					
Geometric	mm		Deformation		
R_i	23	λ	0.82	γ	$0.1°/mm$
R_{outer}	30	ϕ	0.1	Θ_{min}	$6°$
Z_{min}	10	Ω	$0.79°/mm$	r_i	$16mm$
Height	45				

Table 1. Geometric and deformation parameters of phantom.

We use the same element and fitting technique as the real data between initial and deformed times. Our fitting criterion, the tag error, is the magnitude of the vector e, which was used to calculate the SPAMM forces. Fitting can be controlled manually or automatically by increasing the SPAMM strength and boundary strength as the model deforms in order to overcome the stiffness of the elements. All RMS tag errors were reduced to $< 0.2mm$ while the average errors in nodal positions were all reduced to less than 5%. Results are shown in Fig. 6. The color map, seen here and in other figures as grey-scale without any loss of information, is that of the twisting parameter.

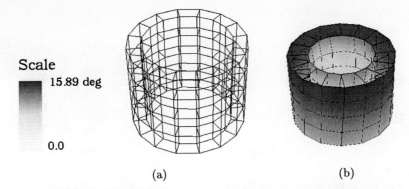

Fig. 6. Validation results: fitting method was applied to a computational, cylindrical phantom. (a) Initial configuration and (b) deformed shape with a color plot of twisting parameter on inner and outer walls.

5.2 Reconstructed Normal RV Wall Motion

We applied our method to a set of 3 orthogonal 1D tagged MRI images of normal ventricles. The tag errors during the model fitting stages are shown in Table 2. Although we capture the motion of the LV in addition to the RV, we concentrate on results for RV deformation which concur with previous studies and show the possibility of providing more detail. For example, one group of researchers measured systolic long axis displacement of tag points in MRI images [17]. Unlike their reporting of average values in certain regions, we can display the spatial and temporal distribution with our model. These researchers reported that the maximum motion (about $25mm$) occured in the basal region of the RV free wall. The color map in Fig. 7 is a plot of absolute axial displacement along the LV long-axis which was prescribed during imaging). This figure shows maximum displacement of about $19mm$ at the RV base and in the RV outflow tract.

Similar to observations by [3], we found significant displacement of the free wall towards the septum and septal wall thickening which contributed to a smaller RV cavity. In a cross-sectional view, the most significant contraction is that of the posterior basal portion towards the outflow portion. Fig. 7 also shows the paths of cardiac material points located at the centers of the elements. Note that these points are different from those used during model fitting. It is apparent that the initial displacement of these points is greater than their final displacement.

We also attempted to plot twisting on the RV wall. The apparently large concentration of twisting in the free wall shown in Fig. 8 results from a large forward displacement in a portion of the wall that is near the model axes rather than an actual twist. Thus, global twisting may not be a helpful parameter to use for the RV because of its non-circular cross-section. However, differences in twisting (i.e., between walls or between levels) may be good indicators of regional deformation.

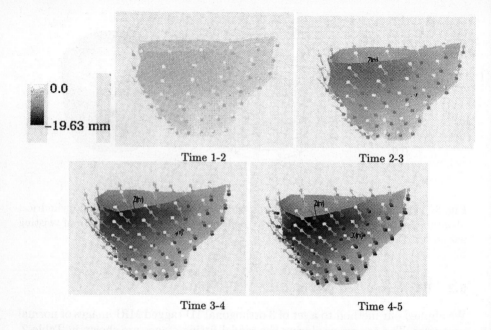

Fig. 7. Color plot of axial displacement on RV as it deforms through 4 time intervals. The paths of RV mid-wall points are shown from time 1 (white) to time 5 (red)

It is too early to conduct a more thorough comparison of our results with those found in literature. At this point we demonstrate the capability of the fitting technique to capture major trends in the deformation of the normal RV and identify areas needing improvement. We plan to validate the model with data from several patients and to identify which parameters derived from the reconstruction are clinically useful.

6 Conclusion

We have developed a novel approach which fits a geometrically complex biventricular model to data from 1D tagged MRI images. In this paper, we validated the fitting technique on a computational phantom with predefined geometry and deformations. The results presented here show possibly useful clinical information about RV contraction. Through this work, we learned that the complicated RV wall motion may be best described with regional deformation parameters, i.e., strains. An in-depth study of these deformations should lead to greater knowledge of normal and abnormal heart wall motion. Our preliminary results of reconstructed normal RV wall motion demonstrate the plausibility of using this method in a clinical setting.

RMS Errors (mm) During Model Fitting				
View and tag orientation	Time 1-2	Time 2-3	Time 3-4	Time 4-5
SA-Vertical	0.235	0.270	0.393	0.364
SA-Horizontal	0.244	0.274	0.361	0.351
LA-Horizontal	0.269	0.278	0.335	0.281

Table 2. Error between model material points and SPAMM stripes during model fitting for each time interval (SA = Short - axis, LA = Long - axis)

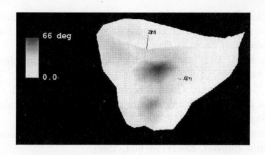

Fig. 8. Color plot of twisting parameter on RV free wall

7 Acknowledgements

This research has been funded by grants from the NSF (Career Award 96-24604), the Whitaker Foundation, and the NIH/NLM (LM06638-01).

References

1. L. Axel, D. Bloomgarden, C.N. Chang, D. Kraitchman, and A.A. Young. SPAMMVU: a program for the analysis of dynamic tagged MRI. In *Proceedings of the Soc. of Magnetic Resonance in Medicine 12th Annual Meeting*, page 724, 1993.
2. L. Axel and L. Dougherty. Heart wall motion: Improved method of spatial modulation of magnetization for MR imaging. *Radiology*, 272:349–50, 1989.
3. D. Barnard and J.S. Alpert. Right ventricular function in health and disease. *Curr Probl Cardiol*, 12:422–29, 1987.
4. C.J. Chuong, M.S. Sacks, G. Templeton, F. Schwiep, and Jr. R.L. Johnson. Regional deformation and contractile function in canine right ventricular free wall. *Am J Physiol*, 260:H1224–1235, 1991.
5. E. Haber, D.N. Metaxas, and L. Axel. Three-dimensional geometric modeling of cardiac right and left ventricles. In *Biomedical Engineering Soc Annual Meeting*, San Diego, California, 1997.
6. J.W. Hurst. *Atlas of the Heart*. Gower Medical, New York, 1988.
7. A.D. McCulloch and J.H. Omens. Non–homogeneous analysis of three–dimensional transmural finite deformation in canine ventricular myocardium. *J Biomechanics*, 24:539–48, 1991.
8. D.N. Metaxas. *Physics-based deformable models: applications to computer vision, graphics, and medical imaging*. Kluwer Academic Publishers, Cambridge, 1996.
9. C.C. Moore, W.G. O'Dell, E.R. McVeigh, and E.A. Zerhouni. Calculation of three dimensional left ventricular strains from biplanar tagged MR images. *Journal of Magnetic Resonance Imaging*, 2:165–75, 1992.

10. P.M.F. Nielsen, I.J. Le Grice, and B.H. Smaill P.J. Hunter. Mathematical model of geometry and fibrous structure of the heart. *J Appl Physiol*, 260:H1365–H1378, 1991.
11. W.G. O'Dell, C.C. Moore, W.C. Hunter, E.A. Zerhouni, and E.R. McVeigh. 3-dimensional myocardial deformations: calculation with displacement field fitting to tagged MR images. *Radiology*, 195:829–35, 1996.
12. J. Park, D. Metaxas, and L. Axel. Analysis of left ventricular wall motion based on volumetric deformable models and MRI-SPAMM. *Med Image Analysis J*, 1(1):53–71, 1996.
13. J.S. Pirolo, S.J. Bresina, L.L. Creswell, K.W. Myers, B.A. Szabo, M.W. Vannier, and M.K. Pasque. Mathematical three-dimensional solid modeling of biventricular geometry. *Annals of Biomed Eng*, 21:199–219, 1993.
14. R.A. Raines, M.M. LeWinter, and J.W. Covell. Regional shortening patterns in canine right ventricle. *Am J Physiol*, 231:H1395–1400, 1976.
15. M.S. Sacks, C.J. Chuong, G.H. Templeton, and R. Peshock. *In vivo* 3-d reconstruction and geometric characterization of the right ventricular free wall. *Annals of Biomed Eng*, 21:263–275, 1993.
16. W.P. Santamore, G.D. Meier, and A.A. Bove. Contractile function in canine right ventricle. *Am J Physiol*, 239:H794–804, 1980.
17. M. Stuber, E. Nagel, S.E. Fischer, M.B. Scheidegger, and P. Boesiger. Systolic long axis contraction of the human myocardium. In *Proceedings of the SMR*, 1995.
18. L.K. Waldman, J.J. Allen, R.S. Pavelec, and A.D. McCulloch. Distributed mechanics of the canine right ventricle: effects of varying preload. *J Biomechanics*, 29(3):373–81, 1996.
19. A.A. Young and L. Axel. Non-rigid heart wall motion using MR tagging. In *Proceedings of the IEEE Computer Society Conference on computer vision and pattern recognition*, pages 399–404, Campaign, Illinois, 1992.
20. A.A. Young, Z.A. Fayad, and L. Axel. Right ventricular mid-wall surface motion and deformation using magnetic resonance tagging. *J Appl Physiol*, 271:2677–88, 1996.
21. A.A. Young, D. L. Kraitchman, L. Dougherty, and L. Axel. Tracking and finite element analysis of stripe deformation in magnetic resonance tagging. *IEEE Trans on Med Imaging*, 14(3):413–21, September 1995.
22. O.C. Zienkiewicz and R.L. Taylor. *The Finite Element Method*. McGraw-Hill, New York, fourth edition, 1989.

Magnetic Resonance Guided Radiofrequency Ablation: Creation and Visualization of Cardiac Lesions

Albert C. Lardo, Ph.D., Henry Halperin, M.D., Christopher Yeung, BA.Sc.,
Pitayadet Jumrussirikul, M.D., Ergin Atalar, Ph.D., Elliot McVeigh, Ph.D.

Johns Hopkins School of Medicine
Departments of Biomedical Engineering, Cardiology, and Radiology
Baltimore, M.D. 21205

Abstract. Current management of atrial fibrillation (AF) refractory to pharmacological therapy involves the creation of lines of conduction block in the atrial tissue either by direct surgical incision or fluoroscopy guided radiofrequency (RF) ablation. While these techniques have been shown to be effective in terminating atrial fibrillation, open heart surgery carries considerable inherent risk and fluoroscopy guided approaches are technically difficult and result in extremely long radiation exposure times. Magnetic resonance (MR) guided ablation therapy may represent a safer and more practical alternative for creating lines of conduction block in patients with AF. We have developed a novel MR compatible system that permits simultaneous high resolution MR imaging, cardiac electrical mapping, and RF energy delivery. This system has, for the first time, made it possible to perform a comprehensive MR guided electrophysiology study including guidance, delivery, and monitoring of cardiac ablation therapy.

Introduction

Atrial fibrillation is a common cardiac arrhythmia that affects over 2 million people in the United States and is characterized by rapid, random, and hemodynamically inefficient atrial contractions that result in 75,000 stokes per year [1]. In patients unresponsive to drug therapy, AF management is achieved by the surgical maze procedure [2] where strategically placed long linear atrial incisions are created to compartmentalize the electrical activity of the atrial chamber and terminate abnormal excitation pathways. While the efficacy of this procedure has been demonstrated [3], the procedure is technically difficult and involves significant operative risk. A less invasive alternative designed to mimic the surgical maze procedure has been attempted using fluoroscopy guided radiofrequency ablation therapy, where electrical energy is deposited into the tissue and localized RF induced hyperthermia results in irreversible cellular destruction and elimination of abnormal electrical propagation pathways. While early experience with this technique appears promising, the success of fluoroscopy guided cardiac ablation is limited by the inability to create and visualize linear and contiguous (incision-like) lesions, which in turn leads to extremely long procedure times, ineffective treatments, and excessive x-ray exposure for both the patient and physician. In light of these limitations, the development of an alternative interventional approach is warranted.

MR guided thermal therapy delivery may be a logical alternative to fluoroscopic techniques as it offers several theoretical and practical advantages including: 1) elimination of patient and physician exposure to ionizing radiation, 2) rapid three-dimensional visualization of cardiac chambers and thermal lesions with high spatial resolution, 3) real time catheter placement with a potential reduction in the number of required surgical lesions and a corresponding reduction in procedure time, 4) simultaneous high resolution imaging, electrical mapping and RF delivery, 5) potential for real time spatial temperature monitoring using temperature sensitive imaging protocols and T1/T2 signal changes in heated tissue, and 6) high resolution atrial imaging to evaluate function and flow dynamics during AF which may provide an assessment of future risk of embolization. We have developed a novel MR compatible hardware system for use with a loopless intracardiac MR imaging catheter previously described by our group [4], to perform a comprehensive MR guided interventional electrophysiology study. While previous studies have described the use of MR guided thermal therapies for the control of abdominal, prostate, and liver tumors, to date no studies have demonstrated the ability to create and visualize cardiac RF ablation lesions using interventional MRI. Accordingly, the purpose of this study was to develop and characterize a novel MR ablation/antenna system capable of high-resolution intracardiac imaging for guidance, delivery, and monitoring of cardiac radiofrequency thermal therapy.

Methods and Materials

Under fluoroscopic guidance, a 3F imaging antenna and a 5F MR compatible ablation catheter were placed in the right atrium and right ventricle of healthy dogs via the right femoral and jugular veins respectively. RF ablation was performed on the posterior wall of the right atrium and the right ventricular apex using a customized MR compatible 4 mm electrode tip catheter and clinical ablation unit (Medtronic Atakar®, Minneapolis, MN) over a range of clinically used powers (10-50W) and a constant duration of 60 sec. Under MR guidance, several RF burns were delivered to both the posterior-lateral wall of the right atrium and right ventricular apex. Catheter and antenna guidance imaging was performed using the cardiac phased array coil in a 1.5T closed system (Signa 5.0, General Electric, Milwaukee, WI) with a gradient echo imaging protocol (TR/TE = 1.0/1.2ms, field of view = 24 cm, slice thickness = 8 mm, 256 x 192 matrix, tip angle = 11 degrees, readout bandwidth = 64 kHz). Following each 60-second burn session, lesion imaging was performed every three minutes with the cardiac phased array coil and antenna using both T1 gradient echo and T2 weighted fast spin echo sequences (TE = 50.8ms, ETL = 8, field of view = 14 cm, slice thickness = 6 mm, 256 x 128 matrix, readout bandwidth = 62.5 kHz) to characterize temporal and spatial MR signal changes of the cardiac tissue following RF injury. To compare the MR lesion appearance and size with the anatomical lesion, the heart was excised immediately following sacrifice and inspected. Lesions in the right atrium and ventricle were photographed and matched with the corresponding lesions from T2 weighted fast spin echo images.

MR Imaging Antenna

The intravascular imaging catheter used in these studies consists of a dipole antenna constructed from a 1.2 mm diameter segment of co-axial semi-flexible cable and MR compatible matching, tuning and decoupling circuitry [4] (Figure 1). The outer conductor of the cable, which is used to carry the MR signal to the antenna circuitry, serves as one pole, while the inner conductor serves as the second pole that receives the MR signal generated following body coil excitation of the slice. Because of the extremely high sensitivity and SNR in the immediate vicinity of the antenna, near microscopic resolution is a possible which is ideally suited for visualization of small thermal RF lesions. This major advantage is in addition to the excellent tissue characterization inherent to MRI.

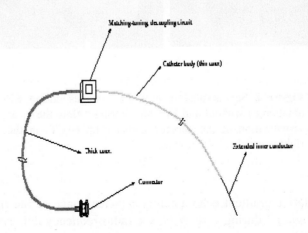

Figure 1 Schematic of the dipole imaging antenna.[4]

MR Compatible Filters

One of the problems associated with simultaneous radiofrequency energy delivery and MR imaging is electromagnetic interference that results in interference with the MR image. While the frequency of the radiofrequency generation unit (550kHz) is well below the 64 MHz proton precession frequency at 1.5 T, higher harmonics of the radiofrequency signal can produce significant image degradation. To overcome this limitation, novel MR compatible filters were designed and constructed to suppress these higher harmonic signals and permit simultaneous RF ablation and electrophysiology monitoring during MR imaging. These multi-stage, low-pass filters consist of a strategic arrangement of electrical components that achieve a cut off frequency of approximately 10MHz. Figure 2 shows an example of the dramatic effect of the RF ablation signal on image quality as the left panel represents the MR image during RF delivery without filtering while the image on the right shows the same slice during RF delivery with filtering. Note there is no evidence of noise or artifact and the tip of the ablation catheter is clearly visible.

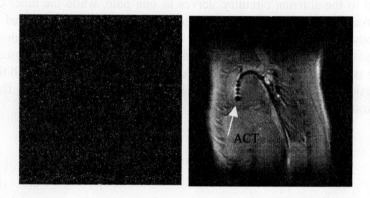

Figure 2 Sagital phased array coil images during RF ablation a) without and b) with filtering. Note the clear visualization of the ablation catheter tip (ACT) in the right ventricle.

Results

A representative gradient echo antenna catheter image of the right atrium is shown in Figure 3 during a 30 W 60 sec radiofrequency delivery (FOV = 14 cm). The MR compatible ablation catheter (AC) is shown on the lateral wall of the right atrium (arrow) directly adjacent to the imaging antenna. Note that the superior vena cava and entire atria is illuminated exclusively by the antenna catheter. Figure 4 shows a post-mortem coronal fast spin echo image

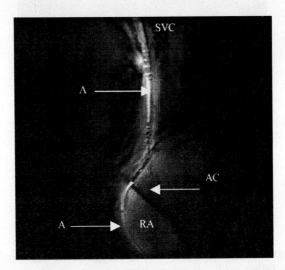

Figure 3 Antenna image showing the placement of the antenna (A) and ablation catheter (AC) in a canine right atrium (field of view = 14cm).

through the atria and ventricle of a dog acquired using the cardiac phased array coil, with the intracardiac antenna coil image shown in the enlarged window "C". The ablated areas of the myocardium can be visualized (arrows) in the intraventricular septum (IVS) and the enlarged area of the RA. Blood in the RA and RV is shown in white. Figure 5 shows a series of fast spin echo images of a right ventricular apex lesion before and after RF three RF burns. The first image of the series represents the baseline image before RF delivery with the arrow indicating the position of ablation catheter. The second image is 5 min following two 10 W 30sec ventricular burns. Note the hyperintense region at the tip of the ablation catheter (arrow). The third image is the same slice imaged 10 min following three 25W 60sec RF burns. The hyperintense region around the ablation catheter tip in the right ventricular apex is more pronounced in both intensity and size.

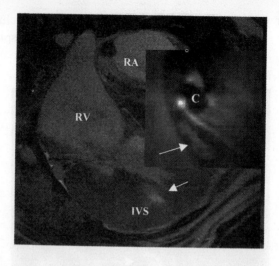

Figure 4 Coronal fast spin echo image of atria and ventricle following RF ablation with the torso and antenna coil "C".

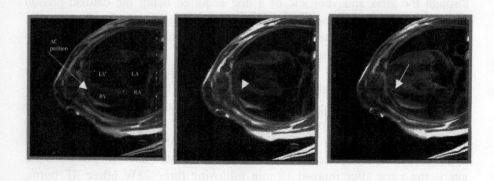

Figure 5 T2 weighted fast spin echo images showing right ventricular apex slices a) at baseline and following 60 sec RF energy delivery at b) 10W and c) 30W. Note the increase in lesion size between b) and c).

Discussion

Over the past several years, MRI guided thermal therapy has slowly evolved from a theoretical research tool to a clinically applied treatment that has shown significant promise as an alternative to traditional invasive surgical procedures and radiology imaging techniques. The ongoing maturity of this exciting interventional tool has largely been driven by applications related to the local control of regional metastic cancer in most major organs. Despite the recent advent of cardiac ablation techniques, which have revolutionized the management of patients with supraventricular arrhythmias refractory to pharmacological therapy, MRI guidance of thermal therapy in the heart has received virtually no attention. This is most likely attributed to the many challenges inherent to interventional MR cardiac imaging, including the geometric complexity of the heart, significant organ motion, presence of high blood flow, and the need for rapid imaging and display. In this study, we describe a system designed to permit MR guided cardiac thermal therapy and thus potentially serve as an alternative to surgical and fluoroscopy guided ablation techniques for atrial fibrillation and other cardiac arrhythmias. These encouraging, but preliminary results indeed indicate that MRI may be used to guide cardiac thermal therapy, although further work is required to determine the direct applicability and utility of this exciting technique.

Conclusions

These preliminary studies have demonstrated that it is possible to perform RF tissue ablation during MR imaging without compromising SNR. The tip of the catheter is clearly defined in gradient echo images and ablation lesions could be visualized in the right atrium and ventricle using T2 weighted FSE imaging with the both the intracardiac antenna and cardiac phased array coil. MR guided ablation may be a logical alternative to fluoroscopy guided techniques that will eliminate radiation exposure and may potentially reduce procedure times by facilitating the creation of linear, contiguous and transmural atrial lesions required for AF termination. Additionally, accurate visualization of the areas of ablation may allow for a reduction in the total number of lesions needed, which may also reduce the reoccurrence of AF.

References

1. Zipes D. Atrial Fibrillation: A tachycardia-induced atrial cardiomyopathy. Circulation 1997;95:562-564.

2. Cox J, Jaquiss R, Schuessler R, Boineau J. Modification of the maze procedure for atrial flutter and fibrillation, II: surgical technique of the maze II procedure. J Thorac Cardiovasc Surg 1995;110:485-495.

3. Haissaguerre M. Right and left atrial radiofrequency ablation catheter therapy of paroxysmal atrial fibrillation. J Cardiovasc Electrophysiol 1996;7:1132-1144.

4. Ocali O, Atalar E. Intravascular magnetic resonance imaging using a loopless catheter antenna. Magn. Reson. Med. 37, 112-118

Human Versus Robotic Organ Retraction During Laparoscopic Nissen Fundoplication

Benjamin Poulose[1], Michael Kutka[1], Mario Mendoza-Sagaon[1], Aaron Barnes[2], Calvin Yang[3], Russell Taylor[3], Mark Talamini[1]

[1] Johns Hopkins University School of Medicine
Department of Surgery
Blalock 665
600 N. Wolfe Street
Baltimore, MD 21287
talamini@welchlink.welch.jhu.edu

[2] Johns Hopkins University
Department of Mechanical Engineering
122 Latrobe Hall
Baltimore, MD 21218

[3] Johns Hopkins University
Department of Computer Science
224 New Engineering Building
Johns Hopkins University
Baltimore, MD 21218

Abstract. Advances in technique and instrumentation have enabled surgeons to perform a growing array of procedures through laparoscopy. However, these efforts have often been compromised by exerting excessive forces during retraction of the structures necessary for anatomical view. Here, we present a comparative study of human and robotic performance in force controlled organ retraction during laparoscopic Nissen fundoplication (LNF). Six female pigs (20-25 kg) were anesthetized, intubated, placed on mechanical ventilation, and pneumoperitoneum (13mm Hg CO_2) was established. A force sensing retractor (FSR) was constructed to record the forces applied in retracting the stomach during dissection of the esophageal hiatus (EH). The FSR was calibrated using known forces and then operated by either human alone or robot under human guidance using the FSR data. The EH was visualized, dissected, and LNF completed. Less force was utilized with robotic (74.3±10.5 grams) versus human (108.9±34.3 grams) retraction (p=0.007) to obtain proper anatomical view of the EH. No significant differences were observed for retraction setup time (robot 14.3±0.8 minutes and human 13.7±9.9 minutes) or hiatal dissection time (robot 14.0±3.0 minutes and human 14.0±6.1 minutes). These preliminary results present our continuing effort to develop and evaluate an automated surgical assistant for laparoscopy. As increasingly advanced, personnel-intensive laparoscopic procedures are performed, robotic retraction may present a superior alternative to human retraction by minimizing the forces exerted on organs yet maintaining excellent anatomical view.

Introduction

The benefits of laparoscopic techniques are being applied to an ever increasing number of general surgical procedures. Patients typically experience less post-operative pain, shorter hospital stay, and return to daily routines faster compared to the same procedures performed by more traditional "open" technique [3, 8, 11]. As an increasing array of more complex, longer duration laparoscopic procedures are performed, the likelihood of iatrogenic injury to the patient also increases. Often, participation of assistants not familiar with laparoscopic techniques is unavoidable in personnel-intensive procedures. A common task relegated to these assistants is the retraction of organs necessary to obtain proper anatomical view. This exposure, critical to both traditional and minimally invasive surgery, is especially important in laparoscopy as surgeons forfeit their primary sense of touch in favor of a more visually based technique. However, once organs are retracted and the proper view established, the camera view is mainly focused on the immediate operative field and not on the retracted organ. Thus, these surgical assistants are regularly entrusted to use an unfamiliar instrument to retract an unseen organ for an extended period of time, increasing the risk of iatrogenic harm. Injury to visceral or vascular structures are serious complications that can result in peritonitis, sepsis, intra-abdominal abscess or hemorrhage. Often, these injuries are not recognized at the time of the laparoscopic procedure, increasing the chance of a fatal outcome [1].

The union of surgical robotics, computer integrated video, and laparoscopy is attempting to transfer time consuming, repetitive tasks from human to robot in an effort to increase safety and improve surgical outcome. Considerable experience has been gained with robotic camera control during laparoscopy, displaying the feasibility and efficacy of using surgical robots in the operating room [5]. In addition, passive systems such as the "Iron Intern" have been developed to hold structures fixed in space during minimally invasive surgery [6]. However, these passive systems are unable to respond to anatomical shifts caused by changes in respiration, organ manipulation, and patient position. Pioneering work in active, force feedback robotic retraction systems will enable neurosurgeons to retract neural tissue with precision and minimal damage [2]. Newer computerized surgical graspers are enabling physicians to obtain tactile information about the tissue, providing critical clinical cues to the laparoscopic surgeon [4]. Experience is lacking regarding the effectiveness of force feedback surgical robotic systems that actively assist surgeons in organ manipulation during laparoscopic general surgical procedures. A surgical robot may be able to minimize iatrogenic injury and maintain anatomical view by sensing the force directly applied to retracted organs and by adjusting itself to maintain a constant retraction force. Here, we present the first comparative study of human and robotic organ retraction during an advanced laparoscopic procedure, the laparoscopic Nissen fundoplication (LNF). We employ a novel force-sensing organ retraction system to measure the forces applied to a retracted structure and to complete the robotic "sensor-effector" loop. These preliminary results and evaluation aid in our development of an automated laparoscopic surgical assistant system.

Materials and Methods

The Force Sensing Retractor (FSR) was developed to measure the force applied to organs during surgical manipulation. A standard laparoscopic retractor (United States Surgical, Norwalk, CT) was modified to create the FSR. Two 350 Ohm polyimide encapsulated constantan strain gauges (Model CEA-06-250-UN-350, Vishay Measurements Group, Raleigh, NC) were bonded to the middle tine of the retractor in a bending beam configuration (Fig. 1). The strain gauges were connected to a strain indicator (Model P-3500, Vishay Measurements Group, Raleigh, NC) which produced positive or negative voltages depending on FSR deflection (Fig. 1). The output of the strain indicator was then routed to a Grass Recorder (Model 7D Polygraph, Grass Instruments, Quincy, MA) and PC for continuous data collection of retraction forces.

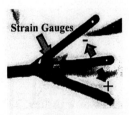

Fig. 1. Gauges bonded to standard organ retractor provide force sensing in main retraction axis

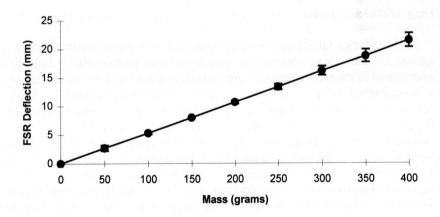

Fig. 2. Linear force response to known masses is confirmed

Before each experiment, the FSR was calibrated using known weights and the linearity of force response to the test weights was confirmed (Fig. 2). A linear equation derived from calibration data was used to determine the force applied to the retracted organ. All forces are presented as mass equivalents in grams.

The LARS robot [10] was developed jointly by Johns Hopkins University and IBM Research to aid surgeons in a wide variety of laparoscopic applications including camera holding and precise instrument control for active assistance during laparoscopic procedures (Fig. 3). LARS possesses 4 degrees-of-freedom (three rotations and one depth of penetration centered at the entry port), image guided camera aiming, and several safety features designed to minimize haphazard movement of instruments within the abdomen. Sensors mounted on the instrument carrier limit the amount of force and torque exerted on the surgical instruments. Should forces or torques exceed safety thresholds, the robot ceases all motion until they are again within safe limits or the operator intervenes.

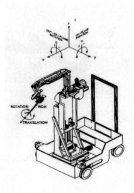

Fig. 3. LARS surgical robot

Six female pigs (20-25 kgs) were premedicated with intramuscular ketamine and general anesthesia was administered with intravenous pentobarbital. The animals were placed in the supine position. An endotracheal tube was placed and connected to a mechanical ventilator (Harvard Apparatus Model 613. Southnatick, MA). A central venous catheter and arterial catheter were placed in the femoral vein and artery, respectively. A Veress needle was inserted into the peritoneal cavity and CO_2 pneumoperitoneum was achieved with a standard insufflator (Olympus Surgical, Olympus America, Inc.) using an intra-abdominal pressure of 13mm Hg. Five 10mm trocars (Ethicon Endosurgery, Cincinnati, OH) were placed as previously described for standard laparoscopic Nissen fundoplication [9]. A 30° laparoscope (Karl Storz Endoscopy, Charlton, MA) was introduced into the umbilical port and standard laparoscopic video equipment was used (Olympus Surgical, Olympus America, Inc). The liver was retracted manually in all experiments, fully exposing the stomach.

For the three pigs undergoing human retraction, the previously calibrated FSR was inserted into the port at the left anterior axillary line and was sutured to the most cephalad portion of the gastric fundus. FSR data collection was confirmed, and the surgical assistant retracted the stomach using the FSR and one additional laparoscopic grasper, exposing the gastro-esophageal junction for dissection. The surgical assistant was blinded to the readings from the FSR.

The remaining three pigs underwent robotic retraction. LARS was brought to the left side of the animal at the level of the left lower extremity. The FSR was placed into the LARS instrument holder and the instrument was advanced into the abdomen via left anterior axillary line port. The FSR was sutured into the most cephalad portion of the fundus, and the camera operator used an additional laparoscopic grasper to expose the esophageal hiatus. In this preliminary experiment, a human operator closed the force feedback loop by monitoring the FSR output and modifying LARS placement as needed to maintain proper anatomical view of the gastro-esophageal junction for dissection. In future studies, this process will be automated by feeding FSR data into the robot's controlling computer, allowing the robot to analyze and change retractor position without human intervention.

In all surgeries, stomach retraction was required during esophageal hiatus dissection, after which the FSR was removed, esophagus mobilized, and standard laparoscopic Nissen fundoplication was performed. In addition to FSR data, retraction setup time (measured as the interval between "first touch" of the FSR and proper hiatal exposure) and total retraction time (time from suturing of FSR to mobilization of the esophagus) were recorded. Ease of retractor placement, retractor maneuverability, anatomical view, and ease of removal were scored on a 1-10 scale (1=worst, 10=best) by the same primary surgeon.

Continuous variables between human and robotic groups were analyzed using the student's t-test. Differences were considered statistically significant at $p<0.05$.

Results

All six laparoscopic Nissen fundoplications were performed successfully and organ retraction data obtained for human and robot control of stomach retraction during esophageal hiatus dissection. The mean force applied during human retraction was 108.9 ± 34.3g with a range of 52.5g to 180.7g. Using robotic retraction of the stomach, the mean force applied was 74.3 ± 10.5g with values ranging from 56.1g to 94.8g ($p=0.007$ compared to human retraction). Represented over time, forces required were markedly less for robotic retraction than for human retraction (Fig. 4). Furthermore, retraction setup time and total retraction time did not differ significantly between human and robotic retraction (Table 1).

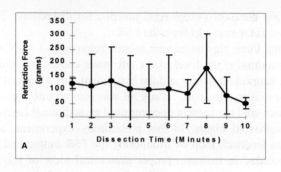
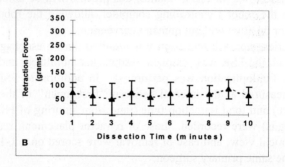
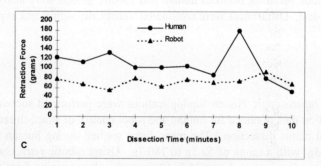

Fig. 4. Panel A shows wide variation in human retraction force with mean of 108.9g (n=3). Panel B displays robotic retraction (n=3) with lower mean force (74.3g) and less variation (p=0.007 vs human retraction). Composite view of human and robotic retraction forces are seen in Panel C (negative axes omitted for clarity in Panels A and B; error bars omitted in C)

Table 1. Retractor setup and hiatal dissection times were similar for human and robot

Parameter	Human (n=3)	Robot (n=3)
Setup (mins)	13.7±9.9	14.3±0.8
Dissection (mins)	14.0±6.1	14.0±3.0

Examining the more subjective measures, human and robotic retraction did not differ regarding ease of retractor placement, retractor maneuverability, anatomical view, and ease of removal (Table 2). In addition, one less surgical assistant was required when using the robot (Fig. 5); the camera holder easily doubled as primary assistant in manipulating the second laparoscopic grasper used to help retract the stomach.

Table 2. Human and robotic retraction afforded similar ease of placement, maneuverability, anatomical view, and ease of removal (1=worst, 10=best)

Parameter	Human (n=3)	Robot (n=3)
Ease of Placement	7	7.7
Maneuverability	7	7.7
Anatomical View	7.7	7
Ease of Removal	8.7	7.7

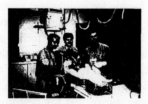

Fig. 5. Robotic retraction of stomach during laparoscopic Nissen fundoplication. With the robot, only two people were needed to complete the surgery versus the usual three person team (in this view, person at far left is adjusting robot and did not assist in surgery)

Throughout the experiment, the LARS robot and FSR performed reliably without significant alteration to standard surgical procedure. Minor changes in port placement were required to provide adequate clearance for full range of motion for the robot. One incident of software difficulty caused the robot to become unresponsive, but safety was maintained simply by loosening the FSR from the robot using a quick-release clamp and removing it from the immediate operative field. The robot was soon rebooted, FSR placed into position again, and the operation continued. Electrocautery caused significant fluctuations in FSR output, but data collection returned to normal immediately after use without the need for re-calibration.

Discussion

Surgical robotic systems present an extremely useful tool to the laparoscopic surgeon. To date, most experience in the pre-clinical and clinical general surgical realms utilizes passive systems to control the laparoscopic camera and to perform rudimentary structure-grasping actions. Progress has been made in developing active robotic force feedback systems for neurosurgical applications [2]. In general surgery, systems have been designed to enhance the laparoscopic surgeon's senses by providing tactile information about the tissue retracted by a laparoscopic grasper [4]. These systems provide an important adjunct to the usual audio and visual information presented to the surgeon. An eventual goal in surgical robotics is to develop a fully automated, active surgical assistant capable of analyzing its actions and responding appropriately and safely. This robot should be designed to have its own intelligence and to perform its function more effectively than a human in the intended task [7]. To develop these systems, not only is a reliable means of obtaining data from the robot's environment needed, but baseline pre-clinical studies must be performed to evaluate these force feedback robotic systems. In this study, we present a unique means of measuring the forces applied directly to retracted organs in a pre-clinical laparoscopic model. This preliminary experiment compares "head to head" human laparoscopic retraction and robotic retraction. From this baseline retraction data, streamlined algorithms can be developed to set operating constraints on active robotic surgical assistants, ensuring patient safety.

In retracting the gastric fundus for esophageal hiatus visualization and dissection, the LARS robot performed better than a human by greatly minimizing the force exerted on the stomach. By keeping retraction forces as low as possible, the risk of direct injury to retracted viscera was minimized. Although the operator of the FSR during human retraction was blinded to the output of the device (and thus could not adjust his performance to achieve a biased result) the results may have differed to a larger extent had he not been aware that his performance was being "measured." Because of this knowledge, the operator may have been more careful than usual in not exerting excessive forces on the retracted organ. Nevertheless, wide variations existed during human retraction (Fig. 4A) that were not observed during robotic retraction (Fig. 4B)--even with operator knowledge of performance monitoring. In these experiments, the LARS robot was manipulated by joystick, utilizing a human viewing the FSR data to complete the force feedback loop to maximize proper anatomic view. With the robot performing organ retraction, forces exerted on the stomach were minimal, with much less variation in force compared to human. This decrease in force variation is likely due to the minimal movement of the FSR and less motion of organs around the robot-controlled FSR. Repositioning the robot occasionally forced the surgical assistant to remove his hand from the camera, resulting in an interruption of the "flow" of the procedure. As the FSR data stream is coupled to the robot's computer and drive motors, we expect to create a fully autonomous robot with an even further decrease in retraction forces, given the robot's ability to make instantaneous adjustments in space. Although force information in this experiment is available in the main retraction axis using data supplied from the center tine of the FSR, a more complete system being developed in our lab utilizes six strain gauges placed on all three tines of the FSR. Using this information, the robot can not only respond to changes in the main axis of retraction, but can also rotate about its longitudinal axis to allow a more human-like movement and further minimize retraction force. This system would also account for the load placed on the side tines of the retractor, which was not measured in this experiment.

Additional data suggest no significant difference between human and robot in retraction setup time and total retraction time. Often, new surgical technologies present large learning curves to the surgeon—possibly compromising efficiency [7]. Here, LARS was easily mated to the FSR, brought to the operating room table, and the FSR inserted into the abdomen without difficulty. Also, robotic retraction and manipulation did not significantly increase the time of surgery as measured by total retraction time. Although a more subjective analysis was used, the anatomical view obtained was fairly consistent when using either human or robotic retraction.

Further uses of the FSR include new applications to increase safety in human laparoscopic retraction and in telerobotic force feedback systems. Since the main laparoscopic view in most procedures is focused on the surgical site and not on retracted organs, the FSR could provide critical information to the human assistant by informing him or her of excessive forces applied on the retracted organ, without disrupting the primary surgeon's view. With the planned integration of FSR data with the LARS robot, a unique telerobotic system for use with force feedback control can be created. This would allow remote or telementoring surgeons full video, audio, and force responsive manipulating capability while many miles away from the operative site.

Recent advances in laparoscopy have enabled the general surgeon to offer the benefits of minimally invasive surgery to a wider range of patients with varied surgical issues. As these procedures increase in complexity and operative time, potential complications and the risk of operator-caused injury also increase. Force sensing laparoscopic instruments present one way to make organ retraction during complex procedures safer. Robotic surgical systems that utilize this force sensing technology for organ retraction may be superior to human retraction by minimizing the force exerted on organs, decreasing chance of iatrogenic injury, and making laparoscopic procedures safer.

References

1. Deziel, D.J.: Avoiding Laparoscopic Complications. Int. Surg. (1994) 79:361-364
2. Fukushima, T., Gruen, P.: Computers and Robotics in Neurosurgery. In: Taylor, R., Lavalee, G., Burdea, G., Moesges, R. (eds.): Computer Integrated Surgery. MIT Press
3. Gadacz, T.R., Talamini, M.A.: Traditional Versus Laparoscopic Cholecystectomy. Am. J. Surg. (1991) 161(3):336-338
4. Hannaford, B., Trujillo, J., Sinanan, M., Moreyra, M., Rosen, J., Brown, J., Leuschke, R., MacFarlane, M.: Computerized Endoscopic Surgical Grasper. Proceedings, Medicine Meets Virtual Reality, San Diego (1998)
5. Kavoussi, L.R., Moore, R.G., Adams, J.B., Partin, A.W.: Comparison of Robotic Versus Human Laparoscopic Control. J. Urol. (1995) 154:2134-2136
6. McEwen, J.A.: Solo Surgery With Automated Positioning Platforms: Concepts and Opportunities for the Integration of Instrumentation with Automated Positioning Systems. Proceedings, New Frontiers in Minimally Invasive and Interventional Surgery, New Orleans (1992)
7. Satava, R.M., Ellis, S.R.: Human Interface Technology. Surg. Endosc. (1994) 8:817-820

8. Soper, N.J., Barteau, J.A., Clayman, R.V., Ashley, S.W., Dunnegan, D.L.: Comparison of Early Postoperative Results for Laparoscopic Versus Standard Open Cholecystectomy. Surg. Gynecol. Obstet. (1992) 174:114-118
9. Talamini, M.A., Mendoza-Sagaon, M., Gitzelmann, C.A., Ahmad, S., Moesinger, R., Kutka, M., Toung, T.: Increased Mediastinal Pressure and Decreased Cardiac Output during Laparoscopic Nissen Fundoplication. Surgery. (1997) 122(2):345-52
10. Taylor, R.H., Funda, J., Eldridge, B., Gomory, S., Gruben, K., LaRose, D., Talamini, M., Kavoussi, L., Anderson, J.: A Telerobotic Assistant for Laparoscopic Surgery. IEEE Engin. Med. Biol. (1995) May/June:279-287
11. Vogt, D.M., Curet, M.J., Pitcher, D.E., Martin, D.T., Zucker, K.A.: Preliminary Results of a Prospective Randomized Trial of Laparoscopic Onlay Versus Conventional Inguinal Herniorraphy. Am. J. Surg. (1995) 169:84-90

A New Laparoscope Manipulator with an Optical Zoom

Etsuko KOBAYASHI, Ken MASAMUN, Takeyoshi DOHI, Daijo HASHIMOTO*

Department of Precision Machinery Engineering, Graduates School & Faculty of
Engineering, The University of Tokyo,
7-3-1, Hongo, Bunkyo-ku, Tokyo 113, Japan
e-mail: etsuko@miki.pe.u-tokyo.ac.jp

*Tokyo Metropolitan Police Hospital

Abstract. This report describes a new type of laparoscope manipulator with an optical zoom. The manipulator was designed with regard to its safety in medical settings. It is based on a five-bar linkage mechanism. Back and forth movements of a laparoscope are achieved by an optical zoom. By using the five-bar linkage mechanism with the optical zoom, the manipulator need never interfere with the surgeon or the patient. However, the problem of the quality of the image created by the zoom lens remained. To address this problem, we used a short laparoscope instead of an ordinary laparoscope. In this way, the manipulator achieved a high quality laparoscope image with a sufficient degree of safety

1. Introduction

Laparoscopic surgery is becoming more popular as a form of minimally invasive surgery [1]. Internal anatomy is observed through the laparoscope and procedures are performed using long forceps that are inserted through trocar sleeves. Compared with open surgery, laparoscopic surgery is more difficult because the surgeon is forced to operate within the limited angle of laparoscopic view and the limited movement of the instruments.

One of the problems in laparoscopic surgery is the fluid manipulation of the laparoscope. Because the surgeon usually uses both hands to manipulate long instruments, it is difficult for the assistant (camera operator) to hold the laparoscope steady and keep the view upright while quickly aiming the scope at the point required by the surgeon.

Several engineers have therefore developed laparoscope manipulators and operator-machine interfaces [2][3][4][5]. The representative manipulator is AESOP (Computer Motion Inc., U.S.A), which has successfully acquired FDA approval as a robot for clinical use. However, laparoscope manipulators developed to date appear to lack adequate safety measures and capacity for sterilization.

Robots for medical use differ from industrial robots in the following four ways [6].
1. These robots contact the human body directly.
2. They are not allowed repeated trial movements.
3. They are designed to operate easily, because the surgeon is not a specialist in operating robots.
4. They have different functions for each medical procedure.

From the above, we concluded that significant improvements in robot design were needed to satisfy the requirements of the operating theater. The close contact between the robot and the patient requires that safety measures be built into both software and hardware. It is preferable for the robot to be mechanically safe and simple with limited range of movement, rather than to have its safety and usefulness achieved only through the use of complicated software.

Therefore, we have developed a laparoscopic manipulator using a five-bar linkage mechanism and optical zooming [7]. This mechanism allows the manipulator to achieve sufficient safety, and allows for sterilization and minimum obstruction. These are the most important factors for medical robots. However, the problem of image quality achieved by the zoom lens remains.

In this paper, we describe the new type of laparoscope manipulator together with an innovative zooming laparoscope.

2 Mechanism of the laparoscope manipulator

We developed the manipulator using a five-bar linkage mechanism (Fig. 1). In this setup, the laparoscope is attached to a holder with two degrees of angular freedom near the insertion site of the abdomen. The manipulator holds the camera end. The manipulator has two degrees of freedom. Its movement in the X-Y plane changes the angle of the laparoscope. A zoom lens substitutes for the back and forth movement of the laparoscope.

To realize the X-Y plane movement of the manipulator, we chose a five-bar linkage mechanism. In this mechanism, the top (P) moves within two degrees of freedom in the X-Y plane by changing the angles of two other links (A and B). Furthermore, we add another link (H) to the top of the manipulator and a parallel link mechanism (links B, D, E and F). Link (H) remains horizontal at any position by the parallel link mechanism. By link (H) changing in length and setting direction, the surgeon can set the holding point (camera end) at the required position before the manipulation, with the manipulator positioned some distance from the insertion point.

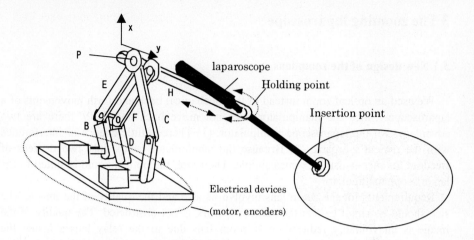

Fig. 1. Mechanism of the manipulator. Because links B, D, E and F make a parallel link mechanism, link H remains horizontal. In this mechanism, all electrical devices can be positioned below.

The advantages of this mechanism are as follows.
1. The manipulator can be placed some distance from the patient's abdomen. As a result the manipulator imposes minimum obstruction on the work of the surgeon and there is little chance of the manipulator coming into contact with the surgeon or the patient.
2. The five-bar linkage mechanism means that the range of movement is limited mechanically. This avoids unexpected movements if the software does not produce accurate responses.
3. A zoom lens substitutes for the back and forth movement of the laparoscope. This minimizes the chance of interference with the organs being examined.
4. Electrical devices such as motors can be positioned below, so that the upper part consists only of simple links. With this mechanism, the upper link is easily removed from the controller, allowing the controller device to be covered with a drape and the linkage part to be sterilized. That is, most parts of the manipulator can be sterilized and only the electrical devices escape sterilization.

We used stepping motors as actuators of our manipulator. The actuators are controlled by a personal computer (PC-9821Xt16, CPU Pentium 166 MHz) with an open-loop design. To avoid the accumulation of error, the angle of the links is measured by the absolute rotary encoders before use as a control. Encoders measure absolutely the angle of the bottom links at all times, and the initial position does not need to be reset after the surgeon moves the manipulator manually or stops it in case of emergency. The size of this manipulator is 300 x 300 mm and the height is a maximum of 400 mm.

3 The zooming laparoscope

3.1 New design of the zoom lens

We used an optical zoom instead of the mechanical back and forth movements of a laparoscope. Since the manipulator does not move back and forth, there are two advantages for the laparoscope manipulator. (1) There is little chance of interference with the patient's organs. (2) Because the manipulator needs only two degrees of freedom, its mechanism becomes simple. Therefore, the optical zoom is suited to the laparoscope manipulator.

Requirements for the zoom lens involve its size and the quality of the image. The size should be small so that the surgeon's work is not obstructed. The quality of the image is unavoidably reduced by a zoom lens due to the relay lenses inside the laparoscope and the zoom lens.

To address this problem, we used a short laparoscope instead of an ordinary laparoscope. Fig. 2 shows the construction of our zooming system and Fig.3 shows its picture. We call it a zooming laparoscope. Our zooming laparoscope system consists of a trocar sleeve with optical fibers for a light guide, a short laparoscope and a zoom lens. There are optical fibers in the trocar sleeve to allow light to pass through it. The short laparoscope is the same length as the trocar sleeve and has only one lens at the tip of it. The length of the short laparoscope is 155 mm and the angle of the field of vision is 80 degrees. The short laparoscope is inserted into the trocar sleeve. For the zoom lens we used two lenses. One is a diameter of 22 mm and the other is 7 mm. By using a cam mechanism to move the lens, we can change its magnification by turning the outer tube. The second tube is used to focus. The long focal depth means that once we have focused appropriately we do not have to focus again when at another angle. Table 1 shows the specifications of the zooming laparoscope.

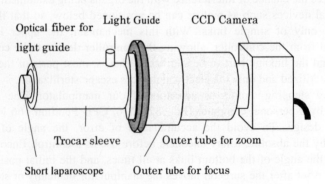

Fig. 2. The construction of a zooming laparoscope

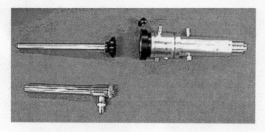

Fig. 3. Zooming laparoscope; left up is a short laparoscope. Left down is a trocar sleeve with optical fibers. Right is a zoom lens.

Table 1. Specifications of the zooming laparoscope.

CCD camera	SK-1057 3CCD (SINKOKOKI)
Magnification	6.0x
Focal depth (0.3 x)	5.61 (mm)
Size: Zoom lens	ϕ 30 x 158 (mm)
Trocar sleeve	ϕ 10 x 155 (mm)
Short laparoscope	ϕ 14 x 135 (mm)
Weight	800 (g)

Merits of the zooming laparoscope are as follows.
1. An ordinary laparoscope contains many lenses. On the other hand, the short laparoscope has only one lens. Therefore, by simplifying the optical system, the quality of the image is vastly improved.
2. Because the short laparoscope never comes close to the organs and its length is the same as the trocar sleeve, it never interferes with forceps movements or with the organs being examined.
3. Because the short laparoscope never closes to the organs, it avoids attaching blood to the tip of the laparoscope.

Therefore, we can realize a laparoscope manipulator with a high quality laparoscope image and a sufficient degree of safety by the zooming laparoscope.

Three manual trials of the zooming laparoscope are done on ordinary cholecystectomy. We confirmed that the zooming laparoscope had sufficient magnification an image quality. Fig.4 shows a comparison of laparoscope image between the zooming laparoscope and an ordinary laparoscope. Left is an image of the zooming laparoscope. The surgeon can see the cystic duct in the same magnification with the ordinary laparoscope.

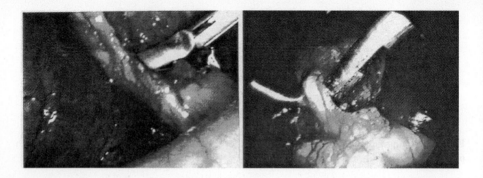

Fig. 4. Laparoscopic images of the cholecystectomy; left is the image of a zooming laparoscope, right is an ordinary laparoscope.

3.2 Automatic control of a zooming laparoscope

We developed an automatic control system for the zoom lens (see Fig.5). We used a DC motor (MINIMO co. ltd. 1016 M006G with Gear head 256:1) and a friction belt. The diameter of it is 10 mm. By turning the friction belt, the outer tube of the zoom lens is turned. The value of this design is its simplicity. There are no complicated mechanical parts such as ball bearings. Therefore, with the motor sealed, the whole mechanism can be sterilized.

Fig. 6 shows a laparoscope manipulator with a zooming laparoscope.

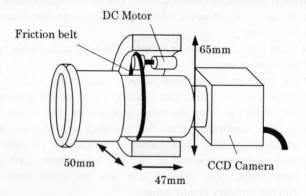

Fig. 5. Automatic control of the zooming laparoscope

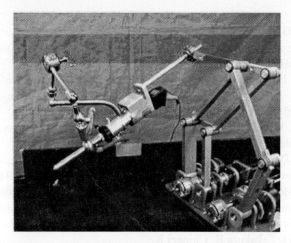

Fig. 6. Laparoscope manipulator with a zooming laparoscope.

4.Discussion

We used a five-bar linkage mechanism for the manipulator. This design provided mechanical safety, minimum obstruction to the work of the surgeon and the capacity for sterilization. Furthermore, by putting another link on top of the five-bar linkage mechanism, the surgeon can set the holding point of the manipulator to optimize the range of movement of the manipulator for each operation.

We developed a new type of laparoscope with a zoom lens. By simplifying the optical system, we were able to achieve a high quality image.

A trocar sleeve containing optical fibers is useful as a light source. When placed in other insertion points, light can be obtained from different directions. It has a lot of possibility. For example, light from the different direction makes the shade and then the surgeon can recognize the distance from a forceps to organs.

5. Conclusion

We have developed a new type of laparoscope with an optical zoom. Coupled with this zooming laparoscope, a manipulator using a five-bar linkage mechanism achieved mechanical safety and high image quality. We are confident that this manipulator meets the essential requirements for medical use.

This study was partly supported by the Research for the Future Program (JSPS-RFTF 96P00801).

REFERENCES
1. Hashimoto D, Hata N, Dohi T: Highly Qualified Laparoscopic Surgery: Gasless 3-D operation and intraoperative graphics navigation. Proc. of Computer Assisted Radiology: 811-816 (1995).
2. Taylor RH, Funda J, Eldridge B, Gomory S, Gruben K, LaRose D, Talamini M, Kavossi L, Anderson J A: Telerobotic Assistant for Laparoscopic Surgery. Computer Integrated Surgery: 581-592 (1995).
3. Sackier JM, Wang Y: Robotically Assisted Laparoscopic Surgery: From Concept to Development. Computer Integrated Surgery: 577-580 (1995).
4. Finlay PA, Ornstein MH: Controlling the Movement of a Surgical Laparoscope. IEEE Engineering in Medicine and Biology Vol.14 No.3: 289-299 (1995).
5. Koseki Y, Masamune K, Kataoka H, Masutani Y, Suzuki M, Dohi T, Hashimoto D: Development of an Endoscope Manipulator System for Laparoscopic Surgery. Proc. of Computer Assisted Radiology: 1049 (1996).Dohi T, Hata N, Miyata K, Hashimoto D, Takakura K, Chinzei K,
6. Yamauchi Y: Robotics in Computer Aided Surgery. Journal of Computer Aided Surgery Vol.1 No.1: 4-10 (1995).
7. Kobayashi E, Masamune K, Suzuki M, Dohi T and Hashimoto D: Development of a laparoscope manipulator using five-bar linkage mechanism. Proceedings of Computer Assisted Radiology and Surgery: 825-830 (1997).

A Newly Developed Stereotactic Robot with Detachable Drive for Neurosurgery

Ken MASAMUNE, L.H. JI, Makoto SUZUKI, Takeyoshi DOHI, *Hiroshi ISEKI, *Kintomo TAKAKURA

Graduate school & Faculty of Engineering, the University of Tokyo
*Dept. of Neurosurgery, Tokyo Women's Medical College
e-mail: masa@miki.pe.u-tokyo.ac.jp

Abstract. This paper describes the development of a needle insertion manipulator for stereotactic neurosurgery. This robot fulfils the requirements of having both a safe mechanical design and the capacity for being sterilized. Many kinds of robots are examined in neurosurgery. Their purpose is the precise positioning of surgical instruments such as biopsy needles, electrodes etc. Some are already available commercially and have been proven useful in the operating theatre. However, their clinical application is limited by specific problems including cost, safety, positioning requirements, maintenance requirements. The main problems have been with the safety of the mechanical design and difficulties with sterilization and disinfecting pre- and post operatively. The manipulator described in this report achieves mechanical safety and has the capacity for cover-sheet-free sterilization. The manipulator has three major components: the main mechanical component (with 6 degrees of freedom), the torque transmission component, and the electric motor, which cannot be sterilized. The electrical parts are detachable. Using this mechanism, we can clearly separate the surgical area from the mechatronics components. In this paper, the basic design and the prototype development and testing are described.

1. Introduction

Since the end of 1980s, many kinds of robotic technologies have been applied to stereotactic surgery, especially neurosurgery [1][2][3][6][7]. MINERVA in Switzerland, and NEUROMATE (IMMI) in France are now currently considered representative of advanced surgical robots for neurosurgery. The main purpose of these robots is the precise positioning of surgical instruments such as biopsy needles, electrodes and X-ray needles [4]. However, even those which are commercially available are limited in their clinical application by the following problems: cost, safety, maintenance requirements and the robot's mass and weight. As safety is the most important concern, our priority was to design a robot that was mechanically safe. The redundant working area of the robot is dangerous not only for the patient but also for the surgeons, even when safety has been built into the software and mechanical movement is slow. The next concern is to address the sterilization and disinfecting problem. It is common practice for advanced medical robots to be covered with sterilized plastic sheets. These are necessary when the robot is used in clinical settings. The reason for the cover sheet is that robots have many electrical parts, which cannot be sterilized because of problems arising during sterilization. Rusting, breakage and malfunction of the robot can result from autoclaving or ethylene oxide gas (EOG) sterilization.

In this paper, the requirements for a medical manipulator and a newly designed needle insertion medical robot for stereotactic neurosurgery are described, with a special focus on solving the sterilization problem.

2. System requirements

Stereotactic neurosurgery requires precise positioning of the insertion instruments, which perform biopsy, inject drugs, or position electrodes. Precision is the main concern, because it is crucial that any functional areas and major blood vessels of the brain be avoided. The acceptable positioning tolerance for stereotactic surgery is about 1-3mm, including distortions due to the imaging system. Stereotactic neurosurgery is usually performed with a frame, which is connected to the bed. The frame builds the absolute reference system to determine the position of insertion of the neurosurgical tools. Before conducting surgery, X-ray, CT and MRI scans are used to define the exact anatomical location of the target, relative to the stereotactic frame.

Considering these requirements, it appeared that the most direct approach was to redesign an industrial robot to position the instruments. Industrial robots are very good at controlling localization, maintaining a constant position, etc. However, significant changes are needed to satisfy the requirements of the operating theatre. Neither the hardware nor the software of industrial robots is designed for surgery and cannot be applied in a medical setting. Therefore, we propose a completely new design, based upon specific clinical demands. Medical robots have different requirements to industrial robots. We listed most important item below.

Safety: Prevention of accidents must be given the highest priority. In particular, safety has to be built into the mechanical design. There should be no possibility of interference with the patient except for the required movements. If there is a power failure when a medical robot is being used, the surgeon must be able to continue the operation manually. In comparison, if there is a power failure in an industrial setting, one can simply wait for the power to return.

Sterilization, Washable structure: The parts which are in direct contact with the patient have to be completely sterile and therefore must be steralizable. Parts without direct human contact can be covered with sterile sheets. However, we prefer to use fewer sheets as the manipulator often tears the sheets, thus breaking the sterile area. After the operation, the manipulator should be disinfected. Therefore the shape and the structure of its mechanism must be simple and easy to wash.

No trial movement permitted: The main purpose of today's surgical robot is basically to remove human tissue (for biopsy, hip prosthesis placement, etc.). Therefore, it is clear that test runs are not permitted.

In addition, we need different functions for each medical procedure. User friendly interfaces are also required.

While we consider the safety of medical robots to be the most important issue, the next major issue is that of sterilization. While most neurosurgical robots have significant safety measures, there is a need for a lot more discussion of the sterilization problem. As long as sterilized plastic cover sheets are used, the robot will remain a 'special' instrument in clinical settings. In the next section we describe the design of our new manipulator, which fulfills the above requirements as a medical robot.

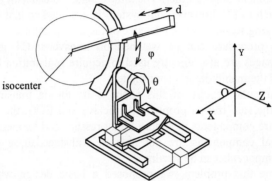

Fig. 1. Principle mechanism of an isocentric needle insertion manipulator

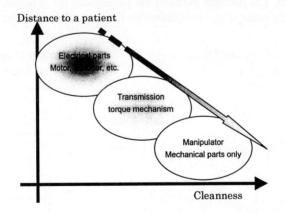

Fig. 2. Level of sterilization of the manipulator

3. A new mechanism

The basic mechanical structure of our robot is the same as our former prototype [3]. The concept behind our manipulator is a motorized stereotactic frame with six degrees of freedom, as shown in Fig. 1. This isocentric structure has the advantage of canceling the positional error in the center point, which is the target. By this structure, the robot avoids collision with the patient's head except for the insertion axis d. Compared to redundant degree of freedom robots, this mechanism is a safety feature built into the robot's design. Having an identical geometrical structure to a conventional stereotactic frame enables the surgeon to operate the robot manually in emergency situations. Furthermore, the reliability of the control is high because all axes are independent of each other. The almost same mechanism are applied to use in other works such as [7], however, our system is designed so that it can be positioned on the CT imaging scanner bed, so the size of the manipulator is restricted. During the operation, the procedure can be watched on transverse CT images without any artifact. CT images are also directly used to acquire registration between the patient coordinate and the manipulator's coordinate.

Another particular feature of this robot is its torque transmission mechanism, which solves the sterilization problem. Autoclave and EOG, the typical sterilization methods, require components to endure high pressure and temperature or acid liquid. Many electrical components are not able to withstand these conditions so only mechanical components can be sterilized.

To overcome this problem, we proposed a basic design whereby we separate mechanical components from electrical components. Fig.2 shows this design concept. This separation means that we can safely bring the mechanical components closer to the surgical area. The distance between the patient and the manipulator is decreased and the risk of the manipulator contaminating the surgical field is also decreased.

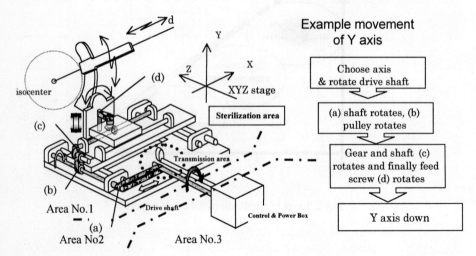

Fig. 3. Mechanism of the needle insertion manipulator and principle of the movement of Y axis

With this design, our new robot can be separated into three parts, two mechanical areas which can be sterilized, and one mechanical and electrical area which cannot be sterilized. Fig. 3 shows a mechanical outline of the manipulator. Area No.1 is the main mechanism. It has 6 degrees of freedom and consists only of mechanical parts. Area No.2 is also assembled with sterilizable mechanical parts, the role of which is to transfer rotating power from the power source Area No.3 to the mechanical area No.1. Area No.3, the power source, includes three pulse motors which cannot be sterilized. In the right side of Fig.3, one example of the moving Y axis is described. The rotating power of each axis is transferred via Area No.2 to the gear transmission system in Area No.1.

We used aluminum for the main parts of the manipulator. The drive shafts and transmission shaft are made of stainless steel (SUS304) to transfer the power. These are all sterilizable materials and are autoclave tolerant. In addition, we can easily separate the XYZ axis and the arc axis for sterilization.

Feed screws are used for the XYZ axis and the insertion axis d. Table 1 shows the specifications of the manipulator. Fig. 4 is a photograph of the first prototype robot.

Table 1. Specification of the manipulator

Mechanism (DOF)	XYZ axis(3), rotation axis(2), insertion axis(1)
Actuator & Feed mechanism	**3 pulse motors** **XYZ, rotation axis**: gear, spline shaft, feed screw for transmission **Insertion axis** : flexible shaft & feed screw or manual
Moving range Depth Rotate axis Latitude axis XYZ stage	 0-110 mm -45 - 45 (deg.) 10-70 (deg.) 0-90(mm)
Weight	7(kg) (including motors)
Size	320(w) x 360(d) x 440(h) mm^3

4. Experimental Result

We checked the movement of each axis and confirmed that the XYZ stage and the d axis moved correctly. The accuracy of the movement was within 1mm for each axis. Of course, by using gears, backlashes were over 5mm, which is not small. The reason for this is the many gears and rubber belts used in the transmission mechanism. However, we plan to use a "one-way movement" and thus backlash will no longer be a problem. In addition, by using CT images, we can check the exact position of the manipulator before the insertion task.

With the arc axis, we could not always confirm its precise and correct movement. Sometimes the pulse motor stopped even though the control signal was sent correctly. This was because of an overload, caused by a manufacturing error, and friction.

Currently we are working on improvements and are manufacturing a new manipulator. For sterilization testing we sterilized each part a minimum of 3 times by autoclaving, and no damage (distortion, rusting etc.) was found. Fig. 5 shows the manipulator installed into the X-ray CT imaging system. It is put on the scanner's bed and its size is small enough to be set in the gantry.

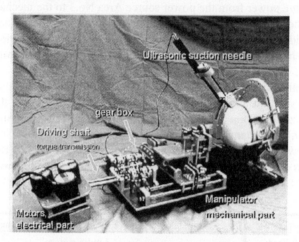

Fig. 4. Overview of the manipulator

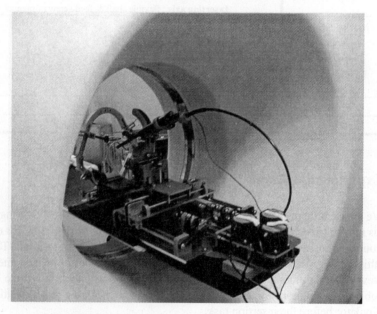

Fig. 5. Manipulator installed in the X-ray imaging system

5. Discussion

Clinically oriented design

Mechanical safety was achieved by using the virtual sphere principle. The size of our manipulator is small enough for it to be settled on the X-ray CT scanner's bed, which increases the precision of positioning. At this operation, this manipulator only does positioning and needle insertion, but not more complex procedures. For safety, redundant movement is not necessary.

Sterilization is the next important problem in the development of medical robotics. In this paper, we suggest our concept of separating mechanical components from detachable electrical components using a transmission shaft. Only the electrical components that are some distance away from the surgical area require covering with drapes. Many medical robots, like the stereoscopic microscope, use plastic cover sheets. However, we consider it is not appropriate to merely use plastic cover sheets for medical robots. This manipulator is only inserting the needle to the target. It seems more complicated task to use such a sterilized cover sheet.

Cost should be also carefully thought about. Much expensive robots are not acceptable to use for such a simple task. Considering the total number of applicable operations and patients in one hospital in one year, only over 100 to 200 operations would require the medical robot. So, it makes no sense to make a large investment in such manipulators for this rate of use. So a low cost is preferable. Because of simple structure, our manipulator is not as expensive as other medical robots when controlling units etc. are included.

Future work

Our immediate priority is to improve the manipulator fabrication. After further experimentation and testing, we are expecting to use it in a clinical setting.

The next stage will probably to develop MRI compatible type using mechanism written above. We succeeded to develop an MRI compatible manipulator for neurosurgery in 1995 [5]. Because of the strong magnetic field in the MRI scanner, we used ultrasonic motors and encoders made of non-ferromagnetic materials to ensure that there was few artifact in the scanned image. However, this manipulator also had a sterilization problem in clinical settings. With these non-ferromagnetic electrical materials, it would be possible to develop an MRI compatible manipulator, because all the materials used already are non-ferromagnetic, except for the motors and a few bearing parts inside the gear transmission shaft.

We have also developed a surgical simulation of needle puncturing [3]. To use this simulation clinically, the registration problem needs to be considered. Registration is required not only between the manipulator and the patient's head, but also between the manipulator and the X-ray image.

6. Conclusion

Mechanical safety is achieved by using the virtual sphere principle. We separated the mechanical components from the electrical components to solve the sterilization problem. We conclude that this prototype is first in demonstrating new principles of how medical robots can be developed, taking full account of safety and sterilization considerations. This research is partly supported by JSPS-RFTF96P00801 program.

References

[1] D. Glauser, H. Fankhauser, M. Epitaux, J.-L. Hefti, A. Jaccottet: Neurosurgical Robot Minerva: First Results and Current Developments, J. of Image Guided Surgery,1:266-272,1995.
[2] F. Badano, et. al., The NEURO-SKILL Robot: a New Approach for Surgical Robot Development, Proc. MRCAS95, pp.318-323, 1995.
[3] K. Masamune, et al., Robots for neurosurgery, Advanced Robotics, Vol.10, No.4, pp.391-401, 1996.
[4] K. Masamune, et al., Development of a CT-guided Neurosurgical Manipulator for Photon Radiosurgery System, CAR97, p.1035, 1997.
[5] K. Masamune, et al., Development of a MRI Compatible Manipulator for Stereotactic Neurosurgery, Image Guided Surgery, 1995.
[6] Yamauchi Y., Ohta Y., Dohi T., Kawamura H., Tanikawa T., Iseki H.: A needle insertion Manipulator for X-ray CT image guided neurosurgery, J.of LST, vol. 5-4, 814-821, 1993.
[7] Kelly PJ, Goerss SJ, Kall BA: Evolution of contemporary instrumentation for computer-assisted stereotactic surgery, Surgical Neurology 30(3):204-15, 1988

Calibration of Video Cameras to the Coordinate System of a Radiation Therapy Treatment Machine

Scott W. Hadley, L. Scott Johnson, and Charles A. Pelizzari

University of Chicago
The Department of Radiation and Cellular Oncology
5841 South Maryland Ave. MC 1105
Chicago, IL 60637
s-hadley@uchicago.edu
www.radonc.uchicago.edu

Abstract. There has been recent interest in using video cameras along with computer vision and photogrammetric techniques to aid in the daily positioning of patients for radiation therapy. We describe here a method to calibrate video cameras to the beam coordinate system of a radiation therapy treatment machine. Standard camera calibration relates the three-dimensional coordinate system of a calibration phantom to the two-dimensional image coordinates. Using a calibration phantom designed for simultaneous X-ray and video imaging, both types of images can be calibrated to a single coordinate system. A series of X-ray images of the calibration phantom is taken using the motion of the treatment machine. Camera calibration parameters derived from these images are used to find a transformation from the coordinate system of the calibration phantom to the beam coordinate system of the treatment machine. This transformation is applied to the video camera calibration to provide a camera calibration directly to the beam coordinates of the machine.

1 Introduction

External beam radiation therapy uses a linear accelerator to produce megavoltage X-rays to deliver a prescribed dose to a tumor deep inside a patient. The linear accelerator is mounted on a gantry which rotates about a horizontal axis. The focal spot of the X-ray beam, for a typical machine, is 100cm from the axis of rotation and traces out a circle in a vertical plane as the gantry rotates. A patient lies on the treatment couch which rotates about a vertical axis. These two axes of rotation allow the beam to enter the patient's body from nearly any direction. Prohibited are those beam directions that would cause the gantry to intersect either the couch or the patient. The *isocenter* of the treatment machine is defined as the point in the room where the axes of rotation of the gantry and couch intersect. The standard convention is to define the isocenter as the origin, the Y-axis as the axis of rotation of the gantry and the Z-axis as the axis of rotation of the treatment couch, see figure 1.

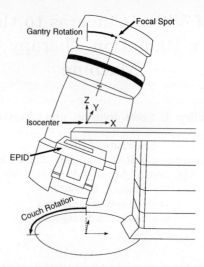

Fig. 1. Diagram of radiation therapy linear accelerator. The gantry houses the linear accelerator and rotates about a horizontal axis. The patient lies on the treatment couch which rotates about a vertical axis. These two axes of rotation intersect at the isocenter. Below the treatment couch is the electronic portal imaging device (EPID) which is attached to, and rotates with, the gantry.

The ideal treatment has the dose from the X-rays delivered to the tumor and little dose to the surrounding normal tissues and organs. Conformal radiation therapy seeks to minimize the dose to normal tissue surrounding the tumor by shaping the aperture of the X-ray beam to match the shape of the tumor in projection. Computer-based treatment planning using computed tomography (CT) images is used to decide how many beams will be used, what aperture they will have and what direction they will enter the body. A physician, on each slice of the CT image, outlines the tumor and any critical structures to be avoided. The 3-D tumor geometry is used to choose a point inside the patient that should be placed at the isocenter of the treatment machine during treatment. Typical conformal treatments use two to six different beam directions chosen to assure coverage of the tumor, exclude critical structures and spread dose to normal tissue over a large volume. The total dose to the tumor is divided into several fractions given once or twice a day. A typical treatment takes several weeks and the patient must be positioned 20 to 40 times.

The most common method of reproducing the position of the patient uses skin marks and isocentric lasers in both the CT room and the treatment room. At the time of image acquisition, the patient is placed on the couch of the CT machine in the pose required for treatment. Lasers mounted on the walls and ceiling trace out orthogonal planes to represent the treatment machine coordinates. A pen is used to trace where the lasers fall on the patient's skin surface. A calibration between the lasers and the CT machine is used to align the laser coordinates to the CT coordinates. A corresponding set of lasers in the treatment room is used to reproduce the position of the patient on the treatment couch.

There are two components to the errors in patient positioning for fractionated radiation therapy. Random errors reflect the inability of a positioning system along with human operators to reproduce the same position day after day. Systematic errors represent a deviation in the planned patient position from the average position. The goal of any system to position the patient is to minimize the random errors and have negligible systematic error. If it were possible to minimize the random error, then measurement of the systematic error could be more accurate and require fewer observations. Several research centers have been working on new techniques both to eliminate systematic errors and reduce random errors.

The position of the patient may be checked, typically once per week, by taking X-ray images of the patient at the time of treatment. An electronic portal imaging device (EPID) is a planar digital imager attached to the gantry to capture an X-ray image as the treatment beam exits the patient. EPID images can be compared to corresponding predicted images computed from the CT and treatment plan data. The three translation and three rotation parameters needed to place the patient in the proper position can be obtained through computer analysis of visible bony anatomy[1]. The major advantage of this method is that the X-ray beams used to treat the tumor also produce the images, which accurately represent the position of the patient relative to the beams. However, it is time consuming and contributes excess dose to normal tissue. Also it is not well suited to use in all sites of the body, for example in breast and lung treatments.

Recently there has been interest in using video cameras and photogrammetric techniques to aid in the daily positioning of patients. The German Cancer Research Center (DKFZ) demonstrated that photogrammetric techniques could track the motion of a patient's head with an accuracy of better than 0.1 mm[2]. The measurements were made relative to the initial position of the photogrammetric phantom and thus can not give an absolute measurement of the position in the treatment machine coordinates. This limits the technique to reducing the random errors in position. Without a calibration to the beam coordinates the systematic error in the patient's position remains unknown.

Recent work at the University of Chicago Department of Radiation Oncology has centered on using a pair of live video subtraction images to reproduce a patient's position in the treatment room[3]. Two video cameras mounted to the wall and ceiling of the treatment room are directed toward the isocenter. On the first day of treatment, images from the two cameras are saved for use as a reference for future positioning. The patient's position is reproduced by comparing live video with the reference image using a subtraction technique. Radiation therapists, while looking at the live video subtraction, interactively move the patient to produce a null image and thus reproduce the previous position. The technique has been shown to be fast and easy to implement in a busy radiation therapy clinic. Its use has facilitated a reduction in the random errors in patient positions. The current system dose not incorporate any type of geometrical calibration and thus cannot be used to measure the systematic positioning error of the patient relative to the beam coordinate system.

A set of video cameras calibrated to the beam coordinate system of the treatment machine could in principle be used to make absolute measurements of the patient position in beam coordinates before each treatment. Geometric information from CT images used for computer based treatment planning could then be directly related to live video images of patients in the treatment room. Such a system could help to reduce both systematic and random errors in patient positioning.

2 Method

Central to our method is a calibration phantom that can be used for both X-ray and video camera images. Our phantom consists of steel ball bearings in a known 3D configuration. The balls are painted white and mounted on black plastic surfaces and thus are easily visible in video images. In the X-ray images, the steel bearings appear as opaque circles, see figure 2. The center of a circle is found by matching a circular template with the edges of the circle in the image. The center of a circle is assumed to be the projection of the center of the spherical ball bearing. The extracted image points and corresponding 3D phantom coordinates are used to estimate the camera parameters using Tsai's method[4].

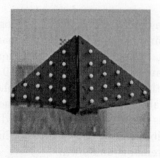 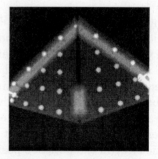

Fig. 2. Digital and X-ray image of the phantom used for camera calibration. Simultaneous images of the phantom tie the two imaging modalities to a common coordinate system.

Two sets of X-ray images are used to estimate the relationship between the calibration phantom and radiation beam coordinate system. The first image set is obtained while rotating the gantry around the stationary phantom. The camera parameters are used to estimate the plane in which the focal spot rotates and the center of rotation, i.e. the isocenter. The second set of images is obtained by rotating the couch, and thus the phantom, while holding the gantry and image plane fixed. This second set of camera calibration parameters is used to estimate the axis of rotation of the couch. One camera/phantom position is common to both sets and is used as a link between the two.

2.1 Camera Model and Calibration

We use Tsai's camera calibration method with both the video and X-ray images. The model includes 6 extrinsic parameters for the translations and rotations needed to express the calibration points in the camera coordinates. We express 3D coordinates with the homogeneous vector $v = [x, y, z, 1]^T$ and use a 4x4 matrix,

$$T_{p,c} = \begin{bmatrix} R & t \\ 0_3^T & 1 \end{bmatrix}, \qquad (1)$$

to represent the transformation from one coordinate system to another. Here, for example, $T_{p,c}$ is a transformation from the phantom to the camera coordinates, where R is a 3x3 rotation matrix, $t = [t_x, t_y, t_z]^T$ represents the translation between the origins and $0_3 = [0, 0, 0]^T$. The camera model is such that the Z-axis of the camera coordinate system is perpendicular to the imaging plane, the X-axis is parallel to the rows of the pixel array, and the Y-axis is parallel to the columns of the pixel array. The 5 intrinsic camera parameters that are estimated include the focal length, f, the image center, $[C_x, C_y]$, horizontal scale factor, s_x, and the radial lens distortion, ρ.

After this first calibration the relationship, between the phantom and camera coordinates and the image plane is well known. At this point, the relationship between the beam coordinates and the phantom remain undetermined.

2.2 Beam Coordinate Estimation

The first step in finding the transformation from the calibration phantom to the beam coordinate system is to locate the isocenter of the treatment machine in the phantom coordinates. A graticule is placed between the image plane and the X-ray source and used to find the X-ray beam direction in the image plane. The image coordinate of the central spot of the graticule, in several calibrated images, is triangulated back to phantom coordinate system and considered the position of the isocenter, t_{iso}.

The set of camera calibration parameters, for the X-ray images, obtained with the calibration phantom held fixed is used to estimate the plane in which the gantry rotates. In the camera coordinate system, the focal spot is located at the origin. Thus let $s = [0, 0, 0, 1]^T$ be the focal spot of a treatment machine from a calibrated X-ray image. First, all focal spots are expressed in the coordinates of the calibration phantom and isocenter, t_{iso}, subtracted off. Using the inverse of the coordinate transformation in Equation 1

$$s_{p_i} = T_{p,c_i}^{-1} s - t_{iso}, \qquad (2)$$

where the subscript i indicates the ith camera position. The plane that best fits the focal spots is determined using single value decomposition (SVD). The result is 3 orthogonal eigenvectors used to form a 3x3 rotation matrix, R_{SVD}, where the eigenvector with the smallest eigenvalue is chosen to be the Y-axis of the new coordinate system. The X- and Z-axes are considered to be arbitrary. After expressing all the focal spots in the new coordinate system, the isocenter is further refined by subtracting off the average Y coordinate of the focal spots, $t_y = [0, \bar{s}_{\text{gy}}, 0, 1]^T$. We denote the phantom-to-gantry transformation using the subscript g for gantry, and p for the phantom,

$$T_{\text{p,g}} = \begin{bmatrix} I_3 & -t_y \\ 0_3^T & 1 \end{bmatrix} \begin{bmatrix} R_{\text{SVD}} & 0 \\ 0_3^T & 1 \end{bmatrix} \begin{bmatrix} I_3 & -t_{\text{iso}} \\ 0_3^T & 1 \end{bmatrix}, \qquad (3)$$

where I_3 is a 3x3 identity matrix. To obtain a transform from the gantry rotation plane to the camera coordinates, $T_{\text{g,c}}$, the inverse of this transformation is used. Next we need only to rotate about the Y-axis so that the axis of rotation of the treatment couch corresponds to the Z-axis.

To model the motion of the treatment couch, the second set of images taken with the X-ray camera held fixed and the calibration phantom rotated with the couch is used. The motion of the treatment couch is modeled by premultiplying the transformation from the home phantom position, p_{h}, to the camera by the inverse of the transform for the rotated phantom position, p_j, to the camera,

$$\begin{bmatrix} R_{\text{p}_{\text{h}},\text{p}_j} & t_{\text{p}_{\text{h}},\text{p}_j} \\ 0_3^T & 1 \end{bmatrix} = T_{\text{p}_j,\text{c}}^{-1} T_{\text{p}_{\text{h}},\text{c}}. \qquad (4)$$

In practice the translation $t_{\text{p}_{\text{h}},\text{p}_j}$ is small, and we ignore it. To find the rotation about the Y-axis, we use the rotation model,

$$R_{Y,\phi_j} R_{Z,\theta_j} R_{Y,\psi_j} = R_{\text{p}_{\text{h}},\text{p}_j}, \qquad (5)$$

and solve the kinematic equations for the angles ϕ_j, θ_j and ψ_j[5]. If the couch rotation were perfect, θ_j would be the rotation angle of the jth couch position and ψ_j would equal $-\phi_j$. Due to errors in the calibration and imperfections in the mechanical rotation in the couch, the rotation angles ϕ_j and ψ_j form a distribution. We use the average over all $-\phi_j$ and ψ_j to obtain a compromise rotation angle $\bar{\psi}$. The resulting transformation,

$$T_{\text{b,g}} = \begin{bmatrix} R_{Y,\bar{\psi}} & 0_3 \\ 0_3^T & 1 \end{bmatrix}, \qquad (6)$$

relates the machine's beam coordinates to the in-plane gantry coordinates. The transformation from machine coordinates to phantom coordinates is then

$$T_{\text{b,p}} = T_{\text{p,g}}^{-1} T_{\text{b,g}}. \qquad (7)$$

This transformation is used to relate both X-ray and video camera calibrations to the machine's beam coordinates.

3 Experiments

We applied this technique to a pair of video cameras mounted to the wall and ceiling of the radiation therapy treatment room. The calibration phantom was placed on the treatment couch and x-ray imaged with 24 gantry angles and two couch rotations. Video image were acquired of the phantom. The phantom was then removed from the table and x-ray images using the graticule were taken from 12 gantry angles. The above technique was applied to the video cameras to obtain the transformation from the beam coordinate system to the video image.

A head phantom was used to test the ability of the system to project information from CT images into the treatment room. A CT image of the head phantom was taken with lead fiducial placed along the laser lines. The center of the lead fiducial were found in the CT image and an isocenter chosen. The head phantom was then carefully positioned on the treatment couch using the isocentric lasers. The position of the fiducial, as seen in the video images, and position as projected from the CT data were compared. Volume rendered images, from the perspective of the video cameras, of the head phantom CT data were prepared using the camera calibration data and compared to the video images.

The ability of the system to accurately track objects was tested as well. A target, similar to the calibration phantom but much smaller, was placed on a machinist translation stage, which has an accuracy of better than 0.02 mm, and translated over a 12.7 mm distance. The position of the target was found my minimizing the distance between the extracted points in the image and the projected points. The magnitude of the known translation was compared to the translation of the estimated position

4 Results

Figure 4 shows the CT image, video images and volume renderings of the head phantom. The fiducial landmarks located in the CT image have been projected into the video image as an "X". The standard deviation of the residual of the projected location of the fiducial and the location extracted from the image by hand was 0.4646 and 1.1419 pixels for the side and top views. The residual for the camera calibration of these two cameras was 0.4146 and 0.3541 pixels respectively. The volume rendered images represent the correct position of the head phantom on the treatment table.

Images of the tracking experiment are shown in figure 4. The magnitude of the known translation was compared to the magnitude of the translation estimated by the calibrated system using linear regression. The slope and intercept of the regressed line was 1.0067 ± 0.0041 and -0.0105 ± 0.0238 respectively.

5 Discussion

The head phantom experiment demonstrates the ability to project information from the CT image into the treatment room. Small differences in the projected

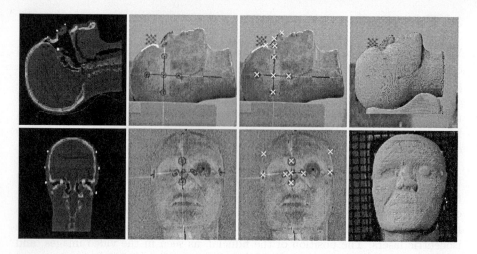

Fig. 3. Demonstration of projecting information from treatment planning CT scan into the treatment room using the calibrated video system. Fiducial landmarks were placed along the laser lines at the time of the CT image, first column. The the location of the fiducial, bright spots in CT image, were projected into the video image, second and third columns. The volume rendered images, fourth column, of the head phantom CT image demonstraits the ability of visualize the correct position, in the treatment room, before the first day of treatment.

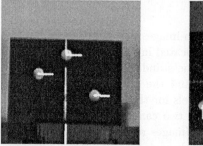 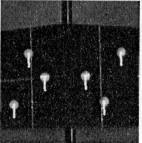

Fig. 4. The target for the tracking experiment consisted of six white spheres mounted to two orthogonal planes. The white lines on the images indicates the position of the spheres in subsequent images. Such a device could be incorporated into CT treatment planning images and, with the calibrated video system, aid in the positioning of patients for radiation therapy.

position of fiducials and their position in the video remain ambiguous. It is possible that the room lasers are not positioned exactly on the isocenter of the machine. Future experiments to determine the absolute accuracy of the video system are planned. The volume rendered images represent the position of the head phantom well. The rendered images do lack photorealism and do not represent how the patient will appear on the treatment couch.

The tracking experiment showed the systems ability to measure the targets position with an accuracy sufficient for radiation therapy. The goal we set for our system is patient positioning within 1 mm and 1 degree of rotation from the planned position. Using such a target incorporated into a bite block may be able to achieve this goal.

6 Conclusion

The potential for video cameras and photogrammetric techniques to aid with patient positioning has been previously demonstrated. This work has been limited to position measurements made relative to the coordinate system of a photogrammetric phantom or reproducing a position from a previous days treatment. These techniques can reduce the random positioning errors but cannot measure the systematic errors.

The technique presented here calibrates video cameras to the coordinate system of the radiation therapy linear accelerator. This would allow photogrammetric techniques to make absolute measurements and thus reduce both systematic and random errors in positioning. Information from CT data can also be accurately projected into live video images to aid human operators in daily patient positioning. Techniques such as these could reduce the systematic error in patient positioning and improve the accuracy of delivering radiation to the patient.

References

1. Kenneth G.A. Gilhuijs, *Automatic verification of radiation treatment geometry*, Ph.D. thesis, University of Amsterdam, 1995.
2. Markus Menke, Frank Hirschfeld, Thomas Mack, Otto Pastyr, Volker Sturm, Wolfgang Schegel , "Photgrammetirc accuracy measurements of a head holder system used for fractionated radiotherapy," *Int. J. Radiat. Oncol. Biol. Phys.*, vol. 29, no. 5, pp. 1147–1155, 1994.
3. B.D. Milliken, S.J. Rubin, R.J. Hamilton, L.S. Johnson, G.T.Y. Chen, "Performance of a video-image-subtraction-based patient positioning system," *Int. J. Radiat. Oncol. Biol. Phys.*, vol. 38, no. 4, pp. 855–866, 1997.
4. Roger Y. Tsai, "A versatile camera calibration technique for high-accuracy 3d machine vision metrology using off-the-shelf TV camera and lenses," *IEEE Journal of Robotics and Automation*, vol. RA-3, no. 4, pp. 323–344, 1987.
5. Paul P. Richard, *Robot Manipulators*, MIT Press, 1984.

An Image Overlay System for Medical Data Visualization

Mike Blackwell[1], Constantinos Nikou[1], Anthony M. DiGioia[1,2], and Takeo Kanade[1]

[1] Center for Medical Robotics and Computer Assisted Surgery,
Carnegie Mellon University, Pittsburgh, PA
{mkb, costa, tk}@cs.cmu.edu   http://www.mrcas.ri.cmu.edu
[2] Center for Orthopaedic Research, UPMC Shadyside Hospital, Pittsburgh, PA
digioia@cor.ssh.edu   http://www.cor.ssh.edu

1 Introduction

Image Overlay is a computer display technique which superimposes computer images over the viewer's direct view of the real world. The positions of the viewer's head, objects in the environment, and components of the display system are all tracked in space. These positions are used to transform the images so they appear to be an integral part of the real world environment. By utilizing semi-transparent display devices, the images can appear to the viewer to be inside of real objects. For example, a 3D image of a bone, reconstructed from CT data, can be displayed to a surgeon inside the patient's anatomy at exactly the location of the real bone, regardless of the position of either the surgeon or the patient. In effect, Image Overlay can provide the viewer "X-ray vision" in a wide variety of applications.

Image Overlay is a form of "augmented reality" in that it merges computer generated information with real world images. In a typical augmented reality system the real world images come from a video camera, which are enhanced with properly aligned computer images and displayed on a computer monitor. The neurosurgical system from Brigham and Women's [6] is an excellent example of this type of system. There are some limitations with typical augmented reality systems, however, which are addressed by Image Overlay. With Image Overlay the surgeon does not need to look away from the surgical field to view the image – it appears within the patient. Also, the real world information is not limited by the resolution or field of view of a camera, since the surgeon views the patient directly. Image Overlay is also distinct from "virtual reality" in that the images are based on real data and are merged at the proper scale and location into the viewer's direct experience of the environment, instead of replacing the viewer's senses with purely virtual data. With Image Overlay the surgeon does not need to wear bulky head gear which would limit his visual acuity – at most the system might require lightweight clear polarized glasses.

We have built two prototype Image Overlay systems to evaluate the technology for applications in the medical domain, especially in areas where improved visualization can reduce the surgical exposure. Target applications include intraoperative tool localization and guidance, as well as surgical education and training. This paper describes the prototype systems and initial experimental results.

2 System Description

An Image Overlay system consists of four basic components:

- Computer graphic workstation,
- Semi-transparent display,
- Position tracking system, and
- Software to correlate positions and transform images.

2.1 Workstation

In order to present a convincing illusion that the computer generated images are part of the environment, the workstation must be able to transform and re-display images in real-time, at least 30 updates per second. We are using an Indigo-II R10K (Silicon Graphics Inc., Mountain View, CA), which handles complex 3D geometric images with ease.

2.2 Semi-Transparent Display

There are several techniques for producing a semi-transparent display. One is to use a standard flat panel liquid crystal display (LCD) with the backlight removed. The result is a display in which one can see through the image (some computer overhead projectors use this technique). The problem with this technique is that the image is typically very dim and the transparency is not high, because LCD panels are not optimized for this purpose. The technique we use is based on a standard computer display monitor coupled with a half silvered mirror or beam splitter glass. The viewer looks directly at the environment through the glass, while simultaneously seeing a reflection of the computer display from the glass, as shown in Figure 1.

The result of the display/mirror combination is a "virtual" image which appears to float below the mirror exactly the same distance as the display sits above the mirror. It is important that the virtual image be positioned such that it appears to lie within the patient, and not too far above or below the region in which the surgeon is working. This is because in order to see the patient clearly the surgeon must focus his eyes on the patient. If the virtual image is located at a different focal distance, the surgeon's eyes must re-focus to see it clearly. If this focal disparity is too great it will lead to eye strain and fatigue. This is the primary cause of "VR sickness" that some people experience with head-mounted displays – the viewer's eyes must focus on the display, which is very close to the eye, but artificial visual cues fool the brain in to thinking that the displayed

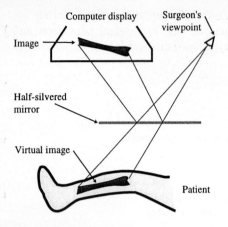 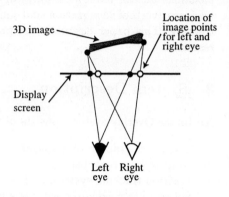

Fig. 1. Using a half-silvered mirror to create a semi-transparent "virtual" display.

Fig. 2. Location of image points on display for each eye to produce stereoscopic effect.

objects are much farther away, leading to a discrepancy. Image Overlay avoids this problem by placing the virtual image within the patient.

The virtual image produced by the display/mirror system is a flat two-dimensional image, exactly the same as the surface of the display. An enhancement to the system is to utilize a stereoscopic technique to produce three-dimensional images [5], [9]. This is done by presenting a slightly different image to the left and right eyes – the different images the eyes would see if looking at an actual 3D scene due to their slightly different positions in space, as shown in Figure 2. There are a number of ways to produce this stereoscopic effect. One is with the Crystal Eyes system (StereoGraphics Corp., San Rafael, CA), in which the left and right eye images are alternated very rapidly on the computer monitor. A pair of "shutter glasses" is synchronized to this alternation, blacking out one lens or the other to ensure the each eye sees the appropriate image. By alternating the images fast enough, no flicker will be detected and the stereoscopic effect will be achieved. Another system (VRex, Elmsford, NY) uses a special polarized film applied to the computer monitor. This film polarizes every other scan line of the monitor in the opposite direction. Coupled with glasses with oppositely polarized lenses, one eye will see the even scan lines, and the other eye the odd scan lines. By simultaneously drawing the left and right eye images to the alternate scan lines, the stereoscopic effect will again be achieved.

2.3 Tracking System

The primary requirements for the position tracking system are that it must be at least as accurate as the spatial resolution of the display system and that it be as fast as the image update time. One such system is the OptoTrak 3020 (Northern Digital, Toronto, ON), which uses three cameras to triangulate the positions of infrared light emitting diodes (LEDs) attached to the objects to be tracked. Other systems include different optical tracking systems (Northern Digital Polaris, Image Guided Technologies FlashPoint), magnetic field trackers (Ascension Flock of Birds, Polhemus FastTrak), mechanical linkages (Faro Arm), or some combination. Whichever system is used, it must be capable of tracking the viewer's eye positions, the display itself, and the patient. For some applications it may also be necessary to track additional objects, such as surgical instruments or structures within the patient.

2.4 Registration and Display Software

The remaining components of an Image Overlay system are a means of properly registering image data to the external environment and software to transform the images so they appear to be part of the environment. Registration is the process of sensing objects in the environment and then corresponding those objects to their counterparts in the image data. There are many ways to achieve registration, but most rely on sensing the three-dimensional shape of objects, using, for example, multiple camera views, digitizing probes, or ultrasound probes. These 3D shapes can then be matched to geometric features in the image data, producing a registration transformation [10].

Once the objects to be displayed have all been transformed in to the same coordinate system via the calibration and registration transformations, they must be displayed so that they appear to the eye exactly as if they existed in their virtual spatial locations. We use the OpenGL graphical libraries to render three-dimensional objects on the two-dimensional display, so this process requires correctly computing the projection matrix. The projection matrix is defined by a viewing frustum with the apex positioned at the eye and the edges passing through the corners of the virtual image, as shown in Figure 3. The viewing frustum differs from that typically used in computer graphics in two ways. First, the frustum is skewed depending on the eye position, since the viewing axis is not necessarily normal to the screen. Second, objects which lie exactly on the virtual image plane will be display in fixed locations regardless of the eye position. For example, if the eye gets closer to the image the object appears to grow larger because it is filling more of the field of view even though it is still drawn the same size. Stereoscopic displays are produced by computing a different projection matrix for each of the two eye positions.

An additional subtlety in the display rendering is that the mirror flips one axis, yielding a left-handed coordinate system. Depending on how the data is represented, this can be accommodated by scaling one of the axes by -1 at some point in the display pipeline.

3 Image Overlay Prototype Systems

In our first Image Overlay prototype the display was built around a 21-inch CRT monitor coupled with a large (1-meter square) half-silvered mirror (Figure 4).

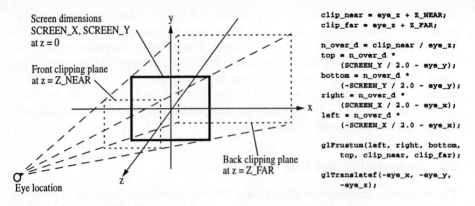

Fig. 3. Viewing frustum for one eye. The physical screen (or virtual image) lies in the XY plane. OpenGL pseudo-code to compute the projection matrix is shown on the right.

The Crystal Eyes stereoscopic system was used to produce 3D images. The OptoTrak system was used to track the display, patient, and viewer's head (with a target attached to the Crystal Eyes glasses). This prototype convinced us that the Image Overlay concept worked, and was the basis for some initial accuracy studies [2]. The prototype also revealed a number of limitations. Foremost was it's size – it was extremely large and cumbersome, difficult to move, hard to calibrate, and impractical for any sort of clinical setting. Another problem was its accuracy. For computational efficiency, the display software assumed that the display was perfectly flat and the pixels evenly spaced. The CRT monitor was in fact fairly curved. The thick glass on the face of the CRT also caused diffraction effects. The curvature and diffraction lead to significant inaccuracies in the system, especially near the edges of the workspace (these effects are analyzed in [4]).

Based on our experiences with the first prototype a new Image Overlay system was recently constructed, pictured in Figure 5. This system is much smaller and easier to move. The display is a high resolution flat LCD panel (Silicon Graphics Presenter 1280). The geometry of the mirror with respect to the display and user's head was carefully chosen to minimize the size of the mirror while still allowing a large field of view. The display/mirror combination is attached to an articulating arm so the system can be easily moved in and out of the surgical field as appropriate. OptoTrak targets are again used to track the head, display, and patient. The system is initially two-dimensional, but we are beginning experimentation with a VRex style stereoscopic display.

The new Image Overlay system is much more suitable for a clinical environment. It's small size and articulation allow it to be easily moved about the OR, so the OptoTrak camera can be positioned to maintain the required line of sight to the tracking targets. Sterilization is addressed by "bagging" the system in sterile plastic draping (similar to that used for surgical microscopes) and at-

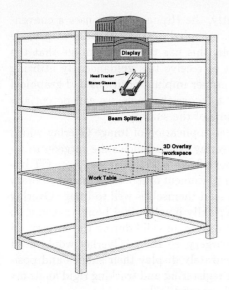
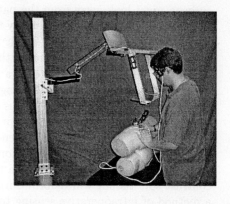

Fig. 4. Configuration of original prototype Image Overlay system.

Fig. 5. The new Image Overlay prototype in a pelvic screw fixation simulation.

taching a sterile disposable OR lamp handle to the display so the surgeon can move it. The mirror is currently glass, but will be replaced by Lexan to prevent breakage if hit by a tool handle (the illusion of the virtual image is good enough that you quickly forget that the mirror is there!).

4 Applications

There are many potential medical applications of the Image Overlay technology. We are focusing on two specific areas, intraoperative guidance and surgical education.

4.1 Intraoperative Guidance

The first clinical application is assisting the surgeon in the proper positioning of the acetabular and femoral prosthetic implant components during a total hip replacement surgery. The Image Overlay system is used in conjunction with the Hipnav system [11], which we are currently using in a pre-clinical trial with a simpler guidance feedback technique. In the Hipnav system the proper locations and orientations of the implant components are determined preoperatively from kinematic and biomechanical simulations based on CT data. During the surgery an Optotrak system is used to track the patient and the surgical tools. A digitizing probe is used to collect points on the pelvis, and these points are matched to the CT data to determine the correct registration transformation. Once the registration is known the Hipnav system can guide the surgeon to properly place the tools, and thus the implants. Currently, the Hipnav system uses a conventional two-dimensional computer display, mounted on the OR wall, to provide guidance to the surgeon. Although simple, this has the disadvantage that the surgeon must look away from the patient to receive this guidance. By utilizing the Image Overlay system to display the proper implant positions and graphical indications such as arrows on which way to move the tools, we can potentially increase the accuracy and decrease the time of the surgery.

Closed reduction of fractures is another application of Image Overlay which we are experimenting with. The Image Overlay system allows the surgeon to visualize the positions and orientations of bone fragments (generated from CT images) and provides guidance for the proper placement of screws or intramedullary rods. Orthopaedic applications in general lend themselves well to Image Overlay for two reasons. First, the applications typically involve rigid bony anatomy, so models built from preoperative data tend to remain valid during the surgery. In contrast soft tissues will deform during surgery, so Image Overlay would need a method of intraoperative sensing to accurately display their shapes and positions. Second, techniques already exist for registering and tracking rigid anatomy using systems such as Optotrak [10] or ultrasound [12].

We are also experimenting with neurosurgical procedures, in particular tumor resection based on MRI data. Using Image Overlay to display the three-dimensional locations of tumors, vessels, and critical areas, the surgeon can plan the craniotomy and approach to minimize the surgical exposure while avoiding the critical areas. Registration is performed via a stereotactic frame which is attached to the patient's head during the scan and in the same position during the procedure. Conceptually, Image Overlay could also be used to display the positions of tools in the brain with respect to the tumor, but questions of overall system accuracy and the deformation of the brain following the craniotomy [3] must be resolved before this can be considered safe or appropriate.

A system very similar to Image Overlay is already being tested clinically in a neurosurgical procedure. The VolumeGraph system [7] from the Tokyo Womens Medical College displays a static three-dimensional image produced from preoperative MRI data, and reflects the image off a half-silvered mirror so the 3D image appears aligned inside of the patient's head. While this system has the same accuracy constraints as Image Overlay, it illustrates that the concept can find clinical utility.

4.2 Surgical Education

Our other main area of research with Image Overlay is in simulations for surgical education. The use of the system is similar to its use in the clinical applications, except a cadaver specimen or plastic phantom is used in place of the patient. Virtually any surgical procedure can be enhanced with the Image Overlay system, allowing the surgeon to directly observe the results of every action. The constraints on the system are greatly reduced for simulations, primarily because the accuracy requirements are reduced. Preoperative data can be collected at as high a resolution as necessary without regard to radiation exposure, or generic preoperative data can be substituted (from the Visible Human data set, for example). Motions of anatomical structures can be estimated or internally instrumented. Registration can be performed by attaching fiducial landmarks to the phantom patient prior to scanning and then recording their positions prior to the procedure. The first procedure we are simulating with Image Overlay is the insertion of an intramedullary rod to reduce a femur fracture, followed by screw insertion to lock the distal end of the rod. In this simulation the surgeon can see and manipulate the two femoral bone fragments, and well as the rod inside of the bone. During distal locking, the position of the distal hole and the trajectories for the screw are displayed in their proper locations.

5 Conclusion

Our experience with the two prototypes has shown that Image Overlay produces a very convincing illusion that the user is really seeing objects "inside" of the patient. Anecdotally, users tell us that the system becomes "transparent" and they quickly forget that it is there (and are surprised when they accidently smash a tool in to the mirror – in the first prototype we resorted to covering the tool tops with foam). While this shows that Image Overlay achieves its desired effect, it also points out a large danger, that the user will tend to believe what he sees, even if it is incorrect. This can be especially problematic when using Image Overlay to observe anatomical structures that aren't otherwise visible – it's main strength – since there may be no other cues to its accuracy.

Inaccuracies can arise from a number of sources: the registration can be incorrect, the patient's anatomy can change from the preoperative data, or the display device can be improperly calibrated. Some of these errors are endemic to all image guided surgical procedures, and are being addressed by several research groups, including ours. Some inaccuracy is more subjective – some users are better able to use the system than others, perhaps due to better stereoscopic perception. We are continuing usability and accuracy studies by having users perform different positioning tasks. The time to complete the task and errors in the final position are measured to characterize both the subjective and objective errors of the system in different configurations [2].

One source of error in our current prototype is the location of the user's eyes. The system tracks the location of glasses that the user is wearing, and then makes assumptions on where the eyeballs lie behind the glasses and that the eyes are looking straight forward. These assumptions will invariably be approximations. While the error is minimized by distance to the display and patient, it still adds to an overall system error. One possible solution that we are exploring is attaching eye pieces, or perhaps just a nose bridge, to the display/mirror device. This would constrain the user's eyes to one position. It would also eliminate the need for the user to wear head gear to track the head, and also allow a reduction in the size of the mirror. The system would then be used like a surgical microscope (a "macroscope" in this case), pulled in to the field of view when required, and pushed away when not needed. This reduces some of the flexibility of the system, but it also simplifies it and improves the accuracy.

Overall, our research has shown Image Overlay to be a promising new data visualization technique with a wide variety of medical applications. Surgical education will probably be one of the first applications of Image Overlay due to the reduced accuracy requirements. Clinical applications will follow, as enhancements to image guided surgical techniques, as the accuracy issues are better understood and addressed.

References

1. W. Bauer, H.J. Bullinger, A. Hinkenjann, O. Riedel: "Planning of Orthopaedic Surgery in Virtual Environments by the Example of Osteotomy Operations," *Interactive Technology and the New Paradigm for Healthcare*, edited by Morgan et al., IOS Press, 1995.
2. M. Blackwell, R.V. O'Toole, F. Morgan, L. Gregor: "Performance and Accuracy Experiments with 3D and 2D Image Overlay Systems," *Proc. Medical Robotics and Computer Assisted Surgery*, 1995.
3. R.D. Bucholz, D.D. Yeh, J. Trobaugh, et al.: "The Correction of Stereotactic Inaccuracy Caused by Brain Shift Using an Intraoperative Ultrasound Device," *CVRMed-MRCAS 97*, pp. 459–466, 1997.
4. M. Deering: "High Resolution Virtual Reality," *Computer Graphics* 26, no. 2, July 1992.
5. D. Drascic, P. Milgram: "Positioning accuracy of a virtual stereographic pointer in a real stereoscopic video world," *SPIE Stereoscopic Displays and Applications II*, Vol. 1457, 1991.
6. W.E.L. Grimson, T. Lozano-Perez, W.M. Wells, et al.: "An Automated Registration Method for Frameless Stereotaxy, Image Guided Surgery, and Enhanced Reality Visualization," *Trans. Medical Imaging*, 1996.
7. H. Iseki, Y. Masutani, M. Iwahara, et al.: "Volumegraph (three-dimensional image-guided navigation), Clinical Application of Augmented Reality in Neurosurgery," *VSMM'96*, 1996.
8. R.V. O'Toole, M. Blackwell, F.M. Morgan, et al.: "Image Overlay for Surgical Enhancement and Telemedicine," *Interactive Technology and the New Paradigm for Healthcare*, vol. 18, pp. 271–273. IOS Press, January 1995.
9. C. Schmandt: "Spatial input/display correspondence in a stereoscopic computer graphics work station," *Computer Graphics*, 17, no. 3, pp. 253–261, July 1983.
10. D. Simon, M. Hebert, T. Kanade: "Techniques for Fast and Accurate Intrasurgical Registration," *Journal of Image Guided Surgery* 1, no. 1, pp. 17–29, 1995.
11. D. Simon, B. Jaramaz, M. Blackwell, et al.: "Development and Validation of a Navigational Guidance System for Acetabular Implant Placement," *CVRMed-MRCAS 97*, pp. 583–592, 1997.
12. J. Tonetti, L. Carrat, S. Lavallée, et al.: "Ultrasound-based registration for percutaneous computer assisted pelvis surgery: Application to iliosacral screwing of pelvis ring fractures," *CAR97*, 1997.

Volumetric Image Guidance via a Stereotactic Endoscope

Ramin Shahidi[1], Bai Wang[1], Marc Epitaux[1], Robert Grzeszczuk[2], John Adler[1]

[1] Stanford University, Department of Neurosurgery, Image Guidance Laboratory,
300 Pasteur Dr., MC: 5327, Stanford, California 94305-5327, USA
{shahidi, bai, mepitaux, adler}@igl.stanford.edu
http://igl.stanford.edu

[2] Silicon Graphics, Inc., Mountain View, California 94943, USA
rg@sgi.com

Abstract. We have developed a surgical setup based on modern frameless stereotactic techniques that enables surgeons to visualize the field of view of the surgical endoscope, overlaid with the real-time and volumetrically reconstructed medical images, of a localized area of the patient's anatomy. Using this navigation system, the surgeon visualizes the surgical site via the surgical endoscope, while exploring the inner layers of the patient's anatomy by utilizing the three-dimensionally reconstructed image updates obtained by pre-operative images, such as Magnetic Resonance and/or Computed Tomography Imaging. This system also allows the surgeon to virtually "fly through and around" the site of the surgery to visualize several alternatives and qualitatively determine the best surgical approach. Moving endoscopes are tracked with infra-red stereovision cameras and diodes, allowing the determination of their spatial relation to the target lesion and the fiducial based patient/image registration.

1. Introduction

Recent developments in computation technology have fundamentally enhanced the role of medical imaging, from diagnosis to computer-aided surgery. Today, Computer assisted methods provide on-the-fly information for dynamic navigation, analysis and inspection of the 3-D image structures during surgical procedures. Moreover, conventional stereotactic techniques, in which the frame of reference is bolted to the skull, are being replaced by frameless systems that incorporate fiducial markers for registration. The combination of these two methods provide the surgeon with interactive and intuitive access to the imaging data, like Magnetic Resonance Imaging (MRI), Computed Tomography (CT) in an ongoing surgical procedure.

The objective of our paper is to describe a system for a real-time 3-D surgical navigation using an operating endoscope. This system allows for the overlay of volumetrically reconstructed patient images onto the view of the surgical field as seen through the endoscope. This technique permits surgeons to navigate around the patient to explore the inner anatomical structures of the patient, thus providing "on-the-fly" volumetric and 2-D information for planning and navigational purposes. The important part of this system is the navigation software, which does not burden the surgeon with the implementation details of the computation model. The graphic interface provides surgeons with an interactive environment, to directly address the problems associated with the task by selecting from a variety of possible visualization capabilities. All other aspects, such as object tracking, are carried out automatically.

2. Background
In the past, the task of correlating preoperative and intraoperative imaging studies was left to the surgeon and depended on his/her knowledge of human anatomy. Stereotaxi was one of the first procedures to effectively corollate preoperative images with the patient's physical anatomy during the operation.

2.1. Frame Based Stereotaxi
Up to recent years, the most common use of stereotaxi was for biopsies, for which a surgical trajectory device and a frame of reference were used [1]. Traditional frame-based methods of stereotaxy defined the intracranial anatomy with reference to a set of fiducial markers, attached to a stereotactic frame [2]. The stereotactic frame-bolted into the patient's skull prior to imaging and worn throughout the duration of the procedure-was used for registering the patient with the pre-operative data [3]. The trajectories prescribed by trigonometric calculations obtained from pre-operative images were interpolated into the operative field using a trajectory enforcement device. This device, placed on top of the frame of reference was used to guide the biopsy tool to the target lesion based on prior calculations [4]. Use of a mechanical frame allowed for high localization accuracy, but caused patient discomfort and limited surgical flexibility. In addition, such surgical techniques did not allow the surgeon to visualize the approach of the biopsy tool to the lesion.

2.2. Two-Dimensional Frameless Image Guided Stereotaxi
There has been an emergence of image-guided techniques for registration that are eliminating the need for the frame all together. The first frameless stereotactic system utilized an articulated robotic arm to register pre-operative imaging with the patient's anatomy in the operating room [5,6,7]. The next step was the use of sonic devices for tracking the instruments in the operating room [8]. A significant evolution of the frameless system was the introduction of Optical Tracking System (OTS) which utilized infra-red diodes and vision-cameras to track a moving object in the operating room [9,10,11,12]. All three systems mentioned above, use externally placed markers on the patient to register pre-operative imaging with the patient's anatomy in the operating room [13]. These frameless methods, however, have limited positional accuracy and use limited image data displays as 2-D views. In addition, they tend to lose their spatial registration with respect to pre-operative data [14]. For example, in neurosurgical applications, the deformation of the brain due to CSF drainage (brain-shift) causes significant errors in the localization of the targeted lesion.

2.3 Three-Dimensional Frameless Image Guided Stereotaxi
In 1994, several groups introduced the concept of intraoperative volumetric image guidance, using various approaches [15,16,17,18]. Volumetric imaging techniques greatly enhance a surgeon's ability to create a plan prior to surgery, to follow it during surgery, and to modify the surgical approach based on intra-operative information. The intraoperative use of 3-D imaging has been limited, due to a lack of computation power. However, recent advances in graphic hardware designs, provides the means for effective utilization of such 3-D images for intraoperative guidance, such as the fusion of preoperative 3-D images with the video images of the surgical site [19,20,21].

3. Overview

The main draw backs of fiberoptic endoscopy are that, it can only display visible surfaces, and can not be used inside an opaque tissue. Virtual endoscopy on the other hand, can make an opaque tissue transparent and look beyond the visible surface. Thus, the correlation of the actual endoscopic video images with the volumetrically reconstructed imaging data, provides precise additional exposure of the pathology and its surrounding tissue during the surgery. A hypothetical scenario of our proposed system's use in the operating room will help to delineate its features.

Prior to obtaining pre-operative images, six markers (fiducials) are placed on the patient. These are small (~1mm), stick-on markers surrounded by pantopaque-filled spheres glued to the skin. Pantopaque is an oil-based, iodine containing X-ray contrast agent that until recently was used for myelograms. The iodine makes the fiducials visible on CT images while the oil base renders it visible on MRI examinations. The image data will be transferred to the SGI Infinite Reality workstation (Silicon Graphics Inc., Mountain View, CA), via the hospital's computer network. The volume will be rendered, and (in the case of multiple imaging modalities) fused. If necessary, the image data will then be segmented to allow detailed visualization in the appropriate anatomic context of the lesion, the vascular structures, and the fiducials. Segmentation of the fiducial markers, the brain, the vascular system (from CTA or MRA) and the surface of the brain will be fully automatic. The segmentation of the lesion (if applicable), however, would only be partly automatic, since the irregular anatomy surrounding lesions are currently too unpredictable for automatic segmentation.

In the operating room, the patient will be positioned in the usual fashion and the registration process will be accomplished using the Optical Tracking System (Image Guided Technologies Inc., Boulder, CO). Optical tracking is a technique that allows a unique detection of flashing objects with known frequencies in 3-D space. Diode markers can also be added to conventional surgical tools (e.g., probes or endoscopes) to enable their tracking in space. Using such tracking techniques, the position of the encoded surgical pointer in 3-D space is automatically recognized. By pointing the encoded surgical probe to the actual markers and moving the computer cursor on the markers' imaging counterparts, registration of the volumetric image and the patient's actual physical anatomy can be accomplished. At this point, since the patient and the 3-D image are registered and the surgical probe can be tracked with respect to the patient, the virtual counterpart of the probe can also be tracked with respect to the 3-D image. A line extending from the displayed image of the probe indicates the trajectory of the planned approach.

Moving the tool, automatically leads to a change in the displayed potential trajectory. This system simplifies the planning of a minimally invasive approach to a direct and interactive task. In addition to displaying the probe's trajectory in 3-D, the location of the infra-red diodes on the probe will determine the precise location and depth of the tool, hence, the precise location and depth of the operative site.

The surgical probe can also be replaced with the diode encoded rigid fiberoptic endoscope (PS Medical, Goleta, CA). The volumetric images of the surgical corridor (focused on the surgical site) are then re-oriented to show the endoscope's virtual birds-eye-view. This information allows the workstation to automatically display the real time 3-D images of the surgical corridor in context, as oriented to the surgical approach. 3-D reformatting uses volume display techniques and allows instantaneous variations of transparency. With this technique, deep as well as superficial structures can be seen in context, considerably enhancing intra-operative guidance. These 3-D virtual endoscopic views can be seen next to the endoscope's actual views.

4. Methods

To incorporate this system, the following steps have been taken: 1) deployment of a fast 3-D Engine for a reconstruction of the medical data, 2) development of various visualization and navigation tools in a user friendly environment, 3) 3-D patient/ image registration and real-time tracking of the surgical tools, and 4) perspective rendering of the localized 3-D data to match the fiberoptic endoscope images.

4.1. Fast Volume Rendering Engine

Direct volume rendering is a technique for displaying sampled scalar or vector fields without fitting any geometric primitives to the data [32,33]. Instead, the volume is sampled directly with a set of rays emanating from the eye, hence the name of the technique: "Ray Tracing" [34,35]. As each ray is traversed, the optical properties along the path are computed. These may include absorption, reflection, refraction, and emission. In addition, it is possible to devise modes that do not have a natural physical interpretation, but which can provide useful information, nevertheless.

In conventional implementations, each ray is traced from the eye to its point of termination before the next ray is considered. However, many newer algorithms [36,37] choose to process the rays simultaneously taking advantage of spatial coherence and the locality of the reference, to dramatically improve performance. This approach is particularly attractive on platforms capable of hardware texture-mapping. Drawing a texture-mapped plane perpendicular to the line of sight produces identical results to sampling a volume with a set of rays under orthographic projection. Similarly, ray casting under perspective projection can be accomplished by drawing a set of texture-mapped concentric spheres centered at the eye (Fig. 1).

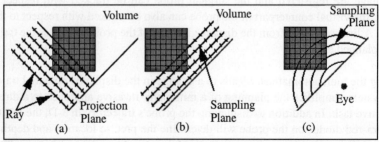

Figure 1: Ray-casting with orthographic projection. a) ray order, b) sampling surface and, c) sampling with perspective projection.

The ray casting method we adopted employs a general framework which unifies the treatment of volumes and geometry. A volume is characterized by both appearance and geometry. The volume's appearance is a collection of voxels, while the geometry is given by a set of 3-D Simplices (Tetrahedra), which define the region of interest. The volume is rendered by polygonizing the geometry into a series of triangles that are texture-mapped with appearance data. This results in a highly flexible approach, allowing us to take full advantage of available graphics hardware. In addition, the technique is flexible enough to allow for many desirable operations such as selecting arbitrarily shaped regions of interest, multi-modality rendering, and rendering both volumetric and surface rendering as embedded geometrical objects.

It is critical that the surgeons be able to interact with the system in a manner that does not hinder their performance. Therefore, the visuals needed for navigation have to be generated at highly interactive rates, which is a hard task to achieve using conventional, software-only solutions. As a result, we have decided to take advantage of the graphic board of SGI-IR Workstation, which conducts many graphical calculations in the hardware, thus substantially increasing the rendering process. Our software is deployed on top of C++, OpenGL, SGI's Inventor and VI Tool-Kits. The speed of our volume rendering varies from 15 frames/sec to 45 frames/sec depending on the data characteristics (between 20MB to 60MB) on a SGI-IR 4xproc.

4.2. Visualization and Navigation Software (Genesis2000)
In addition to the 3-D Engine, a 2-D Engine is implemented in our volumetric navigation software. The 2-D Engine provides the user with orthogonal views (Axial, Sagital, Coronal). The implemented 2-D Engine, however, is capable of displaying the orthogonal view in 3-D as well. By applying six cutting planes to the 3-D Engine, three orthogonal views for axial, Sagital, and Coronal views can be presented. When the 2-D Engine is on slice mode, both cutting planes are enabled. When the 2-D Engine is on non-slice mode, only one cutting plane is enabled, and will cut out everything between the viewer and the plane. When necessary, the 2-D Engine supports a reverse view, by flipping the effective cutting plane area and reversing the view direction. The 2-D Engine can also display non-orthogonal slices (oblique slices). When in slice mode, due to the small gap between the two cutting planes, performance is in real-time. For a 512x512x128 data set, three 512x512 2-D views and 32bit color images can be generated at about 30 frames/second on the SGI-IR.

We have implement various tool boxes to our software package. The main tool boxes are the "Loader" (loading and saving the medical data-sets), the "Basic Tool Box" (histogram, opacity, color, and light adjustments), the "Basic Segmentation Tool Box" (seed-fill, semi-automated contouring, and basic analysis), the "Basic Registration Tool Box" (multimodality and patient/image fusion), and the "Basic Navigation Tools" (viewing, registration and navigation parameters). These tool boxes are used to control the current system's lookup table, in order to interactively update the images that are being modified. The system lookup table is 32bit, i.e., for red, green, blue and alpha. The tool-boxes control every channel of the lookup table separately, so different tissues can be assigned different visualization properties.

The user interface is probably the most crucial part of our system. It is fully conformed towards our surgeon's requirements and was designed taking into consideration their constant feed back. The interface is designed to be intuitive and easy to use. It does not burden the physician with the details of implementing the computational model. All aspects of graphics and analysis are carried out automatically. It also remembers the windowing arrangements for all its users, and it has the ability to save the rendering settings to minimize the initialization time. In order to maintain the simplicity of the interface without losing its functionality, our interface is specifically designed for surgical navigation purposes.

4.3. Registration and Tracking Surgical Instrument

The basic principle involved in tracking the surgical instruments, is triangulation which is used for the recovery of the depth of an indicator from vision-cameras. In our case, the indicators are the infra-red diodes that are being tracked by three infra-red cameras in the surgical space. Using the computer-vision technique, the indicator must be established between features from the three images (from infra-red cameras) that correspond to some physical property in space (infra-red signal). Then, provided that the relative positions of the centers of projection, the effective focal length, the relative orientation of the optical axis, and the sampling interval of each camera are all known, the closest distance of the object to the camera can be calculated [28,29].

The surgical endoscope and other surgical tools must work in synchronisity in order to maintain a dynamic model of the surgical site. Our main challenge was to keep all sensors in a sub-millimeter spatial registration, and maintain a detailed dynamic model of the motion. We had build a special interface so that two or three objects could be tracked at the same time. In addition, we have built an infra-red-based "tracking clip" that can be tracked by infra-red cameras. Our "tracking clip" can be mounted on top of various surgical devices such as an endoscope. For this project, we used the infra-red vision-cameras by Image Guidance Technologies Inc. to track our tracking clip. The orientation of the projection axis and the position of the tip of the endoscope was calculated and extrapolated from the three known points (infra-red diodes) on the tracking clip holding the endoscope.

In order to register the imaging data-set with the patient's physical anatomy, we used six fiducial markers that were glued to the surface of the object during the CT and MR imaging. The object was then moved to the surgical site with the markers still attached. Registration was performed using standard orthogonal views (Axial, Sagital, Coronal) of the image data. For each marker, the technician positioned the tip of the infra-red diode-coded pointer (being tracked by infra-red cameras) on top of each marker, and positioned the computer cursor on top of the marker's imaging counterpart. Based on at least three sets of point pairs (not located in a plane), the registration system computed and forced the transformation matrix to register the patient's stereotactic space and the imaging space. At this point, since the patient and the volume image were registered, one could track the movement of an object around the patient, and the object's virtual counterpart was moved around the volume image with the same exact orientation.

4.4. Volumetric Data Overlay

From the information obtained in section 4.3., the position of the endoscope's lens and its field of view, which is a volumetric conic section, can be obtained. In turn, these data allow the trajectory angles $(\theta_x, \theta_y, \theta_z)$ for the surgical endoscope to be calculated. At this point, if we rotate the 3-D data-set in reverse angle $(-\theta_x, -\theta_y, -\theta_z)$, the viewing projection will be the same as the endoscope's field of view. Thus, by multiplying the viewing projection matrix by the inverse matrix of the actual transformation matrix, the desired viewing angle can be obtained.

An imaginary cone, starting from the tip of the virtual endoscope and parallel to its trajectory axis represents our virtual endoscope's field of view (FOV). 2-D multi-layer modalities can be obtained by moving a vector along the surface of the cone (FOV). Using the parametric equation below, it is possible to calculate all the intersecting points between the cone and the volumetric data-set. Once the contours of the cone are defined, one can calculate all the voxels within the conic section:

$$X = L \cdot \tan\theta \cos\alpha + x_1$$
$$Y = L + y_1$$
$$Z = L \cdot \tan\theta \sin\alpha + z_1$$

Where $R = L \cdot \tan\theta$ is the radius in the base of the cone and y_1, x_1, z_1 are the coordinates of the origin of the cone, and θ is the angle between, the cone's axis and semi-axis. This formula represents a cone with its major axis along the Y axis. To transfer this cone to the image's virtual space coordinates, we multiply [X, Y, Z] by the object's orientation matrix. This orientation matrix is the inverse of the orientation matrix obtained from the transformations of the actual image with respect to the cone. When we increment θ and L, the surface of the cone, as well as the intersection points between the cone and the image are all covered.

The rendering, after this alignment, is accomplished by reformatting a data-set along its common coordinate system to achieve a 2-D image overlay. Using this reformatting information and our 2-D Engine's oblique cutting plane capabilities, it is possible to make cuts - orthogonal to the cone's major axis - one layer at a time. These multimodalities can be observed as "raw" monochromatic images that are orthogonal and parallel to the tip of the trajectory device as it moves through the object.

This conic volume as a "see-through" projection in the 3-D data-set provides volumetric and multi-layer capabilities for the surgeon. With this system, the surgeon will have a choice of various image display mechanisms with our system. He/she can observe the actual endoscopic image and its virtual counterpart next to each other, or overlaid with each other with different blending parameters. Oblique 2-D multimodalities oriented to match the endoscope's trajectory can be displayed next to the 3-D images. With this technique, deep as well as superficial structures can be seen in context, considerably enhancing intra-operative guidance.

5. Results and Discussion

The validation process followed in successive stages. Observing the volumetric data from the endoscope's perspective provided the means for testing the overall accuracy of our navigational system. The screen presentation of the endoscope's view of 3-D objects, were compared to the screen presentation of 3-D virtual objects at various depths. The images obtained from both modalities were compared to observe the differences in spacial occupancy of the anatomical structures. Each step mentioned above was also validated with variations in the field of view of the endoscope.

5.1. Phantom Testing

In order to test our system, we have used a phantom. This phantom (shown in figure 3: second from top, and right image) is a solid plastic mock-up of a skull, containing geometrical structures inside. In the same image the "tracking clip", which was designed and built by our group, is shown holding an endoscope. The geometrical structures consist of a rectangular cube, a cone, a cylinder and a sphere. The phantom also contains spatially fixed 2mm holes, set 10mm apart; and a 100x100mm grid pattern with 1mm grids. There are 6 fiducial markers attached to the surface of the skull, the same as the ones being used during the actual stereotactic surgery. For MR imaging, the phantom is embedded in a water-sealed glass container and the container is filled with water. Once the container is emptied, it can be used for a CT imaging.

Using this phantom a series of feasibility experiments were conducted. The first involved the real time overlay of 3-D CT images with the phantom, using fiducial registration and an optical tracking system. Our initial goal was to simply obtain optimal registration (figure 3: two right images on the bottom). Our second goal was to maintain the spatial registration of the surgical tools (i.e., surgical pointer and endoscope) and the phantom, as the tool moved around and through the object (figure 3: second and third from top, and left image). The third involved perspective volumetric image overlay with the actual endoscopic trajectory views (figure 3: two top images). Subsequent sectioning of the image allowed for a precise quantization of the system's targeting accuracy and image/anatomy overlap at different depths.

5.2. Overall Results

Figure 2, shows the overall performance of our system. There have been 100 random cases studied. In each case, the Least-Square-Mean (LSM) error based on pixel-offsets were measured, and plotted versus the depth of observation, and the field of view of the endoscope. On the top-left of figure 2, the Least-Square-Mean vs. depth is represented on a 3D Plot. It is illustrated that, as the field of view increases, the errors tend to increase on the edge of the reconstructed field; and the deeper the measurements from the tip of the endoscope, the more error is obtained. The best reconstruction results were obtained using the following parameters: the depths of up to 25mm with the observation toward the center of the endoscope's viewpoint. Using these parameters the worst scenario yields less than 1.5mm offset. Over all, we have demonstrated the precision of our reconstruction to be around 3.0mm in the worst case (with FOV equals to 120degrees and at depths of 50mm). In real surgical scenario these errors might increase, due to the intraoperative deformation of tissue.

5.3. Sources of Error

Overall the accuracy of the system is directly dependent on the precision with which the registration is conducted. In addition, the results are also dependent on the amount of lens distortion, its focal length and field of view. Moreover, for any given video image, there is a sampling error that can be estimated as a fraction of the largest extent of the imaged object. For example, the highest resolution image that can be made by a standard NTSC video image is 640x480 pixels. This would give the precision of 1mm/pixel for an object with an extent on the window of 512x512pixels. Thus, the precision of the instrument is also related to the distance of the camera from the object, the film resolution and the lens quality.

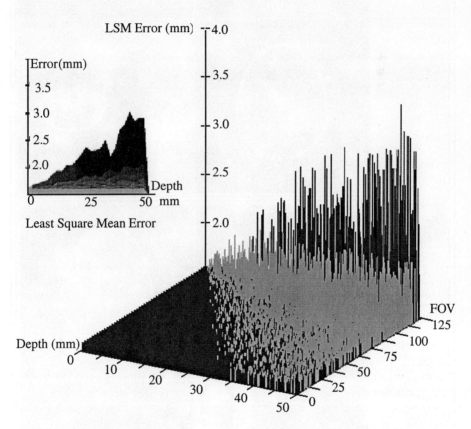

Figure 2: Results of 100 random cases of endoscopic's reconstruction study with variables field of views at different depths.

A lot more testing and statistical analysis are needed to validate the accuracy of our system. Next, we will test our system on deformable phantoms and also cadavers with target lesions inserted in them. Finally, we will test our system in a real surgical scenario, where a volumetric virtual endoscopic updates will be compared with the video images obtained from an endoscope, looking at the patient's physical anatomy.

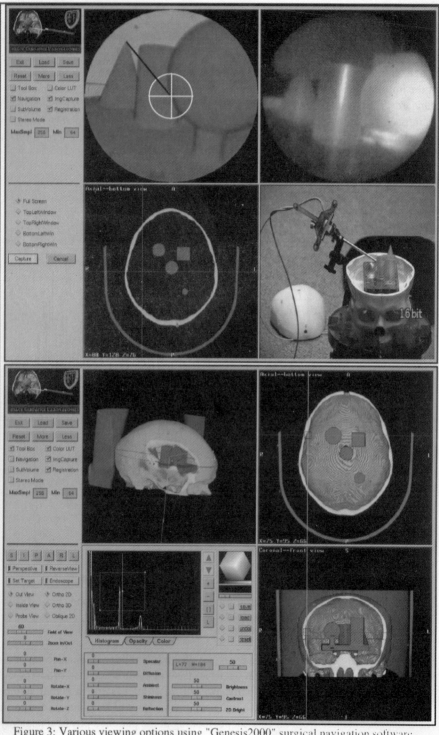

Figure 3: Various viewing options using "Genesis2000" surgical navigation software.

6. Future Work

We are currently working on a multi-step lens calibration to compensate for lens distortion. The first step will be to compensate for the lens curvature. The second step will be the initial calibration stage to automatically incorporate the lens' field of view and focal length into our system. The last step will be an automated matching of the stereoscopic endoscopic images, and the stereoscopic 3-D reconstructed images based on a real-time surface matching of the localized area, as seen through the endoscope. Another project currently under investigation in our lab, is the development of a system which would utilize intra-operative ultrasonic images as sources of the patient data, in order to compensate for intraoperative tissue deformations. Volumetric pre-operative CT or MR imagery can then be spatially deformed (warped) to match the intra-operatively acquired 3-D US images. Such images can then be fused with images from the surgical endoscope or microscope.

References

1. TM. Peters, A. Olivier. "CT-aided stereotaxy for depth electrode implantation and biobsy," Canadian Journal of Neurological Sciences, 10:166-169, 1983.
2. P. Gildenberg, HH. Kaufman, KSM. Murthy, "Calculation of stereotactic coordinates from computed tomography scan," Neurosurgery, 10:580-586, 1982.
3. P. Kelly, B. Ball, S. Goerss, "Results of computer tomography-based stereotactic resection of metastatic intracranial tumors," Neurosurgery 22:7-17, 1988.
4. RJ. Maciunas, RL. Galloway, JW. Latimer. "The Application Accuracy of Stereotactic Frames Neurosurgery," 35(4):682-695, 1994.
5. B. Guthrie and JR. Adler. Frameless Stereotaxy: Computer Interactive Neurosurgery. Perspectives in Neurological Surgery. 2(1):1-22, 1991.
6. WB. Legget, MM. Greenberg, WEJ. Gannon, "The Viewing wand: a new system for three-dimensional CT correlated intraoperative localization," Current Surgery, 1991, 48:674-678.
7. P.F. Hemler, T. Koumrian, J.R. Adler, and B. Guthrie," A Three Dimensional Guidance System for Frameless Stereotactic Neurosurgery," In Proc. of the Fifth Annual IEEE Symposium on Computer-Based Medical Systems, pages 309-314, Durham, North Carolina, 6/92.
8. JW. Trobaugh, WD. Richard, KR. Smith, RD. Bucholz, "Frameless stereotactic ultrasonography: method and applications," Compute Med. Imaging Graph 1994 Jul;18(4):235-246.
9. KR. Smith, KJ. Frank, and RD. Bucholtz. "The Neurostation - A Highly Accurate, Minimally Invasive Solution to Frameless Stereotactic Neurosurgery," Computerized Medical Imaging and Graphics, 18(4):247-256, 1994.
10. P. Cinquin, E. Bainville, C. Barbe, et., al,."Computer Assisted Medical Interventions," IEEE Engineering in Medicine and Biology, pages 254-263, 1995.
11. S. Lavallee, J. Troccaz, P. Sautot, B. Mazier, P. Cinquin, and P. Merloz, "Computer- Assisted Spinal Surgery Using Anatomy-Based Registration. In Computer-Integrated Surgery,' R.H. Taylor et al. (eds), pp 425-449, MIT Press, 1995.
12. LP. Nolte, H. Visarius, E. Arm, F. Langlotz, O. Schwarzenbach, L. Zamorano, "Computer Aided Fixation of Spinal Implants," Jour of IGS, 1:65-73, 1995.

13. HF. Reinhardt. "Neuronavigation: A Ten-Year Review. In Computer-Integrated Surgery," RH. Taylor et al. (eds), pages 329-341, MIT Press, 1995.
14. RD. Bucholtz, DD. Yeh, J. Trobaugh, et., al. "The Correction of Stereotactic Inaccuracy Caused by Brain Shift Using an Intraoperative Ultrasound Device," in Proc. CVRMed-MRCAS'97, pages 459-466, Grenoble, France, 1997.
15. R. Kikinis, l. Gleason, W. Lorensen, W Wells, WE Grimson, T Lozano-Perez, G. Ettinger, S. White, F. Jolesz, " Image Guided Techniques for Neurosurgery," In Proc. VBC 94, pp. 537-540, Rochester, 1994.
16. R. Shahidi, "Applications of Virtual Reality in Stereotactic Procedures: Volumetric Image Navigation via Surgical Microscope" Ph.D. Thesis, Rutgers University, Submitted 1994.
17. W.E.L. Grimson, T. Lozano-Perez, W. M. Wells III, G. J. Ettinger, S. J. White, and R. Kikinis. "An Automatic Registration Method for Frameless Stereotaxis, Image Guided Surgery, and Enhanced reality Visualization," in Proc. IEEE Compt Vis and Patt. Recog., pp. 430-436, 1994.
18. ACF Colchester, J Zhao, CHenri, RL Evans, P Roberts, N. Maitland, DJ Hawkes, DLG Hill, AJ Strong, DG. Thomas, MJ Gleeson, TCS Cox," In Proc. VBC 94, pp. 541-551, Rochester, 1994.
19. R. Shahidi, R. Mezrich, D. Silver, "Proposed Simulation of Volumetric Image Navigation Using a Surgical Microscope," Jour Img Guid Surg, 1:249-265, 1995.
20. A.C.F. Colchester et al. Development and Preliminary Evaluation of VISLAN, a Surgical Planning and Guidance System Using Intraoperative Video Imaging. Med Image Analysis,1(1):73-90, 1996.
21. K. Darabi, KD. Resch, J. Weinert, U. Jendrysiak, A. Perneczky, " Real and Simulated Endoscopy of Neurological Approaches in an Anatomical Model", In Proc., CVRMed-MRCAS, pp. 323-326, Grenoble, France, 1997.
22. Robert A. Drebin, Loren Carpenter, and Pat Hanrahan. "Volume rendering. Computer Graphics" (ACM SIGGRAPH Proceedings), 22(4):65-74, 1988.
23. M. Levoy, "Display of Surfaces from Volume Data", IEEE Computer graphics & Applications 0272-1716/88/0500-0029., 1988.
24. M. Levoy, "A Hybrid Ray Tracer for Rendering Polygon and Volume Data. IEEE Computer graphics & Applications 0272-1716/90/0300-0033., 1990.
25. M. Levoy, "Efficient Ray Tracing of Volume Data", ACM Trans. Graph., 9(3): 245 261, 1990.
26. B. Cabral, N. Cam, J. Foran. Accelerated Volume Rendering and Tomographic Reconstruction using Texture Mapping Hardware. In Proceedings of the 1994 Symposium on Volume Visualization, pages 91-98, 1994.
27. P. Lacroute and M. Levoy, "Fast Volume Rendering Using a Shear-Warp Factorization of the Viewing Transformation," In Proc. of SIGGRAPH '94, Orlando, FL, pages 451-458, 1994.
28. Kortokov E., Henriksen K., Kories R., Stereo Ranging with Verging Cameras, IEEE PAMI, Vol. 12, NO. 12 Dec. 1990.
29. Alvertos N., Brzakovic D., Gonzalez R C., Camera Geometries for Image Matching in 3D Machine Vision: IEEE on Pattern Analysis and Machine Intelligence (PAMI), Vol 11, NO. 9. 9/1989.

The Application Accuracy of the Frameless Implantable Marker System and Analysis of Related Affecting Factors

Qinghang Li, Lucia Zamorano, Zhaowei Jiang, Fernando Vinas and Fernando Diaz

Wayne State University, Department of Neurological Surgery, 4160 John R. Suite 930, Detroit, MI 48201.
E-mail: li@neurosurg.wayne.edu.   Fax: (313) 966-0368

ABSTRACT

The purpose of this study was to determine the application accuracy of a new frameless marker system for interactive intraoperative localization of intracranial lesions. The influence of image quality, registration error, repeatability, and marker distribution on the application accuracy were analyzed and compared. A phantom was mounted with the standard Z-D ring and also implanted with frameless marker system, which randomly distributed on the surface. The phantom was scanned as routine with 1 mm and 2 mm sections. The pixel sizes were used 1.18 x 1.18 and 0.59 x 0.59. The two systems were tested under different image quality and registration. The target point was digitized and the coordinates were recorded and compared with reference points. The difference between two systems were tested with paired t-test. Image data were loaded into a SUN Workstation and registered with NSPS.4.0 software. The coordinate of each fiducial marker was recorded into a file as the reference. The tip of each semi-invasive fiducial marker was digitized to achieve a frameless transformation matrix, and the special points on the Z-D ring were digitized to achieve a frame-based transformation matrix. The differences from the reference points were used as the deviation from "true point". The mean square root (RMS) was calculated to show the sum of vectors. The results of 2 mm section group showed that the registration error of frame-based system is 3.42 ± 0.22 mm and the error of the frameless system is 1.01 ± 0.63 mm (P<0.001). The RMS are 2.57 ± 0.54 mm and 1.53 ± 0.65 mm respectively (P < 0.001). The RMS of error registration (one point off 5 mm) are 5.01 ± 0.26 mm and 2.23 ± 0.13 mm respective (P=0.003). The results of 1mm section group showed that the RMS are 1.20 ± 0.42 mm and 0.90 ± 0.47 mm respectively (P=0.121). The higher the quality (the thinner scan thickness) of image it is, the better the application accuracy will be (P=0.001 and 0.032 respectively). These preliminary results showed that the frameless semi-invasive fiducial marker system can provide clinical acceptable accurate localization as the frame based surgical localization system did. There is no significant difference between the experimental and clinical results. The higher the quality of image it is, the better the application accuracy will be. But there is no significant difference between 1mm sections and 3 mm sections of MRI images.

Key words: Image guided surgery, Application accuracy, stereotactic surgery, frameless and frame based systems,.

1. INTRODUCTION

Stereotactic localization using multimodality of medical images (such as CT or MRI) provides highly accurate intraoperative localization and allows the surgeon to resect a lesion in its entirety while sparing critical areas of the brain. The use of stereotactic frames and rigid pin fixation to the skull have provided extreme levels of mechanical accuracy for surgical localization. As an alternative to conventional stereotaxis, a variety of frameless stereotactic systems have been developed to provide surgical localization intraoperatively, which has eliminated the requirements of a rigid frame that may interfere with access to the operating field (1,3-5). As the use of computer-interactive technologies have become more common in neurosurgery, frameless methods are also widely applied to the neurosurgery and the need for an optimum skull fiducial marker system has increased. Two main fiducial marker system have been developed. Skin marker system is easy to use and sticks on the surface of the skull. However, the motion of the skin during the surgery or other procedures is an important source of affecting factors on the application accuracy. The bone screw marker system is fixed on the skull and more stable during the surgery. It can provide more reliable results for clinical usage. Therefore, it is very important to have a quantitative study to analyze the affecting factors on the application accuracy.

The application accuracy of a surgical localization system is a function of its mechanical accuracy interacting with the selected parameters of imaging studies chosen to visualize the lesion and its related anatomy. However the mechanical accuracy of the system can not represent the application accuracy of this system. It will be significantly worse than the weakest link of localization accuracy in a system, because other errors will be added to it rather than being hidden within it. In the surgical procedure artificial factors are also an important sources of the errors of localization. In addition to the mechanical limitations of the surgical localization system, the errors associated with the many steps of surgical localization (including imaging techniques, point selection, vector calculation, mechanical couplings and adjustments, other system adjustments, registration procedure and techniques, etc.) all contribute to the final clinically relevant error. In order to provide high levels of surgical localization accuracy, all of these error related factors should be controlled and reduced to a extreme low level. Therefore to determine how much distortion of these affecting factors caused during the whole procedure of image guided surgery on the application accuracy of the system is a very important content for this study. Theoretically speaking, the frame-based and frameless surgical localization system should have similar application accuracy. However quantitative comparison between these two system has not been reported. We present our preliminary experience with the use of semi-invasive fiducial markers (Fisher, Freiburg-Leibinger) comparing their application accuracy to that of the ZD stereotactic ring (Fisher-Leibinger, Freiburg, Germany), for the interactive-intraoperative localization of intracranial lesions.

2. MATERIAL AND METHODS

This study was designed to determine the influence of different affecting factors on the application accuracy. The each affecting factor were tested and analyzed. A paired t-test was used to perform statistical analysis

2.1 Experimental Setup

The semi-invasive markers developed with Fisher-Leibinger consist of three parts: a titanium screw, a base, and an insert. Due to the varying thickness of the galea, the titanium bone screws are available in two different lengths, 10 and 18 mm, both with a thread length of 7 mm. The base has in one end a thread to attach to the screw, and a cavity for insert at the opposite end. There are three types of inserts available: a computed tomographic (CT) -angiogram compatible insert, a multimodality image insert, and an intraoperative insert. The CT-angiogram insert is a gold-filled sphere. The multimodality image insert can be filled with different substances, including radioactive isotopes for use with CT, magnetic resonance imaging (MRI), digital angiography (DA), or positron emission tomography (PET) scans. The intraoperative insert has been created to replace the image insert for intraoperative registration. The image inserts are spherical in shape so the center is not accessible for intraoperative registration while the intraoperative insert is flat, and its height corresponds exactly to the center of the spherical image insert.

2.2. Phantom preparation

A phantom was mounted with the standard Z-D ring and also implanted with five semi-invasive screws of the frameless marker system, which randomly distributed on the surface. A steel sphere with diameter of 2 mm was mounted into the phantom as target point. The Phantom was imaged using a Semens Somatom Plus CT scanner (Siemens, Eriangen, Germany). Scan thickness was set at 1 and 2 mm; for each thickness, two kinds of image resolution were used. Pixel sizes are 1.18 x 1.18 and 0.59 x 0.59 respectively. We use 2 mm thickness and pixel size 1.18 x 1.18 image resolution in one group, and 1 mm thickness and 0.59 x 0.59 image resolution in another group to observer if there is a significant difference between the best and the worst image quality conditions. The images were transferred to a stereotactic computer. The Neurosurgical Planning System (NSPS) software developed at Wayne State University was used for image registration. The NSPS runs on a SUN SPARC10 station (Sun Microsystems, Mountain View, California), used to achieve fast calculations to reconstruct volumes from imaging studies. The workstation is connected to the Detroit Medical Center's central computer network, from which images derived from CT and MRI can be transferred. It allows image viewing and manipulation in real-time during preplanning and intraoperatively. The coordinates of target point were recorded and saved into a file as a reference point.

2.3. Surgical localization system

A contact-less, pre-calibrated motion analysis system was chosen to locate the instruments. It can track up to 256 pulsed infrared light emitting diode (LED) markers with a maximum sampling rate of about 3500 markers per second (OPTOTRAK 3020, Northern Digital, Waterloo, CAN). Within a field of view of 1.0 m x 1.2 m at a distance of 2.0 m the camera can locate each LED with an accuracy of 0.15 mm. By attaching at least three markers onto each rigid body its location and orientation in space can be determined. The system is precalibrated, reducing set-up time and allowing the better tolerance to environmental changes. The limitation of the system is the need of a direct viewing between the camera and the LED's. To overcome this limitation we have designed a special holder to allow for different heights and angulations. The OPTOTRAK system has the ability to define several rigid bodies. Each rigid body is assigned a separate dynamic reference. It provides relative coordinates from the camera to any one of these rigid body's dynamic reference on the fly, by attaching to the skull or other rigid body. By calibrating the relative coordinates the transformation matrix is established. This eliminates the need for new matching during neurosurgery procedure. The motion analysis system is controlled by DOS based software running on a personal computer networked with a Unix workstation (SUN Microsystems, Inc. Mountain View, CA) which is used for image data acquisition/reconstruction and real-time instrument visualization. A single monitor provides all information.

2.4. Experimental procedure

In order to determine the influence of the quality of image, a special designed plate mounted with ten semi-invasive markers was used. The distance between each marker was directly measured by a precise vernier calliper. The scan section thickness were 1 mm and 3 mm respectively. After images were transferred into SUN Workstation, NSPS.4.0 software was used to reconstruct the images to form 3 2-D images (i.e. axial, coronal, and sagittal planes). Then, each marker coordinate was digitized 8 times and recorded into a file. The distance between markers from digitized results were compared with the distance that from directly measured. A paired t-test was used to compare the results from two different image quality groups and also from different distance groups.

For each image group, the experiment procedure included the image registrations, which based on the Z-D ring and frameless marker system and the digitization of the target point. In each image group, three times of image registration were finished in order to check the repeatability of the system. In addition, an artificial error registration was also finished by 5 mm differ from the ideal point of the registration in order to observe the influence of artificial error during the image registration. In each registration, the target point was digitized 3 times. The coordinates of each digitization were recorded and save into a file for the off-line statistical analysis. These coordinates were used to compare with the coordinates of the reference point.

2.5. Image Data Acquisition

Interactive image guidance requires the registration of images derived from CT and/or MRI. Those images must be registered to each other and to the patient by using common points of reference, such as anatomical points or fiducial markers.

Before Gadolinium enhanced MRI, we placed five semi-invasive markers (Leibinger-Fisher, Freiburg, Germany) on the phantom. The semi-invasive markers consist on two parts: a base, which is fixed to the head with a very small (2 mm) Titanium screw, and the insert. The threads of the base were firmly screwed to the skull bone, using the pilot hole as a guide. The insert is a 3 mm ball-shaped plastic container, filled with a radio-opaque material, which was designed to be brightly visible on both CT and MRI images, including T-1, proton density, and T-2 weighted images. Once placed, these markers remained on the phantom during the scanning, and thorough the experimental procedure.

In order to determine the influence of the quality of image, a special designed plate mounted with ten semi-invasive markers was used. A MRI T1 sequence was used and the scan section thickness were 1 mm and 3 mm respectively.

2.6. Intraoperative registration and localization

Registration is the process of defining some special points based on the fiducial markers or anatomical landmarks from CT, MRI, or PET scan data and correlating them with these points located on the head of the patient in the real world, in the operating room. The goals are: firstly, to match, or correlate, data from the medical image to the 'real world', which refers to the coordinate space of the surgical instruments. A tracking device is attached to the instruments to continually relay information regarding position to the system. Coordinate matching ensures that any point seen in a medical image corresponds to an actual point in the real world (i.e., the patient's spinal anatomy). Second is to correlate different images with each other. Each imaging modality displays anatomical structures and lesions in a unique way. This benefits the surgeon by providing several different ways to viewing a same anatomical structure, but requires the development of an interactive relationship between the images and the 'real world'. Registration is used to build the relationship and enable the surgeon to use each imaging modality to its greatest advantage for localizing the anatomical structure. Intraoperative digitization through an infrared system is based upon the use of a three-dimensional (3-D) motion analysis system (OPTOTRAK, Northern Digital, Waterloo, Canada). This system is consists of an opto-electronic system with light- emitting diodes (LED). Three infrared sensors track target points defined by several miniature leads mounted on the surgeon's operative instrument, in a predefined relationship, and referred to as a "surgical rigid body or pointer". Another similar rigid body is mounted to the head holder or patient's ring (patient's rigid body). The patient's rigid body is used to tell the system where the real patient is, and the surgical rigid body tells the system the position of the surgical instrument. Then transformation matrix are calculated, the unique coordinate system is set up. Each time the surgeon moves the instrument, three monitors mounted in the room display the instrument's position on previously acquired computer-generated images.

In the image registration the image coordinates of each fiducial marker obtained from the CT scan was recorded into a file as the reference points (absolute image coordinates). In the operating room, the image registration was performed for the semi-invasive fiducial markers and the Z-D stereotactic ring. By touching the tip of each semi-invasive fiducial marker and four points on the Z-D ring to form the appropriate transformation matrix for each system. The image coordinates are matched with the real world patient's anatomy. Frame-based registration was showed in workstation A and frameless registration was showed in workstation B. After the image registration the surgical tracking mode was used to track the surgical instruments. By touching the tip of each semi-invasive fiducial marker with the pointer (surgical rigid body), the system recorded their spatial position, as they were touched by the tip of the probe during the image registration. In this way, the X, Y and Z coordinates of the markers were recorded.

2.7. Statistical analysis

A systematic error analysis was performed comparing the coordinates of target points on the medical images and the coordinates of intraoperatively digitizing target points based on the registration from each surgical localization system. Statistical analysis was performed on the sample of experimental data and sample of 19 patients.

A comparison of the 3-D measurements (x, y, z) of the coordinates of the target point from each experimental data and each patient with the ring and fiducial markers to absolute image coordinates was performed. The ten times repeated measurements for each test using each of method, which allowed for testing of internal consistency of the measurements for each method. Statistical analysis pertaining to various comparisons among methods was performed on the average measurements per study subject.

The mean deviation from the absolute image coordinates were calculated from all 3-D mean measurements (x, y, z) of each experiment data and patient for each methods correlating the ring and fiducial markers-based registration to the absolute image coordinates. Also, the deviation from target point in three direction (anterior-posterior, medial-lateral, and superior-inferior direction) of each experimental data and patient between ring and fiducial measurements were calculated similarly. Therefore, to assess differences among patients per each of the x, y, z measurements a mean square root of the distance between the planes of the three mentioned distances, for the *ith* patient, was calculated as follows:

distance$_{ijk}$ = SQRT $((X_{ij}-X_{ik})^2 + (Y_{ij}-Y_{ik})^2 + (Z_{ij}-Z_{ik})^2)$
where j,k= 1,2,3.

A paired t-test was applied to test for significance of the mean deviation between the frame based and frameless system. A one-sample mean t-test was applied to test for mean significance of distance among the three methods. A paired t-test was used to compare the magnitude of difference of mean distances (Delta values) of the ring-based registration and absolute image coordinates versus the fiducial markers-based registration and absolute image coordinates. To estimate the average mean difference of the distance, a 95% confidence interval (95% CI) was obtained. The semi-invasive fiducial system was compared with the ZD stereotactic ring (Fisher, Freiburg, Germany), which has demonstrated a high level of application accuracy in previous studies. After registered by both system, 119 random points on these 12 patients were collected and compared. A statistical analysis was performed, comparing the error difference between both methods of registration (ring fiducial and the semi-invasive fiducial markers), in determining the position of ten points on the patient's head. For that purpose, we compared the Mean Root Square (RMS), the Mean Error of Localization (MEL), and the Mean Error in 3-D (MED).

The RMS represents the mean of the sum of vectors between two records on one points which is the maximum distance between them. It is calculated as follow:

RMS = SQRT $((X1 - X2)^2 + (Y1 - Y2)^2 + (Z1 - Z2)^2)$

The Mean error of localization (MEL) is determined by calculating the mean of the sum of the scalar distances between the true target and the points achieved by the localization system. This number is based on how far from target each individual attempt was, irrespective of direction. Here we assume that records from Z-D stereotactic frame system as the true target. The mean error of localization takes into account the precision of each individual localization attempt. In this way, the surgeon can reasonably know " what is the greatest distance that this particular device could place me away from my chosen target"? It is calculated as follow:

MEL = ((X1 - X2) + (Y1 - Y2) + (Z1 - Z2)) / 3

The Mean error in 3-D (MED): Using this way is to analyze the error rate in three different dimensions. It reflects the error on a specific dimension, therefore it should be calculated for each axis by the formula

MED = (X1 - X2)/N

3. Results

3.1. The error produced by image and digitization

This affecting factor is defined as the difference between a known distance (precisely measured before the scan procedure) and same distance digitized from medical image. The error is related with the scanner and human digitization. The results are shown in Table 1:

Table 1: The errors produced by image scanner and human digitization in different image quality groups (Mean error ± SD mm)

Distances \ Sections	1 mm	3 mm
25 mm	0.17± 0.19	0.20± 0.21
50 mm	0.19± 0.16	0.25± 0.21
75 mm	0.27± 0.24	0.21 ± 0.14
100 mm	0.21± 0.19	0.24± 0.24

There is no significant differences between 1 mm and 3 mm sections of MRI groups. In varying the distances, there is also no significant difference. For a surgical localization system, this is not a important affecting factor to the application accuracy of the system.

3.2. The application accuracy of the frame-based and frameless surgical localization system

Anteroposterior, lateral, and vertical components of the target coordinate from each digitization were examined individually for their error. The Root-Mean-Square (RMS) was also calculated from these three components. The results are shown in Table 2 and Table 3. There is a significant difference between two systems (P = 0.0001) in low resolution and 2 mm thickness scan images but no significant difference in high resolution and 1 mm thickness image groups (P = 0.121). The image quality also takes a important role on the application accuracy. The higher the quality (the thinner of the scan thickness)of image it is, the better the application accuracy it will be (P = 0.001 and 0.032 respectively) (Figure 1)

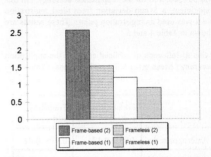

Figure 1. The comparison of application accuracy between frame-based and frameless localization system.(2 = 2 mm thickness of CT scan and 1 = 1 mm thickness of CT scan

Table 2: Comparison of application accuracy between frame-based and frameless localization system (Mean error ± SD mm, CT sections = 2 mm.)

	Frame-based system	Frameless system
Anteroposterior	1.20 ± 0.29	0.76 ± 0.31
Lateral	1.79 ± 0.17	1.03 ± 0.48
Vertical	1.33 ± 0.89	0.45 ± 0.38
RMS	2.57 ± 0.54	1.53 ± 0.65

Table 3: Comparison of application accuracy between frame-based and frameless localization system (Mean error ± SD mm, CT sections = 1 mm.)

	Frame-based system	Frameless system
Anteroposterior	0.34 ± 0.26	0.67 ± 0.41
Lateral	0.48 ± 0.26	0.45 ± 0.32
Vertical	0.98 ± 0.45	0.3 ± 0.12
RMS	1.20 ± 0.42	0.90 ± 0.47

3.3. The influence of artificial errors in the image registration

During surgical procedure if an artificial error in the image registration happened, what kind of effects will be occurred on the application accuracy. In this experiment, a 5 mm deviation from ideal registration point was used as registration point. These results are shown in Table 4 and 5.

Table 4: Influence of artificial error on the application accuracy (Mean error ± SD , CT sections = 2mm)

	Frame-based system	Frameless system
Anteroposterior	1.95 ± 0.17	0.93 ± 0.42
Lateral	1.16 ± 1.14	1.58 ± 0.81
Vertical	2.85 ± 0.43	0.64 ± 0.36
RMS	3.91 ± 0.66	2.01 ± 0.73

Table 5: Influence of artificial err on application accuracy (Mean error ± SD mm, CT sections = 1mm.)

	Frame-based system	Frameless system
Anteroposterior	1.11 ± 0.51	0.39 ± 0.53
Lateral	0.77 ± 0.81	0.63 ± 0.48
Vertical	2.42 ± 0.93	0.61 ± 0.37
RMS	2.92 ± 1.23	1.15 ± 0.07

The artificial errors during the image registration can also directly effect on the clinical application accuracy in the both systems. There is a significant difference between normal registration and artificial error registration in two image quality groups. (P = 0.001 and 0.001 respectively) The frameless localization system has the better application accuracy in the two image quality group. (P = 0.029 and 0.04 respectively) (Figure 2).

3.4. The influence of marker's position on the application accuracy

Generally speaking, markers of frameless system should be distributed as far as possible for the

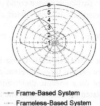
—+— Frame-Based System
---- Frameless-Based System

Figure 2. The influence of artificial error on the application accuracy.

reason of accuracy. However, it is difficult to determine what kind of distribution is the best. We tested two groups of distributions. One is localized around the area 6 x 6 cm, which is close to surgical area and easy to do the registration. Another group is distributed around the whole skull, which is suppose to be more accurate than the local distributed marker group. The results are shown in Table 6 and 7.

Table 6: Influence of marker distribution on the application accuracy
(Mean error ± SD mm, CT sections = 2 mm)

	Local distribution	Whole skull distribution
Anteroposterior	1.01 ± 0.44	0.93 ± 0.42
Lateral	0.47 ± 0.54	1.58 ± 0.81
Vertical	0.41 ± 0.26	0.64 ± 0.36
RMS	1.33 ± 0.37	2.01 ± 0.73

Table 7: Influence of marker distribution on application accuracy (Mean error ± SD mm, CT sections = 1 mm)

	Local distribution	Whole skull distribution
Anteroposterior	0.30 ± 0.15	0.39 ± 0.53
Lateral	0.39 ± 0.16	0.63 ± 0.48
vertical	0.17 ± 0.21	0.61 ± 0.37
RMS	0.58 ± 0.13	1.15 ± 0.07

The local distribution of markers around the lesion has the better application accuracy. (P = 0.001)

4. Discussions

The first affecting factor in the image guided surgery is image factor. After images transformed from scanned and restructured how much distortion occurred? From our results, it seems very small only 0.2mm to 0.3 mm. This deviation generally will not produce a big influence on the application accuracy of the system. The different distances from 25 mm to 100 mm produced a similar error. There is no significant difference between them. In 1 mm and 3 mm sections of MRI groups, it also showed a similar results with no statistically difference. However when thickness increased to 10 mm, the difference is significant. Our results only proved that under 3 mm thickness of section, the application accuracy no significant improved as the thickness reduced.

Theoretically speaking, the frame-based and frameless surgical localization system should have similar clinical application accuracy because the transformation matrix from both systems are calculated by at least three fixed points on the Z-D ring or on the fiducial markers. This is based on rigid body mechanics. The only difference is the points from the Z-D ring are on the ring which have to be fixed to the skull by pins, while the points from fiducial markers are directly fixed to the skull by the screws.

Registration methodology constitutes a basic process in image-guided surgery. The interface surrounding the patient's head (i.e. stereotactic system or fiducial markers) must accurately transfer the target coordinates from CT and MRI to the digitizing system. Conventional stereotactic surgery uses rigid fixation (ring) mounted on the head of the patient by several screws (frame-based stereotaxis). Stereotactic frames have been the standard of clinically accepted levels of accuracy; consequently, any new methodology for registration should be compared against this basic standard. Although they are accepted from the accuracy point of view, the use of stereotactic rings offers several disadvantages. They are uncomfortable for the patient, and logistically they should be placed the same day of the surgery. Furthermore, the stereotactic ring can be displaced from its original position with the possibility of mechanical error on localization, as we have observed in one of our study patients. The longer the ring remains placed on the patient, the risk of this complication is higher; special attention is required to avoid frame dislocation. Additionally, the use of a standard stereotactic ring complicates airway management during surgery, especially during awake procedures. Moreover, standard stereotactic rings are obstructing, limiting the choices of surgical approaches. This is especially true for skull base lesions, or when a combined supra- or infratentorial approach is required.

As an alternative to conventional stereotaxis, a variety of frameless stereotactic systems have been developed to provide surgical localization intraoperatively. They provide a reference interface, allowing for an unobstructed surgical approach and airway management. As of last year several frameless navigational devices have been developed (2,5,6,7-12). Generally, two methods are currently used for frameless stereotaxis; fiducial markers applied to the scalp or semipermanent fiducial markers rigidly fixed to the patient's skull. When fiducial markers attached to the skin are used, the scalp may move relative to the cranial bones, deviating the fiducial points from their intended positions. These skin-attached fiducial markers are useful for some procedures, but do not provide the same level of accuracy obtained with rigid fixation. However, most frameless digitizing systems have been developed using noninvasive fiducial markers attached to the skin.

In order to achieve a higher degree of accuracy with frameless systems, a system of semipermanent fiducial markers has been developed. These markers could be left in place for several days without risk of being displaced, and allow for staged procedures, which are required in epilepsy surgery, for example, or in some skull base tumors.

In this study, we compared semipermanent fiducial marker accuracy with stereotactic frame accuracy, using the frame as the standard of a clinically-acceptable degree of accuracy. Using the same image protocol, the statistical analysis revealed a small significant difference between both methodologies (2.95 ±.45 mm). In order to define which of the two methods is more accurate, we compared each with the absolute image coordinates. Our study showed that the semipermanent fiducial marker system is more accurate than the stereotactic ring (the difference with the absolute image coordinates was 3.35 ±.59 mm for the stereotactic ring, and 1.72 ±.42 mm for the fiducial system). Although the difference between the two methodologies is statistically significant, its clinical implications may not be relevant.

An assessment of differences among the mean differences of various methods per each of the x, y, z coordinates is done by constructing the 95% CI. A mean difference of Z_2-Z_1 (Table 2) was significant, which implies that the significant difference in the distance is possibly due to this. Furthermore, the 95% CI also provides an estimate of the size of $\Box Z$ (i.e. $\Box Z=Z_2-Z_1$) with a probability of 95%. Therefore, fiducial-based registration is more accurate than the stereotactic frame.

We believe that the semi-permanent implantable fiducial marker system represents the next step in the application of stereotactic techniques in neurosurgery. It cannot yet replace traditional frame-based stereotactic surgery when minimal invasion and maximum prediction of target trajectory repeatability is required, like during a biopsy of a deep-seated lesion, functional procedures, or placement of implants. In other words, a function of stereotactic frames that cannot be replaced by the semipermanent fiducial system is its ability to act as an accurate holder and guidance to bring an instrument to a specific target. All frameless passive systems imply an iterative trial error method not acceptable for those procedures. However, this semi-permanent implantable fiducial system is ideal for a far greater range of cases in which frame-based stereotaxis is too limited, such as large centered craniotomies, skull base procedures, lesions where a combined supra-infratentorial approach, or staged procedures are required. In the future, active robotic systems could be used to guide an instrument to a target in a defined trajectory, which may be more precise than that achieved with the stereotactic arc. Interactive image-guided neurosurgery is evolving beyond the limitations placed by the mechanically-based stereotactic frames systems designed at the turn of the century. As new surgical navigational frameless systems are being developed, we anticipate that the semipermanent fiducial markers system are likely to replace other fiducial systems or even the stereotactic ring, introducing a new generation of possibilities in neurosurgery.

6. References

1. Bucholz RD, Smith KR (1993) A comparison of sonic digitizers versus light emitting diode-based location. In Maciunas RJ (ed) Interactive Image-Guided Neurosurgery. AANS Publications Committee, Park Ridge 1993. Pp 179-200
2. Bucholz RD, Ho HW, and Rubin JP.(1993) Variables affecting the accuracy of stereotactic localization using computerized tomography. J Neurosurg 79: 667-673
3. Golfinos JC, Fitzpatrick BC, Smith LR, Spetzler R (1995) Clinical use of a frameless stereotactic arm: Results of 325 cases. J Neurosurg 83: 197-205
4. Heilbrun MP, Mc Donald P, Wiker C, et al (1992) Stereotactic localization and guidance using a machine vision technique. Stereotact Func Neurosurg 58: 94-98
5. Murphy MA, Barnett GH, Kormos DW, Waisemberger J (1993) Astrocytoma resection using an interactive frameless stereotactic wand: An early experience. J Clin Neurosci 1: 3337
6. Kato A, Yoshimine T, Hayakawa T, et al (1991) A frameless, armless navigational system for computer-assisted neurosurgery. J Neurosurg 74: 845-849
7. Li Q.H., Holdener H.J., Zamorano L., King P., Jiang Z.W., and Diaz F.: Computer assisted insertion of pedicle screws. *Lecture Notes in Computer Science 1131*. Eds by Karl Heinz H_hne and Ron Kikinis, page 571-581, 1996.
8. Maciunas RJ, Fitzpatrick JM, Galloway RL, Allen GS. Beyond stereotaxy: Extreme levels of application accuracy are provided by implantable fiducial markers for interactive image-guided neurosurgery. In Maciunas RJ (ed) Interactive Imaged-Guided Surgery. AANS Publications Committee, Park Ridge 1993, pp 259-270
9. Nolte LP, Zamorano L, Jiang Z, Wang Q, Langlotz F, Berlemann U (1995) Image-guided insertion of transpedicular screws: A laboratory set-up. Spine 20: 497-500
10. Takizawa T (1993) Neurosurgical navigation using a noninvasive stereoadapter. Surg Neurol 40: 1-7
11. Watanabe E, Mayanagi Y, Kosugi Y, Manaka S, Takakura K (1991) Open surgery assisted by the neuronavigator, a stereotactic, articulated, sensitive arm. Neurosurg 28: 792-800
12. Zamorano L, Nolte L, Jiang C, Kadi M (1993) Image-guided neurosurgery: Frame based versus frameless approaches. Neurosurgical Operative Atlas 3: 402-422
13. Zamorano L, Nolte L, Kadi M, Jiang Z (1993) Interactive intraoperative localization using an infrared-based system. Neuro Res 15: 290-298
14. Zamorano L, Nolte LP, Kadi AM, Jiang Z (1994) Interactive intraoperative localization using an infrared-based system. Stereotact Funct Neurosurg 63: 84-88
15. Zamorano L, Kadi M, Jiang Z, Diaz FG (1994) Zamorano-Dujovny multipurpose neurosurgical image-guided localizing unit: Experience in 866 consecutive cases of "open stereotaxis". Stereotact Funct Neurosurg 63: 45-51

Multi-level Strategy for Computer-Assisted Transbronchial Biopsy

Ivan Bricault[1], Gilbert Ferretti[2] and Philippe Cinquin[1]

[1] TIMC-IMAG, Institut Albert Bonniot, 38706 La Tronche cedex, France
[2] Department of Radiology, Hôpital Michallon, CHU Grenoble, France
E-mail : Ivan.Bricault@imag.fr

Abstract. The Computer-Assisted Transbronchial Biopsy project involves the registration, without any external localization device, of a pre-operative 3D CT scan of the thoracic cavity (showing a tumor that requires a needle biopsy), and an intra-operative endoscopic 2D image sequence, in order to provide an assistance to a transbronchial puncture of the tumor. Because of the specific difficulties resulting from the processed data, original image processing methods were elaborated and a multi-level strategy is introduced. For each analysis level, the relevant information to process and the corresponding algorithms are defined. This multi-level strategy then achieves the best possible accuracy.

The results presented here demonstrate that it is possible to localize precisely the endoscopic camera within the CT data coordinate system. The computer can thus synthesize in near real-time the CT-derived virtual view that corresponds to the actual endoscopic real view.

1 Introduction

For diagnosing and staging lung cancers in patients, obtaining histological samples is a fundamental step. But many mediastinal tumor formations are invisible during bronchoscopy and not accessible to a transthoracic biopsy. Then a transbronchial needle biopsy is a minimally invasive alternative to surgery, and thus a very valuable procedure [1].

Nevertheless, the transbronchial biopsy procedure involves a "blind" puncture without a direct visual control on the lesion. So, when no specific assistance is provided, it can explain that despite of its potential benefits the transbronchial biopsy remains underutilized [2].

A computer assistance can promote the transbronchial biopsy. The computer can reconstruct 3-D endoluminal views from CT data (*Virtual Bronchoscopy*). When preparing a transbronchial biopsy, virtual views can help a pre-operative planning of an optimal needle trajectory [3].

But virtual bronchoscopy provides only a pre-operative assistance. The aim of *Computer-Assisted Transbronchial Biopsy* is to provide an intra-operative assistance : during the endoscopic procedure, the operator wants to see in real-time the exact virtual view (computed from CT data) that corresponds to the current endoscopic real view, i.e. the virtual view must follow the movements of the fiberoptic camera inside bronchial tree. Thus, the operator benefits from an Augmented Reality technique : extraluminal elements detected on CT are augmenting the endoscopic perception (Figure 1). One can then verify that the needle reaches the tumor, without hurting any critical tissues.

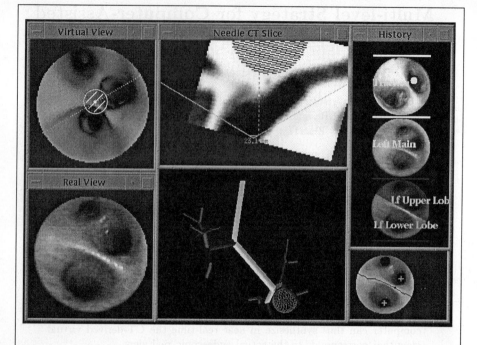

Fig. 1. Computer-Assisted Transbronchial Biopsy – Results. The system achieves an automatic registration between real and virtual bronchoscopy, in order to help guiding the trans-bronchial needle biopsy. – *"Real View"* : The real bronchoscopic video sequence is analyzed in near real-time by the computer. – *Lower right window* : Result of the automatic segmentation of the wall that splits both bronchi. – *"History"* : The computer is able to recognize the different explored bronchi. From top to bottom, each subdivision level encountered is extracted. The bottom view identifies both current bronchi (left upper and lower lobe). – *Lower central window* : The computer tracks the trajectory of the flexible endoscope inside a 3D geometrical model of the bronchial tree. Both current bronchi are located by specific colours. We can see a spherical target defined for the trans-bronchial needle biopsy. – *"Virtual View"* : The system can synthesize a virtual view from CT scan data. The target appears in transparency. Using specific image processing algorithms, the bronchoscopic camera position is automatically computed, so that the virtual view follows the actual camera movements and automatically matches the real view. – *"Needle CT Slice"* : The computer shows the CT slice containing the bronchoscopic center of view and the expected biopsy needle trajectory. The distance to the center of the target is computed.

2   A multi-level strategy

Our approach is based on algorithms able to localize in real-time the fiberoptic camera position inside the CT data coordinate system, using only image processing, and without any external localization device. Because this localization task is difficult, we have developed a specific multi-level strategy. Four levels of image analysis are required in order to achieve a complete localization of the endoscope.

The level-1 analysis follows the endoscope movements inside the tracheo-bronchial tree hierarchy. The aim is to anatomically identify the various explored bronchial subdivisions, in order to help the operator navigate and find a correct path to the biopsy site.

Then, when the operator is in the neighborhood of the lesion, an accurate localization of the endoscope is achieved in levels 2,3,4 in order to guide the biopsy in a safe and accurate manner :
- The level-2 analysis gives an approximative endoscopic localization, producing a virtual view roughly similar to the real view.
- The level-3 analysis generates a precise endoscopic localization, but is restricted to 4 degrees-of-freedom.
- Finally, the level-4 analysis computes an endoscopic localization with 6 degrees-of-freedom (3 translations and 3 rotations entirely define the endoscopic camera position in the CT coordinate system).

2.1 Level-1 : Bronchi anatomical identification

We have achieved the bronchial subdivision image segmentation with mathematical morphology operators, involving dynamics and watershed line computations (see [4] for details).

A 3D geometrical model of the tracheo-bronchial tree allows us to predict the various subdivision relative orientations. During a real endoscopic exploration, it is then possible to identify each bronchus thanks to a comparison between segmented (endoscopic) and expected (CT) subdivision orientations. We need to use only one generic 3D bronchial model for every patients : indeed, our method is robust enough to tolerate the small inter-individual anatomical variations.

Using a digital alpha workstation and 100×100 endoscopic images, the computer can process 2 to 10 images per second. The computer is able to follow an endoscopic exploration up to the fourth level of subdivision.

2.2 Level-2 : Approximative localization

We consider here that the direction of the endoscopic axis of view remains parallel to the bronchial axis. Level-2 registration uses the alignment between CT and endoscopic inter-bronchial walls (see [4] for details). It is a direct localization method that involves no optimization process and that is very fast. The whole procedure, including endoscopic image segmentation and virtual image computation, allows a tracking of camera movements with 0.5 to 2 images per second.

The quality of the real/virtual registration depends on the fitting between CT-defined and segmented inter-bronchial walls, and depends on the parallelism of CT-defined bronchial axis and actual endoscopic axis of view. As we will describe it in the following, when these conditions are not fulfilled, then level-3 and level-4 are useful to reestablish the matching quality.

2.3 Level-3 : four degrees-of-freedom precise localization

We use here a new 2D/2D "daemon-based" [5] registration algorithm, presented in [6]. We still suppose, here, that the endoscope axis remains aligned with the bronchial axis (4 degrees of freedom).

We try to find the virtual view that best matches an endoscopic real view. An initial virtual view is computed from level-2 algorithm. From the translation, rotation and zoom parameters given by real/virtual "daemon-based" registration, we can adjust the estimated endoscope position and then create a new virtual view. Iterating this process can finally give a virtual view very similar to real view : it means that the endoscope is correctly located [6]. We usually achieve the level-3 localization with 2 or 3 iterations only and no more than a few seconds.

2.4 Level-4 : six degrees-of-freedom localization

As level-3 registration involves an intermediate 2D/2D registration step, the camera localization is restricted to four degrees of freedom. In this section, we present a precise six degrees-of-freedom localization that involves a 3D reconstruction of bronchial surface, thanks to a model-based shape-from-shading algorithm.

Motivations Level-3 algorithm needs to be very tolerant against pixel intensity variations. Indeed, when we try to register virtual and real views, we want to consider only the structural information in the images (i.e. the global shape of bronchial subdivisions). Thus our daemon-based algorithm, involving only unitary vectors in the direction of decreasing grey values [6] is very robust regarding lightening conditions : as a characteristic of our multi-level strategy, for a particular analysis level, we select all the relevant information but only the relevant information.

Nevertheless, pixel intensity values are important, because they can reveal a difference between real and virtual optical axis directions : when optical axis direction changes, some parts of the image become darker while others become brighter. As we will demonstrate it in the following, thanks to a "model-based shape-from-shading", we will be able to process these grey value informations, but only because level-3 gives us the necessary pre-registered initial conditions.

In the case of bronchoscopic images, the shape-from-shading problem is very difficult, because we have to tackle major topological ambiguities :

- only a small part of bronchial surface appears in one bronchoscopic image. The information found in the image is not sufficient to solve the topological ambiguities (in particular concerning the image edges, which represent in reality the major part of the image).
- in a bronchial subdivision image, the only visible singular point is a saddle point, so it can not be used for propagation [7]. We should use a propagation from the extremity of both bronchi, but these regions are not correctly visualized (occultation, lightening attenuation).

Furthermore, we have to consider a point light source at finite distance, and a perspective projection. Only few algorithms studied such image construction conditions [8] (but they do not have to tackle topological ambiguities).

Finally, the difficulties encountered for bronchial image 3D reconstruction are numerous and can not be solved by usual shape-from-shading algorithms developed so far.

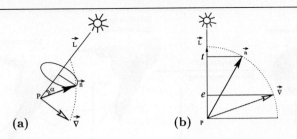

Fig. 2. Using model-based constraints for shape-from-shading. (a) The bronchial surface normal n, corresponding to an endoscopic pixel with intensity equal to $t = \cos(\alpha)$, has an undefined position on the cone forming an angle α with the lightening direction **L**. Knowing the CT surface normal ∇, we can choose **n** as the vector on the cone that is the closest to ∇. (b) **n** can then be computed from t, ∇, and e which is the pixel intensity in the CT virtual image (see text).

Model-based shape-from-shading Our solution comes from the development of a new shape-from-shading algorithm : we use the 3D data about the bronchial surface (coordinates, distance to camera, normal vectors) that are given by the *pre-registered CT model* resulting from level-3. Our algorithm is based on the 3 following points.

(1) CT-derived 3D data allows us to correct lightening attenuation effects. During the synthesis of virtual images, the lightening attenuation is computed from the distance of the bronchial point to light source. Considering any pixel in a real bronchial image, an approximation of this distance to light source is given by the pre-registered 3D CT model. Then we can use the lightening attenuation formula, in order to correct lightening artifacts before processing the image.

(2) CT data allows us to compute real bronchi normals. Let us consider a pixel in a bronchial subdivision real image. Let t be the pixel intensity (from 0.0 to 1.0). If **n** is the unknown normal direction in the corresponding bronchial surface point, and **L** is the light ray direction, then **n** must be such that $t = \mathbf{n} \cdot \mathbf{L}$, but **n** remains undefined (Figure 2a).

Let e be the same pixel intensity in the virtual image, previously registered (level-3) with the real image. We have $e = \nabla \cdot \mathbf{L}$, where ∇ is the normal direction given by the 3D CT model in the corresponding bronchial surface point (Figure 2b).

Then we can decide to choose **n** as the vector, such that $\mathbf{n} \cdot \mathbf{L} = t$, which is *the closest to* ∇. So we can show easily that **n** is defined by

$$\mathbf{n} = \left(t - e\sqrt{\tfrac{1-t^2}{1-e^2}}\right)\mathbf{L} + \sqrt{\tfrac{1-t^2}{1-e^2}}\nabla \quad \text{(Eq.3)}$$

(3) Eq.3 above defines the normal vectors for each pixel in bronchial image. Then the whole surface can be reconstructed, from the center of inter-bronchial wall (its coordinates are given by 3D CT model), propagating surface variations given by normal vectors and using a 3D grid model of the reconstructed surface (3D because of the specificities of the perspective projection).

Level-4 CT/bronchoscopy registration Up to level-3, the optical axis was previously maintained fixed when estimating the camera position. We now want

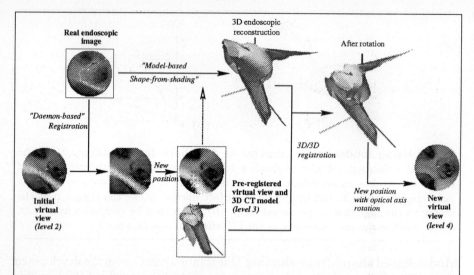

Fig. 3. Principle of level-3-4 CT/bronchoscopy registration. This step of a 6 degrees-of-freedom registration comes from a real execution of our algorithms. We start from a virtual view (for example, issued from level-2 algorithm) that approximatively matches the real view. Then level-3 daemon-based registration gives a pre-registered CT virtual view and 3D model, used for model-based shape-from-shading (in this 3D model visualization, one can recognize three branching partial tubes corresponding to the three bronchial holes visible in the virtual view). A 3D/3D registration between the real reconstructed 3D surface and the CT 3D surface allows us to compute the rotational component, and then to correct the CT point of view by an optical axis rotational adjustment.

to adjust an incorrect optical axis direction estimation, i.e. we want to achieve a full 6 degree-of-freedom CT/bronchoscopy registration.

We use here the 3D bronchial surface resulting from our model-based shape-from-shading algorithm. This endoscopic 3D surface can be compared to CT model 3D surface. A least-squares fitting of these two 3D point sets is achieved; for that purpose, 3D points from each set corresponding to the same light ray are matched. The rotation between CT model surface and endoscopic reconstructed surface, given by this 3D/3D registration step, is then applied to optical axis direction (Figure 3). As a result, the difference between virtual and real optical axis directions decreases.

Such a registration process can be iterated : the level-2 initial virtual view is replaced by the new corrected virtual view, and level-3 and level-4 processings are iterated.

Results Our model-based shape-from-shading method is able to take into account lightening and perspective artifacts, and to solve topological ambiguities, thanks to CT data.

Iterating the Figure 3 localization process, in general only twice, we obtained on real endoscopic images very good localization results, with a computation time being no more than a few seconds. Tests with virtual images show the good results obtained concerning the registration accuracy (Figure 4). We observe

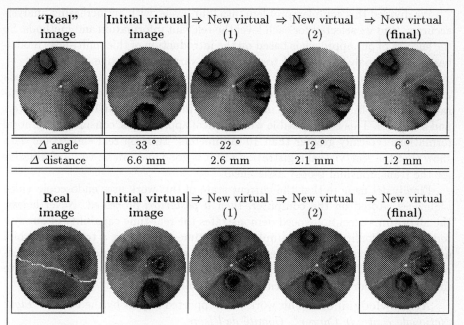

Fig. 4. Level-4 localization results. Each step involves the processing sequence described in Figure 3 (daemon-based registration plus model-based shape-from-shading). *Top : with virtual images.* Here the "real" image is a virtual view from a known position. Expected and computed endoscopic points of view are compared; the difference is quantified by a rotation and a translation parameter (Δ angle and Δ distance). We observe how the localization process is able to correct an important initial misregistration. *Bottom : with a real endoscopic image.* 3 iterations of the localization process are sufficient to obtain a visually very good matching between real and virtual views.

that the achieved precision increases during level-4 process. The demonstrated final precision is sufficient for clinical applications, considering that the tumor diameter is generally greater than 10 millimeters.

A failure can occur if the reference real image or a generated virtual image happen to be not informative enough (for example if the endoscope is too close to the bronchial wall, or if bronchial edges are too partially visualized). Nevertheless, in case of failure, our multi-level strategy leaves the possibility to restrict the analysis to level-2. Furthermore, this level-2 localization can benefit from adjusted parameters (optical axis direction, CT inter-bronchial wall geometry) inherited from a level-3 and level-4 analysis on a previous image with better quality.

3 Conclusion

Computer-assisted transbronchial biopsy is a challenging medical and scientific issue. As far as we know, our prototype system constitutes the first proposed solution : indeed, bronchoscopic data can be hardly processed by most usual computer vision algorithms, because of many specific difficulties.

We divided this complex problem into four levels, with an increasing analysis accuracy, and we selected for each level the relevant information and methods. So the success of our approach is based on the introduction of this multi-level model-based image analysis strategy, together with various innovative algorithms.

With our computer-assisted transbronchial biopsy system, execution speeds are below 5 seconds for level 1 to 4 complete 100×100 image processing. Accuracy, measured by using virtual instead of real images, is about 1 to 2 millimeters and 5 degrees. This is compatible with medical applications, considering tumoral formations typically greater than 10 millimeters. Tests on real endoscopic data show that the real/virtual registration result is good and can be very informative for the transbronchial biopsy assistance.

Finally, let us note that the current state of this work uses endoscopic video sequences, stored on the computer, then *a posteriori* processed. Nevertheless, the algorithms execution speed demonstrates the real-time capability of our system. This is confirmed by preliminary real-time tests using a tracheobronchial anatomical specimen. In the near future, we will proceed into further experiments in clinical conditions, and we will develop dedicated protocols in order to fully evaluate our system efficiency and reliability.

Acknowledgments : This work was supported in part by the French *"Ligue Nationale contre le Cancer", Comité de l'Isère*.

References

1. J. F. Turner and Ko-Pen Wang, "Staging of mediastinal involvement in lung cancer by bronchoscopic needle aspiration," *Journal of Bronchology*, vol. 3, pp. 74–76, 1996.
2. Edward F. Haponik and Deborah Shure, "Underutilization of transbronchial needle aspiration," *Chest*, vol. 112, no. 1, july 1997.
3. H.P. McAdams, P.C. Goodman, and P. Kussin, "Virtual bronchoscopy for directing transbronchial needle aspiration of malignant hilar and mediastinal lymph nodes," in *Radiological Society of North America*, Chicago, 1996.
4. Ivan Bricault, Gilbert Ferretti, and Philippe Cinquin, "Computer-Assisted Bronchoscopy : Aims and Research Perspectives," *Computer Aided Surgery (formerly : Journal of Image Guided Surgery)*, vol. 1, no. 4, pp. 217–225, 1995, [Also in MR-CAS'95 proceedings].
5. Jean-Philippe Thirion, "Fast intensity based non rigid matching," in *Medical Robotics and Computer assisted Surgery*, Baltimore, november 1995, pp. 47–54.
6. Ivan Bricault, "A Fast Morphology-Based Registration – Application to Computer-Assisted Bronchoscopy," in *CVRMed-MRCAS*, J. Troccaz, E. Grimson, and R. Mösges, Eds. march 1997, Lecture Notes in Computer Science, Springer-Verlag.
7. Ron Kimmel and Alfred M. Bruckstein, "Global Shape from Shading," *Computer Vision and Image Understanding*, vol. 62, no. 3, pp. 360–369, november 1995.
8. Takayuki Okatani and Koichiro Deguchi, "Shape Reconstruction from an Endoscope Image by Shape from Shading Technique for a Point Light Source at the Projection Center," *Computer Vision and Image Understanding*, vol. 66, no. 2, pp. 119–131, may 1997.

A Fast, Accurate and Easy Method to Position Oral Implant Using Computed Tomography
Clinical Validations

Guillaume Champleboux[1], Thomas Fortin[2], H. Buatois[3]
Jean Loup Coudert[2], Eric Blanchet[1]

[1] TIMC-IMAG, IAB - Faculté de Médecine de Grenoble
38700 La Tronche, France. Email: Guillaume.Champleboux@imag.fr
[2] Faculté d'Odontologie de Lyon, 69008 Lyon, France
[3] 41 Av. Alsace-Lorraine, 38000 Grenoble, France.

Abstract

This paper presents a simple method and new material which allow transferring results of surgical planning - such as the implant fixture axis - to the surgical site. This method is based on drilling a linear guide in a resin splint corresponding to the fixture axis. A simple mechanical setup links the Computed Tomography (CT) data set with the drilling machine. Since the optimal fixture axis is determined with a software interface, it can be transferred as a linear guide to the resin splint with the drilling machine. Technical validation demonstrates that the accuracy of the method is 0.2 mm in translation and 1 degree in rotation. These results provide a high level of accuracy and clinical validation has begun with several patients. The results for the patients are very satisfactory.

1 Introduction

The objective of a surgical procedure in oral implant treatment is to place a fixture on the jaw bone according to several prosthetic criteria of success such as phonation, appearance and masticatory functions. Computed tomography is used more and more for dental implant surgery planning in order to meet the above criteria of success. The standard method for determining the fixture axis using CT Images consists of the following steps:
- Determination of the prosthesis suprastructure position with a diagnostic cast of the maxilla and mandible.
- CT image acquisition with the materialized prosthesis axis.
- CT-based planning for the fixture axis.
This last step allows taking into account the dimension of the anatomical volume, jaw bone quality, and avoids damaging structures such as dental nerve and sinus. The result is a compromise between the prosthesis axis (materialized) and the ideal axis (computerized) hereby referred to as the optimal axis.
For more details see [1], [2], [3], [4], [5], [6], [7], [8], [9]. the main problem is now to **transfer** the information from the surgical plan to the surgical site.

In this paper a simple and accurate method to place one or several oral implants is briefly decribed (see [10] for more details and an explanation of the principles and methodology of the system. This will be followed by a description of the technical validation of the system. Finally, we conclude with a detailed presentation of the first clinical validation on two patients.

2 Transfer of the optimal axis to the surgical site

Presentation

To our knowledge there is at present no common simple system which allows the transfer of scanner information, i.e., the coordinates of the optimal axis, to the surgical site. After the evaluation of the optimal axis, the clinician has to mentally integrate the geometry of the mouth with the CT scans through the area, and transfer it to the surgical site without any encoded reference. Various solutions have been developed:
- Fortin et al.[3] used a guide drilled into a resin splint to accurately place the implant in the planned position. The guide was drilled thanks to computed planning and a 3D localizer.
- Solar et al.[11] propose an image-guided drill positioning system. These solutions require sophisticated hardware.
- Bauer et al. [12] propose a two parts device made of a holder and a drilling duct to be fixed upon the holder. The holder contains radiopaque markers which link the Scanner with the setup (holder-drilling duct). After the determination of the implant axis thanks to CT images, the drilling duct is therefore processed by stereolithography. The referenced paper do not describe either surgical planning or clinical validation.

Description of the method

The method described herein was reported in [10] and also uses a guide made into a resin splint. The basis is a drilling machine whose configuration can be tuned with 4 degrees of freedom (dof), because an axis in space has 4 dof. To drill the guide it is of primary importance to find a rigid transformation T between the reference coordinate system (RCS) of the scanner R_S - in which the optimal axis is defined - and the RCS of the drilling machine (noted as R_M).

Finding the transformation T between the two RCS.

A mechanical device was built which allows fixing two tubes made of titanium in a defined position. Because these two tubes (called linker tubes) can be linked easily to the drilling machine, the RCS of the drilling machine will be **visible** in the 3D CT data set (see Fig. 1a). It associates the resin splint to a removable mechanical support and provides for removable links which preserve the respective position of the splint and the mechanical support when they are associated. Fixing the two tubes during the molding of the resin splint requires no more than surrounding the tubes with resin inside the device. Once the resin is solid, the separation between the splint and the device is achieved by removing the two shafts (see Fig. 1b). While processing the CT Images containing the track of the tubes, it is possible to define a RCS which is the RCS of the mechanical device

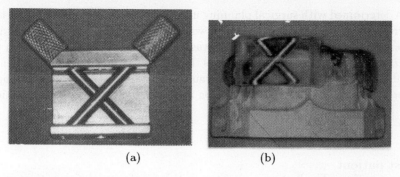

Fig. 1. *(a) Mechanical system for the fixation of the tubes in the resin splint. Device + two titanium tubes + two metallic shafts. (b) Fixation of the tubes in the resin splint*

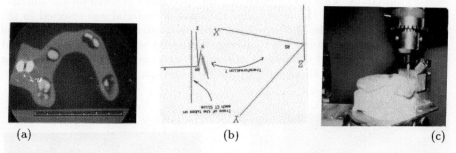

Fig. 2. *(a) CT Image passing though the tubes. (b) The 3D representation showing the RCS of the scanner R_S, the track of the tubes and the RCS of the drilling machine R_M defined by the axes of the tubes. (c) The splint is fixed on the drilling machine and drilled following the fixture axis.*

in the RCS of the scanner, i.e., the transformation between the two essential RCSs is determined (see Fig. 2b).

Drilling the guide.
Once the surgical planning has been done, the resin splint is attached to the device with the two shafts. The whole system is then fixed on the plate of the drilling machine. The system was designed such that the reference RCS of the drilling machine coincides with that defined by the titanium tubes (see Fig. 2c). Currently, for drilling, the tune of the plate is done by hand

Technical validation.
Starting from a "master model" with several teeth missing, a plaster cast was molded. One or more titanium tubes (inner diameter 2mm, length 10 mm) were included in the plaster cast. A resin splint was then molded on the plaster cast with the mechanical system which allows the drilling machine the scanner to be linked. The axes of the implant are also determined with the software used for surgical planning. Validating this technique involved ascertaining whether the

axes determined with surgical planning using CT images were indeed reported on the resin splint. Every time the splint was drilled, the drill entered the titanium tube in the plaster cast. This result was valid for each of the 8 titanium tubes inserted in the 3 different plaster casts. In fact, a 1.8 mm diameter drill entered a 2.0 mm diameter titanium tube. Because the titanium tube is 10 mm long, the error is less than 0.2 mm in translation and less than 1.1 degrees in rotation.

3 Clinical validation

First patient

Presentation. The first case reported in this paper concerns a patient without teeth on the maxilla (see Fig. 3a). A prosthesis study was conducted to place teeth and implants according to the criteria of phonation, appearance and masticatory functions. This led to modeling the placement of teeth on the maxilla. During the molding of the resin splint radiopaque material was inserted in the splint in order to model the prosthesis axes associated with the nine planned teeth. The two linker tubes were added to the splint with the system described above (see Fig. 3b) and CT images of the patient were acquired with the splint in the mouth. The CT slices were 1 mm thick and spaced every millimeter.

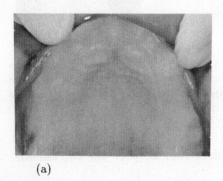
(a)
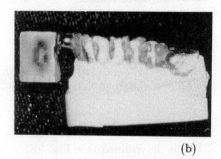
(b)

Fig. 3. *(a) The toothless maxilla of the first patient. (b) The molded resin splint on the cast with the linker tubes inserted. The prosthesis axes are also materialized in the splint*

Surgical planning with a software interface on a workstation. To place a virtual implant on the CT data set, two points must be clicked on two different slices in order to give the direction of the implant. This is done using the tracks of the radiopaque marker in two different slices; thus the initial direction of the virtual implant is known. Reformatted slices are also computed and displayed on the right side. These reformatted slices, both a pseudo-sagittal and a pseudo-frontal slice, allow the determination of the length and the width of the implant. The translation and rotation "push-buttons" are useful to tune the orientation and position of the virtual implant in order to take into account the position of the sinus and the structure of the bone. On the current CT image, the projection of the implant on the plane defined by the CT slice is graphically represented, the perpendicular to the projection is also added. This shows the direction of the implant relative to the curve defined by the bone. When all the criteria are satisfactory, the features of the implant are saved and a new virtual implant can be planned (see Fig. 4).

The track of the later implants are already displayed in another color. This yields the position of an implant relative to the others. Once surgical planning is achieved, the resin splint is fixed on the plate of the drilling machine and drilled according to the several computed postions (see Fig. 5a). Then the two linker tubes are detached from the splint in order to have an adapted surgical guide. Some of the resin is also removed because gum has been cut from the bone and must not hide the bone. With the guide in the mouth the surgeon drills the bone taking into account the feature (diameter and length) of the implant to be positioned, and screws the implant in the drilled hole (see Fig. 5b).

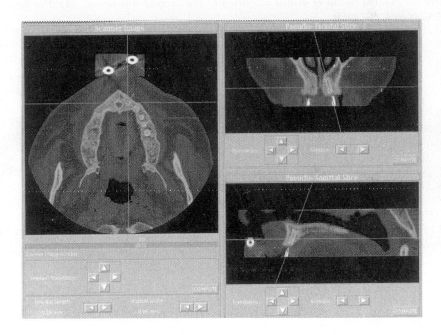

Fig. 4. *The display of the whole interface, current CT slice, tracks of virtual implant, reformatted slices and track of the current implant on these slices.*

Result and discussion. It was possible to fix only eight of the nine planned implants (see Fig. 6a). One failed due to the poor quality of the bone. The results were very good compared to the X-ray control image (see Fig. 6c). Netherthe-less, complete osteointegration must be attained followed by fixing the prosthesis on the implant before results can be declared fully satisfactory. Verification with another scanner was ruled out due to an excessive x-ray dose for the patient over a short period. 3D Images obtained by using marching cube algorithm on the

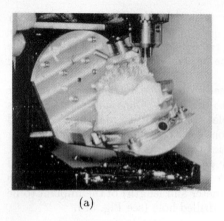 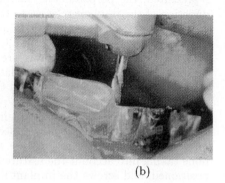

Fig. 5. *(a) The splint is drilled according to the computed positions. (b) The bone is drilled with the guide.*

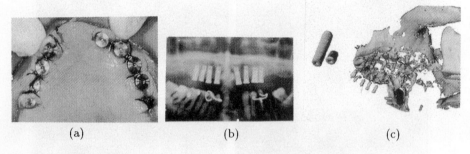

Fig. 6. *(a) The result for eight implants. (b) 3D reconstruction of the bone and the position and feature of the implants.(c) X-ray Image for verification.*

CT data set (see Fig. 6b). are a mean of verification. This tool of visualization must be developed in order to give the surgeon an other mean of work which is already the mental integration of 2D images.

Second patient

The challenge was to place one implant in the posterior localisation of the mandible and to avoid the dental nerve. The steps described for the first patient were followed (see Fig. 7a, 7b, 8a, 8b). Result is very satisfacory. The same conclusion incoming osteointegration and fixation of the prosthesis on the implant remains valid. The the X-ray control image shows good parallelism of the implant and the previous teeth.

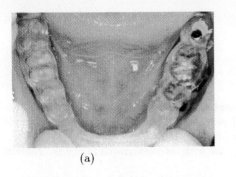 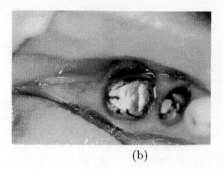

Fig. 7. *(a) The splint in position in the mouth. (b) the site before the surgical act.*

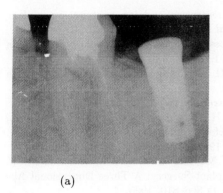 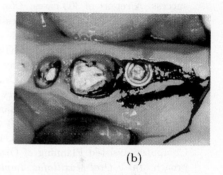

Fig. 8. *(a) X-ray Image for verification (patient 2). (b) The site after the surgical act.*

4 Conclusion and future work

In this paper a fast and accurate system to postion oral implants has been described. Technical validation was conducted, proving that despite possible errors high accuracy is obtained compared with the accuracy of the surgical act when it is done without the surgical guide. It is possible to place several oral implants with an accuracy of 0.2 mm. This technique is now being clinically validated. The use of this system for the first two patients (one with eight implants, the other with one implant) has given very good results (verification is done with an X-ray image). However, before fully satisfactory results can be declared, complete osteointergration must be awaited, followed by fixing the prosthesis on the implant. Using another scanner for verification was ruled out to minimize the patients'exposure to X-ray dose.

Clinical validation continues with a number of different cases. Currently The system has been used by 4 surgeons for 10 patients (34 implants) and results are very satisfactory. Parts of the software need to be improved. It will be possible in the future to recompute slices passing by any plane, i.e., not only the pseudo-sagittal and pseudo-frontal plane. The use of 3D reconstruction images must become easier in order to be able to display in real time and modify implants on these images.

References

1. Jeffcoat M.K. A Dental implant treatment planning tool for low-cost imaging workstations. In *Annual International conference of the IEEE Engineering in Medicine and Biology Society*, volume 13, pages 348–349, 1991.
2. Edge M.J. Surgical placement guide for use with osteointegrated implants. *Journal of Prosthet Dent.*, 57:719 – 722, 1987.
3. T. Fortin, J.L. Coudert, G. Champleboux, P. Sautot, and S. Lavallee. Computer-assisted dental implant surgery using computed tomography. *J. of Image Guided Surgery*, 1(1):53–58, 1995.
4. Bass S.L. The effects of preoperative resorption and jaw anatomy on implant success. A report of 303 cases. *Clin. Oral Impl. Res*, 2:193–198, 1991.
5. Jaffin A. and Berman C. The excessive loss of Branemark fixtures in type IV bone: a 5 analysis. *J. Periodontol.*, 62:2–4, 1991.
6. Weingart D., Hurzler M.B., and Knode H. Restoration of maxillary residual ridge atrophy using Le Fort I osteotomy with simultaneous endosseous implant placement: Technical Report. *Int. J. Oral Maxilofac. Implants*, 7:529–535, 1992.
7. Duyck J., Naert I.E., Van Oosterwyck H., Van der Sloten J., De Coomans M., Lievens S., and Puers B. Biomechanics of oral implant: a review of the literature. *Technology and Health Care*, 5:253–273, 1997.
8. Verstreken K., Van Cleynenbreugel J., Marchal G., Naert I., and Suetens P. Computer-Assisted Planning of Oral Implant Surgery: A Three Dimensional Approach. *Int J Oral Maxillofac. Implants*, 11:806–810, 1996.
9. Th. Fortin, J.L. Coudert, B. Francois, A. Huet, F. Niogret, M. Jourlin, and Ph. Gremillet. Marsupialization of dentigerous cyst associated with forein body using 3D CT images: a case report. *The Journal of Clinical Pediatric Dentistry*, 22(1):29 – 33, 1997.
10. Champleboux G., Blanchet E., Fortin Th., and Coudert J.L. A fast, accurate and easy method to position oral implants using computed tomography. In Lemke H.U., Vannier M.V., Inamura K., and Farman A.G., editors, *Computer Assisted Radiology*. Elsevier Science, 1998.
11. Solar P., Grampp S., Gsellmann B., Rodinger S., Ulm C., and Truppe M. A computer-aided navigation system for oral implant surgery using 3D-CT reconstruction and real time video-projection. In Lemke H.U., Vannier M.V., Inamura K., and Farman A.G., editors, *Computer Assisted Radiology*, pages 884–887. Elsevier Science, 1996.
12. J. Bauer, T. Kaus, T. Gruner, Th. Fleiter, R. Niemeier, and M. Schaich. CT-Data-Based Construction of a dental drilling device. In H.U. Lemke, editor, *CAR'96 (Computer Assisted Radiology)*, pages 958–963. Springer, 1995.

Experimental Protocol of Accuracy Evaluation of 6-D Localizers for Computer-Integrated Surgery: Application to Four Optical Localizers

Fabrice Chassat, Stephane Lavallée, Ph.D.

TIMC Laboratory, Faculté de Médecine, I.A.B., 38706 La Tronche France
e-mail : Fabrice.Chassat@imag.fr

Abstract. This paper describes an experimental protocol in order to evaluate the accuracy of localizers for computer-integrated surgery (CIS), and the result of the evaluation for four commercially available optical localizers (Optotrak, FP5000 , Polaris active and passive). This paper shows that the four systems have static xyz accuracy compatible with most of CIS applications, but they significantly differ when comparing their accuracy of moving rigid bodies.

1 Introduction

In CIS, the six degrees of freedom (6D) localization is used to locate and follow in space the position and orientation of rigid bodies constituted of markers, with respect to a reference rigid body. For example, a localizer can be used to track the tip and the axis of a pointer or surgical tool on pre-operative images (after registration) or to digitize landmarks or surfaces on anatomical structures to track the position of the sensor such as an ultrasound probe, or to measure the relative positions of bones [1, 2, 3],

An extensive list of commercial products existing for localization can be found in [4, 5], but few of them meet the CIS requirements in terms of accuracy (about 1mm in 1m^3), reliability, clinical usability... Four technologies have been used in CIS :

Mechanical technology : Mechanical localizers such as Viewing-Wands^{TM} use a 6-axes coding robot-arm [6, 7]. The main problem of this technology is the global clutter if we need to locate more than one rigid body.

Magnetical technology : Magnetical localizers such as Polhemus^{TM} or Flocks-of-Birds^{TM} use a magnetic source and a receiver of magnetic fields [8]. The problem of this technology is the relative inaccuracy due to metallic objects. At least, those systems imply to use non-ferromagnetic objects in the environment.

Acoustical technology : Acoustical localizers such as Pegasus^{TM} measure the time of flight between emitters and receivers in order to get distance information. Unfortunately, measurements are sensitive to several perturbation such as air movements, parasite reflexions, temperature gradients in space and time [9].

Optical technology : In this category ther are the most usefull localizers for surgery because of their good accuracy and good reliability [10]. However, it is important to notice that optical localizers raise the problem of visibility between the markers that constitute the rigid bodies and the cameras. Some systems use three linear CCD cameras and infrared LEDs plugged in rigid bodies. The position measurement is made by computing the intersection of the three planes corresponding to each camera. Other systems use a classical stereovision principle to locate markers which can be active like LEDs, or passive like retro-reflective spheres or patterns [11]. Each camera gives a three dimension line of view. The intersection of two 3D lines gives a point. For both technologies, rigid bodies transformations are computed from individual markers locations using paired-points matching algorithms [12].

2 Experimental protocol for localizer evaluation

2.1 Intrinsic Accuracy Test (I.A.T.)

Here, we characterize the intrinsic accuracy of the localizer that is important to obtain an upper bound of the useful accuracy. One marker is located with respect to the coordinate system associated with the localizer. An experiment corresponding to this test is presented in Fig.1. We use a 1m motorized linear displacement system which can perform displacements of 0.1mm. And we measure the position of 100 points M_i, where each point is separated from his neighbours M_{i-1} and M_{i+1} by a true distance of 10mm. The x axis is the horizontal displacement (right to left from the cameras at a 1m90 depth to the cameras), the y axis is the depth displacement from 1m90 to 2m90 with respect to cameras, and the z axis is the vertical displacement at a 1m90 depth to the cameras. On each series of 100 points M_i we check that $e_i = ||M_i - M_{center}|| - i.10mm = 0$, where M_{center} is the point corresponding to the middle of the linear displacement system. Then, we calculate for e_i the mean error : $\overline{e} = \frac{1}{N} \sum_{i=1}^{N} e_i$, the rms error : $rms = \sqrt{\frac{1}{N} \sum_{i=1}^{N} (e_i - \overline{e})^2}$, the max error : $Max|e_i|$.

2.2 Relative Rigid Body Accuracy Test (R.R.B.A.T.)

Here we characterize the accuracy of the localizers for the relative measurement between two rigid bodies. They are placed in a common rigid support as represented in Fig.2. With the localizer, we get the transformation matrices T_0 ... T_N from Ref_{body}, which are associated to one rigid body, to Ref_{sensor} which is associated to the other rigid body. Considering (x_i, y_i, z_i) as the coordinates of the origin point of Ref_{body} in Ref_{sensor} we check the stability of those transformation matrices by computing the distances : $d_i = \sqrt{(x_i - \overline{x})^2 + (y_i - \overline{y})^2 + (z_i - \overline{z})^2}$, where $\overline{x}, \overline{y}, \overline{z} = \frac{1}{N} \sum_{i=1}^{N} x_i, y_i, z_i$ between the two systems of reference. Then, stability of the rotation angle α_i between Ref_{body} and Ref_{sensor} is studied. We specified those quantities by calculating the max and rms error on d_i and α_i.

This test is performed with 8 different conditions, with N=100 and the support in a plane roughly parallel to the cameras except for test IV :
I static on identical positions.
II static on different positions.
III hand-holding on identical positions.
IV hand-holding on different positions with a random angle of the support with respect to cameras.
V dynamic in translation at a constant low speed.
VI dynamic hand-holding with circular motions at low speed on, that is to say that the support is making circles very slowly around an axis which is orthogonal to the rigid bodies support.
VII dynamic hand-holding with circular motions at medium speed.
VIII dynamic hand-holding with circular motions at high speed.

2.3 Pivot Repetability Test (P.R.T.)

We are interested in evaluating the accuracy of the determination of the tip of a pointer (attached to a rigid body Ref_{sensor}) with the pivot method [13]. A sapphire sphere is placed at the tip of the pointer and is put in a small hole. We slowly rotate the pointer around the sphere and get 50 positions of Ref_{sensor}, then we find the location of the most invariant point in the coordinate system associated with a rigid body attached to the hole, as presented in Fig.3. The pivot test provides an invariant point with residual errors of the 50 measures: rms_{pivot} and max_{pivot}. The xyz coordinates of this invariant point should be independant of the experiment, thus we repeat the pivot measurements for 20 experiments. So we could measure a mean point and the rms_{repeat} and max_{repeat} deviation from this mean point.

2.4 Surface Digitization Accuracy Test (S.D.A.T.)

To evaluate accuracy of surface digitization, it is first necessary to calibrate the pointer. It is done using the precedent pivot method with N=1000 rotating positions. Then, 100 predefined points of the surface of a plane (which is a 14μm stabilized surface) are collected (see Fig.4). With these points, we fit a least-squares plane and determine the residual distance d_i of each point to the least-squares plane. We study the rms and max error in mm of $|d_i|$.

3 Evaluation of four optical localizers

In this section, we present the results of the experimental protocol that is defined in section 2 for four commercially available optical localizers :
Optotrak^{TM} (Northern Digital Inc. Ontario Canada) which is a system using 3 linear cameras. (This system was acquired in 1992 and never revised.) (Fig.5)
FP5000^{TM} (Image Guided Technologies. Boulder, Colorado USA) which is also a system with 3 linear cameras. (1996). (Fig.6)

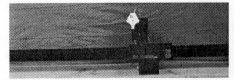

Fig. 1. I.A.T. protocol

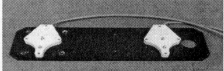

Fig. 2. R.R.B.A.T. protocol

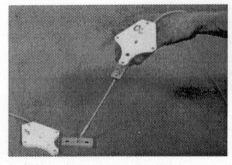

Fig. 3. P.R.T. protocol

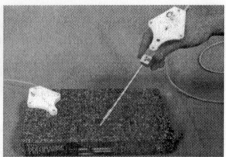

Fig. 4. S.D.A.T. protocol

Active Polaris^{TM} (Northern Digital Inc. Ontario Canada) which is a system using two 2-D cameras. (1997). (Fig.7)

Passive Polaris^{TM} (Northern Digital Inc. Ontario Canada) which is a system using two 2-D cameras. (1997). Passive Polaris is in fact an hybrid system that can track active or passive markers indifferently, but we evaluated only the passive mode of this system. (Fig.7)

All those localizers produce measurements at a frame rate compatible with most of CIS applications. Although, the Optotrak system has high speed measurement capabilities, this was not considered as an important criteria for C.I.S. The size of rigid bodies are roughly similar for the four evaluated localizers.

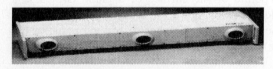

Fig. 5. Optotrak device

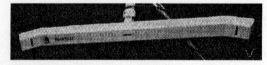

Fig. 6. FP5000 device

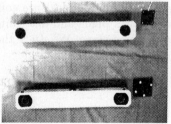

Fig. 7. Polaris devices and rigid bodies (up : Active system, down : Passive system)

Every values concerning distances are in mm, while every values concerning angles are in degrees. The results of the I.A.T. tests are not numerically mentionned but are discussed in the next section. The results of the R.R.B.A.T. tests are in Table 1, results of the P.R.T. are in Table 2, results of the S.D.A.T. are in Table 3.

Table 1. Relative Rigid Body Accuracy Test (distances values are in mm, angle values are in degrees)

		Localizer	Optotrak	FP5000	Polaris Active	Polaris Passive
Static measure	d_{max}	0.288	1.764	1.062	0.624
	rms error on d	0.067	0.408	0.189	0.1431
	α_{max}	0.020	0.337	0.355	0.1484
I	rms error on α	0.009	0.141	0.126	0.0536
Static measure in	d_{max}	1.052	2.825	3.156	0.712
diferents posititons	rms error on d	0.220	0.571	0.653	0.172
	α_{max}	0.071	0.649	0.863	0.150
II	rms error on α	0.026	0.275	0.279	0.055
Static measure in	d_{max}	0.400	1.424	3.253	1.026
hand-holding	rms error on d	0.098	0.331	0.432	0.241
	α_{max}	0.035	0.422	0.578	0.168
III	rms error on α	0.011	0.104	0.204	0.057
Static measure in	d_{max}	0.883	3.035	9.179	2.026
diferents posititons	rms error on d	0.149	0.621	2.073	0.405
in hand-holding	α_{max}	0.050	0.504	0.771	0.388
IV	rms error on α	0.015	0.183	0.240	0.101
Dynamic measure in	d_{max}	1.297	1.820	3.729	2.100
translation at constant speed	rms error on d	0.225	0.415	0.620	0.451
	α_{max}	0.096	0.501	0.796	0.216
V	rms error on α	0.026	0.191	0.260	0.065
Dynamic measure in	d_{max}	0.560	1.855	6.526	1.838
rotation at low speed	rms error on d	0.126	0.337	0.961	0.346
	α_{max}	0.059	0.687	0.585	0.166
VI	rms error on α	0.015	0.236	0.207	0.061
Dynamic measure in	d_{max}	0.575	2.180	9.205	1.839
rotation at medium speed	rms error on d	0.114	0.453	1.161	0.362
	α_{max}	0.059	0.657	0.724	0.166
VII	rms error on α	0.021	0.160	0.202	0.065
Dynamic measure in	d_{max}	0.521	5.100	23.881	1.622
rotation at high speed	rms error on d	0.107	0.628	4.639	0.314
	α_{max}	0.063	1.795	0.811	0.203
VIII	rms error on α	0.024	0.521	0.232	0.080

Table 2. Pivot Repeatability Test, every values are in mm

Localizer	Optotrak	FP5000	Polaris Active	Polaris Passive
Error : max(error max$_{pivot}$)	0.683	9.101	2.201	5.217
mean(rms$_{pivot}$ error)	0.102	0.813	0.385	0.608
Distance : rms$_{repeat}$	0.313	0.492	0.248	0.312
max$_{repeat}$	0.478	0.815	0.434	0.594

Table 3. Surface Digitization Accuracy Test, every values are in mm

Localizer	Optotrak	FP5000	Polaris Active	Polaris Passive
rms distance	0.058	0.709	0.593	0.253
max distance	0.249	1.852	4.819	0.755

4 Discussion

Tests I.A.T. (intrinsic accuracy) : It appears that the Optotrak device is the most accurate system for this test, but all localizers have enough intrinsic accuracy for CIS applications. We can notice for each localizer a maximum error for the displacement in direction y (depth).
Actually, this test only provides a lower bound of errors, the values are indeed in the same range that the linear displacement accuracy that we used.
Tests R.R.B.A.T. (relative accuracy) : To conclude on those tests, we can say that the Optotrak and the Passive Polaris have better accuracy than the two others. The FP5000 gives sufficient accuracy for most of the CIS applications but in some particular applications it is unusable. The Active Polaris, due to its data acquisition protocol (it pulses all the LEDs corresponding to one rigid body and at the next step all the LEDs corresponding to the other rigid body) provides very bad results when we get motion positions and is therefore unusable in those cases. Nevertheless, the relative accuracy in static position of the Active Polaris is similar to the FP5000.
Tests P.R.T. (pivot) : The global results on the different positions of the tip of the pointer are all similar and all good. Optotrak is the only device which is able to have a very stable error. The other devices can make ponctual important errors which do not really influence the final result since it is average on a large number of data.
Tests S.D.A.T. (planar surface) : As for the three others tests, the Optotrak gives the best results. In fact, all results for this tests are acceptable even if the Active Polaris has a maximum error which can raise problems in some cases.
General discussion : According to our results, we can say that those four localizers are raisonnably adapted for surgery, but care should be taken with each one of them. Furthermore, we have noticed that those systems have not the same behaviour for the four tests.
Table 4 presents a synthesis of the most signifiants results for CIS. We made the

table using the results of the I.A.T., R.R.B.A.T.IV, R.R.B.A.T.VI, P.R.T. and S.D.A.T. protocoles. We have chosen to present the results as a mark between + + and - -, using 2*4 differents threshold values for the rms error and max error (T_0, T_0', T_1, T_1', T_2, T_2'). For example, the threshold values for the R.R.B.A.T. IV are (0.2, 1, 0.4, 2, 0.8, 4) in mm.

Table 4. Global results

	Localizer	Optotrak	FP5000	Polaris Active	Polaris Passive
Intrinsec Accuracy Test	y axis	+	0	0	+
Relative Rigid Body Accuracy Test	IV	+ +	0	- -	+
	VI	+ +	+	- -	+
Pivot Repeatability Test		+	+	+ +	+
Surface Digitization Accuracy Test		+ +	0	-	+

5 Conclusion

This paper has presented a generic experimental protocol to evaluate localizer for CIS, and results of the evaluation for four optical localizers.

The experimental protocol is based on the required specifications for CIS applications and consists on four tests : I.A.T. which characterizes the intrinsec accuracy of the localizer, R.R.B.A.T. which characterizes the relative accuracy between two rigid bodies, P.R.T. which evaluates the repeatablity of the localizer to determine the tip of a pointer, and S.D.A.T. which characterizes the accuracy of surface digitization.

The second part of the paper, which is the evaluation using the defined protocol of four optical localizers (Optotrak, FP5000, Polaris active, Polaris passive) allows us to conclude on that the Optotrak is the most appropriated device for CIS if we consider only the global accuracy and robustness, but it is very expensive and its very high weight and size can cause many disagreements. FP5000 has robust measures. Accuracy is fair but sufficient. Nevertheless it is unusable for high-demanding applications. Active Polaris has a rather good accuracy but relative motion of two rigid bodies yield unacceptable errors. This is explained by the acquisition method. Passive Polaris has a good accuracy and is not affected at all by motions of the rigid bodies (due to its data capture principle). However, partial occlusions of markers provide small shifts and many rigid bodies configuration raise missing data.

Acknowledgement : Authors wish to thank Vincent Dessenne, Eric Bainville, Biao Chen and Nicolas Moreau for their contributions to integration and initial tests of localizers. This project is financially suppported by European Project IGOS II (Image Guided Orthopaedics Surgery).

References

1. S. Lavallee, J. Troccaz, P. Sautot, B. Mazier, P. Cinquin, P. Merloz, and J.P. Chirossel. Computer assisted spine surgery using anatomy-based registration. In R. Taylor, S. Lavallee, G. Burdea, and R. Mosges, editors, *Computer Integrated Surgery*, chapter 32. MIT Press, Cambridge, MA, 1996.
2. F. Leitner, F. Picard, R. Minfelde, H.J. Schulz, P. Cinquin, and D. Saragaglia. Computer-assisted knee surgical total replacement. In J. Troccaz, E. Grimson, and R. Moesges, editors, *CVRMed-MRCAS Proc., LNCS Series 1205*, Grenoble, 1997. Springer-Verlag.
3. E. Bainville, P. Chaffanjon, and P. Cinquin. Computer generated visual assistance to a surgical intervention: the retroperitoneoscopy. In *AAAI 94 Applications of Computer Vision in Medical Image Processing, Spring Symposium*, Stanford, USA, 1994.
4. A. Mulder. Human movement tracking technology. http://fas.sfu.ca/cs/people/ResearchStaff/amulder/personal/vmi/HMTT.pub.html, 1994.
5. J. Atha. Current techniques for measuring motion. *Ltf Applied Ergonimics*, pages 245–257, 1984.
6. R. Rohling, P. Munger, J.M. Hollerbach, and T. Peters. Comparison of relative accuracy between a mechanical and an optical tracker for image-guided neurosurgery. *Journal of image guided surgery*, 1(1):30–34, 1995.
7. R. Marmulla, M. Hilbert, and H. Niederdellmann. Immanent precision of mechanical, infrared and laser guided navigation systems for CAS. In K. Inamura H.U. Lemke, M.W. Vannier, editor, *Proceedings of the 11th International Symposium and Exhibition*, pages 863–865. CAR'97, 1997.
8. A.R. Gunkel, W. Freysinger, W.F. Thumfart, and M.J. Truppe. Application of the ARTMA image-guided navigation system to endonasal sinus surgery. In *Computer Assisted Radiology (CAR'95)*, pages 1147–1151, Berlin, 1995. Springer.
9. H.W. When and P.R. Beranger. Ultrasound-Based Robot Position Estimation. *IEEE Transactions on Robotics and Automation*, 13(5):682–692, 1997.
10. K.R. Smith, K.J. Frank, and R.D. Bucholz. The Neurostation: a highly accurate minimally invasive solution to frameless stereotactic neurosurgery. *Computerized Medical Imaging and Graphics*, 18(4):247–256, 1994.
11. A. Colchester, J. Zhao, K. Holton-Tainter, C. Henri, N. Maitland, P. Roberts, C. Harris, and R. Evans. Development and preliminary evaluation of VISLAN, a surgical planning and guidance system using intra-operative video imaging. *Medical Image Analysis*, 1(1):73–90, March 1996.
12. K.S. Arun, T.S. Huang, and S.D. Blostein. Least-squares fitting of two 3-D point sets. *IEEE Trans. Pattern Anal. Machine Intell.*, PAMI-9(5):698–700, 1987.
13. S. Lavallee, P. Cinquin, and J. Troccaz. Computer Integrated Surgery and Therapy: State of the Art. In C. Roux and J.L. Coatrieux, editors, *Contemporary Perspectives in Three-Dimensional Biomedical Imaging*, chapter 10, pages 239–310. IOS Press, Amsterdam, NL, 1997.

Visualization and Evaluation of Prostate Needle Biopsy

Jianchao Zeng, Charles Kaplan[1], John Bauer[2], Isabell Sesterhenn[3], Judd Moul[4] and Seong K. Mun

Imaging Science and Information Systems Center
Department of Radiology, Georgetown University Medical Center
2115 Wisconsin Avenue, NW, Suite 603, Washington, DC 20007

Abstract. Three-dimensional (3-D) computer visualization is playing an increasingly important role in medical imaging applications. Visualization is helpful and important because it provides more flexibility for medical education, training and pre-operative planning, and it offers a better method to evaluate schemes currently used in the clinical environment for their improvements and optimizations. We have developed a 3-D visualization system for prostate needle biopsy simulation. Surface models of the prostate are reconstructed from the digitized pathological tissue images of the real prostate specimens. The needle biopsy of the prostate can be visualized and simulated automatically by the system or interactively by a urologist with a 6 degree-of-freedom (DOF) tracking device. This system has been used to validate the effectiveness of the automatic simulation for the evaluation of prostate needle biopsy. It has also been used to compare the performance of the existing biopsy schemes. In this paper, further experiments are conducted using this visualization system with a total of 107 reconstructed 3-D prostate surface models to evaluate the correlation between tumor volume and positive needle core volume. Preliminary experimental results are also given.

1 Introduction

The screening methods of prostate cancer include prostate specific antigen (PSA) and digital rectal exam (DRE). Based on the screening results, a transrectal ultrasound (TRUS) guided prostate needle biopsy may be recommended which currently is the gold standard for the diagnosis of prostate cancer. Due to the low resolution of the ultrasound images, however, a urologist can hardly differentiate abnormal tissues from normal ones during the biopsy. Therefore a number of schemes have been developed to help urologists in doing the prostate needle biopsy, such as the systematic sextant biopsy [Hodge et al. 1989] and the 5-region [Eskew et al. 1997], which designate locations of needles on the prostate as well as number of needles to use. It is reported that the current biopsy schemes need to be improved in terms of their accuracy in cancer detection [Bankhead 1997]. In addition, since tumor volume plays an extremely important role in helping a physician decide which method to use for the cancer treatment, it is necessary to develop a practical approach for the physician to estimate tumor volume from the positive needle core volumes of the biopsy results. Currently there is no accurate approach available used in the clinical environment.

We have developed a 3-D visualization system that can be used to help physicians solve these problems in prostate needle biopsy. Surface models of the prostate are reconstructed from the digitized pathological tissue images of the real prostate specimens. The needle biopsy of the prostate can be visualized and simulated automatically by the system or interactively by a urologist with a 6 DOF tracking device. Experiments have been conducted using the visualization system to show that the automatic simulation is reliable to be used for the evaluation of prostate needle biopsy by comparing its performance to that of a urologist [Zeng, Kaplan et al. 1998]. This system has also been used to evaluate the existing sextant and 5-region biopsy schemes, and it is shown that the 5-region scheme is performing better than the sextant scheme in terms of the rate of tumor detection, and the amount of positive core volume. In this paper, we conduct further experiments with this system to investigate the correlation between the tumor volume and the positive needle core volume. In section 2, the visualization system is briefly described, followed by the evaluation experiments and the preliminary experimental results in section 3. Conclusions are given in section 4.

2 The 3-D Visualization System

2.1 Reconstruction of the 3-D Prostate Surface Models

As the first step of developing a visualization system for the prostate needle biopsy, 3-D prostate surface models are constructed from the real specimens of prostates with localized cancer, which were resected from the patients and sliced at 4 μm thickness and 2.25 mm intervals. Each slice was then filmed and digitized with a scanning resolution of 1,500 dots per inch, and the contours of key pathological structures, such as urethra and the seminal vesicle as well as the tumors, were extracted by a pathologist. In order to realize real-time visualization performance, surface modeling is used in the model reconstruction process, which is sufficient for the purpose of visualization of prostate needle biopsy. For each structure, the contours are stacked up and interpolation between each pair of contours is performed using a 3-D elastic model-based technique. The interpolation between adjacent contours C1 and C2 is completed by generating a force field that acts on C1 and forces it to gradually move and conform to C2. The

---

[1] Urology Division, Georgetown University Medical Center, Washington, DC 20007
[2] Department of Urology, Walter Reed Army Medical Center, Washington, DC 20307
[3] Department of Genitourinary Pathology, Armed Forces Institute of Pathology, Washington, DC 20306
[4] The Center for Prostate Disease Research, Uniformed Services University of the Health Sciences, MD 20814-4799

volumes of the tumor and the prostate gland are calculated based on each pair of contours of the structures (tumor and prostate gland) after interpolation, which are important parameters for later evaluation experiments. The 3-D model of each structure in the prostate is finally constructed by tiling triangular patches onto the interpolated contours using a deformable surface-spine model which uses a second order partial differential equation to control the deformation of the surface [Xuan et al. 1997]. After a 3-D model is constructed for each structure, a complete 3-D prostate surface model is then constructed by combining the models of all the structures in the prostate. Currently, more than 200 digitized prostate specimens have been acquired, and more than 100 3-D prostate surface models have been constructed on an SGI Onyx Infinite Reality 10000 Workstation.

2.2 Visualization of the Prostate Biopsy

The visualization system is developed using C++ and the object-oriented 3-D visualization development toolkit Open-Inventor on the SGI Onyx Workstation. Graphical user interface is realized based on the Motif toolkit. While menu operations are mostly performed using a two-dimensional (2-D) mouse, the interactive biopsy simulation is mainly carried out using a 6 DOF tracking device (6-D mouse) which is especially integrated in the visualization system. In addition to general visualization functions, such as model manipulation (e.g., rotation, translation and zooming) and model property change (e.g., transparency and color), this system primarily provides functions specific for the prostate needle biopsy. It has two simulation modes: an automatic simulation and an interactive simulation. The whole process of a prostate needle biopsy with any specific scheme can be simulated based on the reconstructed 3-D prostate surface models. In the automatic simulation mode, the locations for needle insertion on the surface of the prostate are calculated automatically by the computer based on the requirement of the specific biopsy scheme. Thirty degrees of angle with respect to the local normal vector of the prostate surface are also calculated automatically for each needle. Needles are then mounted to the positions in the calculated poses. After shooting the needles, the system then detects which needles are hitting the tumors inside the prostate by calculating ray intersection along the needle direction with the tumors. If there is any (the biopsy is then called positive), the system calculates the positive needle core volumes by the amount of intersection and displays the results on the screen. Since this whole process is controlled by the system, it can be finished very quickly, making it possible to apply this simulation to a large number of samples (3-D prostate models) for later statistical analysis if its performance can be validated. Each step of the automatic biopsy simulation process can also be visualized from any perspective by manipulating the 3-D prostate model in real time. Figure 1 shows the needle locations on the prostate for the sextant and 5-region schemes. Figure 2 shows the needles mounted in these locations in their initial poses. Figure 3 shows the side view of the needles after being fired in the prostate. An example of needle biopsy results for both the sextant and 5-region schemes is shown in Figure 4, where the prostate is displayed in semi-transparency for see-through purpose.

 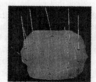

Figure 1 Needle locations calculated for the sextant and 5-region schemes

Figure 2 Needles mounted in their initial locations and poses

Figure 3 Side view of the needles after being fired in the prostate

Figure 4 An example of needle biopsy result for sextant and 5-region

Figure 5 Virtual ultrasound probe and the needle in use

Figure 6 Synthesized ultrasound image with needle path and fired needle

For the interactive simulation, a 6 DOF tracking device is integrated to simulate the ultrasound probe used during actual prostate biopsy procedure. The tracking device consists of an ultrasound transmitter, a controller, and a freely movable receiver device that serves as a tracker. With this device, the system can track both the position (x, y, z) and the orientation angles (Pitch, Yaw, Roll) of the receiver in real time (50Hz). The tracking information is simultaneously used in controlling movement of the virtual ultrasound probe in the visualization system. The synthesized ultrasound images are refreshed in real time to follow the movement of the probe. The ultrasound images show intersectional anatomical slices of the prostate as biopsy guidance for the user (a urologist). With this interactive simulation mode, the urologist can perform a virtual needle biopsy as though he/she is performing a real biopsy on a patient. He/she determines the location for each needle insertion based on a specific biopsy scheme under the guidance of the synthesized ultrasound image. The angle of the needle is fixed with the ultrasound probe, and the upcoming path of the needle is always displayed and overlaid on the ultrasound image so that the urologist knows where the needle will go through inside the prostate. The result of a biopsy is automatically calculated by the system after each biopsy and is displayed to tell the urologist whether the biopsy is positive or negative and how much the positive needle core volume is. Figure 5 shows the virtual ultrasound probe and the needle in use, while Figure 6 shows the corresponding synthesized ultrasound image with needle path and the fired needle.

3 Evaluation and Experiments: Correlation between Tumor Volume and Positive Core Volume

Tumor volume is one of the key parameters to be used for the determination of cancer stage and therapy methods [Tanagho and McAninch 1995]. For example, the therapy for patients with low-stage prostate cancer is currently radical prostatectomy or radiation therapy, while patients with locally extensive cancer are advised to have radiation therapy and surgery is not recommended. It is therefore important for a physician to be able to estimate the tumor volume as accurately as possible, especially when the tumor is still small and non-palpable. Currently there is no practical approach that can help a physician estimate the tumor volume. It is even not sure if it is possible to have such an approach. In this paper, we investigate this possibility by first considering the correlation of the tumor volume to the positive needle core volume. If there is a strong correlation, it suggests that there may be a possibility to estimate the tumor volume from the positive needle core volume. We also investigate the correlation in terms of the PSA values and the race to see if the correlation shows any special features for these special groups of patient.

3.1 Correlation in General Cases

We use 107 3-D prostate models on the needle biopsy visualization system with both sextant and the 5-region. Figure 7 shows a correlation result of tumor volume vs. positive core volume with the sextant biopsy scheme. Table 1 gives the corresponding correlation coefficient and the level of significance. Since the level of significance is 0 which is smaller than 0.01, the correlation is significant between the two volume variables with the sextant scheme. The results with the 5-region scheme are shown in Figure 8 and Table 2, which also indicates that the correlation is significant.

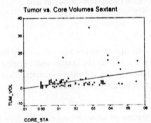
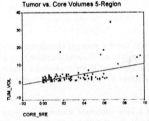

Figure 7 Plot of tumor volume vs. core volume with sextant scheme

Figure 8 Plot of tumor volume vs. core volume with 5-region scheme

Table 1 Correlation coefficient and the level of significance with sextant scheme (Tumor volume not normalized)

Correlations of Tumor vs. Core Volumes Sextant

		CORE_STA	TUM_VOL
Pearson Correlation	CORE_STA	1.000	.440**
	TUM_VOL	.440**	1.000
Sig. (2-tailed)	CORE_STA		.000
	TUM_VOL	.000	
N	CORE_STA	107	107
	TUM_VOL	107	107

**. Correlation is significant at the 0.01 level (2-tailed).

Table 2 Correlation coefficient and the level of significance with 5-region scheme (Tumor volume not normalized)

Correlations of Tumor vs. Core Volumes 5-Region

		CORE_5RE	TUM_VOL
Pearson Correlation	CORE_5RE	1.000	.509**
	TUM_VOL	.509**	1.000
Sig. (2-tailed)	CORE_5RE		.000
	TUM_VOL	.000	
N	CORE_5RE	107	107
	TUM_VOL	107	107

**. Correlation is significant at the 0.01 level (2-tailed).

Volume of a prostate gland may also need to be considered since it can affect on capsular penetration which is also a key factor in determining methods for therapy. A tumor may still be confined to a larger prostate gland while another tumor of the same size has already penetrated the capsule of a smaller prostate gland. To further validate the correlation between the tumor volume and the core volume, we first normalize the tumor volume by the volume of prostate gland, and then investigate its correlation to the positive needle core volume for both the sextant and 5-region schemes. The results are shown in Figure 9 and Table 3, and Figure 10 and Table 4, respectively.

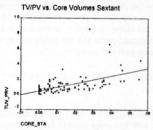
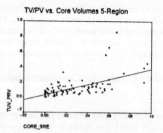

Figure 9 Plot of normalized tumor volume vs. core volume with sextant scheme

Figure 10 Plot of normalized tumor volume vs. core volume with 5-region scheme

Table 3 Correlation coefficient and the level of significance with sextant scheme
(Normalized tumor volume)

Correlations

		CORE_STA	TUV_PRV
Pearson Correlation	CORE_STA	1.000	.585**
	TUV_PRV	.585**	1.000
Sig. (2-tailed)	CORE_STA		.000
	TUV_PRV	.000	
N	CORE_STA	107	107
	TUV_PRV	107	107

** Correlation is significant at the 0.01 level (2-tailed).

Table 4 Correlation coefficient and the level of significance with 5-region scheme
(Normalized tumor volume)

Correlations

		CORE_5RE	TUV_PRV
Pearson Correlation	CORE_5RE	1.000	.635**
	TUV_PRV	.635**	1.000
Sig. (2-tailed)	CORE_5RE		.000
	TUV_PRV	.000	
N	CORE_5RE	107	107
	TUV_PRV	107	107

** Correlation is significant at the 0.01 level (2-tailed).

As can be seen, the results show a stronger correlation between the normalized tumor volume and the positive needle core volume. The correlation coefficients increase by 0.145 and 0.126 for the sextant and 5-region schemes, respectively. Therefore it can be said that the normalized tumor volume (by the volume of prostate gland) shows a better association with the positive needle core volume than the absolute tumor volume alone.

3.2 Correlation by PSA Values

The elevated PSA value is a very important marker to indicate suspicion of prostate cancer. Therefore it may be reasonable to expect that the higher the PSA value the stronger the correlation between the tumor volume and the positive needle core volume. To investigate this possibility, we segment the PSA values into groups and calculate the correlation for each group separately.

(1) Group 1: PSA Values 0-4

The sample size (number of 3-D prostate models) for this group is 16. The results for both sextant and 5-region schemes are shown in Figure 11 and Table 5, and Figure 12 and Table 6, respectively.

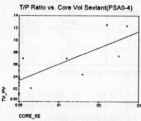
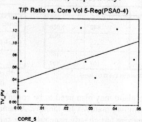

Figure 11 Plot of normalized tumor volume vs. core volume with sextant scheme (PSA0-4)

Figure 12 Plot of normalized tumor volume vs. core volume with 5-region scheme (PSA0-4)

Table 5 Correlation coefficient and the level of significance with sextant scheme (PSA0-4) (Normalized tumor volume)

Correlations

		CORE_SE	TV_PV
Pearson Correlation	CORE_SE	1.000	.788**
	TV_PV	.788**	1.000
Sig. (2-tailed)	CORE_SE	.	.000
	TV_PV	.000	.
N	CORE_SE	16	16
	TV_PV	16	16

**. Correlation is significant at the 0.01 level (2-tailed).

Table 6 Correlation coefficient and the level of significance with 5-region scheme (PSA0-4) (Normalized tumor volume)

Correlations

		CORE_5	TV_PV
Pearson Correlation	CORE_5	1.000	.685**
	TV_PV	.685**	1.000
Sig. (2-tailed)	CORE_5	.	.003
	TV_PV	.003	.
N	CORE_5	16	16
	TV_PV	16	16

**. Correlation is significant at the 0.01 level (2-tailed).

(2) Group 2: PSA Values 4-10

The sample size for this group is 64. The results for both sextant and 5-region schemes are shown in Figure 13 and Table 7, and Figure 14 and Table 8, respectively.

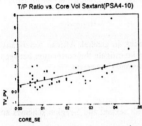

Figure 13 Plot of normalized tumor volume vs. core volume with sextant scheme (PSA4-10)

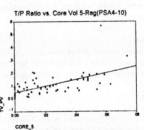

Figure 14 Plot of normalized tumor volume vs. core volume with 5-region scheme (PSA4-10)

Table 7 Correlation coefficient and the level of significance with sextant scheme (PSA4-10) (Normalized tumor volume)

Correlations

		CORE_SE	TV_PV
Pearson Correlation	CORE_SE	1.000	.607**
	TV_PV	.607**	1.000
Sig. (2-tailed)	CORE_SE	.	.000
	TV_PV	.000	.
N	CORE_SE	64	64
	TV_PV	64	64

**. Correlation is significant at the 0.01 level (2-tailed).

Table 8 Correlation coefficient and the level of significance with 5-region scheme (PSA4-10) (Normalized tumor volume)

Correlations

		CORE_5	TV_PV
Pearson Correlation	CORE_5	1.000	.603**
	TV_PV	.603**	1.000
Sig. (2-tailed)	CORE_5	.	.000
	TV_PV	.000	.
N	CORE_5	64	64
	TV_PV	64	64

**. Correlation is significant at the 0.01 level (2-tailed).

(3) Group 3: PSA Values More Than 10

The sample size for this group is 27. The results for both sextant and 5-region schemes are shown in Figure 15 and Table 9, and Figure 16 and Table 10, respectively.

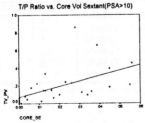

Figure 15 Plot of normalized tumor volume vs. core volume with sextant scheme (PSA>10)

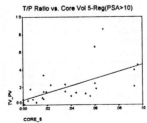

Figure 16 Plot of normalized tumor volume vs. core volume with 5-region scheme (PSA>10)

Table 9 Correlation coefficient and the level of significance with sextant scheme (PSA>10) (Normalized tumor volume)

Correlations

		CORE_SE	TV_PV
Pearson Correlation	CORE_SE	1.000	.531**
	TV_PV	.531**	1.000
Sig. (2-tailed)	CORE_SE		.004
	TV_PV	.004	
N	CORE_SE	27	27
	TV_PV	27	27

** Correlation is significant at the 0.01 level (2-tailed).

Table 10 Correlation coefficient and the level of significance with 5-region scheme (PSA>10) (Normalized tumor volume)

Correlations

		CORE_5	TV_PV
Pearson Correlation	CORE_5	1.000	.618**
	TV_PV	.618**	1.000
Sig. (2-tailed)	CORE_5		.001
	TV_PV	.001	
N	CORE_5	27	27
	TV_PV	27	27

** Correlation is significant at the 0.01 level (2-tailed).

Unfortunately, the results are not as they were expected: the correlation coefficients do not increase with the PSA values. However, at the moment we cannot conclude that there is no direct association between the PSA values and the correlation since the sample sizes are not large enough for some of the groups. Further investigations will be conducted in this respect.

3.3 Correlation by Race

It is recognized that prostate cancer grows differently in different races. In general, African Americans have more chance to grow prostate cancer than Caucasians. In this respect, we investigate the correlation between the tumor volume and the positive needle core volume among African Americans and Caucasians.

(1) African Americans

The sample size for the African Americans is 28. The results for both sextant and 5-region schemes are shown in Figure 17 and Table 11, and Figure 18 and Table 12, respectively.

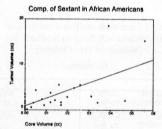

Figure 17 Plot of normalized tumor volume vs. core volume with sextant (African Americans)

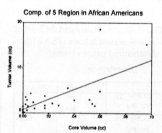

Figure 18 Plot of normalized tumor volume vs. core volume with 5-region (African Americans)

Table 11 Correlation coefficient and the level of sig. with sextant (African Americans)

Correlations

		CORVOL	TUMVOL
Pearson Correlation	CORVOL	1.000	.643**
	TUMVOL	.643**	1.000
Sig. (2-tailed)	CORVOL		.000
	TUMVOL	.000	
N	CORVOL	28	28
	TUMVOL	28	28

** Correlation is significant at the 0.01 level (2-tailed).

Table 12 Correlation coefficient and the level of sig. with 5-region (African Americans)

Correlations

		CORVOL	TUMVOL
Pearson Correlation	CORVOL	1.000	.681**
	TUMVOL	.681**	1.000
Sig. (2-tailed)	CORVOL		.000
	TUMVOL	.000	
N	CORVOL	28	28
	TUMVOL	28	28

** Correlation is significant at the 0.01 level (2-tailed).

(2) Caucasians

The sample size for Caucasians is 77. The results for both sextant and 5-region schemes are shown in Figure 19 and Table 13, and Figure 20 and Table 14, respectively.

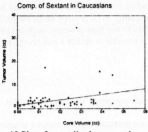
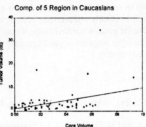

Figure 19 Plot of normalized tumor volume vs. core volume with sextant (Caucasians)

Figure 20 Plot of normalized tumor volume vs. core volume with 5-region (Caucasians)

As expected, the correlation for the African Americans is much stronger than that of the Caucasians. The correlation coefficients increase by 0.295 and 0.250 for the sextant and 5-region schemes, respectively. This may imply that race is an important factor in estimating the tumor volume from the positive needle core volume. Further investigations will be done to confirm this possibility.

3.4 Summary

We have experimentally shown that in general there exists a significant correlation between the tumor volume and the positive needle core volume. This correlation is even stronger between the normalized tumor volume (by the volume of prostate gland) and the positive needle core volume. This result supports the possibility that the

Table 13 Correlation coefficient and the level of sig. with sextant (Caucasians)

Correlations

		CORVOL	TUMVOL
Pearson Correlation	CORVOL	1.000	.348**
	TUMVOL	.348**	1.000
Sig. (2-tailed)	CORVOL	.	.002
	TUMVOL	.002	.
N	CORVOL	77	77
	TUMVOL	77	77

**. Correlation is significant at the 0.01 level (2-tailed).

Table 14 Correlation coefficient and the level of sig. with 5-region (Caucasians)

Correlations

		CORVOL	TUMVOL
Pearson Correlation	CORVOL	1.000	.431**
	TUMVOL	.431**	1.000
Sig. (2-tailed)	CORVOL	.	.000
	TUMVOL	.000	.
N	CORVOL	77	77
	TUMVOL	77	77

**. Correlation is significant at the 0.01 level (2-tailed).

larger the core volume the larger the tumor volume. Since there may be other factors, such as locations of the positive needles, that contribute to the prediction of tumor volume, more controlled experiments will be needed to confirm the cause-and-effect relationships between the positive core volume and the tumor volume.

Due to insufficient data, the correlation between the tumor volume and the positive core volume does not increase with the PSA values. However, this correlation does increase for African Americans in comparison to Caucasians.

4 Conclusions

We have developed a 3-D computer visualization system, and have conducted experiments with a large number of 3-D prostate models using this system. To explore the possibility of estimating tumor volumes from the positive needle core volumes, we have investigated the possible correlation between the tumor volume and the positive needle core volumes with 107 3-D prostate models. A significant correlation is found between these two kinds of volumes, which supports the possibility that the tumor volume may be reasonably estimated from the positive needle core volumes. More controlled experiments will be conducted to confirm the cause-and-effect relationships before we will move forward to develop a mathematical model that can predict and estimate the tumor volumes from the positive needle core volumes. In addition, new prostate models will be reconstructed and used to verify the prediction model of tumor volume, and clinical evaluation will also be conducted.

The 3-D visualization system provides an ideal platform for the simulation and evaluation of prostate needle biopsy. It is also useful for education, especially for visualizing anatomy of prostate, and training of residents and medical students. With the advancement of imaging technologies and improvement of imaging quality, it becomes quite possible to develop an on-line prostate needle biopsy system which provides real time augmented 3-D prostate images to help a urologist to quickly and precisely identify the abnormality in the prostate inside the patient's body. This idea is not limited to the prostate needle biopsy; it may be applied to any type of biopsy, such as kidney biopsy. It may also be applied to other surgeries beyond biopsies, making it possible to realize a real on-site image-guided minimally-invasive surgery system.

References

Bankgead, C.: Sextant biopsy helps in prognosis of Pca, but it's not foolproof. Urology Times, Vol. 25, No. 8, August 1997.

Eskew, A. L., Bare, R. L. and McCullough, D. L.: Systematic 5 region prostate biopsy is superior to sextant method for diagnosing carcinoma of the prostate. J. Urol., **157**: 199, 1997.

Hodge, K. K, et al.: Random systematic versus directed ultrasound guided trans-rectal core biopsies of the prostate. J. Urol., **142**: 71, 1989.

Tanagho, E. A. and McAninch, J. W. (Eds): Smith's General Urology (14th Edition), Appleton & Lange, 1995.

Xuan, J., Hayes, et al.: Surface reconstruction and visualization of the surgical prostate model. SPIE Medical Imaging, 1997.

Zeng, J., Kaplan, C., et al.: Optimizing prostate needle biopsy through 3-D simulation. SPIE Medical Imaging'98, San Diego, February 1998.

Virtual Endoscope System with Force Sensation

Koji IKUTA , Masaki TAKEICHI , Takao NAMIKI

Department of Micro System Engineering, School of Engineering, Nagoya University
Furocho, Chikusa-ku, Nagoya 464-8603, Japan
ikuta@mech.nagoya-u.ac.jp

Abstract. We have developed a Virtual Endoscope System (VES) with force sensation to train inexperienced young doctors and simulate operations that require special technical skills. In this paper, we describe the force simulation mechanism employed by our VES and dynamical models of an endoscope and colon. The force simulation mechanism was developed with the use of four rubber rollers and differential gears. The simple structure of this mechanism enables easy control and stable linear and rotational drive of the endoscope, and we have confirmed its force simulation ability by several experiments. We also developed the dynamical models of an endoscope and colon to calculate reactive force that doctors receive from a colon in real-time, and we confirmed the accuracy of these models by software simulation of endoscopic. We believe this system is adequate for training young doctors in endoscopic insertion.

1. Introduction

Explosive growth of the elderly population is inevitable in the early 21st century, and most patients who require colonoscopic diagnosis are aged persons. Although minimally invasive methods for the diagnosis of internal organs have been developed to reduce pain in current clinical settings, with colonoscopy, both discomfort to the patient and the time required for diagnosis heavily depend on the technical skill of the doctor. Moreover, in some cases, inexperienced doctors have damaged colons in colonoscopic diagnosis. Therefore, a training system in colonoscopic diagnosis for young doctors has been desired.

Accordingly, we propose a Virtual Endoscope System (VES) with force sensation for the repeated training of inexperienced young doctors in colonoscopic insertion and operation. Using information on the patient's internal organs, of the system generates a force sensation to simulate the feeling of an actual operation and diagnosis.

2. Virtual Endoscope System

The total concept of the Virtual Encoscope System is shown in **Fig.1**. The VES consists of the following three main parts.

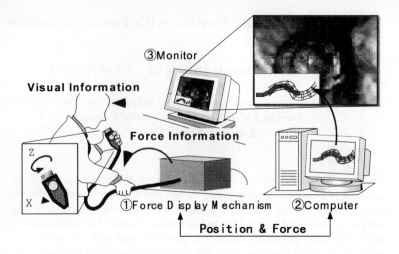

Fig. 1. Virtual Endoscope System with Force Sensation

1) **Force Simulation Mechanism**: Doctors insert and operate the same type of endoscope used in actual diagnosis.
2) **Computer** : a high-speed micro computer calculates the reactive force between the endoscope and digestive tube in real time and controls the VES mechanism.
3) **Monitor** : CT images of the colon are converted into 3D-Computer graphics and displayed on the monitor.

By linking the VES mechanism to the monitor through the computer, the doctor obtains not only visual information but also force sensation according to the position and posture of the endoscope. The insertion of the endoscope in the virtual digestive tube accurately simulates insertion in an actual colon.

The proposed VES has the following features,

1. It can be used with an actual endoscope in various
2. It improves skills through the use of simulated force and visual information
3. It can be used for repeated trainings
4. It can be adapted to simulate any type of data on individual patients or parts

With these features, the system can be used to train inexperienced doctors and simulate operations that require special technical skills.

Force information is a very important aspect in the training of medical skills such as endoscopic operation. However almost all conventional studies have concentrated on the development of visual information from medical image processing, and very few have attempted to simulate the force mechanically. Therefore, in the present study we focused on the realization of a mechanism and a control system for the virtual situation of actual endoscopic operation.

3. Force Simulation Mechanism

3.1 Basic Concept

First, the colon and endoscope are modeled in virtual space according to the procedure to be performed by doctors. When the endoscope touches several points of the colon (**Fig.2**), the basic principle of the dynamics is used to calculate the force at each point as the total force and torque transferred to the doctor's hand. In other words, the force simulation mechanismrecreates the total force and torque and conveys the sensation to the doctor's hand. The force simulation mechanism requires the following specifications:

1. Giving the endoscope two degrees of freedom (infinite linear motion and infinite rotation)
2. Correctly conveying the force and position information calculated in the virtual space to the doctor

To realize these requirements, we developed the mechanism using two components; a "torque-coupled roller mechanism" and "differential gear mechanism."

3.2 Torque-Coupled Rubber Roller Mechanism

To consider operation of the endoscope, the force simulation mechanism must give the endoscope "infinite" linear motion and rotation motion. The simplest mechanism is a torque-decoupled type (**Fig.3(a)**), but this type is seriously flawed by the friction produced by the dormant roller while the other roller drives. Hence, we applied a coupled type (**Fig.3(b)**) to solve this problem. This type consists two rubber rollers mounted on 45° axes to the endoscope. By coordinating the rotating directions of the two rollers, we can cancel the opposing frictional forces when we want to drive and transfer thrust and torque to the endoscope.

Though two rubber rollers can realize both linear and rotary drive, for more stable support we use four rubber rollers; two for the linear drive and two for the rotary drive. Therefore, we can control the force simulation mechanism easily.

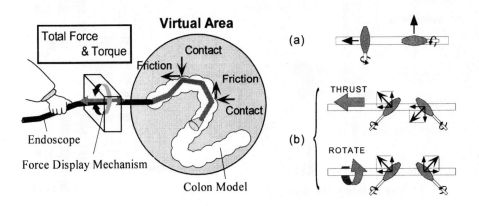

Fig. 2. Concept of Force Simulation System   **Fig. 3.** Two Types of Driving Mechanism

3.3 Introducing Differential Gear

The use of a differential gear offers the following advantages:
1. A reduced number of motors
2. Easier control
3. Reduced friction force between the rollers and endoscope
4. Accurate transfer of thrust and torque to the endoscope

The schematic design of the force simulation mechanism is shown in **Fig.4**. The rotary drive is realized by the upper unit and the linear drive is realized by the lower unit.

In general, a mechanism using four rollers would require the use of four motors. However, it would be complicated to control coupled-type system through the cooperated use of four motors. For this reason we added two differential gears in this mechanism (shown in **Fig.4**) to reduce the number of motors from four to two and simplify the control.

In this mechanism, the function of the differential gear transfers the torque of the motor to the tips of both shafts, and the tips of both shafts rotate in the same direction when a motor drives (**Fig.5(a)**). In this situation, the relation of the rotational velocity between a motor and shafts can be equated as:

$$2\omega_c = \omega_a + \omega_b \tag{1}$$

When the motor is locked (**Fig.5(b)**), eq.(2) is given because ω_c in eq.(1) is equal to zero.

$$\omega_a = -\omega_b \tag{2}$$

Accordingly, the tips of the two shafts can be freely rotated in opposite directions by the external torque (**Fig.5(b)**).

For example, when simulating thrust, the motor of the rotary drive unit stays locked, but the two rollers rotate according to the motion of the endoscope by the function of the differential gear. On the other hand, these rollers produce rotational forces to the endoscope. In theory, however, rotary forces have no effect on the endo-

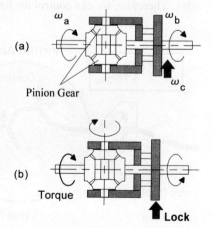

Fig. 4. Concept of Force Simulation Mechanism **Fig. 5.** Basic Motion of Differential Gear

scope since these forces can be cancelled by the feature of the coupled-type driving mechanism. Thus, with the use of the differential gear, frictional forces are lower than those produced with the decoupled-type.

Finally, we explain the correct transfer of thrust and torque from the rollers to the endoscope. According to the eq.(1), the revolution of the motor is always equal to the total revolution of the shaft tips. Therefore, if the revolution of one roller is reduced some obstacle or problem, the revolution of one of the other rollers is increased by the function of the differential gear, and we can correctly transfer the motor power to the endoscope. In this case, the unnecessary force is transferred to the endoscope because it is impossible to cancel the opposing force against the direction we want to drive. In the present system, however, since we designed this mechanism to realize the linear and rotary drive by each unit, we can cancel the unnecessary force by controlling the motor of the other unit.

3.4 Force & Position Sensing

In this system, we applied a six-component-force sensor for measuring forces of six independent DOFs, and we applied two encoders for measuring the position (linear and rotational) of the endoscope.

Since the system in the present study was desingned for training of endoscope insertion using an actual endoscope, we did not attach any measurement devices to the endoscope. Alternatively, we applied the force sensor beneath the mechanism and placed two encoders on the insertion hole for the endoscope (**Fig.6**).

3.5 Adjustable Diameter

To enable application of various types of endoscopes to this mechanism, we made the spaces between the rollers adjustable. Accordingly, this mechanism can be applied to endoscopes hanging in diameter from 8 to 24mm, and with a little improvement, it is applicable to training with catheters of 2～3mm in diameter.

3.6 Prototype (VES-II)

According to the principles we described above, we developed a prototype model called the VES-II. The VES-II is shown in **Fig.6** and a close-up view of the rubber

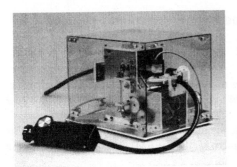
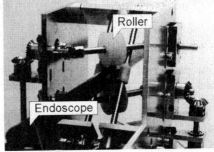

Fig. 6. Force Simulation Mechanism (VES-II)　**Fig.7** Close up View of Rubber Roller Mechanism

roller mechanism is shown in **Fig.7**. The arrangement of the rollers of the VES-II is slightly different from that of the concept seen in **Fig.4**. In fact, they are arranged on concentric circles. By locating rollers concentrically, we can drive the endoscope based on the same principle described above but with greater stability.

4. The Servo System for force simulation

4.1 The control method

First we studied to the realization of a *free mode* and *elastic mode* by operating an endoscope. *Free mode* means a case in which the endoscope does not touch the colon, and *elastic mode* means a case in which the endoscope touches the colon, which acts against it as a spring.

The control system of the VES-II gets force information from the force sensor and calculates the value of the theoretical position of the endoscope. Then it compares the value of the theoretical position with the value of the current position measured, and decides what output voltage to supply to the motor.

4.2 Experiments

The results of the experiments are shown in **Fig.8(a),(b)**.

In **Fig.8(a)**, we see that the reactive force is almost zero.

In **Fig.8(b)**, the reactive force increases as the deformation becomes larger at each of three types of virtual spring stiffness. This figure shows that the measured reactive force diverges from the theoretical line (solid line). This discrepancy occurred because the static friction between the rollers and endoscope was overcome by the operation force of the endoscope. This problem should be solved by fine tuning of control parameters.

In this experiment, we can feel the sensation of pushing a spring, and we can confirm that the endoscope returns to the beginning position where the endoscope began to touch the virtual colon.

5. The dynamical models of an endoscope and colon

5.1 The presupposition condition

The purpose of modeling is to analyze the motion of an endoscope in a virtual space, and to calculate the total reactive force and torque which returns from the colon to the hand of the doctor.

The proposed model defines an endoscope as multiple robotic links. Though this analysis is less accurate than the finite element method (FEM), it requires far less time for calculation.

The presupposition conditions for the modeling can be summarized as follows:

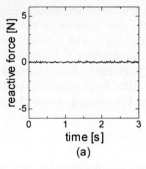 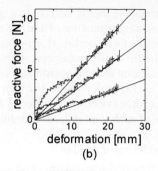

Fig. 8. Force Simulation Ability of The VES- II

1. An endoscope is defined as multiple links, each comprising a rigid arm combined with viscoelastic components.
2. A colon is defined as a viscoelastic circular cylinder with various diameters.
3. Frictional force between the endoscope and colon is considered using a frictional cone as a representation of the inner contact force.

The algorithm of this modeling is constructed under a motion equation used for the analysis of a manipulator. Considering the actual motion of an endoscope and colon, we attempted to simplify the equation by deducting infinitesimal effect elements.

5.2 The modeling of an endoscope

First, we consider a general model of an endoscope and colon which includes all forces of action. An endoscope is defined as an n multiple links model which has $(n-1)$ mobile joints with viscoelastic components. Since a real endoscope is flexible, we consider an endoscope to have the infinite joints. The motion of endoscope is limited by the number of joints. Thus, we must decide the number of joints and the length of one link. As the number of joints increases, the accuracy of the calculated motion improves. The force simulation mechanism requires continuous real-time analysis in virtual space. In other words, it is necessary to compromise and approximate in the range where the doctor can recognize.

Therefore we must find a suitable number of joints to compromise on processing time. Since the direction of the whole endoscope is determined by the displacement and frequency of the tip, the assumption of modeling in the tip is very important. Modeling in the root part is not a severe problem since the motion is very slow. Therefore, our design, the length of each link gradually increases from the tip to the root.

Next we define the degree of freedom of each mobile joint. The joint nearest to the hand has a thrusting and rotating mechanism and the other joints have a rotating mechanism in two rectangular directions. Each joint has a viscoelastic component (**Fig.9**).

Here we derive an equation to formulate this system. Multiple links can be expressed using Newton-Euler's equation of motion as follows.

$$\mathbf{M(q)\ddot{q}} + \mathbf{V(q,\dot{q})} + \mathbf{G(q)} = \sum_{i}^{n} \mathbf{J}_{r_i}^{T}(\mathbf{q})\mathbf{F}_i + \mathbf{T} \tag{3}$$

$$\mathbf{T} = -K[\mathbf{q} - \mathbf{q}_0] - D\dot{\mathbf{q}} \tag{4}$$

$M(q)$ means the inertia matrix. $V(q,\dot{q})$ means the centrifugal force, Coriolis force. $G(q)$ means weight function. Here we explain the first function on the right side of eq.(3). Contact force occurs at n points where the colon wall contacts each mobile joint and the tip of the endoscope. Then contact force vector $\mathbf{F}_i$ is converted into the force of each joint in local coordinates using Jacobian matrix $\mathbf{J}(q)$ systems. Functional force $\mathbf{T}$ of eq.(3) is defined as the sum of the elastic force (elasticity coefficient K) and viscous force (viscosity coefficient D) of a mobile joint. q_0 means the position of the balance of each joint in local coordinates.

5.3 The modeling of a colon

The shape of the colon is defined as a viscoelastic circular cylinder with various diameters. Here we consider the following equation:

$$S(\mathbf{r}) = 0 \qquad (5)$$

$$R = \phi(s) \qquad (6)$$

Curve S expresses the shape as the central curve of the colon model (**Fig.10**).

Setting radius R according to S, we express the three-dimensional shape of the colon with various diameters. These equations are able to correspond to deformation of the colon according to contact force. Moreover, we consider the elasticity coefficient K_d and viscosity coefficient D_d of the surface of the colon wall. The static friction coefficient μ_s and kinetic friction coefficient μ_d are also considered.

5.4 Simplification of model equation

Here we explain the reduction of the terms of the above equations.

First, the deformation speed during insertion of the endoscope is very slow. Thus, the terms $M(q)$ and $V(q,\dot{q})$ in eq.(3) are thought to be sufficiently smaller than the weight of the endoscope or contact force.

Therefore, eq.(3) can be simplified by reducing the terms $M(q)$ and $V(q,\dot{q})$ as follows:

$$G(q) = \sum_{i}^{n} \mathbf{J}_{r_i}^{T}(q)\mathbf{F}_i - K[q - q_0] - D\dot{q} \qquad (7)$$

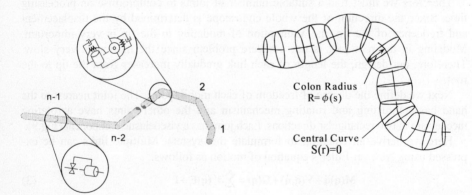

Fig. 9. Endoscope Model   **Fig. 10.** Colon Model

By solving this equation of motion on the short time-interval, the dynamic behavior of the endoscope can be analyzed quasi-dynamically.

The viscous term cannot be omitted to keep a joint angle of each mobile joint. If omitted, the joint angle returns to the previous position of balance at the next moment the contact force is absent.

5.5 Calculation of contact judgment and the contact force

Here we explain the contact judgement between the endoscope and colon.

First, we can calculate the distance between a joint of the endoscope and the central curve of the colon. Then, the geometry of the contact point can be estimated for comparison with the radius R of the colon model.

In the case of contact, the contact force is expressed as follows in the normal coordinates:

$$\mathbf{f}_i = \{-K_d(l_i - R) - D_d\|\mathbf{v}_i\|\} \cdot \frac{\mathbf{v}_i}{\|\mathbf{v}_i\|} \tag{8}$$

where l_i means the distance between the joint and nearest point of the central curve, and $\mathbf{v}_i$ means the velocity vector of a joint in the normal coordinate.

Next, $\mathbf{f}_i$ is divided into vertical and tangential components of the colon on contact points to examine the frictional condition. Supposing vertical vector as $\mathbf{n}_i$, the vertical component of the contact force $\mathbf{f}_{ni}$ and tangential component $\mathbf{f}_{ti}$ are given as follows:

$$\mathbf{f}_{ni} = \mathbf{f}_i \cdot \mathbf{n}_i \quad , \quad \mathbf{f}_{ti} = \mathbf{f}_i - \mathbf{f}_{ni} \tag{9}$$

From these vectors, the frictional condition can be judged.

Here, when the static frictional condition of the endoscope, reactive force $\mathbf{F}_i$ is expressed by of following:

$$\mathbf{F}_i = \mathbf{f}_i \tag{10}$$

Then the kinetic frictional condition, $\mathbf{F}_i$ is expressed by

$$\mathbf{F}_i = \mu_d \|\mathbf{f}_{ni}\| \cdot \frac{\mathbf{f}_{ti}}{\|\mathbf{f}_{ti}\|} + \mathbf{f}_{ni} \tag{11}$$

The difference of each condition of use of the frictional cone is indicated in **Fig.11(a), (b)**, respectively.

After transforming the reactive force in the normal coordinates to one in the local coordinates of each mobile joint by the transform matrix, it is substituted into the equations of motion of the endoscope.

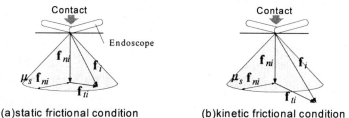

(a) static frictional condition   (b) kinetic frictional condition

Fig. 11. Frictional Cone

5.6 Simulation

We have analyzed the above dynamical models of the endoscope and colon.

Here the endoscope is defined to have five mobile joints. The first joint has a thrusting and rotating mechanism and the other four joints have rotating mechanisms with two degrees of freedom.

We established the central curve of the colon as the shape of the cubical parabola equation according to eq.(9). Then we formed the colon by locating various diameters along the central curve. In this model, the central curve is not deformed but the diameter of the colon is easily deformed, in order to simulate the viscoelastical property of the colon wall.

In this paper, we decided our parameters (*e.g.* the elasticity and viscosity coefficients of the dynamical models) in accordance with the features of the force simulation mechanism. In actuality, however we would like to base our decision on these parameters on the propeties measured from actual endoscopes and organs in the next step.

The result of simulation is shown in **Fig.12**. These graphs indicate the result obtained for an endoscope inserted by constant thrusting force. **Fig.12(b)** shows the variation of position and **Fig.12(c)** the variation of reactive force.

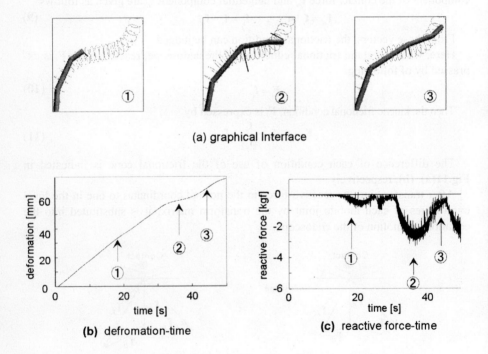

Fig. 12. The Result of Simulation

Although the input thrusting force is constant, the velocity of the tip, a time differential of displacement, varies between 30sec and 40sec in **Fig.12(b)**. This behavior occurs because the endoscope is subjected to substantial reactive force when it contacts colon wall, where the tip must change the direction according to the cubical parabola equation. However, after turning the tip to the direction along the central curve at 40sec, the reactive force decreases (**Fig.12(c)**).

Fig.12(a) shows the graphical interface viewed by the doctor during the procedure. The thick line represents the endoscope and the successive circles depict shape of the colon. The straight thin lines spreading from each joint are the reactive force vectors. The size and direction of force can be visually confirmed.

These results confirm that an endoscope insertion operation could be qualitatively realized using an endoscope and colon model. The simplification of eq.(3) did not influence the reality.

6. Total control system with force sensation

We realized a total system that conveyed to a doctor the actual sensation of inserting an endoscope to the colon by linking a force simulation mechanism (VES-II) with a dynamic model and monitor display connected via a high-speed micro computer (**Fig.13**).

Since the total system can be downsized, a compact desktop training system will be available for general hospitals in the near future.

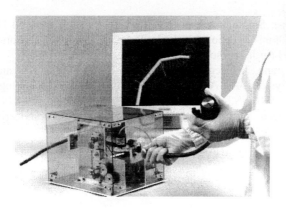

Fig. 13. Total Virtual Endoscope System and Monitor Display

7. Conclusions

We proposed a virtual endoscope system (VES) with force feedback and sensation, and we developed a force simulation mechanism to realize a training system for colonoscopic diagnosis in a virtual digestive tube. It can convey the sensation of reactive force from a digestive tube during insertion.

The dynamical models of both the endoscope and digestive tube were formulated in real-time to calculate the interactional force between them. The force simulation ability of the VES was successfully verified by several experiments.

Acknowledgement

The authors would like to specially thank Dr. Fumio Isaji for his useful advice, as well as Mr. Takahashi, Mr. Senda, Mr. Nakanishi, and Mr. Tachibana for their support during the making of this equipment.

References

1. Koji Ikuta, Takao Namiki, Masaki Takeichi: "Study on Virtual Endoscope System with Force Sensation", Proc. of 2nd Annual Conference of the Robotics Symposia, pp.19-22 1997 (in Japanese)
2. Koji Ikuta, Takao Namiki, Masaki Takeichi: "Study on Virtual Endoscope System with Force Sensation −2nd:Verfication of force sensation and Mathematical model-", Proc. of 15th Annual Conference of the Robotics Society of Japan, pp.19-22 1997 (in Japanese)
3. Shigeo Hirose, Shinichi Amano : The VUTON: High Payload High Efficiency-Holonomic Omni-Directional Vehicle, Proc. Int. Symp. on Robotics Research, pp. 253-260 1993 (in Japanese)
4. K.Mori, A.Urano, J.Hasegawa, J.Toriwaki, H.Annno and K.Ktatada: Virtualized Endoscope System −An Application of Virtual Reality Technology to Diagnostic Aid- ,IEICE* TRANS.INF.&SYST., Vol.E79-D, No.6, pp.809-819, 1996.(*IEICE-Institute of Electronics, Information and Communication Engineering of Japan)

Using Region-of-Interest Based Finite Element Modelling for Brain-Surgery Simulation

Kim Vang Hansen, Ole Vilhelm Larsen

Virtual Centre for Health Informatics
Department of Medical Informatics and Image Analysis
Aalborg University
Denmark

Abstract. Brain surgery simulation requires a mathematical model of the geometric and elastic properties of the entire brain. To allow for realtime manipulation of the model it is necessary to differentiate the level of accuracy between different subparts of the brain model. A Finite Element Model (FEM) of the brain is presented capable of differentiating the spatial and temporal accuracy in different parts of the model. In a user defined region-of-interest around the surgical target point a dynamic FEM model is used to give high accuracy. The remaining parts of the brain is modelled by a static FEM model having less accuracy. The two models are integrated into one model for the entire brain using Condensation. In the context of our early version of a brain surgery simulator we have tested the condensed model versus a full dynamic model of the brain. Promising results concerning spatial error and execution time are shown.

1 Introduction

Surgery simulation [4][1][7][11] have gained growing interest in recent years. The reasons for this are manifold. The success of flight simulators has shown the attainable benefits by letting a trainee practice in a virtual computer environment prior to real world actions [12]. The fast development of computer power now starts to allow interactive manipulation of 3D models representing human organs [4].

The work presented in this paper is motivated from practical needs related to developing a surgery simulator for brain surgery. The aim is to develop a computer-based simulator where a trainee can practice general surgical procedures or where a skilled surgeon can practice surgical details and plan a specific operation prior to performing the specific surgical procedure.

The core of a surgery simulator is a 3D model of the organ of interest and simulation is to a large extent manipulations of the 3D model. One of the fundamental requirements of a surgery simulator is its ability to model deformations of tissue. Surgical procedures often involves pushing around tissue and cutting in tissue which gives rise to deformations of the tissue.

It can be argued that the following three requirements are important in the development of deformable models of human tissue:

- The models should allow for cutting.
- The models should be physically realistic.
- Deformations should be calculated with high speed to allow for real-time simulations.

If cutting should be performed the traditional surface based models can not be used, since these models are empty inside and a cut will not open up for any underlying tissue [1]. Cutting requires volumetric models of the tissue. As a cut is a local procedure, i.e. not effecting the entire organ, the volumetric model must be represented as a local mesh-based model and not as a globally oriented parametric model [5]. The Finite Element Method (FEM) which produces local mesh-based models has been used for different types of surgery simulation, i.e. craniofacial surgery [10], the human leg [1], the liver [4], and the gal bladder [11].

To obtain the most realistic simulation, the model must approximate the physical tissue as well as possible and the deformations should be as similar to deformations of real tissue as possible. We believe that FEM Models, which are models capable of incorporating knowledge of measurable physical properties of tissue, are currently the most promising way to ensure physically realistic deformations.

Real-time simulation is a very challenging requirement. It requires finding the right balance between model size and model accuracy. In brain surgery simulation it is necessary to model the tissue, the blood vessels, nerves, etc. with very high precision, since brain surgery fundamentally is a process of manipulating the details of the brain structure. Models with such a high level of details can only come close to real-time performance if the models are limited in size. In brain surgery simulation it is, however, a problem, that the human brain is a complex organ consisting of several tissue types connected in complicated structural patterns. Surgery at any point in the brain is affected by global properties such as the orientation of the patient relative to the field of gravity, the mass of the brain, the amount of fluid around the brain, the amount of fluid in the internal ventricles, etc., since these properties affect the elastic properties of the brain tissue. Even though brain surgery is almost always performed as minimally invasive surgery, where only a very limited area of the brain is targeted, it is, due to the effect of the global properties, not acceptable to neurosurgeons only to model the area around the target point. It is therefore necessary to develop models for the entire brain, where some parts can be modelled with high precision and other parts with less precision, but still taking into account the elasticity of the brain.

We have previously presented an approach where the model for the entire brain is constructed in order to allow a differentiation of the spatial and temporal accuracy in different parts of the model [8]. The differentiation is obtained by applying a dynamic FEM sub-model with high accuracy to the area around the target point and a static FEM sub-model with less accuracy for the remaining parts. The area with high accuracy is manually pointed out by the user as a special Region-of-interest, ROI. The different models are integrated into one FEM model for the brain using a well known technique called Condensation. In this paper an overview of the approach is given, and through a line of experiments the approach is evaluated in the context of our early version of a surgery simulator. The experiments are focused on the spatial error and the processing time.

In section 2 the FEM models are described and in section 3 integration of the models using condensation is described. Section 4 and 5 describe and present the results related to experiments conducted to show the performance of the method regarding time consumption and accuracy. Section 6 discusses the results and concludes on the work.

2 Modelling by the Finite Element Method

The task of modelling a solid body of matter can be referred to as a continuum problem [9]. In a continuum problem the displacement variable contains an infinitely number of values since it is a function of each generic point in the body. The finite element method reduces the problem to one of a finite number of unknowns by dividing the body into elements and by expressing the displacement field within the element in terms of assumed approximations. Figure 1 shows the discretisation of a solid body into a number of finite elements in the form of tetrahedrons.

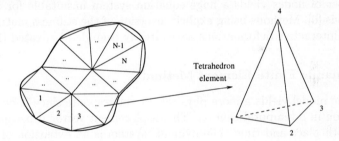

Fig. 1. Discretisation of the continuum problem into discrete 4 node tetrahedrons.

The tetrahedrons are described by 4 nodes, where the displacement field is described by linear interpolation between nodes. In the finite element representation of a problem, the nodal displacement becomes the finite number of unknowns. Using linear elasticity properties (Hooke's law) to define the relation between applied force **f** and the deformation **u** of the modelled body the equation for each element becomes a linear matrix system:

$$\mathbf{K_e u_e = f_e} \quad (1)$$

Since there are 4 nodes in an element each with 3 degrees of freedom **f** and **u** become vectors of [12x1], and **K** the *stiffness matrix* is a [12x12] matrix describing the elastic properties of the element based on material and geometric properties. Thus, for each element it is possible to define different element properties and then assemble the elements into a complex model.

The elements must be assembled in order to find the properties of the overall system modelled by the mesh of elements. The global matrix equations of the system have the same form as the equations for an element, except the fact that they contain many more terms since they include all nodes. The assembly of the global stiffness matrix becomes,

$$\mathbf{K} = \sum_e t(\mathbf{K_e}) \qquad (2)$$

where $t()$ is a transfer function from element to global node numbers.

2.1 Static Finite Element Method

The result of the assembly procedure is a large linear equation system which must be solved with respect to $\mathbf{u}$. Since $\mathbf{u}$ is time independent this system is called a static finite element system

$$\mathbf{K}_{[3N \times 3N]} \cdot \mathbf{u}_{[3N \times 1]} = \mathbf{f}_{[3N \times 1]} \qquad (3)$$

where N is the number of nodes. When modelling large complex structures the number of nodes yields a huge equation system unsuitable for interactive applications [6]. Methods using explicit inversion of the stiffness matrix in order to obtain interactive deformations have already been demonstrated [1].

2.2 Dynamic Finite Element Method

A dynamic model yields a more physical correct response since it describes the deformation in a temporal context. The displacement vector $\mathbf{u}$ becomes a function of both place and time. The dynamic system is an extension of the linear static system where mass and damping is added. The equation to be solved becomes:

$$\mathbf{M}\ddot{\mathbf{u}}_n + \mathbf{C}\dot{\mathbf{u}}_n + \mathbf{K}\mathbf{u}_n = \mathbf{f}_n \qquad (4)$$

where subscript n denotes time $n\Delta t$ where Δt is the size of the time step. $\mathbf{M}$ is the mass matrix, $\mathbf{C}$ is the damping matrix. Assuming lumped masses at the nodes and mass proportional damping then,

$$\mathbf{M}^e_{ii} = \rho \frac{V^e}{4}, \qquad \mathbf{C}^e_{ii} = \alpha \mathbf{M}^e_{ii} \qquad (5)$$

where ρ is the mass density, V^e the element volume, α is a scaling factor and i is the element nodal number (i=1,2,3,4). $\mathbf{M}$ and $\mathbf{C}$ are assembled similar to the stiffness matrix $\mathbf{K}$.

The dynamic equation is solved for $\mathbf{u}$ using *the trapezoidal-rule method* to calculate $\ddot{\mathbf{u}}$ the acceleration and the velocity $\dot{\mathbf{u}}$ [3].

3 Region-of-interest based Finite Element Modelling

To obtain the most precise modelling of the brain for a simulation, the entire brain should be modelled as a dynamic system. This would involve tens of thousands of nodes in the model and for such large models real-time simulation would not be possible.

The main idea behind this paper is to have a user-defined target area for the surgical procedure and then only model a Region-of-interest (ROI) around the target area as a dynamic system. For such small regions real-time simulation is expected to be possible.

As argued in the Introduction the remaining part of the brain is still very important for modelling the target area and can thus not be disregarded. We suggest to model the remaining part as a static model and then, through condensation, integrate the two models into one model.

The integration ensures that the elastic properties of the remaining part effects the dynamic system of the ROI. This means that when pushing tissue around in the target area you not only sense the tissue in the small dynamic model, but also the resistance from tissue in the larger static model. If for example the static models contain non-deformable material like the skull, this will directly be sensed when manipulating tissue in the target area. The information left out to give a simpler system is related to the dynamics of the deformations. The static model can only tell us how the deformation will look eventually after the model have reached a steady state phase, not how the deformation developed over time.

By speeding up of the calculation of the static model real-time simulation is also expected for this model, and thus for the entire condensed model.

Condensation is a technique by which a matrix equation system can be partitioned into several subsystems allowing individual treatment of the subsystems. Condensation is basically done by eliminating some of the nodes from the matrix equation system by pre-calculations [9].

The ROI is described as a dynamic model marked with subscript d

$$\mathbf{M}_d \ddot{\mathbf{u}}_d + \mathbf{C}_d \dot{\mathbf{u}}_d + \mathbf{K}_d \mathbf{u}_d = \mathbf{f}_d \tag{6}$$

The remaining part is modelled using a static model (subscript s).

$$\mathbf{K}_s \mathbf{u}_s = \mathbf{f}_s \tag{7}$$

The complete model ordered with the ROI nodes first:

$$\begin{bmatrix} \mathbf{M}_d & 0 \\ 0 & 0 \end{bmatrix} \begin{bmatrix} \ddot{\mathbf{u}}_d \\ \ddot{\mathbf{u}}_s \end{bmatrix} + \begin{bmatrix} \mathbf{C}_d & 0 \\ 0 & 0 \end{bmatrix} \begin{bmatrix} \dot{\mathbf{u}}_d \\ \dot{\mathbf{u}}_s \end{bmatrix} + \begin{bmatrix} \mathbf{K}_d & \mathbf{K}_{ds} \\ \mathbf{K}_{sd} & \mathbf{K}_s \end{bmatrix} \begin{bmatrix} \mathbf{u}_d \\ \mathbf{u}_s \end{bmatrix} = \begin{bmatrix} \mathbf{f}_d \\ \mathbf{f}_s \end{bmatrix} \tag{8}$$

where subscript ds and sd refer to the interaction between the two models. In expanded form these equations become

$$\mathbf{M}_d \ddot{\mathbf{u}}_d + \mathbf{C}_d \dot{\mathbf{u}}_d + \mathbf{K}_d \mathbf{u}_d + \mathbf{K}_{ds} \mathbf{u}_s = \mathbf{f}_d \tag{9}$$

$$\mathbf{K}_{sd} \mathbf{u}_d + \mathbf{K}_s \mathbf{u}_s = \mathbf{f}_s \tag{10}$$

When equation (10) is solved for $\mathbf{u_s}$ and the result is substituted into (9), we obtain

$$\mathbf{M_d \ddot{u}_d + C_d \dot{u}_d + K_d u_d - K_{ds} K_s^{-1} K_{sd} u_d = f_d - K_{ds} K_s^{-1} f_s}$$

or (11)

$$\mathbf{M_d \ddot{u}_d + C_d \dot{u}_d + \tilde{K} u_d = \tilde{f}}$$

where $\mathbf{\tilde{K} = K_d - K_{ds} \cdot K_s^{-1} \cdot K_{sd}}$ and $\mathbf{\tilde{f} = f_d - K_{ds} \cdot K_s^{-1} \cdot f_s}$. The inversion of $\mathbf{K_s}$ can be done prior to the simulation and will not influence the total complexity of the condensed model.

4 Experimental Design

The experimental work is aimed to measure the spatial error introduced and the processing time involved in computing the deformation.

For the experiments only a simplified model of the brain is used. The very precise model with detailed information about the surface structure, blood vessels, nerves, etc. is still under construction. The deformation used in all experiments is caused by two forces applied on both sides of an opening in the surface pulling the sides apart, see figure 4.

Measuring the spatial accuracy. Assuming that the full dynamic system calculates the correct deformation, it is possible to measure the spatial error of the condensed model by measuring the spatial difference between the result of a deformation for the condensed models and the full dynamic model. The spatial difference is measured as the Euclidean distance between all common nodes in the models, i.e. the nodes in the ROI.

As it is expected that the spatial error is related to the dynamics of the system, the force has been applied to the system in three different ways. As shown in figure 2 the situations are ramp functions with different rise times i.e. 0.5, 1, and 2 seconds. The applied force has been determined experimentally as a force giving realistic deformations of the brain models when viewed in the simulator. The duration of the test is 200 iterations or 10 seconds.

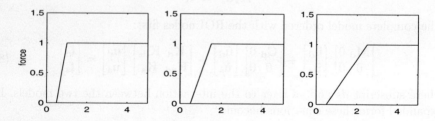

Fig. 2. The forces are ramp functions with a risetime of 0.5, 1 and 2 seconds.

To determine which effect the size of the ROI will have on the accuracy and processing time two setups were made. The full dynamic model contains 799 nodes, setup 1 is a condensed model of 306 nodes and setup 2 contains 228 nodes.

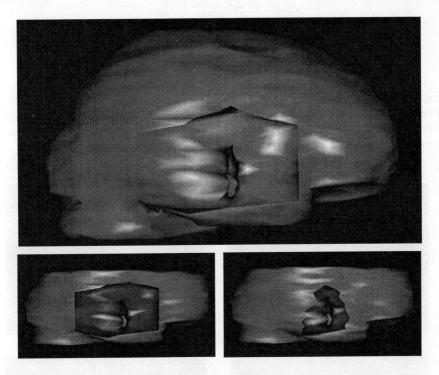

Fig. 3. The models used in the experiments. The full dynamic model (*top*), the condensed model of setup 1 (*left*) and the condensed model of setup 2 (*right*). The dark areas illustrate the dynamic part of the model.

Measuring the time consumption. The time used to calculate the deformation at each time step is measured. Based on the iteration-time a frame rate is calculated.

The remaining test parameters are described in table 1. Since finite element modelling of brain tissue is a fairly new area, the material parameters are not described in literature. As an approximation the brain tissue is modelled with the material parameters of rubber.

The system was implemented on a Silicon Graphics ONYX with four MIPS R10000 processors and a RealityEngine II graphical interface. Notice that the deformations are calculated using a single processor, parallel features are only used to separate rendering from the actual simulation.

Table 1. Parameter settings used during all tests. The rubber lamé constants λ and μ defining the material properties for rubber can be found in [2].

λ	μ	ρ	α	Time step
0.4 $\frac{10^5\ kg}{cm^2}$	0.0012 $\frac{10^5\ kg}{cm^2}$	1.0 $\frac{g}{cm^3}$	0.8	0.05 $sec.$

5 Experimental Results

Figure 4 visualises how the deformation used in the line of experiments develops over time. The cylindrical objects are representing spatulas capable of pushing tissue around. The time spent on the deformation is either 0.5, 1 or 2 seconds depending on the ramp functions in use (see figure 2).

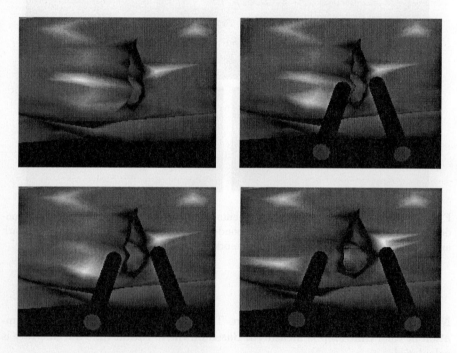

Fig. 4. This figure shows the deformation of the brain model as the forces increase according to the ramp function (figure 2).

Spatial accuracy. Figure 5 shows the mean and max. error for the condensed model with setup 1 compared to the full dynamic model.

We notice that the mean steady state error (above 100 iterations) is below 0.2 mm for all three ramps functions. There are, however, significant differences between the three ramps when looking at the errors occurring shortly after the force has been applied. For ramp 1 and 2 the error rapidly climbs to a peak value of 0.4 and 0.3 respectively. From this peak it is graduately lowered to the steady state error. For ramp 3 it slowly increases until it reaches its maximum value at the steady state error.

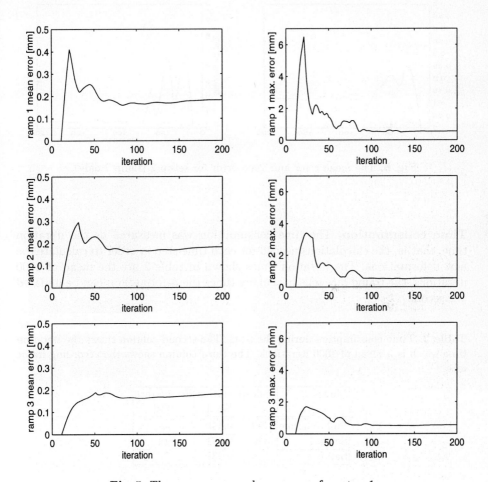

Fig. 5. The mean error and max. error for setup 1.

The maximum error for the condensed model follows a common pattern for the three ramp functions. It peaks shortly after the force is applied with values of approximately 6 mm, 4 mm and 2 mm respectively. Within the next 50 iterations the max. error is lowered to less than 1 mm.

In figure 6 the mean and max errors for the condensed model with setup 2 are shown. Only results with ramp 2 are shown, as all three ramps followed the same pattern represented by ramp 2. The pattern is a performance very close to that of setup 1 but with a minor increase in the max. error. The most significant change is the duration of the time interval where the max error occurs. The max. error has not one but several peaks in the first 100 iterations.

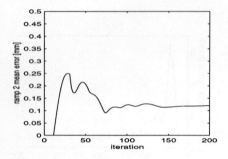 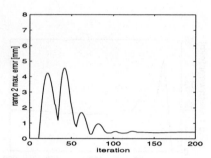

Fig. 6. The mean error and max. error for setup 2 (ramp 2 only).

Time consumption. The time consumption was measured as the iteration time, that is, the calculations needed for each time step in order to calculate the new deformations. The iteration times shown in table 2 are the mean of 1000 iterations, the frame rate tells how many times the deformations can be updated per second.

Table 2. Time consumption during the tests. The second column shows the iteration time which is a mean of 1000 iterations. The third column shows the according frame rate.

Model	nodes	Iteration [sec.]	Frame rate [Hz]
Full dynamic	799	0.440	2
Setup 1	306	0.071	14
Setup 2	228	0.037	27

6 Discussion and Conclusion

Examining the results from the test for spatial accuracy it is characteristic that the condensed model has a very small mean error. The mean performances of the condensed model and the full dynamic model are therefore very similar. The similarity is obtained because the condensation allows the dynamic model to sense the elastic properties of the larger part of the brain modelled by the static model.

Bearing in mind that real-time performance of the simulator is of interest it is important that the condensed model not only gives small mean errors but at the same time a significant reduction in processing time.

The experiments also show where the price for the reduction is being payed. It is in the dynamic properties of the condensed model. The experiments show max errors up to 6 mm shortly after the force has been applied rapidly. These errors are most likely caused by a mis-match between the deformations of the static and the dynamic model shortly after force impact. In the dynamic model the deformation develops over time. In the static model the final result of the deformation is determined at the instant where the force is applied. The deformation of the static model is therefore presented to the dynamic model prior to the point in time where it would have occurred, had it been modelled as a dynamic model.

However, these problems are only significant for abrupt manipulations, and as large max. errors occur together with small mean errors, only few nodes have been affected by the errors. How these max. errors affect the usability of the condensed model in a surgery simulation needs to be further investigated. A preliminary evaluation by the neurosurgeon related to our surgical simulator team calls for no major concern when used in a realistic simulation situation.

The experiments with the condensed model with different sized dynamic sub-models show that it is possible to develop condensed models with very small dynamic parts and still maintain very good spatial accuracy. As the size decreases, the sensitivity to rapid changes in the force is increased.

Concerning time consumption the results closely reflect the complexity of the models. For the very simple brain model (low node density) used in the experiments the condensed models comes close to real-time performance. As the node density for a realistic brain model is expected to be considerably higher, our dream of a real-time simulator can benefit from the ongoing rapid increase in processing power on the computer market.

Based on the line of experiments presented in this paper it can be concluded that a condensed model with both dynamic and static sub-models has interesting properties for use in brain surgery simulation. It allows for the elastic properties of the entire brain to be taken into account when modelling deformation in a Region-of-interest around the surgical target point. The condensed model has a complexity significantly lower than a dynamic model for the entire brain and therefore the processing time is much lower and realtime performance is coming closer.

The next step in developing a simulator for brain surgery is to enhance the physical realism of the model. Material parameters for brain tissue, blood vessels etc. need to be determined, and the appropriate node density must be computed. Once these problems are overcome, a new line of experiments can determine how close we are to realtime simulation with realistic models.

References

1. Morten Bro-Nielsen and Stephane Cotin. Real-time volumetric deformable models for surgery simulation using finite elements and condensation. *Computer Graphics Forum*, 15(3):57–66, 1996.
2. Philippe G. Ciarlet. *Mathematical Elasticity, Volume I: Three-Dimensional Elasticity*. Elsevier Science Publisher B.V., 1988.
3. Robert D. Cook, David S. Malkus, and Michael E. Plesha. *Concepts and Applications of Finite Element Analysis*. John Wiley & Sons, 1989.
4. S. Cotin, H. Delingette, and N. Ayache. Volumetric deformable models for simulation of laparoscopic surgery. In *Computer Assisted Radiology (CAR' 96)*, 1996.
5. S. A. Cover, N. F. Ezquerra, J. F. O'Brien, R. Rowe, T. Gadacz, and E. Palm. Interactively deformable models for surgery simulation. *IEEE Computer Graphics and Applications*, 13:68 – 75, 1993.
6. Sarah F. F. Gibson. 3D ChainMail: a Fast Algorithm for Deforming Volumetric Objects. http://www.merl.com/reports/index.html, 1996.
7. Sarah Gibson et. al. Volumetric object modeling for surgical simulation. *Medical Image Analysis*, 2:121 – 132, june 1998.
8. Kim Vang Hansen, Martin Stumpf Eskildsen, and Ole Vilhelm Larsen. Region-of-interest based finite element modelling of the human brain - an approach to brain-surgery simulation. In *Proceedings of the 14th International Conference on Pattern Recognition, (ICPR'98)*, August 1998.
9. Kenneth H. Huebner. *The Finite Element Method for Engineers*. John Wiley & Sons, 1975.
10. Erwin Keeve, Sabine Girod, and Bernd Girod. Craniofacial surgery simulation. Telecommunications Institute, University of Erlangen-Nuremberg, German, 1996.
11. U. Kuhn, Kühnapfel, H.-G. Krumm, and B. Neisius. The Karlsruhe Endoscopic Surgery Trainer - A "Virtual Reality" based Training System for Minimal Invasive Surgery. *CAR*, 1996.
12. Richard M. Satava. Advanced simulation technologies for surgical education. *Bulletin of the American College of Surgeons*, 81, 1996.

An Image Processing Environment for Guiding Vascular MR Interventions*

R. van der Weide[a], K.J. Zuiderveld[a], C.J.G. Bakker[a], C. Bos[a], H.F.M. Smits[a],
T. Hoogenboom[b], J.J. van Vaals[b], M.A. Viergever[a]

[a]Image Sciences Institute, room E 01.334, University Hospital Utrecht,
Heidelberglaan 100, 3584 CX Utrecht, the Netherlands;
[b]Philips Medical Systems, Best.
email: remko@isi.uu.nl

Abstract. MRI offers potential advantages over conventional X-ray techniques for guiding and evaluating vascular interventions. Image guidance of such interventions via passive catheter tracking requires real-time processing of the dynamically acquired MR slices and advanced display facilities inside the MR examination room. Commercially available clinical MR-scanners currently do not provide this functionality.

This paper describes a processing environment that allows near-real-time MR-guided interventions. Two stand-alone workstations connected to our MR-scanner offer a flexible and fast tool for guiding the interventionist without affecting the stability of the MR-scanner. The paper describes and discusses our approach, including image processing techniques. Results of a phantom balloon angioplasty experiment are presented.

1 Introduction

Magnetic resonance imaging (MRI) offers several advantages over conventional X-ray imaging, and has therefore received interest recently for guiding and monitoring interventional procedures such as biopsies and thermal tumor ablation. Since harmful contrast agents are not required for MR imaging of vasculature, and functional information can be provided, for instance with regard to flow and capillary perfusion, it is potentially also an attractive modality to guide intravascular interventions [1].

Two approaches for image guidance of intravascular MR interventions have been advocated, viz. active [2] and passive tracking. In the latter approach, the catheter is located by processing of the dynamically acquired MR images. This method requires dedicated intravascular devices that are visible in the MR slices,

---

* This study was supported by the Netherlands' Ministry of Economic Affairs (program "IOP Beeldverwerking"). The research was carried out within the framework of the program "Imaging Science", sponsored by the Netherlands' Foundation for Image Sciences, and co-sponsored by the industrial companies Philips Medical Systems, Shell International Exploration and Production, ADAC Europe and Cordis Europe.

but do not contain any conducting material. In order to show the feasibility of MR-guided balloon angioplasty with passive catheter tracking, we developed MR-compatible guide wires and catheters that are locally impregnated with dysprosium oxide [3]. These areas of increased susceptibility cause artifacts depicted by small signal voids in the MR image.

During an MR intervention slices are acquired dynamically, *i.e.* every image is processed and displayed immediately after acquisition. Hence, image processing techniques should allow fast (within 1 sec.) localization of device markers in MR slices. However, commercially available scanners do not support any complex image processing of dynamic scans. Therefore, near-real-time image processing was achieved by building an image processing environment separated from our MR-scanner (Philips Gyroscan ACS-NT15), and connected via Ethernet.

Several other groups followed a similar approach using add-on systems for attaining real-time MR imaging ("MR fluoroscopy") [4–8]. Most of the reported systems were developed to achieve real-time reconstruction or low-level processing of image data, and hence often require specially designed hardware that is dedicated to these tasks. Although these systems can receive, reconstruct and display multiple images per second and thus achieve considerably higher refresh rates, they focus on specific fast sequences like EPI and spirals, where –in contrast with our sequences that supply images at a rate of maximally one per second– reconstruction is a fundamental bottleneck.

Our environment has been developed with the intent to enable passive catheter tracking by rapidly feeding the acquired images to image processing algorithms. Since, we focus on a direct clinical application, the system was designed such that it guarantees stability during *in vivo* MR interventions. It offers sufficient performance for our purposes and flexibility with regard to image processing functionality to be developed. It employs the graphics hardware of low-cost, non-MR-dedicated workstations for fast visualization.

2 Environment

An image processing environment for MR-guided intravascular interventions should meet three requirements:

1. The scanner stability must be preserved. Major modifications to the scanner software are thus not acceptable.
2. The environment must have a high degree of flexibility, allowing new visualization and device tracking algorithms to be easily implemented without affecting the stability of the system.
3. An in-room, MR-compatible display close to the scanner bore is required. Remote control from outside the examination room must be possible.

To preserve the stability of the MR-scanner, a Direct Reconstructor INterface (DRIN) was installed on our scanner. This minor and safe extension to the reconstructor software uses a TCP/IP protocol and allows connected clients to receive either modulus, phase, real and imaginary images in both spatial and frequency domain, including the associated acquisition parameters. We use the local network to connect our systems to the scanner reconstructor.

2.1 Hardware

Our image processing environment consists of two O2 (Silicon Graphics, Inc.) UNIX workstations. One –the "master"– is located in the operator room adjacent to the MR examination room and is equipped with an R10000 processor acting as a client of the DRIN server. The console is a standard color monitor. The workstation ("slave") located in the MR room is a diskless R5000 O2, which boots from the master via Ethernet. It displays on a 13" inch 18-bit 1280×1024 color LCD (Presenter 1280, Silicon Graphics).

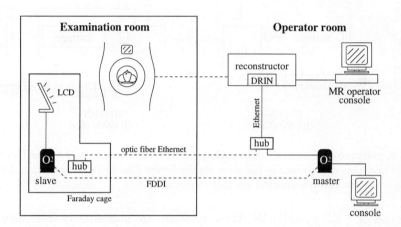

Fig. 1. Hardware environment; O2 workstations communicate via optic fiber connections. Raw image data are first transmitted to the master via Ethernet, and next to the slave via FDDI.

Radio-frequency radiation emitted by the LCD and the slave was avoided to interfere with the MR signal by Faraday caging them (fig. 1). Data communication with the master was established via optic fiber connections. An optic Ethernet connection (10 Mb/s) between both workstations allows booting of the slave with remote control from the master. Image data are transferred from the master to the slave via a much faster optic fiber connection (Fiber Distributed Data Interface (FDDI), 100 Mb/s), which guarantees minimal data transport delay between both systems. Although the slave might also login at the DRIN server for retrieving image data, this would considerably increase Ethernet load, thereby decreasing performance.

2.2 Software

In order to achieve the required stability, flexibility and performance, the implementation was performed by event-driven, object-oriented programming with a Tcl/Tk [9] user interface. Several C++-objects were implemented that encapsulate data receiving from DRIN (**DrinClient**, see fig. 2), communication between the O2 workstations (**Server** and **Client**), image storage (**Storage**), and visualization (**Display**). The **DrinClient** object receives the acquired images in data

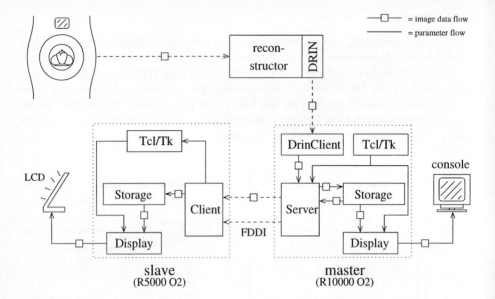

Fig. 2. Software environment; data packages from DRIN are received by the DrinClient object and immediately sent to the slave via the Server–Client FDDI connection. Display parameters are also transmitted via this connection.

packages of 8 KB from DRIN. These packages are immediately transmitted to the TCP/IP-based **Server** object, which distributes them to the connected **Client** objects.

The event-driven approach of Tcl/Tk ensures fast and appropriate handling of interrupts from communication ports. Inter-object communication is also entirely performed by the event mechanism. Since all tracking and visualization algorithms are encapsulated within the object **Display**, extensions and modifications to these algorithms do not involve other objects, thus conserving their stability. This guarantees flexibility and stability of the software. The graphics hardware of the O2 systems is exploited by using the OpenGL library [10].

Events are handled in sequence of priority. In order to achieve a minimal delay between data acquisition and visualization in the MR examination room, events related to image data transfer from DRIN to the slave have a high priority level. Display and storage of newly received images on the master have lower priority and are thus only started after the completion of data transfer to the connected clients.

The slave is controlled from the master by the operator. Therefore, modified display parameters (*e.g.* for window-leveling, zooming) are copied immediately to the slave via the **Server–Client** connection. This guarantees identical displaying on both systems. The Tcl/Tk script interpreter also permits on-the-fly execution of script code on both systems for changing the operation of the systems, which makes them highly flexible and facilitates development, testing and experimenting.

2.3 Image processing

An MR-guided intervention procedure is preceded by a series of scans for (i) localization of the stenosis and specification of the scan planes, (ii) quantification of the pre-operative flow through the stenosis, and (iii) a 2D phase-contrast (2DPC) acquisition with a geometry identical to the dynamic scan series. This 2DPC image brightly depicts the vasculature that the interventional devices are likely to pass (fig. 3a). It is therefore suitable to indicate the positions of the located devices. We call this a "roadmap", similar to the contrast-enhanced roadmap image for conventional X-ray interventions.

The actual intervention is carried out using a dynamic gradient echo technique. Images show small regions of marker-induced decreased signal intensity (fig. 3b). Subtraction of a previously acquired reference image can improve visualization of the device markers (fig. 3c). This operation is available in the graphics hardware of the O2 systems. Motion artifacts reduce the quality of the subtraction, but can be overcome partly by the selection of a new reference image by the operator after a substantial patient movement.

For guidance of the interventionalist during the positioning of the intravascular devices, information on the locations of the markers as contained by the subtraction image should be combined with the morphologic information of the vasculature. Therefore, we first color the roadmap (fig. 3a) red. Next, the subtraction image is inverted, thus yielding white markers, which is finally merged with the roadmap image by applying alpha-blending [11]. We call the result the "overlay" image. All required image processing operations were implemented using the graphics hardware, and thus are very fast.

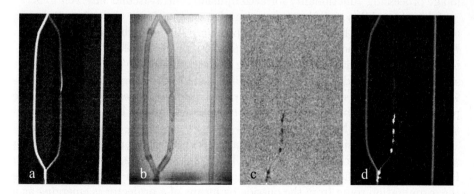

Fig. 3. (a) 2DPC image of a flow phantom, which serves as a roadmap during the intervention; (b) dynamically acquired modulus image containing five dysprosium markers in the lower part of the middle tube; (c) result after subtraction of a reference image; (d) overlay image; in reality, the vasculature is colored red and the markers are white.

3 Results

Our imaging set-up provides near-real-time image guidance of MR interventions with a refresh rate of one image per two seconds. Acquisition of each MR image takes approximately one second. Image data transfer between DRIN and the master takes 0.7 second. The latency introduced by the data transfer to the slave is negligible as a result of the division of the image in small data packages and the fast FDDI connection. Image processing and display takes approximately 0.3 second for a 1024^2 overlay image. Modulus images of a dynamic scan series can also be displayed by the LCD at the scanner front within 0.5 seconds after acquisition, but any image processing of these images is not possible.

Image guidance using the overlay technique was tested during an *in vitro* interventional MR procedure. A 6 mm flexible plastic tube loop with a dilatable stenosis was connected to a flow system and taped onto the forearm of a volunteer. This experiment allowed us to practice a clinical application of MR-guided balloon angioplasty in patients with an obstructed hemodialysis access graft under realistic conditions with regard to patient positioning and sterility issues (fig. 4).

4 Discussion and conclusions

We have demonstrated that near-real-time imaging for MR-guided interventions can be achieved with a stand-alone, non-MR-dedicated workstation containing graphics hardware. Delays introduced by the described image processing and visualization do not considerably decrease refresh rates as compared with those currently achieved for dynamic scan series on a commercially available MR-scanner, whereas these scanners do not provide dynamically available advanced image processing functionality for accomplishing intravascular interventions.

Scanner stability, which is an essential condition for a clinical application, is conserved by the high degree of independence of the developed environment. Flexibility is also achieved by this approach, where development and implementation of visualization and tracking algorithms do not involve the scanner software, and thus do not require modifications by the manufacturer. The environment seems also suitable for the development and testing of new image processing algorithms required for new imaging techniques like perfusion, diffusion and functional MRI.

Visualization inside the MR examination room was accomplished by placing a diskless slave workstation and a LCD in the MR suite, encapsulated in a Faraday cage in order to avoid RF interference. Although visualization inside the examination room from the outside by means of a projector is emerging as a good alternative, it was not considered an appropriate solution for our purposes because of the required image resolution and the specific construction of our MR suite. A second computer outside the MR suite is required for booting of the diskless slave, and for control by an operator. Current image processing is entirely performed by the graphics hardware of both systems.

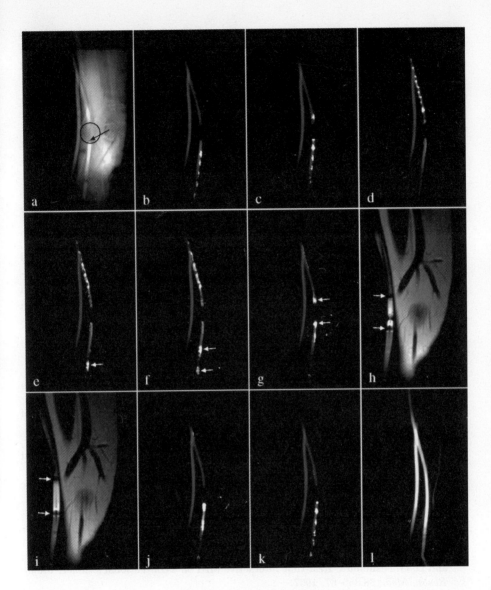

Fig. 4. Results of an *in vitro* MR-guided balloon angioplasty. (a) First modulus image of the dynamic scan series depicting the phantom (two tubes) taped onto a forearm; the stenosis (arrow) in the right tube, which is superimposed on the arm, causes a signal void distally (circle). (b-d) Introduction of the guide wire (seven markers); in the region of the signal void, markers are not visible. (e-g) Introduction and positioning of the balloon catheter (arrows) across the stenosis; the guide wire has been moved further distally in (g). (h,i) Balloon inflation with Gd-DTPA doped water causes the stenosis to dissolve (visualization performed by a spin-echo sequence with a different geometry); markers are indicated by arrows. (j,k) Catheter and guide wire are withdrawn. (l) Post-operatively acquired 2DPC image with recovered tube lumen.

The overlay technique provides morphological information of the patient's vasculature as well as the location of the stenosis and the marker positions of the invasive devices. Therefore, it sufficiently supports image guidance of MR interventions in simple vasculature such as in human limbs. However, three-dimensional coordinates of the tips of these devices are not yet explicitly calculated. This is essential for steering the scanner by automatic modification of the scan plane in order to allow vascular interventions in regions of complex three-dimensional vasculature like the brain. Therefore, advanced tracking algorithms are required, which are currently being developed in our group. As a consequence of the object-oriented programming of the image processing environment we described, incorporation of these algorithms without affecting stability is straightforward. The extra computational capacities of the master might be used by these tracking algorithms, while the slave can focus on rapid visualization.

Our image processing environment has convincingly demonstrated its potential for guiding balloon angioplasty procedures in phantom experiments, and allowed us recently to start the *in vivo* application of MR-guided balloon angioplasty on clinical patients with a hemodialysis access graft obstructed by a stenosis. We expect to successfully perform an MR-guided intervention on a patient within some months.

References

1. F. A. Jolesz and S. M. Blumenfeld. Interventional use of magnetic resonance imaging. *Magn. Reson. Q.*, 10:85–96, 1994.
2. C. L. Dumoulin, S. P. Souza, and R. D. Darrow. Real-time position monitoring of invasive devices using magnetic resonance. *Magn. Reson. Med.*, 29:411–5, 1993.
3. C. J. G. Bakker, R. M. Hoogeveen, W. F. Hurtak, J. J. van Vaals, M. A. Viergever, and W. P. T. M. Mali. MR-guided endovascular interventions: susceptibility-based catheter and near-real-time imaging technique. *Radiology*, 202:273–6, 1997.
4. R. C. Wright, S. J. Riederer, F. Farzaneh, P. J. Rossman, and Y. Liu. Real-time MR fluoroscopic data acquisition and image reconstruction. *Magn. Reson. Med.*, 12:407–15, 1989.
5. R. W. Cox, A. Jesmanowicz, and J. S. Hyde. Real-time functional magnetic resonance imaging. *Magn. Reson. Med.*, 33:230–6, 1995.
6. A. B. Kerr, J. M. Pauly, B. S. Hu, K. C. Li, C. J. Hardy, C. H. Meyer, A. Macovski, and D. G. Nishimura. Real-time interactive MRI on a conventional scanner. *Magn. Reson. Med.*, 38:355–67, 1997.
7. K. Kose, T. Haishi, A. Caprihan, and E. Fukushima. Real-time NMR imaging systems using personal computers. *J. Magn. Res.*, 124:35–41, 1997.
8. A. F. Gmitro, A. R. Ehsani, T. A. Berchem, and R. J. Snell. A real-time reconstruction system for magnetic resonance imaging. *Magn. Reson. Med.*, 35:734–40, 1996.
9. J. K. Ousterhout. *Tcl and the Tk toolkit*. Addison–Wesley Publishing Company, Reading, Massachusetts, 2nd edition, 1994.
10. Jackie Neider, Tom Davis, and Mason Woo. *OpenGL Programming Guide*. Addison-Wesley Publishing Company, April 1995.
11. T. Porter and T. Duff. Compositing digital images. In H. Christiansen, editor, *SIGGRAPH '84 Conference Proceedings (Minneapolis, MN, July 23-27, 1984)*, pages 253–259, July 1984. In Computer Graphics, Volume 18, Number 3.

Fluoroscopic Image Processing for Computer-Aided Orthopaedic Surgery

Z. Yaniv[1], L. Joskowicz[1], A. Simkin[2,3], M. Garza-Jinich[4], and C. Milgrom MD[3]

[1] Institute of Computer Science, The Hebrew Univ., Jerusalem 91904 Israel.
[2] Lab. of Experimental Surgery, Hadassah Univ. Hospital, Jerusalem 91120 Israel.
[3] Dept. of Orthopaedic Surgery, Hadassah Univ. Hospital, Jerusalem 91120 Israel.
[4] IIMAS - Univ. Nacional Autonoma de Mexico, AP 20-726, Mexico 01000 DF.
{zivy,josko}@cs.huji.ac.il, ruskin@vms.huji.ac.il, milgrom@md2.huji.ac.il

Abstract. This paper describes the fluoroscopic X-ray image processing techniques of FRACAS, a computer-integrated orthopaedic system for bone fracture reduction. Fluoroscopic image processing consists of image dewarping, camera calibration, and bone contour extraction. Our approach focuses on bone imaging and emphasizes integration, full automation, simplicity, robustness, and practicality. We describe the experimental setup and report results quantifying the accuracy of our methods. We show that after dewarping and calibration, submillimetric spatial positioning accuracy is achievable with standard equipment. We present a new bone contour segmentation algorithm based on robust image region statistics computation which yields good results on clinical images.

1 Introduction

Current orthopaedic practice heavily relies on fluoroscopic images to perform surgical procedures. Fluoroscopic X-ray images are captured by an image intensifier mounted on a C-arm and viewed on a monitor (Fig. 1). Surgeons rely on the images to determine the relative position and orientation of bones, implants, and surgical instruments. While inexpensive and readily available, fluoroscopy has limitations. The images have a narrow field of view, have poor resolution and contrast, and show significant geometric distortion. Because they are uncorrelated, two-dimensional static views, the surgeon must mentally recreate the spatio-temporal intraoperative situation. Significant skill, time, and frequent use of the fluoroscope are required, leading to positioning errors and complications and to significant cumulative radiation exposure to the surgeon [12].

Recent research shows that computer-aided systems can significantly improve the accuracy of orthopaedic procedures by replacing fluoroscopic guidance with interactive display of 3D bone models created from preoperative CT studies and tracked in real time. Examples include systems for acetabular cup placement [13], for total knee replacement, and for pedicle screw insertion [9, 10].

Flurosocopy can still play an important role in computer-aided surgery systems. By correcting, calibrating, and correlating them, a limited number of enhanced fluoroscopic images can be used for accurate navigation. For example,

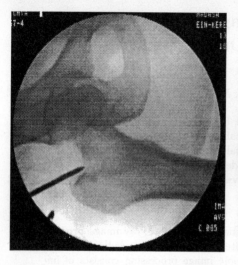
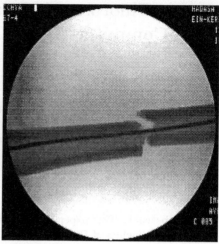

Fig. 1. Fluoroscopic images of a femur fracture with drill bit on the proximal femoral tronchanteric fossa (left), and medial linear fracture with guide wire (right).

[1], [6] and [11, 16] describe systems that use enhanced fluoroscopy and real-time tracking to assist surgeons in distal intramedulary nail locking. They can also be used for registration – establishing a common reference frame between the preoperative CT study and the intraoperative situation.

We are currently developing a computer-integrated orthopaedic system, called FRACAS [7], for closed medullary nailing for bone fracture reduction [2]. FRACAS' goals are to reduce the surgeon's cumulative exposure to radiation and improve the positioning accuracy by replacing uncorrelated static fluoroscopic images with a virtual reality display of spatial bone fragment models created from preoperative CT and tracked intraoperatively in real time. Fluoroscopic images are used to register the bone fragment models to the intraoperative situation and to verify that the registration is maintained.

This paper describes FRACAS' fluoroscopic image processing techniques and experimental results. To correlate the images and use them for accurate registration and navigation, we correct the distortion, determine the fluoroscopic camera parameters, and extract the bone contours. While many methods for these tasks are described in the literature, our method emphasizes integration, full automation, simplicity, robustness, and practicality. It focuses on fluoroscopic bone images and their use in 2D/3D anatomy-based registration. We report experimental results quantifying accuracy, distortion, and camera parameter estimation, and present segmentation results of several sets of clinical images.

2 Problem characteristics

Fluoroscopic images present substantial distortion due to three factors [1, 3, 6, 14]: (1) the image intensifier receptor screen is slightly curved, (2) the surrounding magnetic fields of the Earth and nearby instruments deflect the X-ray beam electrons, and (3) the C-arm armature deflects under the weight of the image intensifier, changing the focal length of the camera. The first effect can be modeled as radial pincushion distortion and is independent of the C-arm location. The second effect yields image translation and spatially variant rotation, and is C-arm orientation dependent. The third effect requires knowing the magnitude of the deflection. The distortion pattern resulting all the three factors is present in all units, including modern ones, and varies from unit to unit and from session to session, with up to 10mm shift on the image edges [14].

Prior to each session, the amount of distortion and the fluoroscopic camera parameters must be determined for predefined C-arm orientations [3]. Usually, the dewarping and camera calibration steps are decoupled [8, 11, 14] and the parameters are obtained by imaging specially designed phantoms. To correct for distortion, a uniform grid of fiducials (e.g. steel balls or holes) is imaged. The location of the fiducial centers in the image and in the model are compared, and a *dewarp map* is computed specifying how to shift each pixel in the image to its real projected location. To obtain the camera characteristics, a parametric pinhole camera model defined by simultaneous equations relating the parameters is used. An object with known fiducial geometry and known location is imaged, and the positions of the image and the geometric points are matched. Solving the set of equations yields the parameter values [15].

Once the images have been corrected for distortion and the camera parameters are know, the next step is contour extraction of relevant anatomical structures. The main difficulties are that the images are noisy, have limited resolution, exhibit non-uniform exposure variation across the field of view, and have varying contrast and exposure from shot to shot. Common image processing techniques [17] yield poor results, with under and over segmentation, high sensitivity to threshold values, and require frequent threshold adjustments.

3 Materials and methods

We use Phillips BV 25 units with 9" field of view in all our experiments. The images were transfered from the fluoroscope's video output port to the computer using a frame grabber with a resolution of 720x560 and pixel size of 0.44mm. We built a custom dewarping grid and calibration object which is fitted via existing screw holes to the image intensifier plate. The design is inexpensive, simple to manufacture, and lightweight, to minimize additional C-arm deflection.

The dewarping grid is a 7mm thick coated aluminum alloy plate with 405 4mm diameter holes uniformly distributed at 10mm intervals machined to 0.02mm precision. It is simpler and cheaper to make than the commonly used steel balls mounted on a radiolucent plate and yields similar results. The calibration object (Fig. 2) is a hollow Delrin^{TM} three-step cylinder with eighteen 5mm diameter steel balls in three parallel planes angularly distributed to avoid overlap in the image. An additional ball in the top circular face marks the center of the object. A rectangular bar, affixed to the bottom of the cylinder, has holes that

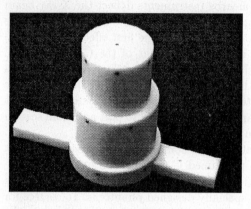 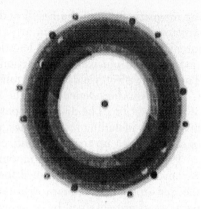

Fig. 2. Calibration object (left) and its fluoroscopic image (right).

allow mounting the object directly on the image intensifier plate. The balls are mounted at heights of 20, 100, and 180mm from the cylinder base, forming circles of 130, 115, and 90mm diameters respectively. The object weights 1.5kg.

To determine the intrinsic accuracy and repeatability error of the system, we acquired five series of images of the dewarping grid at a fixed C-arm orientation and exposure. We observed small relative rigid motion between shots introduced by the frame grabber. We correct for this motion in all our images by shifting the image pixels so that the center of the fluoroscope's circular field of view is always in the same position. Once this shift was corrected, we measured the distances between matching hole centers in pairs of images. For 1389 measurements, the mean error was $mean = 0.038$mm with standard deviation $\sigma = 0.032$mm, minimum $min = 0.001$mm, and maximum $max = 0.227$mm. Since the error is almost an order of magnitude smaller than other errors, we conclude that there is no need to take several exposures and average between them, as done in [14].

4 Image dewarping

Fluoroscopic image dewarping has received considerable attention [3]. It consists of computing a dewarp map from a reference image of a fiducials grid attached to the image intensifier plate and from the known fiducials centers geometric coordinates. The map is obtained in four steps: (1) identify the fiducials in the image from the background, (2) compute the coordinates of each fiducial center to sub-pixel accuracy, (3) pair the image and geometric fiducial centers, and (4) compute for each pairing the correction from the distances between the image and geometric fiducial center coordinates. New undistorted images are produced by computing for each pixel in the distorted image its new location and grayscale value in the undistorted image according to the dewarp map.

Global methods [3, 8] model the distortion across the entire image as a single function (e.g., a bivariate polynomial), whose coefficients are determined by least

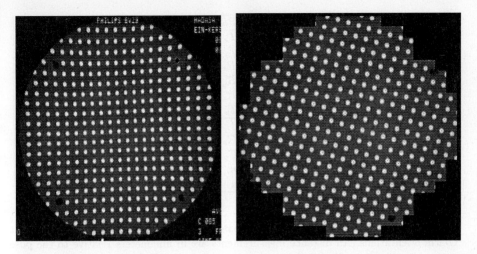

Fig. 3. Fluoroscopic images of the dewarping grid in its original position (left) and in its new position after dewarping (right). Black dots mark detected hole center points.

squares fitting of the image and geometric center coordinates. Local methods [6, 14] model the distortion by tesselating the image field of view into triangles or quadrilaterals for which individual distortion functions are computed. The functions are determined by the distances between the image and geometric fiducial center coordinates, usually by bilinear interpolation. Global methods produce compact maps, but assume that the distortion in the image is smooth and continuous. Local methods make no assumptions on the nature of the distortion and model it more accurately when it varies considerably across the field of view. Recently [3] reported comparable results when using local bilinear interpolation and global 4th-order polynomials.

We chose local bilinear interpolation because of its simplicity, computational efficiency, and generality in modeling unknown distortions. The procedure is simple to use and, unlike some others, does not require any user input for hole segmentation and center identification. The gray-scale value used in hole segmentation is automatically determined by finding the saddle point of the grid image histogram. Empirically, this proved to be an adequate threshold which yielded correct segmentation regardless of exposure setting and C-arm orientation. The center hole coordinates are computed to sub-pixel accuracy by weighted pixel gray scale average. To compute the dewarp map, the program tessellates the field of view into quadrilaterals whose endpoints are the hole center points. It uses the bilinear radial function to compute the undistorted coordinates of each image pixel. The coefficients for each region are obtained by solving a set of eight linear equations expressing the distances from the quadrilateral endpoints. The gray scale value of each new undistorted pixel is also obtained by pixel gray scale value bilinear interpolation. Since the C-arm orientation – its pitch and yaw – influences the dewarp map, we acquire distortion maps for a set of predeter-

Pose angle	Mean	Std Dev	Min	Max
(0, -10)	0.381	0.201	0	0.890
(0, 10)	0.415	0.205	0	0.937
(0, -15)	0.390	0.203	0	0.991
(0, 15)	0.313	0.193	0	0.838
(10, 15)	0.489	0.211	0	0.946
(10,-15)	0.344	0.201	0	0.913
(-10,15)	0.310	0.193	0	0.870
(0, 90)	1.931	0.541	0	2.917
(80, 0)	2.708	0.861	0	4.219
(0, 180)	2.550	0.703	0	3.717

(a) dewarping results

Param	Mean	Std Dev	Min	Max
T_x (mm)	0	0.882	-1.300	1.185
T_y (mm)	0	0.251	-0.317	0.339
R_x (deg)	0	0.342	-0.393	0.348
R_y (deg)	0	0.145	-0.233	0.169
R_z (deg)	0	0.213	-0.407	0.170
T_z (mm)	915.756	15.129	891.825	929.508
f	48.598	0.772	47.433	49.402
C_x	257.544	0.182	257.289	257.760
C_y	203.815	0.085	203.699	203.960
κ	0.00013	0.00001	0.00012	0.00015
s	1.00032	1.00283	1.00165	0.0009

(b) calibration results

Table 1. (a) Distance variation of 348 pairs of furthest center points for different C-arm orientations. All distance measurements are in millimeters relative to the pose angle yaw=$0°$, pitch=$0°$. (b) Calibration parameters nominal values and sensitivity to C-arm orientation. The extrinsic parameters T and R are with respect to a coordinate frame on the center of the image intensifier.

mined orientations. We compute dewarp maps for the most common poses, e.g., anterior-posterior and lateral views, and small angular neighborhoods around them, instead of acquiring many maps for different angular segments and interpolating between them [1,3].

To quantify how sensitive the dewarp map is to changes in C-arm orientations, and thus to determine how many predetermined orientations must be captured, we computed distortion maps at different orientations. Table 1(a) summarizes the results. We observe a significant point center shift of up to 4mm between extreme C-arm orientations and of almost 1mm for orientation of $15°$ apart. To determine the accuracy of the dewarp map function on new images, we acquired an image of the grid attached to the image intensifier cover at a fixed C-arm orientation and computed the dewarp map. Then, we detached the grid, placed it at an arbitrary angle on the cover, acquired a new image, and corrected it with the dewarp map (Fig. 3). We located the image hole centers in the new dewarped image with the hole segmentation routine, and computed a worst case error bound by taking the relative distances between pairs of points that are furthest apart. For 30 measurements, the mean error was 0.104mm, with $\sigma = 0.060$mm, $min = 0.007$mm, and $max = 0.198$mm. Previous studies report similar residual errors after correction.

5 Camera calibration

We use Tsai's [15] 11 parameter pinhole camera model and solution method to model the fluoroscopic camera. Since the parameters are pose dependent, we compute them for the same C-arm orientations as for dewarping. The parameters are the relative position $T = T_x, T_y, T_z$ and orientation $R = R_x, R_y, R_z$ of the pinhole with respect to the imaging plane, the focal length f, the image center location C_x, C_y, and the image scaling and radial distortion coefficients, s and κ. Because the images have been previously corrected, the radial image distortion assumption holds. We could set the parameters $s = 1$ and $\kappa = 0$, but we compute them anyway to further verify the dewarping procedure.

The set of equations relating the parameters are obtained by formulating the transformations from the world coordinate to the camera coordinates, transforming the 3D camera coordinates into 2D coordinates in an ideal undistorted image, and adding radial distortion, shifting, and scale. The equations can be solved in two steps, based on the radial alignment constraint. Following the camera calibration procedure for single view non-coplanar points, the extrinsic parameters R and T, with the exception of T_z, are found by solving a set of linear equations. Based on these values, the remaining parameters are derived. While this method requires at least seven points, we use the least squares method to incorporate more points.

To determine the variation for the different C-arm orientations, we conducted measurements for six extreme orientations. Table 1(b) summarizes the results. Note that the variation in T_z, which measures the distance between the camera pinhole and the image plane, is significant and confirms the deflection of the C-arm [6]. The small radial distortion and scaling deviations show that the dewarping procedure is very accurate. To quantitatively validate the accuracy of the calibration, we imaged the calibration object and computed the calibration parameters. We then constructed the projection matrix and used it to compute the geometric coordinates of the ball centers. For each ball, we computed the distance between the geometric and the image coordinate centers. The mean distance error for 78 measurements is 0.201mm with $\sigma = 0.089$mm, $min = 0.033$mm, and $max = 0.449$mm.

6 Contour extraction

Reliably extracting bone contours in fluoroscopic images is difficult because the images are noisy, have limited resolution, exhibit non-uniform exposure variation across the field of view, and have varying contrast and exposure from shot to shot. The bone structures are surrounded by tissue, contain overlapping contours, and have internal contours. Since our ultimate goal is to register the images with 3D contour models, we aim at obtaining a sufficiently dense set of points, possibly disconnected, on the bone contour with the fewest possible number of outliers.

We ruled out top-down model-based segmentation methods because they are difficult to use for anatomical structures. We considered the three main bottom-up approaches to contour segmentation: edge detection, active contours, and region growing [17]. Our experiments with standard edge detection techniques on actual fluoroscopic images showed that the Marr-Hilderth edge operator is overly sensitive to noise and non-uniform image exposure, producing too many false contours. The Canny edge detector yielded better results but required extensive threshold adjustments for every image, with frequent over and under segmentation. We ruled out the active contours techniques because they cannot detect overlapping contours require an initial guess near the target, and are computationally expensive [1]. The region growing methods yielded better results but created many spurious boundaries because of the non-uniform exposure across the field of view.

We developed a new bone contour segmentation algorithm based on robust image region statistics computation [4]. Its main advantage is that it adaptively sets local segmentation thresholds from a robust statistical analysis of image content. Working on the gradient image, it starts from global threshold setting and performs region growing based on adaptive local thresholds and zero-crossings filtering. Because the algorithm uses both global and local thresholds, it is less sensitive to the exposure variations across the field of view. Pixels are classified into one of three categories, *bone*, *candidate*, or *background*, according to the number of pixels above a predefined percentile, and not according to a prespecified absolute value. The percentile indicates the number of pixels in the gradient image histogram with gray values below (background) or above (bone), with candidate pixels in between. Initial region classification is obtained with global percentile thresholds. To overcome the non-uniform exposure, the classification is adaptively updated with local percentile thresholds over a fixed size window. Filtering the result with the original image zero crossings localizes the contour inside the region. The contour segmentation inputs global and local, upper and lower percentile thresholds, and a window size. It finds edge pixels in four steps:

1. Initial global classification
Compute the gradient image and its histogram. Set the global threshold values according to the given global image percentiles. The gradient image pixels are classified according to the global thresholds as *background* (below the lower threshold), *bone* (above the upper threshold), or *candidate* (between the lower and upper thresholds).

2. Revised local classification
For each *candidate* pixel in the gradient image, place a local window of prespecified size centered at the pixel and compute the local thresholds from its histogram. The pixel label is modified according to the local threshold values.

3. Region growing and small components elimination
Recursively relabel as *bone* all pixels labeled *candidate* with one or more neighboring *bone* pixels (either the four or eight neighboring scheme can be used). Next, remove all connected *bone* pixel components with too few pixels (e.g., less than 50) by relabeling them as *background*. They are most likely noise.

4. Filtering with zero-crossings image
Compute the binary zero-crossings image of the original image and perform an AND operation with the binary labeled gradient image. The labeled gradient image is converted to a binary image by setting *bone* pixels to 1 and *background* pixels to 0. The result are the pixels on the bone contours.

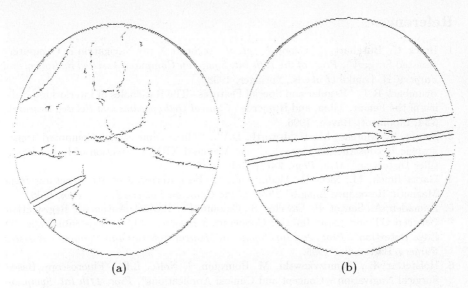

Fig. 4. Extracted pixel contours of the fluorosocopic images in Fig. 1. The contours of the metal tools were also segmented because metal density is higher than bone density.

We conducted a preliminary evaluation of the contour extraction algorithm on three sets of fluoroscopic images taken from actual surgeries. The global and local gradient image threshold percentiles (lower=60%, upper=94.7%, lower=60%, upper=99%), window size (13×13 pixels^2), and number of neighbors ($n = 4$) were kept constant for all images in a session. Fig. 4 shows typical results. Note that there are very few outliers, which can be removed with a simple model-based scheme or by combining segmentation and registration, as in [5].

7 Conclusion

We have presented a practical approach to fluoroscopic image processing consisting of image dewarping, camera calibration, and bone contour extraction. We report experimental results quantifying the accuracy of our setup and methods. We found an intrinsic system accuracy of 0.04mm, average dewarping accuracy of 0.1mm and always below 0.2mm, and average calibration error of 0.2mm and always below 0.45mm. We found significant dependence on the C-arm orientation, with dewarp variations of up to 1mm for angles of $10°$ or more, and as much as 4mm between extreme orientations. Changes in the C-arm deflection have also a significant effect on the calibration parameters. These results match those of previous studies and suggest that submillimetric spatial positioning accuracy is achievable with standard equipment. Preliminary results of the contour segmentation algorithm show good contour tracing and very few outliers. Our current work focuses on registering the extracted bone contours with surface bone models obtained from preoperative CT images and on designing experiments to establish the overall accuracy of our method.

References

1. Brack, C., Burghart, R., Czpof, A., *et. al* "Accurate X-ray Navigation in Computer-Assisted Surgery", *Proc. of the 12th Int. Symp. on Computer Assisted Radiology and Surgery*, H. Lemke *et al* eds., Springer, 1998.
2. Brumback R.J., "Regular and Special Features - The Rationales of Interlocking Nailing of the Femur, Tibia, and Humerus" *Clinical Orthopaedics and Related Research*, **324**, Lippincott-Raven, 1996.
3. Fahrig, R., Moreau, M., Holdsworth, D.W., "Three-Dimensional Computed Tomographic Reconstruction Using a C-arm Mounted XRII: Correction of Image Intensifier Distortion" *Med. Phys.* **24**(7), July 1997.
4. Garza-Jinich, M., Meer P., Medina, V., "Robust Retrieval of 3D Structures from Magnetic Resonance Images" *Proc. of the Conf. on Pattern Recognition*, 1996.
5. Hamadeh, A., Sautot, P., Lavallée, S., Cinquin, P. "Towards Automatic Registration Between CT and X-ray Images: Cooperation Between 3D/2D registration and 2D Edge Detection", *Proc. 2nd Int. Symp. on Medical Robotics and Computer Assisted Surgery*, Baltomore, 1995.
6. Hofstetter, R., Slomczykowski, M. Bourquin, I, Nolte, L.P., "Fluoroscopy Based Surgical Nagivation – Concept and Clinical Applications", *Proc. 11th Int. Symp. on Computer Assisted Radiology and Surgery*, H.U. Lemke *et al.* eds, 1997.
7. Joskowicz, L., Tockus, L., Yaniv, Z, Simkin, A., Milgrom, C. "Computer-Aided Image-Guided Bone Fracture Surgery – Concept and Implementation", *Proc. 12th Int. Symposium on Computer Assisted Radiology and Surgery*, H.U. Lemke *et. al.* eds, Springer 1998.
8. Koppe, R., Klotz, E., Op de Beek, J., Aerts, H., "3D Vessel Reconstruction Based on Rotational Angiography", *Proc. of 9th Int. Symp. on Computer Assisted Radiology*, Springer, 1995.
9. Lavallée, S., Sautot, P., Troccaz, J., Cinquin, P., Merloz, P. "Computer Assisted Spine Surgery: a Technique for Accurate Transpedicular Screw Fixation Using CT Data and a 3D Optical Localizer", *J. of Image-Guided Surgery* 1(1), 1995.
10. Li Q.H., Holdener H.J., Zamorano L., *et. al.* Nolte L.P., Visarius H., and Diaz F., "Computer-assisted transpedicular screw insertion" *Lecture Notes in Computer Science*, Springer, 1996.
11. Phillips R., Viant W.J., Mohsen A.M.M.A., Griffits J.G., Bell M.A., Cain T.J., Sherman K.P. and Karpinski M.R.K., "Image Guided Orthopaedic Surgery - Design and Analysis" *IEEE Transactions on Robotics and Control*, March 1996.
12. Sanders R. "Exposure of the Orthopaedic Surgeon to Radiation", *J. of Bone Joint Surgery* 75 A(3), 1993.
13. Simon, D.A, Jaramaz, B, Blackwell, *et al.* "Development and Validation of a Navigational Guidance System for Acetabular Implant Placement", *Proc. of CVRMed-MRCAS'97*, Lecture Notes in Computer Science 1205, Springer 1997.
14. Schreiner, S., Funda, J., Barnes, A.C., Anderson, J.H., "Accuracy Assessment of a Clinical Biplane Fluoroscope for Three-Dimensionial Measurements and Targeting", *Proc. of SPIE Medical Imaging*, 1995.
15. Tsai, R., "A Versatile Camera Calibration Technique for High-Accuracy 3D Machine Vision Metrology Using Off-the-Shelf TV Cameras and Lenses" *IEEE Journal of Robotics and Automation*, Vol. RA-3, No. 4, August 1987.
16. Viant, W.J., Phillips, R., Griffiths, et al. "A Computer Assisted Orthopaedic System for Distal Locking of Intramedullary Nails", *Proc. of MediMEC'95*, 1995.
17. Woods R.E., and Gonzalez R.C., *Digital Image Processing*, Addison-Wesley, 1992.

Probe Design to Robustly Locate Anatomical Features

Kevin B. Inkpen, Richard J. Emrich, Antony J. Hodgson

Department of Mechanical Engineering
University of British Columbia, Vancouver, BC, Canada

Abstract. Computer-assisted surgical techniques which seek to avoid relying on CT or MRI scans often require intraoperative location of anatomical features. The conventional optoelectronic probe measures a cloud of points on the feature surface, but the resulting location estimate is subject to bias and variation due both to local deformations in the surface and to measurement noise. We compare three probe designs – the conventional point probe, a flat probe and a V-probe – and show that all exhibit strong directional variability when estimating the centre of a quarter arc. We also show that the V-probe design is superior in tests on a 2D image, reducing the variability in localizing a femoral condyle by 50%.

1 Introduction

We are currently developing a technique for computer-assisted total knee replacement (TKR) surgery which does not require preoperative CT scans (similar to [1]). Certain variations of our approach require approximating centres of the posterior portions of the femoral condyles, which have been shown to closely fit spherical surfaces [2]. We propose to pass an optoelectronic digitizing probe over the condylar surfaces and fit a sphere to them, taking the centre of the fitted sphere as the condylar centre. This paper concentrates on the reliability of this latter process. In particular, we wish to characterize the repeatability with which we can define these centres.

Commercially available probes usually have a point or small (about 2 mm diameter) spherical end that touches the subject (see Figure 1). Such probes are versatile in that they can be used define points on surfaces with detailed concave and convex features. In our application, however, the subject surface is generally convex with local flaws that do not represent the ideal sliding surface that we are trying to locate. We suggest alternative probe designs that may be less sensitive to local deformations in the articular surface and may lead to more reliable estimates of the condylar centres. For general registration applications as discussed in [3], the effect of probe design should be considered when the goal is to quickly gather data that accurately constrain a convex feature.

In this paper we investigate using a probe with a flat contact surface to provide data as a series of tangent lines (rather than points) as the probe is swept along a surface. We also investigate the use of a V shaped probe that returns a series of local curvature bisector lines from a similar scan. A best fit 'centre' point of the contour can be found by minimizing an appropriate cost function. At this stage, we are interested in the repeatability of an estimated centre point location found from a single scan of a surface.

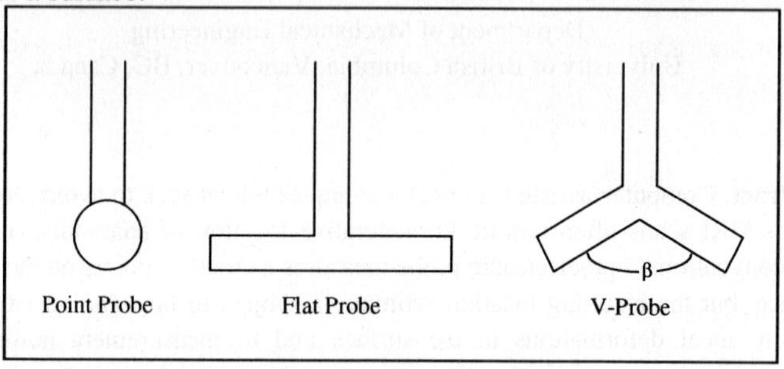

Fig. 1. Different Probe Designs

We simulate 1000 scans each over two different 2D test curves using each probe design and compare the standard deviations from the mean of the resulting estimated centres. We show that the V-probe exhibits significantly less standard deviation, thus better repeatability, than the other two designs.

2 Methodology

We simulated tests of a point probe, a flat probe, and V-probes with a variety of β angles (10° increments from 120° to 170°) on two reference curves:
(1) the circumference of a true quarter arc with a 13 mm radius.
(2) the posterior-distal quadrant of a 2D contour of the lateral condyle of a human femur (~13 mm radius) obtained from a sagittal MRI of a 31 year old female with no significant knee pathology.

For both curves, we simulated sweeping the probes across a 90° range, added measurement noise, and found the best-fit centre point by minimizing an appropriate cost function (see Sections 2.1 - 2.3) using MATLAB's Nelder-Mead simplex method.

For each probe type and each reference curve, we ran 1000 simulated scans which resulted in 1000 estimated centres. We then computed the standard deviation of centre point location as a measure of the repeatability of the probe type.

We simulated the intraoperative process of acquiring points along the curve as a rotation of the probe about the origin (roughly the centre of the curve) with the radius being determined by the requirement that the probe maintain contact with the curve. In practice the surgeon would tend to start with the probe at one end of the curve with zero velocity, sweep through approximately 90°, and come to rest at the end of the curve. We therefore calculated the sampling position vector θ as:

$$\theta = \theta_s + (\theta_f - \theta_s)(1 + \sin(\pi((t/t_s) - 0.5)))/2 \qquad (1)$$

where t is a vector of time steps from t = 0 to total scanning time (t_s) with a step size of (sampling frequency)$^{-1}$. θ_s and θ_f are the start and finish angles of the scanned range. In this study t_s = 1 s, sampling freq. = 60 Hz, θ_s = 90°, and θ_f = 180° for all simulations and all angles are measured positively CCW from the x axis. For the V-probes, the range of θ was reduced to [$\theta_f - (\pi - \beta)/2$] - [$\theta_s + (\pi - \beta)/2$] to ensure that there was no contact outside of the sampled range used for the other probes.

During each simulation, we added white noise with σ = 0.02 radians to each sampling position θ to ensure that we were not always sampling at the same points. We also added white noise with σ = 0.2 mm to all (x,y) coordinate data to simulate the measurement errors of a typical optoelectronic localizer. Assuming a distance of 120 mm from the probe surface to the probe markers, a corresponding white noise with σ = 0.20/120 = 0.0017 radians was added to all angular data.

2.1 Point Probe

To estimate the centre of the best-fit circle, we computed the contact point of the probe to the surface at each sampling position θ and added noise as described above, producing a set of noisy data points (x_p, y_p). With candidate circles defined by their centre coordinates and radius (x_c, y_c, r_c), the point probe cost function 'PPCF' is the sum of squared normal distances from the points to the candidate circle:

$$PPCF = \Sigma \left(r_c - ((x_p - x_c)^2 + (y_p - y_c)^2)^{1/2} \right)^2 \qquad (2)$$

2.2 Flat Probe

For the flat probe, we calculated the contact point between the probe and the surface contour, (x_f, y_f), and the angle of the probe face, (α), at each sampling position θ and added noise. The flat probe cost function 'FPCF' is the sum of squared distances along the lines coperpendicular to both the candidate circle and the flat probe:

$$FPCF = \Sigma \left((x_f - x_t) \sin \alpha + (y_f - y_t) \cos \alpha \right)^2 \qquad (3)$$

where (x_t, y_t) are the co-ordinates of the point on the candidate circle whose tangent is parallel to the probe face.

2.3 V-Probe

At each sampling position θ, the V-shaped probe contacts the surface contour in two places and the centre of any 'local' best-fit circle at this sampling position must lie somewhere along the bisector of the V. As the probe is swept along the surface contour over the scanned range, these bisectors form a set of lines intersecting near the centre of an overall best-fit circle. The angle of each bisector, γ, and a point on the bisector at the apex of the V, (x_v, y_v), form the data set and have noise applied. The cost function 'VPCF' expresses the sum of the squared normal distances between the candidate centre point, (x_c, y_c), and the bisectors:

$$VPCF = \Sigma ((x_v - x_c) \sin \gamma - (y_v - y_c) \cos \gamma)^2 \qquad (4)$$

Note that in this case, we cannot explicitly estimate the radius of the arc.

3 Results

3.1 True Arc

Figures 2 and 3 show the 1000 estimated arc centres for the point probe and 140° V-probes respectively. The results for the flat probe are comparable to the point probe and so are not shown here. Note the extended distribution of these estimates along the axis of symmetry of the arc.

To evaluate the repeatability of each probe design, standard deviations in centre point location were found for two different measures: 'Sym. Axis' is the standard deviation measured parallel to the bisector of the scanned range. 'Perp. Axis' is the standard deviation measured perpendicular to the bisector of the range.

Table 1. Standard deviations of centre point location from true arc

	Sym. Axis (mm)	Perp. Axis (mm)
Point	0.134	0.043
Flat	0.116	0.041
V120	0.137	0.025
V130	0.112	0.027
V140	0.080	0.027
V150	0.070	0.028
V160	0.062	0.030
V170	0.056	0.028

3.2 Posterior-Distal Condyle Image

As in the first test, 1000 scans were simulated with each probe design on the same set of points representing the contour of a sagittal section through the distal femur. All three probe designs proposed a different mean centre point location (See Fig. 4).

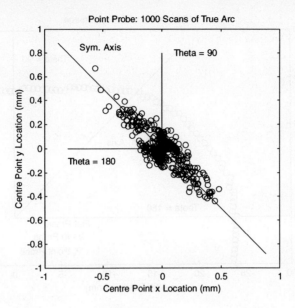

Fig. 2. Point probe: Estimated centre point locations for true arc.

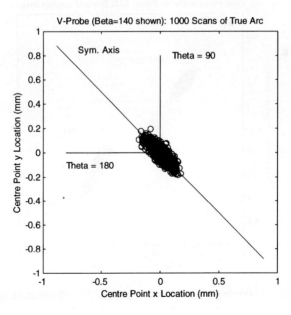

Fig. 3. V140 Probe ($\beta = 140°$): Estimated centre point locations for true arc.

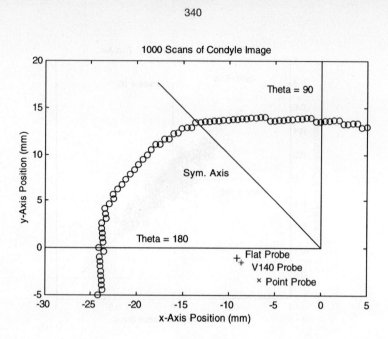

Fig. 4. Average centre point estimation for each probe design on condyle image.

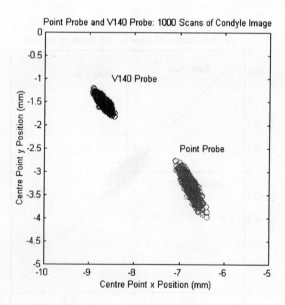

Fig. 5. Distribution of centre point estimates for point and V140 probes on condyle image.

Repeatability of each probe design was calculated again and is shown in Fig. 6.

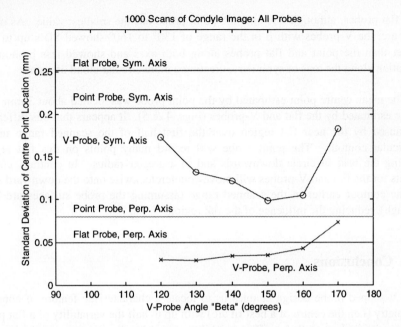

Fig. 6. Standard deviation of centre point location on condyle image, all probe designs.

4.0 Discussion

The extent of the cloud of centre point estimates derived from the true arc indicates sensitivity to measurement noise. All three probes exhibited 2-5X more deviation along the arc's axis of symmetry than perpendicular to it. This can be explained by looking at the cost functions: For the point and flat probes, the circle descriptors involve three parameters (x, y, and r), where negative displacements of (x,y) along the arc's axis of symmetry coupled with increases in radius (r) will cause the least change in cost. For the V-probe, (x,y) are found to minimize the summed distances to the radial data lines (set of bisectors), so displacements in the direction 'most parallel' to the average data line (ie. along the arc's axis of symmetry) will cause the least change in cost. The SD of the flat probe's centre estimate distribution is ~15% lower than that of the point probe, but the V-probe's distributions showed further reductions of 35-50% in SD, showing that it is markedly less sensitive to measurement noise. Increased V-probe angles (β) produced significantly lower standard deviations of the point location along the axis of symmetry but had no significant effect perpendicular to the axis of symmetry.

On the condyle image, all three probes again showed maximum SD along the axis of symmetry of the best fit arc. There is a small difference in SD between the point and flat probes, although this time the point probe has the smallest value. As on the true arc, the V-probes with β in the range of 130° to 160° showed SD's up to 50% lower than the point and flat probes along both axes and showed less pronounced variation along the axis of symmetry, creating a more circular cloud of points.

The mean centre point estimated by the point probe was located about 3 mm from those estimated by the flat and V-probes (Figs. 4 & 5). It appears that this difference is caused by the near flat region over the first half of the scanned range in this particular contour. The point probe will record many points on this flat region, forcing the best fit circle downwards and to a greater radius. In contrast, contact points for the flat and V-probes will move counterclockwise onto the downward slope of the contour earlier in the scanned range (assuming the probe surfaces are large enough), reducing the influence of the flat region.

5.0 Conclusions

The V-shaped probe design enables us to locate a characteristic feature of condylar geometry (i.e., the centre of a best fit arc) with up to half the variability of a flat probe or conventional point probe. The variability of this localization is greatest along the arc's axis of symmetry. We are planning to extend this study to three dimensions, where the V-probe will be replaced by a three-faced pyramidal probe. Such a probe is also likely to have benefits in other registration applications.

Acknowledgements

We thank Dr. Boris Flak of the UBC Department of Radiology for help in obtaining the MRI scan of the knee, Roger Tam of the UBC MAGIC Lab for assistance in converting the image for use in this project, and Robert W. McGraw of the UBC Department of Orthopaedics for discussions on TKR procedure.

References

1. Leitner, F., Picard.F., Minfelde, R., Schulz, H-J., Cinquin P., Saragaglia D.: Computer Assisted Knee Replacement Surgical Total Replacement. In: Troccaz, J., Grimson, E., Mosges, R. (eds): CVRMed-MRCAS '97. Lecture Notes in Computer Science, Vol. 1205. Springer-Verlag, Berlin Heidelberg New York (1997) 627-638.
2. Kurosawa, H., Walker, PS.,Abe, S.,Garg, A., Hunter, T. : Geometry and Motion of the Knee for Implant and Orthotic Design. Journal of Biomechanics (1985); 18 (7): 487 - 499.
3. Simon, D.A., Hebert, M.., Kanade T.: Techniques for Fast and Accurate Intra-Surgical Registration. In: DiGioia, A.M., Kanade, T.,Taylor, R. (eds.): MRCAS '94, Vol. 1. Pittsburgh, Pennsylvania. (1994) 90-97.

Concepts and Results in the Development of a Hybrid Tracking System for CAS

Wolfgang Birkfellner[1]*, Franz Watzinger[2], Felix Wanschitz[2], Georg Enislidis[2], Michael Truppe[3], Rolf Ewers[2] and Helmar Bergmann[1,4]

[1] Department of Biomedical Engineering and Physics, University of Vienna
[2] Clinic of Oral and Maxillofacial Surgery, Medical School, University of Vienna
[3] ARTMA Medizintechnik, Vienna
[4] Ludwig-Boltzmann Institute of Nuclear Medicine, Vienna

Abstract. We present the design and the results achieved in the development of a hybrid magneto-optic tracking system suitable for computer aided surgery. Our approach towards a reliable and accurate hybrid position sensor system that is not entirely dependent on an unobstructed line-of-sight between sensor assembly and patient is the combined use of an optical tracker with a direct current (DC) pulsed electromagnetic tracking system (EMTS). The proposed hybridization method aims at providing both accurate and uninterrupted position data by overcoming the drawbacks of both tracking technologies. Results presented include the preliminary assessment of algorithms for fusion of position data from both sensor systems, for calibrating the EMTS to the environment and for detecting systematic distortions in the DC tracking system caused by ferromagnetic materials in order to improve the reliability of the proposed system.

1 Introduction

Navigation systems employed in computer aided surgery (CAS) are gaining increased acceptance as accurate and reliable tools for interventions where utmost accuracy is necessary [1]. While optical [2, 3, 4] and mechanical systems provide reliable position data, neither of these approaches can be considered perfect. Optical tracking systems (OTS) can be obstructed; the optical contact between patient and camera can break and cause a complete failure of the navigation device. This is not a severe drawback in interventions where the patient is immobilized by a Mayfield clamp or a similar device since only one instrument has to be tracked continuously. Most other interventions make it necessary to track both the patient and the tool. In interventions with a crowded operating field such as cranio- and maxillofacial surgery we consider the line-of-sight requirement to be a restriction forcing the surgeon to modify proven techniques. The usage of electromagnetic tracking systems (EMTS) which are not dependent on a free line-of-sight date back to the beginnings of CAS. The fact that the magnetic

---
* e-mail: wbirk@bmtp.akh-wien.ac.at

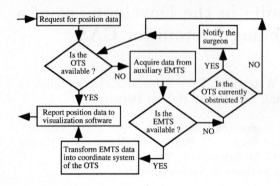

Fig. 1. A flow diagram of the hybrid tracking system. If the optical component of the system is unavailable due to obstruction of the optical path or low sampling rates of the OTS data from the auxiliary sensor system are employed and checked for validity. The methods for registration of the tracking systems and for assessing the data from the EMTS are presented in the paper.

field can be distorted by conductive or ferromagnetic materials in the vicinity of the sensor or the field emitter does, however, limit the usability of these devices for high precision surgical interventions. Experiments showed distortions caused by common surgical tools of 1.5-15 mm and 1-4° [5]. Our approach towards a tracking system that overcomes these problems is to combine a direct current (DC) pulsed electromagnetic system with a highly accurate OTS. In order to ensure the reliability of such a hybrid tracker distortions in the reference field of the EMTS induced by ferromagnetic tools have to be noticed. Earlier work on sensor fusion for head tracking in augmented reality (AR) [6] lacks this feature.

In order to make a hybrid magneto-optic system usable for CAS the following criteria had to be fulfilled:

- assessment of method for registration of the tracking systems in order to report position data in a common coordinate system $\text{Ref}_{\text{optical}}$ (fig. 2).
- development of calibration and registration algorithms for providing sufficient spatial accuracy of both tracking system components (error ≈ 1 - 1.5 mm and 1° in the operating theater).
- methods for ensuring the reliability of the electromagnetic tracker component by checking the validity of the position data acquired from the auxiliary EMTS.

A flow diagram of the data acquisition cycle can be seen in fig. 1. Once a request is being sent from the visualization software the system checks whether it can provide data from the OTS; if the OTS is not available, either due to obstruction of light emitting diodes (LED) or because of low sampling rates, the system requests position information from the electromagnetic component. In this case the hybrid system checks the validity of the readings and forwards the data, which have to be transformed to the coordinate system of the OTS only if the EMTS is not distorted. Therefore the system is able to handle periods of obstruction of the optical sensor component. Furthermore, the system's update rate is given by the sampling rate of the faster of the two systems when both trackers are in an operational state. Since the EMTS used is a DC pulsed system (the

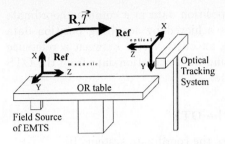
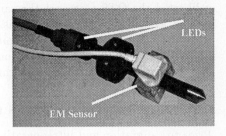

Fig. 2. Sketch illustrating the principle of the hybrid tracking system. The optical tracking system can be registered relative to the EMTS prior to a surgical intervention in order to obtain the transformation parameters **R** and **T**, which merge the coordinate frames of the EMTS and the OTS.

Fig. 3. Stylus setup used for the initial assessment of the hybrid tracking system. A stylus made of non- ferromagnetic materials (carbon fiber and titanium) was equipped with 16 LEDs and an electromagnetic sensor (EM Sensor).

magnetic reference field is produced by coils which are fed by rectangular currents rather than with alternating currents with continuously changing voltage) it is only susceptible to artifacts induced by ferromagnetic metals. Conductive materials do not affect the accuracy of the tracker [5] since the quasistatic magnetic field does not induce eddy currents in conductive materials once the field has been established.

2 Materials and Methods

2.1 Hardware

The tracking systems used for our laboratory investigations are a widely used OTS (Flashpoint 5000, Image Guided Technologies Inc., Boulder, USA) with a spatial accuracy of 0.3 - 1.5 mm [2, 3] and a DC driven EMTS (Flock of Birds, Ascension Technologies Inc, Colchester, USA). According to the specifications the nominal accuracy of the EMTS in an environment containing no ferromagnetic materials is given as 1.8 mm/0.5°, and the spatial resolution is 0.5 mm/0.2°. For data acquisition and implementation of the algorithms an IBM-PC running DOS 6.21 and Borland C++ 5.0 was used. All software routines were implemented in ANSI-C.

2.2 Clinical application and tool design

The hybrid tracking system is planned for further refinement of techniques already in use at our hospital [7]. Fig. 3 shows the carbon fiber stylus which was used for our experiments. It contains 16 LEDs which ensure that position and orientation can be determined accurately by the OTS at all viewing angles. For laboratory tests we attached one EMTS sensor to the tool as shown (fig. 3) and calibrated the OTS to report the same position data in a common coordinate system as the magnetic sensor; this was achieved by acquiring position data from the EMTS sensor and determining an offset vector between a reference LED and the reported sensor position using the orientation data from the OTS and a Monte-Carlo optimization technique.

2.3 Registration of the EMTS to the OTS

Prior to calibration and intraoperative use the coordinate systems $\text{Ref}_{\text{magnetic}}$ and $\text{Ref}_{\text{optical}}$ have to be registered relative to each other. The position readings from the OTS ($\mathbf{p}_{\text{opt}}$) and the EMTS ($\mathbf{p}_{\text{mag}}$) are merged by transforming $\mathbf{p}_{\text{mag}}$ to optical tracker space according to

$$\hat{\mathbf{p}}_{\text{mag}} = \mathbf{R}\mathbf{p}_{\text{mag}} + \mathbf{T} \tag{1}$$

where $\hat{\mathbf{p}}_{\text{mag}}$ denotes the position data obtained from the EMTS in optical tracker space. The transformation parameters $\mathbf{R}$ (a rotation matrix) and $\mathbf{T}$ (the translation vector) were determined by applying a point-to-point registration algorithm based on singular value decomposition (SVD) [8]. The SVD-algorithm was taken from [9].

2.4 Compensation of the influence from the OR environment on the EMTS

For reasons to be discussed later the magnetic field emitter of the EMTS has to be placed below the OR table in a clinical setup. In a previous study on an acrylic skull model we found the distorting effect of the static OR-environment to be significant (6.4±2.5 mm / 4.9±2.0°) [5].

Therefore we implemented a calibration method for compensating the influence of the environment by using a distortion mapping technique [10, 11, 12]. A lookup table (LUT) was used to compensate the distortions caused by the static environment. This was achieved by acquiring accurate position information from the OTS and by correcting each measurement from the EMTS to the proper value. In our laboratory setup the digitizing volume of 200*200*200 mm³ was divided by a grid of 50 mm width. The stylus was placed to the grid positions in magnetic tracker space with an accuracy of ± 1.5 mm. After placing the stylus at these positions the difference vector

$$\mathbf{\Delta}_{ijk_{\text{LUT}}} = \mathbf{R}^{\text{T}} \left(\mathbf{p}_{\text{opt}} - \mathbf{T} \right) - \mathbf{p}_{\text{mag}} \tag{2}$$

was determined. Before being reported to the visualization software the measurements from the EMTS have to be corrected and transformed to optical tracker space by calculating

$$\mathbf{p}'_{\text{mag}} = \mathbf{R} \left(\mathbf{p}_{\text{mag}} + \mathbf{\Delta}_{ijk_{\text{LUT}}} \right) + \mathbf{T} \tag{3}$$

The grid positions in magnetic tracker space are denoted by the indices i, j and k. The grid point associated to a position $\mathbf{p}_{\text{mag}}$ is determined by seeking the closest

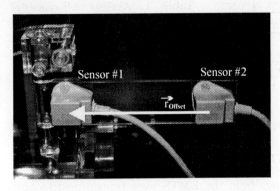

Fig. 4. Setup for detecting distortions in the EMTS. Two fluxgate sensors (Ascension Technologies Inc.) are mounted to a perspex plate (representing a rigid body) on a non-metallic frame. The difference between the true position of sensor #1 and the measured value caused by a ferromagnetic sample was compared to the difference of the measured value $|\|x_1 - x_2\||$ from the known distance $\|r_{\text{Offset}}\|$ of the sensors on the plate.

point on the calibration grid. The optimal value for $\Delta_{ijk_{\text{LUT}}}$ was approximated using a linear interpolation.

A distortion mapping method meeting the high requirements of CAS also has to take into account the error in orientation data. However, calibrating the distortion of the orientation data for the EMTS is too difficult because of the number of measurements necessary. This is illustrated by the fact that authors in [10, 11, 12] have not attempted to correct the orientation distortion. A possible solution to this problem is discussed.

2.5 Automated Assessment of the Accuracy of Position Data obtained from the EMTS

When using an EMTS in a surgical navigation device it is of vital importance to check the correctness of the position data acquired. Unlike the OTS, which fails in the case of obstruction but is highly accurate when a free line-of-sight to the camera bar is provided, the accuracy of the EMTS is affected by systematic errors caused by the high magnetic susceptibility of ferromagnetic materials and by a poor signal-to-noise ratio at greater distances from the emitter.

Our approach to ensure the reliability of acquired data without additional control from the OTS is to mount several sensors onto a rigid body (fig. 4). Due to the complex nature of the magnetic field the variation in field strength caused by a small body (i. e. a surgical tool) or by noisy readings is not shift-invariant. Therefore comparing the known distance r_{Offset} on the rigid body to the measured apparent distance of two sensors in magnetic tracker space is a measure of the accuracy of the EMTS.

EMTS Readings	$|\Delta x|$ [mm]	$|\Delta y|$ [mm]	$|\Delta z|$ [mm]	$\overline{\Delta r}$ [mm]
Uncorrected	1.1 ± 1.0	2.0 ± 1.0	2.8 ± 0.8	3.9 ± 0.9
Corrected	0.7 ± 0.9	1.1 ± 0.8	1.4 ± 0.9	2.2 ± 1.0

Table 1. Average difference of measurements (N=125) from the distortion corrected and uncorrected EMTS data transformed to optical tracker space and the measurements from the OTS.

3 Results

3.1 Calibration of the EMTS

In a first experiment the readings from the EMTS were transformed to optical tracker space using the initial registration parameters $\mathbf{R}$ and $\mathbf{T}$ acquired from uncorrected readings $\mathbf{p}_{i_{\text{mag}}}$. The corrected and uncorrected measurements $\left(\hat{\mathbf{p}}'_{i_{\text{mag}}} \text{ and } \hat{\mathbf{p}}_{i_{\text{mag}}}\right)$ were compared to the data $\mathbf{p}_{i_{\text{opt}}}$ acquired from the OTS, and both the translation errors $|\Delta x|, |\Delta y|$ and $|\Delta z|$ as well as the euclidean error Δr were determined and averaged (table 1).

3.2 Detection of Environmental Distortions

The experimental setup shown in fig. 4 was used to determine the sensitivity of the proposed method for determining the reliability of the position readings from the EMTS with distorting materials like surgical tools present. The complete setup is described in more detail in [5]. The deviation induced by a steel rod (150 mm length, 10 mm diameter) from the known position of sensor #1 was assessed by evaluating

$$\Delta_{\text{det}} = \left| \|\mathbf{x}_2 - \mathbf{x}_1\|_{\text{measured}} - \|\mathbf{r}_{\text{Offset}}\|_{\text{known}} \right| \qquad (4)$$

where $\mathbf{x}_1$ and $\mathbf{x}_2$ denote the readings from sensor #1 and #2, and $\|\mathbf{r}_{\text{Offset}}\|$ is the known distance of the sensors on the rigid body as shown in fig. 4. The difference between the fixed position of sensor #1 and the acquired measurement $\mathbf{x}_1$ was compared to the quantity Δ_{det} (fig. 5). 100 measurements were taken and the difference between the true position of sensor #1 and the acquired value $\mathbf{x}_1$ was plotted together with Δ_{det} as a function of the distance of the ferromagnetic sample to the sensor assembly. The values for the distance sample - sensor were collected into adjacent bins with a width of 50 mm, and the ordinate values were averaged within these bins. It can be seen that an erratic reading of $\mathbf{x}_1$ also induces a deviation Δ_{det} which serves as a measure for the reliability of position data acquired.

In order to avoid artifacts due to Gaussian noise a threshold $\Delta_{\text{det}_{\text{thresh}}}$ for the deviation Δ_{det} was defined. If Δ_{det} exceeded this value the system was considered to be distorted. In 77 % of all cases the EMTS was found to be distorted beyond a limit of 1.0 mm. Several values for the threshold $\Delta_{\text{det}_{\text{thresh}}}$ were used (0.5, 1.0, 1.5 and 2.0 mm) for detecting these cases. The percentage of detected distortions

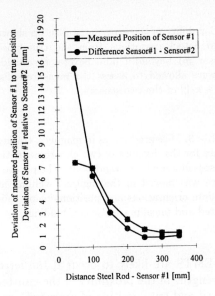

Fig. 5. Deviation from a constant position of electromagnetic sensor #1 induced by a steel rod compared to the deviation of two sensors mounted to a perspex plate as shown in fig. 4. The displacement of the measured value from sensor #1 and quantity Δ_{det} (eq. 4) are shown as a function of the distance between sensor assembly and ferromagnetic sample.

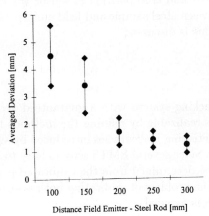

Fig. 6. Averaged error of EMTS sensor readings in cases where the distortion Δ_{det} caused by a steel sample exceede 1 mm and was not detected when using a threshold $\Delta_{det_{thresh}}$ of 1 mm. Associated with each value is the percentage of the 25 cases where undetected distortion ocurred. The x-axis denotes the distance of the ferromagnetic sample from the field emitter. The averaged true error is displayed together with its standard deviation.

as a function of $\Delta_{det_{thresh}}$ is presented in table 2. From these results we concluded that a value of 1 mm would be optimal for $\Delta_{det_{thresh}}$ since the spatial resolution of the EMTS is given as 0.5 mm.

In a further experiment we assessed the accuracy of the measured value $\|\mathbf{x}_2 - \mathbf{x}_1\|_{measured}$ with and without LUT correction by moving the perspex plate shown in fig. 4 to 100 positions at random orientations (table 3). It can be seen that a value of 1.2 mm for $\Delta_{det_{thresh}}$ was realizable in the laboratory experiments.

Furthermore we analyzed the cases where the error induced by the steel sample exceeded 1 mm and was not detected by the mechanism described above. It is straightforward to assume that the performance of the distortion detection methods is poor in cases where the distance from the sensor assembly and the ferromagnetic body exceeds the distance of the two electromagnetic sensors

$\Delta_{det_{thresh}}$	Detection rate (in %)
0.5	87
1.0	67
1.5	39
2.0	28

Table 2. Capability of the experimental setup shown in fig. 4 to detect deviations from the true position of sensor #1 beyond 1 mm. Several thresholds $\Delta_{det_{thresh}}$ were allowed to assess the measured distance $|\|x_1 - x_2\||$ of the two sensors.

EMTS-readings	$\|r_1 - r_2\|$ [mm]	max	min
Uncorrected	102.7 ± 1.0	105.2	100.9
Corrected	103.1 ± 0.6	104.0	102.0

Table 3. Measured values in magnetic tracker space for the distance of two electromagnetic sensors mounted on a rigid body. The perspex plate was moved in the digitizer volume at random orientations and positions using calibrated and uncalibrated sensor readings.

significantly. Erratic readings from the EMTS are likely to occur if the ferromagnetic tool is exposed to high field strengths in the proximity of the emitter. The averaged difference between measured and true position of sensor #1 was assessed as a function of the distance between steel sample and field emitter (fig. 6). A strategy for avoiding these situations is discussed.

4 Discussion

From our results we conclude that a tracking system with a guaranteed accuracy of less that 2 mm euclidean error is realizable by refining the methods for compensating static distortions and for detecting inaccuracies introduced by surgical instruments presented in this paper. Since several EMTS sensors have to be used, five or six degrees of freedom can be determined from the calibrated position readings only. In this configuration the problem of calibrating both position and orientation readings from the EMTS is avoided.

In order to improve the detection rate of invalid readings from the EMTS (fig. 6) it is necessary to physically block the emitter from the events in the operating theater. Mounting the emitter below the OR table and applying the distortion mapping routine appears to be a method for achieving this. Since the magnetic field used for position determination is very weak the operating range of the EMTS is delimited to a sphere of less than one meter in diameter. Outside this volume we have found the influence of the OR inventory to be negligible [5].

A user-friendly surgical tracking system should also be easy to be set up. Our method to perform this is to place the field emitter in a fixed position below the OR table. The influence of the ferromagnetic environment therefore has to be compensated once, whereas the optical component is registered relative to the calibrated EMTS before each intervention by using the methods described.

Some drawbacks of the current design include the difficulty of realizing wireless tracking like in videometric systems [4] although the rather huge number of signal leads from the single magnetometers can be reduced by multiplexing the raw sensor readings. Changing the geometry of the OR-table (for instance by tilting parts of it) would also destroy the registration of the setup.

We conclude that the development of hybrid tracking technologies has the potential to provide a reliable and user-friendly tracking system which promotes the integration of CAS technologies in demanding clinical routine applications.

5 Acknowledgment

We wish to thank A. Gamperl and W. Piller for their help in designing and manufacturing the hardware necessary for the experiments as well as Len Chamberlain (Image Guided Technologies Inc.) and Steve Work (Ascension Technologies Inc.) for their kind advice. Part of this work was supported by the Austrian Science Foundation FWF (Research Grant No. P12464-MED).

References

1. R. H. Taylor, S. Lavallée, G. C. Burdea, R. Mösges (eds.): "Computer-Integrated Surgery - Technology and Applications", MIT Press, Cambridge, (1996).
2. S. A. Tebo, D. A. Leopold, D. M. Long et al.: "An Optical 3D Digitizer for Frameless Stereotactic Surgery", IEEE Comput Graph, 55 - 64, (1996).
3. W. E. L. Grimson, G. J. Ettinger, S. J. White et al.: "An Automatic Registration Method for Frameless Stereotaxy, Image Guided Surgery, and Enhanced Reality Visualization", IEEE T Med Imaging, Vol. MI 15(2), 129-140, (1996).
4. A. C. F. Colchester, J. Zhao, K. S. Holton-Tainter et al.: "Development and preliminary evaluation of VISLAN, a surgical planning and guidance system using intraoperative video imaging", Med Image Anal, Vol. 1(1), 73-90, (1996).
5. W. Birkfellner, F. Watzinger, F. Wanschitz et al.: "Systematic Distortions in Magnetic Position Digitizers", paper accepted for publication in Med Phys.
6. A. State, G. Hirota, D. T. Chen et al.: "Superior Augmented Reality Registration by Integrating Landmark Tracking and Magnetic Tracking", Proceedings of SIGGRAPH 96, in Computer Graphics Proceedings, ACM SIGGRAPH, 429 - 438, (1996).
7. F. Watzinger, F. Wanschitz, A. Wagner et al.: "Computer-Aided Navigation in Secondary Reconstruction of Post- Traumatic Deformities of the Zygoma", J. Craniomaxillofac. Surg. 25, 198 - 202, (1997).
8. K. S. Arun, T. S. Huang, S. D. Blostein, "Least- Squares Fitting of Two 3-D Point Sets", IEEE T Pattern Anal Vol. PAMI-9(5), 698-700, (1987).
9. W. H. Press, S. A. Teukolsky, W. T. Vetterling, B. P. Flannery: "Numerical Recipes in C - The Art of Scientific Computing, Second Edition", Cambridge University Press, (1992).
10. S. Bryson: "Measurement and calibration of static distortion of position data from 3D trackers", SPIE Vol. 1669, 244 - 255, (1992).
11. M. Ghazisaedy, D. Adamczyk, D. J. Sandin et al.: "Ultrasonic Calibration of a Magnetic Tracker in a Virtual Reality Space", in VRAIS '95, March 11-15, 1995, Proceedings, 179 - 188, (1995).
12. M. A. Livingston, A. State: "Magnetic Tracker Calibration for Improved Augmented Reality Registration", Presence Vol. 6(5), 532 - 546, (1997).

Computer-Assisted Interstitial Brachytherapy

W. Freysinger, E. Hensler*, A. R. Gunkel, R. J. Bale**, M. Vogele, A. Martin, T. Auer**, P. Eichberger**,
A. Szankay**, T. Auberger**, K. H. Künzel***, O. Gaber***, W. F. Thumfart, P. H. Lukas**

Clinic of Ear-, Nose-, and Throat Diseases
University of Innsbruck, Anichstr. 35, A-6020 Innsbruck, Austria.
e-mail: Wolfgang.Freysinger@uibk.ac.at
* Clinic of Radiotherapy and Oncology
** Department of Radiology I
*** Institute of Anatomy****
University of Innsbruck
Anichstr. 35, A-6020 Innsbruck, Austria
****Müllerstr. 59, A-6020 Innsbruck, Austria

Abstract:
We present the current state-of-the art of computer-assisted interstitial (fractionated) brachytherapy as a "picture-book" without wanting to give an in-depth presentation of either brachytherapy itself or of otolaryngologic aspects of oncologic treatment. However, our results show that 3D-computer-assisted navigation techniques can successfully be applied in interstitial brachytherapy to exactly plan the hollow-needle's position(s) in order to reach a prospective planning of brachytherapy which exploits the full 3D-information of the modern imagery and incorporates state-of-the-art navigational techniques.

Patients:

All patients were informed about the nature of the treatment and gave their consent to participate in this clinical study. The tumors in the study included metastases of a hepatocellular carcinoma, adenoid cystic carcinoma (2 of the tonsil, 2 of the tongue, 2 of the floor of mouth, and 2 combinations thereof), 1 Schmincke carcinoma caudal of the sphenoid, in the pharyngeal space, and one secondary carcinoma of the tonsil. All together, 25 individual sessions were undertaken.

Materials and Methods:

The general approach is briefly outlined in the following. After an interdisciplinary discussion between the two departments (ENT and ROI) a palliative approach was chosen in all cases. The high-dose-rate brachytherapy is delivered fractionated to place, typically 30 Gy into the tumor, in ideally four sessions. Our approach is to insert the hollow needles every session anew in weekly intervals. Starting with a joint ENT-ROI definition of the optimal tumor target, the access trajectory, the number of needles needed to irradiate the tumor the procedure is defined. This plan implements an optimized patient positioning for treatment. Once the patient positioning is defined it is maintained throughout all sessions of therapy, unless intraoperative changes arise due to unforeseeable circumstances. The patient undergoes 3D-CT scanning (Siemens Somatom +, Germany) in the according position. We do, depending on the location of the tumor and depending on the general conditions of the patient, the scans either with or without general anesthesia. Typically, the patient is hospitalized for three days: at the very fist day of treatment the navigation is prepared: CT-Scanning, and creation of a 3D-reconstruction of the patient on the Allegro workstation (ISG Technologies, Canada), and setup of the Viewing Wand navigation system itself (ISG Technologies, Canada). The second day the intervention takes place under general anesthesia and the third day, to allow sufficient patient recovery and monitoring, the patient is released.

The navigation system:

This well-known 3D-navigation system comprises either a position sensitive mechanical articulated arm (Faro, USA) or the recent IR-LED equipped probes and the optical Polaris digitizer (NDI, USA).The ISG Viewing Wand allows to precisely determine the actual position within the patient's 3D-CT data set; the position is visualized as the origin of a set of crosshairs in the three regular CT views, multiplanar reformats and the 3D-reconstruction. More detailed information about the navigation system and related information can be found elsewhere.[1-5]

Initially, we used the arm itself to perform a real-time positional control of the brachytherapy needle. However, we found that the chance to bend the needles are substantial, especially when attached to the position-sensitive articulated arm. Based on laboratory investigations and cadaver studies we designed a targeting device which is in use now regularly. Moreover, the implementation of the targeting device allows to separate the planning process from surgery in time and space: we now do preplanning with the VBH-mouthpiece and the headholder in conjunction with the targeting device the day before the intervention. The alignment of the whole setup is kept throughout the whole duration of the fractionated brachytherapy unless intraoperative changes have to be made, like alterations of the alignment of the targeting device due to mechanical interferences with the patient etc. (*Nota bene*: this may occur since the planning is without the patient on the Viewing Wand and chest, shoulders or the cranial part of the thorax itself is not imaged!)

The patient fixation system:

The necessary immobilization is achieved by means of the VBH-headholder [6], a registration mouthpiece [7] and the navigation is set up according to a protocol developed in our clinic [8]. The patient immobilization device allows a reproducible and reliable patient fixation [9]; in combination with positional-control elements, the patient positioning can be verified and reliably adjusted for each session. These position control elements are, similar to the main components of the VBH-headholder, stabile fixable hydraulic arms with a sharp tip pointing to 4 well defined and - in the course of the up to 5 weeks lasting brachytherapy - constant patient anatomical features (warts, naevi, scars and so forth). Very recently we have started to treat "mobile" structures with 3D-computer-assisted navigation (i.e. structures related to the neck and the floor of the mouth, etc.). For this purpose we use, partly, whole-body fixation on base of a body-frame (ELEKTA, Sweden) with vacuum cushions and partly an exact fixation of the lower jaw, again and similar to the working principle of the VBH-headholder, based on an individual dental cast of the patient's lower dentition. This has been found to be reliable even in edentulous patients [10]. Pre-interventional planning of the optimum access path is either done by means of a targeting device [11] or intraoperatively [12] either with the mechanical arm to which a standard hollow needle attaches [13] or by insertion of either the arm's probe or the optical probe in the targeting device.

Results and Discussion:

In the cases where a well defined structure is present, the brachytherapy needle can be placed within millimetric accuracy in each of the sessions of the fractionated HDR-brachytherapy sessions. We have achieved an aiming accuracy of better than 2 mm in all spatial directions. In the cases where mobile structures, i.e. soft tissue is involved, accuracy goes down substantially. However, we still are able to substantially improve the repeatability and the availability of intraoperative positional information. As shown in the "picture book" the preplanned targets may be located with millimetric accuracy, constant throughout the sessions of fractionated therapy; in the cases where the tumor is not contained in the bony structures of the skull a needle placement within one centimeter of the preplanned position is possible, c. f. the last patient demonstrated.

Moreover, we have found that the time needed to conclude single session of interstitial brachytherapy may be reduced in special cases from eight hours to three hours.

Our approach represent possibly one of the first clinical approaches to realize interstitial computer-assisted brachytherapy of the whole ENT-head and neck region. Evidently, the best results can be obtained where the malign process is rigidly contained in bony structures, e.g. like a solitary retro-orbital metastasis of a hepatocellular carcinoma. It is necessary to note here that we do not want to give a rigorous treatment on brachytherapy; it is our intention to demonstrate the Innsbruck developments and the current clinical experience.

Conclusions:

As can be seen from the figures, we have already solved major problems and have achieved the key milestones to implement a prospective planning for brachytherapy, essentially by developing a versatile and reliable patient (re-) positioning and fixation device, intraoperative protocols and essential targeting devices for optimizing the placement of hollow needles into a tumor for interstitial brachytherapy.

References:

[1] S. J. Zinreich, S. A. Tebos, D. M. Long, H. Brem, D. E. Mattox, M. E. Loury, C. A. Vander Kolk, W. M. Koch, D. W. Kennedy, R. N. Bryan, Frameless Stereotactic Integration of CT Imaging Data: Accuracy and Initial Applications, Radiology, 188, 735 - 742, 1993.
[2] W. Freysinger, A. R. Gunkel, R. J. Bale, M. Vogele, C. Kremser, G. Schön, W. F. Thumfart, 3D Navigation in ENT surgery, Annals of Otology, Rhinology and Laryngology, in press.
[3] R. J. Bale, M. Vogele, A. Martin, T. Auer, E. Hensler, P. Eichberger, R. Sweeney, W. Freysinger, A. R. Gunkel, W. F. Thumfart, P. H. Lukas, The VBH head holder improves frameless stereotactic brachytherapy of head and neck tumors, Computer Aided Surgery, 2(5), (1997) in print.
[4] W. Freysinger, A. R. Gunkel, W. F. Thumfart, 3D-Gesteuerte interstitielle Brachytherapie in Mundboden und Zungengrund. Annual meeting of the German ENT Society, Hannover, Germany, 20. - 24. Mai 1998.
[5] T. Auer, E. Hensler, P. Eichberger, A. Bluhm, A. Gunkel, W. Freysinger, R. Bale, O. Gaber, W. F. Thumfart, P. Lukas, 3D-Navigation in der interstitiellen stereotaktischen Brachytherapie, Strahlentherapie und Onkologie, 174(2), 82-87 (1998).
[6] R. J. Bale, M. Vogele, W. Freysinger, A. R. Gunkel, A. Martin, K. Bumm, W. F. Thumfart, A minimally invasive head holder to improve the performance of frameless stereotactic surgery. Laryngoscope, 107(3), 373-377 (1997).
[7] A. Martin, R. J. Bale, M. Vogele, A. R. Gunkel, W. F. Thumfart, W. Freysinger, A noninvasive versatile registration device for frameless stereotaxy. Radiology, in print.
[8] W. Freysinger, A. R. Gunkel, W. F. Thumfart, Image-guided endoscopic ENT surgery, European Archives Otol Rhinol Laryngol, 254, 343-346 (1997).
[9] R. J. Bale, M. Vogele, W. Freysinger, A. R. Gunkel, A. Martin, K. Bumm, W. F. Thumfart, A minimally invasive head holder to improve the performance of frameless stereotactic surgery, Laryngoscope, 107(3), 373-377 (1997).
[10] A Martin, Dissertation, University Innsbruck, Austria.
[11] P. Lukas, E. Hensler, T. Auer, A. R. Gunkel, W. Freysinger, R. J. Bale, W. F. Thumfart, Stereotactic Interstitial Brachytherapy with 3D Navigation in Head and Neck Tumors, Radiology 201(P), 233 (1996).
[12] W. Freysinger, A. R. Gunkel, A. Martin, M. Vogele Dreidimensionale computerunterstützte interstitielle rahmenlose stereotaktische Brachytherapie, Oto- Rhino- Laryngologia Nova 6, 334 (1996).
[13] E. Hensler, Th. Auer, O. Gaber, W. Freysinger, R. Bale, W. Thumfart, P. Lukas, Introduction of Computer Assisted Navigation to Radiation Brachytherapy, Computer Assisted Radiology, H. U. Lemke, M. W. Vannier, K. Inamura, A. G. Farman (Hrsg.), Proceedings of the International Symposium on Computer and Communication Systems for Image Guided Diagnostics and Therapy, CAR '96, Elsevier, Amsterdam, p. 1040 (1996).

The picture book:

Intraoperative setup for the ISG "Freehand" System: Sauerwein Brachy therapy unit (left) IR camera (center) and navigation system (right) can be differentiated.

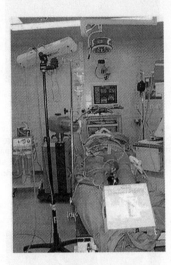

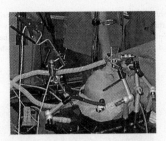

A typical preplanned needle position: left of the crosshair which shows the actual position in the axial data set the ideal target "target" is shown.

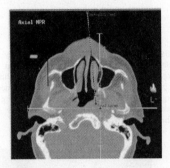

Same as before, but the position sensitive arm is used for intraoperative navigation, i.e. to adjust the targeting device through which the navigation system's probe is guided.

The distance from the targeting device to the tumor center, i.e. the stopping place of the radioactive seed, is shown in axial, coronal, sagittal and a trajectory view of the CT-data set.

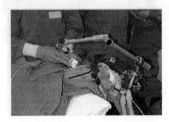

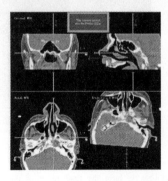

This view shows the setup for the optically probes of the ISG Viewing Wand The components of the holder, the ISG starburst and the ISG probe can be seen; the patient is now anesthetized and ready for needle insertion:

Planning of the brachytherapy session and verification of the actual needle position is done with the immobilized patient in the VBH-headholder; her a CT-based verification of the needle placement is shown.

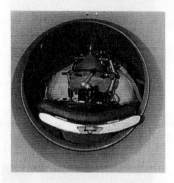

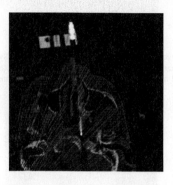

This shows the brachytherapy needle already inserted along the preplanned path with the help of the targeting device; at the moment an endoscopic inspection of the main nasal cavity is performed by the surgeon to check the macroscopic positioning of the needle in the Schmincke-tumor caudally to the sphenoid sinus

The next patient suffered from an adenoid cystic carcinoma of the paranasal sinuses; brachytherapy was performed after enucleation of the eye. In this patient the preplanned needle position is shown here; at the lower left components of the VBH-headholder are shown in a 3D-reconstruction.

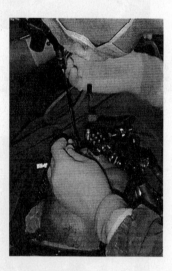

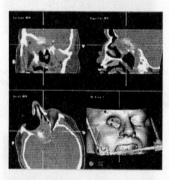

And here the results of two sessions: control CT-slices showing virtually the same positions of session 2

And here we have the final result of the achieved position, compre with the planned position!

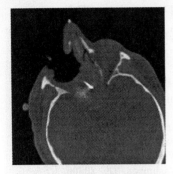

and of session 3:

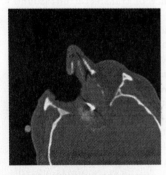

Lastly, some ideas of interstitial brachytherapy in the floor of the mouth (here, we got coincidence between planned and achieved position in the cm-regime). However, positional information was sufficient. This figure is an intraoperative on-line screenshot during the planning session of accessing the posterior aspect of the floor of the mouth with all necessary hints: entry and target point, trajectory.

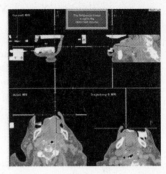

And this is how it looks like intraoperatively from a macro view with all hollow-needles in place. In this patient our new device for reproducible fixation of the lower jaw was used.

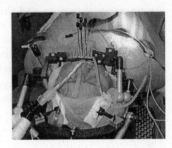

3-D Model Supported Prostate Biopsy Simulation and Evaluation

Jianhua Xuan[1] Yue Wang[2,5] Isabell A. Sesterhenn[3]
Judd W. Moul[4] and Seong K. Mun[5]

[1] University of Maryland Baltimore County, Baltimore 21250, USA
[2] The Catholic University of America, Washington, DC 20064, USA
[3] Armed Forces Institute of Pathology, Washington, DC 20306, USA
[4] Walter Reed Army Medical Center, Washinton, DC 20306, USA
[5] Georgetwon University Medical Center, Washington, DC 20007, USA

Abstract. The diagnosis of localized prostate cancer is carried out by standard core needle biopsies under guidance of transrectal ultrasound imaging of the prostate gland. This paper describes a 3-D model supported virtual environment for prostate cancer diagnosis and biopsy design. A 3-D deformable reconstruction algorithm is developed to define object surface from digitally-imaged surgical specimens. A virtual environment with a multimodal visualization capability is integrated to simulate prostate biopsy protocols. The new system permits an accurate graphical modeling of the object of interest, the localization and quantification of tumors, and the definition of the pathways of biopsy needles. The technique allows the medical experts to probe and manipulate the data in 3-D view space and to evaluate the performance of simulated biopsies subsequently optimize biopsy techniques. Results and analysis of our experiments demonstrate the effectiveness of the individual modular components of the approach. We conclude with an application of the complete framework to a prostate biopsy simulation and evaluation task.

1 Introduction

Graphics-based surgical simulation and planning has phenomenal potential to improve medicine and the health care of mankind. With the advances of three dimensional computed imaging, the information obtained from digital images can be transformed into a computer-synthesized display that facilitates visualization of underlying disease patterns and spatial relationships. In particular, reconstructed 3-D computer models of human organs are used for surgery planning, simulation, image-guided therapy, and treatment assessment. We have advanced from rendering anatomy to aid diagnosis through interactive visualization of complicated or hidden anatomic structures and relationships to planning surgery and to simulate or assist surgery directly. New, more accurate and cost-effective surgical procedures have become possible by integrating computerized graphical models with medical images. For example, image-guided minimally invasive surgery are now streaming into clinical practice carrying medical visualization from diagnosis applications directly to patient care.

The incidence of prostate cancer has increased over the past 10 years with approximately 317,000 American males being diagnosed with prostate cancer in 1996. Prostate cancer has overtaken lung cancer as the most prevalent malignancy in males and is now the second most common cause of cancer death in men. As a result of this rising incidence rate, it is of great interest to study early detection and treatment of this disease. Improved screening programs, prostate-specific antigen (PSA) radioimmunoassay, and increasing awareness of prostate cancer have resulted in a dramatically increased overall detection rate, particular for organ-confined tumors. However, due to the highly variable behavior of the prostate cancer and the lack of appropriate technologies, the complex disease patterns such as the volume, distribution, and multicentricity of the prostate cancer have not been incorporated into the staging and biopsy techniques. On the other hand, the treatment of localized prostate cancer has constantly advanced in surgical removal as well as the preservation of potency and continence, and radiation therapy over the past decade. Particularly, a number of new techniques in radiation therapy are being developed, such treatments as conformal radiation, proton therapy, combinations of radiation and hormone therapy, and radioactive seed implantation. It is of great interest in radioactive seed implantation to treat prostate cancer, since techniques of image-guided radiation therapy (ultrasound at present) can provide more accurate placements of these radioactive seeds within the prostate.

To increase early detection rate and deliver effective treatments of prostate cancer, we develop an image-guided biopsy simulation system with advanced image analysis and computer graphics techniques. Three-dimensional (3-D) computerized prostate models are reconstructed with an accurate 3-D representation of all internal anatomical structures of the prostate (e.g., urethra, seminal vesicles, ejaculatory ducts, etc.). The prostate needle biopsy simulation system is then implemented by an interactive 3-D visualization system with various realistic imaging probes and needles for examination and path planning. With an accurate 3-D prostate model, realistic imaging probes and needles provided by our virtual simulation system, a surgeon can sit in front of the computer to plan better needle paths and further to practice the actual biopsy procedure before he/she actually performs on a patient. More importantly, by analyzing outcomes of this simulation, we can validate the effectiveness of various biopsy techniques in prostate cancer detection and tumor volume estimation.

2   3-D Prostate Modeling

Surgical prostate specimens from patients with biopsy-proven prostate cancer are sectioned into $4\mu m$ sections at $2.5mm$ intervals, and each prostate specimen usually consists of $10 - 15$ such slices. All slices are then digitized by using a Leafscan 45 Scanner at a resolution of 1500 dpi. Slices of each prostate specimen are aligned by a feature-based manual registration performed by pathologists using Photoshop. Finally digital images are stored on CDROMs as our prostate database. Contour extraction and segmentation are conducted manually by pathologists on Photoshop guided by microscopic section information. The regions of interest are the prostate capsule, surgical margins, urethra, seminal vesicles, ejaculatory ducts, carcinomas, and all areas of PIN .

Reconstruction of the prostate model is achieved by using a new deformable surface-spine model described as follows: A deformable spine (axis) of the prostate model is determined from its contours, then all the triangular finite elements are contracted to the spine through expansion/compression forces radiating from the spine while the spine itself is also confined to the surfaces. The surface refinement is governed by a second-order partial differential equation from Lagrangian mechanics, and the refining process terminates when the energy of this dynamic deformable surface-spine model reaches its minimum [2]. Figure 1(a) shows a complete reconstructed 3-D prostate model rendered with all anatomical structures such as the prostate capsule, urethra, seminal vesicles, ejaculatory ducts and carcinomas.

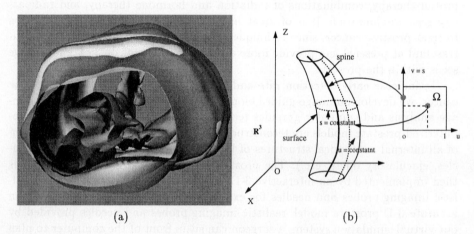

Fig. 1. (a) Reconstructed prostate model. (b) Mathematical model.

We define the surface and spine as geometric mappings from material (parametric) coordinate domains into three-dimensional (3-D) Euclidean space $\Re^3$. The strain energy $\mathcal{E}$ can be found to characterize the deformable material of either the surface or spine, which will be discussed in the next section as an instance of the spline function. Then the continuum mechanical equation

$$\mu \frac{\partial^2 \mathbf{x}}{\partial t^2} + \gamma \frac{\partial \mathbf{x}}{\partial t} + \frac{\delta \mathcal{E}(\mathbf{x})}{\delta \mathbf{x}} = \mathbf{f}(\mathbf{x}), \qquad (1)$$

governs the non-rigid motion of the surface (spine) in response to an extrinsic force $\mathbf{f}(\mathbf{x})$, where μ is the mass density function of the deformable surface (spine) and γ is the viscosity function of the ambient medium. The third term on the left-hand side of the equation is the variational derivative of the strain energy functional $\mathcal{E}$, the internal elastic force of the surface (spine).

The deformable energy of surface $\mathbf{x}(u,v,t)$ can be definned by

$$\mathcal{E}_{surface}(u,v,t) = \int_0^1 \int_0^1 (w_{10} \left|\frac{\partial \mathbf{x}}{\partial u}\right|^2 + 2w_{11} \left|\frac{\partial \mathbf{x}}{\partial u}\right| \times \left|\frac{\partial \mathbf{x}}{\partial v}\right| + w_{01} \left|\frac{\partial \mathbf{x}}{\partial v}\right|^2$$
$$+ w_{20} \left|\frac{\partial^2 \mathbf{x}}{\partial u^2}\right|^2 + 2w_{22} \left|\frac{\partial^2 \mathbf{x}}{\partial u \partial v}\right|^2 + w_{02} \left|\frac{\partial^2 \mathbf{x}}{\partial v^2}\right|^2) \, du dv, \quad (2)$$

where the weights w_{10}, w_{11} and w_{11} control the tensions of the surface, while w_{20}, w_{22} and w_{02} control its rigidities (bending energy). The deformable energy of spine $\mathbf{x}(u,t)$ is given by

$$\mathcal{E}_{spine}(s,t) = \int_0^1 (w_1 \left|\frac{d\mathbf{x}}{ds}\right|^2 + w_2 \left|\frac{d^2\mathbf{x}}{ds^2}\right|^2) \, ds. \quad (3)$$

The weight w_1 controls the tension along the spine (stretching energy), while w_2 controls its rigidity (bending energy).

To couple the surface with the spine, we enforce $v \equiv s$, which maps the spine coordinate into the coordinate along the length of the surface as shown in Figure 1(b). Then we connect the spine with surface by introducing following forces on the surface and spine respectively [3]:

$$\mathbf{f}_{surface}^a(u,s,t) = -(a/l)(\bar{\mathbf{x}}_{surface} - \mathbf{x}_{spine}) \quad (4)$$
$$\mathbf{f}_{spine}^a(s,t) = a\,(\bar{\mathbf{x}}_{surface} - \mathbf{x}_{spine}) \quad (5)$$

where a controls the strength of the forces; $\bar{\mathbf{x}}_{surface}$ is the centroid of the coordinate curve ($s = $ constant) circling the surface and defined as $\bar{\mathbf{x}}_{surface} = \frac{1}{l}\int_0^1 \mathbf{x}_{surface} \left|\frac{\partial \mathbf{x}_{surface}}{\partial u}\right| du$, where l is the length given by $l = \int_0^1 \left|\frac{\partial \mathbf{x}_{surface}}{\partial u}\right| du$. In general, the above forces coerce the spine staying on an axial position of the surface. Further, if necessary, we can encourage the surface to be radially symmetric around the spine by introducing the following force:

$$\mathbf{f}_{surface}^b = b(\bar{r} - |\mathbf{r}|)\hat{\mathbf{r}}, \quad (6)$$

where b controls the strength of the force; $\mathbf{r}$ is the radial vector of the surface with respect to the spine as $\mathbf{r}(u,s) = \mathbf{x}_{surface} - \mathbf{x}_{spine}$, the unit radial vector $\hat{\mathbf{r}}(u,s) = \mathbf{r}/|\mathbf{r}|$, and $\bar{r}(s) = \frac{1}{l}\int_0^1 |\mathbf{r}|\frac{\partial \mathbf{x}_{surface}}{\partial u} du$, as the mean radius of the coordinate curve $s = $ constant. Also, it is possible to provide control over expansion and contraction of the surface around the spine. This can be realized by introducing the following force:

$$\mathbf{f}_{surface}^c = c\hat{\mathbf{r}}, \quad (7)$$

where c controls the strength of the expansion or contraction force. The surface will inflate where $c > 0$ and deflate where $c < 0$.

Summing the above coupling forces in the motion equation associated with surface and spine, we obtain the following dynamic system describing the motion of the deformable surface-spine model:

$$\mu \frac{\partial^2 \mathbf{x}_{surface}}{\partial t^2} + \gamma \frac{\partial \mathbf{x}_{surface}}{\partial t} + \frac{\delta \mathcal{E}_{surface}}{\delta \mathbf{x}} \tag{8}$$

$$= \mathbf{f}^{ext}_{surface} + \mathbf{f}^{a}_{surface} + \mathbf{f}^{b}_{surface} + \mathbf{f}^{c}_{surface} \tag{9}$$

$$\mu \frac{\partial^2 \mathbf{x}_{spine}}{\partial t^2} + \gamma \frac{\partial \mathbf{x}_{spine}}{\partial t} + \frac{\delta \mathcal{E}_{spine}}{\delta \mathbf{x}} = \mathbf{f}^{ext}_{spine} + \mathbf{f}^{a}_{spine}, \tag{10}$$

where $\mathbf{f}^{ext}_{surface}$ is the external force applied on the surface and $\mathbf{f}^{ext}_{spine}$ the external force applied on the spine.

Both the finite difference method and the finite element method can be used to compute the numerical solution to the surface $\mathbf{x}_{surface}$ and spine $\mathbf{x}_{spine}$. Finite difference method approximates the continuous function $\mathbf{x}$ as a set of discrete nodes in space. A disadvantage of the finite difference approach is that the continuity of the solution between nodes is not made explicitly. The finite element method, on the other hand, provides continuous surface (or spine) approximation by approximating the unknown function $\mathbf{x}$ in terms of combinations of the basis functions. In finite element method, we first tessellate the continuous material domain, (u, v) for the surface and s for the spine in our case, into a mesh of m element subdomains D_j, then we approximate $\mathbf{x}$ as a weighted sum of continuous basis functions $\mathbf{N}_i$ (so-called shape functions): $\mathbf{x} \approx \mathbf{x}^h = \sum_i \mathbf{x}_i \mathbf{N}_i$, where $\mathbf{x}_i$ is a vector of nodal variables associated with mesh node i. The shape functions $\mathbf{N}_i$ are fixed in advance and the nodal variables $\mathbf{x}_i$ are the unknowns. The motion equation can then be descritized as

$$\mathbf{M} \frac{\partial^2 \mathbf{x}}{\partial t^2} + \mathbf{C} \frac{\partial \mathbf{x}}{\partial t} + \mathbf{K} \mathbf{x} = \mathbf{F}, \tag{11}$$

where $\mathbf{x} = [\mathbf{x}_1^T, ..., \mathbf{x}_i^T, ..., \mathbf{x}_n^T]$, $\mathbf{M}$ is the mass matrix, $\mathbf{C}$ the damping matrix, $\mathbf{K}$ the stiff matrix, and $\mathbf{F}$ the forcing matrix. $\mathbf{M}$, $\mathbf{C}$, and $\mathbf{F}$ can be obtained as follows:

$$\mathbf{M_j} = \int\int_{E_j} \mu \mathbf{N}_j^T \mathbf{N}_j du dv, \quad \mathbf{C_j} = \int\int_{E_j} \gamma \mathbf{N}_j^T \mathbf{N}_j du dv, \quad \mathbf{F_j} = \int\int_{E_j} \mathbf{N}_j^T \mathbf{f}_j du dv. \tag{12}$$

To compute $\mathbf{K}$, we have the following equation:

$$\mathbf{K}_j = \int\int_{E_j} (\mathbf{N}_b^T \beta \mathbf{N}_b + \mathbf{N}_s^T \alpha \mathbf{N}_s) du dv, \alpha = \begin{bmatrix} w_{02} & w_{22} \\ w_{22} & w_{20} \end{bmatrix}, \beta = \begin{bmatrix} w_{01} & 0 & 0 \\ 0 & w_{11} & 0 \\ 0 & 0 & w_{10} \end{bmatrix} \tag{13}$$

where $\mathbf{N}_b = [\frac{\partial^2 \mathbf{N}}{\partial u^2}, \frac{\partial^2 \mathbf{N}}{\partial u \partial v}, \frac{\partial^2 \mathbf{N}}{\partial v^2}]^T$, $\mathbf{N}_s = [\frac{\partial \mathbf{N}}{\partial u}, \frac{\partial \mathbf{N}}{\partial v}]^T$.

The Deformable Surface Element

The deformable surface consists of a set of connected traingular elements chosen for their capability to model a large range of topological shapes. Barycentric coordinates in two dimensions are the natural choice for defining shape functions over a triangular domain. Barycentric coordinates (L_1, L_2, L_3) are defined by the following mapping with material coordinates (u, v):

$$\begin{bmatrix} u \\ v \\ 1 \end{bmatrix} = \begin{bmatrix} u_1 & u_2 & u_3 \\ v_1 & v_2 & v_3 \\ 1 & 1 & 1 \end{bmatrix} \begin{bmatrix} L_1 \\ L_2 \\ L_3 \end{bmatrix}, \qquad (14)$$

where $(u_1, v_1), (u_2, v_2)$, and (u_3, v_3) are the coordinates of three vertex locations of the triangle.

We use the 9 degree-of-freedom (dof) triangular element which includes the position and its first parametric partial derivatives at each triangle vertex. The shape functions of the first node in a 9 dof triangle are [4]:

$$\mathbf{N}_1^{9^T} = \begin{bmatrix} N_1 \\ N_2 \\ N_3 \end{bmatrix} = \begin{bmatrix} L_1 + L_1^2 L_2 + L_1^2 L_3 - L_1 L_2^2 - L_1 L_3^2 \\ c_3(L_1^2 L_2 + 0.5 L_1 L_2 L_3) - c_2(L_1^2 L_3 + 0.5 L_1 L_2 L_3) \\ -b_3(L_1^2 L_2 + 0.5 L_1 L_2 L_3) + b_2(L_1^2 L_3 + 0.5 L_1 L_2 L_3) \end{bmatrix}. \qquad (15)$$

The triangle's symmetry in Barycentric coordinates can be used to generate the shape function for the second and third nodes in terms of the first. To generate $\mathbf{N}_2^9$ use the above equations but add a 1 to each index so that $1 \to 2$, $2 \to 3$ and $3 \to 1$. The $\mathbf{N}_3^9$ functions can be obtained by adding another 1 to each index. Note that the shape functions for 9 dof triangle do not guarantee C^1 continuity between adjacent triangular elements. In [4], a 12 dof triangular element can be made C^1 continuous by adding a 1 dof on each edge of the triangle, see [5] for the detail. An alternative to have C^1 continuous triangular element is to use a 18 dof element which include the nodal location, its first and second partial derivatives evaluated at each node [6]. In this paper we use 9 dof triangular element although the extension to 12 or 18 dof triangular element is straight-forward.

The Deformable Spine Element

The finite element of the spine has 4 dofs between two nodes located at the ends of the segment. The dofs at each node correspond to its position and tangent. The spine segment can be approximated as the weighted sum of a set of Hermite polynomials: $\mathbf{x} \approx \mathbf{x}^h(s) = \sum_{i=0}^{3} \mathbf{x}_i N_i$, where $N_i, i = 0, ..., 3$ are given as follows:

$$\begin{aligned} N_0 &= 1 - 3(s/h)^2 + 2(s/h)^3, \\ N_1 &= h(s/h - 2(s/h)^2 + (s/h)^3), \\ N_2 &= 3(s/h)^2 - 2(s/h)^3, \\ N_3 &= h(-(s/h)^2 + (s/h)^3), \end{aligned} \qquad (16)$$

where h is the parametric element length.

3-D prostate models can be interactively visualized by the state-of-the-art graphics toolkit, object-oriented *OpenInventor*. With a sophisticated set of various kinds of lights, 3-D manipulators, and color and material editors, etc., we can examine the 3-D prostate model in any viewpoint and interactively walk through it to better understand relationships of anatomical structures of the prostate and its tumors.

3 Needle Biopsy Simulation

The diagnosis of both the clinically palpable and the non-palpable prostatic lesion requires tissue diagnosis. Biopsy is required in all patients with suspected prostatic malignancy. Conventional techniques are usually performed with digital rectal guidance. The use of digital biopsy can only be performed when a palpable area of abnormality is identified. However, with small lesions, this is not an accurate technique. Thus, for diagnosis of non-palpable lesions or of small and subtly palpable ones, ultrasound guided biopsy can be performed accurately, safely and quickly. Transperineal biopsy and transrectal biopsy are two common approaches that can be utilized in the prostate cancer diagnosis. Fig. 2(a) shows the diagram of transrectal biopsy whose procedure will be simulated. Under ultrasound guidance, the needle is placed through the guide into the lesion (Fig. 2(b)).

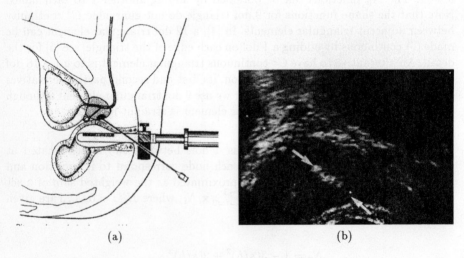

Fig. 2. (a) Diagram of the prostate needle biopsy, (b) the ultrasonic image.

In this section, we first describe an image-guided needle biopsy simulation system implemented with a real-time imaging probe and a needle tracking system. Then we implement a systematic needle biopsy simulation system which enables us to validate various blind biopsy techniques by comparing their cancer detection rates.

3.1 Image-Guided Needle Biopsy Simulation

The image-guided needle biopsy simulation system simulate the clinical procedures of prostate cancer biopsy in the following two steps:
(i) Examining the prostate using the ultrasound-like probe: Different ultrasound-like imaging probes are simulated to provide axially and/or longitudinally oriented sectional images for efficiently planning needle pathways.
(ii) Defining the needle paths and performing simulated biopsy: Needles with or without triggers are constructed and simulated to perform actual biopsy on 3-D computerized prostate models according to the planned needle pathways, see Figure 3 (a).

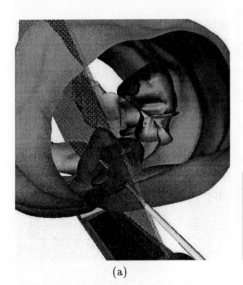

	SRSCB	S5RB	SRSCB+S5RB
T1c (24%)	10 (77%)	9 (69%)	10 (77%)
T2 (76%)	37 (88%)	33 (79%)	38 (90%)

(a) (b)

Fig. 3. (a) 3-D view of the needle biopsy simulation, (b) Clinical stage and positive biopsy distribution.

3.2 Systematic Needle Biopsy Simulation

In 1989, Hodge *et al.* proposed the technique of six random systematic core biopsy (SRSCB) of the prostate gland. The technique has gained acceptance by urologists for detection of carcinoma of the prostate (CaP) since then. With the image-guided needle biopsy simulation system we can verify the validity of the SRSCB technique in detecting prostate cancer and possibly recommend new biopsy technique to increase the detection rate. We have implemented both SRSCB and systematic 5-region biopsy technique (S5RB) in our simulation system.

In this simulation, we have reconstructed 55 computerized prostate models of prostate specimens taken from patients and performed biopsy techniques on them. The simulation results are shown in Figs. 4 and 5, where the detection probability of each needle can be calculated to indicate the clinical importance. Fig. 3 (b) gives the clinical stage and positive biopsy in 55 patients, where T1c means small tumor and T2 means large tumor. By correlating the simulation results with clinical data such as PSA we can evaluate the biopsy strategies for detection of prostate cancer. In addition, the prostate biopsy simulation system can show the biopsy procedure in 3-D space to record and analyze various causes of hit or miss in individual cases.

	# of Positive Cores	% of Total Cores
L–Base	13	10%
L–Mid	23	17%
L–Apex	27	20%
R–Base	7	5%
R–Mid	29	22%
R–Apex	34	26%
Total	133	

(a)   (b)

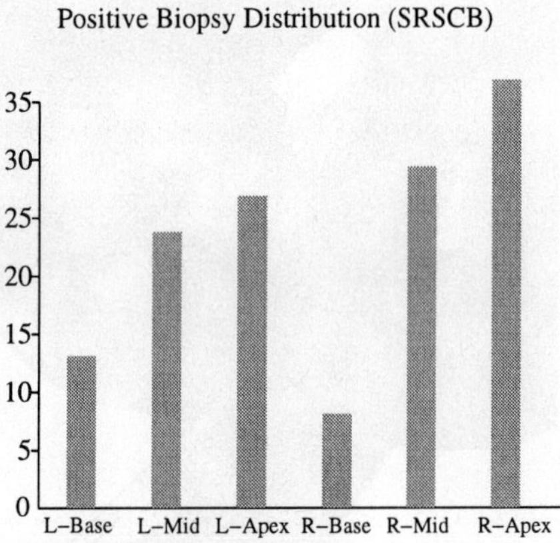

Fig. 4. Positive biopsy distribution (SRSCB): (a) table, (b) histogram.

4 Conclusion

In this paper, we have developed a vitual environment for prostate needle biopsy simulation using advanced image analysis and computer graphics techniques. 3-D computerized prostate models are first reconstructed from microscopic images of surgical prostate specimens. Computer simulation systems are then implemented to simulate both image-guided and systematic prostate needle biopsy

	# of Positive Cores	% of Total Cores
L–Base	12	12%
L–Apex	14	14%
M–Base	2	2%
M–Apex	30	31%
R–Base	13	13%
R–Apex	26	27%
Total	97	

(a)　　　　(b)

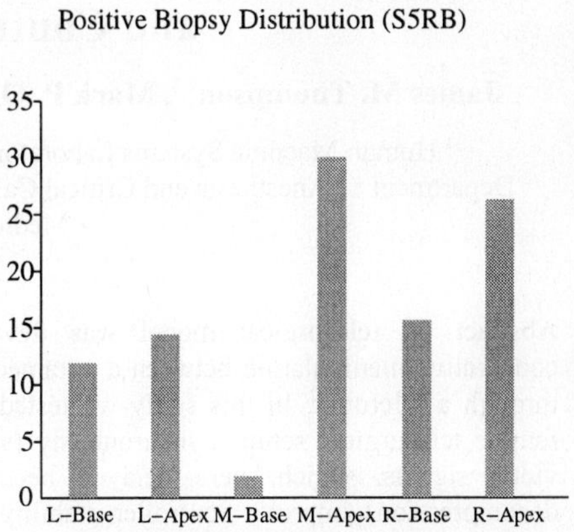

Fig. 5. Positive biopsy distribution (S5RB): (a) table, (b) histogram.

techniques with interactive visualization and manipulation capabilities. With such a simulation environment, a surgeon can better plan needle paths in 3-D space in order to increase cancer detection rate. Simulation results on various prostate needle biopsy techniques have also demonstrated that we can validate the effectiveness of different biopsy techniques in prostate cancer detection by analyzing the simulation outcomes.

References

1. A. Chiarodo, "National Cancer Institute roundtable on prostate cancer: Future directions," *Cancer Res.* vol. 51, pp. 2498-2505, 1991.
2. J. Xuan, I. Sesterhenn, W. Hayes, Y. Wang, T. Adali, M. Freedman, and S. K. Mun, "Surface reconstruction and visualization of surgical prostate models," *Medical Imaging*, Newport Beach, Feb. 1997.
3. D. Terzopoulos, A. Witkin, and M. Kass, "Symmetry-seeking models and 3D object reconstruction," *Int. J. Computer Vision*, vol. 1, pp. 211-221, 1987.
4. Zienkiewicz, *The Finite Element Method*, The Third Edition, McGraw-Hill Book, 1967.
5. G. Celniker and D. Gossard, "Deformable curve and surface finite-elements for free-form shape design," *Computer Graphics*, Vol. 25, No. 4, pp. 257-266, July 1991.
6. T. McInerney, and D. Terzopoulos, "A dynamic finite element surface model for segmentation and tracking in multidimensional medical images with application to cardiac 4D image analysis," *Computerized Medical Imaging and Graphics*, vol. 19, no. 1, pp. 69-83, 1995.

Human Factors in Tele-inspection and Tele-surgery: Cooperative Manipulation under Asynchronous Video and Control Feedback

James M. Thompson[1,2], Mark P. Ottensmeyer[1], and Thomas B. Sheridan[1]

[1] Human Machine Systems Laboratory, Massachusetts Institute of Technology
[2] Department of Anesthesia and Critical Care, Massachusetts General Hospital and Harvard Medical School

Abstract. A telesurgical model was developed for simulation experiments evaluating cooperative manipulation between a paramedic local to the patient and a physician operating through a telerobot. In this study we tested the hypothesis that sending the signals from a remote telesurgical setup asynchronously (sending the telemanipulator signals ahead of the video signals, which were delayed because of the time it took for compression / decompression) improve controller stability and favorably affect task performance by the medical team. We found essentially no difference in task performance between the synchronous and asynchronous transmission of the telesurgical signals when the physician operated the laparoscope and the assistant operated the laparotomy tools. But with asynchronous transmission we found a significant improvement (31% to 60%) in task completion time when the physician operated any of the laparotomy tools.

1. Introduction

The purpose of this project is to evaluate telesurgery from a human factors engineering viewpoint. In particular it focuses on two interrelated problems:

1). Cooperative manipulation between a paramedic local to the patient and a physician operating through a telerobot.

2). Coping with time delay in both visual and force feedback.

In our first series of experiments, using synchronously transmitted video and telemanipulator signals, we found that the time delay made operation of the laparoscopic tools by the surgeon extremely difficult.

In the experiments reported here we asked the question: Does sending the signals from a remote telesurgical setup asynchronously (sending the telemanipulator signals ahead of the video signals, which were delayed because of the time it took for compression / decompression) improve controller stability and favorably affect task performance by the medical team.

Though the use of communication systems in medicine is not new, the use of a high bandwidth audio and video link has recently been applied to the diagnosis and treatment of the patient. Still, there are numerous situations where the bandwidth is not sufficient for the simultaneous transmission of teleoperator control signals, real time video signals and audio signals. In such a case, it is common to employ CODEC (compression and decompression) boards for the transmission of the video signals. Standard videoconferencing equipment over ISDN and fractional T1 phone lines currently use this technology for video conferencing calls. Video compression and decompression imposes a time delay, and combined with the time delay imposed by the communication system produces a total time delay that adversely affects the task completion time of currently proposed telesurgical systems.

Investigators have shown that teleoperator users start to use a "move and wait" strategy as the closed loop time delay increases above 0.1 seconds [1,2]. In our first series of experiments, we found that the synchronous transmission of video and telemanipulator signals (our model of 600 ms video delay plus a 600 ms communication delay) resulted in a total round trip time delay that seriously affected task performance time and resulted in a "move and wait" strategy when the surgeon operated the laparoscopic tools. In this current set of experiments we explore the hypothesis that sending the signals from a remote telesurgical setup asynchronously would improve controller stability and possibly favorably affect task performance by the surgical team.

2. Methods

The experimental system is presented in Figure 2.1 and described below.

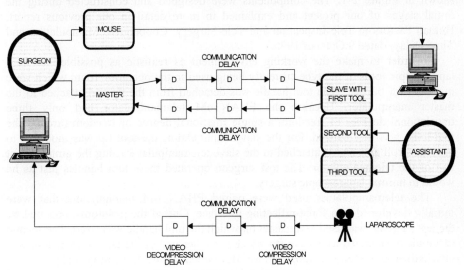

Figure 2.1 Telesurgical System

2.1 Telemanipulator and Tools

The telemanipulator and tools are important in enabling the surgeon to diagnose and treat the trauma patient in the remote environment. One needs to be able to control a laparoscope for viewing, and be able to manipulate a hemostat (to be used as a blunt probe or to grasp intra-abdominal contents), scissors and a gripper / clip applicator (for clamping the bleeding vessel).

2.2 Telesurgical System: Time Delay

In a telesurgical system one is faced with two types of time delays: (1) delay associated with the transmission of the signals from the teleoperator over a communication link, and (2) the delay due to the video compression and decompression because of a communication bandwidth limit.

The transit time for signals sent over communication channels depend on the medium (e.g. ISDN, satellite) and the traffic over that medium. With an ISDN setup, the typical round trip delays are in the order of 600 ms [3]. The distance can also be a factor. Researchers reported a 1.4 second round trip delay in a teleoperator connection between Tokyo and Washington, D.C. [4].

There is also a delay associated with the video compression and decompression needed when unlimited bandwidth is not available. Current video conferencing equipment that uses ISDN lines requires approximately 300 ms for the video compression and subsequent decompression for one way transmission. The components of these delays are shown in Figure 2.1.

2.3 Experimental Apparatus

Our experimental set-up is intended to model the telesurgical system described in the previous section. In particular, our set-up for the asynchronous experiments is as shown in Figure 2-1. The components were designed and constructed during the initial stages of our project and explained in more detail in our previous report, Human Factors in Tele-Inspection and Tele-Surgery: Cooperative Manipulation and Time Delay, dated 9 October 1995.

In order to make the working environment as realistic as possible, we used laparoscopic tools of the type currently being used in the operating room which were modified for our use. The tool handle was detached from the tip and attached to the master manipulator. Because the PHANToM telemanipulator had only three translational degrees of freedom, a single rotational degree of freedom (around the tool axis) was mechanized. For the slave manipulator, the tool tip was modified to provide a roll axis and is attached to the slave telemanipulator using the gimble wrist end of the telemanipulator. The test surgeon operated these tool handles just as he would in normal laparoscopic surgery.

The telemanipulators used were paired PHANToM manipulators that were initially developed as a force-reflecting interface. One of the phantoms, operated by the test surgeon, was used as a master on which the tool handle was fixed. The second manipulator operated as a slave (to which the other end of the laparoscopic tool was attached). The control software used was developed as part of the project [5].

The audio / visual system consisted of microphones and headsets, cameras and displays and a two-way communications setup. Thus both audio and video were available to both the surgeon and assistant. We used two matched headphone / boom microphone systems connected through a pre-amp / amplifier to the audio delay boards. A CCD camera was used for the laparoscope.

We used a Prime Image A/V mainframe with two video delay boards and a 2 channel audio board to generate the audio and visual delays. This was connected to our camera, monitors and audio communication equipment and used to model the transmission line and video compression / decompression delays.

The video images were recorded with a Video Hi-8 recorder and routed to the two video monitors and VHS recorder through a Silicon Graphics Galileo video board.

We used the same surgical laparoscopic simulators designed and constructed for our first series of experiments. The simulator used for our experiments was modeled after laparoscopic training simulators [6,7] which has four surgical incision sites for trocar insertion and has a clear side wall for recording the experiments with a camcorder.

In our experimental setup, the surgeon operated a mouse pointer that was superimposed over the image from the surgical site and was used by the surgeon as a visual tool to direct the actions of the assistant. This video overlay was generated by a Silicon Graphics Indigo2 Extreme workstation using the Galileo video card.

2.4 Experimental Surgical Tasks Used

Grasp and Transfer Experiments

This experiment evaluated the ability of the surgical team to control the hemostat and to work together to perform a task. The performance time was defined as the time it takes for the surgeon – assistant team to transfer 6 clips from one location to the other and back.

Hemostasis

In this experiment we evaluated the use of the clip applicator / hemostat and the scissors by the surgical team (surgeon and assistant). We started with a model of the neurovascular bundle (a nerve, artery and vein usually travel together) made up of tan, blue and red rubber bands. The task completion time was measured as the time it took the team to correctly place the hemostat / clipper completely around the related vessel (with the exclusion of adjacent structures), clip off the vessel, and then to cut the redundant vessel with the scissors.

2.5 Experimental Subjects

The test surgeon throughout these preliminary experiments was an experienced emergency room physician and anesthesiologist. The assistants were engineering graduate students. These were the same individuals that were tested in the first set of experiments run the previous year.

2.6 Data Recording

The experiments were recorded to a VCR deck using a high fidelity Sony Camcorder. The first author later reviewed these videotapes and the task completion times were recorded for each of the individual experiments.

2.7 Experimental Design: Synchronous and Asynchronous Transmission

In our first set of experiments we buffered the telemanipulator signals while the video signal was being processed, then sent both the video and telemanipulator signals simultaneously (synchronous) over the transmission link. In our second set of experiments we immediately sent the telemanipulator signals over the transmission link without waiting for the video signals (which needed 0.6 second round trip for the video compression-decompression) which resulted in asynchronous transmission of video and telemanipulator signals.

3. Results

The results for the individual tool combinations for each experiment are presented in Figures 3.1 to 3.4 and discussed in the following sections of this paper.

In general, we found that when the surgeon operated the laparoscope there was a slight improvement in task completion time when the task was performed with asynchronous (as compared to synchronous) video and telemanipulator feedback signals. When the surgeon used any of the other tools, we found a dramatic improvement in task completion time when the signals were sent asynchronously, for both the 0.6 second and 1.2 second delays.

3.1 Grasp and Transfer Experiments

There were two physician / assistant tool combinations for this experiment. In the first scenario, the physician operated the scope through the teleoperator while the assistant operated the two hemostats. In the second scenario, the surgeon operated one of the hemostats while the assistant operated the laparoscope and the other hemostat. As in our first series of experiments, we found that task completion time is lowest (better performance) when the surgeon operated the laparoscope rather than operating one of the hemostats. We found this to be the case in all six experiments in which we varied the time delays for both the video and telemanipulator signals.

In our second set of experiments we studied the effect of asynchronous video and telemanipulator signal transmission on task completion time with various time delays. The results show a significant improvement in task completion time with asynchronous (as compared to synchronous) signal transmission. The results for the experiments with no transmission time delays are shown in Figure 3.1.

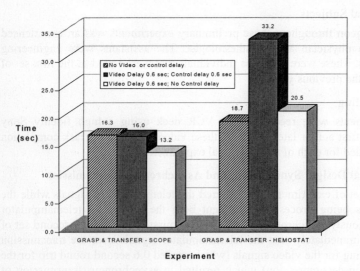

Figure 3.1. Grasp and Transfer Experiments: Performance times for asynchronous and synchronous signals with no transmission time delay. ("Grasp & Transfer – Scope" means that the surgeon operated the laparoscope in the Grasp & Transfer experiment)

The results for a transmission time delay of 0.6 seconds are presented in Figure 3.2.

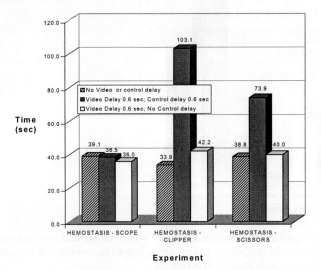

Figure 3.2. Grasp and Transfer Experiments: Performance times for asynchronous and synchronous signals with a 0.6 second transmission time delay. ("Hemostasis – Scope" means that the surgeon operated the laparoscope in the Hemostasis experiment)

3.2 Hemostasis Experiments

There were three physician / assistant tool combinations for this experiment, a laparoscope, clipper / hemostat, and a scissors. In the first scenario, the physician operated the scope through the teleoperator, while the assistant operated the clipper and the scissors. In the second scenario, the surgeon operated the clipper / hemostat while the assistant operated the laparoscope and the scissors. In the third scenario the physician operated the scissors while the assistant operated the laparoscope and the clipper. As in our first series of experiments, task completion time is lowest (better performance) when the surgeon operated the laparoscope rather than operating one of the other tools. We found this to be the case in all six experiments in which we varied the time delays for both the video signals and the telemanipulator signals.

In our second set of experiments we studied the effect of asynchronous video and telemanipulator signal transmission on task completion time with various time delays. Our results, which are presented below for each time delay, also showed a significant improvement in task completion time with asynchronous (as compared to synchronous) signal transmission, except when the physician operated the laparoscope. The results for the experiments with no transmission time delays are shown in Figure 3.3. The results for a transmission time delay of 0.6 seconds are presented in Figure 3.4.

4. Discussion

In this second series of experiments in our telesurgery project we attempted to

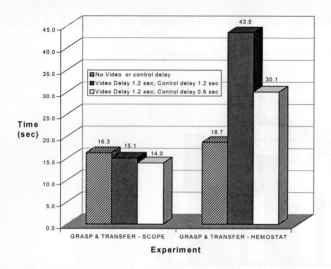

Figure 3.3. Hemostasis Experiments: Performance times for asynchronous and synchronous signals with no transmission time delay. ("Grasp & Transfer – Scope" means that the surgeon operated the laparoscope in the Grasp & Transfer experiment)

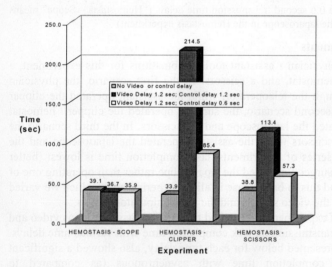

Figure 3.4. Hemostasis Experiments: Performance times for asynchronous and synchronous signals with a 0.6 second transmission time delay. ("Hemostasis – Scope" means that the surgeon operated the laparoscope in the Hemostasis experiment)

test the hypothesis that sending the signals from a remote telesurgical setup asynchronously (sending the telemanipulator signals ahead of the video signals, which were delayed because of the compression / decompression it required) would improve controller stability and favorably affect task performance by the surgical team.

We had interesting results. There was essentially no difference in task performance between the synchronous and asynchronous transmission of the telesurgical signals when the physician operated the laparoscope. But we found a significant improvement (31% to 60%) in task completion time when the physician operated any of the laparotomy tools with asynchronous transmission when compared to synchronous transmission.

The results when the physician operated the laparoscope can be easily explained. Degradation in team performance resulting from the effects of time delay (controller instability) is reduced by several factors. First, because the laparoscopic output is an entire field, the person controlling the laparoscope needs to be less sophisticated. Secondly, because the surgeon knows the contents of the surgical field, and what task sequence needed to be performed, he/she is more efficient in minimizing movements (stabilizing field of view) of the laparoscope. In essence, the control of the laparoscope was fairly passive as compared to the operation of the laparoscopic tools.

The significant improvement in task completion time (for asynchronous as contrasted to synchronous transmission) when the surgeon operated the laparoscopic tools can be explained by looking at the effect of time delay on stability of the telemanipulator system. The main advantage with asynchronous transmission probably resulted from the increased stability of the telerobotic manipulator because of the decreased time delay seen by the controller. In the case of synchronous transmission (Figure 2.1), since the telemanipulator signals were sent with the video signals, the controller had an additional delay due to the time it took to compress and then decompress the video signals. The controller delay was

$$T_d = D_c + D + D_d$$

where: T_d is the total delay seen by the controller
D_c is the delay due to video compression
D is the delay due to signal transmission (e.g. phone line)
D_d is the delay due to video decompression

In the case of asynchronous transmission (Figure 2.1), the telemanipulator signal was sent ahead of the video signal and the controller delay was then:

$$T_d = D$$

where: T_d is the total delay seen by the controller
D is the delay due to signal transmission (e.g. phone line)

We see that the controller had a smaller time delay in the asynchronous mode, which made it more stable and easier for the physician to operate the tools.

The main disadvantage with asynchronous transmission was that the operator did not receive the force feedback information at the same that he received the video input. The results of our experiments seem to suggest that the improvement in performance because of the more stable controller more than offset the degradation in performance due to the asynchronous force feedback and visual image seen by the physician.

5. Conclusions

In this second series of experiments in our telesurgery project we attempted to test the hypothesis that sending the signals from a remote telesurgical setup asynchronously (sending the telemanipulator signals as quickly as possible, ahead of the video signals, which are necessarily delayed because of the compression / decompression required) improves controller stability and favorably affects task performance.

We found essentially no difference in task performance between the synchronous and asynchronous transmission of the telesurgical signals when the physician operated the laparoscope and the assistant operated the laparotomy tools. But with asynchronous transmission we found a significant improvement (31% to 60%) in task completion time when the physician operated any of the laparotomy tools.

This is an important finding that can be applied to any situation which involves the cooperative actions of an expert operating a remote telemanipulator system (that is limited by bandwidth considerations) and a non-expert person operating some tools at the local site (where the telemanipulator slave is working).

References

1. Ferrell, W. R. and Sheridan, T. B.: Supervisory control of remote manipulation. *IEEE Spectrum* 4, no. 10, (1967):81-88.
2. Black, J.:. Factorial study of remote manipulation with transmission time delay. *Master's thesis, MIT, Engineering Projects Lab, Department of Mechanical Engineering*, Dec. 1970.
3. Zydacron, Inc.: ZydApp2 User's Guide for software release 1.1, February:87.
4. Mitsuishi, M., Watanabe, T., Nakanishi, H., Hori, T., Watanabe, H., and Kramer B.: A tele-micro-surgery system with co-located view and operation points and a rotational-force-feedback-free master manipulator. *Second Annual International Symposium on Medical Robotics and Computer Assisted Surgery:* (1995):111-118.
5. Hu, J., Ren, J., Thompson, J. M., and Sheridan, T. B.: Fuzzy sliding force reflecting control of a telerobotic system. *Proceedings of IEEE Conference on Fuzzy Systems,* September 1996.
6. Bailey, R. W., Imbembo, A. L., and Zucker, K. A.: Establishment of a laparoscopic cholecystectomy training program. *The American Scientist:* 57(4), (1991):231-236.
7. Muntzer, M.: A cheap laparoscopic surgery trainer. *Annals of the Royal College of Surgeons of England*: 74:256-257. 6. Bailey, R. W., Imbembo, A. L., and Zucker, K. A. (1991). Establishment of a laparoscopic cholecystectomy training program. *The American Scientist:* 57(4), (1992):231-236.

Computer Assisted Coronary Intervention by Use of On-line 3D Reconstruction and Optimal View Strategy

S.-Y. James Chen and John D. Carroll

Cardiology Division, Department of Medicine
University of Colorado Health Sciences Center
james@stbernard.uhcolorado.edu, jcarroll@rigel.uhcolorado.edu

Abstract. A novel method has been developed for on-line reconstruction of the 3D coronary arterial tree based on a pair of routine angiograms acquired from any two arbitrary viewing angles using a single-plane or biplane imaging system. An arterial segment of interest (*e.g.*, coronary stenosis) is selected on the projection of reconstructed 3D coronary model. Afterwards, the process of optimal view strategy is employed resulting in foreshortening, overlap, and composite maps relative to the selected arterial segment by which any computer-generated projection associated with the gantry orientation can be previewed. By use of the three maps, the views with minimal foreshortening and vessel overlap for the selected arterial segment of interest can be determined to guide subsequent angiogram acquisitions for interventional procedure. More than 200 cases of coronary arterial systems have been reconstructed. A validation confirmed the accuracy of 3D length measurement to within RMS 3.1% error using 8 pairs of angiograms of intra-coronary catheter wire of 105 mm length.

1 Introduction

Many endeavors of computer assisted techniques for estimation of the three-dimensional (3D) coronary arteries from biplane projection data have been reported [1]-[7]. These methods were based on the known or standard x-ray geometry of projections, placement of landmarks, or the pre-determined vessel shape and on iterative identification of matching structures in two or more views. Other knowledge-based or rule-based systems have been proposed for 3D reconstruction of coronary arteries by use of of a vascular network model [8]-[12]. Because the rules or knowledge base were organized for certain specific conditions, it is not likely to generalize the 3D reconstruction process to arbitrary projection data. In [13], the 3D coronary arteries were reconstructed from a set of x-ray perspective projections by use of an algorithm from computed tomography. Due to the motion of heart, only a limited number of projections can be acquired. Therefore, accurate reconstruction and quantitative measurement are not easily achieved.

The linear approach of closed-form solution for the general 3D reconstruction problem based on 2D projections was a significant development in [14]-[19]. Unfortunately, actual data are always corrupted by noise or errors and the linear approach based techniques may not be sufficiently accurate from noisy data. Hence, optimal estimation has been explicitly investigated. In [20]-[25], a two-step approach was proposed for an optimal estimation of 3D object structures based on maximum-likelihood and minimum-variance estimation. Preliminary estimates computed by the linear algorithm were used as initial estimates for the process of optimal estimation.

In this paper, an on-line 3D reconstruction technique is proposed to accurately reconstruct the coronary arterial trees based on two views acquired from routine angiograms at arbitrary orientation using a single-plane or biplane imaging system. The reconstructed patient-specific 3D coronary arterial tree is used to facilitate the determination of optimal view strategy.

2 On-line 3D Reconstruction of Coronary Arterial Tree

After routine cardiac catheterization is initiated, a standard coronary arteriogram is completed in two standard views: one injection in a biplae system and two injections in a single-plane system. With the acquired two angiogram sequences, a pair of images were chosen corresponding to the same or close acquisition time instance (*e.g.*, end-diastole or end-systole) in the cardiac cycles for 3D reconstruction process. The proposed method of on-line 3D reconstruction consists of three major steps: (1) identification of 2D coronary arterial trees and feature extractions, (2) determination of transformation defining the spatial relationship of the acquired two views, and (3) calculation of 3D coronary arterial structures.

2.1 Recognition of 2D coronary arteries

A semi-automatic system [24] based on the technique of deformation model and segmentation technique was employed for identification of the 2D coronary arterial tree in the given angiograms. The identified centerlines and the branching relationships are used for construction of the vessel hierarchy in each angiogram by their labeling according to the appropriate anatomy and connectivity among the primary and secondary coronary arteries. The labeling process on the coronary tree is performed automatically by traversing the identified vessel centerlines and associated bifurcations, and finally results in a vessel hierarchically <u>directed</u> <u>graph</u> (digraph) containing a set of nodes with corresponding *depth levels* and two types of arcs (descendant and sibling arcs) defining the coronary anatomy. In the hierarchical digraph, each node represents a vessel in the coronary arterial tree, and the *descendent arc* connects the nodes between the vessel and its branch. If a vessel has multiple branches, the nodes associated with these branches are connected as a linked list by *sibling arcs* according to the branching locations relative to the ascendant vessel. With the constructed hierarchical digraph, bifurcation points, directional vectors, and diameters are then calculated for all of the coronary arterial bifurcations, and the results are saved into the nodes associated branching vessels in the hierarchical digraph.

2.2 Determination of transformation defining the spatial relationship of two views

The spatial relationship between the employed two views can be characterized by a transformation in the forms of a rotation matrix $\boldsymbol{R}$ and a translation vector $\boldsymbol{t}$ with the x-ray source (or focal spot) served as the origin of 3D coordinate space. The geometrical relationship between the two views can be characterized by $[x_i', y_i', z_i']^T = \boldsymbol{R} \cdot ([x_i, y_i, z_i]^T - \boldsymbol{t})$. In the first view, let (u_i, v_i) denote the image coordinates of the i-th object point, located at position (x_i, y_i, z_i). We have $u_i = Dx_i/z_i$, $v_i = Dy_i/z_i$, where D is the perpendicular distance between the x-ray focal spot and the image plane. Let (ξ_i, η_i) denote the scaled image coordinates, defined as $\xi_i = u_i/D = x_i/z_i$, $\eta_i = v_i/D = y_i/z_i$. The second projection view of the employed single-plane imaging system can be described in terms of a second pair of image and object coordinate systems $u'v'$ and $x'y'z'$ defined in an analogous manner. Scaled image coordinates (ξ_i', η_i') in the second view for the i-th object point at position (x_i', y_i', z_i') are given by $\xi_i' = u_i'/D' = x_i'/z_i'$, $\eta_i' = v_i'/D' = y_i'/z_i'$.

In our previously proposed method [24][25], the transformation was calculated based on the identified bifurcation points of the 2D coronary arterial trees in the two views and can be only effective to the images acquired from the biplane systems (or a single-plane system without table movement) during the acquisition. In this paper, a new 3D reconstruction technique is presented by incorporation of the bifurcation points and the vessel directional vectors of bifurcations. This new technique can be utilized adequately in both single-plane and biplane environments. The proposed method can also be employed to obtain accurate results of 3D reconstruction even when the table is moving during the injection or with the ECG-triggered mode disabled in acquisitions. For 3D reconstruction, the required prior information (*i.e.*, the intrinsic parameters of each single-plane imaging system) include: (1) the distance between each focal spot and its image plane, SID (focal-spot to imaging-plane distance), (2) the pixel size, p_{size} (*e.g.*, .3 mm/pixel), (3) the distance $\overline{ff'}$ between the two focal spots or the known 3D distance between two points in the projection images, and (4) iso-center distance (with respect to which the rotary motion of the gantry arm rotates) relative to the focal spot.

To calculate the transformation, the objective function was defined by minimization of (1) image point errors in term of the square of Euclidean distance between the 2D input data and the projection of calculated 3D data points and (2) directional vector errors between the 2D vessel directional vectors and the projection of calculated 3D vessel directional vectors. Given the set of 2D bifurcation points and directional vectors extracted from the pair of images, an "optimal" estimates of the transformation and 3D bifurcation points were obtained by minimizing:

$$\min_{R,t,\hat{p}',v'} \mathcal{F}(R,t,\hat{P}',\hat{v}') = \sum_{i=1}^{n}(\hat{\xi}'_i - \frac{\hat{x}'_i}{\hat{z}'_i})^2 + (\hat{\eta}'_i - \frac{\hat{y}'_i}{\hat{z}'_i})^2 + \left(\hat{\xi}_i - \frac{c_1 \cdot p'_i + t_x}{c_3 \cdot p'_i + t_z}\right)^2$$
$$+ \left(\hat{\eta}_i - \frac{c_2 \cdot \hat{p}'_i + t_y}{c_3 \cdot \hat{p}''_i + t_z}\right)^2 + \|\hat{v}_i - [R^{-1} \cdot \hat{v}'_i]_{xy}\|^2 + \|\hat{v}'_i - [\hat{v}'_i]_{x'y'}\|^2, \quad (1)$$

where n denotes the number of pairs of corresponding points extracted from the two images and $\hat{P}$ and $\hat{P}'$ denote the sets of 3D position vectors of bifurcation points $\hat{p}_i = (\hat{x}_i, \hat{y}_i, \hat{z}_i)$ and $\hat{p}'_i = (\hat{x}'_i, \hat{y}'_i, \hat{z}'_i)$, respectively, $\hat{\nu}_i$ and $\hat{\nu}'_i$, denote the respective 2D vessel directional vectors of bifurcations in each views, and $\hat{v} = \{\hat{v}_1, \hat{v}_2, \ldots, \hat{v}_n\}$ and $\hat{v}' = \{\hat{v}'_1, \hat{v}'_2, \ldots, \hat{v}'_n\}$ denote the calculated 3D vessel directional vectors of bifurcations in two views, and $[\hat{v}_i]_{xy}$ and $[\hat{v}'_i]_{x'y'}, i = 1, \ldots, n$, denote the calculated 2D projection vector at bifurcation on the image planes, c_k denotes the respective kth column vectors of matrix R, and R^{-1} is the inverse matrix of R.

2.3 Calculation of 3D coronary arterial tree

After the transformation (R, t) that defines the two views is obtained, this information will be used for establishing the point correspondences on 2D vessel centerlines in the pair of images and calculating 3D morphologic structures of coronary arterial tree. The calculated transformation in conjunction with the epi-polar constraints were employed as the framework for establishing the point correspondences on the vessel centerlines based on the two identified 2D coronary arterial trees [24]. Since the information of relative orientations and locations of two cameras is known (*i.e.*, in term of a transformation calculated previously), the correspondences of image points can be solved by employing "epi-polar constraints" theory [26].

With the point correspondences on 2D vessel centerlines (ξ_j, η_j) and (ξ'_j, η'_j) and the transformation (R, t), the 3D vessel centerline points of coronary arteries (x_j, y_j, z_j) can then be calculated [24][25]. To recover the morphology of the 3D arterial lumen, the contour points on each circular lumen cross section centered at (x_i, y_i, z_i) are calculated. The normal vector at the plane spanned by the cross section is parallel to the tangent vector at point (x_i, y_i, z_i) on the vessel skeleton (or 3D vessel centerline). For any cross section of vessel segment, it can be modeled as a circular disk centered at (x_i, y_i, z_i) with diameter d_i. Then the 3D lumen surface is easily represented by filling up the polygons between every two consecutive circular disks.

3 Determination of Optimal Views

The reconstructed 3D coronary arterial tree can be rotated to any selected viewing angle yielding multiple computer-generated projections to determine for each patient which standard views are useful and which are of no clinical value due to excessive overlap. Therefore, the 3D computer assistance provides means to improve the quality and utility of the images subsequently acquired. When an arbitrary computer-generated image is produced, the gantry information defining the current projection is calculated in the form of left anterior oblique/right anterior oblique (LAO/RAO) and caudal/cranial (CAUD/CRAN). These gantry angles are defined in a spatial coordinate system with the iso-center as the origin. The LAO/RAO angulation is defined on the y-z plane, while the CAUD/CRAN angulation is defined on the x-z plane. With the spatial coordinates, the position of focal spot (x_f, y_f, z_f) can be formulated by use of two rotations $R_x(\alpha)$ and $R_y(-\beta)$ as,

$$[x_f, y_f, z_f] = [x_n, y_n, z_n] \cdot R_x(\alpha) R_y(-\beta) \qquad (2)$$

where $(x_n, y_n, z_n) = (0, 0, D_{fc})$ denotes the neutral position of focal spot (or anterior-posterior (AP) view with $0°$ LAO and $0°$ CAUD, D_{fc} is the distance between iso-center and focal spot (which is provided by manufacture), R_x and R_y denotes the rigid rotations with respect to x-axis and y-axis, and α and β denote the LAO and CAUD angles, respectively.

Let $p_i, i = 0, 1, \ldots, m$ denote the points along the centerline of a 3D vessel l. Let $l_j = [l_{j_x}, l_{j_y}, l_{j_z}]^t$, $j = 1, 2, \ldots, m$ denote the vectors associated with individual sections between p_{j-1} and p_j. The functions $\mathcal{S}(\alpha, \beta, l)$ and $\mathcal{O}(\alpha, \beta, l)$ in term of gantry orientation (α and β angles) for evaluation of degrees of foreshortening and overlap with respect to the selected arterial segment l can be defined as follows:

$$\mathcal{S}(\alpha, \beta, l) = \sum_{j=1}^{m} \| l_j \cos(\theta_j) \|^2 = \sum_{j=1}^{m} (l_j \cdot z_p)^2 \qquad (3)$$

$$\mathcal{O}(\alpha, \beta, l) = \mathcal{N}\left(\left\{\sum_{i=1}^{n}\sum_{j=1}^{m_i} \Pi(\hat{l}_j^i)\right\} \cap \left\{\sum_{k=1}^{m} \Pi(l_k)\right\}\right) / \mathcal{N}\left(\sum_{j=1}^{m} \Pi(l_j)\right) \qquad (4)$$

subject to the constraints pertinent to the achievable gantry angles of imaging system (which depend on different manufacture designs)

$$-120° < \alpha < 120°, \quad -60° < \beta < 60°,$$

where "$\cdot$" denotes the inner product and θ_j is the angle between the directional vector l_j and projection vector $z_p = [-\cos(\alpha)\sin(\beta), -\sin(\alpha), \cos(\alpha)\cos(\beta)]^t$, and where $\hat{l}_j^i$ denotes the j-th segment of the i-th artery (consisting of m_i segments) in the coronary tree (consisting of n coronary arteries), $\Pi(\cdot)$ denotes the operator projecting an artery segment onto the image plane in the forms of a pixel-based array, $\cap$ denotes the intersection operator, and $\mathcal{N}(\cdot)$ is the function that counts the number of pixels onto the pixel-based array. On the basis of Eqs. (3) and (4), the composite function $\mathcal{V}(\alpha, \beta, l) = \mathcal{S}(\alpha, \beta, l) \oplus \mathcal{O}(\alpha, \beta, l)$ can be derived which incorporates the measurements of foreshortening and overlap by a fusion operator $\oplus$. Based on the function $\mathcal{V}(\alpha, \beta, l)$, a set of gantry angles $(\tilde{\alpha}, \tilde{\beta})$'s which minimize the vessel foreshortening and overlap relative to the artery l can be determined and utilized to acquire subsequent views for diagnostic or therapeutic procedure during coronary intervention.

4 Experimental Results

The accuracy of the proposed method was evaluated by use of 8 pairs of angiograms containing a Johnson & Johnson catheter guide wire with markers of 15 mm inter-distance. Images were acquired from Philips Integris H 3000 at various viewing angles. Eight markers (in terms of 2D points) along with the wire (in term of a 2D curve) were first identified manually on both images. With the identified marker points, the transformation that characterized the two views was calculated. Afterwards, the 3D catheter guide wire was reconstructed by use of the proposed technique. The length of catheter wire was calculated resulting in root-mean-square 3.1% error relative to the actual length 105 mm.

The total processing time varies from 7 to 10 minutes including image transfer (3 - 4 minutes) and all the computational processing (4 - 6 minutes). Angiograms of more than 200 cases acquired from a single-plane or biplane system have been completed for 3D reconstruction. The transformation was determined without the need of calibration object, and the 3D coronary arterial trees were reconstructed including left coronary , right coronary, and bypass graft systems. Among these studies, one example was chosen for demonstration in this paper. In Figs. 1(a) and 1(b), a pair of angiograms of LCA tree acquired from a biplane imaging system are shown. The reconstructed 3D left coronary arterial tree was obtained and viewed at gantry angulation $31.6°$ LAO and $49.3°$ CAUD after the process of 3D reconstruction was employed where the arterial segment (9.8 mm) of interest near the left coronary circumflex artery was manually marked as shown in Fig. 1(c).

With the selected arterial segment (*i.e.*, corresponding to a lesion), the process of optimal strategy was applied resulting in the estimates of foreshortening, overlap, and composite maps as shown in 1(d), 1(e), and 1(f). Each map consists of four quadrants characterizing the gantry orientations in terms of (LAO, CRAN), (RAO, CRAN), (RAO, CAUD), and (LAO, CAUD), respectively. Due to the mechanical limitation, the moving range of the gantry arm is confined from $120°$ LAO to $120°$ RAO and from $60°$ CRAN to $60°$ CAUD. The degrees of foreshortening and overlap in the respective maps are characterized by 5 different regions with individual shaded gray levels. The composite map is defined based on a fusion scheme such that the measures of foreshortening serve as the basis superimposed with the measures of overlap.

By use of the maps as shown in Figs. 1(d)-(f), any computer-predicted projection can be "previewed" accompanied with the estimates of foreshortening and overlap by pointing at any location in the map. Figs. 2(a)-(c) show three typical examples of unappreciated views. The remaining two views as shown in Figs. 2(d) and (e) demonstrate no vessel overlap and 0% foreshortening with respect to the selected arterial segment of interest, which can be utilized for acquiring subsequent images to facilitate further clinical diagnosis.

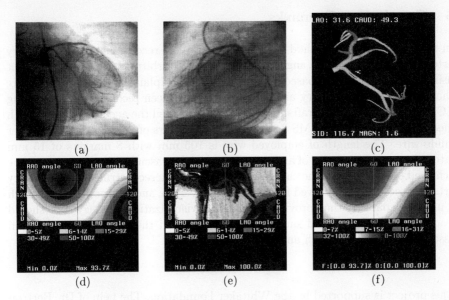

Fig. 1. (a)(b) The employed first ($0°$ LAO, $16°$ CAUD) and second views ($89°$ LAO, $1°$ CAUD) of left coronary artery angiograms. (c) The selected segment of interest (9.8 mm) with 17% foreshortening based on gantry angulation ($31.6°$ LAO, $49.3°$ CAUD). The foreshortening map (d), the overlap map (e), and the composite map (f) resulting from (d) and (e) illustrate various degrees of respective overlap, foreshortening, and combination relative to the selected arterial segment.

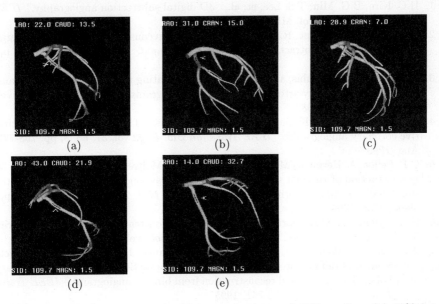

Fig. 2. Unappreciated views: (a) 0% foreshortening and 27% overlap, (b) 45% foreshortening and no overlap, and (c) 18% foreshortening and 40% overlap. (d)(e) Views with 0% foreshortening and no vessel overlap adequate to be utilized for subsequent image acquisitions.

5 Concluding Remarks

In this paper, a novel method is proposed for on-line reconstruction 3D coronary arterial tree from routine angiograms acquired at arbitrary angles and without using calibration objects based on a single-plane or biplane imaging system. More than 120 cases of coronary arterial systems have been reconstructed including LCA, RCA, and bypass grafts. A validation confirmed the accuracy of 3D length measurement to within RMS 3.1% error using 6 pairs of angiograms of catheter guide wire. The length of employed wire is 105 mm with 8 markers of 15 mm inter-distance. The choice of an optimal view of the vasculature of interest can be achieved on the basis of the capability of rotating the reconstructed 3D coronary arterial tree with the derived foreshortening, overlap, and composite maps. Such a unique capability thus provides an optimal visualization strategy that should lead to more efficient and successful diagnostic and therapeutic procedures in assessment of lesion length and diameter narrowing.

Acknowledgment

This project is supported by the Whitaker Foundation. The help of Dr. Bertron M. Groves in providing some angiograms and Keith E. Hellman in providing graphical user interface for image transfer is greatly appreciated.

References

1. H.C. Kim, B.G. Min, T.S. Lee, et. al., "3D digital subtraction angiography," *IEEE Trans. Med. Imag.*, vol. MI-1, pp. 152-158, 1982.
2. K.L. Parker, K.L. Pope, R. van Bree, et. al., "3-d reconstruction of moving arterial beds from digital subtraction angiography," *Comput. Biomed. Res.*, vol. 20, pp. 166-185, 1987.
3. K. Kitamura, J.M. Tobis, and J. Sklansky, "Estimating the 3D skeletons and transverse areas of coronary arteries from biplane angiograms," *IEEE Trans. on MI*, vol. MI-7, pp. 173-187, 1988.
4. T. Saito, M. Misaki, K. Shirato, and T. Takishima, "Three-dimensional quantitative coronary angiography," *IEEE Trans. on Bio. Eng.*, vol. 37, no. 8, pp. 768-777, Aug. 1990.
5. C.P. Pellot, A. Herment, M. Sigelle, P. Horain, H. Maitre, and P. Peronneau, "A 3d reconstruction of vascular structures from two x-ray angiograms using an adapted simulated annealing algorithm," *IEEE Tran. on Med. Imag.*, vol. 13, no. 1., pp. 49-60, Mar. 1994.
6. N. Guggenheim, P.A. Doriot, et al., "Spatial reconstruction of coronary arteries from angiographic images," *Phys. in Medic. & Biol.*, vol. 36, pp. 99-100, 1991.
7. A. Wahle, E. Wellnhofer, I. Mugaragu, H.U. Sauer, H. Oswald, and E. Fleck, "Assessment of diffuse coronary artery disease by quantitative analysis of coronary morphology based upon 3-d reconstruction from biplane angiograms," *IEEE Trans. on MI*, vol. 14, no. 2, pp. 230-241, 1995.
8. S. Stansfield, "ANGI: A rule based expert system for automatic segmentation of coronary vessels from digital subtracted angiograms," *IEEE Trans. on PAMI*, vol. 8, no. 2, pp. 188-199, 1986.

9. C. Smets, F. Vandewerf, P. Suetens, and A. Oosterlinck, "An expert system for the labeling and 3d reconstruction of the coronary arteries from two projections," *Int. J. Card. Img.*, vol. 5, no. 2-3, pp. 145-154, 1990.
10. G. Coppini, M. Demi, R. Mennini, G. Valli, "3D knowledge driven reconstruction of coronary trees," *Medical & Bio. Eng. & Comp.*, pp. 535-542, 1991.
11. D. Delaere, C. Smets, P. Suetens, G. Marchal, and F. Van de Werf, "Knowledge-based system for the 3d reconstruction of blood vessels from two angiographic projections," *Med. Biol. Eng. Comput.*, vol. 29, no. 6, pp. ns27 - ns36, Nov. 1991.
12. I. Liu and Y. Sun, "Fully automated reconstruction of 3-d vascular tree structures from two orthogonal views using computational algorithms and production rules", *Optical Engineering*, vol. 31, no. 10, pp. 2197-2207, Oct. 1992.
13. A. Rouge, C. Picard, D. Sanit-Felix, et al., "3-d coronary arteriography," *Int. J. of Card. Img.*, vol. 10, pp. 67-70, 1994.
14. H. C. Longuet-Higgins, "A computer algorithm for reconstructing a scene from two projections," *Nature*, vol. 293, no. 10, pp. 133-135, September 1981.
15. R. Y. Tsai and T. S. Huang, "Uniqueness and estimation of 3D motion parameters of rigid objects with curved surfaces," *IEEE Trans. on PAMI*, vol. 6, no. 1, pp. 13-27, Jan. 1984.
16. J.Q. Fang, T.S. Huang, "Some experiments on estimating the 3-d motion parameters of a rigid body from two consecutive image frames," *IEEE Trans. on PAMI*, vol. 6, pp. 547-554, Jan. 1984.
17. J. Philip, "Estimation of 3-d motion of rigid objects from noisy observations," *IEEE Trans. on PAMI*, vol. 13, pp. 61-66, 1991.
18. C. E. Metz and L. E. Fencil, "Determination of three-dimensional structure in biplane radiography without prior knowledge of the relationship between the two views: Theory," *Medical Physics*, 16 (1), pp. 45-51, Jan/Feb 1989.
19. L. E. Fencil and C. E. Metz, "Propagation and reduction of error in three-dimensional structure determined from biplane views of unknown orientation," *Medical Physics*, 17 (6), pp. 951-961, Nov/Dec 1990.
20. J. Weng, T.S. Huang, and N. Ahuja, "A two-step approach to optimal motion and structure estimation," *Proc. IEEE Workshop Computer Vision*, pp. 355-357, 1987.
21. J. Weng, N. Ahuja, and T. Huang, "Closed-form solution and maximum likelihood: a robust approach to motion and structure estimation," *Proc. IEEE Conf. Computer Vision and Pattern Recognition*, pp. 381-386, 1988.
22. J. Weng, T.S Huang, N. Ahuja, "Motion and structure from two perspective view: algorithms, error analysis and error estimation," *IEEE Trans. on PAMI*, vol. 11, pp. 451-476, Jan. 1989.
23. J. Weng, N. Ahuja, T.S. Huang, "Optimal motion and structure estimation," *IEEE Trans. on PAMI*, vol. 15, no. 9, pp. 864-884, 1993.
24. S.-Y. J. Chen, K.R. Hoffmann, J.D. Carroll, "Three-dimensional reconstruction of coronary arterial tree based on biplane angiograms," *Proceedings of SPIE Medical Imaging: Image Processing*, vol. 2710, Newport Beach, California, pp. 103-114, 1996
25. S.-Y. J. Chen and C.E. Metz, "Improved determination of biplane imaging geometry from two projection images and its application to 3D reconstruction of coronary arterial trees," *Medical Physics*, vol. 24, no. 5, May 1997, pp. 633-654.
26. B.K.P. Horn, Robot Vision, The MIT Press, McGraw-Hill Book Company, 1986.

A Robotic Approach to HIFU Based Neurosurgery

Brian L Davies, Sunita Chauhan and Mike J S Lowe

Dept. of Mechanical Engineering,
Imperial College of Science, Technology and Medicine,
Exhibition Road, London SW7 2BX.

Email: b.davies@ic.ac.uk

Abstract. The use of robotics in surgical interventions not only has the potential for minimally invasive surgical procedures but can improve performance and result in reduced operative time and post-operative trauma/recovery. This paper describes the concept of a robotic based High Intensity Focused Ultrasound system as a neuro-surgical tool for the destruction of subcortical lesions. A novel multi-transducer applicator system is proposed in order to minimise the effects of off-focal hot-spots and cavitation. Analytical models have been developed for simulating the acoustic field of the multi-transducer system. The models predict the interactive field effects from specific spatial configurations of the probes with respect to each other and to the target. Finally, the design aspects for a robotics based dedicated manipulator for HIFU-based brain surgery have been explored, together with those predicted from a laboratory system.
Keywords: Neurosurgery, Surgical Robots, Ultrasound Surgery, Treatment Planning

1 Introduction

Because of its complex anatomy and vital functionality, brain tissue surgery has always remained a formidable medical challenge. The need to devise precise and minimally invasive surgical methods is, therefore, more demanding for the brain than for any other organ or part of the human body. A widely used and well-established technique for neuro-surgery, particularly for point-in-space applications such as taking tissue biopsy, is stereotactic surgery. This method has been adopted by other treatment disciplines as well, (for instance in radiation therapy and surgery, in seed implantation in the brain, etc.) because it gives accurate registration of surgical tools. The disadvantage is that they are invasive and the reference base-frame needs to be clamped/screwed to the patient's skull, both in the pre-operative and intra-operative stages. Moreover, the frame may obstruct access to the surgical site or constrain the motion of the tools. To alleviate these problems, frame-less techniques have recently been introduced. These frame-less techniques however, can be less accurate and are presently in the developmental stage.

To avoid the risks involved in open brain surgery, efforts are being made world wide to develop minimally invasive surgical methods such as Computer Assisted Surgery

(CAS) and robotic surgery. Surgical targets in stereotatic surgery, and in most contemporary CAS procedures, are usually not under direct real-time vision. However, tool trajectories may be guided by registering and projecting their position onto 3-D reconstruction on the computer monitor screen during the operation. It is difficult to use these indirect vision methods to achieve precise micro-surgical manipulations with appropriate hand-eye co-ordination. Robotic techniques are more accurate, and require less operating time than human actions, particularly in tasks requiring repetitive actions.

In traditional open surgery, there is a need to create an access wound in the tissue. The surgical process involving opening the tissue may cause anatomical shifts, apart from making the procedure invasive. For brain tissue, in particular, these incisions may prove fatal in some cases. Also, the opening of the *dura* may cause severe loss of blood and cerebrospinal fluid, which in turn may result in large pressure changes and motion of the brain tissue. These risks are more severe if the lesions are bigger in size and/or are deep-seated. To minimise these complications, it is desirable to devise minimally invasive or non-invasive means of surgery.

Recently, **H**igh **I**ntensity **F**ocused **U**ltrasound as a non-invasive surgical modality has shown promising results, particularly in the areas of urology and oncology [1,2]. HIFU surgery is based upon the thermal effects of ultrasound and is beneficial if well-controlled thermal doses (without cavitation) can be administered in desired locations. It is necessary to study the requirements of each specific case and to decide upon the safety limits by considering the effects of all the exposure parameters involved in the treatment planning phase, prior to actual surgery/irradiation. In order to study the behaviour of the ultrasonic beam, as it traverses through the tissue, computer models have been developed and simulation results are presented in this paper.

In the case of brain tissue which is encased in the bony envelope of the skull, a direct application of the ultrasound energy is difficult because bone reflects a large amount of the incident energy. Therefore, it is necessary to create access craniotomies of considerable size in order to place the applicators directly on the *dura mater* (via an appropriate acoustic couplant). This however, should not introduce any risk because the external skull can be grafted and sutured and the whole procedure is still non-invasive to the sensitive brain tissue.

1.1 A New Multiple Probe Approach

It is necessary to minimise the effects of cavitation at high intensity levels as desired for tissue ablation and to avoid the off-focus hot-spots that are inherent in conventional HIFU systems and electronic arrays. To achieve this, a method is proposed in this paper for using separate multiple probes to simultaneously ablate the target from different angles. This ensures that the total required power is divided into low intensity beams. The probe selection, its dimensions and the applicator power play a crucial role in making the system minimally invasive. The concept of providing the required thermal dose from well spaced multiple probes favours minimal access. Thus two or three small craniotomies will be required, which can be planned in safe regions on the skull surface and for which appropriate focal lengths can be chosen. This will be advantageous only if the surgery system is designed to avoid constructive interference outside the composite focal region of the participating beams, thus avoiding hot-spots in the normal tissue regions. Moreover, the dimensions of the focal region should be planned in such a manner that it is confined well-within the abnormality. This may be particularly difficult to achieve in the case of small lesions. Alternatively, the probe may need to be scanned over the whole volume of the lesion when the lesion is larger than the composite focus. The development of such a system, which requires robotic techniques to simultaneously move and focus the probes, is the underlying aim of the present research and will be described in the following sections.

Ultrasound provides an indirect form of surgery in which the cutting formats are not straightforward (in contrast to the case of well defined surgical cuts using routine clinical tools e.g. knives, scalpels, scissors etc.). It is thus necessary to study the beam characteristics in terms of power, size and shape when it propagates through the tissue. For this purpose, mathematical models have been developed. These predict the interactive field resulting from the joint effect of multiple transducers in a variety of spatial configurations and excitation conditions. The models developed at Imperial College are summarised below. Validation work and parametric studies of transducer properties and positions along with the field modifications by introducing a diagnostic probe coaxially at the center of one of the surgical probes (for online feedback) will be reported elsewhere.

2 Computer Simulations

Models for predicting the beam patterns generated by a focused transducer are well established [3]. They typically make use of integrals of the fields due to point sources or plane waves. In our models, we exploit the point source approach which is formalised by Huygen's principle and the Fresnel Kirchoff's diffraction theory [3] and we extend the concept to incorporate the interactive field of multiple transducers. Field characteristics of an ultrasonic transducer such as the radial and transverse power amplitude, intensity profiles, beam plots at any point in the field both for two dimensional (cylindrical wave equation) and three dimensional (spherical) coordinates can be studied by using these models. The results in this paper were obtained using the two dimensional model. The software is written in such a way that almost all the field parameters can be entered as desired (for instance, the size and shape of the probe, the frequency of operation, focal length, velocity in the sound medium, axial and radial distance, number of Huygen's pts per mm etc.). This flexibility is necessary in order to understand the effects of individual variables on the beam characteristics. The co-ordinate system, showing three probes in a plane for the 2-D calculations are illustrated in fig.1. The model assumes plane strain in the plane of fig.1, so that each point in this plane represents a line source. The probes are arranged so that they produce a confocal superimposed focus within the target region. The multi-transducer model is initially developed for three probes only, but can be extended to any desired number within the defined co-ordinate system. The overall field distribution obtained from the interference of individual probes is given by complex summation of individual potentials and then plotting the absolute value of the sum, solving the wave equation for cylindrical 2-D calculations for the constituent probes. The acoustic pressure amplitude p(r,t) at any arbitrary point P(r,θ) in the field at a distance r from the source and time t is given by [3]:

$$p(r,t) = A\sqrt{\frac{2\lambda}{\pi r}} \cdot e^{i(\omega t - kr)} \qquad (1)$$

where, λ is the wavelength of sound, ω is the angular frequency, k is the wave number and A is an arbitrary constant. Only the wave travelling in the positive z-direction has been considered (fig.1). For large *r*, the cylindrical wave can be approximated as a plane wave with pressure amplitude decreasing as $1/\sqrt{r}$. The intensity, in terms of pressure amplitude is calculated as:

$$I = \frac{p^2}{\rho \cdot c} \qquad (2)$$

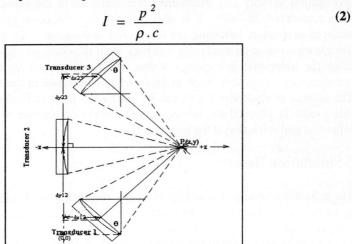

Fig.1. The planner co-ordinate system used for modelling the three transducer system.

The spatial configurations (location & orientation) of all of the probes can be separately entered and thus the corresponding effects of individual probes on the composite intensity/beam profiles can be studied. Initially, a linear propagation of sound waves is assumed in a homogenous and loss-less medium for the purpose of calculating the field parameters. In practice, biological tissue is not homogenous and the ultrasound energy is attenuated due to reflection, refraction, scattering and absorption during its passage to the target. The fraction of the incident energy that is absorbed gives rise to the desired focal hot-spot for ablation. The original model has been extended in two ways: first to incorporate the attenuation effects ($e^{-\alpha x}$) as a function of propagation distance(x) and second to calculate tissue temperature rise by solving Pennes' bio-heat equation (expressed for one dimension):

$$\rho.c(\frac{dT}{dt}) = \kappa(\frac{d^2T}{dx^2}) + \omega.c_b(T_a - T_b) + q \qquad (3)$$

where T is the tissue base temperature, T_a is the local arterial blood temperature, T_b is the local venous temperature, c_b is the Sp. heat of blood, c is the Sp. heat of the tissue, ρ is the tissue density, ω is the blood perfusion rate, q is the volumetric heat generation rate and κ is the thermal conductivity of the tissue. The effects of blood perfusion during short ablation periods are assumed to be negligible ($\omega = 0$). With this assumption, the temperature elevation in the exposed area was computed by adding the effects from individual Huygen's sources, similar to the calculation of field intensities in the previous models.

The model was further extended to include the effects of heterogeneity of the brain tissue as seen by the propagating ultrasound wave. The acoustic properties of grey and white matter are found to be widely different [4]. The interface of various layers has been considered as a straight line for the given size of the probes. This is a preliminary approach to the practical *in vivo* situation and only the differences in propagation velocity and attenuation characteristics of the constituent media have been considered. Initially, it is also assumed that the beam propagates from one medium to another following refraction and attenuation only. It is assumed that there is no acoustic internal reflection back from the skull, which is quite reasonable since the individual low energy beams, in the domain of selected focal length, becomes very feeble after the joint focus, as will be shown in the simulation results. The number of absorption layers can be inputted as desired. Further development of this model is planned to include curved interfaces together with the effects of reflection and refraction at the boundaries.

3 Simulation Results

The simulation results obtained by using the specifications of transducers operating at a resonance frequency of 1.88 MHz, 25.4 mm active aperture and focused at 63.5 mm have been presented in fig.2 and 3. The transducer specifications are those used in an experimental study to validate the acoustic field model, which will be reported elsewhere. Fig.2 shows the field computations for a particular spatial arrangement. Here the probes are considered to be positioned on an arch of radius equal to the focal length and oriented in the plane of the arch at an angle of 35^0 with respect to the middle probe, such that they produce a superimposed confocal area. The intensity is plotted as a dimension-less ratio, with maximum intensity at the focus normalised to unit intensity at the source. In fig.2(a), intensity variation along axial and radial dimensions in a loss-less medium has been illustrated. Fig.2(b) shows the temperatures produced in the exposed area by considering power absorption in the medium. For temperature estimations, the base temperature is taken as 37.6^0 C considering an absorption coefficient of 0.7 dB/cm/MHz$^{1.1}$ as suggested for human soft tissue [4,5]. The plots clearly show that for a two sec pulse, a highly focused region of 65^0 C average is produced whilst the off-focus regions are at about 42^0 C. These results are ideal for very localised ablation of tumours etc. Thus, it is possible to predict the temperature elevation in the focal region as well as throughout the irradiation field (region of interest) of the probes.

The simulation results of fig. 3 show the effects of absorption of the acoustic beam during its passage through biological media. Fig.3 (a) and (b) depict a comparison of the axial beam intensities in a loss-less medium and with those in an absorbing medium (with a=0.7 dB/cm/MHz$^{1.1}$) for a single probe. As is evident from these results, the joint focus is smaller in size, the overall intensity is lower and the focal peak shifts towards the surface (transducer face) when absorption effects are introduced. The axial beam characteristics through multi-layered tissue are shown in fig 3(d). Fig. 3(c) shows the schematic of the field composed of three layered tissue and the corresponding axial beam trace is shown in 3(d) for typical layer thickness and absorption coefficients lying in the range of grey and white matter (1.08 - 1.93 dB/cm at 1.88 MHz). Depending upon the ultrasonic characteristics of the medium in the path of constituent probes, the focal region may change its geometrical characteristics (location, size and shape) and field intensity values as compared to that predicted in either a loss-less medium or homogeneous absorbing medium. By pre-operative estimations of the type and depth of tissue layers, in the path of individual acoustic beams emanating from constituent probes, it is possible to predict field modifications. Further developed model would be used to determine optimum positions and treatment according to location of tumour.

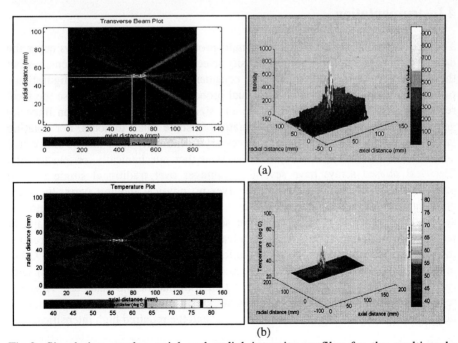

Fig.2. Simulation results: axial and radial intensity profiles for the multi-probe system in a loss-less medium (a); and temperature predictions (b) for a medium with α=1.19dB/cm at 1.88 MHz, base temp. =37.6 for 2s exposure.

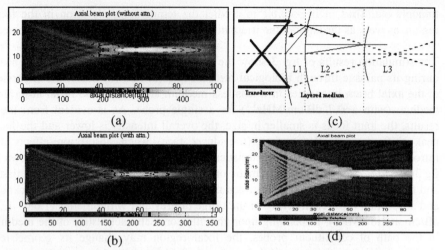

Fig.3. Predicted axial beam plots: in a loss-less medium (a) and in a homogenous absorbing medium (b) with a = 0.7 dB/cm/MHz$^{1.1}$; 3-layered medium schematic (c) and beam plot calculated for L1=20mm, α=1.93dB/cm; L2=40mm, α=1.09dB/cm; L3=30mm, α=1.19dB/cm.

4 Instrumentation

The size of the superimposed foci of a multi-probe system may not always cover the desired target. The frequency and intensity selection govern the foci dimensions but they cannot be varied indefinitely. By considering various spatial configurations, power inputs and frequencies of individual probes, it is possible to diffuse the focal region for slight modifications in shape and size with an overall effect on intensity generation. This may suffice for the ablation of some small tumours. For ablating larger lesions, it therefore, becomes necessary to mutually scan all the individual beams together, over the area of interest, either mechanically or electrically. Electrical phased arrays have several advantages over traditional single focused probes such as: electronic scanning involves no physical moving parts, the focal point can be changed dynamically to any location in the scanning plane and the system can generate a wide variety of scan formats for heating any shape of target. However, the most critical disadvantage is the formation of constructive interference zones which produce pseudo foci beyond the actual focal region. Other inherent disadvantages include: increased complexity of scanning electronics (particularly for large arrays), higher cost of transducers and scanners. Also the requirement of a large number of elements and greater complexity will result in large apertures to achieve high quality images and the required high intensities.

The procedure of mechanical scanning of the focused beams over the abnormality, however, will become more complex in the case of multiple probes. The problem can be segregated into two steps: Firstly, it is required to exactly match the foci of multiple beams such that they intersect within the target boundaries and secondly to maintain the co-ordinated focusing while they are being scanned. The second stage will be more difficult to implement, because of the motion constraints (the probes are not free to move as in the case of extra-corporeal methods but have to be seated and scanned within fixed craniotomies). This would require complex and precise manipulation strategies through the use of robotic techniques. A schematic diagram of the ultrasound surgical system is shown in fig.4.

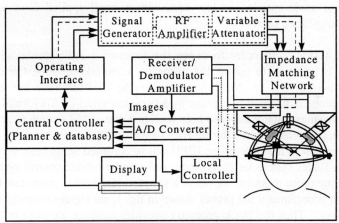

Fig.4. Robotic HIFU Neurosurgery System

Time gated, high intensity continuous sinusoidal bursts are applied by a radio-frequency power generator and are then fed to the transducers via a variable attenuator. Depending upon the specific application and tissue under investigation, the attenuation levels and time settings are varied. The transducers are also impedance matched with the r.f-generator circuitry for an efficient energy transfer. The transducers are coupled to the tissue of interest by the use of a couplant assembly which comprises fluid infusers/diffusers to regulate and control the amount of couplant in order to minimise the effect of abnormal pressure build-up of couplant over the sensitive tissue, while mechanically scanning the target.

4.1 Design aspects of the manipulator system

Surgical Robots. The Mechatronics in Medicine Group at Imperial College (IC) has a long-standing research activity in Robots for Surgery. Special-purpose systems have been produced for Prostatectomies and for Prosthetic Knee Replacement [6,7] It is felt that industrial robots, designed for their large reach envelope, are less suitable than special-purpose systems which can be designed to be simple, small and light to suit the specific task. Robots in Industry are required to be caged away from human contact for safety, which is clearly not practicable for surgery. For this reason, industrial robots have often been used in neurosurgery to position a fixture next to the head and then be locked off, unpowered, whilst the surgeon used the fixtures to carry out manual interventions. This was felt to be safer than using the industrial robot to actively remove the tissue and it was quite clear that the surgeon, and not the robot, was in-charge of the procedure. The only special-purpose neurosurgery robot to be used clinically (Minerva) was a large structure, which, although very accurate, was very complex and expensive [8]. The IC general approach to surgery robots is to use a small special-purpose active robot mounted upon a larger " gross positioning" robot which can be locked off, unpowered, once the active robot is in approximately the right location. By this means, the active robot can be made simple and low cost, with a small applied force and motion capability to enhance safety.

Motorised HIFU. In order to sweep the focus of a HIFU probe and ablate a volume, it is common to mount the probe on a motorised, three Cartesian axes, system. Alternatively, an electronic array may be used to adjust the focal depth, whilst the probe is scanned in a plane by a two-axes system. A hydraulic powered, plastic 3-axes manipulator has also been used in a closed MR system to provide real-time imaging of ablated tissue during HIFU ablation [9].

The IC approach to multiple-probe HIFU can be achieved in its most versatile form by use of a 3-axes system for each probe, and using a robotic control system for co-ordinating the probe motions. However a simpler, lower cost system can be used for a number of procedures if the probes shown in fig. 1, are rigidly mounted together in a single block. Thus the block geometry provides accurate focusing of the probes, whilst a simple 3-axes system sweeps the combined focus through a volume. In practise the probes typically require an offset angle of 35 degrees to each other and so the combined block becomes large. Whilst in some aspects of neurosurgery a large skull flap can be removed, which can allow access for the block via a flexible couplant bag interposed between the dura and the probe. However, the range of these applications is limited in neurosurgery, although there are potential benefits for many other areas, such as tumour ablation in the liver or the prostate.

4.2 The Neurosurgery HIFU Robot

In its most widely applicable form, the neurosurgery robotic system has been designed to position each of the 3 probes independently at any of 3 burr (entry) holes on the skull. This is achieved by a modified form of stereo-tactic frame (Fig. 5) in which the normal diametral arch has been replaced by 3 quarter-arches, joined at the top swivel-point so that each is motorised and free to rotate independently around the base-ring. The 3 probes are located on a probe- mount which can be driven along each quarter-arch. Thus any probe-mount can be located at the computer co-ordinates of any selected burr-hole on the skull, where it can be locked in position to facilitate safety. The probe-mount also serves as a fixture to facilitate burr-hole drilling.

Each probe-mount has 3 powered axes of motion: a pitch, a yaw and an in/out relative to the pitched/yawed mount (Fig 6). The tip of the mount carries the HIFU probe, to which is attached a flexible bag containing the coupling medium. The 3 axes of each probe motion allow its focus to be located anywhere within the target. A robotic control system co-ordinates the 9 motors of the 3 probes, to allow the 3 foci to overlap at a precise position which can also be swept anywhere in the brain. Alternatively the foci can be juxtaposed to give a larger region of heating. This 3 probe system requires the small, low-powered motors to have co-ordinated motions, but can provide total versatility in positioning and sweeping the probe focus. As commented in the previous section, however, simpler, cheaper systems are possible for particular procedures which require a less flexible approach.

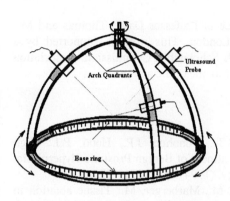 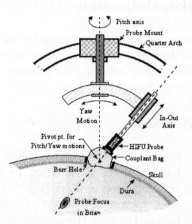

Fig.5. Modified Head frame. **Fig.6.** Schematic diagram of motions of a single probe.

5 Conclusion

The use of High Intensity Focused Ultrasound as a surgical modality is highly promising for minimally invasive procedures e.g. as required in neuro-surgery and may also result in a totally non-invasive treatment for other disciplines, which do not require any access wounds e.g. for surgery requiring abdominal access. However, it is necessary to undertake detailed studies in order to understand the interaction of highly intense ultrasound beams with biological tissues, normal and abnormal, in terms of a well-defined mathematical understanding. Numerical models enable the prediction of the after-effects of pre-defined exposures leading to planning of safer treatments. Simulation studies using a multi-transducer approach have been presented in this paper. The aim with this configuration is to minimise the effects of hot-spots in the off-focal areas in comparison to a single transducer.

Further experimental investigations are being carried out in order to study the attenuation effects in mammalian tissue *in vitro*. It is recognised that these are preliminary predictions and it is required to further explore the physical phenomena such as non-linear propagation, scattering effects from tissue heterogeneities & curved tissue boundaries and dynamic changes in tissue characteristics during the process of irradiation in order to simulate actual *in vivo* situations. The design and development of appropriate instrumentation for the precise, accurate and complete irradiation of a defined tissue volume is equally important. In the case of the multi-probe system, mechanical scanning of the joint focus in the target area (for ablating bigger tumours) is a crucial aspect of the instrument design. To achieve this a mechanical mechanism for robotic based HIFU system as described in this work, has been designed and developed at Imperial College. Further improvements with appropriate safety considerations are being carried out.

Acknowledgements

The authors wish to acknowledge the advice of Professor David Thomas and Mr. Neil Kitchen of Queen Square hospital, London. This work is supported by a scholarship award from the Commonwealth Scholarship Commission, Association of Commonwealth Universities, Govt. of UK to one of the authors.

References

1. Bihrle, R., Foster, R.L., Sanghvi, N.T., Donohue, J.P., Hood, P.J.: High Intensity Focused Ultrasound for the treatment of Benign Prostatic Hyperplasia: early united states experience. J. Urology. (1994) 151, 1271-1275.
2. Madersbacher, S., Kratzik, C., Susani, M., Marberger, M.: Tissue ablation in Benign Prostatic Hyperplasia with high intensity focused ultrasound. J. Urol. (1994) 152, 1956-1961.
3. Kino, G.S., Acoustic Waves: Devices, Imaging & Analog Image Processing, Prentice Hall Inc., New Jersey (1986).
4. Fry, F.J., Kossoff, G et al.: Threshold Ultrasonic Dosages for Structural Changes in the Mammalian Brian, J. Acous. Soc. Am. (1970) 48, 1413-1417.
5. Robinson, T.C. and Lele, P.P.) An Analysis of Lesion Development in the Brain and in Plastics by High Intensity Focused Ultrasound at Low MHz Frequencies, J. Acous. Soc. Am. (1972) 51, 1333-1351.
6. Harris, S.J., Mei, Q., Arambula-Cosio, F. et al.: A Robotic procedure for transuretheral resection of prostate, In Proc. MRCAS'95, Baltimore,USA, Nov.4-7(1995), 264-271.
7. Harris, S., Jakopec, M., Davies, B.L.: Interactive pre-operative selection of cutting constraints, and interactive force controlled knee surgery by a surgical robot, proceedings of MICCAI conf. Oct.11-13 (1998) Boston.
8. Glauser G., Flury P., Epitauz M., Piquet Y.,and Burckhardt C.: Neurosurgical operation with the dedicated robot Minerva, IEEE, EMBS Magazine, March(1993), 347-351.
9. Cline, H.E., Hynynen, K., Watkins, R.D., et al.: A Focused Ultrasound system for MRI guided ablation, Radiology (1995) 194, 731-737.

Virtual Surgery System Using Deformable Organ Models and Force Feedback System with Three Fingers

Naoki SUZUKI [1], Asaki HATTORI [1], Akihiro TAKATSU [1], Takahiro KUMANO [2], Akio IKEMOTO [2], Yoshitaka ADACHI [2], Akihiko UCHIYAMA [3]

[1] Institute for High Dimensional Medical Imaging, Jikei University School of Medicine
4-11-1, Izumihoncho, Komae-shi, Tokyo 201-8601, Japan
nsuzuki@jikei.ac.jp, hat@tkd.att.ne.jp, takatsu@jikei.ac.jp
[2] Suzuki Motor Corporation R & D Center
2-1, Sakura-namiki, Tsuzuki-ku, Yokohama, Kanagawa 224-0046, Japan
{kumano, ikemoto, adachi}@yrd.suzuki.co.jp
[3] School of Science and Engineering, Waseda University
3-4-1, Okubo, Shinjuku-ku, Tokyo 169, Japan
uchiyama@uchiyama.comm.waseda.ac.jp

1. Abstract

We aimed to develop a virtual surgery system capable of performing surgical maneuvers on elastic organs, the structure of which has been obtained from a patient. We tried to manipulate three dimensional (3D) organs as elastic models by hand or surgical tools in real time in a virtual environment. And we tried to obtain the sense of touch by using force feedback device with manipulator attached to the thumb, forefinger and middle finger of the operator.

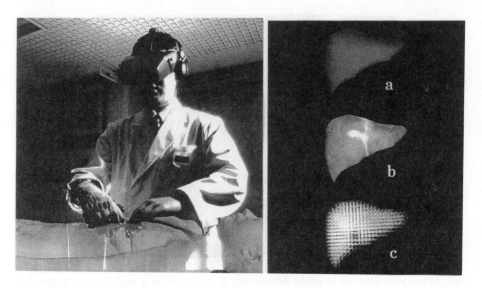

Fig.1.(upper left) A typical scene of the operator performing a surgical simulation.
Fig.2.(upper right) Structure of the deformable organ model of a liver. Fig.2b is the reconstructed liver with a texture mapping of autopsied liver tissue. Fig.2c is inner structure of the reconstructed liver model. The liver model was filled with 1880 spheres.

2. Method

2-1. VR surgery simulation system

We wanted to devise a system that would allow pushing, pinching, or incising of soft tissue models in the surgical simulation. When a large incision is made, the inner structures of an organ, such as blood vessels, are also likely to be incised or deformed. Our system therefore had the following requirements. At first, the simulation should performed as real time simulation and the image should be real. That is, the system have to represent the accurate and detailed shape of the patient's organ and to deform the organ according to physical and anatomical knowledge. Second, the organ model should be performed quantitative deformation with accuracy including the organ's inner structures. In the real time simulation, user is able to manipulate (push, pick, pinch, incise and excise) the organ model by hand or with surgical tools in virtual space. And we need to devise a system to connect easily to the force feedback device and to obtain values for force feedback.

The image generation in our system is performed by an Onyx Reality Engine2 (Silicon Graphics Cray Inc). We thought that it is difficult at present to perform the calculations of organ structure with the compiled anatomical structure for the finite element method in real time due to speed limits of the processor. It is also difficult to divide human structures automatically into finite elements. We have proposed a so-called "sphere-filled model" to produce an elastic organ model. In this model, a mass composed of small spheres fills the inside of a 3D organ model. Organ models are reconstructed from contour organ sets obtained from 3D data sets using CT or MRI. We fill the inside of the organ with some element spheres. All element spheres have the same radius, and are placed at a face-centered cubic lattice. The external force applied to the organ model displaces some of these spheres, which in turn displace the spheres surrounding them until ultimately the shape of the entire organ is deformed. The magnitude and direction of the force generated when the spheres are moved, determines their return to their original position, allowing the force-feedback system to generate a sense of touch.

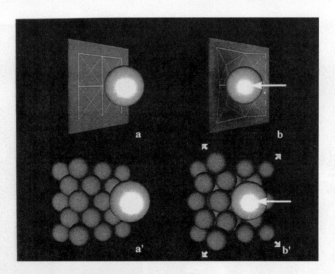

Fig.3. The basic behavior of model deformation. If external force is applied to the model, it is deformed by the movement of each element sphere.

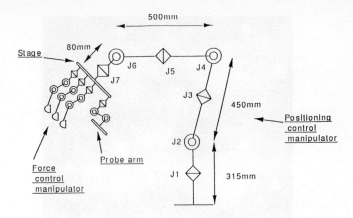

Fig.4. The block diagram of the design of the force feedback device system. The locations of joints and relational location of motion controlled manipulators are seen in the schema.

2-2. Force feedback device

We tried to develop a force feedback device which gives the user the sense of touch as if actual contact were being made with the organ. However, in the field of surgical simulation, there are some important points to be considered when a force feedback device is designed. One is how to measure the movement of the operator's hand with high accuracy. Another is how to give the operator's hand a realistic sensation of the virtual environment. To satisfy these requirements, the development of a high performance force feedback system is anticipated. We designed and built a sixteen degrees-of-freedom (DOF) force feed back device for manual interaction with virtual environments.

The features of the device manufactured for our virtual surgery system are summarized as follows.
At first, the force feedback system is composed of two types of manipulators, a force control manipulator and a motion control manipulator. And we tried to design three force control manipulators, those are attached to the end of the motion control manipulator. Second, both ends of each force control manipulator are attached to the thumb, forefinger and middle finger of the operator. In addition, the force control manipulator has a joint structure with minimal inertia and less friction. And the motion control manipulator has a mechanical stiffness should be realized in the system to complete surgical maneuvers without stress. Fig.4 shows the block diagram of the design of the force feedback device system. The locations of joints and relational location of motion controlled manipulators are seen in the schema.

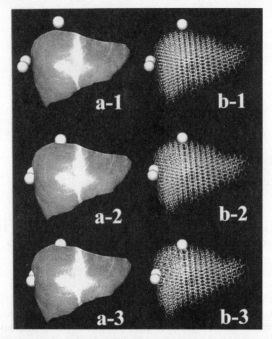

Fig.5. The response of the deformable liver model to variations in force. Fig. 5a-1 to a-3 shows the performance of the model when it was pushed by three fingers. Fig. 5b-1 to b-3 show the condition of spheres of the model.

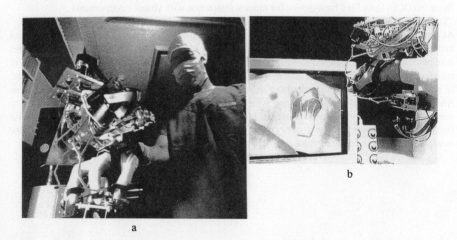

Fig.6. The appearance of the force feedback system. The operator's thumb, forefinger and middle finger are attached to the distal part of the motion controlled manipulators.

3. Results

Fig. 1 shows a typical scene of the user performing a surgical simulation with our system. In this image the 3D image which the user observes with a head mount display (HMD) is composited to clear the user's works. In this case the user is not using the force feedback system which we developed, and is instead using a cyberglobe which is commercially available. Using the liver as an example, the structure of our deformable organ model is shown in Fig. 2a ,2b and 2c. Fig. 2a and 2b are the reconstructed liver model by the sphere filled model. The liver contours are obtained from the 3D data set of MRI with a 4 mm slice in a 4 mm pitch and 1880 spheres fill this liver model. The surface of the liver model was wrapped with surface images of autopsied liver tissue using a texture mapping method to obtain a realistic appearance for the simulation (Fig.2b). In this simulation the surface texture can be easily changed to color code by the user (Fig.2a). Fig. 2c shows the spheres that fill the liver. In this image the spheres were displayed with the wire frame image and the liver surface were eliminated.Fig. 3 show the basic behavior of model deformation. If external force is applied to the object, each element sphere is pressed and moved in turn (Fig.3b'). The entire object is deformed (Fig.3b). Fig. 5 show the response of the deformable liver model to variations in force. Fig. 5a-1 to a-3 shows the performance of the model when it was pushed by three fingers. The white ball indicates the object that pushed the surface of the model liver. Fig. 5b-1 to b-3 show the condition of spheres of the model. These images were displayed at 10-12 frames/s. And there was no significant difference in delay in image generation. Fig. 6a,b shows the appearance of the force feedback system. A surgeon attached his right arm to the device. The operator's thumb, forefinger and middle finger are attached to the distal part of the motion controlled manipulators. By the combination of sphere-filled model and force feedback device, it was possible to manipulate a model liver with 1880 spheres at a speed of about 10 frame/s. The rate of image generation is about 10 fold slower than the responsiveness of the force feedback device. We had to interpolate the magnitude of force when it was supplied to the force feedback device in order to create a realistic sense of touch.

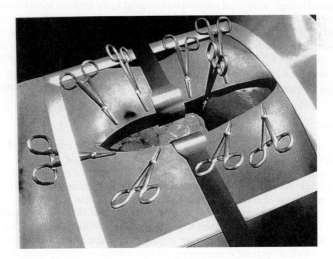

Fig.7. A simulation of open surgery in the abdominal region. Forceps, abdominal retractor and surgical knife are used in the simulation.

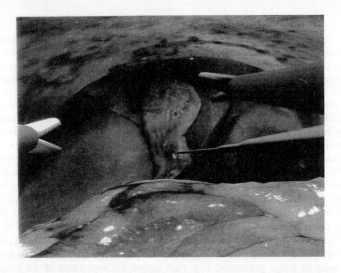

Fig.8. A simulation of laparoscopic surgery in the abdominal region with the same data set used for the open surgery in Fig.7.
In this image the 3D image which the operator observes with a head mount display (HMD) is composited on the image of the user.

This speed was not changed when the operator touched the organ model with one finger or three fingers. One of the benefits of the sphere-filled model is that there is no difference in calculation time when the number of outer forces is different. Fig. 7 shows a simulation of open surgery in the abdominal region. Forceps, abdominal retractor and surgical knife are used in this simulation. Data from the patient was reconstructed from the MRI data set and the skin and organ surfaces were texture mapped (skin surface, patient's surface image; liver and intestines, Image of autopsied specimen) to increase the reality in the virtual environment. When the view point, field of vision and surgical tools are changed, laparoscopic surgery can be performed. Fig. 8 shows laparoscopic surgery in the abdominal region with the same data set used for the open surgery in Fig. 7. It is possible to incise the organ surface with an electric knife and to pinch the liver with forceps.

4. Conclusion

By filling the object model with element spheres, containing a relatively with high speed manipulation for controlling deformation was achieved. This method is suitable for real-time simulation and quantitative deformation of tissues. We are also albe to point out a few merits of this method. In the sphere-filled model, no matter how complicated the shapes of the organ of interest may be, organ models can be constructed by the same operation. In our virtual surgery system, it is possible to perform surgical maneuvers at a speed approaching that of the actual procedure, with a sense of touch. We have applied this system to surgery in the abdominal region in this paper and we plan to extend the region of application to other organs and various types of surgery. This surgical experience, in which a patient's morphological characteristics are reproduced in a virtual environment, will allow the establishment of a new method of clinically applicable surgery as well as an educational innovation, in the near future.

References

1. Thomas H. Speeter: Three Dimensional Finite Element Analysis of Elastic Continua for Tactile Sensing: The International Jounal of Robotics Reserch, 11 No. 1:1-19, February 1992.
2. Robb, R.A, D.P. Hanson: The ANALYZE software system for visualization and analysis in surgery simulation. In: Computer Integrated Surgery, Eds. Steve Lavalle, Russ Taylor, Greg Burdea and Ralph Mosges, MIT Press, 1993.
3. Suzuki. N, Takatsu. A, Kita. K,Tanaka. T, Inaba. R, Fukui. K: Development of an 3D image simulation system for organ and soft tissue operations.: Abstract of the World Congress on Medical Physics and Biomedical Engineering 1994; 39a: 609.
4. Suzuki. N, Hattori. A, Takatsu. A: Medical virtual reality system for surgical planning and surgical support.: J. Comput. Aided Surg., 54-59, 1(2), 1995
5. Robb, R.A., D.P. Hanson, J.J. Camp: Computer-aided surgery planning and rehearsal at Mayo Clinic. Computer, 29(1):39-47, 1996.
6. Suzuki. N, Kawakami. K, Hattori. A, Takatsu. A.: Abdominal surgery planning using medical virtual reality system.: CAR '96 1996; 1058
7. S.Cotin, H. Delingette, M. Bro-Nielsen, N. Ayache, J.M. Clement, V. Tassetti, J. Marescaux: Geometric and Physical Representations for a Simulator of Hepatic Surgery: Health Care in the Information Age, Eds:H.Sieburg, S.Weghorst, K.Morgan, IOS Press and Ohmsha, 1996.
8. Dwight A. Meglan, Rakesh Raju, Gregory L. Merril, Jonathan R. Merril, Binh H. Nguyen, Shankar N. Swamy, Gerald A. Higgins: The Teleos Virtual Environment Toolkit for Simulation-Based Surgical Education: Health Care in the Information Age, Eds:H.Sieburg, S.Weghorst, K.Morgan, IOS Press and Ohmsha, 1996.
9. Naoki Suzuki, Asaki Hattori, Shinya Kai, Akihiro Takatsu: Surgical planning system for soft tissues using virtual reality: In: Medicine Meets Virtual Reality, Eds: K.S.Morgan et al.,pp.159-163, IOS Press, 1997.

A Modular Surgical Robotic System for Image Guided Percutaneous Procedures

Dan Stoianovici Ph.D.[1,2], Louis L. Whitcomb Ph.D.[2],
James H. Anderson Ph.D.[4], Russell H. Taylor Ph.D.[3], and
Louis R. Kavoussi M.D.[1]

[1] James Buchanan Brady Urological Institute, Johns Hopkins Medical Institutions
[2] Department of Mechanical Engineering, Whiting School of Engineering
[3] Department of Computer Science, Whiting School of Engineering
[4] Department of Radiology, Johns Hopkins Medical Institutions

- Johns Hopkins University -

Abstract. This paper presents a robotic system for precise needle insertion under radiological guidance for surgical interventions and for delivery of therapy. It is extremely compact and is compatible with portable X-ray units and computer tomography scanners. The system presents a modular structure comprising a global positioning module, a miniature robotic module, and a radiolucent needle driver module. This system is the newest member of a growing family of modular surgical robots under development. The system may be operated stand-alone under joystick control making it readily adaptable to any operating room, or under full image guided computer control.

1 Introduction

Needle access required for percutaneous surgery is presently preformed in the operating room by manually inserting the needle under single-view fluoroscopic radiological guidance. This procedure is challenging; it requires extensive experience due to the lack of three-dimensional information of the inter-operative X-ray imager.

To overcome this problem several researchers investigated the use of robotic systems to assist in needle placement. Potamianos and Davies [3], [4] proposed a stereo-pair of two x-ray views registered to a common fiducial system with a five degree of freedom (DOF) passive linkage equipped with position encoders to position a passive needle guide. Bzostek et al. [1] used an active robot (LARS [8]) for similar purposes. These systems successfully addressed difficult issues of image-to-robot registration and provided convenient means for defining target anatomy. In their present state of development, however, these robotic systems are expensive and their size makes them cumbersome for routine use in the operating room.

In contrast, our group recently reported the development of a simple, non-computerized system, PAKY [5], which based on a minimal approach offered immediate application in the operation room. PAKY is a radiolucent needle driver actuated by an electrical motor. A passive arm connected to the operating table supports the driver. The surgeon uses the usual technique of "Superimposed Needle Registration" [5] to manually orient the driver and therefore the needle. PAKY is then locked into the desired orientation and needle insertion is manually controlled from a joystick. The records of twelve patients who underwent percutaneous nephrolithotomy using PAKY demonstrated that the calyx chosen by the surgeon was accessed on the first attempt in each case [2].

The PAKY device was the first member of a growing family of surgical robotic modules under development at Johns Hopkins University. This paper reports on the second member of this family, a remote center of motion (RCM) actuator module called the "MINI-RCM" and its integration and operation with the PAKY module.

In the attempt to simplify the orientation procedure, increase accuracy, reduce radiation exposure, and achieve PAKY's compatibility with advanced imaging equipment (i.e. computerized tomography) our group developed the MINI-RCM. This module integrates both with PAKY and with a variety of additional end effectors presently under development. Hardware development of the MINI-RCM is completed and pre-clinical testing of the system is in progress. A general presentation of this new system, MINI-RCM & PAKY, is outlined next.

2 Robotic Design

A schematic of the system MINI-RCM & PAKY for radiological needle insertion is presented in Figure 1. This modular system comprises the needle driver PAKY, a low dof robot (MINI-RCM), and a passive arm.

The trocar needle used for percutaneous procedures is loaded into the needle driver PAKY. The needle driver presents a radiolucent construction providing unimpeded X-ray imaging of the anatomical target. An electrical motor integrated into the driver's fixture provides automated needle insertion. The driver is constructed of acrylic, making it inexpensive to manufacture as a sterile disposable part [6].

The MINI-RCM is an extremely compact robot utilizing the RCM principle of the LARS robot reported by Taylor et al [8]. In contrast to LARS, the MINI-RCM employs a chain transmission rather than a parallel linkage. This provides unrestricted rotations about the RCM point, uniform rigidity of the mechanism, and eliminates singular points. In order to accommodate different end-effectors, the MINI-RCM includes an adjustment of the location of the RCM point. Due to this adjustment the two axes of rotation (R1 about y direction and R2 about x direction, Figure 1) may be non-orthogonal (79 deg to 90 deg). This special scheme renders a miniaturized RCM design: the robot may be folded into a $171 \times 69 \times 52mm$ box and it weighs only $1.6Kg$.

The needle is initially placed into the driver PAKY such that its tip is located at the remote center of motion of the MINI-RCM (RCM Point in Figure 1). For this purpose PAKY is equipped with a visible laser diode whose ray (Laser

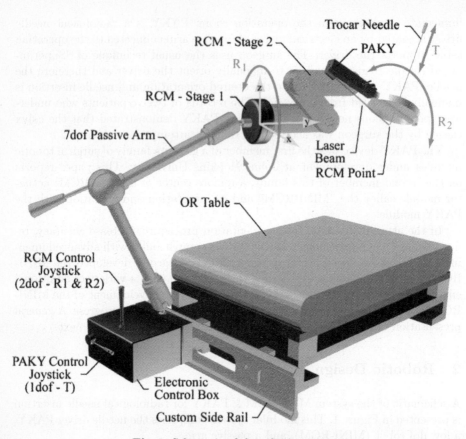

Fig. 1. Schematic of the robotic system

Beam in Figure 1) intersects the needle at the RCM point, thus helping the surgeon position the needle into the driver. The robot presents two motorized DOF implementing the rotations R1 and R2 about the RCM point (needlepoint). At present, the PAKY & MINI-RCM robotic assembly is supported by a passive 7 DOF passive arm which may be locked at the desired position by depressing a lever. A custom rigid rail is mounted on the side of the operating room fluoroscopic table (Figure 1) to provide a sturdy base for the robotic arm. This is critical in order to provide a fixed reference frame for the robotic system and maintain needle trajectory under the insertion force.

A photograph of this modular system presenting the PAKY needle driver supported into the MINI-RCM robot is presented in Figure 2. The laser beam used for needle positioning may be observed at its point.

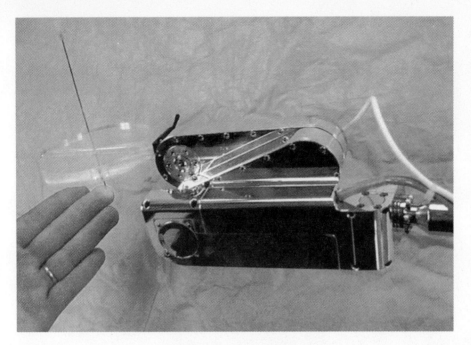

Fig. 2. MINI-RCM & PAKY robot

3 Operation Principle

Inserting a needle at an arbitrary location requires six DOF. If the skin insertion site of the needle is prescribed, however, one may observe that only two rotations are necessary in order to orient the needle and only one translation is necessary to insert it. Therefore, a total number of three DOF are necessary and sufficient to aim any anatomical target while initially positioning the needle tip at the desired skin entry point.

The proposed robotic system is used as follows: Using the laser beam mark the surgeon initially positions the needle into the driver such that its tip is located at the RCM point. Then, the surgeon chooses the skin entry site and using the passive arm he/she manipulates the system such that the needlepoint is located as desired while the orientation of the needle is arbitrary. The system is locked by depressing the lever of the positioning arm. This operation does not require X-ray imaging.

The two-rotational RCM stage is then employed to precisely orient the needle such that its axis extends into the desired target, based on radiological data. During this orientation stage the tip of the needle pivots about the skin entry point, the RCM point. When accurately oriented the needle insertion is performed using the needle driver PAKY.

The procedure may be performed in two modes: manual or automatic.

The manual mode is well suited for immediate utilization of the device in surgical procedures: it uses the portable x-ray fluoroscopy machine (C-Arm)

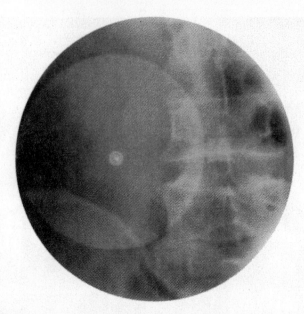

Fig. 3. PAKY's needle superimposed over a calyx of the kidney

available in the operating room, does not require additional computers or personnel, and represents an extension of the current surgical practice while increasing performance and safety. This approach employs a two-axis joystick controlling the RCM and a one-axis joystick controlling needle insertion (R1 & R2, T in Figure 1). A velocity control loop regulates the speed of the motors by using velocity feedback obtained from the optical encoder position signals. In this operation mode the surgeon uses "Superimposed Needle Registration" [5] to orient the needle: from the joystick the surgeon orients the needle such that in fluoroscopy it appears as a single point superimposed over the desired anatomical target (Figure 3). Then, imaging from a lateral view, needle insertion is controlled from PAKY's joystick under continuos monitoring. The RCM provides fine adjustment of needle orientation increasing accuracy and reducing radiation exposure for the patient [7]. Concurrently, the joystick control of the system separates the surgeon's hands from the radiation field.

PAKY's radiolucency, the low profile of the RCM robot, and the maneuverability of the gross positioning arm are features that make this system compatible with advanced imaging devices such as computerized tomography scanners. The proposed system is used in conjunction with such a complex imager to automatically perform needle orientation and insertion based on complex imaging and registration techniques, which are subject of future development.

Clinical testing for the evaluation of the MINI-RCM & PAKY has been commenced at the Johns Hopkins Hospital. The robot was controlled manually using the joysticks for needle orientation and insertion. X-ray fluoroscopy from a C-Arm was used. Initial observations revealed the ease of accurate needle

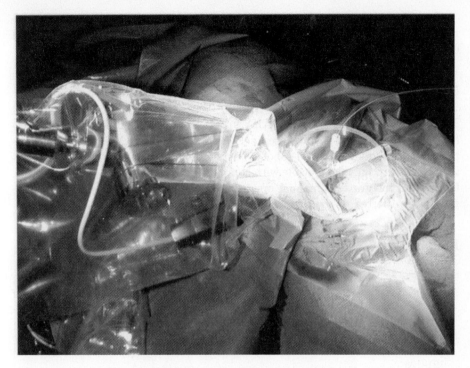

Fig. 4. MINI-RCM & PAKY in clinical use

alignment as compared to the stand-alone PAKY system. A photograph of the MINI-RCM & PAKY performing a percutaneous access procedure is presented in Figure 4. The needle is placed into the collecting system of the kidney and an access wire is passed through.

4 Safety Features

Safety is essential for surgical robots. The proposed system addresses safety by employing a low DOF robot, by decoupling needle orientation from the needle insertion, and by using non-backdrivable transmissions.

As previously presented, percutaneous needle access implies only 3 DOF. Our system implements all and only these DOF, such that the system has a minimal architecture and restricts arbitrary movements.

Furthermore, needle orientation and insertion are implemented by different mechanisms, which are independently activated by safety buttons on the joysticks. For needle alignment the surgeon activates only the MINI-RCM and orients the needle using the two-dimensional joystick while the needle pivots around the skin insertion site. When properly aligned, the RCM is deactivated. Needle insertion is then enabled by activating PAKY. Using this scheme, the system prevents the needle to be inserted before being properly aligned and prevents changes of orientation while inserting it.

In addition, the robot uses worm transmissions rendering a non-backdrivable mechanism. This preserves robot's configuration when deactivated or in the event of a power failure.

5 Conclusion

The proposed system extends PAKY's performance and capabilities for performing image-guided needle access by employing a low DOF RCM robot. The particular design of the RCM robot renders miniaturization and versatility making this system fully compatible with complex imaging equipment. Concurrently, the system integrates a manual operation mode such that the system may be rapidly transferred to the surgical setting.

References

1. Bzostek, A., Schreiner, S., Barnes, A.C., Cadeddu, J.A., Roberts, W., Anderson, J.H., Taylor, R.H., Kavoussi, L.R.: An automated system for precise percutaneous access of the renal collecting system. Lecture Notes in Computer Science, Vol. 1205. Springer-Verlag, Berlin Heidelberg New York (1997) 299–308
2. Cadeddu J.A., Stoianovici D., Chen R.N., Moore R.G., Kavoussi L.R.: Stereotactic mechanical percutaneous renal access. Journal of Endourology, Vol. 12, No. 2, (1998) 121–126
3. Potamianos, P., Davies, B.L., and Hibberd, R.D.: Intra-operative imaging guidance for keyhole surgery methodology and calibration. Proc. First Int. Symposium on Medical Robotics and Computer Assisted Surgery, Pittsburgh, PA. (1994) 98–104
4. Potamianos, P., Davies, B.L., and Hibberd, R.D.: Intra-operative registration for percutaneous surgery. Proc. First Int. Symposium on Medical Robotics and Computer Assisted Surgery, Baltimore, MD. (1995) 156–164
5. Stoianovici, D., Cadeddu, J., A., Demaree, R., D., Basile, H., A., Taylor, R., H., Whitcomb, L., L., Sharpe, W. N. Jr., Kavoussi, L., R.: An Efficient Needle Injection Technique and Radiological Guidance Method for Percutaneous Procedures. Lecture Notes in Computer Science, Vol. 1205. Springer-Verlag, Berlin Heidelberg New York (1997) 295–298
6. Stoianovici, D., Cadeddu, J., A., Demaree, R., D., Basile, H., A., Taylor, R., H., Whitcomb, L., L., Kavoussi, L., R.: A Novel Mechanical Transmission Applied to Percutaneous Renal Access. Proceedings of the ASME Dynamic Systems and Control Division, DSC, Vol. 61 (1997) 401–406
7. Stoianovici, D., Cadeddu, J., A., Whitcomb, L., L., Taylor, R., H., Kavoussi, L., R.: A Robotic System for Precise Percutaneous Needle Insertion. Thirteen Annual Meeting of the Society for Urology and Engineering, May 1998, San Diego, CA (1998) 5–6
8. Taylor R.H., Funda J., Eldridge B., Gruben K., LaRose D., Gomory S., Talamini M., Kavoussi L.R., Anderson J.: A Telerobotic Assistant for Laparoscopic Surgery. IEEE Engineering in Medicine and Biology Magazine, Vol. 14, (1995) 279–287

Optimum Designed Micro Active Forceps with Built-in Fiberscope for Retinal Microsurgery

Koji Ikuta[1], Takashi Kato[1], and Satoru Nagata[2]

[1] Department of Micro System Engineering, School of Engineering, Nagoya University,
Furo-cho, Chikusa-ku, Nagoya 464-8603, Japan
ikuta@mech.nagoya-u.ac.jp
kato@bio.bmse.mech.nagoya-u.ac.jp
http://www.bmse.mech.nagoya-u.ac.jp

[2] Department of Ophthalmology, Shiga University of Medical Science, Tsukiwa-cho,
Seta, Otsu, Shiga 520-2192, Japan
nagata@sums.shiga-med.ac.jp
http://www.hitl.washington.edu/people/nagata

Abstract. A new concept of eye microsurgical system is proposed. The final goal of our research project is not only improving surgical instruments but also establishing a total surgical system applicable to today's most difficult microsurgery at the bottom of an eyeball. The new prototype of micro forceps, which has a joint to enlarge the surgical area and also has a built-in thin optical fiberscope to increase the dexterity of retinal microsurgery, was designed as the first step of a long range research plan. Since this micro active forceps is equipped with thin optical fiber inside the stem to obtain a lateral view of the retina, drastic improvement of fine operations can be achieved. And the design of active joint and end-effector were optimized theoretically.

1 Introduction

Microsurgery is the most attractive but most difficult surgical treatment at present. Many fields in medicine have been developing special tools along with special surgical skills. Nowadays, it is claimed there is a great demand for various kinds of microsurgery using micro system technology.

Demand for eye microsurgery is especially clear for the engineer to understand. Eye microsurgery on the retina needs extremely difficult and special skills. Related issues cover general aspects of all kinds of microsurgery. Therefore, technology developed for this subject could be easily generalized to other medical fields.

This paper reports a contribution from micro technology as the first step of a long-term and systematic research plan[1,2].

2 Problems of Today's Eye Microsurgery on the Retina

In this chapter, we would like to explain the representative method of conventional retinal microsurgery and also refer to problems resulting from the characteristics of instruments in use.

2.1 Eye microsurgery at present

Let's start with a brief introduction of current eye microsurgery. Fig. 1 shows today's microsurgery of an eyeball[3]. The retina and thin membrane on the eye ground are operated. A highly trained skillful surgeon handles special forceps under a binocular microscope while a light guide is controlled to illuminate the small surgical area.

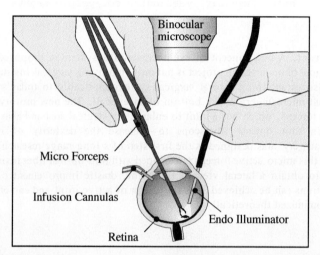

Fig. 1. Conventional eye microsurgery on the retina. A surgeon and an assistant work together looking at indirect retinal top view via binocular microscope. Illumination is also provided from microscope but it is not sufficient for the operation.

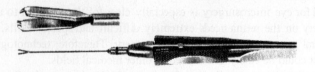

Fig. 2. Example of forceps-type conventional micro instrument for eye microsurgery. Length of the thin metal tube (neck) is about 30 mm and diameter of that is about 1 mm.

2.2 Problems

This surgical method and instrumentation entail two serious issues as follows.

1) *Limitation of operational approach*

The conventional forceps is the straight bar type as shown in Fig. 2 which is maneuvered via a small hole which acts as a pivot on the upper half of the sclera. Thus the working space of the tip of micro forceps is quite limited (only the bottom half of eyeball can be reached). The situation above is explained by Fig. 3.

2) *Limitation of visual information*

Only a top view image through the cornea by a binocular microscope is available. It is extremely difficult to grasp the depth and the distance information between the forceps' tip and the retina. Sometimes the retina has been seriously damaged by young doctors' mistakes.

3. Approach Concepts

Before describing technological articles, we would like to describe our concept of research approach and the development policy.

Our final goal is not only improving surgical tools but also establishing a new microsurgical system applicable to today's most difficult microsurgery. In this kind of research, people on the engineering side should be devote great attention to the *interface between the new technology and its users*. It is needless to say that the users here mean medical doctors.

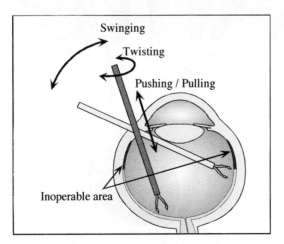

Fig. 3. Limitation of operational area by conventional forceps. The hole on the cornea acts as a pivot of rotational motion.

Unfortunately, there has been much misunderstanding of developments in the medical engineering field. Even though the technology itself may be excellent, it would never be used if medical doctors were displeased with it. It is obvious that the main cause of above unhappy cases lies on the miscommunication between engineers and doctors.

Another big reason is conservatism in medicine. Most surgeons like to keep their own skills cultivated through long periods of clinical training. It is extremely difficult to break out of this closed situation. One solution, the authors think, would be *a drastic improvement of instrumentation while preserving the continuity of operational skills*.

Based on above considerations, we decided to start with the improvement of tools such as micro forceps as the first step. The second step will be the total system as shown in Fig. 11, which will be described later.

4 Micro Active Forceps

The mechanisms and handling methods of micro active forceps made for trials in our laboratory are described in this chapter.

The term *"active"* used here does not mean that electrical devices, i.e. actuators, control each mechanism, but that positive approaches to and observations of the diseased part are possible with articulated forceps with a fiberscope. It is based on the belief that the continuity between the surgeon's skill and surgical instruments should be given particular consideration in microsurgical technologies.

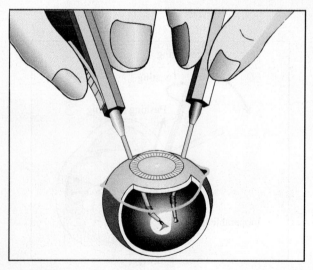

Fig. 4. Overview of the prototype. The angle of the end-neck is adjusted after the first insertion, then fixed by the lock mechanism while the surgeon works upon the tissue.

4.1 Design concepts of prototype

The basic features of developed Micro Active Forceps (MAF) may be summarized as follows:

1) *Active joint with lock mechanism* to make the end-effector approach the diseased part flexibly and address the upper part of eyeball from the inside,

2) *Micro gripper* to grasp fine tissue on the retina,

3) *Built-in optical fiber scope with light guide* to obtain lateral images during operation,

4) *One hand operation* for all tasks is possible,

5) *Solo surgery* is possible, because a surgeon can undertake two-arm operation (bimanual) using two micro active forceps.

Fig. 4 shows the overview of the prototype, and the basic design is described as Fig. 8.

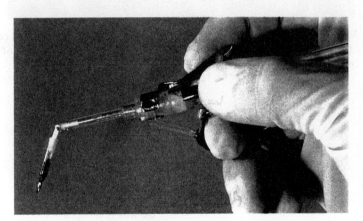

Fig. 5. Maneuver of MAF-II. The bending angle of the end-neck is adjusted by the middle finger and is held by the thumb via the lock mechanism. Then the gripper is worked stably by a forefinger. Each finger's force is transmitted via the nylon wire.

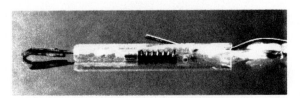

Fig. 6. A close-up view of the end-neck. The guide tube of the micro fiberscope is equipped obliquely. The lateral images of another instrument's tip and retina are obtained through the optical fiber.

Firstly, a mechanism verification model, named MAF-II, was made by hand (Fig. 5 and 6). The shaft diameter is 3 mm and micro optical fiberscope (diameter is 0.4 mm with 2000 pixels) is set at 30 degrees on the tip of the forceps to obtain lateral images of the retina. The feasibility and maneuverability of the MAF-II was verified experimentally, which is explained in a later section.

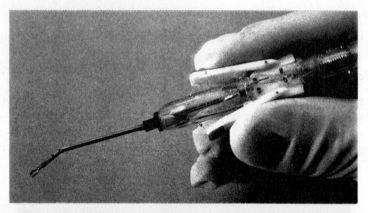

Fig. 7. Maneuver of MAF-III. Both the gripper and the bending angle are controlled simply by two fingers. The shape of the prototype comes to be similar to that of conventional forceps.

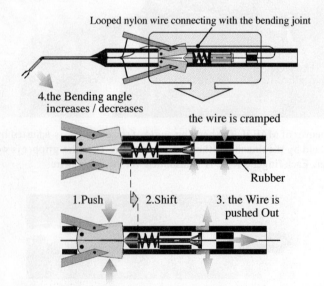

Fig. 8. Basic design of MAF. To earn the bending angle of the joint, the cramped point of looped wire is pushed out by knocking the knob just like the lead of a mechanical pencil.

As the next step of trial production, the MAF-III was made, in which the diameter of the shaft has been thin downed (Fig. 7). 1.4 mm of diameter is close to the size of today's micro instruments. Further miniaturization of the diameter in the next step is possible by using state of the art micro fabrication technology. An active bending joint and micro gripper can be operated by one hand via thin micro wire running through the body of MAF. The bending angle of the active joint and the micro gripper are separately maneuvered by a forefinger and a thumb respectively.

4.2 Mechanical design of the end-neck

In this section, let us examine the required kinematic conditions of the end-neck of MAF. There are two important factors that characterize motions of the tip against the surgical point: *length of the end-neck* and *bending angle of the active joint*. Both design parameters must be optimized. So we started by determining the bending range, and also examined the length of the end-neck.

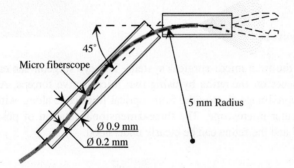

Fig. 9. The bending range of the active joint. Maximum bending angle (45 degrees) depends on the permitted bending radius of a fiberscope runs inside the stem.

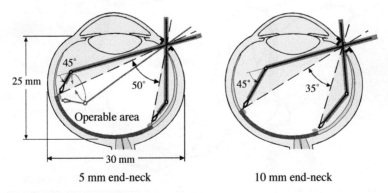

Fig. 10. Operable area of the retina under conditions of two different length of the end-neck, 5 mm and 10 mm.

4.2.1 Determination of bending angle

The bending angle of an active joint mostly depends on the permissible bending radius (PBR) of the built-in fiberscope. The diameter of the fiberscope is 0.2 mm and PBR is 5 mm, and the inside diameter of the neck is 0.6 mm.

Considering sizes above as Fig. 9, the bending angle was assigned to the following range: $0° \leq \theta \leq 45°$.

4.2.2 Length of the end-neck

Next, the optimum length L of the end-neck was examined. It is considered to be in the sphere of $5 \text{ mm} \leq L \leq 10 \text{ mm}$. Where 5 mm is due to the mechanical limitation, while 10 mm is due to the size of an eyeball (25 mm depth). Compared to the conventional forceps, MAF with 10 mm or more longer end-neck have no effect on enlargement of the operable area of the retina.

Fig. 10 shows the comparison with operable ranges of the retina under conditions of 45 degrees of bending angle. It is obvious that the operable area by 5 mm end-neck is larger than that by 100 mm end-neck. So the optimum length of the end-neck should be fixed at 5 mm.

4.3 Total system

Fig. 11 shows the total micro surgical system. The eye surgeon can easily grasp and pick up fine tissues on the retina by using two micro active forceps. A superimposed lateral microscopic image is provided from optical fiberscope along with the top view image by binocular microscope. The three-dimensional relation of positions between the tip of MAF and the retina can be clearly understood.

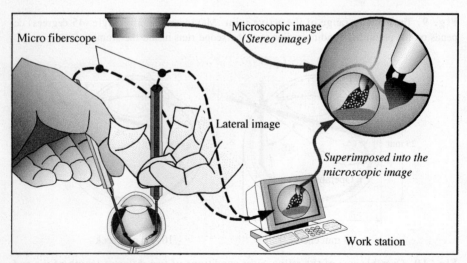

Fig. 11. Proposed total system of retina surgery using micro active forceps with superimposed lateral image.

5 Experimental Evaluation

A preliminary experiment using pig's eyeball was conducted (Fig. 12). The micro active forceps was inserted through the cornea.

There were two main aims as follows:
1) Confirmation of maneuverability of the prototype,
2) Validity of lateral monitoring via fiberscope.

The blood capillary on the retina was grasped softly by the micro gripper. Fig. 13 shows the real lateral image via an optical fiberscope. The distance between the micro gripper and a thin blood capillary can be readily sensed. A surgeon can see both the top view and the lateral view as in Fig. 14.

One hand operation without an assistant was also verified successfully.

Feasibility and maneuverability were verified by eye micro surgeon. The optimization and improvement of the instrument are underway.

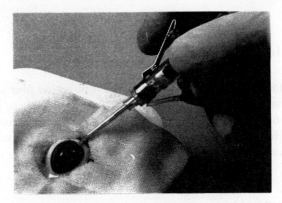

Fig. 1 2. Maneuverability test using a pig's eyeball.

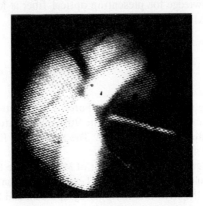

Fig. 13. Lateral image via optical fiber scope. Micro gripper is handing blood capillary on the retina.

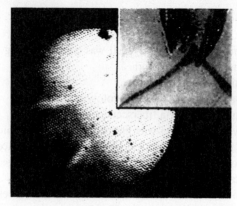

Fig. 14. The microscopic top view image is superimposed on the lateral view image via micro fiber scope.

6 Conclusions

A micro active forceps with micro gripper and built-in optical fiber scope was developed for eye microsurgery on the retina. In addition, a total system, including a new display system able to see the lateral inside view of the tip, was proposed and tested. The maneuverability and feasibility of the prototype was verified experimentally. One-hand operation was also demonstrated.

Acknowledgments

We would like to acknowledge for presenting optical fiber at Mr. Utsumi of Mitsubishi Cable Co. Ltd. and Mr. Narita of Nippon Cable co. Ltd.

References

1. Ikuta, K., Kato, T., Nagata, S.: Micro Active Forceps with Optical Fiber Scope for Intra-Ocular Microsurgery. In: Proceedings of The 9th Annual International Workshop on MEMS '96. IEEE Catalog No. 96CH35856. The Institute of Electrical and Electronics Engineers, Inc. (1996) 456 - 461
2. Ikuta, K., Kato, T., Nagata, S.: Development of Micro Active Forceps with Built-in Fiber Scope for Intra-Ocular Microsurgery. In: Lemke, H.U., Vannier, M.W., Inamura, K. (eds.): Proceedings of the 11th International Symposium and Exhibition on CAR '97. International Congress Series, No. 1134. Elsevier Science B.V., Amsterdam Lausanne New York Oxford Shannon Tokyo (1997) 914 - 919
3. Nagata, M., Ogino, N., Okinami, S., Matsumura, M. (eds.): Ophthalmic Microsurgery 3rd edition. Medical Information Express, Tokyo Osaka (1993)

Gauging Clinical Practice: Surgical Navigation for Total Hip Replacement

James E. Moody Jr.[1]; Anthony M. DiGioia, MD[1,2]; Branislav Jaramaz[1,2]; Mike Blackwell[2]; Bruce Colgan[1]; Constantinos Nikou[2]

[1]Center for Orthopaedic Research, Shadyside Medical Center, 5200 Centre Avenue, Suite 309, Pittsburgh, PA 15232, TEL (412) 623-2673, FAX (412) 623-1108
{moody, branko, colgan}@cor.ssh.edu

[2]Center for Medical Robotics and Computer Assisted Surgery, Robotics Institute, Carnegie Mellon University, Pittsburgh, PA 15213
{digioia, mkb, costa}@cmu.edu

Abstract. HipNav is a hip implant navigation and guidance system which helps surgeons plan acetabular implant orientation preoperatively, and guides them intraoperatively to achieve this intended plan. Through this process, these technologies are used to measure, gauge, and quantify current clinical practice. With HipNav, surgeons plan and execute the procedure in the 3-D realm with accurate patient models, taking advantage of anatomic information normally lost through traditional planning methods. During surgery HipNav tracks the alignment tool with respect to the pelvis, compensating for any pelvic motion, thereby ensuring an accurate measurement of alignment and placement according to the plan.

This past year has seen the system move out of the developmental laboratory setting and into the operating room environment. In addition to its primary clinical function as a surgical assist device, through its measurement and tracking capabilities HipNav has likewise emerged as a powerful research tool. With HipNav we are now able to measure, for example, how the pelvis moves during surgery, how cup placement shifts during the press fit process, and how well traditional implant guides and strategies compare with new strategies based on more complete patient-specific models.

HipNav is still an emerging technology and a continually evolving system. However, data collected to date through the HipNav project have provided new insight into aspects of the total hip replacement process, challenging commonly held assumptions concerning acetabular alignment. Most importantly, HipNav has indications for some areas of established practice that may benefit from reexamination.

1 Introduction

Although many factors may contribute to dislocation following total hip replacement (THR) surgery, one of the most common negative influences is the malposition of the acetabular portion of the implant [3], [4]. A non-optimal placement can lead to impingement between the rim of the acetabular cup and the neck of the femoral component. This impingement acts as a fulcrum, such that any attempted motion beyond this point will result in subluxation or even dislocation. In less severe cases malposition can accelerate the wear of the polyethylene liner, generating debris which, in turn, can contribute to early implant loosening or failure[8], [12].

Clearly, the best strategy is to place the acetabular component to minimize or completely avoid the potential for impingement during routine activities of daily living [2], [7]. However, current methods do not provide clinicians with adequate tools to develop optimal implant placement strategies, nor do they provide the means by which the desired plan can be reliably implemented.

The traditional planning method of using a single anterior-posterior X-ray with a transparent template overlay is inherently inaccurate for alignment in that much 3-D information is eliminated during the projection to a 2-D radiograph. Also, this technique does not take into account functional pelvic positions unique to the patient. For instance, pelvic pitch varies significantly as a person moves from a standing to a sitting position; the range of this pitch can differ significantly between patients. These are factors that should be considered in the operative plan.

Current practice of acetabular implant placement relies on a rigid mechanical guide attached to the component insertion tool. This guide may work satisfactorily if the surgeon can ascertain that the pelvis is precisely and securely placed in the known orientation for which the guide was designed. However, precise and repeatable pelvic alignment in an operating room environment is not easily achieved, if even possible, without extensive external fixation. A mechanical implant guide does not account for any deviation in pelvic position, nor does it correct for any peculiarities resulting from the patient's unique anatomical structure or natural posture [6].

Until now there has not been a mechanism by which the implant tool could be accurately oriented to the pelvis. To this end we have developed HipNav, a system coupling a preoperative planner with an intraoperative navigation system. Our approach uses accurate 3-D patient pelvic models to assist surgeons in determining and achieving the optimal acetabular implant orientation, regardless of pelvic motion and orientation on the operating room table.

Inherent in the HipNav system are powerful tracking and measurement utilities. Aside from its intended clinical use we can take advantage of these capabilities to measure and quantify various aspects of the THR procedure.

2 System

Previous papers have described components of the HipNav system and its validation in great detail [1], [11]. However, a brief system overview and examination of our methodology is necessary to provide an adequate insight to our approach and findings.

2.1 HipNav Components

HipNav is comprised of three functional components:
- A preoperative planner.
- A range-of-motion simulator.
- An intraoperative navigation and guidance system.

The preoperative planner presents a 3-D surface model of the patient's pelvis to the surgeon, who can then specify the implant size and location. Figure 1 shows an example of the implant placement screen in which the acetabular implant is modeled as a sphere, thus the orthagonal cross sections appear as circles. The surface model in this particular example depicts only the right half of a pelvis. The centroid of the implant appears as a small dot in the center of the acetabulum. For any given point in the pelvis, simulated sagittal and coronal CT views are presented along with the traditional transverse CT view. These three orthogonal views follow the center of the implant spheroid: as the implant is moved the views adjust accordingly. Thus, the surgeon can fine-tune implant placement along all three axes.

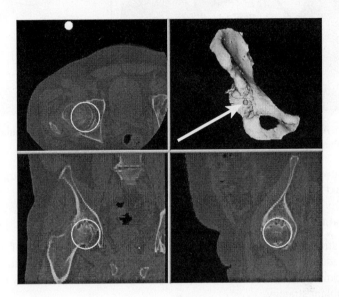

Figure 1: The implant placement screen of the HipNav planner. The arrow indicates the centroid of the spherical implant model.

Once the size and location of the implant are determined, the implant can then be oriented through the orientation utility. Coupled with this utility is the second functional component of HipNav, the range-of-motion simulator. The simulator dynamically predicts impingement for various leg motions given the size, geometry, and orientation of the implant components selected. Thus, the surgeon can optimize the plan (adding more version, for example) to adjust away from an orientation which might otherwise be predisposed to impingement.

A portion of the orientation utility screen is presented in Figure 2, showing both a pelvis with simulated implant in a test orientation, and the resulting predicted functional range of motion.

The third component of HipNav is the intraoperative navigation and guidance system (IOS). Optical tracking hardware monitors the locations and orientations of the data point collection probe and the implant insertion tool. Early in the surgical procedure an optical tracking target is rigidly attached to the pelvis, and after the calibration and registration processes all components can be located and tracked within the operating field accurately and in real time. IOS couples this tracking capability with the

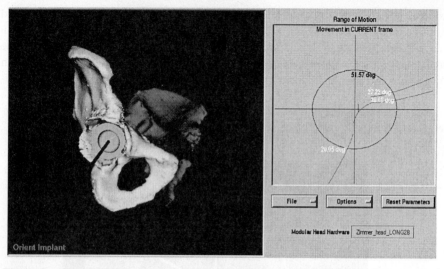

Figure 2: A sample implant orientation and resulting range-of-motion simulation from the HipNav planner.

patient's own preoperative plan and presents this information to the surgeon via various context relevant displays throughout the entire procedure.

2.2 Data Preparation

In preparation for a HipNav case, lateral standing and sitting X-rays of the pelvis are taken in addition to the standard anterior-posterior view. From this lateral series the surgeon can estimate a functional range of pelvic motion, which usually has an impact on the implant strategy.

A CT scan of the pelvis is also performed, from which 2-D contours are extracted, and ultimately a 3-D surface model is constructed. Examples of these models were shown in Figures 1 and 2. The models are also used by the intraoperative system.

2.3 Definition of the Anterior Pelvic Plane

Given the wide variation in pelvic structure and disposition between patients it is imperative to have a simple but robust definition for orientation against which rotations and translations can be described. HipNav measurements are based on what we call the "anterior pelvic plane" (a concept independently proposed by Lewinnek [5]). Assuming a symmetric pelvis, the anterior pelvic plane is simply the plane defined by the most anterior points on the pubic tubercles and on the anterior superior iliac spines. To illustrate, if a pelvic model were held against a window it would touch at these points, and the plane defined by the window would be coincident with the anterior pelvic plane. Conceptually simple, the anterior pelvic plane has these advantages:

- It is intuitive, as it is nearly vertical in a standing person.
- Since it is anatomically based it can be easily measured by physical exam.
- It can be precisley measured in X-rays.
- It is easily determined in 3-D reconstructions.

Conversely, implant manufacturer guidlines typically refer to a pelvic coronal plane, the definition and determination of which is somewhat more subjective.

2.4 Data Collection Devices

HipNav's tracking system[1], capable of sub-millimeter accuracy, can measure the exact position and orientation of optical targets in the operating room. When these targets are attached to various tools, they then become position measuring devices in addition to their primary purpose. Data from these measurement devices can be collected automatically by the system, by the surgeon via a foot pedal, or by the system engineer at the console. All data are logged for intraoperative use as well as for postoperative analysis.

HipNav makes use of three such measurement devices: a point probe, an implant insertion tool, and the patient's own pelvis.

The Point Probe. The point probe (a.k.a, the data probe, or wand) is a specialized optical target with an integral stainless steel probe tip. Point data collection is achieved by the surgeon placing the tip of the data probe on a desired spot and striking a foot pedal to record the position. Point data contains no orientation information, just location coordinate measurements.

The Pelvis as a Measurement Tool. Once equipped with an optical target the pelvis becomes trackable both in location and in orientation. The target is rigidly fixed, therefore any motion in the pelvis results in target motion. The registration process (as described in the Methodology section) is performed so that the target/pelvic motion can be related to the computer's internal model.

A Trackable Implant Tool. The trackable alignment implant tool is simply the appropriate manufacturer's standard implant tool and mechanical guide to which an optical target has been securely affixed. Although its intended function is to set the alignment during press fit we use this now-trackable tool to collect abduction/flexion measurements in three different situations:

- We can measure alignment strategies before press fit.
- We can track the actual change in cup orientation during the press fit process.
- We can measure any effects of post-insertion steps. For example, we can detect any change due to the insertion of fixating screws, or any change resulting from the seating of the acetabular liner.

3 Methodology

The previous section introduced the measurement tools and described the types of measurements each can take. This section focuses on the different classes of measurements (gathered from any combination of the above devices), how they are measured, what the data show, and what conclusions (if any) can be inferred from the data.

---

[1] OPTOTRAK, Northern Digital Incorporated, Ontario.

3.1 Registration

Using the data probe the surgeon is prompted to collect a series of points from designated locations on the surface of the pelvis, in effect creating a "point cloud" in computer memory. Since the pelvic model and the cloud of points are both based on the same physical pelvis, these two representations can be permuted until a precise surface match is found. Once this registration process is complete the conversion from the pelvic model to the operating room is well understood so that any measurements taken in the OR can be accurately mapped onto the computer model [9], [10].

3.2 Pelvic Position Tracking

Natural Pelvic Orientation vs. the Theoretical Neutral. The patient is positioned on the OR table in an attitude typical for a posterolateral approach: The patient is stabilized with a series of anterior and posterior blocks and a bean bag. The non-operative leg is secured to the table in approximately 45 degrees of flexion. The pelvis is now in the baseline position, and once the optical target is attached this position is recorded as the baseline neutral position. In the theoretical (or "ideal") neutral position assumed by mechanical guides the anterior pelvic plane would be perpendicular to the surface of the OR table, and parallel with its long axis.

Table 1 shows the deviation from theoretical neutral of the baseline (or natural) neutral position for each of the HipNav patients. Roll is defined as a rotation about the superior-inferior axis, pitch as a rotation about the lateral axis, and yaw as a rotation about the anterior-posterior axis of the pelvis.

We do not draw any direct conclusions from these data except that they demonstrate a wide variation in natural neutral positions. The best use of such data is in evaluating assumptions held in current practice.

For example, if it could be determined that current planning techniques are valid provided the actual pelvis is within $\pm 5°$ on all axes of the theoretical neutral alignment, then only three of the 15 cases in Table 1 for which data are available would be in the tolerable range. This is, of course, a hypothetical example contrived just to show how such data might be used. It also makes the naive assumption that the same neutral position can be maintained throughout the surgical procedure.

Pelvic Motion. HipNav monitors pelvic position throughout the surgery. In our current protocol a starting, or baseline, position is measured as soon as the optical target has been attached. Pelvic position measurements are subsequently taken after any large force has been applied to the pelvis. We typically take measurements after the femoral head has been removed, after reaming and after press fit, and we take an additional series during the final prosthetic range of motion tests.

The most intuitive representation of the motion data is an animated sequence. Figure 3 shows a sampling of frames from such a sequence for a representative HipNav case. In this particular example only the right half of the pelvis was actually reconstructed from CT data. In the interest of clarity this hemi-pelvis was reflected to produce a realistic-looking pelvic image.

The white outline represents the theoretical neutral orientation.

Figures 3a, 3b, and 3c (the left column) represent the pelvis in "relaxed" positions, i.e., where no force is being applied so the torso can return to a neutral state. Figures

Table 1. Natural Pelvic Orientation - Deviation from Theoretical Neutral

CASE #	ROLL	PITCH	YAW
1	17.4	-4.0	-2.3
2	n/a	n/a	n/a
3	-4.2	1.9	0.5
4	n/a	n/a	n/a
5	21.4	-13.7	5.7
6	n/a	n/a	n/a
7	-9.6	-6.6	6.5
8	18.5	4.6	5.4
9	5.7	0.9	-1.1
10	-6.4	-1.7	-4.4
11	2.0	3.7	1.5
12	3.4	-0.9	-1.1
13	5.1	-1.6	-1.4
14	-7.8	2.2	-6.5
15	10.8	3.8	9.1
16	3.3	9.2	7.5
17	4.5	14.8	-3.3
18	-4.8	2.7	-11.1

3d, 3e, and 3f (the right column) show examples of pelvic motion during the prosthetic range of motion tests in which some force is being applied to the leg.

These images illustrate very convincingly that although the patient is secured and stabilized the pelvis moves significantly. Even more provoking is the realization that when forces are removed the pelvis often does not return to the same neutral position. This demonstrates that the concept of a single neutral position is not realistic.

3.3 Measurement of Placement Strategies

The implant tool is used to measure cup abduction and flexion once the reaming process has been completed. The alignment implant tool is oriented according to some strategy, whether it is the manufacturer's mechanical guide according to the manufacturer's directions, the surgeon's preference based on his or her own experience and knowledge of anatomical cues, or even a new technique as described in a research paper. Once the tool is aligned according to a given scheme the true resulting abduction and flexion can be measured. Table 2 lists the measurements from the first 10 Hip-Nav cases for two strategies (relying on the mechanical guide according to the manufacturer's guidelines, and relying on the surgeon's own experience and anatomical cues). The "HipNav" column contains the planned orientations, and in most cases this is what the surgeon chose to attempt for the final placement.

It is interesting to note that in all cases even though the same surgeon both planned the case and performed the operation there were sometimes significant differences in the preoperative plan and the surgeon's intraoperative strategy. Part of this is due to the limited anatomical cues visible at the incision site, especially with heavier patients.

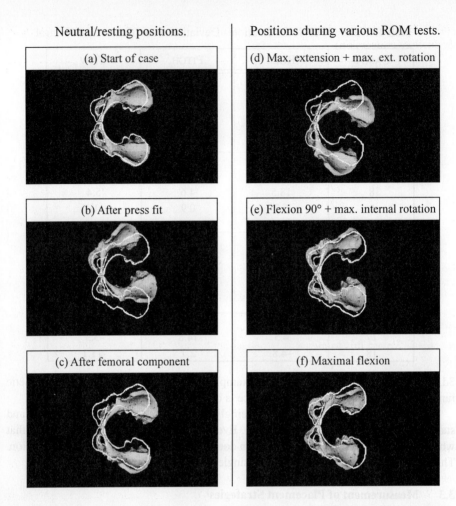

Figure 3: Representative snapshots of pelvic motion during a typical THR. The white outline indicates the ideal orientation as required by mechanical alignment guides.

3.4 Cup Motion

The last column in Table 2 lists the measured orientation of the actual implant placement. Compare this to the planned orientation in the previous column.

This shows that one of the most difficult tasks in the procedure is keeping the implant on an accurate course during press fit, even with the benefit of computer guidance. The implant is typically two to four millimeters larger than the prepared site. But because of tight fit and variances in bone density and quality the cup has a tendency to bind and torque during press fit.

Also, with a slightly rounded striking head on the pressfit tool it is difficult for surgeons to strike directly along the axis. Any off-center impact generates rotational forces about the moment arm defined by the insertion tool, contributing to cup rotation.

We are currently studying this phenomenon in greater detail, expecting that it will

Table 2. Acetabular Implant Strategies; Final Position.(Measurements listed as abduction/anteversion)

CASE #	GUIDE	SURGEON	HIPNAV	FINAL
1	40/-9	50/16	48/19	48/26
2	42/-2	48/24	54/20	51/27
3	41/9	54/26	54/20	61/24
4	n/a	56/23	53/16	54/22
5	48/-7	48/16	55/21	52/16
6	43/19	54/37	56/23	58/33
7	36/1	45/32	56/23	47/20
8	44/3	51/21	54/20	48/20
9	44/20	54/33	56/23	53/16
10	44/5	54/28	54/20	52/27

lead to better implant tool designs and techniques. With HipNav technology we can test the effectiveness of any improvements.

Cup motion can also result from post- press fit procedures. The implant insertion tool can be fitted with an adapter which fits snugly into the acetabular component liner (hooded or standard). From this the final abduction and flexion measurements are recorded. We use this to measure any cup orientation change due to the optional insertion of fixating screws, or even from the force of seating the liner itself.

4   Conclusions

We acknowledge that the subject pool is still too small to yield statistically rigorous clinical conclusions; likewise, the time period has been too brief to attempt any meaningful outcomes analysis. Even so, HipNav has convincingly demonstrated that commonly held assumptions regarding acetabular implant practice should be re-examined.

We have also shown that as a research tool HipNav provides many measurement utilities enabling investigation into varied aspects of total hip replacement:

- HipNav can be used to evaluate new tool designs. Our current data suggest that press fit tools that can deliver forces focused along the main axis may result in better cup placement. HipNav can be used to assess the effectiveness of the tool by tracking the press fit progress and measuring the final orientation.
- HipNav can be used to develop and evaluate new alignment strategies. We expect that new strategies will emerge, either based on new combinations of anatomical landmarks, or hybrid approaches employing mechanical guides with anatomical landmarks. HipNav can be used to measure how these strategies perform in actual practice.
- HipNav can be used to develop accuracy requirements. HipNav can predict how deviations from alignment strategy assumptions affect functional range of motion, thereby helping to establish guidelines for safe practice.
- Intraoperatively, HipNav can be used to measure final implant placement, and can predict potential problems while they can be corrected.

- HipNav research provides a means to disseminate new strategies and information to a wider surgical audience.

5 References

1. Blackwell M, Simon D, Rao S, DiGioia A: Technical report. Design and evaluation of 3-D pre-operative planning software: application to acetabular implant alignment. Carnegie Mellon University, 1996.
2. Daly PJ, Morrey BF: Operative correction of an unstable total hip arthroplasty. J Bone Joint Surg 74A: 1334-1343, 1992.
3. Hedlundh U, Sanzen L, Fredin H: The prognosis and treatment of dislocated total hip arthroplasties with a 22 mm head. J Bone Joint Surg 79B: 374-378, 1997.
4. Khan MAA, Brakenbury PH, Reynolds ISR: Dislocation following total hip replacement. J Bone Joint Surg 63B: 214-218, 1981.
5. Lewinnek GE, Lewis JL, Tarr R, et al.: Dislocations after total hip replacement arthroplasties. J Bone Joint Surg 60A: 217-220, 1978.
6. McCollum DE, Gray WJ: Dislocation after total hip arthroplasty: Causes and prevention. Clin Orthop 261: 159-170, 1990.
7. Ohlin A, Balkfors B: Stability of cemented sockets after 3-14 years. J Arthroplasty 7: 87-92, 1992.
8. Robinson RP, Simonian PT, Gradisar IM, Ching RP: Joint motion and surface contact area related to component position in total hip arthroplasty. J Bone Joint Surg 79B: 140-46, 1997.
9. Simon D, Hebert M, Kanade T: Techniques for fast and accurate intrasurgical registration. J Image Guid Surg 1: 17-29, 1995.
10. Simon DA: Fast and accurate shape-based registration. Technical Report, #CMU-RI-TR-96-45. Carnegie Mellon University, 1996.
11. Simon DA, Jaramaz B, Blackwell M, et al.: Development and validation of a navigational guidance system for acetabular implant placement. First Joint Conference of CVRMed and MRCAS. Grenoble, France, Springer 583-592, 1997.
12. Yamaguchi M, Bauer T, Hashimoto Y: Three-dimensional analysis of multiple wear vectors in retrieved acetabular cups. J Bone Joint Surg 79A: 1539-1544, 1997.

Adaptive Template Moderated Spatially Varying Statistical Classification

Simon K. Warfield, Michael Kaus, Ferenc A. Jolesz, and Ron Kikinis

Surgical Planning Laboratory, Harvard Medical School,
Department of Radiology, Brigham and Women's Hospital, 75 Francis St., Boston, MA 02115
{warfield,kaus,jolesz,kikinis}@bwh.harvard.edu   http://splweb.bwh.harvard.edu:8000

Abstract. A novel image segmentation algorithm was developed to allow the automatic segmentation of both normal and abnormal anatomy. The new algorithm is a form of spatially varying classification (SVC), in which an explicit anatomical template is used to moderate the segmentation obtained by k Nearest Neighbour (k-NN) statistical classification. The new algorithm consists of an iterated sequence of spatially varying classification and nonlinear registration, which creates an adaptive, template moderated (ATM), spatially varying classification (SVC).

The ATM SVC algorithm was applied to several segmentation problems, involving different types of imaging and different locations in the body. Segmentation and validation experiments were carried out for problems involving the quantification of normal anatomy (MRI of brains of babies, MRI of knee cartilage of normal volunteers) and pathology of various types (MRI of patients with multiple sclerosis, MRI of patients with brain tumours, MRI of patients with damaged knee cartilage). In each case, the ATM SVC algorithm provided a better segmentation than statistical classification or elastic matching alone.

Keywords: template moderated segmentation, elastic matching, nearest neighbour classification, knee cartilage, neonate, brain, tumour

1 Introduction

The segmentation of structures or types of tissue from medical images is still a difficult problem. In particular, the segmentation of pathology often requires intensive manual interaction to achieve good, or even acceptable, segmentations. Our goal was to develop a generally applicable segmentation algorithm that could aid in the automation of medical image analysis tasks by successfully segmenting both normal anatomy and common types of pathology.

A strategy of feature detection and classification (spectral segmentation) has been widely used for the identification of tissue types. When spatial information (such as shape and spatial relationships between structures) is significant, a variety of deformable models have been proposed. Some segmentation problems can be solved simply by feature identification and classification. In this case, there is no need to make use of an anatomical template, and the segmentation is a straightforward process. Similarly, some segmentation problems can be solved by matching deformable models directly to the image data [1, 2, 3]. Here we deal with those segmentation problems for which feature identification and classification, or matching deformable models alone, are insufficient.

These different segmentation strategies are often complementary, both in the tasks where they succeed and in the tasks where the fail. For example, classification is often successfully applied for the global segmentation of major tissue types. Deformable models have been successfully applied to the localization of particular anatomical structures. Tissue classification is unsuccessful when different structures to be identified have the same or overlapping spectral properties. Deformable models often need accurate initialization and are usually optimized for particular structures (sometimes with a single closed boundary), and can fail in the presence of abnormal anatomical variability (or even in the presence of normal but highly variable structures, such as the cortex). Optimization strategies have usually been driven by local gradient information which is often insufficient to distinguish particular structures of interest.

We developed a new algorithm, ATM SVC, by embedding a traditional multiple feature k-NN classification into a higher dimensionality problem space. The additional dimensionality is derived from an anatomical template, and acts to moderate the statistical classification. In the special case of the classification problem involving separable classes with nonoverlapping anatomy accurately described by the anatomical model, the ATM SVC solution is the same as the original k-NN classification problem. In the common case involving some spectral overlap, the ATM SVC resolves the ambiguity of the feature space with anatomical context.

ATM SVC integrates an individualized explicit anatomical model with statistical classification. This allows the generation of a spatially varying classification, so that spectral overlap can be remedied through spatial information. In turn this generates a classification of the data which is a more reliable and robust source of information than the raw imaging data for the fast nonlinear registration to operate upon, allowing more accurate nonlinear registration than is possible from greyscale image data alone. By iterating these steps, we have found it possible to segment normal and abnormal anatomy from a range of locations in the body.

2 Method

Our algorithm iterates between a classification step to identify tissues and an elastic matching step to align a template of normal anatomy with the classified tissues. The template of anatomy is used to modify the classification to produce a spatially varying, rather than global, classification. The steps are iterated to improve the final segmentation. Figure 1 illustrates the ATM SVC algorithm.

2.1 The ATM SVC algorithm

When we come to segment a particular patient, several steps are involved in the initialization of data for the algorithm. We choose to represent normal anatomy with a 3D volumetric digital template. The template consists of a 3D volume with each voxel labelled according to the anatomical structure present [4]. Initialization involves the application of feature detection or image enhancement algorithms to construct images that have improved contrasts for the structures of interest (e.g. nonlinear diffusion for noise smoothing [5], local structure enhancement), the execution of an initial alignment

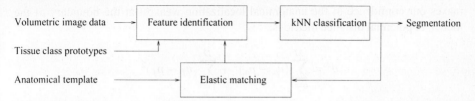

Fig. 1. Schema for Adaptive Template Moderated Spatially Varying Classification. Initialization consists of image acquisition, tissue class prototype selection and linear registration of a template of normal anatomy to the image data. Feature identification is problem dependent and often the image data alone is used. Local filtering strategies for feature enhancement can be motivated by the anatomical template. The anatomical template is converted into a set of features describing anatomical localization with a distance transform. A segmentation based upon these features is done with k-NN classification. The segmentation is then put through a feedback path that is used to refine the segmentation. A fast elastic matching algorithm is used to refine the alignment of the template of normal anatomy to the classified patient data. The anatomical localization is recomputed with the refined atlas, and the process is iterated.

strategy to align the template to the patient scan, and the selection of prototype voxels for tissue classes of interest to allow the construction of a statistical model for the distribution of features for each tissue class.

The initial alignment strategy depends upon whether the anatomy to be aligned is rigid or piecewise rigid, and examples are presented in Section 3. For brain MR, the usual rigid registration techniques are suitable, and we have used volumetric alignment of classified data sets [6]. For the knee joint, we use a piecewise rigid registration by manual alignment of each of the bones.

Spatially Varying Classification The k-Nearest Neighbour (k-NN) classification rule is a technique for nonparametric supervised pattern classification. Efficient techniques for k-NN classification have been developed [7, 8, 9]. Distance is measured with a distance metric appropriate to the problem domain. The main characteristic of the ATM SVC algorithm is to use Euclidean distance in a modified feature space.

We have a template aligned with the data. If this template was precisely aligned and modelled all of the structures present (including pathology) there would be no need for further segmentation. We would just use the model directly. However, the initial alignment of the template captures only global scale, rotation and translation parameters, and local shape differences remain. The relevant local shape differences may require more than one iteration of elastic matching to capture, particularly in the presence of pathology that distorts the patient anatomy significantly away from the normal anatomy of the template.

In order to improve the segmentation, we make use of the approximately aligned template to create a spatially varying classification. The template is used to provide anatomical localization for the classification. We can consider a range of confidence in our anatomical localization, ranging from the regions we have reason to suspect are far away from the anatomical structure, to those regions we suspect are very likely to be the anatomical structure. The nature of the misalignment of the nonlinear registration makes our confidence in the anatomical localization weakest at the boundary of the model. A potential distance metric is:

$$d^2 = \sum_{a=1}^{M}(v_a - p_a)^2 + \sum_{f=1}^{D}(v_f - p_f)^2$$

where we have added M features of spatial information to the usual D features, and $(v_a - p_a)^2$ represents the difference in anatomical localization of the voxel to be classified and the prototype. Qualitatively, when v and p are from the same anatomical region, v_a and p_a will vary together, leading to a small addition (ideally zero) to the overall distance, and so the distance will be mainly determined by the original features. When v and p are from different anatomical regions, v_a and p_a will vary differently, leading to a large change to the overall distance, causing the distance to be large irrespective of the values of the original features.

We generate anatomical localization features by converting each of the structures of an aligned template into a distance map. We model the uncertainty of anatomical localization, which depends upon the size of the potential error in elastic matching. A straightforward model of error is to use a penalty of 0 where labels for the matched structure is present, and increase the penalty linearly or quadratically with distance from the anatomical template until saturating it. When better error bounds on the anatomical localization are known, they can be directly incorporated by modifying the penalty in the relevant regions.

Nonlinear Registration We achieve fast nonlinear registration with an elastic matching algorithm based upon that of Dengler [10]. The goal of the matcher is, given a source data set $g_1(x)$ and a target data set $g_2(x)$, to find a deformation vector field $u(x)$ such that the function $g_1(x - u(x))$ is as similar to the function $g_2(x)$ as possible.

The basic method of computing u is: for a fixed value of x, consider the problem of finding the value of u that minimizes

$$E_x(u) = \int w(x' - x)(g_2(x') - g_1(x' - u))^2 dx'.$$

The resulting value of u is taken as the value of $u(x)$. Here, w is a window function whose width determines the size of the region used to compute $u(x)$.

We compute a classification, and use the classification to update the template alignment. The updated template is then used to generate a new anatomical localization and used to compute a new classification. For the segmentation problems described in Section 3, the algorithm converges to a satisfactory segmentation around five or fewer iterations of this process.

2.2 Summary

The ATM SVC algorithm generates a sequence of segmentations $s^{(j)}$ given both a (multi-modality) data set g and an anatomical template t. The classification of a particular voxel v from a set of training prototypes P with classes $w_i, i \in 1..C$ for C

classes, is determined with a modified k-NN estimate $P(w_i|v) = \frac{k_i}{k}$,

$$s^{(j+1)}(v) = \max_i P^{(j)}(w_i|v) = \max_i \frac{k_i^{(j)}}{k^{(j)}} = \max_i \frac{\#N_{v,w_i}^{(j)}}{\#N_v^{(j)}} .$$

N_v is the subset of prototypes (drawn from the set of training prototypes P), with distance less than or equal to the distance to the kth nearest prototype, d_k. The ATM SVC algorithm differs from the usual k-NN classification by modifying the set of k nearest prototypes, at each iteration, in a manner that depends upon the anatomical template. The usual distance metric is extended to be

$$N_v^{(j)} = \{p \in P : d_k^2 \geq \sum_{f=1}^{D}(v_f - p_f)^2 +$$

$$\sum_{a=1}^{M}(m(t^{(j)}(v_a)) - m(t^{(j)}(p_a)))^2\} ,$$

where N_{v,w_i} is the subset of N_v which consists of prototypes of class w_i, and $\#$ is the cardinality operator for counting the number of elements in a set. D is the dimensionality of the feature space derived from g, M is the number of spatial localization features derived from the anatomical template, $m(t^{(j)}(v_a))$ is the saturated distance transform of structure a of the anatomical template $t^{(j)}$ at voxel v, and

$$t^{(j)}(v) = t^{(j-1)}(v - u^{(j)}(v))$$

where $u^{(j)}(v) = u$ represents the nonlinear registration of the anatomical template $t^{(j-1)}$ to the data g and is obtained by minimizing the elastic matching constraint.

3 Results

In this section the application of ATM SVC to segmentation problems involving both normal anatomy and pathology is presented. For each of these problems, segmentation with a global (non-spatially varying) classification was also carried out (either k-NN classification [9] or the EM algorithm [11]) and a visual comparison was made. In each case the spatially varying classification generated by ATM SVC better reflects the underlying anatomy than global classification techniques.

Classification of Cortical and Subcortical Grey Matter from MR of Neonates In the developing brain rapid changes in the amount of cortical grey matter occur. These changes can be studied with MR imaging [12]. However, because the brain is still developing, the signal intensity characteristics of different parts of the brain can be quite similar, making it difficult to apply conventional classification techniques.

We applied the ATM SVC algorithm to this problem with the goal of improving the segmentation of cortical grey matter and subcortical grey matter. These have similar intensity ranges, but different spatial locations, and accurate measurement of cortical grey matter is a clinically interesting problem. Figure 2 illustrates the improvement in the segmentation that is achieved with ATM SVC.

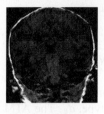 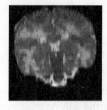 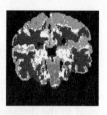 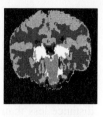

(a) Single slice of baby brain SPGR MR

(b) Single slice of baby brain T2 weighted MR

(c) k-NN classification

(d) ATM SVC classification

Fig. 2. MRI of baby brain, k-NN classification and ATM SVC segmentation. Cortical grey matter is shown in light grey, and subcortical grey matter is shown as white. The quantification of cortical grey matter is a clinically important problem, but it is difficult to distinguish from subcortical grey matter because of the similarity of MR intensity. The ATM SVC algorithm allows the spatial distribution of grey matter to be modelled, and as shown, generates an improved segmentation of cortical and subcortical grey matter over that of k-NN classification alone.

Segmentation of Brain MR of Patients with Multiple Sclerosis White matter lesions appear in the brain of patients with multiple sclerosis and evolve over time. During the lifetime of a lesion some parts of the lesion develop signal intensity characteristics that overlap those of normal grey matter on conventional spin echo MR images [13]. A conventional spin echo MR image was segmented using a statistical classification with intensity inhomogeneity correction using the EM segmentation method of Wells et al. [11], and a spatially varying classification of a slice from a brain MR scan of a patient with multiple sclerosis. Comparison of the segmentations indicated ATM SVC improved the segmentation of normal white matter, the lesions and the grey matter over that of statistical classification alone.

Brain Tumour Segmentation A comparison of manual and ATM SVC segmentation of a brain tumour was carried out. An SPGR MRI of a patient was obtained and segmented with an interactive volume editing segmentation routine (requiring about 60 minutes of operator time). Independently, the SPGR MRI was segmented using ATM SVC (requiring about 5 minutes of operator time, for initial alignment of the template and for prototype selection). The results of the segmentations were very similar. On a voxel to voxel comparison the agreement was over 85%. The primary differences were due to over-smoothing of the boundary of the tumour in the manual segmentation.

Segmentation of Knee Cartilage from MRI ATM SVC was compared with manual outlining for the segmentation of knee cartilage from MRI of a patient with a focal cartilage defect. ATM SVC provided a close match of the cartilage segmentation to the cartilage seen in the MR, particularly in the region of the defect [14]. A quantitative assessment was carried out and the use of the ATM SVC was found to greatly reduce the variability of the segmentation (Table 1).

Observer	1	2	3	4	ATM SVC
C.V. (%)	7.2	9.6	6.6	7.0	3.9

Table 1. Coefficient of variation of volume of manual and ATM SVC femoral cartilage segmentation. Four experts segmented a single MR image with a single focal defect, 5 to 10 times on separate occasions over a period of one month. One of the experts also carried out repeated initializations of the automatic segmentation, so the variability induced in the segmentation by differences in initialization could be determined. The volume of the femoral cartilage was recorded, and the coefficient of variation of the volume for each of the experts and the automatic segmentation is shown. The use of the ATM SVC was found to greatly reduce the variability of the segmentation.

4 Discussion and Conclusion

We have developed a new algorithm which is an adaptive template moderated spatially varying statistical classification. The examples presented in Section 3 demonstrate that ATM SVC can achieve better segmentations than either statistical classification or nonlinear registration alone for the illustrated problems. These problems involve both normal anatomy and also certain types of pathology. The ATM SVC algorithm may fail when structures to be segmented have similar characteristics in all features and are also not spatially distinct. When the structures to be segmented have similar characteristics in all features the classification is strongly dependent upon the spatial localization that can be derived from the nonlinear registration (that is the point of the ATM SVC algorithm). The classification is then strongly dependent upon the boundaries identified by elastic matching. If the structures to be segmented have a boundary that cannot be discerned by elastic matching, the segmentation in the region of the boundary can be wrong, up to the size of the error of the spatial localization.

Related work has examined different types of adaptation in the classification problem. The segmentation of tissue classes in the presence of intensity inhomogeneity and variation of intensity over time was the motivation for the development of an adaptive tissue classification algorithm by Wells et al. [11]. This method iteratively adapts a model of intensity inhomogeneity to drive a tissue classification algorithm. This has the advantage of making it possible to classify patient scans without per-patient prototype selection. For the ATM SVC, we do per-patient training and iterate the classification with respect to an adaptive anatomical model. For the examples of Section 3, we have found it unnecessary to explicitly include estimation of intensity inhomogeneity, although it would be straightforward to incorporate.

An alternative modification to the usual classification model is to use a spatially varying a priori probability field. Kamber et al. [15] built a probabilistic spatially varying a priori model which was successful at reducing the number of false positives in a lesion classification problem. However, this algorithm did not adapt the spatially varying model to the particular patient being segmented and consequently was not able to reduce the number of false negative lesion classifications.

Acknowledgements This investigation was supported (in part) by a Postdoctoral Fellowship from the National Multiple Sclerosis Society (SW).

References

[1] S Solloway, CE Hutchinson, JC Waterton, and CJ Taylor, "The use of active shape models for making thickness measurements of articular cartilage from MR images.", *Magn Reson Med*, vol. 37, no. 6, pp. 943–952, 1997.
[2] D. Louis Collins, *3D Model-based segmentation of individual brain structures from magnetic resonance imaging data*, PhD thesis, McGill University, 1994.
[3] Arun Kumar, Allen R. Tannenbaum, and Gary J. Balas, "Optical Flow: A Curve Evolution Approach", *IEEE Transactions On Image Processing*, vol. 5, no. 4, pp. 598–610, April 1996.
[4] Ron Kikinis, Martha E. Shenton, Dan V. Iosifescu, Robert W. McCarley, Pairash Saiviroonporn, Hiroto H. Hokama, Andre Robatino, David Metcalf, Cynthia G. Wible, Chiara M. Portas, Robert M. Donnino, and Ferenc A. Jolesz, "A Digital Brain Atlas for Surgical Planning, Model Driven Segmentation, and Teaching", *IEEE Transactions on Visualization and Computer Graphics*, vol. 2, no. 3, pp. 232–241, September 1996.
[5] G. Gerig, O. Kübler, R. Kikinis, and F. A. Jolesz, "Nonlinear Anisotropic Filtering of MRI Data", *IEEE Transactions On Medical Imaging*, vol. 11, no. 2, pp. 221–232, June 1992.
[6] Simon Warfield, Ferenc Jolesz, and Ron Kikinis, "A High Performance Computing Approach to the Registration of Medical Imaging Data", *Parallel Computing*, 1998, To appear in Parallel Computing.
[7] Richard O. Duda and Peter E. Hart, *Pattern Classification and Scene Analysis*, John Wiley & Sons, Inc., 1973.
[8] Jerome H. Friedman, Forest Baskett, and Leonard J. Shustek, "An Algorithm for Finding Nearest Neighbors", *IEEE Transactions On Computers*, vol. C-24, no. 10, pp. 1000–1006, October 1975.
[9] Simon Warfield, "Fast k-NN Classification for Multichannel Image Data", *Pattern Recognition Letters*, vol. 17, no. 7, pp. 713–721, 1996.
[10] Joachim Dengler and Markus Schmidt, "The Dynamic Pyramid – A Model for Motion Analysis with Controlled Continuity", *International Journal of Pattern Recognition and Artificial Intelligence*, vol. 2, no. 2, pp. 275–286, 1988.
[11] W. M. Wells, R Kikinis, W. E. L. Grimson, and F. Jolesz, "Adaptive segmentation of MRI data", *IEEE Transactions On Medical Imaging*, vol. 15, pp. 429–442, 1996.
[12] Petra Hüppi, Simon Warfield, Ron Kikinis, Patrick D. Barnes, Gary P. Zientara, Ferenc A. Jolesz, Miles K. Tsuji, and Joseph J. Volpe, "Quantitative Magnetic Resonance Imaging of Brain Development in Premature and Mature Newborns", *Ann Neurol*, vol. 43, no. 2, pp. 224–235, February 1998.
[13] Simon Warfield, Joachim Dengler, Joachim Zaers, Charles R.G. Guttmann, William M. Wells III, Gil J. Ettinger, John Hiller, and Ron Kikinis, "Automatic identification of Grey Matter Structures from MRI to Improve the Segmentation of White Matter Lesions", *Journal of Image Guided Surgery*, vol. 1, no. 6, pp. 326–338, 1995.
[14] Simon Warfield, Carl Winalski, Ferenc Jolesz, and Ron Kikinis, "Automatic Segmentation of MRI of the Knee", in *ISMRM Sixth Scientific Meeting and Exhibition*, April 18–24 1998, p. 563.
[15] M. Kamber, D. L. Collins, R. Shinghal, G. S. Francis, and A. C. Evans, "Model-based 3D segmentation of multiple sclerosis lesions in dual-echo MRI data", in *SPIE Vol. 1808, Visualization in Biomedical Computing*, 1992, pp. 590–600.

Automatic Quantification of MS Lesions in 3D MRI Brain Data Sets: Validation of INSECT

Alex Zijdenbos[1], Reza Forghani[1,2], and Alan Evans[1]

[1]McConnell Brain Imaging Centre and [2]Department of Neurology and Neurosurgery,
Montreal Neurological Institute, Montréal, Canada
{alex,reza,alan}@bic.mni.mcgill.ca
http://www.bic.mni.mcgill.ca

Abstract. In recent years, the quantitative analysis of MRI data has become a standard surrogate marker in clinical trials in multiple sclerosis (MS). We have developed INSECT (Intensity Normalized Stereotaxic Environment for Classification of Tissues), a fully automatic system aimed at the quantitative morphometric analysis of 3D MRI brain data sets. This paper describes the design and validation of INSECT in the context of a multi-center clinical trial in MS. It is shown that no statistically significant differences exist between MS lesion load measurements obtained with INSECT and those obtained manually by trained human observers from seven different clinical centers.

1 Introduction

Although the use of magnetic resonance imaging (MRI) as a qualitative clinical diagnostic tool in the study of multiple sclerosis (MS) has been established for well over a decade, it is only in recent years that its quantitative analysis is attracting interest. This attention is driven by, among other things, the increased use of MRI as a surrogate marker in clinical trials aimed at establishing the efficacy of drug therapies [1, 11]. A landmark study in this respect was the interferon beta-1b trial [15], which showed a correlation between MRI measured lesion load (quantified using manual boundary tracing) and clinical findings. This study clearly shows that manual tracing can be used to measure MRI lesion load with sufficient accuracy to detect a clinical effect; however, the disadvantages of this method are that it is very labour-intensive and that it suffers from high intra- and interrater variabilities.

A number of researchers have shown that computer-aided techniques are able to not only reduce operator burden, but also the inter- and intrarater variability associated with the measurement [5, 13, 26]. However, considering that the amount of MRI data to analyze in present-day clinical trials is often on the order of hundreds or thousands of scans, even minor manual involvement for each scan is an arduous task. The development of fully automatic analysis techniques is desirable to further reduce both the operator time requirements and the measurement variability.

At the McConnell Brain Imaging Centre (BIC), we have developed INSECT (Intensity Normalized Stereotaxic Environment for Classification of Tissues), a system aimed at the fully automatic quantification of tissue types in medical image data. This system has been used to automatically quantify MS lesion load in over 2000 MRI scans, acquired in the context of a large-scale, multi-center clinical trial [22]. Clearly, the thorough validation of results obtained using such an automated technique is crucial for its acceptance into clinical practice. Crucial elements of such validation studies are the assessment of accuracy and reproducibility. In the case of INSECT, results obtained on the same data are perfectly reproducible, which is a considerable advantage over manual lesion delineation. The fact that the analysis is reproducible does however not imply that its results are also accurate. The main focus of this paper is the validation of the accuracy of INSECT for the quantification of MS lesion load in MRI.

2 Methods

This section gives a brief overview of the INSECT processing pipeline, followed by a description of the validation studies performed to assess its accuracy for the automatic quantification of MS lesion load.

2.1 Image Processing

Fig. 1 shows the general architecture of INSECT. The central module of this system is the registration of the data with, and resampling into, a standardized, stereotaxic brain space based on the Talairach atlas [2, 21]. The registration component is preceded by a number of preprocessing algorithms aimed at artifact reduction, and followed by postprocessing algorithms such as intensity normalization and tissue classification. Each of these image processing components is briefly described here.

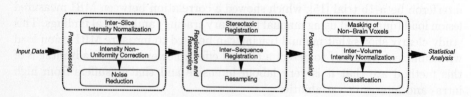

Fig. 1. INSECT flow diagram.

Inter-Slice Intensity Normalization: intensity variation between adjacent slices, an artifact generally attributed to eddy currents and crosstalk between slices, is a common problem in MRI [17, 24, 25]. INSECT employs a correction method in which the scaling factor between each pair of adjacent slices is estimated from local (pixel-by-pixel) correction factors [25]. *Intensity Non-Uniformity Correction:* low-frequency spatial intensity variations, predominantly caused by electrodynamic interactions with the subject and inhomogeneity of the RF receiver coil sensitivity [8,17,18], are a major source of errors in the computer-aided, quantitative analysis of MRI data. A number of researchers have proposed algorithms to correct for this type of artifact [3,10,20,23,25]. INSECT employs a method developed in our institute [20], which was shown to be accurate and robust [19]. *Noise Reduction:* edge-preserving noise filters are often able to improve the accuracy and reliability of quantitative measurements obtained from MRI [12,26]. INSECT relies on anisotropic diffusion, a filter commonly used for the reduction of noise in MRI [7,16]. *Stereotaxic Registration:* this is accomplished by the registration of one of the image modalities to a stereotaxic target, using an automated 3D image registration technique [2]. This method minimizes, in a multi-stage, multi-scale approach, an image similarity measure between these two volumes as a function of a 9 parameter (3 translations, 3 rotations, 3 scales) linear geometric transformation. The stereotaxic target used at the BIC is an average T_1-weighted scan of 305 normal volunteers [2,4,6]. *Inter-Sequence Registration:* processing multi-modal (multi-feature) data typically requires the individual data volumes to be in exact spatial register, i.e., the feature values obtained from each modality at a specific voxel location should all reflect the same location in physical brain space. Since patient motion between different acquisitions is common, all scans of a patient or subject are explicitly registered with each other using the same technique as described for stereotaxic registration, with parameter values tailored to, in particular, the registration of a T_2-weighted scan to a T_1-weighted scan. *Resampling:* following stereotaxic and inter-scan registration, all data volumes are resampled onto the same voxel grid using trilinear interpolation. *Masking of Non-Brain Voxels*: for the application described herein, a standard brain mask, defined in stereotaxic space, is used. The fact that this 'average' brain mask may not accurately fit the individual brain does not affect the quantification of MS lesions, which are typically situated in the white matter well away from the cortical surface. *Inter-Volume Intensity Normalization:* given that all volumes at this stage are stereotaxically registered, they can be normalized using the same technique as described for the correction of inter-slice intensity variations (see [25]). In this case, a single, global intensity scale factor is estimated from the voxel-by-voxel comparison of each volume with a stereotaxic intensity model. *Tissue Classification:* for this application, INSECT employs a back-propagation artificial neural network (ANN) [26], which has been trained once to separate MS lesion from background (non-lesion). The classifier uses six input features, being the T_1-, T_2-, and PD weighted MRI volumes, as well as three (white matter, gray matter, CSF) SPAMs (Statistical Probability of Anatomy Maps), derived from normal human neuroanatomy (see [9]).

In order to process mass amounts of data, INSECT allows the user to specify this type of processing 'pipeline' using a high-level script language. During execution, each individual processing stage is submitted to a load-balancing queue, which distributes the job over a network of interconnected workstations. This results in efficient mass-production using a high degree of (coarse-grain) parallelism.

2.2 Validation

The accuracy of INSECT has been assessed by means of two validation studies, in which automatic results were compared against those obtained from trained observers. *I. Independent Validation*: a total of 10 axial slice triplets (T_1-, T_2- and PD-weighted), each acquired from a different MS patient and at a different scanner, were selected from the data acquired for a multi-center clinical trial. Selection was such that the data reflect a reasonable range of lesion load and spatial distribution. The slices were extracted from data which was registered with and resampled into the BIC standard Talairach $1mm^3$ isotropic brain space. These data were distributed to seven different institutes for evaluation (see the acknowledgements), with the specific request to manually label all MS lesion pixels in each image triplet and return the binary label maps to the BIC. *II. BIC validation*: MS lesions were identified, using manual tracing, by four raters from the BIC community on a total of 29 MRI volume triplets (T_1-, T_2-, and PD-weighted). The raters, who all had substantial previous familiarity with neuroanatomy, were supervised by R.F. and trained for at least a month prior to data analysis. The criteria for lesion delineation were established by R.F. based on existing literature (e.g. [14]) and in collaboration with local neurologists and neuroradiologists.

The primary objective of this validation study is to test the hypothesis that there is no statistically significant difference between automatic and manual measurements, i.e., that the automatic lesion quantification can be seen as yet another expert manual measurement. In the following, the total lesion load (TLL) obtained automatically (INSECT) is compared with those obtained manually (human expert) using z-scores, correlation coefficients, and analysis-of-variance (ANOVA). For the ANOVA, the treatments, or groups, of the analysis are the various manual and the automatic measurements, and the MRI data sets are the subjects. A one-way ANOVA shows whether the mean measurements (over subjects) of the treatments are equal.

3 Results and Discussion

3.1 Independent Validation

An example of the labeled lesion scans obtained in the independent validation study is shown in Fig. 2. This figure clearly illustrates the variability present amongst different expert observers.

Fig. 3 shows the total lesion load, for each of the 10 slices included in the independent validation study, both obtained manually (mean ± sd over 7 raters) and automatically. Since the measurement variance increases with lesion size, the vertical axis shows the cubic root of the TLL, which converts the volumetric TLL

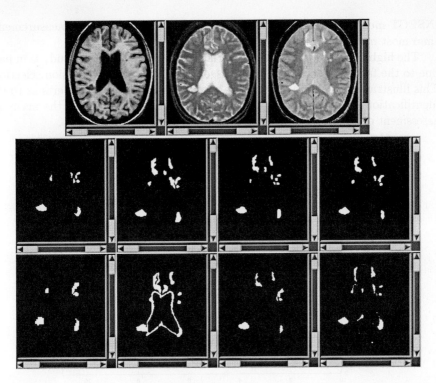

Fig. 2. Source MRI data (*top row, from left to right*: T_1-, T_2-, and PD-weighted image), (*second and third row*) labeled lesions obtained from 7 sites, and INSECT-obtained lesion map (*bottom right*), for slice data set # 10 (cf Fig. 3 and Table 1).

measurement to a 'lesion diameter' (this was only done for illustration purposes; all calculations are done on the original, non-transformed data). Table 1 shows these data in tabular form including the z-scores and associated p-values, for each slice, of the automatic TLL with respect to the mean and sd of the manual TLL. Clearly, the INSECT TLL is not significantly different from the average manual TLL, and is within one standard deviation from the mean on 9 out of 10 data sets. This is confirmed by the ANOVA on these data: F=1.03, p=0.42, indicating that none of the treatment groups is significantly different from any of the others. The interrater coefficient of variation (sd/mean over 10 slices) for the manual measurements is 44±20% (mean±sd).

As expected from these data, the correlation coefficient calculated between INSECT TLL and the average manual TLL is also very high: $r = 0.93$, $p < 0.0001$. It is also interesting to look at the correlations, over these 10 slices, between each pair of measurements. This is done in Table 2, which shows the significance levels of these correlations. From this table, it is clear that INSECT TLL measurements correlate significantly which the measurements made by any and all of the sites, whereas this is true for only 3 out of 7 sites. In other words,

INSECT measurements correlate on average better with manual measurements than most manual measurements correlate with each other.

The high interrater coefficient of variation obtained from this study is in part due to the fact that each of the sites used their own criteria for lesion selection. This illustrates that there is considerable disagreement among experts as to the identification of MS lesions on MRI, which in general confounds the accuracy assessment of computer-aided techniques.

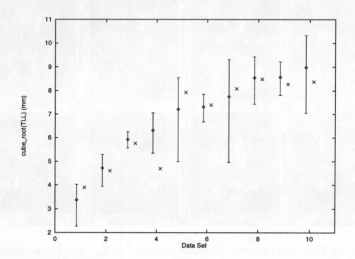

Fig. 3. Manual (mean ± sd) and automatic TLL measurements for each slice. The slices have been ordered with respect to mean manual TLL, which corresponds to the order used in Table 1. In order to obtain uniform variance accross data sets, the vertical axis shows 'lesion diameter' ($\sqrt[3]{TLL}$).

3.2 BIC Validation

Fig. 4 shows the data obtained from the 29-volume BIC validation (cf Fig. 3). effiche z-scores calculated from the data shown in Fig. 4 show that the INSECT TLL is within two standard deviations from the mean manual for 21 out of 29 (72%) volumes, and within one sd for 14 volumes (48%). Although there are a number of volumes for which the INSECT TLL deviates from the average manual TLL, overall this is not significant, as is shown by ANOVA: F=0.09 (p=0.97). Similar to the results obtained in the independent validation, the correlation coefficient calculated between INSECT TLL and average manual TLL is high: $r = 0.95$, $p < 0.0001$. In this case, the pairwise correlations between measurements are all highly significant ($p < 0.0001$). The inter-rater coefficient of variation (sd/mean) of the manual TLLs over the 29 volumes is 27±16% (mean±sd), showing the reduction in variability (down from 44±20%) when all raters adhere to the same lesion selection criteria.

Table 1. Manual (min, max, mean, sd, cv) and INSECT-based lesion volume measurements. Also reported are the z-scores and associated p-values of INSECT versus manual.

Slice Data Set	Manual (mm³)					INSECT		
	min	max	mean	sd	cv	mm³	z	p
1	0	82	38	27	70	59	0.77	0.44
2	43	168	105	43	41	97	-0.17	0.86
3	161	251	208	36	17	191	-0.48	0.63
4	140	442	252	99	39	103	-1.50	0.13
5	153	919	374	250	67	499	0.50	0.62
6	295	555	391	94	24	404	0.14	0.89
7	256	1235	465	343	74	528	0.18	0.86
8	403	893	624	214	34	611	-0.06	0.95
9	485	929	630	153	24	567	-0.41	0.68
10	394	1495	725	375	52	588	-0.37	0.71

Table 2. The significance of the correlation, over 10 slice data sets, between all combinations of manual and automatic measurements.

Site	INSECT	Site 1	Site 2	Site 3	Site 4	Site 5	Site 6	Site 7
1	***	-	*	***	****	****	*	***
2	**	*	-	*	*	n.s.	n.s.	**
3	**	***	*	-	****	**	*	**
4	****	****	*	****	-	***	*	**
5	**	****	n.s.	**	***	-	n.s.	**
6	*	*	n.s.	*	*	n.s.	-	n.s.
7	**	***	**	**	**	**	n.s.	-

$*p < 0.05$, $**p < 0.01$, $***p < 0.001$, $****p < 0.0001$

Based on the visual inspection of the 'outlier' volumes, where the INSECT TLL measurement was significantly different from the distribution of the manual measurements, a number of points can be made: 1) Many of the outliers occur in volumes with small amounts of lesion (see Fig. 4). If the image volume contains many small lesions and/or the image quality is poor, the human raters tended to be somewhat conservative in their measurements. 2) In the same circumstances, different human raters often identified different lesions on the same data set. 3) The criteria for lesion identification that INSECT implicitly uses, are necessarily not identical to those used by the human raters. By studying individual cases and longitudinal scan sequences, we were able to confirm that, although its measurements may deviate from the average manual measurements, INSECT was very consistent (see Fig. 5). In clinical trials, this type of reproducibility is crucial for determining treatment efficacy.

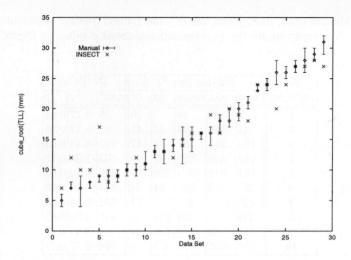

Fig. 4. Manual (mean ± sd) and automatic TLL measurements for each volume. The volumes have been ordered with respect to mean manual TLL. In order to obtain uniform variance accross data sets, the vertical axis shows 'lesion diameter' ($\sqrt[3]{\text{TLL}}$)

4 Conclusion

Validation studies of INSECT, a fully automatic system for the mass quantitative analysis of MRI data, focused on the detection of multiple sclerosis lesions, have been presented. These studies consistently show that there is high degree of agreement between automatically and manually detected lesion load in MRI. Using ANOVA, no statistically significant differences between automatic and manual lesion volume measurements were found. Since INSECT is accurate as compared with expert opinion and eliminates intra- and interobserver variability, it is a valuable tool for the evaluation of drug therapies in large-scale clinical studies.

Acknowledgements

The authors would like to express their gratitude to the people who have manually labeled MS lesions on the validation data sets. For the independent validation, these are: *Dr. Frederik Barkhof*, Dept. of Radiology, Free University Hospital, Amsterdam, The Netherlands; *Dr. Massimo Filippi*, Clinica Neurologica, Ospedale San Raffaele, Milan, Italy; *Dr. Joseph Frank*, Laboratory of Diagnostic Radiology Research, NIH, Bethesda, MD, U.S.A.; *Dr. Robert Grossmann*, Dept. of Radiology, University of Pennsylvania, Philadelphia, PA, U.S.A.; *Dr. Charles Guttmann*, Dept. of Radiology, Brigham and Women's Hospital, Boston, MA, U.S.A.; *Dr. Stephen Karlik*, Dept. of Diagnostic Radiology & Nuclear Medicine, University of Western Ontario, London, Ontario, Canada; and *Dr. David Miller*, Institute of Neurology, Queens Square, University of London, London, U.K. For the BIC validation: *Hooman Farhadi, Reza Forghani, Dana Small,* and *Dr. Selva Tekkök*. The authors also thank *Dr. Gordon Francis* and *Dr. Denis Melançon* for their assistance in establishing the criteria for lesion delineation.

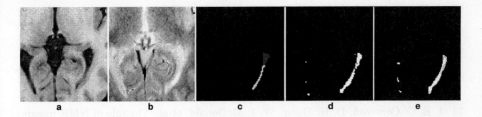

Fig. 5. a and b: T_1- and PD-weighted MRI; c: manual labeling at baseline scan (average of 4 raters); d: INSECT labeling at baseline; e: average INSECT labeling (over a series of 9 scans, taken 3 months apart). The brightness in the 'average' lesion labelings is proportional to the frequency of voxel selection. Panel c shows that, on the baseline scan, at most 2 of the 4 raters identified what INSECT labeled as a large, elongated lesion (d). However, panel e shows that INSECT consistently identified that same lesion on 9 consecutive quarterly scans. This volume corresponds to data set # 5 in Fig. 4.

References

1. F. Barkhof, M. Filippi, D. H. Miller, P. Tofts, L. Kappos, and A. J. Thompson. Strategies for optimizing MRI techniques aimed at monitoring disease activity in multiple sclerosis treatment trials. *Journal of Neurology*, 244(2):76–84, Feb 1997.
2. D. L. Collins, P. Neelin, T. M. Peters, and A. C. Evans. Automatic 3D intersubject registration of MR volumetric data in standardized Talairach space. *Journal of Computer Assisted Tomography*, 18(2):192–205, Mar./Apr. 1994.
3. B. M. Dawant, A. P. Zijdenbos, and R. A. Margolin. Correction of intensity variations in MR images for computer-aided tissue classification. *IEEE Transactions on Medical Imaging*, 12(4):770–781, Dec. 1993.
4. A. Evans, M. Kamber, D. Collins, and D. MacDonald. An MRI-based probabilistic atlas of neuroanatomy. In S. D. Shorvon et al., editors, *Magnetic Resonance Scanning and Epilepsy*, chapter 48, pages 263–274. Plenum Press, 1994.
5. A. C. Evans, J. A. Frank, J. Antel, and D. H. Miller. The role of MRI in clinical trials of multiple sclerosis: Comparison of image processing techniques. *Annals of Neurology*, 41(1):125–132, Jan. 1997.
6. A. C. Evans, S. Marrett, P. Neelin, et al. Anatomical mapping of functional activation in stereotactic coordinate space. *NeuroImage*, 1:43–53, 1992.
7. G. Gerig, O. Kübler, R. Kikinis, and F. A. Jolesz. Nonlinear anisotropic filtering of MRI data. *IEEE Transactions on Medical Imaging*, 11(2):221–232, June 1992.
8. R. M. Henkelman and M. J. Bronskill. Artifacts in magnetic resonance imaging. *Reviews of Magnetic Resonance in Medicine*, 2(1):1–126, 1987.
9. M. Kamber, R. Shinghal, D. L. Collins, G. S. Francis, and A. C. Evans. Model-based 3-D segmentation of multiple sclerosis lesions in magnetic resonance brain images. *IEEE Transactions in Medical Imaging*, 14(3):442–453, Sept. 1995.
10. C. R. Meyer, P. H. Bland, and J. Pipe. Retrospective correction of intensity inhomogeneities in MRI. *IEEE Transactions on Medical Imaging*, 14(1):36–41, Mar. 1995.
11. D. H. Miller, P. S. Albert, F. Barkhof, G. Francis, J. A. Frank, S. Hodgkinson, F. D. Lublin, D. W. Paty, S. C. Reingold, and J. Simon. Guidelines for the use of magnetic resonance techniques in monitoring the treatment of multiple sclerosis. *Annals of Neurology*, 39:6–16, 1996.

12. J. R. Mitchell, S. J. Karlik, D. H. Lee, M. Eliasziw, G. P. Rice, and A. Fenster. Quantification of multiple sclerosis lesion volumes in 1.5 and 0.5T anisotropically filtered and unfiltered MR exams. *Medical Physics*, 23(1):115–126, Jan. 1996.
13. J. R. Mitchell, S. J. Karlik, D. H. Lee, and A. Fenster. Computer-assisted identification and quantification of multiple sclerosis lesions in MR imaging volumes in the brain. *Journal of Magnetic Resonance Imaging*, pages 197–208, Mar./Apr. 1994.
14. I. E. C. Ormerod, D. H. Miller, W. I. McDonald, et al. The role of NMR imaging in the assessment of multiple sclerosis and isolated neurological lesions. *Brain*, 110:1579–1616, 1987.
15. D. W. Paty, D. K. B. Li, UBC MS/MRI Study Group, and IFNB Multiple Sclerosis Study Group. Interferon beta-1b is effective in relapsing-remitting multiple sclerosis. *Neurology*, 43:662–667, 1993.
16. P. Perona and J. Malik. Scale space and edge detection using anisotropic diffusion. *IEEE Transactions on Pattern Analysis and Machine Intelligence*, 12(7):629–639, July 1990.
17. A. Simmons, P. S. Tofts, G. J. Barker, and S. R. Arridge. Sources of intensity nonuniformity in spin echo images. *Magnetic Resonance in Medicine*, 32:121–128, 1994.
18. J. G. Sled and G. B. Pike. Standing-wave and RF penetration artifacts caused by elliptic geometry: an electrodynamic analysis of MRI. *IEEE Transactions on Medical Imaging*, 1997. (submitted).
19. J. G. Sled, A. P. Zijdenbos, and A. C. Evans. A comparison of retrospective intensity non-uniformity correction methods for MRI. In *Proceedings of the 15th International Conference on Information Processing in Medical Imaging (IPMI)*, pages 459–464, Poultney, VT, USA, June 1997.
20. J. G. Sled, A. P. Zijdenbos, and A. C. Evans. A nonparametric method for automatic correction of intensity nonuniformity in MRI data. *IEEE Transactions on Medical Imaging*, 17(1), Feb. 1998.
21. J. Talairach and P. Tournoux. *Co-planar Stereotaxic Atlas of the Human Brain: 3-Dimensional Proportional System - an Approach to Cerebral Imaging*. Thieme Medical Publishers, New York, NY, 1988.
22. H. L. Weiner. Oral tolerance for the treatment of autoimmune diseases. *Annual Review of Medicine*, 48(48):341–51, 1997. 75 refs, Review.
23. W. M. Wells III, W. E. L. Grimson, R. Kikinis, and F. A. Jolesz. Adaptive segmentation of MRI data. *IEEE Transactions on Medical Imaging*, 15(4):429–442, Aug. 1996.
24. D. A. G. Wicks, G. J. Barker, and P. S. Tofts. Correction of intensity nonuniformity in MR images of any orientation. *Magnetic Resonance Imaging*, 11(2):183–196, 1993.
25. A. P. Zijdenbos, B. M. Dawant, and R. A. Margolin. Intensity correction and its effect on measurement variability in the computer-aided analysis of MRI. In *Proceedings of the 9th International Symposium and Exhibition on Computer Assisted Radiology (CAR)*, pages 216–221, Berlin, Germany, June 1995.
26. A. P. Zijdenbos, B. M. Dawant, R. A. Margolin, and A. C. Palmer. Morphometric analysis of white matter lesions in MR images: Method and validation. *IEEE Transactions on Medical Imaging*, 13(4):716–724, Dec. 1994.

Computer-Aided Diagnostic System for Pulmonary Nodules Using Helical CT Images

K.Kanazawa[1], Y.Kawata[2], N.Niki[2], H.Satoh[3]
H.Ohmatsu[4], R.Kakinuma[4], M.Kaneko[5], K.Eguchi[6], N.Moriyama[4]

[1] Dept. of Information Engineering, Takuma National College of Technology
[2] Dept. of Optical Science, University of Tokushima, Japan
[3] Medical Engineering Laboratory, Japan
[4] National Cancer Center Hospital East, Japan
[5] National Cancer Center Hospital, Japan
[6] National Shikoku Cancer Center Hospital, Japan

Abstract. In this paper, we present a computer assisted automatic diagnostic system for lung cancer that detects nodule candidates at an early stage from helical CT images of the thorax. Our diagnostic system consists of analytic and diagnostic procedures. In the analysis procedure, we extract the lung and the blood vessel regions using the fuzzy clustering algorithm, then we analyze the features of these regions. In the diagnosis procedure, we define diagnostic rules utilizing the extracted features which support the determination of the candidate nodule locations.

1 Introduction

According to figures of cancer incidence in Japan, mortality from cancer is increasing annually with the present rate for cancer prevailing in a quarter of all deaths. Among cancerdeath causes, lung cancer is the most common one, accounting for 21.4% of all male cancer deaths cases in Japan. A possibility of opposing the lung cancer is its detection and treatment at an early stage of growth. As a conventional method for the mass screening process, chest X-ray films have been used for lung cancer diagnosis. Since the chest X-ray films are two-dimensional projection images, the overlapping of bone and organs shadows results in disturbing the detection of small lung cancer nodules at early stage.

Recently, chest CT images obtained by helical CT scanner which can make a wide range measurement of the lung region in a short time have drawn interest in the detection of suspicious regions[1]-[3]. However, mass screening based on helical CT images leads to a considerable number of images to be diagnosed which is time-consuming and makes its use difficult in the clinic. In order to increase the efficiency of the mass screening process, our group is working towards a computer-aided diagnosis system for pulmonary nodules detection based on helical CT images. We have already developed a prototype computer-aided diagnosis (CAD) system to automatically detect suspicious nodules from chest CT images and alert physicians attention. The ingredients of the system are the image analysis and the image diagnosis parts. The first part consists of the following procedures; extraction of the lung area, reduction of the partial volume effect and beam hardening, extraction of the region of interest (ROI), and feature extraction from each ROI. The second part procedures detect suspicious nodules and alert physicians attention by applying their proposed diagnosis rules. In this paper, we describe our algorithm of computer-aided diagnosis for pulmonary nodules and we show the performance of the prototype CAD system by using image data of 450 cases.

2 Diagnostic Algorithm

2.1 Image Analysis Procedure

The prototype CAD system is designed to detect the candidates of lung cancer from helical CT images consists of two procedures; image analysis procedure and image diagnosis procedure. The input to this system is helical CT image acquired under the specified measurement conditions shown in Table.1. These images are reconstructed at 10mm increment by using an 180 linear interpolation algorithm and a matrix size of 512×512 pixels with 12 bits quantization. From every patient we collect 35 images with the above mentioned measurement conditions. The diagnostic algorithm is applied to each slice image from upper to lower lung sequentially.

The first procedure of the system deals with the extraction of lung area, the reduction of the partial volume and the beam hardening effects, the extraction of the region of interest(ROI), and finally the feature extraction of ROI.

[Step1] Extraction of the Lung Fields

The lung fields are mostly occupied by air, CT value of the pixels within the lung fields are lower than CT values of the lung wall. Firstly, the original image is transformed to a binary image using a gray-level thresholding algorithm with a threshold value t. Secondly, we eliminate the binary regions, external to the body, trachea and stomach. The tracheal regions are determined as isolated regions which locate at the central region of the body, and the stomachic region are determined as isolated regions which can not exist on the upper slice image. The edges of the remainder regions are defined as the lung contour, the regions within the lung contour are defined as the initial lung fields.

However, this thresholding technique excludes the lung boundary with high CT values from the real lung fields. In order to avoid this problem the lost parts are compensated by using curvature at the boundary of the initial lung fields contour. Therefore, we replace the contour with rapidly changing curvature with a straight line.

[Step2] Analysis of the Lung Fields

As shape of the lung fields and the structures in the lung are seen differently, according to the position of the lung in each slice, the diagnostic parameters have to be adjusted appropriately. Therefore, we classify the lung into four sections based on the area and the shape of the extracted lung regions as shown in Fig.1. In this process, the border between sections is detected through extracting the lung fields sequentially slice by slice.

[Step3] Reduction of the Artifacts

Structures in the lung, such as blood vessels and nodules, are individually defined by a segmentation process. However, the helical CT images involve artifacts by the beam hardening effect and the partial volume effect. These artifacts affect the ROI extraction procedure and present bad extraction result. These artifacts are reduced by a simple technique which used to smooth the lung field's image based on mathematical morphology operation. Then, we apply a smoothing method to the extracted lung images and we subtract this smoothed image from the original image in the lung area. These procedure is used as pre-segmentation process.

[Step4] Extraction of ROI

The interesting organs in the lung, such as blood vessels and nodules, are segmented within the lung fields obtained using fuzzy clustering method. The lung field images are segmented into two clusters, air cluster and other organs cluster. To obtain the binary regions of ROI, firstly, the gray-weighted distance transformation is applied to the segmented image, to which we apply the threshold algorithm in order to eliminate pixels lower than the threshold distance k. Secondly, we apply an inverse distance transformation to extract the ROI. The small size regions contained in the organs clusters are eliminated by this procedure.

The artifacts are reduced by the morphological method described in the previous step, however, the artifact near the circumference of the lung fields are not removed satisfactorily. Thus, to remove such artifacts, we use surface curvatures described in [3]. The ROI tend to be the convex and hyperbolic surface regions on the intensity surfaces. To extract convex and hyperbolic surface regions the calculated curvatures signs are utilized. The signs of these surface curvatures segment the intensity surface into eight basic viewpoint-independent surface types, such as peak surface ($K > 0$ and $H < 0$), flat surface ($K = 0$ and $H = 0$), pit surface ($K > 0$ and $H > 0$), minimal surface ($K < 0$ and $H = 0$), ridge surface ($K = 0$ and $H < 0$), saddle ridge ($K < 0$ and $H < 0$), valley surface ($K = 0$ and $H > 0$), and saddle valley ($K < 0$ and $H > 0$). Since it is difficult to decide whether K and H are zero or not, the four surface types including flat surface, minimal surface, ridge surface, and valley surface are not assigned in practical experiments. In this step, we consider the following surface types regions as ROI; pit surface, saddle ridge, and saddle valley surface types. We apply this extraction method using surface curvatures to the regions where artifacts tend to arise. To put it in the concrete, we extract two lung fields with different threshold values, this extraction method is applied to the different region between the two lung fields.

[Step5] ROI Feature Extraction

Most of the extracted ROI are blood vessel regions. We need to identify ROI as blood vessels or nodules. Thus, we give attention to shape, gray value and position of each ROI. This step extracts the features of each ROI. The following features are considered; F_a : Area, F_t : Thickness, F_c : Circularity, F_g : Gray-level, F_v : Variance of gray-level, F_l : Localization, F_h : Variance of gradient, F_p : **Distance from the lung wall**.

F_a is the number of the pixels of each ROI. F_t is the maximum gray-weighted distance in each ROI, F_c is the rate of occupation inside the circumscribed circle, F_g is the mean CT number of the pixels, F_v is the variance of the CT numbers, F_l is the rate of the isolation, F_h is the variance of the gradient on the boundary of each ROI, F_p is the minimum distance between the circumscribed circle's center of each ROI and the lung wall. The contour of the lung wall is defined as the section of lung contour which cuts out the mediastinal contour.

2.2 Image Diagnosis Procedure

The second procedure of our prototype system detects suspicious region and alerts physicians attention by applying their proposed diagnosis rules. Three diagnostic rules are constructed based on the following medical knowledge;

Point 1 : Lung cancer shape is generally spherical, and is seen as a circle on the cross section. Contrariwise the shape of blood vessels running parallel to the slice image are generally oblong.

Point 2 : The thickness of the blood vessel becomes smaller as its position approaches the lung wall, however the thickness of the lung cancer is generally larger than the ordinary thickness of the blood vessels at each position.

Point 3 : Since the peripheral blood vessels are too small to be seen in the helical CT image and are difficult to recognize, shadows contacting the lung wall are generally nodules or partial volume artifacts.

Point 4 : The gray values of blood vessels running vertical with respect to the slice image are generally higher than the same sized cancer in helical CT images with the specified measurement conditions for mass screening.

Point 5 : The values of pixels of the cancer region are comparatively uniform.

We define the diagnostic rules combining features of ROI to detect suspicious nodules. The diagnostic rules are classified into following three types;

[RULE 1] : **Regions for elimination**

We eliminate the current ROI if the following conditions are satisfied.

(1) Our diagnostic algorithm aims to detect cancer with diameter over 4mm. A ROI with Thickness F_t under 2.0 (corresponding to approximately 4mm) is eliminated.
(2) A ROI for which the percentage of Circularity F_c is under 20% is eliminated as a blood vessel region according to Point 1.
(3) In case where bone exists in the adjacent slice images at the location for the current ROI, we eliminate this ROI as a shadow of a partial volume artifact arising from bone.

[RULE 2] : **Detection of nodules in case of non-contact with the lung wall**

In this rule, we quantify the likelihood of the lung cancer utilizing the extracted features for each ROI. Here we define three quantities as follows;

Roundness : We think that the likelihood of lung cancer for each ROI depends on Circularity F_c. Roundness is in proportion to Circularity F_c.

Size : The area generally becomes larger with distance from the lung wall. We assume the basic thickness which is varied in proportion to Position F_p, and we define Size as the ratio of F_t to the assumed thickness.

Intensity : The cross section of a blood vessel running vertical to the slice image displays high CT values according to Point 4. Thus, Intensity becomes smaller as the gray value F_g becomes large compared with the average value of lung cancer.

Furthermore, we define a likelihood index for lung cancer as follows;

Diagnosis index = Roundness × Size × Intensity

We classify the current ROI as a nodule candidate if this index is over a threshold.

[RULE 3] : Detection of nodules in case of contact with the lung wall

Shadows contacting the lung wall are ordinarily suspicious as described by Point 3, however these shadows can involve the artifact values which are caused by the partial volume effect. Here three characteristics can be observed, nodules have a convex shape inside the lung, artifacts are oblong along the lung wall and the gradient around nodules is higher than artifacts. Therefore to distinguish between nodules and artifacts, we define two indices of Convexness and Contrast as follows;

Convexness : For the three pixel dilation area outside the current ROI, we count the number of pixels which are higher than the average value F_g, and similarly count the number of pixels which are lower than the F_g. We define the Convexness as ratio of these numbers.

Contrast : We define the Contrast as the difference between the average values of the current ROI and the low intensity area outside this ROI.

2.3 Application of Diagnostic Algorithm

This section presents the application of our diagnostic algorithm to Helical CT images concretely width example of result.

Fig.2 presents the process of extraction of lung fields.

Fig.3 presents the extraction process of ROI. Fig.3(a) is the extracted lung fields. The result of the artifacts reduction shows in Fig.3(b), and the Fig.3(c) is the segmented image by using the fuzzy clustering method. Fig.3(d) shows the result of the surface segmentation by using surface curvatures. In Fig.3(e) the defined color-code corresponding to each surface type is as follows, peak surface is white, pit surface is green, saddle ridge is blue and saddle valley is red. Fig.3(e) is the finally extracted ROI. Then, we extract three type ROI as shown in Fig.3(f) using the threshold distance $k = 0.25(green), 1.5(orange), 3.0(red)$ (corresponding to approximately 0.5mm, 3mm, 6mm).

Fig.4 is an example of detection result. In the original image Fig.4(a) which involves four lung cancers where yellow-colored circle indicate. Fig.4(b) presents the result of the diagnosis, our results show nodule candidates as red-colored regions. Our system was able to detect all lung cancers nodules candidates.

3 Experimental Results

To evaluate the performance of the prototype CAD system, the system was applied to the helical CT images of 450 subjects (total: 15,750 slice images). These data were collected in trial mass screening which has been carried out since 1993 in Japan. All data are diagnosed by three expert physicians with the criterion as shown in Table.2.

Table.3 shows the comparative results between the physicians and the prototype CAD system. "definite" are definitive nodules which need further examinations, and the physicians considered these nodules highly suspicious for malignancy. "suspicious" are the nodules also need further examinations, however, the radiologists considered these nodules less likely malignancy compared to the nodules with "definite". A total of 230 nodules were detected by the three physicians. Here we separate each shadow into six groups according to the physician's judgment and the number of physicians who detected it. In this experiment, our system separates all detected nodule candidates into two clusters. The highly suspicious nodules are classified as "Class 1", and other detected shadows are classified as "Class 2". As a result, all the "definite" nodules and the "suspicious" nodules which were identified by the three physicians were detected perfectly as "Class 1". Then, 42 "suspicious" nodules were detected by two of the physicians, these nodules have been classified by CAD system as 36 of them in "Class 1" and 5 in "Class 2", but one nodule was not detected. Then, 167 "suspicious" nodules were detected by one of the physicians, these nodules have been classified by CAD system as 117 of them in "Class 1" and 28 in "Class 2", but 22 nodules were not detected. The sensibility for 230 nodules was 90% (including "Class 2").

Table.4 shows the comparative results between three physicians diagnosis by agreement and the CAD system. CAD system could not detect one nodule which was detected by two physicians also could not detect 5 nodules which have been detected by one of physician as "suspicious". In comparison with these results, the number of the nodules which have been detected by one of the physicians decreased considerably. This fact means that at least one physician changed his judgment, and these nodules are difficult to be detected. 5 cases of 6 false negative cases are involved width such nodules. The sensibility for 120 nodules was 95% (including "Class 2").

Table.5 shows the comparative result between one physician and CAD system. In Table.5, physician A diagnosed 102 of 120 nodules which were detected by agreement. He detected 80 nodules as "definite" or "suspicious", 13 nodules as "non malignant", and 9 nodules were not detected. CAD system detected 85 nodules as "Class 1"($\approx$"definite"), 12 nodules as "Class 2"($\approx$"suspicious"), and 5 nodules were not detected. The sensibility of the CAD system ranks with expert physician.

4 Conclusion

We have developed a computer assisted automatic diagnosis system for pulmonary nodules using helical CT images. We applied it to image data from 450 patients. Experimental results of our CAD system have indicated good performance when compared with physician diagnosis. Currently, we are carrying out the clinical field test program using the CAD system since '97 June. In the field test, first, a physician diagnoses the CT images without the results of CAD system, and after, the same physician diagnoses the same images referring the CAD results. Then, we compare the former and later physician's diagnostic results, and we evaluate the effectiveness of our CAD system for lung cancer screening.

References

1. M.L.Giger, K.T.Bae, and H.MacMahon: "Computerized Detection of Pulmonary Nodules in computed Tomography Images", Invest Radiol, vol.29, no.4, pp.459-465, 1994.
2. K.Kanazawa, K.Kubo, N.Niki, H.Satoh, H.Ohmatsu, K.Eguchi, N.Moriyama: "Computer Aided Screening System for Lung Cancer Based on Helical CT Images", Visualization in Biomedical Computing, Lecture Notes in Computer Science 1131, Springer, pp.223-228, 1996.
3. Y.Kawata, K.Kanazawa, S.Toshioka, N.Niki, H.Satoh, H.Omatsu, K.Eguchi, N.Moriyama: "Computer Aided Diagnosis System for Lung Cancer Based on Helical CT Images", Lecture Notes in Computer Science 1311, Image Analysis and Processing, Springer, pp.420-427, 1997.

Table.1 Measurement condition of the helical CT images.

Beam Width	10mm
Table Speed	20mm/s
Tube Voltage	120kV
Tube Current	50mA
Scan Duration	15sec

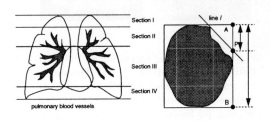

Fig.1. Section classification of the lung

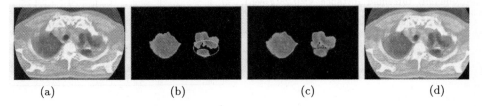

Fig.2. Results of the extraction of the lung fields: (a) Original image; (b) Application of thresholding algorithm; (c) Correction of the lung contour; (d) Extracted lung fields.

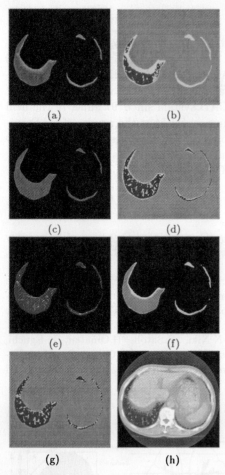

(a) (b) (c) (d) (e) (f) (g) (h)

Fig.3. Results of the extraction of ROI: (a) Extracted lung fields image; (b) Thresholding result; (c) Artifact reduction results; (d) Segmentation result using fuzzy clustering method; (e) Surface segmentation result by using surface curvatures; (f) Extracted lung fields by using different two threshold values; (g) Extracted ROI; (f) Three types ROI using different threshold distance k=0.25(green), k=1.5(orange) and k=3.0(red).

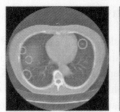 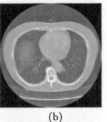

(a) (b)

Fig.4. An example of detection result.

Table.2 Criterion of judgment.

Judgment E	definite malignant lesion
Judgment D	suspicious malignant lesion
Judgment C	non malignant lesion
Judgment B	normal case

Table.3 Comparison between physicians and the CAD system's results.

		Physician	CADsystem		
	Drs.	Nodules	Class1	Class2	FN
E	by 3 Drs.	1	1	0	0
	by 2 Drs.	2	2	0	0
	by 1 Dr.	8	8	0	0
D	by 3 Drs.	10	10	0	0
	by 2 Drs.	42	36	5	1
	by 1 Dr.	167	117	28	22
	Total	230	174	33	23

Table.4 Comparison between agreemental results and the CAD system

		Physician	CADsystem		
	Drs.	Nodules	Class1	Class2	FN
E	by 3 Drs.	1	1	0	0
	by 2 Drs.	2	2	0	0
	by 1 Dr.	8	8	0	0
D	by 3 Drs.	10	10	0	0
	by 2 Drs.	36	30	5	1
	by 1 Dr.	63	49	9	5
	Total	120	100	14	6

Table.5 Comparison between physician A and the CAD system.

			Physician A			CADsystem		
	Drs.	Nds	E,D	C	FN	C1	C2	FN
E	by 3 Drs.	0	1	0	0	1	0	0
	by 2 Drs.	1	2	0	0	2	0	0
	by 1 Dr.	7	6	1	0	7	0	0
D	by 3 Drs.	9	9	0	0	9	0	0
	by 2 Drs.	32	30	2	0	26	5	1
	by 1 Dr.	51	32	10	9	40	7	4
	Total	102	80	13	9	85	12	5

Enhanced Spatial Priors for Segmentation of Magnetic Resonance Imagery

Tina Kapur[1][**], W. Eric L. Grimson[1], Ron Kikinis[2], and William M. Wells[1,2]

[1] MIT AI Laboratory, Cambridge MA, USA
tkapur@ai.mit.edu
http://www.ai.mit.edu/~tkapur
[2] Brigham & Womens Hospital, Harvard Medical School, Boston MA, USA

Abstract. A Bayesian, model-based method for segmentation of Magnetic Resonance images is proposed. A discrete vector valued Markov Random Field model is used as a regularizing prior in a Bayesian classification algorithm to minimize the effect of salt-and-pepper noise common in clinical scans. The continuous Mean Field solution to the MRF is recovered using an Expectation-Maximization algorithm, and is a probabilistic segmentation of the image. A separate model is used to encode the relative geometry of structures, and as a spatially varying prior in the Bayesian classifier. Preliminary results are presented for the segmentation of white matter, gray matter, fluid, and fat in Gradient Echo MR images of the brain.

1 Introduction

The automatic segmentation of anatomical structures from medical images such as MRI or CT will likely benefit from the exploitation of four different kinds of knowledge: *intensity models* that describe the gray level appearance of individual structures (e.g. fluid appears bright in T2-weighted MRI), *relative geometric models* that describe the relative geometry of structures in a subject-specific reference frame (e.g. femoral cartilage is attached to the subject's femur), *shape models* that describe the shape of individual structures in a subject-independent reference frame (e.g. the brain-stem is tube-like), as well as *imaging models* that capture the relevant characteristics of the imaging process.

EM-Segmentation, a segmentation method for MRI images [1], employed Gaussian intensity models for the different tissue classes, and used an imaging model to account for some distortions of the signal that are unique to the MRI process. The work reported here continues along that theme, with two key parts. The first contribution is the addition of a regularizer to the *imaging model* used in the EM-Segmentation algorithm. Regularization combats salt-and-pepper noise

---

[**] The authors would like to thank Martha Shenton for contributing data for this paper. W. Wells received support for this research in part from NIMH Research Scientist Development Awards K02 MH-01110 and R29 MH-50747 (Martha Shenton, PI) and from a Whitaker Foundation Biomedical Research Grant (W. Wells, PI). R. Kikinis received partial support from: NIH: RO1 CA 46627-08, PO1 CA67165-01A1, PO1 AG04953-14, NSF: BES 9631710 and Darpa: F41624-96-2-0001.

common in clinical scans. Previous implementations of EM-segmentation deal with this noise effectively by pre-processing the images with structure-preserving intensity smoothers, particularly gradient-limited diffusion methods [2, 3]. These methods are quite effective, but computationally costly, and not trivial to adjust. We leverage the Bayesian flavor of EM-Segmentation and regularize via a *prior* distribution on the labeling, without incurring undue additional computational cost. Specifically, we model the prior distribution as a Markov Random Field (MRF), and recover its Mean Field (MF) solution using the Expectation-Maximization algorithm. While MF approximations of MRFs have previously been used in computer vision, we believe that the reported work is novel in its use of this prior in conjunction with the EM-Segmentation algorithm.

In the second component, we propose an algorithm that leverages geometric relationships between structures for segmentation purposes. We observe that some structures can be directly segmented from medical images by using methods from low-level computer vision, e.g. skin surface is reproducibly segmented from head MRI using a combination of thresholding, connectivity, and morphological operations. Other structures, such as the brain tissue in head MRI, do not have as salient a combination of intensity and topology as the skin, and are harder to segment using low-level methods. We propose a "coarse to fine" strategy in feature (structure) space – a strategy in which the easily identifiable ("coarse") structures are first segmented automatically and their geometry is then used to bootstrap the segmentation of other ("fine") structures in the image. We present an implementation of this strategy in the form of a *relative geometric prior* (prior distribution on the geometry of "fine" structures, given the geometry of "coarse" structures), and integrate it into the EM-Segmentation algorithm along with the regularizing MRF prior summarized earlier.

Combining the two components, the contribution of this paper may be summarized as the enhancement of the EM-Segmentation algorithm using two priors: an MRF prior to encode piecewise-homogeneity of labels, and a spatial prior to encode the relative geometry of structures.

2 Background on EM Segmentation

Expectation-Maximization (EM) The EM algorithm is an iterative scheme for estimating the parameters of a model that maximize the likelihood of the observed signal. The key step in applying the EM algorithm is to identify a set of *hidden* variables, such that it becomes possible to directly compute the maximum-likelihood estimate of the model using the values of the observed variables and these hidden variables. Once the hidden variables are identified, and the model parameters initialized, the EM algorithm alternates between estimating the hidden variables (as the expected values of the hidden variables using the estimates of the model parameters; the E-step) and the model parameters (as the maximum-likelihood estimates of the model given the observed and hidden variables; the M-step). Each iteration improves the model estimate [4], and the EM algorithm converges to a local minimum of the likelihood function.

EM-Segmentation Segmentation of MRI images is a challenging problem due to the presence of a non-linear gain field attributable to inhomogeneities in the imaging equipment. The EM-Segmentation algorithm [1], approached the segmentation of MRI images as a *maximum likelihood* estimation problem and used the Expectation-Maximization algorithm [4] to simultaneously estimate the class label and gain at each voxel that maximize the likelihood of the observed signal.

The observed MRI signal was modeled as a product of the true signal generated by the underlying anatomy, and the non-linear gain artifact. Using this assumption, an iterative, supervised, Expectation-Maximization style segmentation algorithm was developed that treats the underlying label classes as hidden variables and alternates between estimating those classes (E-step) and the maximally probable gain field (M-step).

In this algorithm, intensity data is log-transformed, thus converting the multiplicative gain field to an additive bias field. Observed log intensity, Y_{ij}, at each pixel is modeled as a normal distribution, independent of all other pixels:

$$p(Y_{ij}|\Gamma_{ij} = k, \beta_{ij}) = N(Y_{ij} - \beta_{ij}; \mu_k, \sigma_k) , \qquad (1)$$

where $N(x; \mu, \sigma)$ is the Gaussian distribution, with mean μ and variance σ^2; Y_{ij} is the observed log intensity at pixel location (i, j); Γ_{ij} is tissue class corresponding to intensity Y_{ij}; μ_k, σ_k are the mean and standard deviation in intensity for tissue class k; β_{ij} is the bias field at pixel location (i, j). The method used a spatially stationary prior probability on the tissue labels Γ:

$$P_{stat}(\Gamma) = \prod_{ij} p_{stat}(\Gamma_{ij}) \qquad (2)$$

where $p_{stat}(\Gamma_{ij})$ is the prior probability that a given voxel belongs to a particular tissue class. This prior probability is constant through the iterations. The bias field β is modeled as a multi-dimensional zero mean Gaussian random variable, to characterize its spatial smoothness.

The E-step computes the posterior tissue class probabilities, W_{ijk} (posterior probability of pixel ij belonging to tissue class k), when the bias field is known:

$$W_{ijk} = \frac{p(Y_{ij}|\Gamma_{ij} = k; \beta_{ij})p_{stat}(\Gamma_{ij} = k)}{\sum_m p(Y_{ij}|\Gamma_{ij} = m; \beta_{ij})p_{stat}(\Gamma_{ij} = m)} . \qquad (3)$$

The M-Step computes the value of the bias field β that maximizes the average likelihood of observation, as $\beta = FR$, where $R_{ij} = \sum_k \frac{W_{ijk} * (Y_{ij} - \mu_k)}{\sigma_k^2}$, and F is a linear operator that can be approximated by smoothing filters. This step is equivalent to a MAP estimator of the bias field when the tissue probabilities W are known. Detailed derivations of these steps can be found in [1].

In the next two sections, we preserve this EM framework for iterating between tissue classification and bias field estimation, and present two different methods for computing spatially varying priors on tissue class to enhance the spatially stationary prior shown in Equation 2 and used in Equation 3 of the E-step.

3 Addition of Markov Prior

As noted, EM-Segmentation [1] uses a spatially stationary prior on tissue class, i.e. at each iteration, the prior probability that a voxel belongs to a particular tissue class remains constant, and is independent of the labels of voxels in its neighborhood. In this work, we incorporate a Markov prior on tissue class, under which the prior probabilities at a voxel are influenced by the labels in its immediate neighborhood. This prior model acts as a regularizer and biases the solution towards piecewise-homogeneous labelings. Such a regularizing prior is useful in segmenting scans corrupted by salt and pepper noise.

MRF priors have been used in computer vision to model smoothness as well as different textures (e.g., [5]). Typical solvers for MRFs include Gibbs sampling [6], the Metropolis algorithm [7], Iterated Conditional Modes (ICM) [8], and Mean-Field (MF) methods [9]. ICM solvers have been used for the segmentation of medical images [10,11].

MRF Formulation: We describe the reformulation of the prior distribution on the tissue labels Γ (from Equation 2) as a Markov Random Field to represent the piecewise homogeneity and the local compatibility of different tissues. The MRF parameters are obtained from manually labeled training data, and its Mean Field solution is recovered using the EM framework of the previous section.

Some notation: $S = \{S_{ij} | 1 \leq i \leq m, 1 \leq j \leq n\}$ is the lattice on which the MRF is defined, and each site of this lattice – referred to as either S_{ij} or simply ij – corresponds to the pixel location (i,j) in the image. $N = \{N_{ij} | 1 \leq i \leq m, 1 \leq j \leq n\}$ defines the neighborhood system for the MRF, where N_{ij} refers to the four neighbors of pixel ij that share an edge with it, i.e. $N_{ij} = \{S_{i,j-1}, S_{i,j+1}, S_{i-1,j}, S_{i+1,j}\}$.

The tissue labels $\Gamma = \{\Gamma_{ij} | S_{ij} \in S\}$ are modeled as an MRF with the neighborhood system N on the lattice S. Γ_{ij} is a discrete-valued random-vector drawn from the set $\{[100\ldots0]^T, [010\ldots0]^T, \ldots [000\ldots1]^T\}$, and assigning the value $[0\ldots1\ldots0]^T$ (with a 1 in the kth position) to Γ_{ij} is equivalent to assigning the kth tissue class to the pixel ij in the image. Γ satisfies the Markov condition, given by: $P(\Gamma_{ij}|S \setminus S_{ij}) = P(\Gamma_{ij}|N_{ij}), \forall ij$, which means that the value of each random variable Γ_{ij} in the field depends only on its four neighbors.

The Hammersley-Clifford theorem established the Markov-Gibbs equivalence and states that the probability of a particular configuration γ of any MRF Γ can be computed using the Gibbs probability of its clique potentials (a clique is a subset of nodes of S that are each others neighbors) over N:

$$P(\Gamma = \gamma) = \frac{1}{Z} e^{-\sum_c V_c(\gamma)} \quad . \tag{4}$$

Here V_c is a clique potential which describes the prior probability of a particular realization of the elements of the clique c.

The spatially stationary prior on the labeled image Γ, given by Equation 2, may be interpreted as an MRF on the image lattice with zeroth order cliques, i.e. there is no interaction between lattice sites. We impose local spatial coherence on the labeling Γ by using first-order cliques. Clique potentials are computed using an Ising-like model derived from training data, i.e., the prior probability of tissue classes k and l occuring adjacent to each other is computed from manually labeled images. Thus, the prior probability on the labeling, $P_{mrf}(\Gamma)$, is not spatially stationary; it interacts with the labels in its neighborhood system.

Computing the field configuration with the maximum Gibbs probability is computationally intractable, so we use a Mean Field approximation to the general Markov model. We approximate the values of the field Γ at neighboring sites by their statistical means, and rewrite $P_{mf}(\Gamma)$, a Mean Field approximation to $P_{mrf}(\Gamma)$, as a product of single site probabilities $p_{mf}(\Gamma_{ij}, N_{ij})$:[1]

$$P_{mf}(\Gamma) = \prod_{ij} p_{mf}(\Gamma_{ij}, N_{ij}) \ , \tag{5}$$

where the single site probability $p_{mf}(\Gamma_{ij}, N_{i,j})$ is written as a product of the single-site prior $p(\Gamma_{ij})$ and the probability of each clique involving pixel ij:

$$p_{mf}(\Gamma_{ij}, N_{ij}) = \frac{1}{Z} p(\Gamma_{ij}) \cdot P_{h-}(\overline{\Gamma}_{i,j-1}) \cdot P_{h+}(\overline{\Gamma}_{i,j+1}) \cdot P_{v-}(\overline{\Gamma}_{i-1,j}) \cdot P_{v+}(\overline{\Gamma}_{i+1,j}) \tag{6}$$

where $\overline{\Gamma}_{ij}$ is a continuous MF approximation to Γ_{ij}, $\cdot$ is component-wise vector multiplication, and Z is a normalizing constant. Equations 5 and 6 describe a general model for a discrete first-order pseudo-Ising MRF, using a particular mean-field approximation. To apply this model we must choose specific representations for p and each of the four neighborhood terms P_{h-}, P_{h+}, P_{v-}, and P_{v+}. In addition we need to supply values for the mean field $\overline{\Gamma}$ in Equation 6.

Using MRF Prior on Tissue Classes in EM Framework: We incorporate the model into the EM framework in the following way: For the single site probability p we use the independent stationary prior, P_{stat}, that was formerly used in the work described in Section 2. For each of P_{h-}, P_{h+}, P_{v-}, and P_{v+}, we use a model based on the empirical joint probability of neighboring pixels. For $\overline{\Gamma}$ we use the estimates on per-pixel tissue probability produced by the previous iteration of the EM segmentation algorithm as described in [1].

Since the basic EM segmentation algorithm is already computing such tissue probabilities, the net effect is a simple modification to the E-step that relates tissue co-occurrence statistics to the tissue probabilities that were computed on neighboring pixels in the previous iteration.

Since Γ is a random variable drawn from unit vectors, we may write the probability distribution modeled by P_{h-} as a linear form $P_{h-}(g) \equiv \Lambda_{h-} g$, where Λ_{h-} is a k x k matrix, where k is the number of tissue classes in the training data, and its mn^{th} element $\lambda_{h-,mn}$ gives the prior probability of tissue class m and n occuring as a horizontal pair in the image, with the left pixel in the pair being tissue class n and the right one being m. The distributions P_{h+}, P_{v-}, and

---
[1] A different tractable MRF model for brain segmentation, using an Iterated-Conditional-Modes solver has been explored in [10].

P_{v+}, and the corresponding Λ's are defined in a similar fashion. We use this representation for the neighborhood probabilities in Equation 6 since it may be directly evaluated on the more general vectors $\overline{\Gamma}$.

4 Addition of Relative Geometric Prior

In this section we describe the second component of our work: a method that leverages geometric relationships between structures for segmentation purposes. The motivating observation is that while some structures are easily segmented using low-level computer vision methods (*primary* structures), there are structures whose segmentation is facilitated by knowledge of their spatial layout (geometry) relative to other structures (*secondary* structures).

Summary of Method: In order to use the relative geometry information for segmentation of a secondary structure in a given image, we first *identify a set of primitives* in terms of which to define its local geometric relationship to one or more primary structures. For example, the *distance* between points on the outside surface of structure P and the closest points on the inside surface of structure B is a primitive that describes local relative geometry of the two surfaces. Next, we *construct the relative geometric model* from training (segmented) images. In order to do this, a random variable is defined for each primitive, and segmented images are used to construct an empirical joint probability distribution over these random variables. This probability distribution serves as a model of the relative geometric relationship between the primary and secondary structures in question. For example, if one primitive is the distance between the *outer* surface of P and the outer surface of S, and another is the distance between the *inner* surface of P and the outer surface of S, then two random variables d_1 and d_2 are defined, one for each primitive relationship, and an empirical joint probability distribution for d_1 and d_2 is constructed from the segmented images. This joint serves as the relative geometric model for structures P and S. Following the construction of the model, we *segment primary structures* in the given image using appropriate algorithms. Finally, we use the geometric model as a *prior on the spatial layout* of the secondary structure, conditioned on the geometry of the segmented primary structures and used the EM-Segmentation algorithm to segment the secondary structure in question.

Note that this method is profitably used for the segmentation of a pair of structures in which one is a primary structure and the geometric relationship between the pair is informative (in an information theoretic sense). If either constraint is violated (neither of the structures is primary, or the relationship is uninformative), this method does not help the resulting segmentation.

Previous Work: A similar relative geometric prior was used in a traditional Bayesian classifier to segment femoral cartilage from Knee MRI images [12]. Also, this work is similar in spirit to landmark based segmentation [13], and different in its detection of a *dense* set of features as the landmarks.

Example Usage of Method to Segment Brain Tissue from MRI Images

We observe that the skin surface and the ventricles are easily segmented in head MRI images, and use those as primary structures for segmentation of brain tissue (white matter and gray matter); the relationship between brain tissue and these primary structures is well described using two primitives: ds, the distance to the inside skin surface, and dv, the distance to the outside ventricle surface.

Next, we detail the algorithm for constructing the aforementioned empirical geometric model, and its usage with the EM-Segmentation algorithm for segmentation of white matter.

Empirical Joint Density Estimation: Example images in which the skin, the ventricles, and white matter have been manually labeled by experts are used to construct a non-parametric estimate for this joint density function. In particular, chamfer distance transforms[14] are computed for the inside skin surface and for the outside ventricle surface. These chamfer maps are used to find ds_i and dv_i, the distance to skin and ventricle surfaces for all pixels i that are labeled white matter, and the values are histogrammed jointly. The histogram is normalized to obtain an empirical estimate of the joint density of ds and dv for white matter. Note that instead of histogramming the values of the random variables, methods such as Parzen Windowing [15] could be used effectively for density estimation.

Usage with EM-Segmentation: The class conditional density is thus:

$$P(ds_i, dv_i | x_i \in WM) \tag{7}$$

where x_i are the spatial coordinates of the ith data pixel; WM is the set of all pixels belonging to white matter; S is the set of all pixels belonging to the skin; V is the set of all pixels belonging to the ventricles; ds_i is short for $ds_i(S)$, which is the distance from x_i to the inside surface of the skin; dv_i is short for $dv_i(V)$, which is the distance from x_i to the outside surface of the ventricles.

Bayes rule allows us to express the posterior probability that a pixel should be classified as white matter based on observations of its intensity and spatial relation to the skin and the ventricles ($P(x_i \in WM | ds_i(S), dv_i(V), I_i)$) as a product of the prior probability that a given pixel belongs to white matter ($P(x_i \in WM)$) and the class conditional density $P(ds_i(S), dv_i(V), I_i | x_i \in WM)$ as follows:

$$P(x_i \in WM | ds_i, dv_i, I_i) = \frac{P(ds_i, dv_i, I_i | x_i \in WM) P(x_i \in WM)}{P(ds_i, dv_i, I_i)} \tag{8}$$

where I_i is the intensity at x_i, and the other terms are as in Equation 7. This expression may be rewritten assuming independence between the intensity at a pixel and its spatial relationship to skin and ventricles as:

$$P(x_i \in WM | ds_i, dv_i, I_i) = \frac{P(ds_i, dv_i | x_i \in WM) P(I_i | x_i \in WM) P(x_i \in WM)}{P(ds_i, dv_i, I_i)} \tag{9}$$

The first term in the numerator is the class conditional density for the model parameters, and is estimated using the method described above. The second term is a Gaussian intensity model for tissue class, obtained from samples of white matter intensity. The third term is the prior probability that a pixel belongs to white matter, computed as a ratio of white matter volume to total head volume in a segmented scan. The denominator is a normalization factor.

This spatial probability distribution (Equation 9) can be used either in conjunction with the Mean-Field prior of Section 3, or by itself, instead of the spatially stationary prior in the E-step of the EM-Segmentation algorithm.

The above method is repeated to obtain a segmentation of gray matter.

5 Results

We have used the work presented in this paper to classify several images from different Gradient Echo brain MRI scans. Two examples are described here.

Gradient Echo Brain MRI with MF: Figure 1 shows the results of EM Segmentation using a Mean-Field prior on a sagittal slice of a Gradient Echo brain MRI. In the left column of the figure, the top image is the gray scale slice with additive white noise. The second image, provided as a baseline, is its classification (gray – gray matter, white – white matter, black – air/csf, red – skin/fat) that was obtained using a standard MAP classifier. The third image in the first column is the classification obtained using EM Segmentation with a spatially stationary prior, and the fourth image is the classification obtained using EM Segmentation with a Mean Field prior. Notice that the segmentation that uses the Mean-Field prior is much less fragmented compared to the segmentation that uses only the spatially stationary prior. Since each of these segmentations is obtained by thresholding the respective weights (W_{ijk} from Equation 3) associated with each tissue class, the middle and the right column of the figure show the weights for each tissue class (gray matter, white matter, csf/air, skin/fat) when the spatially stationary prior and Mean-Field prior are used, respectively. Again, the point to note is the lack of fragmentation when the MF prior is used.

Gradient Echo Brain MRI with MF and Conditional-Spatial Priors: Figure 2 shows the results of EM Segmentation using a Spatial-Conditional prior in conjunction with a Mean-Field prior on a coronal slice of a Gradient Echo brain MRI. In the left column of the figure, the top image is the grayscale slice. The second image, provided as a baseline, is its classification (gray – gray matter, white – white matter, black – air/csf, red – skin/fat) that was obtained using a standard MAP classifier. The third image in the first column is the classification obtained using EM Segmentation with a spatially stationary prior, and the fourth image is the classification obtained using EM Segmentation with Spatial-Conditional and Mean Field priors. Notice that the segmentation that uses the relative spatial priors is much less fragmented, and shows improved distinction between skin and brain tissue, as well as in the segmentation of white matter in the brain stem, compared to the segmentation that uses only the spatially stationary prior. Since each segmentation is obtained by thresholding the respective weights (W_{ijk} from Equation 3) associated with each tissue class, the middle and the right column of the figure show the weights for each tissue class (gray matter, white matter, csf/air, skin/fat) when the spatially stationary prior and Mean-Field prior are used, respectively. Again, the point to note is the lack of fragmentation due to the MF prior, and the improved distinction between brain tissue and skin as well as improved segmentation of white matter.

6 Discussion

Tradeoff between Prior and Observation: A characteristic of Bayesian methods is the delicate balance that needs to be maintained between the influence of the prior term and fidelity to the observed data. If the degree of faith in the prior term is high (i.e. it models the underlying phenomenon accurately) and the observation noisy, then conflicts between the prior and the observations are resolved in favor of the prior. In contrast, if there is negligible noise in the observations, then the prior can be discarded altogether, giving rise to a priorless or maximum-likelihood solution. Unfortunately, it is often the case that the prior term is somewhat accurate, and the data is somewhat noisy i.e. it is not as clear how the two terms should be traded off in Bayes rule. The art of maintaining this balance is colloquially referred to as "tweaking the Bayesian fudge factor" and is arguably crucial to the success of the resulting algorithm.

Empirically speaking, in our case, the relative importance of the regularizing (Markov) prior is inversely proportional to the signal to noise ratio (SNR) in the MRI scan. Since SNR in MR scans is directly proportionally to imaging parameters such as the strength of the ambient magnetic field, we weigh the prior by these parameters. For example, a scan acquired with a 0.5 Tesla magnet is segmented using a higher weight on the MRF prior, as compared with a scan acquired using a 1.5Tesla magnet.

How best to characterize the weighing scheme for the geometric prior is less obvious. It would not be unreasonable, however, to measure the variation of the geometric prior model across individuals and assign a relative importance that is inversely proportional to that measure of variance. As a side-effect of this process, the variance in the relative geometric model could be used to characterize which structures this method is best suited for, and analyze its failure modes. Unless better schemes become apparent, this is the approach we plan to take for characterizing the importance of the geometric prior in classification.

Moving onto 3D: Since the images we are dealing with are inherently 3D volumes, the natural next step is to extend the reported priors by a dimension. While the 3D extension of the regularizing prior is simple to conceptualize and implement, the extension of the geometric prior to 3D will require a convention for normalizing images from different subjects, so that the prior usefully encodes information across a population. The Tailarach coordinate system is a popular normalization method and a possible choice for us.

References

1. W.M. Wells III, R. Kikinis, W.E.L. Grimson, and F. Jolesz. Adaptive segmentation of mri data. *IEEE Transactions on Medical Imaging*, 1996.

2. P. Perona, T. Shiotan, and J. Malik. Anisotropic diffusion. *Geometry-Driven Diffusion in Computer Vision*, pages 73–92, 1994.
3. R. Whitaker and G. Gerig. Vector-valued diffusion. In B.M. ter Haar Romeny, editor, *Geometry-Driven Diffusion in Computer Vision*, pages 93–133, 1994.
4. A.P. Dempster, N.M. Laird, and D.B. Rubin. Maximal likelihood form incomplete data via the em algorithm. *RoyalStat*, B 39:1–38, 1977.
5. S.Z. Li. *Markov Random Field Modeling in Computer Vision*. Springer-Verlag, 1995.
6. S. Geman and D. Geman. Stochastic relaxation, gibbs distributions, and the bayesian restoration of images. *PAMI*, 6(6):721–741, November 1984.
7. N. Metropolis, A.W. Rosenbluth, A. N. Rosenbluth, A.H. Teller, and E. Teller. Equation of state calculations by fast computing machines. *J. Chem. Phys.*, 21(6):1087–1092, 1953.
8. J. Besag. On the statistical analysis of dirty pictures. *RoyalStat*, B-48(3):259–302, 1986.
9. D. Geiger and F. Girosi. Parallel and deterministic algorithms from mrfs: Surface reconstruction. *PAMI*, 13(5):401–412, May 1991.
10. K. Held, E. Rota Kopps, B. Krause, W. Wells, R. Kikinis, and H. Muller-Gartner. Markov random field segmentation of brain mr images. *IEEE Transactions on Medical Imaging*, 16:878–887, 1998.
11. D. Vandermeulen, X. Descombes, P. Suetens, and G. Marchal. Unsupervised regularized classification of multi-spectral MRI. In *Proceedings of the Fifth Conference on Visualization in Biomedical Computing*. SPIE, 1996.
12. T. Kapur, P.A. Beardsley, S.F. Gibson, W.E.L. Grimson, and W.M. Wells III. Model based segmentation of clinical knee mri. In *IEEE International Workshop on Model Based 3D Image Analysis*, 1998.
13. D. Collins, T. Peters, W. Dai, and A. Evans. Model based segmentation of individual brain structures from mri data. In R. Robb, editor, *Proceedings of the First Conference on Visualization in Biomedical Computing*, pages 10–23. SPIE, 1992.
14. G. Borgefors. Distance transformations in digital images. *Computer Vision, Graphics, and Image Processing*, 34:344–371, 1986.
15. R.O Duda and P.E. Hart. *Pattern Classification and Scene Analysis*. John Wiley and Sons, 1973.

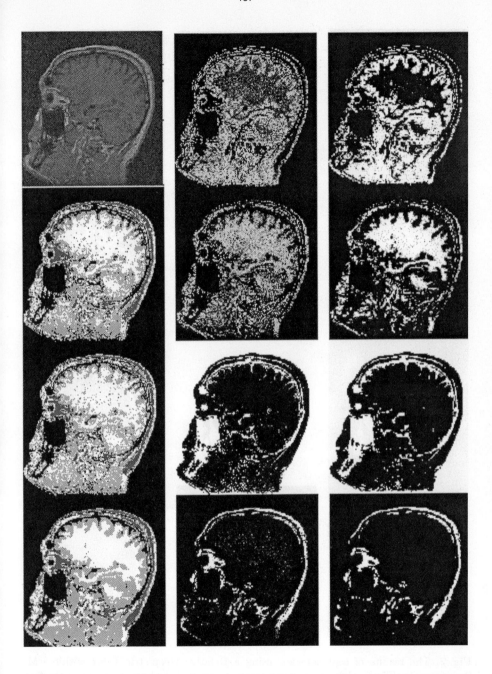

Fig. 1. The results of segmentation using an MRF Prior within EM-Segmentation. The top left image is the input image, and the bottom image in the first column is its segmentation. The middle colum shows the weights W_{ijk} (for gray matter, white matter, air/csf, skin respectively) upon convergence of the EM-Segmentation algorithm with spatially stationary priors. The right column shows the weights when the MRF prior is used with EM-Segmentation. See the text for a discussion of the results.

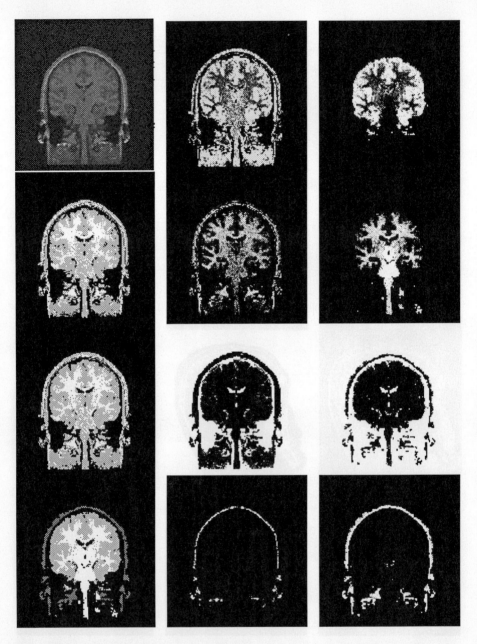

Fig. 2. The results of segmentation using a Relative Geometric Prior within EM-Segmentation. The top left image is the input image, and the bottom image in the first column is its segmentation. The middle colum shows the weights W_{ijk} (for gray matter, white matter, air/csf, skin respectively) upon convergence of the EM-Segmentation algorithm with spatially stationary priors. The right column shows the weights when the geometric prior is used with EM-Segmentation. See the text for a discussion of the results.

Exploring the Discrimination Power of the Time Domain for Segmentation and Characterization of Lesions in Serial MR Data

[1]Guido Gerig, [1]Daniel Welti, [2]Charles Guttmann, [3]Alan Colchester and [1]Gábor Székely

[1]Swiss Federal Institute of Technology
Communication Technology Laboratory
ETH-Zentrum, CH-8092 Zurich, Switzerland
[2]Brigham and Women's Hospital, Harvard Medical School, Boston
[3]University of Kent at Canterbury, Kent, England

gerig@cs.unc.edu, dwelti@vision.ee.ethz.ch
(Long version of this paper: http://www.vision.ee.ethz.ch → Publications)

Abstract. This paper presents a new methodology for the automatic segmentation and characterization of object changes in time series of three-dimensional data sets. The purpose of the analysis is a detection and characterization of objects based on their dynamic changes. The technique was inspired by procedures developed for the analysis of functional MRI data sets. After precise registration of serial volume data sets to 4-D data, we applied a new time series analysis taking into account the characteristic time function of variable lesions. The images were preprocessed with a correction of image field inhomogeneities and a normalization of the brightness function over the whole time series. This leads to the hypothesis that static regions remain unchanged over time, whereas local changes in tissue characteristics cause typical functions in the voxel's time series. A set of features are derived from the time series and their derivatives, expressing probabilities for membership to the sought structures. These multiple sources of uncertain evidence were combined to a single evidence value using Dempster Shafer's theory. Individual processing of a series of 3-D data sets is therefore replaced by a fully 4-D processing. To explore the sensitivity of time information, active lesions are segmented solely based on time fluctuation, neglecting absolute intensity information.

The project is driven by the objective of improving the segmentation and characterization of white matter lesions in serial MR data of multiple sclerosis patients. Pharmaceutical research and patient follow-up requires efficient and robust methods with high degree of automation. Further, an enhanced set of morphometric parameters might give a better insight into the course of the disease and therefore leads to a better understanding of the disease mechanism and of drug effects.

The new method has been applied to two time series from different patient studies, covering time resolutions of 12 and 24 data sets over a period of roughly one year. The results demonstrate that time evolution is a highly sensitive feature to detect fluctuating structures.

1 Introduction

Serial magnetic resonance imaging of patients becomes attractive due to the minimal invasive image acquisition, the speed-up in scanning and therefore patient time, and the high spatial and tissue resolution. The time series reveal information about significant changes of diseased anatomical regions, about the changes as an effect of a drug or radiotherapy treatment, or about subtle morphological changes caused by a neurophysiological disease. The temporal sampling thus not only provides information about morphological but also functional changes.

A typical analysis of this type which is routinely applied is the analysis of functional MRI data sets. A patient is stimulated with a specific time pattern of visual, auditory or motor activity. Brightness changes due to local changes in the oxygenation state of blood are expected to show a similar time pattern and can be detected by a correlation of the stimulus function with the time series of each pixel. Here, the signal processing aims at finding the best discrimination between noisy steady state signals and signals correlated with the stimulus [1]. The processing most often assumes that a patient doesn't move during the examination, although slight object motion due to breathing, pulsation of the heart and swallowing is unavoidable. It has been shown that a sub-voxel correction of 3-D motion [2] can considerably improve the voxel-based time-series analysis.

Pharmacological studies or patient follow-up and monitoring, are different. Time frequency is not in the range of seconds, but can be days, months or even years. The study of a tumor change in relation to chemotherapy or radiotherapy, for example, typically requires time intervals of weeks till months. In schizophrenia, temporal changes are studied over long periods by imaging a patient with yearly scans.

The development of a new segmentation technique is driven by the motivation to get a better understanding of the disease process in multiple sclerosis (MS). Research in MS already demonstrated the power of using serial imaging [3]. Drug development for multiple sclerosis uses serial MRI as one measurement among other diagnostic features to study the temporal changes of white matter lesions in the central nervous system. A series of patients is divided into two groups getting either placebo or the new drug. Patients are scanned in intervals of 1, 2 or 4 weeks during a period of about one year. The significance of tests is increased by multi-center studies, collecting image data from various hospitals using a standardized MR protocol. Image data are examined by radiologists, evaluating each scan in relation to the previous one to visually assess the occurrence of new lesions. A quantitative analysis of the total lesion load and of the single lesions is performed using interactive user operated segmentation tools. A typical study often comprises up to several thousands of 3-D data sets. The manual outlining of lesions in large number of series of 2-D slices is not only time consuming but also tedious and error prone. Errors for the segmentation of small structures are often in the range of the volume of the observed structures.

Automated image segmentation systems have been proposed by several groups [4-7]. They consist of well-designed sequences of processing steps, including preprocessing, bias-field correction, feature-space clustering of multi-echo MRI data

[8], and a matching of a statistical anatomical atlas [9, 10] to solve ambiguities of statistical classification. As a result, they present a significantly improved reproducibility and therefore a reduced inter- and intra-rater variability and allow an efficient processing of large amount of data.

Previous segmentation methods mostly intend to segment lesions from single data sets, not taking into account the significance of correlation in the time domain. In radiological examination on the light-box, however, experts use previous scans of patients to decide about significant changes. An early attempt to consider the correlation in the time domain was presented by Metcalf et al. [11] by proposing a 4-D connected component labeling on registered segmented label images. The procedure serves as a postprocessing filter applied after individually segmenting the data sets, removing insignificant lesion candidates which appear only at one time point, or eliminating 4-D lesion patterns with volume below a predefined threshold. The aim still was an improved lesion segmentation, although the 4-D connectivity additionally could give access to time domain information.

So far, temporal changes in signal intensity patterns of multiple sclerosis lesions have not been used to improve and simplify the processing of time series. Guttmann [3] presented a seminal paper on characterizing the evolution of lesions in serial MR data, suggesting to use this valuable information for image processing. The present paper will *explore the time domain information* inherently given by serial MR data sets. The major question in research of disease mechanisms or drug studies is most often not a segmentation of static tissue or static lesions but of temporal changes. We claim that dynamic changes in lesion voxels can be detected by analyzing the time series of each voxel, assuming perfectly registered and normalized data sets. Although the ultimate goal will be a spatio-temporal analysis of the 4-D data sets, this paper only focuses on evaluating the discrimination power of the temporal domain.

Besides exploring time domain as a new feature for segmentation, we are working towards extracting a rich set of morphometric parameters. These include temporal information to analyze the time course of the disease, to understand time correlations of lesion groups and lesion patterns, to determine the lesion load versus time, and finally to combine the results with anatomic atlas information to describe major spatial categories (periventricular, deep white matter, cortical) of lesions. Scientific visualisation of dynamic changes will be important to visually assess the disease course of individual patients.

The paper is organized as follows. Section two shortly describes the preprocessing including bias correction and image brightness normalization, and the combination of serial 3-D to 4-D data sets. The new time series analysis is explained in section three. Section four presents results obtained with data sets from different pharmaceutical studies.

2 Combination of serial 3-D data to 4-D data

Individual magnetic resonance volume data sets acquired in weekly to monthly time intervals can be combined to 4-D $(x,y,z;t)$ data sets, which allows the application of time-series analysis of single voxels.

Registration The serial data sets obtained from the Brigham and Women's Hospital Boston (cf. section 4.1) have been registered by the INRIA research group using crest-line extraction and matching [12]. A second serial data set presented in this paper is processed by the KUL research group using the MIRIT registration software package [13] which maximizes the mutual information between corresponding voxel intensities. Both registration methods work fully automatically. The transformation matrices are input to a geometric transformation which performs trilinear interpolation.

Image brightness normalization and bias correction The corruption of the image brightness values by a low-frequency bias field often occurs in MR imaging and impedes visual inspection and intensity-based segmentation. A mathematical model for bias correction using parametric bias field estimation was proposed in [14]. We assume the original scene to be composed of tissue regions with homogeneous brightness only degraded by noise. The estimation of the parametric bias field is formulated as a non-linear energy minimization problem. Input parameters are the statistics (mean, standard deviation) of expected categories. Using the same set of input parameters for each data set from series of volume images results in a combination of bias correction and brightness normalization. The presence of strong striping artifacts on one of the data sets required a two step procedure by first correcting for brightness changes between individual slices and then for the 3-D bias field [15].

Result of Preprocessing The normalization of brightness and correction of inhomogeneity artifacts results in sets of corrected 3-D data sets. After registration, they are combined to form 4-D data sets. Picking a voxel and visualizing its time course gives a good impression of the quality of the preprocessing. We assume that the signal intensity of white matter should remain constant (figure 1b), whereas voxels representing active lesions would show considerable changes (figure 1c-e).

3 Time series analysis to detect fluctuating lesions

Bias correction, image brightness normalization and spatial registration of serial 3-D image data results in 4-D $[x,y,z;t]$ data sets. The preprocessing yields a spatial and intensity-based normalization of the time series. Therefore, we can assume that static tissue will not change brightness over time, whereas voxels which are part of fluctuating lesions will depict typical variations. Each voxel can be considered as a time series, suggesting the application of methods for

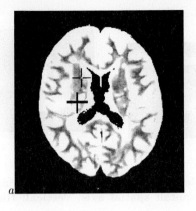
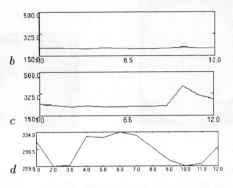

Fig. 1. Time series of voxels for healthy white matter (b) and typical lesions (c,d). Horizontal axis: time, vertical axis: MR intensity. Image (a) illustrates a typical MR slice presenting white matter lesions. The positions of the voxel generating the constant time series (b) is marked with a thin cross, the lesion time series (c) with the thick cross. Plot d represents a time series of another lesion voxel.

one-dimensional signal processing. The signal analysis shows similarities to the postprocessing of functional magnetic resonance data (fMRI), but there is one significant difference. Functional MRI is measured by a repetitive stimulation of a certain task, which allows a comparison of the stimulation function with the time series of each image pixel, most often using correlation techniques. The time course of MS lesion voxels, on the other hand, does not follow a fixed pattern and can only be characterized by a dynamic fluctuation of image brightness.

3.1 Visualization of brightness changes

The time course of lesion voxels can be studied by providing two-dimensional images of arbitrary profiles through 3-D image data versus time. The displays illustrate fluctuations of profiles over a typical time period of one year (Fig. 2. Tissue boundaries in general show very small spatial displacements which can be explained by elastic tissue deformations, whereas some boundaries in the vicinity of lesions can demonstrate larger deformations due to a mass effect (see Fig. 2b lower middle). A characteristic feature for lesion time series is a continuous fluctuation with time, presenting increasing and decreasing time changes or both.

Based on observations of typical time series of lesion voxels we developed features that describe fluctuations. The set of features will be used for discriminating between static tissue and active lesions.

Brightness Difference: A simple calculation determines the minimum and maximum brightness for each time series and calculates the absolute difference $\Delta I = |I_{max} - I_{min}|$. This feature measures the maximum contrast change of a time series within the observed time period (Fig. 3a).

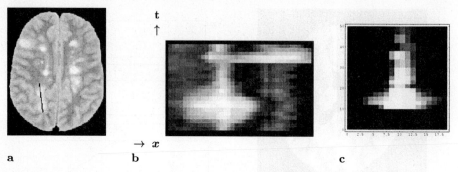

Fig. 2. Visualization of spatio-temporal lesion evolution. a Original image with profile, b space-time display (horizontal: spatial axis, vertical: time axis) and c other typical lesion evolution.

Statistical measures: Mean, standard deviation and variance form a set of statistical features expressing the temporal variation of brightness around the mean value. We expect much higher variance for lesion voxels than for static tissue (3b,c,d).

Signs of fluctuation around mean: The features discussed so far do not consider the temporal pattern or the frequency of fluctuations. We therefore determine the number of zero-crossings of the zero-mean time series and evaluate the time length of positive and negative segments. A noisy static signal will generate a large number of sign changes with small segments, whereas large fluctuations will generate a small number of long segments (3e,f,g).

Time derivatives: The gradient of the time function provides information about the rate of change, both for decreasing and increasing events. Fig. 2 illustrates that lesions often appear with a large brightness change. We used the minimum and maximum gradient as features for our lesion analysis (3h). The attributed time will be further used for displaying temporal evolution (see results).

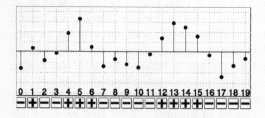

Evaluation of sign changes of zero-mean time series: Analysis of the sequence of signs: Nr. of "segments" (7), maximum (5), minimum (1) and average segment length (2.86).

3.2 Evidence accumulation by combining uncertain measurements

The multiple features derived by signal processing provide probabilistic maps of the likelihood to characterize the sought structures (Fig. 3a-h). Each of this features is inherently uncertain, and they must somehow be combined to derive

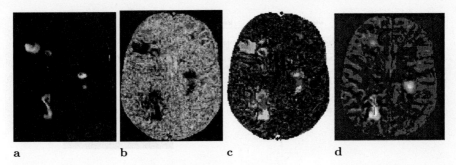

Fig. 3. 2-D cuts of 3-D feature maps: Variance (**a**), Nr. of zero-crossing segments (**b**), length of maximum segment (**c**), and maximum absolute time gradient (**d**)

a measurement which incorporates different properties of the typical temporal pattern of a lesion. A pooling of evidence from different knowledge sources will strengthen beliefs in some cases and erode beliefs in others, even handling contradictory evidence. The following analysis assumes that the features are independent, although this might not be strictly true. A combination of probability measures can be accomplished by using Dempster-Shafer's theory. To get around the computational complexity of the original DS method [16,17], we used binary frames of discernment (BFOD) as proposed by [18]. Details describing the choice of confidence factor functions (cf), basic probability assignments (cfa) and the combination rules can be found in the long paper version (http://www.vision.ee.ethz.ch). The design of these functions and probabilities represents a crucial step. However, our tests with the analysis of very different serial data sets showed that only minor parameter adjustments were necessary. The initial design and training was based on a comparison of the resulting feature maps with segmentation results produced by statistical classification followed by manual corrections.

The Dempster's combination rule is associative and commutative, so that the final probability does not depend on the order in which evidence is combined (Fig. 4a).

The combined 3-D data set is again probabilistic, with a value range of $[0, \cdots, 1]$ (Fig. 4b). A binary segmentation, for example for three-dimensional graphical visualization (Fig. 4c), is obtained by choosing an appropriate threshold either by visual inspection of overlay images or by comparing the segmentation output to hand-segmented training data. Tests with multiple data sets and visual inspection showed that the choice of the final threshold was not critical and revealed very similar results within a range of thresholds, provided a careful design of the cf-functions and bpa assignments.

4 Results

The new segmentation system has been applied to two time series from different patient studies. A first study carried out at the Brigham and Women's hospital

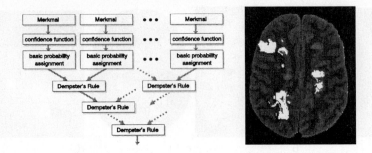

Fig. 4. Combination of fuzzy features by Dempster's rule (left) and segmented active lesions on 2-D slice (right).

covers 40 patients with 24 brain scans, with a fixed sequence of scanning intervals of one, two and 4 weeks. Another study currently analyzed in the European BIOMORPH project [19] comprises 12 serial imaging sessions of 40 patients, each imaging session delivering multiple MR protocols (PD,T1,T2). The data sets are preprocessed as described in section 2 and analyzed using the signal processing methods described in section 3.

4.1 Brigham and Women's Hospital data sets

The image data sets were acquired on a GE Signa 1.5 Tesla using a double echo spin echo pulse sequence (TR 3000ms, TE 30/80ms) half Fourier sampling (0.5 NEX). 54 slices with 3mm slice distance and thickness and 256x256 pixels result in voxel dimensions of 0.96x0.96x3 mm3. The time series includes 24 data sets acquired over a period of 50 weeks with a specific time protocol: weekly scans for 10 weeks followed by every other week scans for 16 weeks and monthly scans for 24 weeks. We could use 23 out of the 24 scans for our analysis. The unequally spaced time image series was converted into a regularly sampled sequence by linear interpolation.

The 3-D visualizations (Fig. 5) display the time course of lesion evolution, coded as a color map ranging from 1 to 23. Additionally, the processing results in a quantification of the temporal evolution of the total lesion load, measured relative to the first image data set. Please remind that the procedure *only measures time changes* and excludes voxels that remain unchanged, thus providing information that is different from the conventional total lesion load over time.

4.2 BIOMORPH data sets

Image data are acquired on a Philips T5 magnetic resonance scanner, 1.5 Tesla, using a double echo spin-echo pulse sequence with TR 2816ms and TE 30/80ms). 24 axial slices 256x256 were measured, with voxel dimensions 0.9x0.9x5.5mm3. 12 scans are measured over a period of 56 weeks: 11 scans with approximately 4 weeks intervals and a last scan with a 13 week interval. This unequally spaced time image series was converted into a regularly sampled sequence by linear interpolation.

Figures 6 and 7 illustrate the segmentation result, again attributing the segmented lesions with the time of appearance.

5 Summary and Conclusions

We present a new image processing system for the time series analysis of serial data sets representing time series. The purpose of this project was the exploration of the discrimination power of the time axis, which is most often not directly used for the segmentation of structures. On purpose, we excluded any absolute scalar or multi-spectral information about structures as most often used for the voxel-wise segmentation of lesions from MRI by multi-dimensional thresholding and statistical clustering. Here, we exclusively analyzed the time series of each voxel to demonstrate the additional information obtained by taking into account the temporal evolution of brightness.

The paper describes the development of a the image analysis techniques for segmentation of fluctuating structures from 4-D data sets. Analyzing the time series of each voxel, we derive a set of statistical and structural features each of which discriminates static tissue from changes in the time function. The extraction of each feature creates a probability map for the presence of the sought structure. The multiple probabilities from the different evidence sources are combined using The Dempster-Shafer theory. We selected this technique because it allows to combine different sources of evidence by considering not only the probability of the occurrence of a feature, but also of the absence and of the ignorance about the measurements. The design of the confidence factor functions and the transformation of confidence factors into basic probabilities represent a decisive step which is comparable to supervised training in statistical classification. Test showed that once trained, these settings can be used for other data sets as well since measurements do not directly depend on absolute intensity values. Further, brightness and contrast of our data sets are normalized in the preprocessing step.

The analysis of normalized 4-D data sets is automatic and takes about 10 minutes processing time (SUN Ultra 1 with 128Mb). The results were visually compared with results from alternative segmentation methods and revealed a surprisingly good sensitivity and specifity to MS lesions. However, we have to keep in mind that our analysis so far is *only based on time series information of one MR echo*. We can expect an even higher sensitivity if multi-echo information could be embedded, and if we would combine the time series analysis with the segmentation of spatial structures. So far, data was inspected by clinical experts by evaluating overlays of the segmented lesions with the original MR scans (Fig. /reffig:dem-com). A quantitative validation and tests with more serial data sets is currently in process and a necessary part of the BIOMORPH project [19]. This project also plans to implant simulated lesions in 4-D data sets to be used as a validation standard. However, we can conclude from visual evaluation that temporal changes represent a highly significant feature for the identification of active lesions and should be considered for future analysis. Further, temporal evolution and the detection of time changes are the most important features for pharmaceutical studies and research, as the goal most often is the evaluation of changes due the disease process or a drug treatment. Besides detection of lesion voxels, our method reveals the time of appearance and disappearance as attributes to each voxel. A dynamic visualization of this temporal information allows the detection of groups and patterns of lesions which show a similar time course. If additionally combined with anatomical atlas information to link lesion positions to anatomy, we would get a new insight in the MS disease process and hopefully a new understanding of the disease mechanism.

Currently, we are extending the time-series analysis by spatial analysis to develop a spatio-temporal description of fluctuating lesion patterns. We will also include information from multiple spectral MR channels (PD, T1, T2, FLAIR) to replace the scalar by vector-valued measurements.

Acknowledgment

The European Union and the Swiss funding agency BBW are acknowledged for supporting this research in the international project on Brain Morphometry (BIOMORPH, EU-BIOMED2 project no BMH4-CT96-0845). We would like to thank Ron Kikinis and Ference Jolesz, Brigham and Women's Hospital, for providing a serial MR data set from a study supported by NIH (contract no. N01-NS-0-2397). Philip Thirion and Nicholas Ayache, INRIA Sophia Antipolis, are acknowledged for providing a registered time series. We thank Dirk Vandermeulen and Frederick Maes, KUL Belgium, for registering a serial data set as part of the BIOMORPH project. Dr. Kappos and Dr. Radü from the University Hospital Basel are acknowledged for helping with their expertise and for making research funding available.

References

1. P.A. Bandettini, A Jesmanowicz, E.C. Wong, and J.S. Hyde, *Processing strategies for time-course data sets in functional MRI of the human brain*, Magnetic Resonance in Medicine, 30:161-173, 199
2. D.L.G. Hill, A. Simmons, C. Studholme, D.J. Hawkes, and S.C.R. Williams, *Removal of stumulus corelated motion from echo plana fmri studies*, In Proc. Soc. Magn. Res. 3rd annual meeting, page 840, 1995
3. Charles R.G. Guttmann et al., *The Evolution of Multiple Sclerosis Lesions on Serial MR*, AJNR 16:1481-1491, Aug 1995
4. R. Kikinis, M.E. Shenton, G. Gerig, J. Martin, M. Anderson, D. Metcalf, Ch.R.G. Guttmann, R.W. McCarley, B. Lorensen, H. Cline, F.A. Jolesz, *Routine Quantitative Analysis of Brain and Cerebrospinal Fluid Spaces with MR Imaging*, JMRI (Journal of Magnetic Resonance Imaging), Vol. 2 No. 6, pp. 619-629, Nov/Dec 1992
5. A.C. Evans, J.A. Frank, J. Antel, and D.H. Miller, *The role of MRI in clinical trials of multiple sclerosis: Comparison of image processing techniques*. Annals of Neurology, 1996. In press.

6. A. Zijdenbos, A. Evans, F. Riahi, J. Sled, H.-C. Chui, and V. Kollokian, *Automatic quantification of multiple sclerosis lesion volume using stereotaxic space*, In forth Int. Conf. on Visualization in Biomedical Computing (VBC), Hamburg, Germany, 1996, pp. 439-448
7. M. Kamber, R. Shinghal, D.L. Collins, G.S. Francis, and A.C. Evans, *Model-based 3-D segmentation of multiple sclerosis lesions in magnetic resonance brain images*. IEEE Transactions in Medical Imaging, 14(3):442-453, Sept. 1995
8. G. Gerig, J. Martin, R. Kikinis, O. Kübler, M. Shenton and F. A. Jolesz, *Unsupervised tissue type segmentation of 3D dual-echo MR head data*, image and vision computing, IPMI 1991 special issue, vol. 10 No. 6, pp. 349-360, July/August 1992
9. S. Warfield et al., *Automatic Identification of Gray Matter Structures from MRI to Improve the Segmentation of White Matter Lesions*, Journal of Image Guided Surgery, Vol. 1, No. 6, June 1996, pp. 326-338
10. Johnston et al., 1996, Segmentation of multiple sclerosis lesions in intensity corrected multispectral MRI. IEEE TMI 15(2):154-169.
11. Labeling of 4D structures in registered 3-D segmentations (exact reference to be added)
12. J-P. Thirion, *New feature points based on geometric invariants for 3d image registration*, Int. Journal of Computer Vision, 18(2):121-137, May 1996
13. F. Maes, A. Collignon, D. Vandermeulen, G. Marchal, and P. Suetens, *Multi-Modality Image Registration by Maximization of Mutual Information*, IEEE Trans. on Medical Imaging, 16(2), pp. 187-198, April 1997
14. Christian Brechbühler, Guido Gerig, and Gabor Székely, *Compensation of spatial inhomogeneity in MRI based on a multi-valued image model and a parametric bias estimate*, Visualization in Biomedical Computing Proc. VBC'96, Lecture Notes in Computer Science, No. 1131, Springer, pp. 141-146, Sept. 1996
15. M. Styner and G. Gerig, *Evaluation of 2D/3D bias correction with 1+1ES-optimization*, Technical Report Image Science Lab, ETH Zurich, TR-179, 1997
16. Glenn Shafer, *A Mathematical Theory of Evidence*, Princeton, NJ: Princeton University Press, 1976
17. J. Gordon, and E.H. Shortliffe, *The Dempster-Shafer Theory of Evidence*, in: B.G. buchanan and E.H. Shortliffe (Eds.), Rule-Based Expert Systems, pp. 272-292, Addison-Wesley, 1985
18. Robert J. Safranek, Susan Gottschlich, Avinash C. Kak, *Evidence Accumulation Using Binary Frames of Discernment for Verification Vision*, Actions on Robotics and Automation, Vol. 6, No. 4, August 1990
19. European project on Brain Morphometry (BIOMORPH, EU-BIOMED2 project no BMH4-CT96-0845, 1996-1998

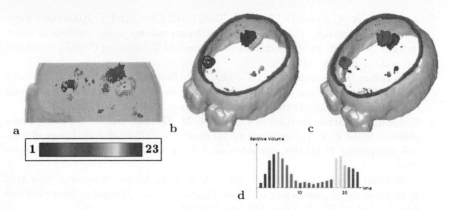

Fig. 5. Three-dimensional display of lesions segmented from the Brigham and Women's data set. (a) Side-view with transparent intracranial cavity. (b) Time of appearance, (c) time of disappearance. (d) Plot of total volume estimates versus time. Remember that the method analysis only fluctuations and excludes static portions of lesions. The color represents the time of appearance or disappearance, respectively, coded from 1 to 23.

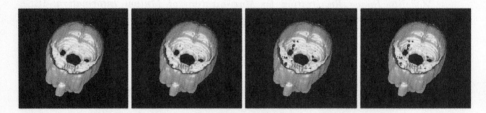

Fig. 6. Three-dimensional renderings of time evolution resulting from the 4-D analysis of the BIOMORPH data set. The images represent weeks 0, 28, 36 and 40.

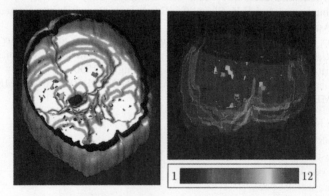

Fig. 7. Three-dimensional displays of lesions segmented from the BIOMORPH data set, top and side view of lesions and intracranial cavity. The color represents the time of appearance, coded from 1 to 12).

Reconstruction of the Central Layer of the Human Cerebral Cortex from MR Images

Chenyang Xu[1], Dzung L. Pham[1,4], Jerry L. Prince[1,2,3],
Maryam E. Etemad[2], and Daphne N. Yu[2]

[1] Electrical and Computer Engineering, [2] Biomedical Engineering, [3] Radiology,
The Johns Hopkins University, Baltimore MD 21218, USA.
[4] Laboratory of Personality & Cognition, GRC/NIA/NIH, Baltimore, MD 21214, USA.

Abstract. Reconstruction of the human cerebral cortex from MR images is a fundamental step in human brain mapping and in applications such as surgical path planning. In a previous paper, we described a method for obtaining a surface representation of the central layer of the human cerebral cortex using fuzzy segmentation and a deformable surface model. This method, however, suffers from several problems. In this paper, we significantly improve upon the previous method by using a fuzzy segmentation algorithm robust to intensity inhomogeneities, and using a deformable surface model specifically designed for capturing convoluted sulci or gyri. We demonstrate the improvement over the previous method both qualitatively and quantitatively, and show the result of its application to six subjects. We also experimentally validate the convergence of the deformable surface initialization algorithm.

1 Introduction

Reconstruction of the human cerebral cortex has many research and clinical uses, including applications in human brain mapping, functional imaging, and neurosurgical path planning. It is a difficult problem because of imaging noise, partial volume averaging, image intensity inhomogeneities, extremely convoluted cortical structures, and the requirement to preserve anatomical topology. Preservation of topology is important for morphometric analysis, surgical path planning, and functional mapping where a representation consistent with anatomical structure is required. During the last decade, there has been a considerable amount of work in obtaining a surface representation of the cortex [1–6]. Most reported methods, however, either require extensive manual interaction [5] or are capable of reconstructing only the visible cortex [1–4].

In [6], a hybrid system combining fuzzy segmentation, isosurfaces, and deformable surface models was presented for reconstructing the central layer of the cortex from magnetic resonance (MR) images (see Sect. 2). This method suffers from several problems, however. First, if intensity inhomogeneities are present in the acquired images, the segmentation used may yield inaccurate results. Second, it was not known whether the iterative process used to initialize the deformable surface would converge in general since it was only applied to one subject. Third, the traditional deformable surface model

---

This work was partially supported by the NSF Presidential Faculty Fellow Award MIP93-50336 and a Whitaker Foundation graduate fellowship.

used in [6] has difficulties converging to boundary concavities, resulting in the loss of deeply convoluted sulci or gyri in the surface reconstruction.

In this paper, we present several improvements over the method presented in [6] for reconstructing the central layer of the entire human cerebral cortex. We address the problems of the previous method by using a fuzzy segmentation algorithm which is robust to intensity inhomogeneities, experimentally validating the convergence of the initialization algorithm, and using a deformable surface model specifically designed for capturing convoluted sulci or gyri. In Sect. 2, we briefly review the method reported in [6]. In Sect. 3, we describe the segmentation and deformable surface algorithms used in our new cortex reconstruction method. In Sect. 4, we present and discuss the results of applying our method to six different subjects.

2 Background

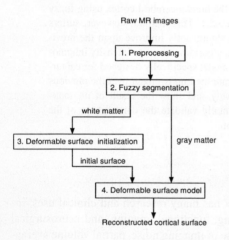

Fig. 1. Overview of cortical surface reconstruction method.

The method reported in [6] has four major steps as illustrated in Fig. 1. After the MR data (T1-weighted image volumes with voxel size $0.9375 \times 0.9375 \times 1.5$mm) are acquired, the images are preprocessed to remove extracranial tissue, cerebellum, and brain stem. Each volume is then interpolated to isotropic voxels. Next, a fuzzy c-means clustering algorithm (FCM) is used to segment the preprocessed data into three tissue classes: cerebrospinal fluid (CSF), gray matter (GM), and white matter (WM). As a result, each tissue is represented as a fuzzy membership function. The use of a fuzzy segmentation offers robustness to noise and partial volume averaging effects and removes the dependency on raw image intensity in later steps.

Once the images have been segmented, an initial estimate of the GM/WM interface is obtained before refinement to the final central layer. Obtaining an initial surface near the desired cortical surface is important because it provides a good starting position for deforming the surface, yields a proper initial parameterization of the deformable surface, significantly reduces the reconstruction time, and improves the reconstruction results. This is accomplished by applying the following operations to the WM membership function. First, hippocampal formations are manually removed, regions around the brain stem are manually filled, and ventricles are automatically filled in the WM membership function. An automatic iterative algorithm is then applied to the WM membership function to ensure that the resulting initial surface has a topology equivalent to a sphere. This algorithm consists of the following steps:

1. Compute isosurface on WM membership function at 0.5.
2. Extract largest connected mesh in the isosurface and remove singular points from the connected mesh.
3. Compute Euler characteristic χ on the extracted mesh. If $\chi < 2$, median filter the WM membership function, recompute isosurface at 0.5 and go to Step 2. If $\chi = 2$, then the surface topology is equivalent to a sphere, and the initialization is complete.

The final output of this process is a smoothed version of the GM/WM interface with the desired topology.

After the initialization is obtained, a traditional deformable surface model [7, 8] is used to refine the initial surface to the central layer of the gray matter.

3 Methods

In this section, we describe two major improvements upon the method described in Sect. 2. The standard FCM segmentation used in the previous method is replaced with an adaptive segmentation that is robust to intensity inhomogeneities. In addition, instead of using a traditional deformable surface model, an enhanced model is used that allows a more accurate reconstruction of the cortex.

3.1 Adaptive Fuzzy C-Means Segmentation

MR images may have intensity inhomogeneities caused by nonuniformities in the RF field during acquisition. The result is a slowly varying shading artifact over the image that can produce errors in intensity-based segmentation methods like FCM. These errors could potentially cause certain regions of the reconstructed cortex to shift into the WM or CSF. In [9], an adaptive fuzzy c-means algorithm (AFCM) was proposed for segmenting 2-D images that are corrupted by intensity inhomogeneities. Using an iterative algorithm, AFCM simultaneously computes fuzzy membership functions for each tissue class, the mean intensity of each tissue class (called the centroid), and an estimate of the inhomogeneity, which is modeled as a gain field. It was shown in [9] that AFCM achieves significantly lower error rates than FCM when segmenting images corrupted by intensity inhomogeneities. Thus, in order to make the cortical surface reconstruction method robust to inhomogeneities, we use AFCM instead of FCM to obtain fuzzy segmentations of the MR brain images into classes of GM, WM, and CSF.

We now briefly describe the steps of AFCM for 3-D images. Details of its derivation for 2-D images are provided in [9]. Let $y(\mathbf{x})$ be the observed image intensity at $\mathbf{x}$, $u_k(\mathbf{x})$ be the membership value at voxel $\mathbf{x}$ for class k such that $u_k(\mathbf{x}) \geq 0$ and $\sum_{k=1}^{K} u_k(\mathbf{x}) = 1$, c_k be the centroid of class k, and $g(\mathbf{x})$ be the unknown gain field to be estimated. K, the total number of classes, is assumed to be 3. The steps for AFCM are as follows:

1. Provide initial values for centroids, $c_k, k = 1, \ldots, K$, and set the gain field $g(\mathbf{x})$ equal to one for all $\mathbf{x}$.
2. Compute memberships as follows:

$$u_k(\mathbf{x}) = \frac{\|y(\mathbf{x}) - g(\mathbf{x})c_k\|^{-2}}{\sum_{l=1}^{K} \|y(\mathbf{x}) - g(\mathbf{x})c_l\|^{-2}} \quad (1)$$

for all $\mathbf{x}$ and $k = 1, \ldots, K$

3. Compute new centroids as follows:

$$c_k = \frac{\sum_\mathbf{x} u_k^2(\mathbf{x}) g(\mathbf{x}) y(\mathbf{x})}{\sum_\mathbf{x} u_k^2(\mathbf{x}) g^2(\mathbf{x})}, \quad k = 1, \ldots, K \qquad (2)$$

4. Compute new gain field by solving the following space-varying difference equation for $g(\mathbf{x})$:

$$y(\mathbf{x}) \sum_{k=1}^{K} u_k^2(\mathbf{x}) c_k = g(\mathbf{x}) \sum_{k=1}^{K} u_k^2(\mathbf{x}) c_k^2 + \lambda_1 (g(\mathbf{x}) * H_1(\mathbf{x})) + \lambda_2 (g(\mathbf{x}) * H_2(\mathbf{x})) \qquad (3)$$

where $H_1(\mathbf{x}) = d_x * \check{d}_x + d_y * \check{d}_y + d_z * \check{d}_z$ and $H_2(\mathbf{x}) = d_{xx} * \check{d}_{xx} + d_{yy} * \check{d}_{yy} + d_{zz} * \check{d}_{zz} + 2(d_{xy}*d_{xy}) + 2(d_{yz}*d_{yz})$. The operators d_x, d_y, d_z are finite differences along the axes of the image volume, and $d_{xx} = d_x * d_x$, $d_{yy} = d_y * d_y$, $d_{zz} = d_z * d_z$, $d_{xy} = d_x * y$, and $d_{xz} = d_x * d_z$ are second order finite differences. Here we have used the notation $\check{f}(i) = f(-i)$. The symbol '$*$' denotes the discrete convolution operator.

5. If the algorithm has converged, then quit. Otherwise, go to Step 2.

Convergence is defined to be when the maximum change in the membership functions over all pixels between iterations is less than 0.01. In Step 4 of the algorithm, λ_1 and λ_2 are parameters that control the expected smoothness of the inhomogeneity. These parameters were determined empirically, and have demonstrated robustness to inaccurate selection. The gain field $g(\mathbf{x})$ in Step 4 was computed using a multigrid algorithm (see [9]).

3.2 Deformable Surface Model

The method reported in [6] used a combination of traditional external forces and unconstrained pressure forces for the deformable surface model. The traditional external forces are computed by minimizing certain energy functions derived from the data [7, 8]. A deformable surface model using such external forces, however, has difficulties in progressing into boundary concavities [10]. Unconstrained pressure forces, proposed in [11, 8], can help push the deformable surface into boundary concavities. However, a deformable surface under unconstrained pressure forces can often behave arbitrarily and cause the surface to intersect itself. Recently, Xu and Prince [10] developed a new external force model, called *gradient vector flow* (GVF). The GVF external force field has a large capture range and is capable of forcing the deformable surface into boundary concavities. In this section, we give a brief overview of GVF used in this paper and describe our improved deformable surface model by using a combination of GVF and a constrained pressure force as its external forces.

The GVF field $\mathbf{v}(\mathbf{x})$ where $\mathbf{x} = (x, y, z) \in \mathbf{R}^3$ is defined as the equilibrium solution of the following system of partial differential equations

$$\mathbf{v}_t = \mu \nabla^2 \mathbf{v} - (\mathbf{v} - \nabla u_{\text{gm}}) |\nabla u_{\text{gm}}|^2 \qquad (4)$$

where $\mathbf{v}_t$ denotes the partial derivative of $\mathbf{v}(\mathbf{x};t)$ with respect to t, and $\nabla^2 = \frac{\partial^2}{\partial x^2} + \frac{\partial^2}{\partial y^2} + \frac{\partial^2}{\partial z^2}$ is the Laplacian operator (applied to each spatial component of $\mathbf{v}$ separately), and u_{gm} is the GM membership function. When GVF is computed on thick edges, such as in the GM membership function, the resulting GVF field converges to the center of the thick edge.

We use a combination of GVF and a constrained pressure force to provide external forces for our deformable surface. The resulting external force is given by:

$$\mathbf{F}_{\text{ext}}(\mathbf{x}) = [<\mathbf{v}(\mathbf{x}), \mathbf{n}(\mathbf{x})> + C(\mathbf{x})]\mathbf{n}(\mathbf{x}) \qquad (5)$$

where $\mathbf{v}(\mathbf{x})$ is the GVF field, $\mathbf{n}(\mathbf{x})$ is the outward normal vector of the surface at $\mathbf{x}$, $<\cdot,\cdot>$ is the inner product of two vectors, and $C(\mathbf{x})$ is a constraint field on the pressure force (defined below). Since the component of the external force in the tangent plane will only affect the parameterization of the surface but not its shape, we project $\mathbf{v}(\mathbf{x})$ onto the normal direction at surface position $\mathbf{x}$. Thus, the internal force is solely responsible for controlling the surface parameterization while the external force is solely responsible for deforming the surface towards the feature of interest.

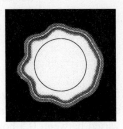

Fig. 2. Example of a deformable contour converging to the center of a simulated GM.

The constrained pressure force is similar in concept to the signed pressure force used in [12]. Unlike the unconstrained pressure force mentioned earlier, the constrained pressure force behaves more conservatively and is less subject to the self-intersection problem. It is used to increase the speed of convergence as well as reconstruction accuracy. The constraint field $C(\mathbf{x})$ is designed to turn off the pressure force once the surface enters the GM and leaves the surface under the influence of GVF external forces only. $C(\mathbf{x})$ is defined to be:

$$C(\mathbf{x}) = \begin{cases} 0 & \text{if } |2u_{\text{wm}}(\mathbf{x}) + u_{\text{gm}}(\mathbf{x}) - 1| < \delta \\ 2u_{\text{wm}}(\mathbf{x}) + u_{\text{gm}}(\mathbf{x}) - 1 & \text{otherwise} \end{cases}$$

where $u_{\text{wm}}(\mathbf{x})$ and $u_{\text{gm}}(\mathbf{x})$ are white matter and gray matter membership functions, and δ is a threshold to control the width of the gray matter region where the pressure force is disabled. δ is chosen to be 0.5 in our experiments. To help understand the behavior of the external forces, we apply a 2D deformable contour, a 2D analog to deformable surfaces in 3D, using external forces defined in (5) on a phantom simulating WM and GM of the brain. In Fig. 2, WM is depicted as the white region in the center and GM is depicted as the surrounding gray ribbon. The initial deformable contour is the circle shown in black and the final converged contour is shown in white. Note that the final contour indeed converges to the center of the simulated GM.

4 Results

The described cortex reconstruction method was applied to MR brain images from six subjects, four taken from the Baltimore Longitudinal Study on Aging [13]. Using an

Table 1. Euler characteristics of surfaces generated for six subjects at different iterations.

Iteration(s)	0	1	2	3	4	5	6	7	8	9	15	20
Subject 1	-757	-49	-6	2	–	–	–	–	–	–	–	–
Subject 2	-1010	-56	-14	-4	-2	-2	-2	-2	0	2	–	–
Subject 3	-666	-50	-16	-12	-4	-2	0	0	2	–	–	–
Subject 4	-860	-66	-24	-8	-6	-2	-2	-2	2	–	–	–
Subject 5	-192	-75	-40	-27	-22	-19	-17	-16	-14	-12	-4	2
Subject 6	-462	-26	-12	-6	0	2	–	–	–	–	–	–

SGI O2 workstation with a 174 MHz R10000 processor, the total processing time per subject varied between 4.5 and 6.5 hours. The time required for manual interaction varied between 0.5 hours and 1 hour for a trained operator. AFCM required approximately 1 hour. The automated steps in GM/WM interface estimation take about 0.5 hours which produces a mesh with between 200,000 and 400,000 vertices. Because of the large number of vertices in the mesh, it takes the deformable surface algorithm about 3 hours to produce the final reconstructed surface. Note that both AFCM and the deformable surface algorithm are fully automated steps.

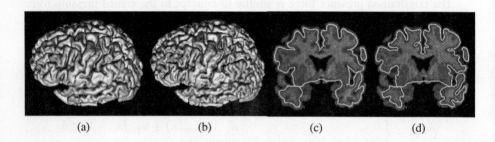

(a)   (b)   (c)   (d)

Fig. 3. Surface rendering of reconstructed cortical surface from one study using (a) the previous method, and (b) the current method. The coronal slice across the anterior commissure superimposed with the cross section of the corresponding reconstructed cortical surface using (c) the previous method, and (d) the new method.

The application of the method to multiple subjects allowed a preliminary validation of the convergence of the deformable surface initialization algorithm (see Sect. 2). In all six cases, the topology of the surface converged to the correct topology in less than 20 iterations. The result is shown in Table 1. Note that an Euler characteristic of 2 implies that the surface has a topology equivalent to a sphere and that a value smaller than 2 implies that the surface has one or more handles (like the handle of a coffee cup). The smaller the Euler characteristic is, the more handles a surface has. From the results, we observe that the median filter used in the iterative process effectively eliminated handles on the surface and that the Euler characteristic was nondecreasing with each iteration.

In Figs. 3(a) and 3(b), we show the surface rendering of the reconstructed cortical surface from one subject using the previous and the new methods. Notice that although the two surfaces look similar overall, the new method seems to maintain more details. In Figs. 3(c) and 3(d), we show the coronal slice across the anterior commissure superimposed with the cross section of the corresponding reconstructed cortical surface using the previous and the new methods. It is apparent from this view that the new method yields more accurate results.

The accuracy of the previous and new methods were also compared quantitatively by computing landmark errors. A trained operator identified five landmarks on the central cortical layer for each hemisphere. The landmarks are located on the root of the central sulcus (CS), the crown of the post-central gyrus (PCG), the most anterior point of the temporal lobe (TL), midway along the calcarine fundus (CALC), and the medial frontal gyrus (MFG). The landmark error was then computed as the minimum distance between the given landmark and the surface. Table 2 shows the results of landmark errors using the previous and the new methods for two hemispheres. On average, the new method offers an improvement of approximately 25% over the previous method.

Table 2. Landmark errors comparison (in *mm*)

Method	CS_1	CS_2	PCG_1	PCG_2	TL_1	TL_2	$CALC_1$	$CALC_2$	MFG_1	MFG_2	Mean	Std
Previous	1.9	2.6	0.7	0.7	0.5	1.3	1.0	0.4	0.9	1.0	1.10	0.68
New	0.5	2.1	0.7	0.4	0.5	1.4	0.7	0.4	0.5	1.1	0.83	0.55

In Fig. 4, we show where the reconstructed cortical surfaces intersect coronal slices taken through the anterior commissures of each subject. These figures show that the surfaces reside on the central cortical layer and that buried gyri (such as the insula) are found. It should be noted that isolated closed 2-D contours appearing in these images are actually part of the 3-D surfaces, which are topologically equivalent to spheres. Although most gyri are properly modeled, certain regions, such as the superior temporal gyrus, are sometimes not found accurately. We are considering further improvements to correct these deficiencies and to further decrease the need for manual interaction.

Acknowledgments

The authors would like to thank Dr. R. Nick Bryan, Dr. Christos Davatzikos, and Marc Vaillant for their support in this work. They would also like to thank Dr. Ron Kikinis and Dr. Susan Resnick for providing MR data.

References

1. A. M. Dale and M. I. Sereno. Improved localization of cortical activity combining EEG and MEG with MRI cortical surface reconstruction: A linear approach. *J. Cogn. Neuroscience*, 5(2):162–176, 1993.
2. D. MacDonald, D. Avis, and A. C. Evans. Multiple surface identification and matching in magnetic resonance images. In *SPIE Proc. VBC '94*, volume 2359, pages 160–169, 1994.

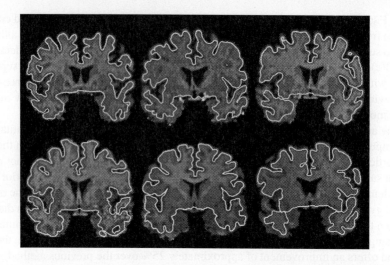

Fig. 4. From left to right and top to bottom, the coronal slice across the anterior commissure for subjects 1 to 6 superimposed with the cross section of the corresponding reconstructed cortical surface.

3. S. Sandor and R. Leahy. Towards automated labelling of the cerebral cortex using a deformable atlas. In *Information Processing in Medical Imaging*, pages 127–138, 1995.
4. C. Davatzikos and R. N. Bryan. Using a deformable surface model to obtain a shape representation of the cortex. *IEEE Trans. Med. Imag.*, 15:785–795, December 1996.
5. H.A. Drury, D.C. Van Essen, C.H. Anderson, C.W. Lee, T.A. Coogan, and J.W. Lewis. Computerized mappings of the cerebral cortex: A multiresolution flattening method and a surface-based coordinate system. *J. Cogn. Neuroscience*, pages 1–28, 1996.
6. C. Xu, D. L. Pham, and J. L. Prince. Finding the brain cortex using fuzzy segmentation, isosurfaces, and deformable surface models. In *the XVth Int. Conf. Inf. Proc. Med. Imag. (IPMI)*, pages 399–404. Springer-Verlag, 1997.
7. M. Kass, A. Witkin, and D. Terzopoulos. Snakes: Active contour models. *International Journal of Computer Vision*, 1(4):321–331, 1987.
8. L. D. Cohen and I. Cohen. Finite-element methods for active contour models and balloons for 2-D and 3-D images. *IEEE Trans. on Pattern Anal. Machine Intell.*, 15(11):1131–1147, November 1993.
9. D. L. Pham and J. L. Prince. An adaptive fuzzy c-means algorithm for image segmentation in the presence of intensity inhomogeneities. In *SPIE Medical Imaging '98: Image Processing*. SPIE, Feb. 21-27, 1998. to appear.
10. C. Xu and J. L. Prince. Snakes, shapes, and gradient vector flow. *IEEE Trans. on Image Processing*, pages 359–369, March 1998.
11. L. D. Cohen. On active contour models and balloons. *CVGIP: Image Understanding*, 53(2):211–218, March 1991.
12. T. Kapur, E. Grimson, W. Wells, and R. Kikinis. Segmentation of brain tissue from magnetic resonance images. *Medical Image Analysis*, 1(2):109–127, 1996.
13. N. W. Shock, R. C. Greulich, R. Andres, D. Arenberg, P. T. Costa Jr., E. Lakatta, and J. D. Tobin. Normal human aging: The Baltimore longitudinal study of aging. U.S. Governement Printing Office, Washington, D.C., 1984.

Regularization of MR Diffusion Tensor Maps for Tracking Brain White Matter Bundles

C. Poupon[1,2], J.-F. Mangin[1], V. Frouin[1], J. Régis[3],
F. Poupon[1], M. Pachot-Clouard[1], D. Le Bihan[1] and I. Bloch[2]

[1] Service Hospitalier Frédéric Joliot, Commissariat à l'Energie Atomique,
91401 Orsay Cedex, France, e-mail : cpoupon@shfj.cea.fr
[2] Ecole Nationale Supérieure des Télécommunications, 75013 Paris, France
[3] Service de Neurochirurgie Fonctionnelle et Stéréotaxique,
La Timone, Marseille, France

Abstract. We propose a new way for tracking brain white matter fiber bundles in diffusion tensor maps. Diffusion maps provide information about mobility of water protons in different directions. Assuming that diffusion is more important along axons, this information could lead to the direction of fiber bundles in white matter. Nevertheless, protocoles for diffusion image acquisition suffer from low resolutions and instrument noise. This paper is essentially dedicated to the design of a Markovian model aiming at the regularization of direction maps, and at the tracking of fiber bundles. Results are presented on synthetic tensor images to confirm the efficiency of the method. Then, white matter regions are regularized in order to enable the tracking of fiber bundles, which is of increasing interest in functional connectivity studies.

1 Introduction

During the last decade, the wide development of magnetic resonance imaging (MRI) has led to the design of a lot of segmentation methods dedicated to brain structures. For instance, the cortex, the white matter and the deep nuclei can be efficiently extracted from standard T1-weighted inversion-recovery MRI. Nevertheless, in spite of the $1mm$ resolution reached by most of the MR sequences, the fiber bundles embeded in white matter can not be tracked.

Therefore, few image analysis methods have been dedicated to brain white matter. Skeletonization has been proposed in [1] to analyze its complex convoluted shape. Simulations of information transmission have been proposed in [2] to detect inter-hemispheric connections. However, white matter organization is of increasing interest in the neuroscience community. For instance, a tension-based mechanism has been recently hypothesized as an explanation of the cortex folding pattern [3]. Moreover, connectivity between different brain areas is a crucial information to infer the brain functional organization. The recent advent of very fast MR sequences, like the echo-planar technique, has opened a new field of modalities which give access to this kind of information. Diffusion imaging implies the acquisition of a great amount of images from which water mobility in different directions is inferred. Assuming that this mobility is more important along axons than in any other direction, the fiber direction can be computed for each voxel of the white matter. Hence, fiber bundles can be tracked throughout the whole brain white matter which is the scope of this paper.

In this paper, we try to explain what kind of information is contained in diffusion maps, and we propose a way of representing tensor information about fiber orientation. Second, we present a Markovian model designed to regularize fiber orientation images. Finally, the behavior of this model with synthetic and real data is described.

2 Diffusion tensor imaging (DTI)

2.1 Diffusion process

In brain tissues, molecules are submitted to a Brownian motion in time that is macroscopically a diffusion process. In the case of an isotropic liquid, the probability that a molecule moves from a distance r during the time t follows a Gaussian law with a variance $var(r) = 6Dt$ where D is the diffusion coefficient that characterizes the mobility of molecules. In anisotropic environments, the mobility is different along each direction of space. Hence, diffusion is a tridimensional process which can be modeled by a second order tensor. The matrix $[D]$ is symmetric, positive and real, i.e. represents a quadratic form. The diffusion coefficient in any direction $\vec{d}$ is given by the tensorial dot product (equation 1). $[D]$ is an intrinsic property of the tissue [4][5][6][7].

$$\delta = \vec{d}^T [D] \vec{d}, \text{ with } [D] = \begin{pmatrix} D_{xx} & D_{xy} & D_{xz} \\ D_{yx} & D_{yy} & D_{yz} \\ D_{zx} & D_{zy} & D_{zz} \end{pmatrix} \qquad (1)$$

2.2 Contents of DTI : reading the raw data

Acquisitions have been done on a GE SIGNA $1,5T$. Imaging acquisition parameters were as follows: 52 axial slices, $3mm$ slice thickness, 128×128 in plane-resolution with a $1.875mm$ size. The six coefficients of $[D]$ are represented in figure 1 for a slice. Some large bundles, such as the corpus callosum or the cortico-spinal fibers, are highlighted in the raw images because they are colinear with one image axis. For instance, an hypersignal (white zone) on the D_{xx} coefficient slice shows an important diffusion process in the x axis, in the corpus callosum, whereas the D_{yy} and D_{zz} coefficient slices present a very low signal at the same location, revealing a lack of diffusion in these directions.

It must be noted that it is very hard to understand the information of the tensor by looking at images of the 6 coefficients of the tensor.

2.3 Visualizing tensor information

It is not easy to read simultaneously 6 images and it would be easier to understand the diffusion if they were gathered in one image. With this aim, we compute the eigen system $\{(\vec{e}_1, \lambda_1), (\vec{e}_2, \lambda_2), (\vec{e}_3, \lambda_3) / \lambda_1 > \lambda_2 > \lambda_3\}$ associated to the tensor $[D]$, for each voxel. A fiber bundle has a strong anisotropy, and a local tensor of that bundle has a first eigen value λ_1 much greater than the others. The diffusion of water protons is the most important along the direction $\vec{e}_1$. A basic idea to represent the information contained in a tensor map is to detect the strongly anisotropic voxels and to represent, in such voxels, the eigen vector $\vec{e}_1$ by a cylinder. An alternative is to represent an ellipsoïd, the axis of which have lengths equal to the 3 eigenvalues of the tensor. But, the visualization in

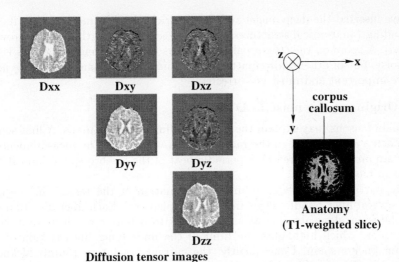

Fig. 1. *Slices of a brain diffusion tensor map; the 6 coefficients are represented, and a T1 MRI gives the corresponding anatomy.*

3D is more complicated for a large set of ellipsoïds. Several factors of anisotropy can be found in the litterature [8][6], but we have decided to choose a basic one (equation 2). A fully anisotropic tissue has a factor 1.0 since $trace[D] = \lambda_1$, and an isotropic tissue has a factor 0.0 since $\lambda_1 = \lambda_2 = \lambda_3$.

$$a = \frac{3}{2}\left(\frac{\lambda_1}{trace([D])} - \frac{1}{3}\right) \qquad (2)$$

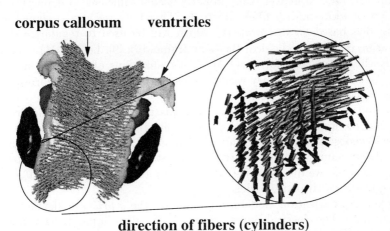

Fig. 2. *Representation of the main directions of diffusion with small cylinders*

Figure 2 gives a result of that simple method applied to a volume of interest around the corpus callosum. Each direction of fiber is represented by a small cylinder which axis is colinear to $\vec{e_1}$ direction and which length is proportional to the anisotropy factor. A threshold on anisotropy has been done to get only directions of the most anisotropic tissues. We clearly observe the corpus callosum.

We have inserted the deep nuclei and the ventricles in this image to help its understanding (anatomical structures have been segmented with a region growing method). A zoom on the corpus callosum shows that this image of vectors is not very noisy, but in other white matter areas which are less anisotropic, the noise is more important and must be corrected.

2.4 Origins of the noise in DTI

Two main reasons may explain the noise in diffusion tensor maps. A first source of artifacts can be found in the motion of the ventricles. The measurements of tensor are probably blurred by a periodic beat of the cerebro-spinal fluid (CSF) related to blood flow.

Second, partial volume effect blurs the estimation of the tensor, in the case where several fiber bundles cross into one simple voxel. Each fiber direction will favor diffusion along its own axis. This leads to a tensor much more difficult to interpret, which highlights the limit of the underlying linearization of the diffusion phenomenon. Consequently, the current resolution (3mm thickness) will not allow the tracking of very thin bundles. All those sources of noise led us to develop a Markovian random field approach for regularizing maps of potential directions of bundles.

3 Markovian regularization: the spaghetti plate model

3.1 Markovian assumption

Let us consider a voxel of white matter where the fibers follow direction $\vec{d}$. Since fibers can not end up inside white matter, we have to find neighboring voxels, forwards and backwards, with similar fiber directions (or perhaps the boundary of white matter). Moreover, this property seems sufficient to define the whole geometry of white matter fiber directions. Therefore, we have designed Markovian models based on this property which will be used to regularize the fiber orientation image in a classical Bayesian framework [9]. Let $\vec{d}(M)$ denotes the putative fiber direction for voxel M. The realizations of the random variable $\vec{d}(M)$ of the field are unitary vectors. Each variable state space corresponds to all directions of the 3D space.

We call this class of models the spaghetti plate models because the deep local minima of the underlying energy look really like this. Hence, the role of the data will be to choose the spaghetti plate corresponding to the underlying white matter geometry namely endowed with the highest proton mobility along spaghetti. In the following, we discuss different types of interaction potentials $V_S(\vec{d}(M))$ leading to spaghetti plate models.

The whole regularization model has to combine the *a priori* model on geometry with the data. The classical Bayesian approach leads to minimizing a sum of two terms:

$$E = \sum_{M \in Volume} V_S(\vec{d}(M)) + \alpha \sum_{M \in Volume} V_D(\vec{d}(M)) \qquad (3)$$

where $V_D(\vec{d}(M))$ should be a function inversely proportional to the mobility of water protons in direction $\vec{d}(M)$ (α is a weight).

3.2 Interaction potentials

If we have a synthetic look at the global appeareance of the fiber bundles in the brain, one may think about a spaghetti plate. When not enough cooked, spaghetti stay pasted together and form some bundles of a few spaghetti. The spaghetti of a same bundle bend under the action of water. The whole packets of spaghetti leads to a plate of interlaced bundles. It is important to notice that a spaghetti not enough cooked cannot have a strong local curvature. Thus, when we move forward along the spaghetti, the direction $\vec{d}$ of the spaghetti can be only slightly modified. This property is used to give a mathematical expression to the spaghetti plate model. Let $\vec{d}(M)$ denotes the putative fiber direction for voxel M. When we consider the set of voxels M of a direction map of spaghetti, we can write the global energy of the spaghetti configuration by adding all the local potentials (equation 4).

$$E_S = \sum_{M \in Volume} V_S(\vec{d}(M)) \quad (4)$$

Let us consider the figure 3.1. For all the neighbors N of the voxel M contained in a solid angle β (forward and backward) which axis is in the potential direction of spaghetti (or fibers) of the voxel M, we compute the angle $\theta(M,N) = \left(\vec{d}(M), \vec{d}(N)\right)$. If all those neighbors N belong to the same bundle, then the angles $\theta(M,N)$ have to be small. The first idea consists in using all $\theta(M,N)$ to give an expression of the "spaghetti" potential $V_S(\vec{d}(M))$ at M (equation 5):

$$V_S(\vec{d}(M)) = \sum_{N \in \mathcal{V}(M) \cap N^{26}} \left| \cos^{-1}\left(\vec{d}(M).\vec{d}(N)\right) \right| \quad (5)$$

where $\mathcal{V}(M)$ is a cone of apex M, direction $\vec{d}(M)$ and aperture angle β, and N^{26} is the 26-neighborhood. Using such a conic neighborhood discards the influence of voxels which could belong to bundles with other directions. The aperture β of the solid angle which defines the neighborhood is set typically to $45°$. In order to allow a range of quasi-equivalent potential for low angles, we finally used the angle cosine rather than a linear function (equation 6). Other choices could be investigated in the future.

$$V_S(\vec{d}(M)) = - \sum_{N \in \mathcal{V}(M) \cap N^{26}} |\cos(\theta(M,N))| \quad (6)$$

Figure 3.2 shows an example of the generation of a spaghetti plate given by this model. The spaghetti directions have been initialized randomly. The energy made up by the sum of $V_S(\vec{d}(M))$ over the whole image has been minimized, using a deterministic algorithm. Voxels outside the image are discarded from the conic neighborhood, which means that no constrain on fiber direction is induced by white matter boundary. Three of the spaghetti have been isolated to point out their low local curvature.

Then, we have built a synthetic object to simulate the case of two noisy orthogonal bundles locally tangent. The image to process is given in figure 4.1a. A deterministic minimization of the energy stemming from the model 6 has been

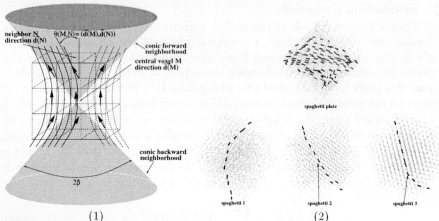

Fig. 3. (1)*Schematic representation of the conic neighborhood of a voxel. (2)Generation of spaghetti by minimization of the energy corresponding to model 6.*

performed ($\beta = 60°$) to get the image given in figure 4.1b. This example points out the weaknesses of the model. The model 6 considers all the neighbors in the cone. The effect of regularization and smoothing may be too important in the case of small bundles or at the interface of two large tangent bundles with very different orientations. This over-regularization effect can be overcome if a fixed number of neighbors is selected in both half-cones.

Let us write $\mathcal{V}^b(M)$, the subset of the neighborhood $\mathcal{V}(M)$ with the best neighbors:
$\mathcal{V}^b(M) = \mathcal{V}^b_{forward}(M) \cup \mathcal{V}^b_{backward}(M)$ where $\mathcal{V}^b_{forward}(M)$ (respectively $\mathcal{V}^b_{backward}(M)$) is made up by the b forward (respectively backward) 26-neighbors with lowest angles $\theta(M,N)$ (equation 7).

$$V_S(\vec{d}(M)) = - \sum_{N \in \mathcal{V}^b(M)} |cos(\theta(M,N))| \qquad (7)$$

The same test as in figure 4.1 has been performed with $b = 4$, leading to good results (figure 4.2).

The local minima of this energy are spaghetti plates, and there can be a huge number of configurations. Among these, we should be able to determine the closest configuration to the white matter geometry. That is the role of a second potential of attachment to the data.

3.3 Data influence

Indeed, we want to select the spaghetti plate with the highest global diffusion. It is possible, with the local tensor $[D(M)]$, to give the value of that diffusion in any direction $\vec{d}$, using the tensorial dot product (equation 1). Then we use equation 8 for the potential $V_D(\vec{d}(M))$:

$$V_D(\vec{d}(M)) = -\vec{d}(M)^T[D(M)]\vec{d}(M) \qquad (8)$$

3.4 Using anisotropy

The spaghetti model 7 does not take into account local variations of the anisotropy in the neighborhood of a voxel M, so that a voxel N with nearly isotropic tensor acts upon its neighborhood, whereas this voxel N does not contain any fiber. One solution to avoid this problem is to weight each term of the potential $V_S(\vec{d}(M))$ corresponding to the neighbor N by the anisotropy $a(N)$ (equation 9). Tests on the synthetic image figure 4.3a reveals that the effect is very important on the ridges of rectangular fibers (figure 4.3b), because these lines include few points of the bundle in their conic neighborhood. The anisotropy balancing clearly prevents such effects (figure 4.3c).

$$V_S(\vec{d}(M)) = - \sum_{N \in \mathcal{V}^b(M)} a(N) |cos(\theta(N))| \qquad (9)$$

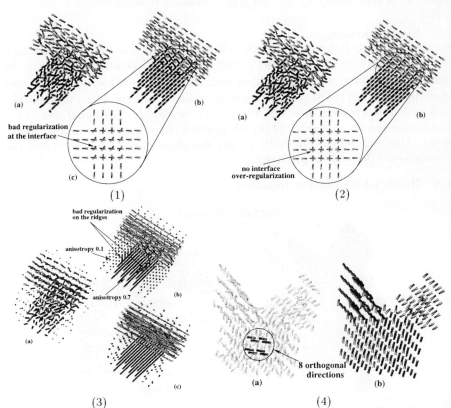

Fig. 4. (1)*Over-regularization at the interface of 2 perpendicular bundles with model 6; (2)Result of energy minimization of the model 7 considering the 4 best neighbors in each half-cone; (3)Introduction of the anisotropy in the spaghetti model 9. (4)Synthetic tensor Y-shaped object with 8 arbitrary misplaced directions; (a) start image, (b) result of regularization with model 9.*

4 Results

4.1 Minimization of the energy

The direction map of our Markovian random field has to be initialized not too far from the solution to speed-up the convergence. The direction of each voxel M is set to have the greatest diffusion, namely to the $\vec{e}_1(M)$ unit eigen vector direction computed from the tensor $[D(M)]$.

The space of variation of the directions $\vec{d}(M)$ is the 3D continous space. To be sure to try uniformly every direction of that space, we have sampled a unit sphere and we test, for each voxel M, all the sampled directions. The sampling of the unit sphere (typically 652 directions) is based on an iterative algorithm starting from an icosahedron and giving a uniform distribution of directions.

The global energy of the model is a linear combination of the "spaghetti" model energy and of the data attachment energy. We have to balance the influence of data by the weight α. The choice of the factor α depends on the value of the mean trace in anisotropic areas, typically 2.0×10^{-9} in white matter, and on the mean spaghetti energy. Since our initialization is not so far from the searched minimum of that energy E, we used a deterministic ICM algorithm to minimize E [10].

4.2 Synthetic image

We have explicitly put 8 local directions in an Y structure at $90°$ of the direction of the bundle to see if the model corrects them efficiently (figure 4.4(a)). To simulate noisy data, we have modified each direction $\vec{d}(M)$ within a $60°$ solid angle around $\vec{d}(M)$. The parameters of the model 9 with the 4 best neighbors in each cone are as follows: $\alpha = 0.5$, $\beta = 45°$, 652 uniformly distributed directions. The bundle has an anisotropy of 0.7 whereas the environment has an anisotropy of 0.1. After convergence of ICM, we get the result (figure 4.4(b)), where the directions are perfectly regularized.

4.3 Brain white matter bundles

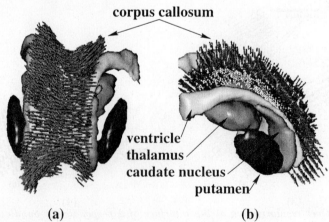

Fig. 5. *Regularization of the corpus callosum*

We have tested our algorithm on brain white matter to regularize fiber bundles. We have chosen some regions of interest around the corpus callosum (figure

5) and around the pyramidal pathways (6) which gather thalamo-parietal and cortico-spinal fibers. In such thick bundles, local angular deviation never overruns $30°$, hence an aperture $\beta = 45°$ is sufficient to follow a fiber. The parameter α has been empirically set to 10^9. For representing only anisotropic bundles, we have weighted the length of every cylinder (representing a fiber direction) by its anisotropy, as before. The mean anisotropy is 0.7 in the corpus callosum and 0.5 in the pyramidal bundle.

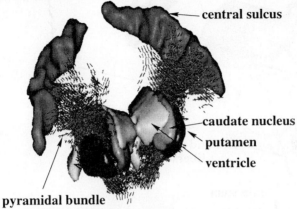

Fig. 6. *Regularization of the pyramidal pathways*

With such regularized images, we are now able to track a fiber direction. two points. For a given voxel M, we look forwards (respectively backwards) for the best neighbor N and we propagate throughout white matter. For instance, we have tracked one fiber direction of the pyramidal pathways. This direction belongs to the cortico-spinal buncle which goes from the primary motor areas inside precentral gyrus until the brain stem passing through the internal capsule (figure 7).

5 Conclusion

We have proposed a new method for tracking brain white matter fiber bundles in diffusion tensor maps. Diffusion maps provide the mobility of water proton in any direction of the 3D space. This information is used to determine the direction of maximum diffusion which is assumed to be that of a fiber bundle. However, diffusion maps are blurred by instrument noise and low resolution. In order to regularize them, we have developed a Markovian framework based on a spaghetti plate model.

Some tests on synthetic tensor images led us to improve the basic model to get a robust algorithm. Then, the regularization process has been implemented on a human brain image. It takes approximately 1 hour on a SPARC-ULTRA-30 station, but a reasonable computation time can be expected with a code-optimized version. Regions of interest around the corpus callosum and the pyramidal pathways have been selected to show results. Finally, an algorithm for tracking single fibers has been developed to give the best path of water diffusion from a given point.

In the future, we plan to correlate such information on brain connectivity with studies of functional connectivity using fMRI, which is a question of increasing interest in brain mapping studies.

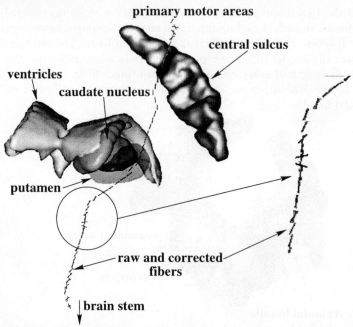

Fig. 7. *The regularization allows the tracking of a fiber direction from primary motor area until the brain stem.*

References

1. M. Naf, O. Kubler, R. Kikinis, M.E. Shenton, and G. Szekely. Characterization and Recognition of 3D Organ Shape in Medical Image Analysis Using Skeletonization. In IEEE/SIAM, editor, *IEEE/SIAM Workshop on Mathematical Methods in Biomedical Image Analysis*, 1996, pp. 139–150.
2. J.F. Mangin, J. Régis, and V. Frouin. Shape bottlenecks and conservative flow systems. In IEEE/SIAM, editor, *IEEE/SIAM Workshop on Mathematical Methods in Biomedical Image Analysis*, 1996, pp. 319–328.
3. D.C. Van Essen. A tension-based theory of morphogenesis and compact wiring in the central nervous system. *Nature*, vol. 385, 1997, pp. 313–318.
4. D. Le Bihan. Molecular Diffusion Nuclear Magnetic Resonance Imaging. *Magnetic Resonance Quaterly*, vol. 7, no. 1, 1991, pp. 1–30.
5. D. Le Bihan. *Diffusion and Perfusion Magnetic Resonance Imaging*, chapter A-2-IV, pp. 50–57. Raven Press, Ltd., New-York, 1995.
6. C. Pierpaoli, P. Jezzard, P.J. Basser, A. Barnett, and G. Di Chiro. Diffusion Tensor MR Imaging of the Human Brain. *Radiology*, vol. 201, 1996, pp. 637–648.
7. J. Mattiello, P.J. Basser, and D. Le Bihan. The B Matrix in Diffusion Tensor Echo-Planar Imaging. *Magnetic Resonance Magazine*, vol. 37, 1997, pp. 292–300.
8. C. Pierpaoli and P.J. Basser. Toward a Quantitative Assessment of Diffusion Anisotropy. *Magnetic Resonance Magazine*, vol. 36, 1996, pp. 893–906.
9. S. Geman and D. Geman. Stochastic Relaxation, Gibbs Distributions, and the Bayesian Restoration of Images. *IEEE PAMI*, vol. 6, no. 6, 1984, pp. 721–741.
10. J. Besag. On the statistical analysis of dirty pictures. *Journal of the Royal Statistical Society, Series B (Methodological)*, vol. 48, no. 3, 1986, pp. 259–302.

Measurement of Brain Structures Based on Statistical and Geometrical 3D Segmentation

Miguel Ángel González Ballester, Andrew Zisserman, and Michael Brady

Robotics Research Group, Dept. of Engineering Science
University of Oxford, Oxford OX1 3PJ, UK
{magb,az,jmb}@robots.ox.ac.uk

Abstract. In this paper we present a novel method for three-dimensional segmentation and measurement of volumetric data based on the combination of statistical and geometrical information. We represent the shape of complex three-dimensional structures, such as the cortex by combining a discrete 3D simplex mesh with the construction of a smooth surface using triangular Gregory-Bézier patches. A Gaussian model for the tissues present in the image is adopted, and a classification procedure which also estimates and corrects for the bias field present in the MRI is used. Confidence bounds are produced for all the measurements, thus obtaining bounds on the position of the surface segmenting the image. Performance is illustrated on multiple sclerosis phantom data and on real data

1 Introduction

The segmentation of three-dimensional structures is fundamental to medical vision applications. Voxel-based [16], slice-based [1,12,14], and deformable 3D surface methods [6,15,18] have been proposed, the latter being preferred because of the intrinsically three-dimensional nature of the data sets and the flexibility of having a surface segmenting the objects in it. The shapes of some structures to be segmented, such as the brain cortex, poses an additional problem, since the shape representation must be able to cope with such complexity.

Often, and central to this article, in clinical studies the size of the effect to be studied is small relative to the voxel size. This is the case, for example, when analysing the time evolution of multiple sclerosis lesions during drug treatment or patient therapy [4], and also when assessing differences in brain asymmetry associated with schizophrenia [5,7]. Accuracy becomes critical, necessitating confidence bounds for every measurement obtained from the data sets. To provide clinically meaningful results, the width of the confidence interval should be significantly smaller than the size of the anatomical effect to be studied. To this end, we describe a method for 3D segmentation from volumetric data combining both a statistical model of the tissues present in the image and a geometric template of the expected shape, and we explain how volume measurements, together with confidence intervals, are obtained from it. Following [11] and [20], the voxel intensities corresponding to a certain tissue type are modelled as a Gaussian distribution with small variance. Two main problems arise when using this model to classify voxels into tissue types, namely corrupting bias fields, and partial volume effects. Both are addressed in our method, which estimates and corrects for the bias field and regards partial volumes as an indicator of boundary location.

Complex biological shapes require a shape modeling technique that is powerful enough to capture sufficient detail, flexible enough to be adapted easily to segment the data, and able to construct higher-level shape descriptors. We use the simplex mesh [6] in an initial step, followed by the construction of a smooth surface using triangular Gregory-Bézier patches [17]. Segmentation of the data is guided by the probabilities computed in the statistical classification, a set of forces implemented on the simplex mesh, and a template of the expected shape built by applying a principal component analysis (PCA) to a set of pre-segmented structures.

The following section describes the statistical model and the bias correction algorithm used to classify the voxels and to detect partial volume effects. Next, the shape representation model, fitting process, and error bound computation are explained. Finally, a set of results are shown for phantom and real data.

2 Statistical model

A Gaussian distribution with small variance centred on an intensity value is used to model the image intensities corresponding to each tissue type. Ideally, this model should suffice to establish a classification of the voxels into tissue types, but real MR acquisitions pose two problems, namely corrupting bias fields, which modify the intensity of a same tissue voxel depending on its location, and partial volume effects due to the presence of more than one tissue type in a single voxel.

The intensities present in a MR image are often corrupted by a multiplicative, spatially varying bias field [9,11]. Many techniques have been proposed to deal with this problem [2,8,19], and the one we use is described in [11], being a modification of the method introduced by Wells and Grimson [20]. The technique uses the E-M algorithm to estimate iteratively the bias field and, for each of the voxels in the image, the probability that it belongs to each tissue type. Tissue types are modelled as Gaussian distributions, and a zero-mean Gaussian model is also assumed for the bias field. Figures 1A and 1B show a slice of a MRI and its corresponding corrected image. The estimated bias field is shown in figure 1C.

An image segmentation into tissue classes can be obtained by assigning to each voxel the tissue type for which its probability is highest, that is, has maximum likelihood. However, in some cases, the maximum likelihood is still small, typically because the intensity value of the voxel after bias correction does not fit well to any of the tissue distributions. These voxels are regarded as containing several tissues, that is, exhibit the partial volume effect (PVE) [16]. Intuitively, voxels belonging to the boundaries between tissues are likely to be most affected. Indeed, we can consider low maximum likelihood voxels as good candidates for boundary voxels. Figure 1D shows the segmentation using explicit Gaussian tissue models for grey matter and white matter, together with a uniform extra class to cater for background and CSF [11]. PVE voxels are coloured white.

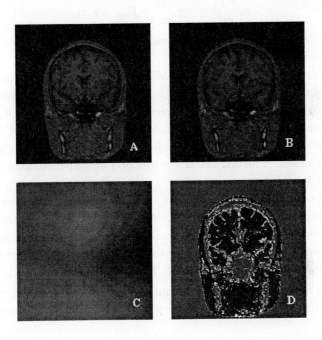

Fig. 1. A) Original slice; B) corrected slice; C) estimated bias field; D) segmentation using a tissue model for white matter and grey matter, plus a uniform class for CSF, air, and other tissues (PVE voxels are coloured white).

3 Geometrical 3D segmentation

Geometrical segmentation aims to detect the outer surface of the structure to be segmented. The advantage of such techniques is that they enable the specification of prior knowledge about the expected topology and shape of the structure by including an initial average model and a description of the allowed variability in shape [3,18]. We use the simplex mesh [6] technique for 3D segmentation, then construct a continuous, smooth surface by means of triangular Gregory-Bézier patches [17]. Prior knowledge is included by applying a principal components analysis (PCA) on the nodes of the simplex mesh, as described later.

A simplex mesh is a discrete shape model, formally defined as a set of 3-connected nodes. A framework in which a simplex mesh is used to segment volumetric data is described in [6]. A set of internal forces model properties of the structure, such as its elastic behaviour or constraints on continuity of the normals of the nodes; similarly, external forces are implemented and make the model converge towards the target volumetric data. The mesh is initialised and subjected to these forces following Newtonian dynamics:

$$m\frac{d^2 P_i}{dt^2} = -\gamma \frac{dP_i}{dt} + F_{int} + F_{ext},$$

where m is the mass unit of a vertex, P_i is the position of the ith node at time t, and γ is a damping factor.

Several operations enhance the flexibility of the simplex mesh when segmenting three-dimensional data. Some can be applied to alter the topology of the mesh, so rendering it suitable for complex shapes or for scale-space approaches to segmentation. Additionally, the density of the mesh is updated by a refinement process which increments the number of nodes in areas where a high level of detail is required. A further attractive property of simplex meshes is that they are dual to triangulations.

Prior knowledge about the expected shape of the structure to be segmented can be introduced into the model by acting on the internal forces that drive the fitting process, but this is not a very flexible method. Marais [13] has developed a scheme in which a PCA is applied to the nodes of a set of meshes segmenting the same structure in different patients. The result of this process is an average mesh $\bar{M}$ and a set of eigenvectors containing the n principal modes of variation, $\nu_1, \ldots, \nu_n$. Other meshes are then expressed in terms of these elements:

$$M = \bar{M} + \sum_{i=1}^{n} \alpha_i \nu_i$$

This process not only limits the amount of information required to describe an object (the set $\alpha_1, \ldots, \alpha_n$ of coefficients), but also restricts the allowed variability in shape, so avoiding unwanted excessive deviations from the average model. Although the simplex mesh has the advantages enumerated above, it is intrinsically not smooth, posing problems for volume estimation of smooth, highly convoluted surfaces, such as the cortex. To address this problem, a triangulation is built from the simplex mesh by adding a vertex in the centre of each face of the mesh and updating its position to the nearest data point in the direction of the normal of the face, by means of a local search. Then, smooth triangular Gregory-Bézier patches on each triangle are used to build a G1-continuous surface (continuity in the tangent plane) passing through the nodes of the simplex mesh, without the need to use interpolating polynomials of very high degree.

Triangular Gregory-Bézier (tGB) patches [17] are tricubic surfaces in barycentric coordinates, defined by 15 control points (refer to Figure 2):

$$GB(u,v,w) = u^3 P_0 + v^3 P_1 + w^3 P_2 +$$
$$12u^2vw P_{211} + 12uv^2w P_{121} + 12uvw^2 P_{112} +$$
$$3u^2v(1-w)P_{01} + 3uv^2(1-w)P_{02} + 3v^2(1-u)wP_{11} +$$
$$3(1-u)vw^2 P_{12} + 3u(1-v)w^2 P_{21} + 3u^2(1-v)w P_{22}$$

where $0 \leq u,v,w \leq 1, u+v+w = 1$ and:

$$P_{211} = \frac{wP^v_{211} + vP^w_{211}}{w+v}, P_{121} = \frac{uP^w_{121} + wP^u_{121}}{u+w}, P_{112} = \frac{vP^u_{112} + uP^v_{112}}{v+u}$$

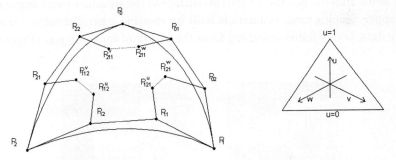

Fig. 2. Triangular Gregory-Bézier patch, defined by 15 control points. A G1-continuous mesh of tGB patches is used to interpolate the nodes of the simplex mesh and its corresponding normals.

The tGB interpolation process leaves one free control point in each of the edges of the triangulation, thereby enabling an even closer fit to the data. Several fitting strategies are being developed, namely local minimisation of distances from points inside a particular patch to the nearest data points, global minimisation of all the distances in the mesh, and a hybrid scheme where distances are minimised in a certain patch and its neighbouring patches up to a certain level, weighting the contribution of the neighbours as a function of the distance.

A desirable property of tGB patches is that analytic formulae for local position and derivatives are available, enabling the computation of shape descriptors based on differential geometric quantities, such as curvature. In a similar vein, the surface area and volume enclosed by a simplex mesh can be computed analytically using the divergence theorem. The availability of these measures is important in the development of quantitative shape descriptors applicable to medical structures, which is one of the most important ongoing lines of research in medical imaging.

4 Edge search and confidence bounds

We assume that PVE voxels correspond to boundary voxels. This information initiates the simplex mesh, which looks for the closest boundary voxel when updating its nodes. This search samples the neighbouring voxels in the direction of the normal of the node, by means of fast, local, 1-D searches, similar to those used in [1]. The same mechanism is used when computing distances from patch points to data points in the process of fitting tGB patches to the simplex mesh.

Due to the partial volume effect, boundary transitions from one tissue to another can occupy more than one voxel. The location of the boundary can thus be bounded by this volume, i.e. from pure voxels of one tissue to pure voxels of another tissue. This interval defines the confidence bound for the measurement. Two simplex meshes and tGB surfaces are computed, representing the upper and lower bounds on the position of the real surface of the structure being segmented. The upper simplex mesh estimate is built by creating a parallel surface tangent to the data points found searching from the centre of each polygon (Figure 3).

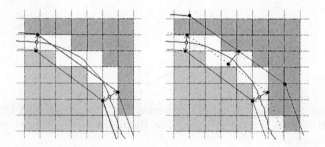

Fig. 3. 2D illustration of the 3D construction of the upper estimate on surface location using the simplex mesh. Upper and lower estimates on the location of the vertices of the mesh are obtained by local searches approximating to the nearest non-PVE voxel (left). Then, the position of the centre of the polygon (line in 2D) is updated to the nearest data point and a parallel surface is built (right).

5 Results

Several experiments have been performed in order to assess the performance of the method. Initially we used synthetic MRI data sets to validate the working of the program and to demonstrate that the tGB patches gave upper and lower bounds on volumes that are far tighter than those using voxel counting or the refined simplex mesh; [10] provides details and the imaging protocols that we simulated. Then we experimented with a phantom consisting of a group of shapes made from paraffin wax and embedded within an agarose gel. By measuring the density of the wax, the true volume can be derived from the weight within a confidence interval of 2% [16]. The phantoms simulate the size and shape of multiple sclerosis lesions, which are usually small relative to the MR acquisition resolution. Simplex mesh segmentation with low density, tGB fitting, and simplex mesh refinement volume measures were obtained. The results again show that the best volume bound estimates are from the use of a mesh of tGB patches interpolating the simplex mesh. It is worth noting that, although the refinement method of the simplex mesh improves the volume measurement significantly, the use of a continuous surface results in a much better estimate. These results are typical of the ones we have achieved with simulated and phantom data [10].

More recently, we have begun to test the method on an in-vivo T1-weighted MRI data set consisting of 124 slices of 256x256 voxels of size $0.781251 \times 0.78125 \times 1.7 mm^3$ (TE=9000ms, TR=24000ms). In this case, no ground truth about the volume of the object to be segmented is available; for this reason we scanned the volunteer twice, the second time with his head rotated through about $20 - 30°$ (Figure 4). Results are given for the left ventricle of the patient.

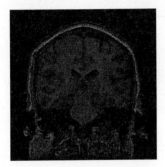 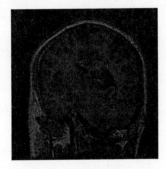

Fig. 4. Slice 56 of the MRI acquisitions used for the study: normal (left) and rotated(right). Note the significant rotation of the right image.

The data set is first bias corrected assuming only one tissue encompassing white matter and grey matter, plus a uniform class modelling the rest of tissues plus CSF and air. Probability maps for the different tissues are generated, and a pre-segmentation labels voxels with a probability smaller than 95% of belonging to one of the tissues as PVE voxels (see Figure 1). A simplex mesh is fitted to the data using the information of the map to guide it. Two meshes are fitted to obtain an upper and a lower bound (*sm U* and *sm L*) of the location of the surface. The numbers of vertices for the fitted refined mesh are 1538 (771 polygons), and 1558 for the rotated set (781 polygons). A set of tGB patches is then built (*tGB U, tGB L*). For the sake of comparison, voxel-based segmentations were performed and validated by an expert using a thresholding tool and setting two thresholds in order to obtain upper and lower bounds (*voxel U* and *voxel L*). Volume measurements are shown in Tables 1 and 2.

	straight	rotated
smU	12192	11100
voxel U	10090	9770
tGB U	9454	9574
tGB L	7835	7998
sm L	7373	7483
voxel L	7314	7162

	straight	rotated
sm	4819	3617
voxel	2776	2608
tGB	1619	1576

Table 1: Measured vol. (mm^3) of left ventricle (initial and rotated).

Table 2: Width of confidence interval (upper bound - lower bound).

Figure 5 shows the upper and lower bounds on the volume of the ventricle, and Figure 6 shows the width of the confidence interval. There are two points to note about Figure 6. First, the confidence interval is significantly smaller for the tGB model, and second, the interval is almost invariant to the patient head rotation.

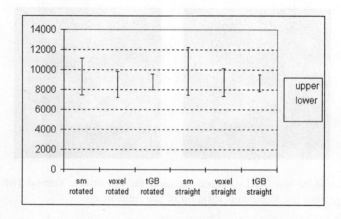

Fig. 5. Volume estimates for the left ventricle (mm^3), with the conditions indicated in the tables above, and for the original and rotated configurations. The vertical bars show the difference between the upper and lower volume estimates.

6 Future work

The method currently forms a framework for the segmentation and measurement of MRI data, leading to the estimation of two surfaces representing an upper and a lower bound on the location of the real surface. We are progressing towards estimating the most probable location of the surface inside the interval. PVE voxels can be modelled as weighted mixtures of two distributions on intensities. Using information about the neighbouring tissues, their distributions, and the intensity of the voxel, a probability distribution function (pdf) on the proportion

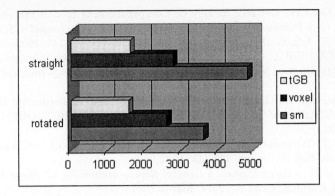

Fig. 6. Width of the confidence interval in the original and rotated condition. The best results are obtained by using a mesh of tGB patches interpolating the simplex mesh. Note that the results for the tGB patches are almost invariant to patient head rotation.

of each tissue present in the voxel can be computed. In turn, this will yield a pdf on the measurement so that both a mean/mode and a standard deviation can be computed.

The flexibility of the shape model is being investigated. A mesh consisting of a set of G1 continuous tGB patches leaves one degree of freedom on each edge connecting two patches. These free control points are currently set to minimise fluctuations on the surface, but a method that minimises the least-squares distance between the patch and target data points is being implemented. This scheme could be modified to minimise the difference between the proportions of each tissue in a voxel estimated as described above, and the proportions derived from the intersection of the tGB patches with each voxel.

Volume is by no means the most sensitive shape descriptor, and more sophisticated descriptors, suitable for medical applications, are being developed. The availability of a smooth continuous surface segmenting the object enables geometrical descriptors such as curvature to be computed and bounded. The segmentation method sketched in this paper shows an improvement over other existing techniques, in the sense that the confidence intervals are significantly narrower. An in-depth study is under way to assess whether this technique will be able to provide clinically valid measurements from MRI for problems such as segmentation of multiple sclerosis lesions or schizophrenia studies, where the size of the effect to be studied is small relative to the voxel size.

7 Bibliography

[1] Blake A., Curwen R., Zisserman A. A Framework for Spatiotemporal Control in the Tracking of Visual Contours. *IJCV*, 11(2):127-145, 1993.

[2] Brechbühler CH., Gerig G, Szekely G. Compensation of Spatial Inhomogeneity in MRI Based on a Parametric Bias Estimate. *Lecture Notes in Computer Science* 1131, Proc. VBC'96, Eds: Karl H. Hoehne and Ron Kikinis, pp. 141-146, 1996.
[3] Cootes T.F., Hill A., Taylor C.J., Haslam J. The Use of Active Shape Models for Locating Structures in Medical Images. *Image Vision and Computing*, vol. 12, no. 6, jul. 94.
[4] Colchester A.C.F., Gerig G., Crow T., Ayache N. and Vandermeulen D. Development and Validation of Techniques for Brain Morphometry (BIOMORPH). In *Proc. CVRMED'97*.
[5] Crow T.J. Temporal Lobe Asymmetries as the Key Etiology of Schizophrenia. *Schizophrenia Bulletin* 16, pp. 433-443, 1990.
[6] Delingette H. *Simplex Meshes: a General Representation for 3D Shape Reconstruction*. INRIA research report no. 2214. March 1994.
[7] DeLisi L.E., Tew W., Xie S., Hoff S.L., Sakuma M., Kushner M., Lee G., Shedlack K., Smith A.M., Grimson R. A Prospective Follow-up Study of Brain Morphology and Cognition in First-Episode Schizophrenic Patients: Preliminary Findings. *Biol. Psychiatry* 38, pp. 349-360, 1995.
[8] Gilles S., Brady M., Thirion J.P., Ayache N. Bias Field Correction and Segmentation of MR Images. Visualization in Biomedical Computing, Proceedings of VBC'96, vol. 1131 of *Lecture Notes in Computer Science*, pp. 153-158, Ed. Springer Verlag, 1996.
[9] González Ballester M.A. *Computer-Aided MRI-Based Analysis of Brain Morphology*. DPhil transfer report, University of Oxford, July 1997.
[10] González Ballester M.A., Zisserman A., Brady M. Combined Statistical and Geometrical 3D Segmentation and Measurement of Brain Structures. *Proc. Workshop on Biomedical Image Analysis*, Santa Barbara, Ca., 1998.
[11] Guillemaud R., Brady M. Estimating the Bias Field of MR Images. *IEEE Transactions on Medical Imaging*, vol. 16, no. 3, pg. 238, 1997.
[12] Kass M., Witkin A., Terzopoulus D. Snakes: Active Contour Models. *Proceedings of ICCV*, pp. 259-268, 1987.
[13] Marais P. In preparation.
[14] Marais P., Guillemaud R., Sakuma M., Zisserman A., Brady M. Visualising Cerebral Asymmetry. *Lecture Notes in Computer Science* 1131, Proc. VBC'96, Eds: Karl Heinz Hoehne and Ron Kikinis, pp. 411-416, 1996.
[15] McInerney D., Terzopoulos T. A Finite Element Model for 3D Shape Reconstruction and Nonrigid Motion Tracking. In *Proceedings of the Fourth Int. Conf. on Computer Vision (ICCV'93)*, pp. 518-523, 1993.
[16] Röll S.A., Colchester A.C.F., Summers P.E., Griffin L.D. Intensity-Based Object Extraction from 3D Medical Images Including a Correction for Partial Volume Errors. *Proceedings of BMVC*, pp. 195-204, 1994.
[17] Schmitt F., Chen X., Du W.H. Geometric Modelling From Range Image Data. *Proceedings of Eurographics'91*, pp. 317-328, Ed. Elsevier, 1991.
[18] Székely G., Kelemen A., Brechbühler C., Gerig G. Segmentation of 2-D and 3-D Objects from MRI Volume Data Using Constrained Elastic Deformations of Flexible Fourier Contour and Surface Models. *Medical Image Analysis*, vol. 1, no. 1, pp. 19-34.
[19] Van Leemput K., Vandermeulen D., Suetens P. *Automatic Segmentation of Brain Tissues and MR Bias Correction Using a Digital Brain Atlas*. Technical report, Kathoelieke Universiteit Leuven, Leuven, Belgium, Jan. 1998.
[20] Wells III W.M., Grimson W.E.L., Kikinis R., Jolesz F.A. Adaptive Segmentation of MRI Data. *IEEE Transactions on Medical Imaging*, vol. 15, no. 4, pp. 429-442, 1996.

Automatic Identificaiton of Cortical Sulci Using a 3D Probabilistic Atlas

Georges Le Goualher[1,2], D. Louis Collins[1], Christian Barillot[2], and Alan C. Evans[1]

[1] McConnell Brain Imaging Center, Montréal Neurological Institute,
McGill University, Montréal, Canada
georges@bic.mni.mcgill.ca,
WWW home page: http://www.bic.mni.mcgill/users/georges

[2] Laboratoire Signaux et Images en Médecine, Université de Rennes, France

Abstract. We present an approach which performs the automatic labeling of the main cortical sulci using *a priori* information for the 3D spatial distribution of these entities. We have developed a methodology to extract the 3D cortical topography of a particular subject from *in vivo* observations obtained through MRI. The cortical topography is encoded in a relational graph structure composed of two main features: arcs and vertices. Each vertex contains a parametric surface representing the buried part of a sulcus. Points on this parametric surface are expressed in stereotaxic coordinates (*i.e.*, with respect to a standardized brain coordinate system). Arcs represent the connections between these entities. Manual sulcal labeling is performed by tagging a sulcal surface in the 3-D graph and selecting from a menu of candidate sulcus names. Automatic labeling is dependent on a probabilistic atlas of sulcal anatomy derived from a set of 51 graphs that were labeled by an anatomist. We show how these 3D sulcal spatial distribution maps can be used to perform the identification of the cortical sulci. We focus our attention on the peri-central area (including pre-central, post-central and central sulci). Results show that the use of spatial priors permit automatic identification of the main sulci with a good accuracy.

keywords: active model, probabilistic atlas, cerebral cortex, sulci, MRI.

1 Introduction

Cortical sulci and gyri define *gross* anatomical landmarks on the surface of the cerebral cortex. Several studies have suggested that some major functional areas can be located with respect to these anatomical landmarks, allowing *a priori* localization of functional areas. The most important illustration of such an anatomo-functional correlation comes from the observation that the central sulcus delimits the sensory area (located on its posterior gyrus, known as the postcentral gyrus) from the motor area located on its anterior gyrus (precentral gyrus). Such *a priori* knowledge of functional localization is incorporated in many neurological applications (neurosurgery, for example). However, high inter-individual variability of the cortical topography (associated with the intrinsic complexity of the 3D cortical fold patterns) make the identification of these landmarks a tedious task. We know that variability of the cortical topography is due to gross brain shape differences between individuals, but also to structural deformation of the cortex. This deformation appears in particular when a sulcus (generally associated with a continuous cortical fold) is decomposed in several apparently independent folds on another subject. Similarly, generally connected adjacent sulci can be sometimes disconnected. Finally, tertiary sulci seem to have random patterns. Processes that are used by experts to perform the identification of cortical folds mix both structural and spatial *a priori* knowledge on the most likely structural patterns of the cortical sulci and their most likely location. Recently, probabilistic brain atlas methodology has been introduced to deal with the intrinsic brain shape variability [1]. This methodology allows the construction of 3D probability maps representing the normal spatial variability of the main anatomical structures. In this paper, we study the use of such a 3D probabilistic atlas of the main sulci, computed from 51 brains, to perform the identification of the cortical folds based on spatial priors.

In the following we describe our methodology to extract a 3D representation of the cortical topography from 3D MRIs. By working systematically in a standardized brain coordinate system, we are allowed to study the 3D spatial variability of the extracted cortical sulci. These probabilistic maps provide us with *a priori* knowledge on the localization of the main sulci and can be used to assist in the identification of the main cortical sulci. Here, we particularly focus our attention on the identification of the sulci of the peri-central area (precentral, central and postcentral sulcus).

2 Background

For several years now, an increasing interest has been given to both the segmentation of the cortical topography as well as its automatic labeling. The range of image processing and pattern recognition methodologies applied to these tasks are wide, leading to a difficult classification or comparison. We have chosen to first make a distinction between methodologies that model the cortical topography of a single subject without labeling individual sulci, from methodologies that attempt to identify specific cortical patterns.

2.1 Representation of the Cortical Topography

The goal of the cortical topography modeling is to represent explicitly each cortical fold and the organization of these entities (connection, adjacency). At this step it is particularly convenient to distinguish between :

– modeling of single *versus* all cortical folds
– modeling of exterior trace *versus* median surface

Existing methods can be classed of crossovers between these two subgroups :

- modeling of exterior trace of all cortical folds [2][3][4]
- modeling of the median surface of a cortical fold [5][6]
- modeling of the median surface of all the cortical folds [7] [8] [9]

Considering the fact that more than 2/3 of the total cortical surface is buried within the cortical folds, it is of the utmost importance to model the median surface of the sulci, not only the superior trace. This kind of modeling allows a better understanding of the cerebral cortex topography by showing patterns that previously were only observable form *post mortem* subjects.

2.2 Automatic Identification of the Cortical Topography

Identification of the cortical folds can be proposed through the atlas matching paradigm [10] [2] [4]. In this methodology a brain model (where all anatomical structures have been labeled) is matched to a studied brain. Identification of anatomical structures on the studied brain is then realized by transferring the labels contained in the model to the studied brain through the recovered non-linear warping. However the considerable inter-subject structural variability of the cerebral cortex topography is not sufficiently well-modeled to allow accurate labeling of individual sulci by this methodology [11]. In particular the basic hypothesis (one to one correspondence between each voxel of the brain model and the studied brain) on which the elastic warping method is based in not verified for the cortical topography.

More complete *a priori* information about the normal cortical topography is needed to perform a correct identification of the cortical folds. Both statistics about structural patterns of the cortical fold (information which can be seen as being independent from a coordinate system) and information regarding the spatial localization of the cortical folds are necessary to perform a correct identification. In [12] [3] [13] such informations are used to perform the identification of 6 main sulci. Knowledge is expressed in the form of heuristics that are defined for each of the sulci. Recognition is performed as a search through the combination of automatically extracted sulcus patterns that best match a heuristic model (note that heuristics have to be defined for each sulcus of interest). The weakness of this application stems from the fact that the recognition is performed in a sequential manner (recognition of the central sulcus, followed by the research of the pre-central sulcus, ...), a method that seems to differ from the constant accept/reject trial hypothesis as performed by an expert. Another promising application has been developed by Mangin et al. [8]. In this application the cortical topography is modeled as the realization of a random graph. Recognition is performed through graph matching between a model graph containing information about the normal variability of the cortical topography and the corresponding graph of the studied subject brain. The methodology used is based on the structural pattern recognition paradigm where information about the structural decomposition of an object is used to automatically performed its identification. While the structural knowledge on the main sulci is explicitly used in this application, spatial priors (which represent also important knowledge to drive the recognition problem) are poorly used. In fact, in this application only a bounding box defines the *a priori* localization of each sulcus. Moreover, the matching method, based on a simulated annealing algorithm, is computationally intensive and requires the adjustment of numerous *ad hoc* parameters.

From our knowledge, few methods have been based on the use of spatial priors (however refer to[14]), and of these only a few sample brains are used to estimate the 3D probability maps of the sulci. Also, it is not well known if a good labeling of cortical sulci can be performed through this simple use of spatial priors.

The method we propose here to assist the labeling of the cortical folds consists of assigning to each automatically extracted cortical fold, the sulcus' name for which the associated 3D probability map is maximum, given the location of the actual fold. This involves *i)* the extraction of an explicit representation of the cortical topography composed of a set of folds and junctions between these entities; *ii)* the computation in a standardized 3D stereotaxic space in order to compute the sulcal probability maps and link the actual 3D spatial position of a cortical fold with these computed probability maps. The method we have used to solve *i)* can be classified as a method which *models the median surface of all the cortical folds* (refer to section 2.1) and will be described in the following section. The second point (*ii*) is solved by using an automatic linear matching algorithm which transforms each brain into a standardized stereotaxic space. 3D sulcal distributions are then computed in this common referential frame. Resulting 3D maps (computed from 51 brains) are then used to identify the cortical folds. Results show colored extracted 3D cortical topography graphs, where each color corresponds to a specific sulcus name.

3 Modeling of the Cortical Topography

We describe here the method used to extract the cortical topography from a 3D MRI.

3.1 Preprocessing

The goal of the preprocessing is to extract the brain tissues, namely the Grey Matter (GM) and the White Matter (WM). An artificial neural network classifier is applied to identify GM/WM/CSF tissue types [15] on 3-D MRI, after correction for 3-D intensity non-uniformity[16]. The classification method uses spatial priors on the location of each tissue type. This last condition implies that all computations must be carried out in common referential frame. Therefore, we use an automatic registration program which uses a 3-D cross-correlation approach to match the single MRI volume with the intensity average of 305 MRI brain volumes previously aligned into standardized stereotaxic space [17]. The registered volumes are then resampled on a 1 mm^3 voxel grid. A geometric surface representing the brain cortical surface is automatically extracted using iterative minimization of a cost function [18]. This last step separates voxels belonging to the brain from those located in the cerebellum. All following computations are carried out within the standardized stereotaxic space (refer also to section 4).

3.2 Processing

Detection of each Sulcus Exterior Trace The method we have used to detect the exterior traces of cortical sulci combines morphological closing (dilatation followed by an erosion) [19] to fill the interspace between adjacent walls of a sulcus and curvature analysis in the cerebral cortex. We have previously shown that the sign of the mean curvature was a good indicator to separate the sulci from the gyri (refer to [20]). By detecting the voxels which have a positive curvature on the bounding hull of the brain we are able to detect the superior traces of the sulci. We apply a thinning method (refer to [21]) in order to reduce this set of voxels to a set of curves and junctions between curves. We obtain at this step the superior traces of the sulci.

Detection of each Sulcus Median Surface We then model each of these curves with our active ribbon method in order to extract the median surface of each sulcus [22].To summarize, the active ribbon method consists of modeling each curve by a spline and subjecting it to a set of forces designed such that the active model will move smoothly from the initial superior trace of the sulcus toward the bottom of the sulcus. The second step of the active ribbon method consists of modeling the successive loci of this active curve , from its initial position towards its final position, by an active surface which converges toward the actual median surface of the fold. The active ribbon method allows for the retrieval of a parametric surface representing the median surface of each fold of the cerebral cortex.

3.3 Encoding of the Cortical Topography

The representation of the cortical topography is directly derived from these results :

$$G_{CT} = \{F, J\}$$

where G_{CT}, the Graph representing the Cortical Topography of a particular subject, is composed of F a set of f folds (one or several folds may constitute a sulcus as defined by an anatomist) and J a set of j junctions (see examples on figure 2).

4 Computation of 3D sulcal probabilistic maps

As said previously, all computations are realized in the same brain-based coordinate system after application of the automatic linear matching algorithm used during the preprocessing (refer to section 3.1). The coordinate system is defined as follows :

- $(0, \vec{x}, \vec{y}, \vec{z})$: where 0 the origin of the coordinate system is the anterior commisure (AC) ; $\vec{x}, \vec{y}, \vec{z}$ are oriented like the brain referential frame defined by Talairach [23], with $\vec{x}$ left-right axis, $\vec{y}$ the postero-anterior axis and $\vec{z}$ the inferior-superior axis.
- (sx, sy, sz) : linear scaling factors. In order to reduce the spatial variability of brain structures due to gross brain size differences, all brains are fit into the same bounding box after registration (refer to [17]).

An anatomist has identified 16 main sulci on 51 extracted cortical topography graphs. These sulci were : (a) the Central Sulcus and (b) the Sylvian Fissure; (c) the Superior, (d) the Middle, and (e) the Inferior Frontal Sulci; (f) the Ascending and (g) the Horizontal Rami of the Sylvian Fissure, as well as (h) the Incisura (located between these other two rami); (i) the Olfactory Sulcus as well as (j) the Sulcus Lateralis, (k) the Sulcus Medialis, (l) the Sulcus Intermedius, and (m) the Sulcus Transversus (all found along the orbitofrontal surface of the brain); (n) the Precentral and (o) the Postcentral Sulci; and finally (p) the Intraparietal Sulcus.

By averaging the labelings of a structure, a continuous 3-D probability field (0.00-1.00 at each voxel) can be constructed for each identified structure. This average is known as a Statistical Probability Anatomy Map (SP_AM)[24].

5 Sulcus Identification Using a Probabilistic Atlas

5.1 Estimation of a Pertinent Probability Threshold

To define this threshold we study the overlap between adjacent SP_AMs. Illustrations of such overlaps with respect to a selected threshold can be seen on the figure 1.

We conclude that a probability threshold of value $p_{thresh} = 0.1$ yields a minimal overlap between adjacent SP_AMs.

5.2 Identification

Identification is performed as follows: for each automatically extracted fold we can compute the probability that this fold belongs to each computed SP_AM. We then have a probability vector:

$$\vec{p} = [p(\theta_0), \ldots, p(\theta_{m-1})] \tag{1}$$

where m is the number of computed SP_AMs, θ_i is a sulcus name. We then find the maximum element of this vector, let say $p(\theta_k)$, and apply the following rule:

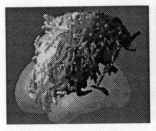 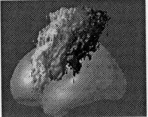 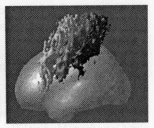

Fig. 1. From left to right : 3D iso-surfaces of the sulcal distribution (computed from 51 subjects) for the precentral, central and postcentral sulci thresholded at different levels. **Left** image is obtained with a probability threshold $p_{thresh} = 0.001$. All the voxels which have a value superior to this threshold are kept. As the minimum non-zero probability value is 1/51, all non-zero locations of probability maps are kept. One can see the important overlap between these adjacent SP_AMs. **Middle:** $p_{thresh} = 0.05$. **Right:** $p_{thresh} = 0.1$. One can see the null overlap when taking this threshold. Note that with this threshold, all the voxels kept belong to the same sulcus on at least 6 different subjects upon 51. (*note that the brain model, displayed at 50% of its original size, is only used to figure the orientation*)

if $p(\theta_k) \geq p_{thresh}$
then affect the name θ_k to the corresponding fold
else
affect *unknown name* to the corresponding fold

Results for the identification of 4 brains are shown on figure 2. Almost all parts of superior, middle and inferior frontal sulcus are correctly identified. Only a few small portions of the central, precentral and postcentral sulci are incorrectly identified. This of course has to be interpreted with the caveat that the anatomist's labeling may not be *correct* for secondary or tertiary sulci.

6 Conclusion

The used of spatial priors to identify cortical sulci has been shown to give a very promising initial guess on the labeling of the main cortical sulci. This illustrates an application of the probabilistic atlas paradigm. When extended to all cortical sulci, the use of spatial priors allows to give a vector of initial probabilities for each possible sulcus name for each cortical fold. Even if the simple sulcus name assignment we have presented based on maximum of probability of sulcal spatial distributions will not be always sufficient to give an exact labeling (due to the density and high variability of sulcal pattern), this methodology considerably decreases the state space of the sulcus recognition problem and gives an initialization for a more complex structural probabilistic matching algorithm which could include knowledge on the most likely structural pattern for each cortical fold or knowledge on admissible sphape deformations [25]. We are now working on the design of such an algorithm.

7 Acknowledgments

The authors are grateful to the Region Council of Brittany (France) for their financial support of this work. They express their appreciation for support from the Canadian Medical Research Council (SP-30), the McDonnell-Pew Cognitive Neuroscience Center Program, the U.S. Human Brain Map Project (HBMP), NIMH and NIDA. This work forms part of a continuing project of the HBMP-funded International Consortium for Brain Mapping (ICBM) to develop a probabilistic atlas of human neuroanatomy.

References

1. J.C. MAZZIOTA, A.W. TOGA, A.C. EVANS, P. FOX, and J. LANCASTER. A probabilistic atlas of the human brain : theory and rationale for its development. *Neuroimage*, 2:89–101, 1995.
2. S. SANDOR and R. LEAHY. Surface-based labeling of cortical anatomy using a deformable atlas. *IEEE Transactions on Medical Imaging*, 16(1):41–54, Feb 1997.
3. N.ROYACKKERS, H. FAWAL, M. DESVIGNES, M. REVENU, and J.M. TRAVERE. Feature extraction for cortical sulci identification. In 9th *Scandinavian conference on image analysis*, volume 2, pages 110–121, June 1995.
4. G. SUBSOL, J.P. THIRION, and N. AYACHE. Application of an automatically build 3D morphometric atlas: Study of cerebral ventricle shape. In Karl Heinz Hohne and Ron Kikinis, editors, *Visualization in Biomedical Computing (VBC)*, pages 373–382. LNCS 1131, Sept 1996.
5. G. LE GOUALHER, C. BARILLOT, Y. BIZAIS, and J-M. SCARABIN. 3D segmentation of cortical sulci using active models. In *SPIE Proceedings of Medical Imaging : Image Processing*, volume 2710, pages 254–263, 1996.
6. Marc VAILLANT, Christos DAVATZIKOS, and R.Nick BRYAN. Finding 3D parametric representations of deep cortical folds. In *Workshops on Math. Methods in Biomedical Image Analysis*, pages 151–159, 1996.
7. G. SZEKELY, Ch. BRECHUHLER, O. KUBLER, R. OGNIEWICKZ, and T. BUDINGER . Mapping the human cerebral cortex using 3-D medial manifolds. In *SPIE Visualization in Biomedical Computing*, volume 1808, pages 130–144, 1992.
8. J.F.MANGIN, J. REGIS, I. BLOCH, V. FROUIN, Y. SAMSON, and J. LOPEZ-KRAHE. A MRF based random graph modelling the human cortical topography. In *CVRMed*, pages 177–183, Nice, France, April 1995. LNCS 905.
9. Gabriele LOHMANN, Frithjof KRUGGEL, and D.Yves VON CRAMON. Automatic detection of sulcal bottom lines in MR images of the human brain. In *Information Processing in Medical Imaging (IPMI)*, pages 369–374. LNCS 1230, 1997.
10. R. BAJCSY and S. KOVACIC. Multiresolution elastic matching. *Computer Vision, Graphics, and Image Processing*, 46:1–21, 1989.
11. D.L. COLLINS, G. LE GOUALHER, R. VENUGOPAL, Z. CARAMANOS, A.C. EVANS, and C. BARILLOT . Cortical constraints for non-linear cortical registration. In K.H. Höene, editor, *Visualization in Biomedical Computing*, pages 307–316, Hamburg, Sept 1996.

12. H. FAWALL. *Contribution à l'étude d'une base de connaissances adaptée à la définition des sillons du cortex cérébral humain*. PhD thesis, Université de Caen, 1995.
13. M. DESVIGNES, N. ROYACKKERS, H. FAWAL, and M. REVENU. Detection and identification of sulci on 3D MRI. In *Human Brain Mapping*, volume 4, page S410, 1997.
14. F. KRUGGEL. Automatical adaptation of anatomical masks to the neocortex. In *Proceedings of the 1th International Conference CVRMed*, volume LNCS 905, France, April 1995.
15. A. ZIJDENBOS, A.C. EVANS, F. RIAHI, J. SLED, J. CHUI, and V. KOLLOKIAN. Automatic quantification of multiple sclerosis lesion volume using stereotaxic space. In *Visualisation in Biomedical Computing (VBC)*, pages 439–448. 4th International Conference, LNCS 1131, september 1996.
16. John G. SLED, Alex P. ZIJDENBOS, and Alan C. EVANS. A non-parametric method for automatic correction of intensity non-uniformity in MRI data. *IEEE Transactions on Medical Imaging*, 17(1):87–97, February 1998. submitted December 1996.
17. D.L. COLLINS, P. NEELIN, T.M. PETERS, and A.C. EVANS. Automatic 3D intersubject registration of MR volumetric data in standardized Talairach space. *Journal of Computer Assisted Tomography*, 18(2):192–205, March, April 1994.
18. D.MACDONALD, D. AVIS, and A.C. EVANS. Multiple surface identification and matching in Magnetic Resonance Images. In *Visualization in Biomedical Computing (VBC)*, volume 2359, pages 160–169, Rochester, 1994.
19. J. SERRA. *Image analysis and mathematical morphology*. Academic Press, London, 1982.
20. G. LE GOUALHER, C. BARILLOT, L. LE BRIQUER, and Y. BIZAIS. 3D detection and representation of cortical sulci. In *Computer Assisted Radiology, CAR'95*, 1995.
21. G. MALANDIN, G. BERTRAND, and N. AYACHE. Topological segmentation of discrete surfaces. In *IEEE Conference on Computer Vision and Pattern Recognition*, pages 444–449, 1991.
22. G. LE GOUALHER, C. BARILLOT, and Y. BIZAIS. Modeling cortical sulci using active ribbons. *International Journal of Pattern Recognition and Artificial Intelligence*, 11(8):1295–1315, 1997.
23. J. TALAIRACH and P. TOURNOUX. *Co-planar stereotactic atlas of the human brain: 3-Dimensional proportional system: an approach to cerebral imaging*. Georg Thieme Verlag, Stuttgart, New York, 1988.
24. A.C EVANS, D.L. COLLINS, C. HOLMES, T. PAUS, D. MACDONALD, A. ZIJDENBOS, A. TOGA, P. FOX, J. LANCASTER, and J. MAZZIOTA. A 3D probabilistic atlas of normal human neuroanatomy. In *Human Brain Mapping*, volume 4, page S349, 1997.
25. A. CAUNCE and C.J. TAYLOR. 3D point distribution models of cortical sulci. In *ICCV*, Bombay, India, january 1998.

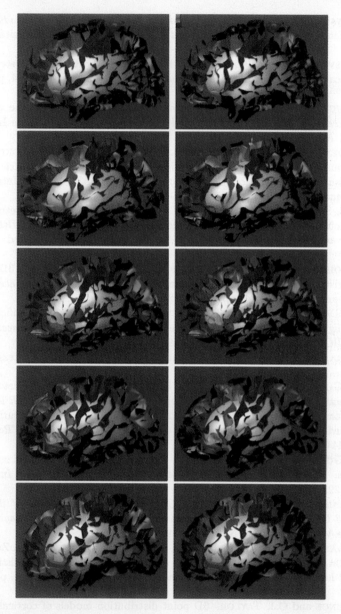

Fig. 2. from top to bottom : 5 different subjects. **left** : automatic labeling using spatial priors, **right** : associated manual labeling by an anatomist; magenta : central sul.; red : sylvian fiss.; **frontal lobe** : yellow:precentral s.; mustard: superior frontal s.; red : middle frontal s.; violet : inferior frontal s.; green : ascending ramus of the syl. fiss.; **antero-inferior part of the frontal lobe** : yellow : horizontal ramus of the syl. fiss.; green : intermedius fronto-orbital s.; blue : lateralis front.-orb. sul.; **parietal lobe** : blue : postcentral s.; green : intraparietal s.; black : unknown; (*note that the brain model, displayed at 50% of its original size, is only used to figure the orientation*)

Segmentation and Measurement of the Cortex from 3D MR Images

Xiaolan Zeng[1], Lawrence H. Staib[1], Robert T. Schultz[2], and James S. Duncan[1]

[1] Departments of Electrical Engineering and Diagnostic Radiology,
[2] Child Study Center,   Yale University, New Haven, CT, 06520-8042

Abstract. The cortex is the outermost thin layer of gray matter in the brain; geometric measurement of the cortex helps in understanding brain anatomy and function. In the quantitative analysis of the cortex from MR images, extracting the structure and obtaining a representation for various measurements are key steps. While manual segmentation is tedious and labor intensive, automatic, reliable and efficient segmentation and measurement of the cortex remain challenging problems due to its convoluted nature. A new approach of coupled surfaces propagation using level set methods is presented here for the problem of the segmentation and measurement of the cortex. Our method is motivated by the nearly constant thickness of the cortical mantle and takes this tight coupling as an important constraint. By evolving two embedded surfaces simultaneously, each driven by its own image-derived information while maintaining the coupling, a final representation of the cortical bounding surfaces and an automatic segmentation of the cortex are achieved. Characteristics of the cortex such as cortical surface area, surface curvature and thickness are then evaluated. The level set implementation of surface propagation offers the advantage of easy initialization, computational efficiency and the ability to capture deep folds of the sulci. Results and validation from various experiments on simulated and real 3D MR images are provided.

1 Introduction

A significant amount of the recent anatomical MRI studies on the human brain have been focused on the cerebral cortex. The cerebral cortex is the outermost layer of gray matter in the brain. It is composed of columns of neurons, aligned perpendicularly to the cortical surface, that serve as basic units of information processing in the brain. Cortical surface area is likely to be proportional to column number and therefore surface area should be related to functional capacities. In addition, regional cortical thickness and gray matter volume may relate to functional capacities, and alteration in each of these features has been suspected in specific neuropsychiatric disorders([17]). In the quantitative analysis of these features of the cortex, segmentation is the first step.

The cerebral cortex is characterized by its convoluted surface. Due to this convoluted nature, the segmentation of the cortex must be considered in 3D. For example, although the cerebral cortical layer is about 3mm thick([1]), an oblique 2D slice that happens to be approximately parallel to a particular sulcus will give the appearance of a much thicker structure. Only by going through the neighboring slices can we get complete information to perform segmentation. Slice by slice manual tracing of the cortex is extremely tedious and labor intensive, hence automatic, reliable and relatively efficient segmentation which enables automated measurement is a highly desirable goal.

1.1 Related work

There has been a large amount of work devoted to automatic 3D segmentation. One type of approach uses region-based methods, which exploit homogeneity in images. Following the work of Geman & Geman[7], Markov Random Field(MRF)-based methods have been widely used. For example, a multispectral voxel classification method was used in conjunction with connectivity to segment the brain into different tissue types from 3D MR images[2]. Material mixture models were also used for the segmentation problem. Region-based methods typically require further processing to group segmented parts into coherent structure(s). Moreover, quantitative measurement of features other than volume does not follow immediately.

A typical alternative strategy is boundary finding, of which active contour methods are of special note. They rely mainly on gradient features for segmentation of structures. For instance, a 3D deformable surface model using the finite-element method was used to segment 3D images[3]. One concern regarding this type of method is that close initialization has to be provided in order to achieve good final results. Also, the need to override the local smoothness constraint to allow for significant protrusions (which is highly desirable in order to capture the sulcal folds) remains a problem.

An iterative algorithm was presented by MacDonald *et al.* for simultaneous deformation of multiple surfaces to segment MRI data with inter-surface constraints and self-intersection avoidance, where surface deformation was formulated as a cost function minimization problem[13]. This method was applied to 3D MR brain data to extract surface models for the skull and the cortical surface. This approach takes advantage of the information of the interrelation between the surfaces of interest. However, drawbacks lie in its extremely high computational expense, and the difficulty of tuning the weighting factors in the cost function due to the complexity of the problem.

Teo *et al.*[19] used a system that exploited knowledge of cortical anatomy, in which white matter and CSF regions were first segmented, then the connectivity of the white matter was verified in regions of interest. Finally a connected representation of the gray matter was created by a constrained growing-out from the white matter boundary. The focus of this work was to create a representation of cortical gray matter for functional MRI visualization.

Davatzikos *et al.* [4] introduced the concept of a ribbon for modeling the outer cortex in cross-sectional brain images and then extended the model into 3D[5]. A deformable surface algorithm was constructed to find the central layer of the cortex. Based on this parameterization, the cortical structure was characterized through its depth map and curvature map. This method explicitly used the structural information of the cortex. However, close initialization and significant human interaction are needed to force the ribbon into sulcal folds.

2 Our Approach

The cortical layer to be recovered has an nearly constant thickness and is bounded by two surfaces: the CSF/gray matter boundary and gray/white matter boundary. Across each surface, there is a local difference in the gray level values, while in between the two surfaces there is a homogeneity of certain voxel statistics. For our purposes, the cortical layer is defined completely by its bounding surfaces and the homogeneity in between. Following our earlier work[20], we propose a new approach of coupled surfaces propagation via level set methods for the segmentation and measurement of the cortex. By evolving two embedded surfaces simultaneously, each driven by its own image-based information while maintaining the coupling, we are able to achieve an automatic and robust segmentation of the cortex, and simultaneously obtain a representation of the inner and outer cortical surfaces from which surface area can be calculated. Furthermore, curvature and thickness maps are easily obtained from this coupled level set formulation.

2.1 Image information derivation

In order to capture the notion of homogeneity inside the cortical layer, we have designed an image gray level-based local operator to obtain the likelihood of each voxel lying on the outer and inner cortical surfaces respectively, instead of using the gradient information alone. This model can potentially be extended to make use of a vector of registered parametric images (such as T1, T2 and PD MR images) or images from different modalities.

At each voxel site s, a small neighborhood around s is drawn(see Figure 2). Now given a possible boundary with normal direction θ, dividing the neighborhood into parts $R1$ and $R2$, the probability that s lies on the boundary between tissue A and tissue B is:

$$p_{AB}(\theta) = p(R1 \in TissueA) \cdot p(R2 \in TissueB) \quad (1)$$

Given an estimation θ^* of θ, we can use $p_{AB}(\theta^*)$ as a measure of the likelihood that s lies on the boundary between tissue A and tissue B.

One way of estimating θ^* is to first generate the vector $P = [p(\theta_1), p(\theta_2), ..., p(\theta_k)]^T$, and θ^* is then the one which corresponds to the element of largest magnitude in vector P. Here we make the assumption of a single parametric image X, in which voxels belonging to tissue A are independently drawn from a Gaussian distribution $G(\mu_A, \sigma_A)$, and voxels belonging to tissue B are independently drawn from $G(\mu_B, \sigma_B)$. We have

$$p_{AB}(\theta) = \prod_{r \in R1} \frac{1}{\sqrt{2\pi}\sigma_A} e^{-\frac{(X_r - \mu_A)^2}{\sigma_A^2}} \cdot \prod_{t \in R2} \frac{1}{\sqrt{2\pi}\sigma_B} e^{-\frac{(X_t - \mu_B)^2}{\sigma_B^2}} \quad (2)$$

In Figure 1, we show an example of the result from our local operator. The local operator was applied to images after we reduced the effects of MR inhomogeneity by correcting using a simple fixed map. The map was determined manually by sampling tissue types throughout the field to decide the average inhomogeneity. Note that more complicated MR image models ([7],[11],[10]) can be used to calculate $p(\theta)$.

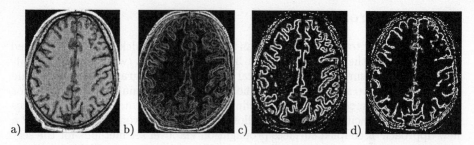

Fig. 1. Results from our local operator compared to image gradient. (a): axial slice from the original 3D brain images; (b): result from gradient operator; (c): result from our local operator $p_{BC}(\theta^*)$, B= gray matter, C=white matter; (d)$p_{AB}(\theta^*)$, A= CSF, B=gray matter.

2.2 Level set method

Level set methods ([18],[14],[15]) are powerful numerical techniques for analyzing and computing interface motion. The essential idea is to represent the surface (in our case) of interest as a front $\gamma(t)$, and embed this propagating front as the zero level set of a higher dimensional function Ψ defined by $\Psi(x,t) = d$, where d is the signed distance from position x to $\gamma(t)$. An Eulerian formulation is produced for the motion of this surface propagating along its normal direction with speed F, where F can be a function of the surface characteristics (such as the curvature, normal direction etc.) and the image characteristics (e.g. the gray level, gradient etc.) The equation of the evolution of Ψ, inside which our surface is embedded as the zero level set is then given by $\Psi_t + F \mid \nabla \Psi \mid = 0$.

The major advantages of using this method over other active contour strategies include the following. First, the evolving level function $\Psi(x,t)$ remains a function; however the propagating front $\gamma(t)$ may change topology, break, merge (this allows the flexibility of the initialization in image segmentation) and form sharp corners as Ψ evolves. Second, the intrinsic geometric properties of the front may be easily determined from Ψ. For example, at any point of the front, the normal vector is given by $n = \nabla \Psi$.

2.3 Coupled surfaces propagation, speed term design

In solving the problem of segmenting the cortex, we consider two moving interfaces describing the inner and outer cortical bounding surfaces respectively. Starting from inside the inner cortical surface (i.e. inside the white matter), with an offset in between, the interfaces propagate along the outward normal direction and stop at the desired place, while maintaining the distance between them.

Embedding each surface as the zero level set in its own level function, we have two equations:

$$\Psi_{in_t} + F_{in} \mid \nabla \Psi_{in} \mid = 0 \qquad (3)$$
$$\Psi_{out_t} + F_{out} \mid \nabla \Psi_{out} \mid = 0 \qquad (4)$$

where F_{in} and F_{out} are functions of the surface normal direction, image-derived information and distance between the two surfaces. The coupling is embedded in the design of F_{in} and F_{out}. At places where the distance between the two surfaces is within the normal range, the two surfaces propagate according to the image-based information. Where the distance between the two surfaces is out of the normal range, the distance imposes a constraint on the propagation of the surfaces.

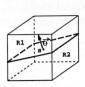 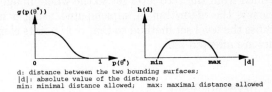

Fig. 2. A local operator to derive image information.

Fig. 3. Functions g and h used in speed term design.

The motivation behind using the coupling constraint between the two surfaces is to make the image information on the partner surface available to the other, thus improving the segmentation result. For example, due to volume averaging, in some regions of the image, the inner cortical boundary may not be well defined while the CSF appears clearly. A single surface approach might result in the inner cortical surface collapsing into CSF. However with the coupling constraint, a minimum distance from the inner cortical surface to CSF is maintained, thus preventing the inner surface from going into CSF. There are also cases near structures such as eye sockets where the CSF can not be observed. While a single surface will grow into these foreign structures, the coupled surfaces approach stops the propagation of the outer cortical surface using the information from the inner cortical surface. (see Figure 9)

With the level set implementation, we have a natural way to establish a correspondence between the points on the two evolving surfaces through distance, which is evaluated without extra computational expense. Recall that the value of the level function of a front at any point is simply the distance from this point to the current front, which is calculated as the shortest distance from this point to all the points on the front[18]. In our case of two moving surfaces, for any point on the inner moving surface, the distance to the outer moving surface is the value Ψ_{out} at this point, and vice versa for the point on the outer moving surface. Hence, we write

$$F_{in} = g(p_{BC}(\boldsymbol{\theta}^*))h(\Psi_{out}) \tag{5}$$
$$F_{out} = g(p_{AB}(\boldsymbol{\theta}^*))h(\Psi_{in}) \tag{6}$$

where g and h are the functions as shown in Figure 3, and A, B, C denote CSF, gray matter and white matter respectively.

Function g maps larger likelihood to slower speed, i.e., as the likelihood gets larger, g tends to zero, while as the likelihood gets to near zero, g tends to a constant. Function h penalizes the distance off the normal range. As the distance goes out of normal range, h goes to zero. Thus, each surface moves with constant speed along the normal direction and slows down when either the image-based information becomes strong or the distance to the other surface moves away from the normal range. Each surface finally stops when the image-derived information is strong enough or the distance to the other surface is out of the normal range. The speed term only has meaning on the front, i.e. the zero level set. It is then extended from the zero level set to the whole image grid[18]. For computational efficiency, the algorithm is implemented using a narrow band method, which modifies the level set method so that only points close to the current propagating fronts are affected [20].

2.4 Measurement

With coupled surfaces propagation via the level set method, it is easy to perform various measurements on the cortical layer with little extra computational expense. Whole brain volume, cortical gray matter volume, white matter volume, cortical surface area, cortical surface shape and cortical thickness maps are among the features most interesting in the study of brain structure and function. Different combinations of the above measurements may help in determining the pathobiology of various neuropsychiatric disorders. We now discuss one by one the above measurements from our coupled surfaces formulation.

Volume With the signed distance function Ψ, the level set formulation keeps track of the inside and outside of the current moving front. Once the evolution of the coupled surfaces is completed, the cortical gray matter voxels are those that lie inside the outer cortical surface while outside the inner cortical surface. In the same fashion, non-brain tissue voxels will be the ones that are outside the outer cortical surface, and voxels of white matter will lie inside the inner cortical surface except for subcortical gray matter and ventricles. Because the signed distance based measures are more accurate than the voxel size based measures, we can obtain a partial volume segmentation on the data set, instead of a binary segmentation. In other words, if the distance from a voxel to the measured cortical boundary is less than the voxel size in width, the voxel is considered to contain multiple tissue types.

Surface area A marching cubes algorithm[12] is performed on the signed distance functions, Ψ_{in} and Ψ_{out}, to extract the embedded zero level sets, in this case the inner and outer cortical surfaces, when the evolution is completed. The surfaces are realized using a triangular representation. Surface area is then calculated as the sum of the areas of the triangles.

Surface curvature and shape index As discussed above, one advantage of the level set implementation is that geometric properties of the propagation front are easily calculated[18]. In our case of surfaces propagating in 3D space, there are many choices for the curvature of the front (for formal definitions of the curvatures, refer to [6]), including mean curvature, κ_M, and Gaussian curvature, κ_G. Both may be conveniently expressed in terms of the level set function Ψ: $\kappa_M = \{\sum_{(i,j,k) \in C}((\Psi_{ii} + \Psi_{jj})\Psi_k^2 - 2\Psi_i\Psi_j\Psi_{ij})\}/\{2(\Psi_x^2 + \Psi_y^2 + \Psi_z^2)^{3/2}\}$, and $\kappa_G = $

$\{\sum_{(i,j,k)\in C}(\Psi_i^2(\Psi_{jj}\Psi_{kk}-\Psi_{jk}^2)+2\Psi_i\Psi_j(\Psi_{ik}\Psi_{jk}-\Psi_{ij}\Psi_{kk}))\}/(\Psi_x^2+\Psi_y^2+\Psi_z^2)^2$, where $C=\{(x,y,z),(y,z,x),(z,x,y)\}$ is the set of circular shifts of (x,y,z).

The maximum principle curvature, κ_1, and the minimum principle curvature, κ_2, are related to Gaussian and mean curvatures through the following formulas: $\kappa_1 = \kappa_M + \sqrt{\kappa_M^2 - \kappa_G}$, and $\kappa_2 = \kappa_M - \sqrt{\kappa_M^2 - \kappa_G}$. We adopt the classification of surfaces by Koenderink[8] using the numerical relationship between the two principal curvatures. A shape index function is defined as $si = \frac{2}{\pi}arctan((\kappa_1+\kappa_2)/(\kappa_1-\kappa_2))$, which classifies the surfaces into nine types as show in Figure 7. With the shape index, gyri (mostly ridges) and sulci (mostly ruts) are automatically identified. Further potential uses of the shape index includes the definition of an atrophy index (sulci widen with age).

Thickness map As discussed above, the value of the level function of a front at any point is the distance from this point to the current front. Also recall that the inner and outer cortical surfaces are the zero level sets of Ψ_{in} and Ψ_{out}. Thus, for any point on the outer cortical surface, the absolute value of Ψ_{in} at the point is simply the distance from the point to the inner cortical surface. Using this measure, we obtain a thickness map between the inner and outer cortical surfaces, which can be used to study the normal thickness variations across different regions of the brain, and also the abnormalities in brain structures.

3 Experimental Result

3.1 Result on simulated MR data with ground truth

We first present our segmentation results on the simulated MR brain images provided by the McConnell Brain Imaging Center at the Montreal Neurological Institute(http://www.bic.mni.mcgill.ca/). The images are generated using an MRI simulator[9], that allows users to independently control various acquisition parameters and obtain realistic MR images. The ground truth of the phantom is provided in the form of membership functions of each voxel belonging to different tissue types, such as the skull, CSF, gray matter and white matter.

The simulated data we tested our algorithm on were T1 images of a normal brain, with the following parameters: voxel size= $1mm^3$, noise= 3%, intensity non-uniformity= 0%. Starting from the unedited images, no further user interaction is needed after the specification of several pairs of concentric spheres as initialization. The spheres grow out and automatically lock onto the inner and outer cortical surfaces. As long as the spheres are placed inside the white matter, the algorithm is robust to starting position. Measurement of the volume is then done as described in the previous section; we use a binary segmentation in this experiment.

To evaluate the segmentation result we apply several measures defined as follows. For any tissue type T in the region of interest, we denote the voxels of tissue type T recovered from our 3D algorithm as V_a and the voxels that are mostly of tissue type T according to the phantom(i.e. the value of tissue T membership function is greater than 0.5) as V_e. We denote the overlap of V_a and V_e as V_{ae}, and the part that is in V_a but not in V_e as $V_{ae'}$. A *true positive(TP) rate* is then defined to be the size of V_{ae} relative to the size of V_e, while the *false positive(FP) rate* is defined to be the ratio of the size of $V_{ae'}$ to the size of V_e.

We also define the *volume ratio* to be the volume of all the voxels segmented as of tissue type T by our algorithm to the total partial volume of tissue type T specified by the phantom(partial volume voxels contribute in only part of the voxel size).

%	whole brain	cortical gray matter1	cortical gray matter2	white matter
TP rate	92.3	93.5	92.4	92.4
FP rate	2.0	5.9	6.0	3.3
volume ratio	96.3	103.9	102.7	98.1

Table 1. Comparison of our volume measurements with the phantom ground truth. whole brain: total brain tissue(white+gray matter); cortical gray matter1: on the frontal 49 Coronal slices; cortical gray matter2: on the top 56 Axial slices;

Table 1 shows our measurement results over 4 types: total brain tissue (including white and gray matter), cortical gray matter in selected slices and the white matter. Since the algorithm is designed specifically for the nearly constant thickness of the cerebral cortex, it recovers only part of the gray matter in the brain stem and the cerebellum where the constant thickness constraint is not satisfied. These regions account for most of the errors in the TP rate and *volume ratio* for the whole brain tissue. Since no ground truth regarding the structural information is provided for the phantom, we compare the cortical gray matter volume on selected slices: frontal 49 Coronal slices and top 56 Axial slices(where there are only white matter and cortical gray matter). The average errors of the TP and FP rates are around 6% to 7%, and the *volume ratio* error is within 4%. For the white matter, the errors for the TP, FP rates and *volume ratio* are also low. These results show that our algorithm performs well in isolating the brain from non-brain tissues and in segmenting the cortex from simulated data.

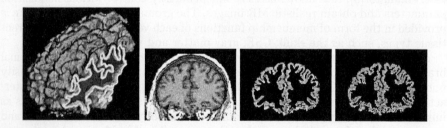

Fig. 4. 3D volume rendering of the cortex from our 3D algorithm with oblique cutting planes. The convoluted thin bright ribbon is the cortical gray matter captured on the cutting plane.

Fig. 5. Coronal slices from 3D images; left: original image; middle: cortical gray matter from manual tracing; right: cortical gray matter from our 3D algorithm.

3.2 Result on real MR data

We then tested our algorithm on frontal lobes of 7 high resolution MRI data sets(SPGR, 2NEX, $1.2 \times 1.2 \times 1.2 mm^3$ voxels) from a randomly chosen subset of young adult autistic and control subjects from our ongoing studies, to measure frontal lobe volume, gray and white matter volume, cortical surface area, surface curvature and cortical thickness. After preprocessing to reduce the effects of the MR bias field inhomogeneity using a simple standard nonlinear map (which is also a step before expert manual tracing), we used a single plane to isolate the part of the 3D image that contained the frontal lobe, and then ran the coupled surfaces algorithm on this part of the image to isolate the brain tissue and segment the cortex(see Figure 6). The frontal lobe was then defined independently in the left and right hemispheres as all tissue anterior to the central sulcus. Sub-cortical nuclei were excluded from our definition of the frontal volume.

Figure 4 shows a 3D volume rendering of the cortical gray matter of a frontal lobe resulted from our algorithm. In Figure 5, 2D Coronal slices of the same result are shown. Over the 7 frontal lobes, the TP and FP rates (compared to manual tracing) of the whole frontal lobe averaged 94.1% and 2.1% respectively, which demonstrated that our algorithm nicely isolated the brain tissue from the non-brain tissue. The average TP and FP rate for the gray matter (measured on 2 slices) in the frontal lobe were 86.7% and 20.8%. As we see in Figure 5, the expert tracing tended to be more aggressive in defining the gray/white matter boundary, which resulted in the relatively larger value of the FP rate. As a second way to analyze the utility of the volume measurements from our algorithm, we compute the reliability statistics on the volume measurements[16]. There was strong agreement between the algorithm and the expert on the volume of the frontal lobe (Pearson r = .991; intraclass correlation coefficient [ICC] = .901). The algorithm systematically estimated the frontal lobe volume to be less than the expert tracer (mean difference = 4%), and this accounts for the lower ICC than Pearson coefficient. Similarly, for gray matter volume of the frontal lobe there was also good agreement (Pearson r = .96).

The outer and inner cortical surfaces captured by the algorithm were masked using the frontal lobe volume information to retain only the parts of the surfaces that are from the frontal lobe as defined above. The average outer and inner cortical surface areas over the 7 frontal lobes are $48800mm^2$ and $63200mm^2$ respectively. Figure 7 shows the outer and inner cortical surfaces of a frontal lobe colored with their shape indices. As we can see, most parts of the gyri are automatically identified as ridge while most parts of the sulci are identified as rut, which coincides with our knowledge of the cortical structure.

The average cortical thickness of the 7 frontal lobes ranged from $3.2mm$ to $3.6mm$, which matches data from postmortem studies([1]). The cortical thickness map displayed in Figure 8 also shows an interesting pattern of information, with gyral crowns represented as thicker than sulcal troughs. This also is in good agreement with postmortem data ([1]). In addition, the primary motor strip and immediately adjacent premotor areas generally appear to contain thicker cortical gray matter than middle frontal areas, and this too is in agreement with known regional variations in cortical thickness ([17],[1]).

Assessing the relationships between surface areas and volumes, we see that the total inner surface area of the frontal lobe correlated quite strongly with the total outer surface area (r = .82). Inner and outer surface areas also predicted total gray matter volume (r's = .76 and .85, respectively). The imperfect relationships suggest some measurement error, but also the possibility that surface area adds unique information beyond that provided by gray matter volume.

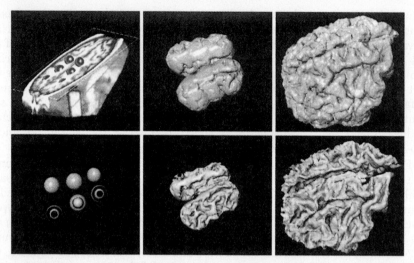

Fig. 6. Propagation of the outer(pink) and inner(yellow) bounding surfaces. left: pairs of concentric spheres(only the outer ones are shown at the top) as initialization in unedited 3D MR brain images(frontal part); middle: intermediate step; right: final result of the outer and inner cortical surfaces of the frontal lobe.

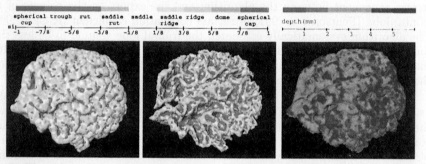

Fig. 7. The outer and inner cortical surfaces of a frontal lobe colored with the specified spectrum representing shape index(si).

Fig. 8. The outer cortical surface colored with cortical thickness.

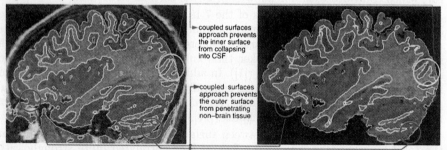

Fig. 9. Single vs. coupled surfaces approach. left: surfaces resulting from single surface approach on a sagittal slice of original image (finding the inner and outer surfaces separately); right: surfaces resulting from the coupled surfaces approach on a sagittal slice of the expert tracing result.

Similarly, average gray matter thickness of the frontal lobe was assessed. These measurements were not significantly correlated with gray matter volume (r = .25) or surface areas (inner = -.38; outer = -.10), suggesting that thickness is nearly a constant and provides unique biological information.

3.3 User interaction and speed issue

Minimum user interaction and computational efficiency have always been two important issues in the problem of segmenting and measuring the cortex. For an expert to manually isolate the non-brain tissue alone (using computer-assisted manual tracing slice by slice) takes 3 to 4 hours. The manual tracing of cortical gray matter is even more time consuming. The multiple surface method of Macdonald et al.[13], could only be computed at medium resolution due to the computational expense. Davatzikos and Bryan[5] report that the "ribbon" algorithm was a fairly computationally demanding iterative procedure; while manual placement of the initial cortical surface and a multi-scale formulation could decrease the computational load (no processing time was given). The initialization for our algorithm only requires the user to specify several pairs of concentric spheres in the white matter, which can be done with several mouse clicks. It should be emphasized that neither the number nor the placement of the spheres affects the accuracy or the reproducibility of the final result. For a 3D image ($1.2 \times 1.2 \times 1.2 mm^3$ in voxel size) of the whole brain, the algorithm runs in about 1 hour on a R10000 SGI Indigo2 machine. **Skull-stripping, segmentation and measurement of the cortex are done simultaneously.** Comparatively, to our knowledge our algorithm outperforms other related techniques with respect to user interaction and computational efficiency.

4 Summary and Future Directions

In this paper, we presented a new approach to the segmentation and measurement of cortical structure which is of great interest in the study of the structural and functional characteristics of the brain. Motivated by the fact that the cortex has a nearly constant thickness, we model the cortex as a volumetric layer, which is completely defined by the two bounding surfaces and the homogeneity in between. Starting from easily initialized spheres, and driven by image-derived information, two interfaces evolve out to capture the inner and outer cortical boundaries, thereby segmenting out the cortical gray matter from the white matter, as well as isolating the brain tissue from the non-brain tissue. Cortical gray matter volume and cortical surface area (both inner and outer) are then measured. Due to the coupled level set implementation, the cortical surface curvature and cortical thickness map are also easily obtained. As seen from various experiments, our algorithm is automatic, accurate, robust and relatively computationally efficient.

Future directions of our research include the following: volume measurement on the sub-voxel level, possible use of a vector image data set, and testing on image data of abnormal brains.

Acknowledgment   This work was supported in part by NIH grant NINDS R01 NS35193, NSF grant IRI-9530768, and NIH grant NICHD 5 P01 HDIDC 35482.

References

1. S.M.Blinkov and I.I.Glezer. *The Human Brain In Figures and Tables. A Quantitative Handbook.* Chapter X, pp182. Basic Books,Inc., Plenum Press, 1968.
2. H.E.Cline, W.E.Lorensen, R. Kikinis, and F.Jolesz. Three-dimensional segmentation of MR images of the head using probability and connectivity. *J. Comput. Assist. Tomogr.*, 14(6):1037-1045, Nov./Dec. 1990.
3. L.D.Cohen and I.Cohen. Finite-Element methods for active contour models and balloons for 2-D and 3-D images. *IEEE Trans. Pattern Anal. Machine Intell.*, 15(11):1131-1147, Nov, 1993.
4. C.A.Davatzikos and J.Prince. An active contour model for mapping the cortex. *IEEE Trans. Med. Imag.*, 14(1):65-80, March, 1995.
5. C.Davatzikos and R.N.Bryan. Using a deformable surface model to obtain a shape representation of cortex. *IEEE Trans. Med. Imag.*, 15(6):785-795, 1996.
6. M.P.DoCarmo. *Differential Geometry of Curves and Surfaces.* Prentice-Hall, New Jersey, 1976.
7. D.Geman and S.Geman. Stochastic relaxation, Gibbs distribution and Bayesian restoration of images. *IEEE Trans. Pattern Anal. Machine Intell.*, 6:721-741, 1984.
8. J.J.Koenderink and A.J.van Doorn. Surface shape and curvature scale. *Image and Vision Computing,* 10(8):557-565, 1992.
9. R.K.-S.Kwan, A.C.Evans and G.B.Pike, An Extensible MRI Simulator for Post-Processing Evaluation, *Visualization in Biomedical Computing* vol. 1131, pp 135-140, Springer-Verlag, 1996.
10. S.Lakshmanan and H.Derin. Simultaneous Parameter Estimation and Segmentation of Gibbs Random Fields Using Simulated Annealing. *IEEE Trans. Pattern Anal. and Machine Intell.*, 11(8):799-810, 1989.
11. R.Leahy, T.Hebert and R.Lee. Applications of Markov Random Fields in medical imaging. *Information Processing in Medical Imaging.* pp:1-14. Wiley-Liss Inc, 1991.
12. W.Lorenson and H.Cline. Marching Cubes: A High Resolution 3D Surface Construction Algorithm. *Proc. SIGGRAPH,* 21(4):163-169, July 1987.
13. D.MacDonald, D. Avis and A.E.Evans. Multiple Surface Identification and Matching in Magnetic Resonance Images. *Proc. SPIE* 2359:160-169, 1994.
14. R.Malladi, J.A.Sethian and B.C.Vemuri. Shape modeling with front propagation: a level set approach, *IEEE Trans. on Pattern Analysis and Machine Intelligence,* 17(2):158-174, Feb, 1995.
15. R.Malladi, R.Kimmel, D.Adalsteinsson, G.Sapiro, V.Caselles and J.A. Sethian. A geometric approach to segmentation and analysis of 3D medical images. *Proc. MMBIA,* 1996.
16. R.T.Schultz and A.Chakraborty. Magnetic resonance image analysis. In E. Bigler (Ed.), *Handbook of Human Brain Function: Neuroimaging,* pp:9-51. New York: Plenum Press, 1996.
17. L.D.Selemon, G.Rajkowska and P.S.Goldman-Rakic. Abnormally High Neuronal Density In The Schizophremic Cortex, A Morphometric Analysis Of Prefrontal Area 9 and Occipital Area 17. *Arch Gen Psychiatry,* vol52:pp805-828, Oct 1995.
18. J.A.Sethian. *Level set methods:evolving interfaces in geometry, fluid mechanics, computer vision and materials science.* Cambridge University Press, 1996.
19. P.C.Teo, G.Sapiro and B.A.Wandell. Creating connected representations of cortical gray matter for functional MRI visualization. *IEEE Trans.Med. Imag.*, 16(6):852-863, 1997.
20. X.Zeng, L.H.Staib, R.T.Schultz and J.S.Duncan. Volumetric layer segmentation using coupled surfaces propagation. *Proc. IEEE Conf. on Computer Vision and Pattern Recognition,* pp:708-715, Santa Barbara, California, June, 1998.

A Biomechanical Model of Soft Tissue Deformation, with Applications to Non-rigid Registration of Brain Images with Tumor Pathology

Stelios K. Kyriacou and Christos Davatzikos

Neuroimaging Laboratory
Department of Radiology
The Johns Hopkins University School of Medicine
Baltimore, MD 21287

Abstract. The finite element method is applied to the biomechanics of brain tissue deformation. Emphasis is given to the deformations induced by the growth of tumors, and to the deformable registration of anatomical atlases with patient images. A uniform contraction of the tumor is first used to obtain an estimate of the shape of the brain prior to the growth of the tumor. A subsequent nonlinear regression method is used to improve on the above estimate. The resulting deformation mapping is finally applied to an atlas, yielding the registration of the atlas with the tumor-deformed anatomy. A preliminary 2D implementation that includes inhomogeneity and a nonlinear elastic material model is tested on simulated data as well as a patient image. The long-term scope of this work is its application to surgical planning systems.

Keywords: brain atlas, registration, biomechanics, inverse methods

1 Introduction

Much attention has been given by the medical imaging community to the modeling of normal brain anatomy. Among others, applications of anatomical modeling include computational neuroanatomy [1, 2], surgical path planning [3], and virtual medical environments [4]. However, little attention has been given to modeling anatomical abnormalities. In this work we describe steps toward the development of a system which simulates soft tissue deformation in the brain caused by the growth of tumors. The main application of our work is currently in the non-rigid matching of brain atlases to brains with pathologies for the purposes of pre-operative planning. In particular, brain atlases can provide a wealth of information on the structural and functional organization of the brain, and ultimately on the response of different brain regions to therapeutic procedures such as radiotherapy. Since they are derived from normal brains, however, brain atlases must be adapted to the pathology of each individual brain. This necessitates the development of a realistic model for the mechanics of tissue deformation due to the growth of a tumor.

Recently, investigators have presented, among other topics, 2D and 3D finite element models of brain dynamics (see for example, Bandak et al. [5] and other references in the same journal issue). In the area of quasistatic brain mechanics, Nagashima and coworkers (see for example [6]), as well as Neff and coworkers [7], used 2D finite element analysis combined with poroelastic theory to allow for the movement of fluids through the brain, and a linear material and linear strains for the elastic deformations, to model edema, and hydrocephalus.

Here, we develop a method for simulating quasi-static brain mechanics, specifically investigating the growth of a brain tumor and the resulting brain deformations. Our goal is to manipulate brain atlases, which are based on normal subjects, by accounting for structural changes occurring with tumor growth and thus facilitate neurosurgical simulations for pre-operative planning and training.

2 Methods

We are using a plain stress finite element method i.e. we assume that there is zero stress in the direction normal to our section. Our model incorporates the parenchyma, the dura and falx membranes, and the ventricles.

2.1 Constitutive models and parameters

In this preliminary work, we assume that both white and gray matter and the tumor tissue are nonlinear elastic solids. The elastic properties are based on the incompressible nonlinearly-elastic neo-Hookean model with $w = \mu(I_1 - 3)$, where w is the strain energy function, μ is the material constant. $I_1 = tr\mathbf{C} = \lambda_1^2 + \lambda_2^2 + \lambda_3^2$, since $\mathbf{C}$, the Right Cauchy Green strain tensor, under a coordinate system that is based on the principal directions, may be written as: $\mathbf{C} = \text{diag}(\lambda_1^2, \lambda_2^2, \lambda_3^2)$, where λ_i, $i = 1, 2, 3$ are the three principle stretches. A stretch is defined as deformed length over original length.

We use a value of 3 kPa for the white matter μ, which, for rather small values of strain [8], corresponds to a Young's modulus of 18 kPa (a value that lies in the range of moduli given by Metz et al. [9]). In addition, we use a value of 30 KPa for the gray matter and tumor tissue μ, 10 times higher than the white matter one.

2.2 Normalization of the image

Given a brain image that contains a tumor we would like to explore methods capable of calculating the origin of the tumor (the position where it started growing). We use a two-part method to perform this normalization of the image. The first part is based on simple contraction of the tumor shape, which effectively reverses the process of the tumor growth, while the second part uses the results of the first part and makes refinements based on nonlinear regression. The two parts of our method are explained in the following sections.

The application of this method shrinks the tumor to a small mass (ideally infinitesimal), resulting in an estimate of the normal state of the brain before the tumor growth. A normal-to-normal atlas matching procedure [10] could then be applied at this point, since two "normal" brain images are involved. Finally, the reverse procedure can grow the tumor back to its current configuration, deforming the surrounding structures accordingly. So, the final image will be a brain map that has been deformed so as to fit the patient data.

Simulation of tumor contraction In the first part, reduction of the tumor size is simulated by uniform contraction. We apply the contraction through a uniform negative strain (usually around -0.6 to -0.9) inside the tumor, which reduces its average diameter to approximately four tenths to one tenth of the original size respectively.

Simulation of tumor enlargement Tumor enlargement simulation is useful for two cases: 1) to create simulated tumor data for the validation of our contraction and 2) to function as the "forward" model in the nonlinear regression/optimization (see next paragraph). In the first case, the tumor seed, a circular mass of diameter about 1 cm, is initially placed somewhere in the brain image. In the second case, the tumor seed created by the contraction run is used instead. The subsequent tumor growth is achieved by uniform expansion, similar to the contraction case above.

Nonlinear regression The second part for the tumor-bearing image normalization is based on an inverse finite element technique (in effect a nonlinear regression) required for the estimation of the original position of the brain tumor. ABAQUS [11] is used for the FEM and the Marquardt algorithm [12] is used for the nonlinear regression. We should note that the first part, the contraction, provides a mapping that may be used in itself as a rather simple image normalization map.

Since many parameters are unknown in the initial configuration, and solving for all of them might be too expensive, we have decided to optimize only the most important ones and just use a reasonable estimate for the rest of the initial parameters. For example, the undeformed shapes of the ventricles are assumed to be known from the contraction part. The shape of the tumor seed is also assumed to be the same as the one resulting from the contraction step. Three scalar parameters are considered unknown and are optimized through this inverse approach: the x and y coordinates of the centroid of the tumor seed shape and the expansion factor required for the seed to reach the tumor size observed in the final images. The errors that the regression routine minimizes against are the distances d_i (an N-sized vector) of the calculated tumor nodes from the experimental (observed) tumor boundary, as well as the distances of the nodes on the calculated ventricles from the experimental ventricular shapes, with N being the number of nodes on both tumor and ventricles. So our cost function f is: $f = \sum_{i=1}^{N} d_i^2$.

3 Results

Figure 1 depicts a simulated tumor case so that the performance of the normalization could be evaluated. The small circular black outline in panel A shows the original tumor seed before the simulated tumor expansion takes place. After the data extraction and mesh creation phase, a mesh is obtained which is overlayed in panel A. By running ABAQUS with the loads, material properties, and boundary conditions, we obtained the deformed mesh/image in panel B. The simulated tumor of panel B was then treated as the starting point for applying the contraction part described in Section 2.2. Panel C was produced after we applied the contraction method with a suitable contraction strain found by trial and error to give an approximately same size tumor seed as the one we started with (panel A). Both the finite element (deformed) mesh and the resulting image are shown. Ideally, we would like this image to be similar to the original image of Panel A since we are using some features of it, in particular the ventricle shapes, in our regression part. Finally, panel D is the combination of the image in panel B and the ventricle outlines that correspond to the results from the nonlinear regression. Good agreement is observed.

Figures 2, and 3 represent results of applying the contraction and subsequent regression to an actual patient tumor-bearing CT image and to the related atlas images. Figure 2 gives the regression results. Panel A shows the patient image with a white outline denoting the tumor. Panel B is the superposition of the deformation mapping given by the contraction strain of -0.60, and the subsequent regression, on the original image.

Figure 3 displays the atlas manipulations for the regression results. Panel A is the original atlas [13]. Panel B presents the warped atlas using the method described in [10] by using the overall size of the brain and ventricles. Panel C presents the image of panel B deformed with the finite element deformation mapping to obtain an atlas that has the characteristics of our patient tumor image. The vertical white lines in both panels B and C have been added to illustrate the mid-line shift due to the tumor. Finally, panel D is the patient image with a few of the structures of the atlas in panel C superimposed. In particular, most of the thalamic structures, the putamen, the claustrum, the cortex, and the ventricles have been included.

4 Discussion

The tumor contraction is easy to apply but it assumes among other things that at the post-tumor configuration, the residual stresses in the tissue are zero, something obviously not true since the tissue has already been deformed by the tumor. The regression part does not have this drawback but at the same time it does

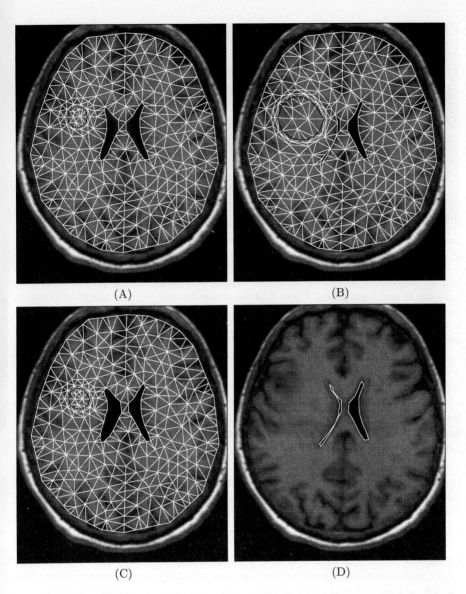

Fig. 1. Normalization of a simulated tumor: (A) the original image and mesh with the simulated tumor seed. (B) the deformed image and mesh due to a "uniform" expansion of the tumor seed. (C) The contracted image and mesh. This image corresponds to panel A. Note that the right ventricle (left side of image) is slightly larger than the corresponding one in A due to our neglect of residual stresses. (D) The ventricle outlines given by the regression overlayed on the deformed image of panel B to point out the correspondence.

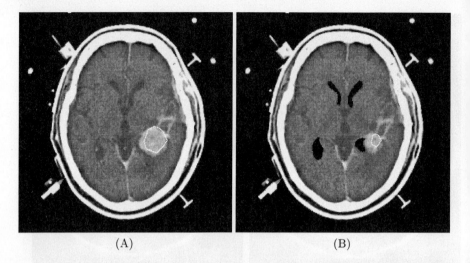

Fig. 2. Regression results for an actual tumor: CT image from a patient (panel A) with the tumor highlighted. Panel B is the image created by deforming the image in panel A based on the regression finite element mapping. Note that the slight mismatch between the tumor and its outline in panel A was needed to combat imperfections in our automatic mesh generation scheme due to the ventricle being very near the tumor.

need the undeformed configuration of the ventricles before the tumor expansion; currently this is provided by the contraction phase. We plan to overcome this limitation by using statistical information on ventricular shapes and sizes for the age and sex of the particular patient. Also we may be able to utilize the inherent symmetry of the brain for structures relatively distant to the tumor.

Our work is currently being extended from 2D to 3D. The 3D brain volume is first segmented and the finite element mesh is then created with an automatic mesh generator, Vgrid, provided by F. Kruggel at the Max-Planck-Institute of Cognitive Neuroscience, Leipzig, Germany. Results will soon be published in a separate article.

In summary, we have shown the utility of the contraction as well as the regression techniques as a means to perform image to atlas registration for patients with localized brain deformations due to mainly tumor enlargement. The technique has potential applications in radiotherapy pre-surgical planning.

5 Acknowledgments

We would like to thank Dr. Don Long (Department of Neurosurgery, The Johns Hopkins Hospital), ISG Technologies (Toronto, Canada), and a grant from the American Cancer Society for partial financial support as well as Drs. R. Nick Bryan (JHU, now at NIH), and James Zinreich (JHU) for many helpful discussions, and Dr. Jeffery Williams (Department of Neurosurgery, The Johns Hopkins Hospital) for providing the CT images.

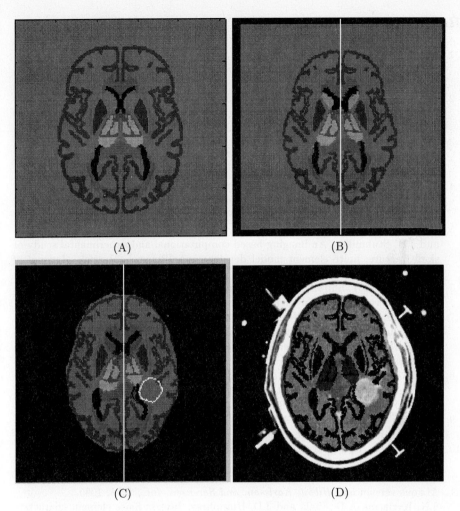

Fig. 3. Regression results for an actual tumor – atlas manipulations: (A): The original atlas slice. (B): The atlas slice warped in overall registration with the patient's image. (C): The deformation of the atlas in panel B based on the inverse of the finite element mapping of figure 2. The white outline represents the position of the tumor in the patient's image. (D): Here we have superimposed some of the atlas structures from the deformed atlas of panel (C) on the image of figure 2, panel A. Panels B and C have been enhanced with the addition of a vertical white line to better visualize the midline shift changes.

References

1. M.I. Miller, G.E. Christensen, Y. Amit, and U. Grenander. Mathematical textbook of deformable neuroanatomies. *Proc. of the National Academy of Sciences*, 90:11944–11948, 1993.
2. C. Davatzikos, M. Vaillant, S. Resnick, J.L. Prince, S. Letovsky, and R.N. Bryan. A computerized approach for morphological analysis of the corpus callosum. *J. of Comp. Assisted Tomography*, 20:88–97, Jan./Feb. 1996.
3. M. Vaillant, C. Davatzikos, R.H. Taylor, and R.N. Bryan. A path-planning algorithm for image guided neurosurgery. *Proc. of CVRMed II - MRCAS III*, pages 467–476, March 1997.
4. J. Kaye, D.N. Metaxas, and F.P. Primiano, Jr. A 3d virtual environment for modeling mechanical cardiopulmonary interactions. *CVRMed-MRCAS'97 Lecture Notes in Computer Science, Grenoble, France*, 1997.
5. F.A. Bandak, M.J. Vander Vorst, L.M. Stuhmiller, P.F. Mlakar, W.E. Chilton, and J.H. Stuhmiller. An imaging-based computational and experimental study of skull fracture: finite element model development. [Review] [31 refs]. *Journal of Neurotrauma*, 12(4):679–88, 1995.
6. T. Nagashima, T. Shirakuni, and S.I. Rapoport. A two-dimensional, finite element analysis of vasogenic brain edema. *Neurol Med Chir (Tokyo)*, 30(1):1–9, 1990.
7. R.P. Subramaniam, S.R. Neff, and P. Rahulkumar. A numerical study of the biomechanics of structural neurologic diseases. *High Performance Computing–Grand Challenges in Computer Simulation Society for Computer Simulations, San Diego*, pages 552–60, 1995.
8. K.K. Mendis, R.L. Stalnaker, and S.H. Advani. A constitutive relationship for large deformation finite element modeling of brain tissue. *Journal of Biomechanical Engineering*, 117(3):279–85, 1995.
9. H. Metz, J. McElhaney, and A.K. Ommaya. A comparison of the elasticity of live, dead, and fixed brain tissue. *J Biomech*, 3(4):453–8, 1970.
10. C. Davatzikos. Spatial transformation and registration of brain images using elastically deformable models. *Comp. Vision and Image Understanding*, 66(2):207–222, May 1997.
11. Abaqus version 5.5. *Hibbit, Karlsson, and Sorensen, Inc., USA*, 1995.
12. S.K. Kyriacou, A.D. Shah, and J.D. Humphrey. Inverse finite element characterization of the behavior of nonlinear hyperelastic membranes. *ASME Journal of Applied Mechanics*, 64:257–62, 1997.
13. WL Nowinski, RN Bryan, and R. Raghavan (Eds.). *The Electronic Clinical Brain Atlas on CD-ROM*. Thieme, 1997.

Building Biomechanical Models Based on Medical Image Data: An Assessment of Model Accuracy

Wendy M. Murray[1], Allison S. Arnold[2], Silvia Salinas[2],
Mahidhar M. Durbhakula[2], Thomas S. Buchanan[3], and Scott L. Delp[2]

[1] Biomedical Engineering Department, Case Western Reserve University & Rehabilitation Engineering Center, MetroHealth Medical Center, 2500 MetroHealth Dr., Cleveland, OH 44109-1998, U.S.A.
wmm@po.cwru.edu

[2] Departments of Biomedical Engineering and Physical Medicine & Rehabilitation, Northwestern University & Sensory Motor Performance Program, Rehabilitation Institute of Chicago, Room 1406, 345 East Superior St., Chicago, IL 60611, U.S.A
{asarnold, s-salinas, m-durbhakula, s-delp}@nwu.edu

[3] Mechanical Engineering Department, University of Delaware, Newark, DE 19716, U.S.A.
buchanan@me.udel.edu

Abstract. The goals of this work were to (i) establish a method for building subject-specific biomechanical models from medical image data, (ii) construct a subject-specific model of the elbow, and (iii) quantify the accuracy of soft tissue excursions estimated from the model. We developed a kinematic model of the elbow joint and its surrounding musculature from magnetic resonance images of a 6'4" male cadaver specimen in one limb position. Moment arms estimated from the model (i.e., the changes in muscle-tendon lengths with elbow flexion angle) were compared to moment arms measured experimentally from the same specimen. In five of the six muscles studied, the model explained 84%-94% of the variation in the experimental data. Model estimates of peak elbow flexion moment arm were within 13% of the experimental peaks. Our results suggest that subject-specific musculoskeletal models derived from medical image data have the potential to substantially improve estimates of soft tissue excursions in living subjects.

1 Introduction

Quantification of soft tissue excursions that occur during movement is important for the planning of orthopaedic surgical interventions, such as tendon transfers and osteotomies. Surgeons frequently introduce changes in muscle force- and moment-generating properties by modifying the length and moment arm of a muscle. Although these changes are usually intended to improve function (e.g., tendon transfer surgeries which enhance hand grasp function in persons with spinal cord injury), they can leave patients with weak or dysfunctional limbs if the muscle fibers are too long or too short postoperatively to generate active force or if the moment arms of the muscles are compromised. Predicting the biomechanical consequences of surgical alterations, therefore, requires detailed knowledge of the soft tissue lengths and excursions before and after the intervention.

Muscle-tendon lengths and moment arms are commonly estimated in cadaver specimens (e.g., [1, 2]) or using nominal biomechanical models (e.g., [3, 4]). However, it remains unclear whether "averaged" experimental data or generic models accurately represent populations that have not been studied in anatomical preparations, such as children or individuals with pathologies (e.g., bone deformities or muscle contracture). Because patients undergoing surgical reconstructions of musculoskeletal structures frequently fall into this category, methods that enable soft tissue excursions of individual subjects to be estimated *in vivo* are needed.

Computer-generated three-dimensional (3D) reconstructions from computed tomography (CT) or magnetic resonance (MR) images provide an accurate, non-invasive method to quantify musculoskeletal anatomy in living subjects [5, 6]. However, accurate measurements of muscle-tendon excursions from medical image data would require extensive imaging protocols to capture the orientations and positions of the muscles in several different joint positions. The combination of medical imaging and graphics-based musculoskeletal modeling is a promising alternative for estimating muscle-tendon lengths and moment arms in living subjects. For instance, a 3D reconstruction of a limb in one joint position can be animated by making basic assumptions about joint kinematics and musculotendon travel with joint rotation. This hybrid method would drastically reduce the time, expense, and data processing concerns that currently limit the applications of 3D reconstructions of medical image data. However, methods for creating subject-specific biomechanical models need to be established. Also, it is critical to demonstrate the accuracy of any model before it can be used to guide patient-specific treatment decisions.

The specific aim of this study was to create a biomechanical model of the elbow joint and its surrounding musculature from MR images and to quantify the accuracy of muscle moment arms estimated using the model. Because a muscle's moment arm determines its change in length over a range of motion [7], our assessment of moment arms in this study also provides a rigorous test of our model's capacity to estimate muscle-tendon lengths and excursions.

2 Methods

A 3D reconstruction of the upper extremity harvested from a 6'4" male cadaver specimen was created from MR images, and a kinematic model of the elbow joint and its surrounding musculature was constructed based on the 3D surface models of the muscles and bones. To determine the accuracy of the model over a range of elbow flexion, moment arms of the brachioradialis, biceps, extensor carpi radialis longus (ECRL), brachialis, pronator teres, and triceps estimated from the model were compared to the moment arms determined experimentally from the same specimen. We also compared the moment arms of the 6'4" specimen to the moment arms estimated from a 5'0" specimen to quantify differences that might be observed between individuals of different sizes and to provide some context for evaluating the errors of our model.

2.1 Construction of the 3D Surfaces

Axial and sagittal images of the upper extremity specimen were obtained using a GE Signa MRI Scanner (Series 2, 1.5T). Five overlapping series of T1-weighted spin-echo images were collected (Table I). In four of the image series, the specimen was scanned in the transverse plane from the proximal scapula to the wrist joint with the elbow fully extended and the forearm pronated approximately 60°. In the fifth series, sagittal images of the elbow joint were obtained with the elbow flexed approximately 30° and the forearm pronated 60°. All series were scanned in contiguous 3 mm slices using an extremity coil, except for the proximal humerus which was scanned using a license plate surface coil. To facilitate registration of the images, multiple Vitamin E capsules were secured to the specimen at the axilla of the upper arm, the distal humerus, and the proximal forearm.

Table 1. MR Imaging Protocols

	DISTAL FOREARM	ELBOW JOINT (AXIAL)	MID-HUMERUS	PROXIMAL HUMERUS	ELBOW JOINT (SAGITTAL)
Pulse Sequence (ms)	TR = 316 TE = 16	TR = 400 TE = 16	TR = 400 TE = 16	TR = 500 TE = 16	TR = 300 TE = 15
Matrix	256x128	256x128	256x128	256x128	256x256
FOV (cm)	28x28	28x28	28x28	40x40	20x20
NEX	1.5	1.5	1.5	1.5	2
# Slices	72	63	65	87	35

Boundaries of the humerus, radius, ulna, the long head of the biceps, the brachialis, the brachioradialis, the ECRL, the pronator teres, and the lateral head of the triceps were identified manually in individual slices. A 3D surface representing each anatomical structure was created from the two-dimensional boundaries in serial images. Muscle attachment sites on the bones were identified by placing markers within the images. Three-dimensional surface models of the Vitamin E capsules visible in each series were also created. The homogeneous transformations between overlapping series of images were calculated from the centroids of the Vitamin E capsules using a least-squares algorithm [8].

2.2 Development of the Kinematic Model

The bone and muscle surfaces obtained from the MR images were used to construct a kinematic model of the elbow joint and its surrounding musculature (Fig. 1). Elbow flexion-extension was modeled as a uniaxial hinge joint with its axis passing through the centers of the capitulum and trochlear groove [9, 10, 11, 12]. The center of the capitulum was estimated from a sphere that was fit to its surface. Similarly, the center of the trochlear groove was estimated by fitting a circle to the trochlear groove. Elbow flexion was defined from full extension (0° flexion) to 130° flexion.

The lines of action of the elbow muscles were represented in the model as a series of points connected by line segments. Origin and insertion points were defined based on the centroids of the muscle attachment sites on the bones. Due to the curvature of the humeral shaft, the calculated centroid of the brachialis origin did not lie on the bone surface. This point was translated anteriorly to place the origin on the surface of the humerus. Because the scapula was not imaged, an effective origin for the biceps was defined along the intertubercular sulcus. Similarly, because the hand was not imaged, an effective origin of ECRL was defined on the distal radius.

In addition to origin and insertion points, intermediate 'wrapping' points were defined as a function of elbow flexion angle. The locations of the wrapping points in full extension were based on the 3D muscle surfaces. As the elbow was flexed, wrapping points that were a shorter distance from the axis of rotation than both of a muscle's attachment sites were removed from the path because a recent anatomical study has shown that the shortest distance between the flexion-extension axis and an elbow muscle's attachment sites indicates peak moment arm [13]. For the triceps, wrapping points were added to the path during flexion to model the tendon of the triceps wrapping over the olecranon process of the ulna. We constrained the models of the muscle-tendon paths so that introducing or removing an intermediate point did not cause an instantaneous change in moment arm or muscle-tendon length. Intermediate 'via' points were also defined, and remained in the model over the entire range of motion to prevent the paths from penetrating bone surfaces. The via points in the model had no substantial effects on the estimated moment arms. Moment arms were estimated with the model using the partial velocity method [14].

2.3 Determination of Muscle Moment Arms from Tendon Displacement Data

Elbow flexion moment arms were estimated experimentally in both the 6'4" male specimen and a 5'0" female specimen. Using the tendon displacement method [7], moment arm (ma) was calculated as the partial derivative of muscle-tendon length ($\partial \ell$) with respect to elbow flexion angle (θ). That is,

$$ma = \frac{\partial \ell}{\partial \theta} \qquad (1)$$

The shoulder joint was disarticulated, the skin and fascia proximal to the wrist joint were removed, and the muscles were prepared as described previously [2]. The upper extremity was mounted on a horizontal surface, supported at the humeral head and the medial epicondyle. Elbow flexion angle was measured with an electrogoniometer (Penny and Giles Biometrics, United Kingdom). Tendon displacement measurements were made by connecting each muscle to a Celesco PT101 position transducer (Celesco Transducer Products, Canoga Park, CA) with a wire and slowly moving the forearm through approximately 120° of elbow flexion. The forearm was maintained in neutral (0° pronation/supination) during moment arm measurements.

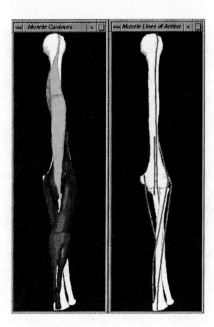

Fig. 1. Computer graphics reconstruction on the 6'4" male specimen (*left*), illustrating the 3D muscle and bone surfaces, and the kinematic model of the elbow joint (*right*), where muscle lines of action were represented as a series of points connected by line segments

The outputs of the position transducer and the electrogoniometer were sampled at 15 Hz. Five trials of tendon displacement vs elbow flexion angle were collected per muscle. The numerical derivative of each trial was digitally filtered using a second order Butterworth filter with a cut-off frequency of one radian^{-1}. The five filtered derivatives were averaged to estimate moment arm. Moment arms were estimated between 20° - 120° flexion for the elbow flexors and 30° - 120° flexion for triceps.

2.4 Assessment of the Accuracy of the Model

The moment arm vs elbow flexion angle curves estimated using the MR based model were quantitatively compared to the moment arms determined experimentally for the large male specimen. For each muscle, the correlation coefficient and the root mean square (RMS) error between the model estimate and the anatomical data were calculated. The square of the correlation coefficient denotes the variation in the experimental data that is accounted for by the model. The RMS error is a measure of the average, absolute value of the difference between the model estimate and the experimental data. That is,

$$RMS = \sqrt{\frac{1}{N} \sum_{i=1}^{N} \left(ma_i^D - ma_i^M\right)^2} \quad (2)$$

where N is the number of data points, ma_i^D is the ith value of the experimental data, and ma_i^M is the corresponding value of the model moment arm. We also compared the model estimate of peak moment arm to the peak from the experimental data. Quantitative comparisons between the experimental data from the 6'4" and 5'0" cadaver specimens provided a means to evaluate the significance of the model errors.

3 Results

The MR based model captured the salient features of the experimental data. In five of the six muscles studied, the correlation coefficients between the model curves and the experimentally determined moment arms were greater than 0.9, and the model explained 84%-94% of the variation in the data (Fig. 2). RMS errors of the model ranged from 3 mm to 7 mm (Fig. 3), and the model estimates of peak elbow flexion moment arms were within 13% of the peaks estimated experimentally (Fig. 4).

Errors in the moment arms from the MR model were generally smaller than differences between the 6'4" male specimen and the 5'0" female specimen. For instance, the errors in the model estimates of peak moment arms were substantially smaller than the differences between peaks in the large and small specimens (Fig. 4). However, for four muscles (biceps, brachialis, pronator teres, and triceps), the model RMS errors were comparable to the differences between the experimental data sets (Fig. 3). For pronator teres and triceps, this occurred because there were only small differences between the moment arms from the 5'0" female and the 6'4" male (Fig. 5, compare differences in PT and TRI curves to differences in BRD curves). In contrast, the model RMS errors for biceps and brachialis were relatively large because the model estimates were shifted versions of the experimental curves (Fig. 2B). If the model estimates of biceps and brachialis moment arms were shifted by -20°, the model's RMS errors would decrease to 2 mm and 4 mm, respectively. Similarly, given a -20° angular shift, the correlation coefficients would increase from 0.916 to 0.998 (biceps) and from 0.783 to 0.987 (brachialis). Thus, the model estimates of biceps and brachialis moment arms could be significantly improved if the source of the angular discrepancy between the model and the experimental data could be identified and addressed.

Of the six muscles evaluated, the brachialis model yielded the least accurate estimate of muscle moment arm. Unlike the other muscles, peak moment arm was not estimated to within 10% by the model, and the model explained only 61% of the variation in the brachialis experimental data. Brachialis has a broad origin on the humerus, and the discrepancy between model and experimental curves may be due to limitations in (i) representing muscles with broad attachments with single origin or insertion points or (ii) obtaining accurate experimental estimates of moment arms from muscles with broad attachment sites.

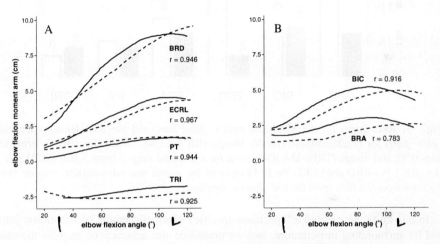

Fig 2. (A). Elbow flexion moment arms of brachioradialis (BRD), ECRL, pronator teres (PT), and triceps (TRI) estimated with the MR based model (*dashed lines*) and estimated using the tendon displacement method in the same cadaver specimen (*solid lines*). (B). Elbow flexion moment arms of biceps (BIC) and brachialis (BRA) estimated with the MR based model (*dashed lines*) and estimated using the tendon displacement method (*solid lines*). With the exception of the brachialis, the correlation coefficients (r) between the model estimates and the anatomical data were greater than 0.9

4 Discussion

Orthopaedic surgical procedures frequently alter the lengths and moment arms of muscles; however, they are planned with little quantitative data that describe muscle function before surgery, or how muscle function might be altered postoperatively. While generic musculoskeletal models have provided some useful clinical insights (e.g., [15]), the accuracy and reliability of generic models for estimating soft-tissue excursions in individuals of different sizes, ages, and pathologies has not been tested.

We believe the development of accurate, time-effective and cost-effective methods to build subject-specific biomechanical models from medical images could provide important insights needed to design and implement more effective surgical procedures.

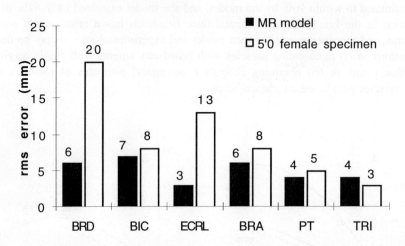

Fig. 3. RMS errors for the MR based model (*filled bars*) and the 5'0" female specimen (*white bars*) for brachioradialis (BRD), biceps (BIC), ECRL, brachialis (BRA), pronator teres (PT), and triceps (TRI). The RMS error for the model ranged from 3 mm (ECRL) to 7 mm (BIC). For BRD and ECRL, the RMS error of the model was substantially smaller than the error from the data from the 5'0" female specimen

In this study, we created a "specimen-specific" kinematic model of the elbow joint and its surrounding musculature, and we quantified the accuracy of muscle moment arms estimated using the model. The model was developed from a minimal set of medical image data—a 3D reconstruction of an upper extremity specimen in a single joint position. Nevertheless, the model was able to capture the salient features of elbow flexion moment arms determined experimentally on the same specimen. Clearly, previous studies which characterized elbow joint kinematics [9, 10, 11, 12] and identified the determinants of peak elbow flexion moment arm [13] guided the development of our model and contributed to the success of our approach. It may be more difficult to develop accurate models of joints with more complex kinematics and muscle-tendon paths, such as the shoulder or the knee, or to characterize joint kinematics *a priori* in a patient with bone deformities. Not surprisingly, the largest source of error in our moment arm estimates was the variation in the moment arms with elbow flexion angle. Further investigation of how muscle-tendon paths change with joint motions *in vivo* would improve the reliability of biomechanical models constructed from a minimal set of medical images.

The results of our study suggest that subject-specific models could greatly improve estimates of soft-tissue excursions in living subjects. Few investigators have attempted to quantify differences in moment arms across differently sized specimens, and most existing musculoskeletal models represent an adult male of average stature.

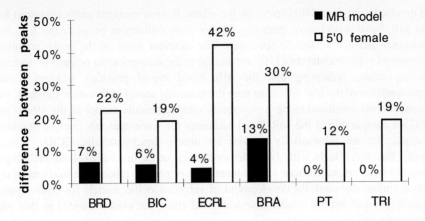

Fig 4. Differences between peak moment arms estimated with the MR based model and determined experimentally from the 6'4" male specimen (*filled bars*) and differences between the peak moment arms of the two cadaver specimens (*white bars*). Differences between peaks are expressed as a percentage of the experimentally determined peak from the male specimen. For each muscle, the MR based model provided a more accurate estimate of peak moment arm compared to the specimen of different anthropometric dimensions

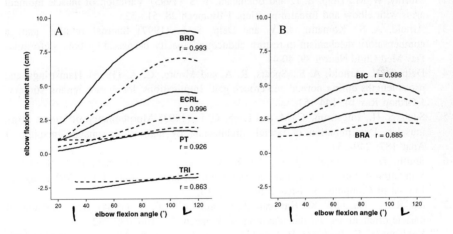

Fig 5. (A). Elbow flexion moment arms of brachioradialis (BRD), ECRL, pronator teres (PT), and triceps (TRI) determined experimentally from the 5'0" female specimen (*dashed lines*) and from the 6'4" male specimen (*solid lines*). (B). Elbow flexion moment arms of biceps (BIC) and brachialis (BRA) determined experimentally from the 5'0" female specimen (*dashed lines*) and from the 6'4" male specimen (*solid lines*). There are substantial differences in moment arm magnitudes between the two specimens for BRD, ECRL, BIC, and BRA, but not for the PT and TRI

In this study, we found that errors in the elbow flexion moment arms estimated from the MR based model were generally smaller than differences between the 6'4" male specimen and a 5'0" female specimen. The moment arms of the most commonly referenced experimental data [16] are similar to the moment arms of the 5'0" specimen in our study, indicating that the MR based model provides a more accurate representation of the 6'4" specimen than the generally accepted literature standard. Peak moment arms estimated using a commonly cited kinematic model of the elbow joint [17] are comparable to the MR based estimates for some muscles (biceps, brachialis, triceps), but are substantially smaller for others (brachioradialis, ECRL, pronator teres). For individuals with bone deformities or other musculoskeletal pathologies, moment arms estimated from experimental data or generic models are likely to be even less accurate. Although the development of subject-specific models for diverse patient populations will require considerable additional effort, the work presented in this paper represents an important first step.

References

1. Delp, S. L., Ringwelski, D. A. and Carroll, N. C. (1994) Transfer of the rectus femoris: Effects of transfer site on moment arms about the knee and hip. J Biomech 27, 1201-1211
2. Murray, W. M., Delp, S. L. and Buchanan, T. S. (1995) Variation of muscle moment arms with elbow and forearm position. J Biomech 28, 513-525
3. Arnold, A. S., Komattu, A. V. and Delp, S. L. (1997) Internal rotation gait: a compensatory mechanism to restore abduction capacity decreased by bone deformity. Dev Med Child Neurol 39, 40-44
4. Delp, S. L., Arnold, A. S., Speers, R. A. and Moore, C. A. (1996) Hamstrings and psoas lengths during normal and crouch gait: Implications for muscle-tendon surgery. J Orthop Res 14, 144-151
5. Scott, S. H., Engstrom, C. M. and Loeb, G. E. (1993) Morphometry of human thigh muscles. Determination of fascicle architecture by magnetic resonance imaging. J Anat 182, 249-257
6. Smith, D. K., Berquist, T. H., An, K. N., Rob, R. A. and Chao, E. Y. S. (1989) Validation of three-dimensional reconstructions of knee anatomy: CT vs MR Imaging. Journal of Computer Assisted Tomography 13, 294-301
7. An, K. N., Takahasi, K., Harrigan, T. P. and Chao, E. Y. (1984) Determination of muscle orientations and moment arms. J Biomech Eng 106, 280-282
8. Veldpaus, F. E., Woltring, H. J. and Dortmans, L. J. (1988) A least-squares algorithm for the equiform transformation from spatial marker co-ordinates. J Biomech 21, 45-54
9. Chao, E. Y. and Morrey, B. F. (1978) Three-dimensional rotation of the elbow. J Biomech 11, 57-73
10. Gerbeaux, M., Turpin, E. and Lensel-Corbeil, G. (1996) Musculo-articular modelling of the triceps brachii. J Biomech 29, 171-180
11. London, J. T. (1981) Kinematics of the elbow. J Bone Joint Surg 63-A, 529-535

12. Shiba, R., Sorbie, C., Siu, D. W., Bryant, J. T., Derek, T., Cooke, V. and Wevers, H. W. (1988) Geometry of the humeroulnar joint. J Orthop Res 6, 897-906
13. Murray, W. M. (1997) The functional capacity of the elbow muscles: Anatomical measurements, computer modeling, and anthropometric scaling. Ph.D. Dissertation Northwestern University, Evanston, IL
14. Delp, S. L. and Loan, J. P. (1995) A graphics-based software system to develop and analyze models of musculoskeletal structures. Comput Biol Med 25, 21-34
15. Delp, S. L. and Zajac, F. E. (1992) Force- and moment-generating capacity of lower-extremity muscles before and after tendon lengthening. Clin Orthop 284, 247-259
16. An, K. N., Hui, F. C., Morrey, B. F., Linscheid, R. L. and Chao, E. Y. (1981) Muscles across the elbow joint: A biomechanical analysis. J Biomech 14, 659-669
17. Amis, A. A., Dowson, D. and Wright, V. (1979) Muscle strengths and musculo-skeletal geometry of the upper limb. Eng Med 8, 41-47

Modelling of Soft Tissue Deformation for Laparoscopic Surgery Simulation

G. Székely, Ch. Brechbühler, R. Hutter, A. Rhomberg and P. Schmid

Swiss Federal Institute of Technology, ETH Zentrum, CH-8092 Zürich, Switzerland

Abstract. Virtual reality based surgical simulator systems offer a very elegant solution to the development of endoscopic surgical trainers. While the graphical performance of commercial systems already makes PC-based simulators viable, the real-time simulation of soft tissue deformation is still the major obstacle in developing simulators for soft-tissue surgery. The goal of the present work is to develop a framework for the full-scale, real-time, Finite Element simulation of elastic tissue deformation in complex systems such as the human abdomen. The key for such a development is the proper formulation of the model, the development of scalable parallel solution algorithms, and special-purpose parallel hardware. The developed techniques will be used for the implementation of a gynaecologic laparoscopic VR-trainer system.

1 Introduction

Endoscopic operations have recently become a very popular technique for the diagnosis as well as treatment of many kinds of human diseases and injuries. The basic idea of endoscopic surgery is to minimise damage to the surrounding healthy tissue, normally caused in reaching the point of surgical intervention for the more inacessible of internal organs. The relatively large cuts in open surgery can be replaced by small perforation holes, serving as entry points for optical and surgical instruments. The small spatial extent of the tissue injury and the careful selection of the entry points result in a major gain in patient recovery after operation.

The price for these advantages is paid by the surgeon, who loses direct contact with the operation site. The necessary visual information is mediated by a specialised camera (the endoscope) and is presented on a screen. While preliminary systems experimenting with stereo optics are already available, today's surgery is usually performed under monoscopic conditions. Due to geometrical constraints posed by the external control of the surgical instruments through the trocar hull, the surgeon loses much of the manipulative freedom usually available in open surgery.

Performing operations under these conditions demands very special skills of the surgeon, which can only be gained with extensive training. The basic optical and manipulative skills can be learned today by using inexpensive, traditional training devices. These training units allow one to learn navigating under monoscopic visual feedback, as well as to acquire basic manipulative skills. In this way the surgeon becomes accustomed to completing a particular task, but because the real-life effect is lost, gets only a limited training range in dexterity and problem solving. Additionally, the organs used by these units are generally made of foam, hence realistic surgical training is impossible. And while experiments on animals are sometimes used for testing new surgical techniques, practical as well as ethical reasons strongly restrict their use in everyday surgical training.

Virtual reality based surgical simulator systems offer a very elegant solution to this training problem. A wide range of VR simulator systems have been proposed and implemented in the past few years. Some of them are restricted to purely diagnostic endoscopical investigations [15, 13, 14], while others, for example, allow the training of surgical procedures for laparoscopic [12, 11, 16, 24, 25], arthroscopic [10, 18], or radiological [26] interventions.

While the graphical performance of commercial systems already renders PC-based simulators possible [15], the real-time simulation of soft tissue deformation is still the major obstacle while developing simulator systems for soft-tissue surgery. Different methods in use for deformation modelling include:

- Free-form deformation techniques of computer graphics [20, 22] use parametric interpolative models (as polynomial models, splines, or superquadrics, e.g.) for deformation estimation of solid primitives. While analogy to physical deformation processes is not always obvious, such techniques have become very popular in surgical simulators [24, 19] due to the resulting fast deformation calculation.
- Different more or less justified simple physical analogies have also been used for tissue deformation modelling. Most popular are mass-spring models [11, 25, 21] but other alternatives like space-filling spheres have also been implemented [27].
- Elastically deformable surface models introduced in computer graphics and computer vision [23] calculate surface deformations by solving the linear elasticity equations using different numerical techniques. These methods allow simulation of tissue deformation based on physical principles [12]. Full 3D extensions of these techniques [16, 17] already represent the first attempts for Finite Element based tissue deformation modelling.

The Finite Element Method (FEM) is a very common and accurate way to solve continuum-mechanical boundary-value problems [1, 8]. In the case of biological tissue, we have to deal with large deformations and also with anisotropic, inhomogeneous, and nonlinear materials. Furthermore, organs and surgical instruments interact, therein leading to numerical contact problems. Nonetheless, provided an adequate formulation is chosen, even in these cases the FEM is a very powerful tool.

Unfortunately, Finite Element calculations are notoriously slow, making them not very appealing for real-time applications like endoscopic surgery simulations. Accordingly, tissue deformation for surgical training systems is, up to now, only calculated by the FEM for fairly simple physical systems [9, 16, 17].

The goal of the presented work is to develop a framework for the full-scale real-time Finite Element simulation of elastic tissue deformation in complex systems such as the human abdomen. The key for such a development is the proper formulation of the model (see Section 2), the development of scalable parallel solution algorithms (see Section 4) as well as dedicated parallel hardware (see Section 3). The developed techniques will be used for the implementation of a gynaecologic laparoscopic VR-trainer system.

2 Elastomechanical Modelling

To enable the virtual reality simulation of surgical operations, we must achieve the following:

- Calculation of realistic deformations and contact forces of the organs
- Performance of the calculations in real-time
- Stable calculations for the time range of the entire simulation

2.1 Explicit Finite Element Formulation

A continuum can be described mathematically with the following set of partial differential equations, satisfied for each material point:

$$\mathrm{div}\sigma + \mathbf{f} = \rho\ddot{\mathbf{u}} \quad \text{(momentum equations)} \tag{1}$$

$$\mathrm{div}(\rho\dot{\mathbf{u}}) + \dot{\rho} = 0 \quad \text{(continuity equation)} \tag{2}$$

$$\sigma = f_1(\epsilon) \quad \text{(constitutive law)} \tag{3}$$

$$\epsilon = f_2(\mathbf{u}) \quad \text{(strain formulation)} \tag{4}$$

where σ is the Cauchy stress tensor, ϵ is the strain tensor, $\mathbf{f}$ is the vector of the volume forces, $\mathbf{u}$ stands for the displacements, and ρ is the density. A superposed dot denotes a derivative with respect to time.

Within the FEM a body is subdivided by a finite number of well defined elements (hexahedrons, tetrahedrons, quadrilaterals, e.g.). Displacements and positions in the element are interpolated from discrete nodal values. A trilinearly interpolated hexahedron consists of eight nodes lying in the corners. Figure 2(left) shows a 2D set of elements. Neighbour elements share some nodes. For every element the equations (1)–(4) can be formulated resulting in the following discrete system of differential equations:

$$\mathbf{M}\ddot{\mathbf{u}} + \mathbf{C}\dot{\mathbf{u}} + \mathbf{K}\delta\mathbf{u} = \mathbf{f} - \mathbf{r}, \tag{5}$$

where $\mathbf{M}$ is the mass matrix, $\mathbf{C}$ is the damping matrix, $\mathbf{K}$ is the incremental stiffness matrix, $\mathbf{u}$ is the vector of the nodal displacements, $\mathbf{f}$ are the external node forces, and $\mathbf{r}$ are the internal node forces. All these matrices and vectors may be time dependent.

One possibility to solve equations in (5) is a quasi-static manner [3, 5]. In this case the dynamic part of the equations is neglected ($\ddot{\mathbf{u}} = \dot{\mathbf{u}} = 0$) and the solution is reached iteratively. Within every iteration a huge set of linear algebraic equations has to be solved. In problems with large deformation and contact interactions the iteration hardly converges and a stable simulation over several minutes is nearly impossible.

Otherwise, the dynamic equations have to be integrated with respect to time [5]. The time integration of the equations can, in principle, be performed using implicit or explicit integration schemes. Using the implicit method, the solution has to be calculated iteratively at every discrete time step, like in the quasi-static problem. Contrary, the explicit time integration can be performed without iteration and without solving a system of linear algebraic equations. This integration scheme is only conditionally stable; that is, only very small time steps lead to a stable solution [4]. An estimation for the critical time step is made by $\Delta t = \frac{\Delta L}{c}$, where c is the maximal wave propagation speed in the medium and ΔL is the smallest element length of the model. In the case of our model of an uterus and its adnexes, this equation leads to 10'000 time steps per second ($\Delta t = 100 \, \mu s$).

These short time steps increase the computational effort but lead to a very stable contact formulation. The disadvantage of this method — that many steps have to be taken — is not so significant since each step is much less time consuming than in an implicit algorithm.

Because of the considerations mentioned above, and based on several numerical tests, we decided to solve the problems with an explicit Finite Element formulation. Unfortunately, this integration scheme is not as accurate as the implicit one and time discretisation errors will usually accumulate. In the next section we will show a way of avoiding this problem.

2.2 Element Formulation / Constitutive Equations

The most time consuming part in the explicit formulation is the computation of the internal element forces (see Section 2.3), including the calculation of stresses and strains. These state variables are related to well defined reference configurations. In the following we have to distinguish the updated and the total Lagrange formulation.

Within the updated Lagrange formulation a state is related to the last successfully calculated configuration. Here, strains are usually of an incremental form. This leads to an accumulation of discretisation errors and in consequence to the above mentioned lack of accuracy. Additionally, an incremental strain formulation (even in the case of elastic materials) usually leads to remaining deformations in a stress free state after a load cycle [6,7]. These errors drastically influence the robustness of a simulation and have to be eliminated.

When a total Lagrange formulation is chosen every state is related to the initial configuration. In this case absolute strain formulations have to be considered (e.g., Green-Lagrange or Hencky). Even with the explicit time integration scheme this leads to an exact static solution, i.e., when the transient terms have been eliminated by damping effects. Contrary to incremental strain formulations, these strains lead to correct results after a load cycle and no error accumulation occurs.

These considerations suggested to use a hyperelastic material law. The Mooney-Rivlin law for nearly incompressible materials leads to an elegant Finite Element formulation and is frequently used in biological tissue modelling. The Mooney-Rivlin material law is a first attempt, and will probably be replaced by a neo-Hookean law, completed with an appropriate damping model.

2.3 Volume Integration

To obtain the internal forces of an element we have to solve the following integral:

$$f_i^I = \int_{V^0} F_{il} B_k^I S_{kl} dV^0 , \tag{6}$$

where repeated subscripts imply summation over the range of that subscript. f_i^I are the internal forces in direction i of node I of the element, F_{il} are the components of the deformation gradient, B_k^I are the derivatives of the interpolation functions with respect to coordinate k, S_{kl} are the components of the 2nd Piola-Kirchhoff stress tensor and V^0 is the initial volume of the element.

Commonly, this integral is evaluated by a numerical 8-point quadrature. That is, the integrand will be computed with respect to 8 different integration points, and the eight values are added with a well defined weighting factor. This computation is very time consuming.

The reduced volume integration is a method to circumvent this overhead [2]. Within this scheme the integrand has to be calculated just once for each element. Considering only the mean strains within an element, some deformation modes (hourglass modes) are not influenced by the resulting forces. These modes have to be controlled with additional stabilisation forces (hourglass control):

$$f_i^I = F_{il} B_k^I S_{kl} V^0 +^{stab} f_i^I . \tag{7}$$

A shortcoming of commonly used formulations for the stabilisation forces is their incremental character. Obviously, this leads to accumulated time integration errors and to incorrect results after load cycles. Consequently we formulate these forces with respect to the initial configuration. This method leads to very stable results even in cases of large deformations. Furthermore, no integration errors will be accumulated.

If Finite Elements are not distorted in the initial configuration absolute formulations have an additional advantage. Many multiplications can be saved, and even the hourglass control needs considerably fewer multiplications.

3 Design of a real-time FEM Computation Engine

The only way to provide the necessary computational power for the real-time solution of complex Finite Element systems is to build a parallel computer which supports fully parallel algorithms for the explicit time integration scheme. Algorithmic design as described in Section 4 below allows to scale the computation to the necessary speed with the selection of an appropriate number of processor units or processing elements (PE). The section summarises the basic requirements and design principles for implementing special-purpose, parallel hardware to perform explicit Finite Element calculations.

3.1 Performance Requirements

Computation Once the necessary FE calculations and the corresponding parallel algorithms are determined, we have to analyse the performance requirements in detail to find out what kind of computer is needed to satisfy our demands.

Analysis of optimised explicit Finite Element algorithms shows that approximately 700 floating point operations per element are needed in each time step. Additional computation time has to be reserved for collision detection and handling. This leads to 10 MFLOPS (Million Floating Point Operations Per Second) per element for the chosen time step of $100\,\mu s$. For 2000 elements, a total of 20 GFLOPS sustained are needed.

This amount of computational power is much too high for a state of the art workstation. Implicit FE calculation can be implemented well on vector-supercomputers, since the main task is to solve huge sparse systems of linear equations [28, 29]. However, the time steps and the vectors of the explicit method are too short, therefore a high performance parallel machine is needed.

The latest processors are able to deliver >300 MFLOPS with optimised programming, so 64 of these will meet our demands. As Finite Element calculations have a tendency to become unstable, accurate computation using double precision floating point operations is necessary. During the time steps, data has to be sent and received with minimal processor involvement, requiring that very light weight protocols be used.

Communication There are three different types of communication: exchange of forces, collision detection and handling, and data transfer to the graphics engine. For a FE model with 2000 elements on a $4 \times 4 \times 4$ processor machine, 5600 force vectors have to be exchanged each time step. This results in a communication bandwidth of 1.35 GByte/s. This is a huge number, but the fact that data only has to be transferred between neighbours eases our requirements.

In collision communication, we note that only part of the surface nodes are potentially colliding with other parts of the FE model, and only about 300 vectors have to be exchanged for a 2000 element model (72 MByte/s).

Finally, the information for all the surface nodes must be sent to the graphics engine. This takes place once every 40ms, but to avoid adding too much latency to the system, data should be sent in a shorter time (20 time steps) . On this basis, 18 MByte/s have to be sent to the graphics engine interface.

3.2 Parallel Processing Architecture

According to the previous algorithmic considerations, a three-dimensional mesh of processors can be optimally used, where every processing element (PE) is

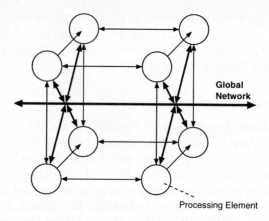

Fig. 1. 3D Communication Architecture

connected to its six neighbours (Figure 1). Every PE calculates a cube of the whole FE model, so it has to exchange data from the faces of its cube with PEs that share the same faces. In addition there are also edges and corners, where data has to be shared among processors that are not connected by a direct channel. Such data has to be routed through other PEs. This is actually no drawback, since in most cases the intermediate PEs have also data to transmit to the same target PE, so they just add their values before transmitting the received data block.

Local Communication To achieve the necessary low latency, we have to exploit the specialties of our communication pattern. If data has to be exchanged between processors, it must be communicated in every time step. Fortunately it is known at programming time which data values have to be sent, in what order, and to which destination. Secondly, when the elements are assigned to the processors, only those processors with elements sharing nodes on the common face of the cubes have to exchange data (collision detection is an exception to this). Bearing this in mind, the best way to provide sufficient communication bandwidth with low latency and minimal software overhead is to use point to point communication and to transmit pure data without additional address information. There is no need for routing information when point to point channels are used, and sending only data values minimises software overhead on the sender side. But the data still has to be recognised by the receiver. The address information, however, of the data is implicitly given by the order within the time step it is sent. It is known at compile time which values have to be exchanged, so the tool that partitions the elements also sets up the order in which data values are sent and received.

Global Communication Communication takes place mostly between neighbours, although data for collision detection has to be exchanged between two processors that may be far away within the mesh. Part of these data values has to be broadcast to all other processors. Additionally, several processors can send and receive data at the same time.

Routing such data through the local channels is very inefficient. Bandwidth is used that is needed for local communication. The routing may consume processor time which can be better utilised for FE calculation and routing through several PEs increases latency to an unacceptable level. Therefore, such messages are better sent over a global network over which any PE can exchange data with all others. Data must be identified, thus packets of data must be sent with information concerning the receiver as well as an identification.

4 Partitioning the Model for Parallel Computation

Explicit FE computation suggests element-wise parallelism, decomposing the spatial domain. Each element is mapped to exactly one processor, and one processor computes the internal forces of several elements (see Figure 2 left). Whenever elements residing on different processors share common nodes, these

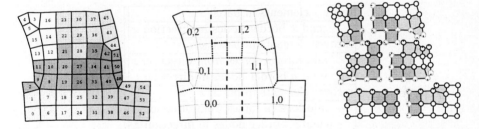

Fig. 2. *Left:* A small 2D model serves for illustrating the concepts on paper. The six different shades of gray illustrate an arbitrary assignment of elements to 2×3 processors. *Middle:* The coordinates of the processors to which parts of the model (groups of elements) are assigned. Dashed lines show x borders, dotted lines y borders. *Right:* The model is partitioned in submodels. Grey shades indicate batches for recovery, arrows mark nodes on the border

nodes must be represented on all involved processors. The resulting force acting on such a distributed node emerges from the communication among the contributing processors, which treat the foreign forces like external forces, adding them to their own.

4.1 Parallel Computation

Due to the inherently 3D nature of the problem, 3D processor networks appear to be the optimal topology for a multiprocessor architecture. PEs are are labelled with "coordinates", which generally do not correspond to geometric coordinates (see Figure 2 middle).

The mapping of elements to processors should balance the computational load while minimising the demand for communication bandwidth.

A force acting on a node must be applied exactly once. This is inherently given for inner forces (from recovery). Inertial and gravity forces are applied only on one PE, where the node is circled black in Figure 2(right). Other nodes (circled gray) initialize forces to 0.

The mapping defines the sequence of computation and communication which have to run on the parallel computer. To make effective use of the parallel architecture, the load should be balanced among the single processors, and waiting for data from other processors should be minimised. The procedure sketched below aims at this goal. The term "recovery" means determining the interior reaction forces within one element (eqn. (6)).

The summation over all elements is split into four phases with communication interlaced between them. Nodes on the x border are marked with a horizontal arrow. Before sending in direction x, all elements with such a node must be computed; they are in batch x, and the figure shows them shaded in a darker gray. While the forces are being transferred, elements in the y batch (lighter gray) are recovered. (No z batch exists in the 2D illustration.) The remaining elements are local to the PE; they belong to the "inner" batch (white).

recover elements in batch x
send x border nodes in direction x
recover elements in batch y
add foreign forces from direction x
send y border nodes in direction y
recover elements in batch z
add foreign forces from direction y
send z border nodes in direction z
recover elements in "inner" batch
add foreign forces from direction z

When possible, the recovery of some "own" elements is computed between sending partially assembled node forces in some direction and using the foreign forces from said direction.

4.2 Collision Detection

The next part is collision detection, which uses the global network for data transfer. We adopt an approximation to collision detection that is commonly used with the FEM. This method only determines which nodes of one contact partner, the slave, penetrate any face of the other contact partner, the master. Flipping the roles of master and slave and averaging will balance this obvious asymmetry. To save time on collision detection, the dynamic behaviour of the model is taken into account. Elements do not move faster then 10 cm/s, so if two elements are 2 cm apart, the earliest time they can touch is 100 ms or 1000 time steps away. A collision between these elements cannot take place within the next 1000 time steps and therefore needs no attention. Secondly, the system is built in a hierarchical manner. Every PE first checks bounding boxes with every other PE, before checking for collisions on an element level.

Thus collision detection takes the following steps:

- Every 1000 time steps all bounding boxes are compared.
- If close enough bounding boxes are detected, the corresponding PEs establish a communication channel to exchange the displacements of nodes that may be involved in collisions.
- During the next 1000 time steps, the displacements of these nodes are sent to and received from the other PEs. Collisions are detected and each PE determines the consequences for its nodes. Because these computations are symmetrical, all force vectors generated by collisions sum to zero.

Since the communication channels are only redefined every 1000 time steps, software overhead is minimised.

5 Conclusion

Explicit Finite Element analysis leads to very stable simulations even in the case of large deformations and contact problems. The use of a total Lagrange formulation increases the stability and eliminates integration errors in the static solution. Reduced integration decreases the calculation costs by a factor of 5–7 and nevertheless leads to very stable and sufficiently accurate results when the stabilisation forces are calculated with respect to the initial configuration.

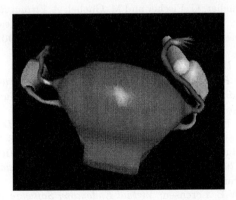

Fig. 3. Deformation of the fallopian tubes with a blunt probe.

Appropriately designed parallel algorithms enable implementation of the explicit integration method on a large, 3-dimensional network of high-performance processor units, allowing the subsequent usage of these techniques even in real-time surgery simulator systems. The usefulness of the developed methods have been demonstrated with the simulation of deformations of the uterus' fallopian tubes during diagnostic gynaecological laparoscopy (see Figure 3). The implementation of the complete laparoscopic simulator system including the construction of the specialised FEM computational engine is in progress.

References

1. K.J. Bathe: *Finite Element Procedures*, Prentice Hall, Englewood Cliffs, New Jersey 1996
2. T. Belytschko and S. Ong: *Hourglass Control in Linear and Nonlinear Problems*, Computer Methods in Applied Mechanics and Engineering, **43**:251–276, 1984
3. M.A. Crisfield: *Non-linear Finite Element Analysis of Solid and Structures - Volume 1: Essentials*, John Wiley & Sons, Chichester 1991
4. D.P. Flanagan and T. Belytschko: *Eigenvalues and Stable Time Steps for the Uniform Strain Hexahedron and quadrilateral*, Journal of Applied Mechanics, **51**:35–40, March 1984
5. E. Hinton: *NAFEMS - Introduction to nonlinear Finite Element Analysis*, Bell and Bain Ltd., Glasgow 1992
6. M. Kojic and K.J. Bathe: *Studies of Finite Element Procedures-Stress Solution of a Closed Elastic Strain Path with Stretching and Shearing Using the Updated Lagrangian Jaumann Formulation*, Computers & Structures, **26**(1/2):175–179, 1987
7. S. Roy et al.: *On the Use of Polar Decomposition in the Integration of Hypoelastic Constitutive Laws*, International Journal of Engineering Science, **30**(2):119–133, 1992
8. O.C. Zienkiewicz and R.L. Taylor: *The Finite Element Method*, McGraw-Hill Book Company, London 1994
9. M.A. Sagar, D. Bullivant, G.D. Mallinson, P.J. Hunter and I.W. Hunter: *A Virtual Environment and Model of the Eye for Surgical Simulation*, Comp. Graphics **28**:205–212, 1994
10. R. Ziegler, W. Mueller, G. Fischer and M. Goebel: *A Virtual Reality Medical Training System*, Proc. 1st In. Conf. on Comp. Vision, Virtual Reality and Robotics in Medicine, CVRMed'95, Nice, Lecture Notes in Comp. Sci., **905**:282–286, Springer-Verlag, 1995
11. U.G. Kühnapfel, H.G. Krumm, C. Kuhn, M. Hübner and B. Neisius: *Endosurgery Simulations with KISMET: A flexible tool for Surgical Instrument Design, Operation Room Planning and VR Technology based Abdominal Surgery Training*, Proc. Virtual reality World'95, Stuttgart, 165–171, 1995
12. S.A. Cover, N.F. Ezquerra and J.F. O'Brian: *Interactively Deformable Models for Surgery Simulation*, IEEE Comp. Graphics and Appl. **13**:68–75, 1993
13. D.J. Vining: *Virtual Endoscopy: Is It Really?*, Radiology, **200**:30–31, 1996
14. : R. Satava: *Virtual Endoscopy: Diagnosis using 3-D Visualisation and Virtual Representation*, Surgical Endoscopy, **10**:173–174, 1996
15. A.M. Alyassin, W.E. Lorensen: *Virtual Endoscopy Software Application on a PC*, Proc. MMVR'98: 84–89, IOS Press, 1998
16. S. Cotin, H. Delingette, J.M. Clément, M. Bro-Nielsen, N. Ayache and J. Marescaux: *Geometrical and Physical Representations for a Simulator of Hepatic Surgery*, Proc. MMVR'96:139–151, IOS Press, 1996
17. M. Bro-Nielsen and S. Cotin: *Real-time volumetric deformable models for surgery simulation using Finite Elements and condensation*, Comp. Graphics Forum **15**(3):57–66, 1996

18. S. Gibson, J. Samosky, A. Mor, C. Fyock, E. Grimson, T. Kanade, R. Kikinis, H. Lauer, N. McKenzie, S. Nakajima, H. Ohkami, R. Osborne and A. Sawada: *Simulating Arthroscopic Knee Surgery using Volumetric Object Representations, Real-Time Volume Rendering and Haptic Feedback*, Proc. CVRMed'97:369–378, Springer-Verlag, 1997
19. C. Basdogan, Ch-H. Ho, M.A. Srinivasan, S.D. Small, S.L. Dawson: *Force interactions in Laparoscopic Simulations: Haptic Rendering of Soft Tissues*, Proc. MMVR'98:385–391, IOS Press, 1998
20. A.H. Barr: *Global and Local Deformations of Solid Primitives*, Computer Graphics **18**(3):21–30, 1984
21. M. Bro-Nielsen, D. Helfrick, B. Glass, X. Zeng, H. Connacher: *VR Simulation of Abdominal Trauma Surgery*, Proc. MMVR'98:117–123, IOS Press, 1998
22. T.W. Sederberg and S.R. Parry: *Free-Form Deformation of Solid Geometric Models*, Computer Graphics **20**(4):151–160, 1986
23. D. Terzopoulos, J. Platt, A. Barr and K. Fleischer: *Elastically Deformable Models*, Computer Graphics **21**(4):205–214, 1987
24. Ch. Baur, D. Guzzoni and O. Georg: *Virgy: A Virtual Reality and Force Feedback Based Endoscopy Surgery Simulator*, Proc. MMVR'98:110–116, IOS Press, 1998
25. M. Downes, M.C. Cavusoglu, W. Gantert, L.W. Way and F. Tendick: *Virtual Environments for Training Critical Skills in Laparoscopic Surgery*, Proc. MMVR'98:316–322, IOS Press, 1998
26. J.K. Hahn, R. Kaufman, A.B. Winick, Th. Carleton, Y. Park, R. Lindeman, K-M Oh, N. Al-Ghreimil, R.J. Walsh, M. Loew, J. Gerber and S. Sankar: *Training Environment for Inferior Vena Caval Filter Placement*, Proc. MMVR'98:291–297, IOS Press, 1998
27. N. Suzuki, A. Hattori, T. Ezumi, A. Uchiyama, T. Kumano, A. Ikamoto, Y. Adachi, A. Takatsu: *Simulator for virtual surgery using deformable organ models and force feedback system*, Proc. MMVR'98:227–233, IOS Press, 1998
28. V.E. Taylor: *Application-Specific Architectures for Large Finite-Element Applications*, PhD Thesis, Dept. El. Eng. and Comp. Sci., Univ. of California, Berkeley, CA, 1991
29. C. Pommerell: *Solution of large unsymmetric systems of linear equations*, PhD Thesis, Department of Electrical Engineering, ETH Zürich, 1992

A Colour Image Processing Method for Melanoma Detection

O. Colot[1], R. Devinoy[2], A. Sombo[2], D. de Brucq[2]

[1]PSI-LCIA, INSA de Rouen, Place E. Blondel, 76131 Mont-Saint-Aignan Cédex, France.
[2]PSI-La3I, Université Rouen, Place E. Blondel,76821 Mont-Saint-Aignan Cédex, France.
Olivier.Colot@insa-rouen.fr

Abstract.

In this paper, we propose a method dedicated to classification between benign and malignant lesions in Dermatology in the aim to help the clinicians for melanoma diagnosis[1].
The proposed methodology reduces the very numerous informations contained in the digitized images to a finite set of parameters giving a description of the colour and the shape of the lesions.
The whole process is shared in three steps: preprocessing, segmentation and classification of the lesions.
The proposed method was applied on a data base of 38 lesions (20 benign lesions and 18 malignant lesions) in the aim to assess the feasability of the proposed method.
The good classification rate obtained with the method is discussed and later tests to engage are underlined.

1. Introduction

Melanoma is an increasing form of cancer in the world. It has increased twice times for 15 years in Canada and it is 3% in the USA at this time.
The rate of clinicians visual investigations gets at 65% of good detection at the very best. In particular, it is very difficult to distinguish some atypical lesions - which are benign - from melanoma because they have the same properties according to the well known ABCDE rules used by dermatologists [1].
There is a visual inspection problem for the atypical class. The unnecessary excision is often practise for these lesions.
The variability of colours and shapes can lead to different interpretation by different dermatologists. So, there is a variability and a no reproductibility of the diagnosis. Different lesions are given in Figure 1.
However, melanoma is well suited for image processing because it is on the skin. Some researches [2-9] have shown the advantages to use image processing in dermatology.

---

[1] This work is supported by the french *Ligue Nationale contre le Cancer*.

Furthermore, the image processing by computer ensures the reproducibility of the analysis. However, the essential difficulty is to design robust and relevant parameters to ensure the separation between melanoma and benign lesions, in particular the atypical lesions (benign) which can be clinically mistaken for melanoma.

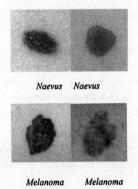

Naevus   Naevus

Melanoma   Melanoma

Fig. 1. Some lesions

At first, the lesion border is the first feature to identify. It is the first step of the processing to engage in order to extract informations about the lesion. So, the border extraction or identification is a critical step in computerized vision analysis in skin cancer as pointed out in [2]. Then, the segmentation step which takes place in any classification processing has to be really accurated.

As discussed in an early review [8], *computer image analysis in skin cancer is in its infancy*. The different developed approaches give results which are more or less accurate, efficient or reliable. It appears that in general each method needs a standarized image acquisition in order to be efficient. However, that is theoretical. Even you take care with the image acquisition conditions, there always exists deviations from standard conditions you define and you need to take them into account in the late image processing. We precise the preprocessing rules of our approach in section 2 where the deviations in image acquisition are taking into account and corrected before the image segmentation step.

The segmentation of coloured images does not involve as numerous studies as grey level image segmentation. In [4] an automatic colour segmentation algorithm is proposed for identification of skin tumor based on the use of six colour spaces. They apply a principal component transform in order to perform the border identification. We develop a multi-model approach too, but with different colour models leading to the definition of a 14-dimensional model of a colour image. This is proposed in section 3.

The whole process is then closed with the classification step developed in section 4.

The dermatologists use slides for lesion images storage and visual inspection for comparison. So, we based our processing on the use of such an information material. We digitalize the slides with a 35mm film scanner Nikon LS-1000.

2. Preprocessing

The preprocessing step is necessary because the images are noisy, the lighting conditions and the acquisition conditions are quite different from one slide to another. Futhermore, the images contains bright pixels due to local lighting conditions and local photometric properties of the lesions. So, we have developed a preprocessing technique which allows a photometric fitting in the aim to improve the images before the segmentation and the classification steps.The colorimetric fitting model or photometric corrective model we propose allows to have the safe skin around the lesion as close to a reference as possible.

In the aim to preserve the dynamics of the R, G and B values, we use a linear transformation on the safe skin area and on the lesion area.

The fitting model is written as it follows:

$$\begin{cases} R' = \dfrac{R - \overline{R_S}}{\sigma_{RS}} \times \sigma_{Rref} + \overline{R}_{Sref} \\ G' = \dfrac{G - \overline{G_S}}{\sigma_{GS}} \times \sigma_{Gref} + \overline{G}_{Sref} \\ B' = \dfrac{B - \overline{B_S}}{\sigma_{BS}} \times \sigma_{Bref} + \overline{B}_{Sref} \end{cases} \qquad (1)$$

where R' (respectively G' and B') is the transformation of a R value of one pixel, $\overline{R}_S$ (respectively $\overline{G}_S$ and $\overline{B}_S$) is the mean of R in the safe skin to be fitted, $\overline{R}_{S\,ref}$ (respectively $\overline{G}_{Sref}$ and $\overline{B}_{Sref}$) is the mean of R in the reference safe skin σ_{RS} (respectively σ_{VS} and σ_{BS}), is the standard deviation of R in the safe skin to be fitted and σ_{Rref} (respectively σ_{Gref} and σ_{Bref}), is the standard deviation in the reference safe skin.

Figure 2 shows the results of the colorimetric corrective model applied to a same lesion taken with three different acquisition conditions.

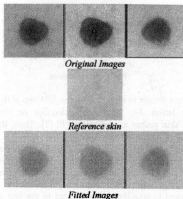

Original Images

Reference skin

Fitted Images

Fig. 2. Photometric correction

3. Segmentation

So as to obtain geometric and colorimetric informations on a lesion, it is necessary to run a segmentation process which will allow to extract the pixels belonging to the lesion from the image. The segmentation process we have developed is based on the cooperation between a segmentation in regions and a segmentation based on edge detection [10]. So, we consider there exists two kinds of pixels in the image:

1. pixels which belong to the safe skin
2. pixels which belong to the lesion.

So, we consider the image is made of two populations. The problem can then be viewed as a problem of two-hypotheses test:

1. *Hypothesis H_S*: the pixel (i,j) is a pixel in the safe skin
2. *Hypothesis H_L*: the pixel (i,j) is a pixel in the lesion

where i and j are the coordinates such as $i \in \{1,...,N\}$ and $j \in \{1,...,M\}$ and $N \times M$ is the image dimension. Under these considerations, we compute a threshold obtained by means of the use of the *Entropy Maximization Principle* (EMP) [11] that is the coarse segmentation. So, we obtain a first region of pixels which surely belong to the safe skin and a second region of pixels which surely belong to the lesion.

To define the contour of the lesion as well as it is possible, it is necessary to perform a local approach, what we call the fine segmentation task. For that, a variable Z is defined from an observation vector Y with 14 components built with the following different colour models for any pixel (i,j):

1. the RGB model (3 parameters)
2. the rgb model (3 parameters)
3. the HIS model (3 parameters)
4. the Faugeras model (5 parameters)

The choice of a colour model is often arbitrary. The modelling we adopt take into account different sources of information. We can consider we have nothing less than a fusion of different sources.
A variable Z is obtained from the projection on the direction linking the two conditionnal means computed in the coarse segmentation step. We compute the means and the covariances of the vector Y under each hypothesis. We replace the mathematical expected values by statistical means under the hypothesis H_S and under the hypothesis H_L, that is to say:

$$\begin{cases} E(Y/H_S) \approx m_S = \frac{1}{Card_S} \sum_{(i,j) \in G_S} Y(i,j) \\ Cov(Y/H_S) \approx \Gamma_S = \frac{1}{Card_S - 1} \sum_{(i,j) \in G_S} (Y(i,j) - m_S)^T (Y(i,j) - m_S) \end{cases} \quad (2)$$

and:

$$\begin{cases} E(Y/H_L) \approx m_L = \frac{1}{Card_L} \sum_{(i,j) \in G_L} Y(i,j) \\ Cov(Y/H_L) \approx \Gamma_L = \frac{1}{Card_L - 1} \sum_{(i,j) \in G_L} (Y(i,j) - m_L)^T (Y(i,j) - m_L) \end{cases} \quad (3)$$

We consider that Y follows a Gaussian distribution such as:

$$f(Y) = \frac{1}{(2\Pi)^{n/2} (\det \Gamma)^{1/2}} \exp\left[-\frac{1}{2}(Y-m)^T \Gamma^{-1}(Y-m)\right] \quad (4)$$

The logarithm of the likelihood $\frac{f(Y/H_S)}{f(Y/H_L)}$ gives:

$$\ln \frac{f(Y/H_S)}{f(Y/H_L)} = \frac{1}{2}\left\{ \ln\left[\frac{\det \Gamma_L}{\det \Gamma_S}\right] - \left[(Y-m_S)^T \Gamma_S^{-1}(Y-m_S) - (Y-m_L)^T \Gamma_L^{-1}(Y-m_L)\right] \right\} \quad (5)$$

Let U be the n-dimensional unit vector giving the direction of the centres of gravity such as:

$$U \triangleq \frac{m_S m_L}{\|m_S m_L\|} \quad (6)$$

Let be T the estimator to choose between the two hypotheses H_S and H_L. It is based on the computation of the scalar product $\langle .,. \rangle$ of the vector Y of observation and the direction of the centres of gravity, that is to say:

$$T(Y(i,j)) = \sum_{l=1}^{n} U_l Y_l(i,j) = \langle U, Y(i,j) \rangle \quad (7)$$

Under the hypothesis H_S, T is a Gaussian estimator with the mean:

$$E(T(Y)/H_S) \approx \sum_{l=1}^{n} U_l m_{S,l} \quad (8)$$

and with the variance:

$$V(T(Y)/H_S) \approx U^T \Gamma_S U \quad (9)$$

Under the hypothesis H_L, we obtain the same formula where L stands for S.
If we compute the projection of the observations on the direction of the conditional means of the two classes (class C_L of pixels belonging to the lesion and class C_S of pixels belonging to the safe skin) we define a cut-off direction U. In the sequel, we consider centered and reduced variables and define the normalized observation vector Y'.
For any pixel in the image, we define a variable Z such as:

$$Z = P_U(Y) = \langle Y, U \rangle = Y_1 u_1 + ... + Y_n u_n \qquad (10)$$

Because of the geometrical structure of the lesions, we have developed a radial search for the contour localization using the variable Z (see the Figure 4) for m orientations of angle θ_m. The aim is to locate the contour point in each direction $\overleftarrow{d_{\theta_m}}$ of angle θ_m.
Let us note that the separation between the lesion and the safe skin can be inside a blurred zone.

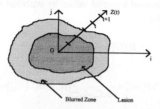

Fig. 3. Radial search principle

Let G_L and G_S be respectively the center of gravity of the lesion and the center of gravity of the safe skin region. In each region, we can consider that the variable Z varies around a mean value given as a straight line. The two defined straight lines (one per region) are quite parallel.
Let us consider the following quadratic cost function:

$$\Phi = \sum_{t \in S} \left(Z(t) - \hat{Z}_s(t) \right)^2 + \sum_{t \in L} \left(Z(t) - \hat{Z}_L(t) \right)^2 \qquad (11)$$

where $\overline{Z}_s$ is the expectation of the variable Z in the safe skin and $\overline{Z}_L$ the expectation of the variable Z in the lesion.

So, we compute the estimation $\hat{a}$ of the slope a and we have then the equations of the two straight lines:

$$\begin{cases} \hat{Z}_s(t) = \hat{a}(t - \overline{t}_S) + \overline{Z}_S \\ \hat{Z}_L(t) = \hat{a}(t - \overline{t}_L) + \overline{Z}_L \end{cases} \qquad (12)$$

The optimal separation between the lesion and the safe skin is obtained by defining a straight line of separation at the middle of the two previous lines. The equation of this straight line is:

$$\hat{Z}_{Sep}(t) = \hat{a}(t) - \frac{1}{2}\hat{a}(\overline{t}_L + \overline{t}_S) + \frac{1}{2}\left(\overline{Z}_L + \overline{Z}_S \right) \qquad (13)$$

The edge point is then defined as the first point cutting the separation line when one runs along this line from the safe skin side towards the lesion side. We give in figure 4, the behaviour of the variable Z according to a given direction θ and the different straight lines we have obtained. To illustrate the segmentation process, we give in figure 5 the results of the edge location obtained on some lesions.

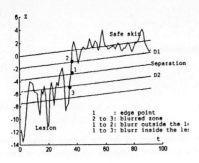

Fig. 4. Edge point location

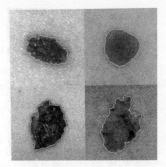

Fig. 5. Contours of different lesions

4. Classification

For the classification, we propose 12 primitives - geometric as well as photometric - which are robust and relevant.
The different parameters are:
1. The compactness of the shape.
2. The expanse.
3. The mean deviation from the gravity center.
4. The regularity of the contour.
5. The lengthening
6. The blurred surface quantization.
7. The homogeneity of R.
8. The symetry of R.
9. The homogeneity of G/R.
10. The symetry of G/R.
11. The deviation between the mean r on the safe skin and the mean of r on the lesion.
12. The deviation between the mean b on the safe skin and the mean of b on the lesion.

The homogeneity is defined as the sum of the transitions clear zone/dark zone and dark zone/clear zone of C (C=R or C= G/R) when the lesion is discribed horizontaly and vertically. The dark zone is defined as the third darker area of C in the lesion and the clear zone is defined as the third clearer area of C in the lesion.
The colour symetry is given by: $s_C = \frac{|\overline{d_D} - \overline{d_C}|}{\overline{d_G}}$ where $\overline{d_D}$ is the mean distance of the darker pixels to the gravity center and $\overline{d_C}$ is the mean distance of the clearer pixels to the gravity center. $\overline{d_G}$ is the mean distance to the gravity center. Let us note that the homogeneity and the symetry are indexes of polychromy.
These parameters or primitives derives from clinical features or are original features. It is possible to increase the number of primitives but only robust and efficient parameters are needed in a classification step.
Let be L the whole set of lesions built with the set L_B of benign lesions and the set L_M of malignant lesions.
We consider the benign lesions as the reference group for which the mean and the standard deviation are computed for each of the q primitives, with $q=12$. So, for a lesion l_i in L_B, we define a vector X_i of dimension q, such as :

$$X_i \stackrel{\Delta}{=} [x_{i1} \quad x_{i2} \quad ... \quad x_{iq}] \quad (14)$$

Let be m_{Bj} and σ_{Bj} the mean and the standard deviation for the jth primitive computed on the whole subset L_B of benign lesions. So :

$$m_{Bj} = \frac{1}{n_B} \sum_{l_i \in L_B} x_{ij} \quad \text{and} \quad (\sigma_{Bj})^2 = \frac{1}{n_B} \sum_{l_i \in L_B} (x_{ij} - m_{Bj})^2 \qquad (15)$$

where n_B = CardL_B is the number of lesions in L_B. Then, we consider the reduced matrix:

$$X' = \begin{bmatrix} Y'_1 & Y'_2 & \ldots & Y'_q \end{bmatrix} \qquad (16)$$

built with the centered-reduced vectors defined as it follows:

$$Y'_j = \frac{Y_j - m_{Bj}}{\sigma_{Bj}} \qquad (17)$$

A *Principal Components Analysis* (PCA) applied to the results obtained for the benign lesions, gives q principal axes e_j of dimension q which allow to build q new uncorrelated primitives. We define then q principal components W_j, on the whole set of all the lesions.

$$W_j = X'.e_j^{tr} \qquad (18)$$

These q vectors allow to build the matrix W which consists of the results obtained on the whole set L of the lesions:

$$W \overset{\Delta}{=} \begin{bmatrix} w_{11} & w_{12} & \ldots & w_{1q} \\ w_{21} & w_{22} & \ldots & w_{2q} \\ \ldots & \ldots & \ldots & \ldots \\ w_{n1} & w_{n2} & \ldots & w_{nq} \end{bmatrix} \qquad (19)$$

where the scalar w_{ij} is the value of the jth primitive for the ith lesion. We want to distinguish the malignant lesions from the benign lesions by the use of the new q primitives e_j. A malignant lesion is defined as a lesion for which one or several primitives are far from those obtained on the benign lesions.
Let be Hyp the matrix defined by $n \times q$ elements Hyp_{ij} as it follows:

$$Hyp_{ij} = \begin{cases} 1 & \text{if} \quad c_{ij} > m_B(e_j) + k\sigma_B(e_j) \\ -1 & \text{if} \quad c_{ij} < m_B(e_j) + k\sigma_B(e_j) \\ 0 & \text{else} \end{cases} \qquad (20)$$

with $k \in \aleph$.
If Hyp$_{ij}$=1, then the lesion l_i is hyper for the primitive j. If Hyp$_{ij}$=-1, then the lesion l_i is hypo for the primitive j and if Hyp$_{ij}$=0, then the lesion l_i is indifferent for the primitive j.
The parameter k gives the authorized deviation from the mean. In the Gaussian case, it gives the error probability. Taking a weak value for k leads to an important rate of false alarm. Unlikely, a big value for k can induce no detection. In practice, k=3 (Probabilty of false alarm is 0,27%) is a well-suited value.
The more relevant primitives to distinguish the melanoma from benign lesions are those which detect the more numerous malignant lesions and which detect the lesions that others do not detect. The selection of these primitives is based on the principle of overlap [12]. A primitive P_j overlaps a primitive P_i when lesions which are considered Hyper or Hypo by P_i are considered Hyper or Hypo by P_j too. A primitive overlaps another one if it gives at least the same information. At the end, there are d primitives among q which are kept for classification.

5. Results

We have applied the classification process on a set of 38 lesions: 20 benign lesions (naevi) and 18 malignant lesions (melanoma). If we take the max or min values of the d primitives, it appears that the two populations of lesions have a quite different behaviour (see Fig. 6). The two thresholds T_{low}=-3 and T_{high}=+3, allow to detect the melanoma.

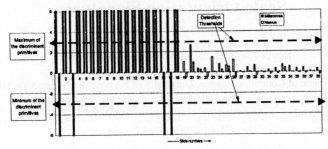

Fig. 6. Melanoma detection with the method Hyper-Hypo

6. Conclusion

The method we have developed does not depend on a standard of acquisition conditions. The robustness of the segmentation and the robustness of the primitives used for the classification seem to be real. Futhermore, the feasability in benign and malignant lesion discrimination are quite possible according to our first results (100% of melanoma detected ; 0% of non-detection or false alarm). However, we have engaged with dermatologists a prospective study in the aim to increase our data base, in particular to increase the number of melanoma. So, we have engaged a test on about 300 slides of benign and malignant lesions.

Acknoledgments

We thank Professor P. Joly and Professor Ph. Lauret of Charles Nicolle's Hospital for their expert opinion.

References

1. Friedman, R.J. : Early Detection of Melanoma: the Role of Physician Examination and Self Examination of tne Skin. CA. 35 (1985) 130-151.
2. Golston, J.E., Moss, R.H., Stoecker, V. : Boundary Detection in Skin Tumor Images: an Overall Approach and a Radial Search Algorithm. Pattern Recognition. 23 (1990) 1235-1247.
3. Cascinelli, N., Ferrario, M., Bufalino, R. : Results obtained by using a Computarized Image Analysis System designed as an Aid in Diagnosis of Cutaneous Melanoma. Melanoma Res. 2 (1992) 163-170.
4. Umbaugh, S.E., Moss, R.H., Stoecker, V. : An automatic color segmentation algorithm with application to identification of skin tumor borders. Comp. Med. Imag. Graph. 16 (1992) 227-236.
5. Scott, E. : Automatic Color Segmentation Algorithms with Application to Skin Tumor Feature Identification. IEEE Engineering in Medicine and Biology. (1993) 75-82.
6. Schindewolf, T., Stolz, W., Albert, R., Abmayr, W., Harms, H. : Classification of melanocytic lesions with color and texture analysis using digital image processing. Anal. Quant. Cytol. Histol, 15 (1993) 1-11.
7. Schindewolf T., Schiffner, R., Stolz, et al. : Evaluation of different image acquisition techniques for computer vision system in the diagnosis of malignant melanoma. J. Am. Acad. Dermatol. 31 -1 (1994) 33-41.
8. Hall, P.N., Claridge, E., Morris Smith, J.D. : Computer screening for early detection of melanoma - is there a future? British Jal of Derm. 132 (1995) 325-338.
9. Colot O., Joly, P., Taouil, K., et al.: Analysis by means of image processing of benign and malignant melanocytic lesions. European Journal of Dermatology. 5 (1995) 441.
10. de Brucq D., Taouil, K., Colot, O., et al. : Segmentation d'images et extraction de contours pour l'analyse de lésions dermatologiques. Proc. Of the 15th Colloque GRETSI, Juan-les-Pins, France (1995) 1205-1208.
11. Kapur, J.N. : A new method for gray-level picture thresholding using entropy of the histogram. CVGIP 29 (1985) 273-285.
12. Hopcroft, J.E., Ullman, J.D. : Introduction to automata theory, languages and computation. Addison Wesley (1979).

Abnormal Masses in Mammograms: Detection Using Scale-Orientation Signatures

Reyer Zwiggelaar[1] and Christopher J. Taylor[2]

[1] Division of Computer Science, University of Portsmouth, Portsmouth, UK
reyer@sis.port.ac.uk
[2] Wolfson Image Analysis Unit, University of Manchester, Manchester, UK
ctaylor@man.ac.uk

Abstract. We describe a method for labelling image structure based on scale-orientation signatures. These signatures provide a rich and stable description of local structure and can be used as a basis for robust pixel classification. We use a multi-scale directional recursive median filtering technique to obtain local scale-orientation signatures. Our results show that the new method of representation is robust to the presence of both random and structural noise. We demonstrate application to synthetic images containing lines and blob-like features and to mammograms containing abnormal masses. Quantitative results are presented, using both linear and non-linear classification methods.

1 Introduction

We are interested in labelling important structures in images. We assume that the position of these structures is unpredictable and that they will be embedded in a background texture. Real examples of this class of problem are ariel images - containing structures of interest such as roads, rivers and trees, and medical images containing blood vessels, ducts and focal abnormalities (e.g. tumours).

We describe an approach based on the construction of a scale-orientation signature at each pixel. This provides a very rich description of local structure which is robust and locally stationary. Given this description, standard statistical classification methods can be used - we give results for both linear and non-linear approaches for synthetic and real medical data.

2 Scale-Orientation Signatures

The Recursive Median Filter (RMF) is one of a class of filters, known as sieves, that remove image peaks or troughs of less than a chosen size [1]. They are closely related to morphological operators [8]. By applying sieves of increasing size to an image, then taking the difference between the output image from adjacent size sieves, it is possible to isolate image features of a specific size. Sieves have been shown to have desirable properties when compared to other methods [4] of constructing a scale space [2]. In particular the results at different positions on the same structure are similar (local stationarity) and the interaction between adjacent structures is minimised.

2.1 Describing Local Structure

For 2-D images, a 1-D RMF can be applied at any chosen angle, by covering the image with lines at this angle, ensuring that every pixel belongs to only one line. By performing 1-D Directional Recursive Median Filtering (DRMF) at several orientations, a scale-orientation signature can be built for each pixel. The signature is a 2-D array in which the columns represent measurements for the same orientation, the rows represent measurements for the same scale, and the values in the array represent the change in grey-level at the pixel, resulting from applying a filter at the scale and orientation corresponding to the position in the array. The grey-level changes are measured with respect to the image filtered at the next smaller scale at the same orientation.

Fig. 1 shows scale-orientation signatures for pixels located on synthetically generated structures. For instance, the response of the DRMF to a binary blob will result in a signature which has values at only one scale and is equal for all orientations (Fig. 1a). For a binary line the resulting signature is highly scale and orientation dependent, with the minimum scale related to the width of the line, and the maximum scale related to the length of the line (Fig. 1b). When the structures get more realistic, such as the Gaussian lines and blobs shown in Fig. 1 c and d, the signatures become slightly more complicated, but the overall shape remains similar. For blob-like structures the centre pixel gives a very characteristic signature, where the scales at which information is present in the signatures are related to the diameter of the structure. This is also true for pixels on the backbone of linear structures, for which the minimum scale in the signatures is related to the width of the linear structure, the maximum scale related to length, and the orientation at which this maximum occurs indicates the direction of the linear structure. Although the signatures for non-centre pixels are not identical they are usually very similar (compare the columns of signatures for each structure in Fig. 1). This local stationarity property is useful for pixel classification. The largest differences occur for the blob-like structures - there is a continuous change between the signatures from the centre of the blob-like structure to the extreme edge with small changes for pixels near the centre and relatively large changes towards the edge of the structure.

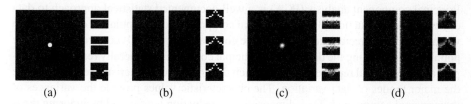

(a) (b) (c) (d)

Fig. 1. Some synthetic examples of multi-scale DRMF signatures, where the larger four images show (a) a binary blob, (b) a binary linear structure, (c) a Gaussian blob and (d) a Gaussian linear structure. The twelve smaller images are the scale-orientation signatures for the centre pixel (top), for a pixel at the extreme edge of the structure (bottom) and for a pixel in between these two extremes (middle). In the smaller scale-orientation signature images, scale is on the vertical axis (with the finest scale at the bottom) and orientation on the horizontal (the background grey-level is zero, i.e. only positive values are present in the DRMF signatures).

2.2 Noise Aspects

To show the effects of noise some example structures and scale-orientation signatures are shown in Fig. 2. The signal to noise ratio (SNR) is increased from left to right from infinite (i.e. no noise present) to 25%. It is clear that the signatures remain stable for signal to noise ratios larger than 0.5. but even below this value certain features in the signatures remain stable, with a band of values across all orientations between two distinct scales. Also note that in the noisy signatures a substantial change occurs at the smaller scales, which are characteristic of the noise that is present in the images. This behaviour of the scale-orientation signatures in the presence of noise, together with the effect shown in Fig. 1, makes it possible to obtain robust classification of pixels.

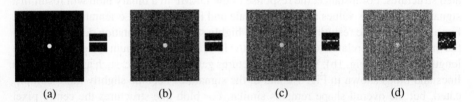

Fig. 2. Some synthetic examples of multi-scale DRMF signatures to indicate the effect of noise on the scale-orientation signatures (the same format as in Fig. 1 is used and only the signature for the centre pixel is shown) ,where the signal to noise ratio is ∞ (a), 1.0 (b) , 0.5 (c) and 0.25 (d).

3 Statistical Modelling

A brief description of the linear and non-linear modelling techniques used in our experiments are discussed in this section.

3.1 Principal Component Analysis

Principal component analysis (PCA) is a well documented statistical approach to data dimensionality reduction [3]. The principal components of a population of observation vectors are the characteristic vectors of the covariance matrix (**C**) constructed from the population. Projecting the data into its principal components generally results in a compact and meaningful representation in which the first few characteristic vectors describe the major modes of data variation. The characteristic values provide the variances of the principal components. Data dimensionality reduction is achieved by ignoring those principal components which have zero or small characteristic values.

3.2 Linear Classification

The objective of the work is to classify pixels, that is to label each pixel as belonging to a certain type of image structure. Since any method is likely to be imperfect it is useful to explore a range of compromises between false negative errors (poor sensitivity) and false positive errors (poor specificity). This can be achieved conveniently by constructing a probability for each pixel. The starting point is an observation vector, $\mathbf{x}_i$, for each pixel i, describing properties relevant to the classification task. For each class, ω_j (e.g. normal or abnormal), the mean, $\mathbf{m}_{\omega_j}$, and covariance, $\mathbf{C}_{\omega_j}$, of the observation vectors is estimated from a training set of signatures in which every pixel has been annotated with the appropriate class by an expert. The probability density of obtaining an observation vector $\mathbf{x}_i$ for a pixel of class ω_j is given by $p(\mathbf{x}_i|\omega_j)$ which can be calculated from $\mathbf{m}_{\omega_j}$ and $\mathbf{C}_{\omega_j}$ assuming a Gaussian distribution. Applying Bayes theorem, a probability image for class ω_j (e.g. abnormal) is found by calculating, for each pixel $P(\omega_j|\mathbf{x}_i)$. Detection can be performed by thresholding the resulting probability image. Different values of the threshold will result in different compromises between true positive and false positive errors. The detection performance as the threshold is varied can be summarised conveniently using Receiver Operating Characteristic (ROC) curves [5].

3.3 Non-Linear Classification

To assess the non-linear aspects of the scale-orientation signatures a basic back-propagation artificial neural network (ANN) was used [6]. The same network was used in all experiments. The architecture comprised an input layer of the 132 components (12 orientations × 11 scales) of the the scale-orientation signatures, two hidden layers and the output layer comprising three units for the synthetic data and two units for the mammographic data (these numbers were used to obtain a direct comparison with the linear classification which provides three and two class probabilities, respectively). The network was fully connected between the second hidden layer (10 units) and both the output layer and the first hidden layer (23 units). The connections between the input layer and the first hidden layer were, however, more restricted. The information from one scale (summed across all orientations) or one orientation (summed across all scales) was connected to each of the units of the first hidden layer.

4 Test Data

To assess the potential of the scale-orientation signatures for the classification of structures in images two different datasets were used: one synthetic, the other derived from real mammographic data. In both cases the datasets were divided into three equal sized subsets - facilitating a training, validation (only used for the non-linear classifier) and test set.

The synthetic data consisted of three separate datasets of 12288 scale-orientation signatures each (see Fig. 2d for a typical example). Each dataset contained equal numbers of signatures obtained from Gaussian linear structures, Gaussian blob-like structures and texture background (which was based on a combination of Gaussian and shot noise). The signatures were extracted from the top 5% of brightest pixels (before noise was added) from 768 images. All the samples were given class expectation values which could be used to determine the mean square error for a certain network.

The second dataset used in our experiments was drawn from mammograms. The signatures were extracted from 54 mammograms of which half contained an abnormality (a spiculated lesion). The available data was separated into three datasets, each comprising signatures from 18 mammograms. The resulting mammographic data comprised three separate datasets of 2700 scale-orientation signatures, each containing equal numbers of "normal" and "abnormal" signatures. The "abnormal" signatures were taken from the annotated central mass while the "normal" signatures were randomly selected from the normal mammograms.

5 Classification of Synthetic Data

We present results for classifying the synthetic data into three classes, using both linear and non-linear classifiers.

A principal component model was trained for every synthetic training data set. The first five principal components cumulatively explained approximately 49%, 60%, 64%, 69% and 73% of the training set variance respectively. A linear classifier was used to classify each signature in the datasets as belonging to the class of linear structure, blob-like structure or the texture background as described in Sec. 3.2. This information was used to obtain class probabilities.

For this data the ANN had three output neurons for the three classes; linear structures, blob-like structures and background texture. The class expectation values used were 0.90 for class samples and 0.05 for non-class samples. The three expectation values were thus directly comparable to the probabilities obtained using a linear classifier with their sum equal to 1.0. The optimal network was found (as described in Sec. 3.3) and used to obtain the expectation values which were used for classification of the data.

Classification accuracy was assessed by producing ROC curves as shown in Fig. 3. There is no difference between the use of the full scale-orientation signature and the reduced dimensionality representation. A sensitivity of 80% is obtained at a false positive rate of 0.15.

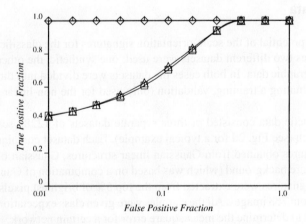

Fig. 3. Synthetic signature classification results for linear classification (△), PCA model based linear classification (□) and non-linear classification (◊).

The ANN performs almost perfect classification which compares very favourable with the linear classifier. 80% sensitivity is achieved at a false positive rate of 0.000013 and 98% sensitivity at 0.00005.

6 Classification of Mammographic Data

The classification of the mammographic data is into two classes, either abnormal mass or non-mass. Again both classification based on linear and non-linear methods are investigated and compared. In addition, application of the approach to images is discussed, with a typical example illustrating the differences in results leading to free response operating characteristic (FROC) curves and the number of false positives as a function of probability threshold.

A principal component model was trained on the mammographic data (individual results for the three datasets were similar). The first five principal components cumulatively explained approximately 31%, 49%, 57%, 62% and 66% of the training set variance respectively. A linear classifier was used to classify pixels as mass/non-mass. The resulting ROC curves are shown in Fig. 4, indicating the effect of using the full signatures or the first 17 principal components (using the principal component model to explain 85% of the variation in the data) in the dataset. Using the full signatures, slightly worse results are obtained. For the results based on the first 17 principal components a sensitivity of 80% is obtained at a false positive fraction of 0.25.

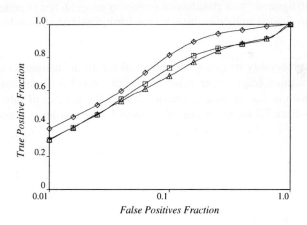

Fig. 4. Mammographic signature classification results for linear classification (△), PCA model based linear classification (□) and non-linear classification (◇).

In this case the ANN had two output neurons for the two classes, mass and non-mass. Again, every sample was given class expectation values. In this case 0.9 for mass samples and 0.1 for non-mass samples. The same approach as in Sec. 5 was followed to obtain ROC curves. The results are shown in Fig. 4 which show that a sensitivity of 80% was achieved at a false positive rate of 0.10.

6.1 Region Classification

An example of a spiculated lesion with central mass is shown in Fig. 5a. A class probability image resulting from the full scale-orientation signatures and a linear classifier is shown in Fig. 5b, results from the first 17 principal components and a linear model are shown in Fig. 5c, and from he non-linear classifier in Fig.5d. This shows that the mass is detected by all three approaches. It should be noted that the area (i.e. the region of pixels) detected has an improved overlap with the annotated region when going from full signature linear model (Fig. 5b), principal component linear model (Fig. 5c) to full signature non-linear model Fig. (5d).

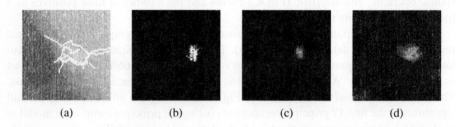

(a)   (b)   (c)   (d)

Fig. 5. Example of applying the linear and non-linear classification approach to a section of a mammogram. (a) original mammogram (b) original mammogram with central mass and spicules annotated (c) full signature linear classification probability image (d) first 17 principal component based linear classification probability image (e) non-linear classification probability image.

The class probability images where obtained for all the mammograms in dataset. Region classification (region size equal to 10 mm) was based on these images and results are shown in Fig. 6. At a sensitivity of 80% the number of false positives per image reduces from 7.5 for linear classification to 3.2 for non-linear classification.

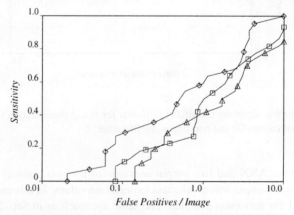

Fig. 6. FROC mammographic region classification results for linear classification ($\triangle$), PCA model based linear classification ($\square$) and non-linear classification ($\diamond$).

7 Discussion and Conclusions

We have described a principled method for the classification of pixels based on scale-orientation signatures which provide a compact description of local structure. Linear and non-linear aspects of scale-orientation signatures can be used for the labelling of structures in images. It is possible to classify pixels into several classes such as linear structures, blob-like structures or background texture.

For the synthetic data sets the results obtained using the ANN are considerably better for unseen data than the classification using a linear approach implying better generalisation. At a sensitivity of 80% the false positive rate reduces from 0.15 for the linear method to 0.000013 for the ANN.

When comparing the linear and non-linear classification results for the mammographic data it is clear that allowing for non-linear behaviour of the scale-orientation signatures provides as overall improvement. At a sensitivity of 80% the false positive rate improved from 0.25 to 0.10. When applied to images the results show an overall better performance for the non-linear modelling approach. For region classification at a sensitivity of 80% the number of false positives per image reduces from 7.5 for linear classification to 3.2 for non-linear classification. These results are comparable with methods presented in the literature [7, 9].

Results for both synthetic and mammographic data indicate that the non-linear aspects of the scale-orientation signatures provide additional information which improves the classification results. Using the non-linear technique described the detection of spiculated lesions is improved.

The approaches described for the classification of structures in images could be improved by the normalisation of the scale- orientation signatures to provide a better classification of the various structures, although some specificity may be lost.

References

1. J.A. Bangham, T.G. Campbell, and R.V. Aldridge. Multiscale median and morphological filters for 2d pattern recognition. *Signal Processing*, 38:387–415, 1994.
2. R. Harvey, A. Bosson, and J.A. Bangham. The robustness of some scale-spaces. In *Proceedings of the 8th British Machine Vision Conference*, pages 11–20, Colchester, UK, 1997.
3. I.T. Jolliffe. *Principal Component Analysis*. Springer Verlag, 1986.
4. S.N. Kalitzin, B.M. ter Haar Romeny, and M.A. Viergever. Invertible orientation bundles on 2d scalar images. In *Lecture Notes in Computer Science*, 1252:77–88, 1997.
5. C.E. Metz. Evaluation of digital mammography by roc analysis. *Excerpta Medica*, 1119:61–68, 1996.
6. University of Stuttgart. *Suttgart Neural Network Simulator*. User Manual, Version 4.1, 1995.
7. N. Petrick, H.-P. Chan, B. Sahiner, M.A. Helvie, M.M. Goodsitt, and D.D. Adler. Computer-aided breast mass detection: false positive reduction using breast tissue composition. *Excerpta Medica*, 1119:373–378, 1996.
8. P. Soille, E.J. Breen, and R. Jones. Recursive implementation of erosions and dilations along discrete lines at arbitrary angles. *IEEE Transactions on Pattern Analysis and Machine Intelligence*, 18(5):562–567, 1996.
9. W.K. Zouras, M.L. Giger, P. Lu, D.E. Wolverton, C.J. Vyborny, and K. Doi. Investigation of a temporal subtraction scheme for computerized detection of breast masses in mammograms. *Excerpta Medica*, 1119:411–415, 1996.

Detecting and Inferring Brain Activation from Functional MRI by Hypothesis-Testing Based on the Likelihood Ratio

Dimitrios Ekatodramis, Gábor Székely and Guido Gerig

Swiss Federal Institute of Technology
Communication Technology Laboratory
ETH-Zentrum, CH-8092 Zurich, Switzerland
{ekato,szekely,gerig}@vision.ee.ethz.ch

Abstract. For the measure of brain activation in functional MRI many methods compute a heuristically chosen metric. The statistic of the underlying metric which is implicitly derived from the original assumption about the noise in the data, provides only an indirect way to the statistical inference of brain activation. An alternative procedure is proposed by presenting a binary hypothesis-testing approach. This approach treats the problem of detecting brain activation by directly deriving a test statistic based on the probabilistic model of the noise in the data. Thereby, deterministic and parameterized models for the hemodynamic response can be considered. Results show that time series models can be detected even if they are characterized by unknown parameters, associated with the unclear nature of the mechanisms that mediate between neuronal stimulation and hemodynamic brain response. The likelihood ratio tests proposed in this paper are very efficient and robust in making a statistical inference about detected regions of brain activation. To validate the applicability of the approach a simulation environment for functional MRI is used. This environment also serves as a testbed for comparative study and systematic tests.

1 Introduction

The human brain has a highly complex functional organization. Functional MRI techniques are specialized to code information about neurophysiological mechanisms of the brain in the image contrast. The analysis of functional MRI data aims at providing detailed maps depicting neuronal brain activation due to a specific sensory stimulation, so called *activation maps*.

Most analysis methods compute a metric upon which brain activation in functional MRI data is detected. This metric arises from a heuristically posed question, like *'how well does a model correlate with the time series data?'*, or *'what is the amount of signal power in the time series at the stimulation frequency?'*. Answers to these questions indirectly lead to the conclusion about brain activation being present or not. In fact, a direct solution to the problem posed in functional MRI is the answer to the basic question *'is brain activation present or not?'*. We present a binary hypothesis-testing approach to answer this question. For this, we make the assumption that each time series measurement represents either the hemodynamic response signal buried in noise or just pure noise. This binary hypothesis can be denoted as

$$H_1 : \text{Measurement} \equiv \text{Signal+Noise}$$
$$H_0 : \text{Measurement} \equiv \text{Noise}$$

The signal may be a deterministic and parameterized model for the hemodynamic response, while the noise is characterized by a probabilistic model.

Validation of functional MRI results can be performed by comparison with findings using different modalities such as PET, MEG or EEG on the same person. Until now the exact nature of the transient behavior between onset of sensory stimulation, neuronal activation and hemodynamic response of the brain, remains unclear. This implies that validation can never become complete, since any underlying model or assumption in the analysis does not accurately represent the physical nature of functional MRI experiments. We present an environment where the hemodynamic response and the experimental parameters of a functional MRI experiment can be simulated in a realistic manner. Artificially produced data sets are necessary to evaluate the reliability of analysis methods that are applied on real data with similar experimental conditions.

2 Methods

2.1 Binary Hypothesis Testing

Having made an observation (time series) with functional MRI, one is faced with the necessity of making a binary decision between the two hypotheses H_1 (signal present) and H_0 (signal not present). Once a rule is selected to decide which of the two hypotheses is true for the present observation, the procedure is referred to as binary hypothesis testing. We present the Neyman-Pearson test as a binary hypothesis-testing approach.

The Likelihood Ratio and the Neyman-Pearson Test. Interpreting the hypotheses H_1 and H_0 as a known source output (signal or '0') which has gone through some probabilistic transition mechanism (addition of noise), the measurement can be described by a random variable $\boldsymbol{X}$. Then the likelihood ratio $\Lambda(\boldsymbol{x})$ provides the test

$$\Lambda(\boldsymbol{x}) = \frac{p_{\boldsymbol{X}|H_1}(\boldsymbol{x})}{p_{\boldsymbol{X}|H_0}(\boldsymbol{x})} \underset{H_0}{\overset{H_1}{\gtrless}} \gamma \qquad (1)$$

to decide which of the two hypotheses is true for a particular observation $\boldsymbol{x}$ ([13]). The likelihood ratio is the ratio of the probability density functions of the measurement $\boldsymbol{X}$, assuming that H_1 or H_0 is true, respectively. For the likelihood ratio tests in this paper we determine the threshold γ using the Neyman-Pearson criterion. According to this criterion the false alarm probability P_f (deciding for H_1 when H_0 is true) is constrained to a specified value α, while the detection probability P_d (deciding for H_1 when H_1 is true) is maximized for this constraint. Under the assumption of Gaussian white noise it is shown by Van Trees [13] that the threshold γ is then determined by solving the equation

$$P_f = P[\Lambda(\boldsymbol{x}) > \gamma | H_0] = \int_\gamma^\infty p_{\Lambda|H_0}(\lambda) d\lambda = \alpha \qquad (2)$$

where $p_{\Lambda|H_0}(\lambda)$ denotes the probability density function of the likelihood ratio under H_0. Note that for a likelihood ratio test based on the Neyman-Pearson criterion (Neyman-Pearson test), the false alarm probability P_f and therefore the statistical inference is completely specified by the constraint α for P_f. Therefore, whenever a Neyman-Pearson test can be designed, the user himself can determine the statistical inference to result from the binary decision problem.

Detection of Known Time Series Signals. A time series can be viewed as a series or collection of samples or observations taken from a continuous time signal. Having made an observation of a time series, we can make the following binary hypothesis:

$$\begin{array}{llll} H_1 & : & Y_i = s_i + n_i, & i = 1, \cdots, N \\ H_0 & : & Y_i = n_i, & i = 1, \cdots, N \end{array} \qquad (3)$$

Under H_1 we assume that the Y_i of the observed time series consist of samples s_i of a known signal which is corrupted with additive Gaussian white noise. The noise samples n_i are assumed to be members of a Gaussian white noise process with zero mean and variance σ_n^2. They are statistically independent. The samples s_i can be thought of representing the model time series of the hemodynamic brain response. H_0 makes the assumption that the Y_i of the observed times series consist of pure noise samples of the same type. N indicates the number of samples in the observed time series. The assumption of Gaussian white noise allows to formulate the likelihood ratio test

$$\sum_i y_i s_i \underset{H_0}{\overset{H_1}{\gtrless}} \gamma \qquad (4)$$

By using equation (2) for the determination of the threshold γ according to the the Neyman-Pearson criterion we obtain

$$\gamma = \sigma_n \sqrt{2 \sum_i s_i^2} \cdot \text{erf}^{-1}(1 - 2\alpha) \qquad (5)$$

where α is the constraint for the false alarm probability P_f and erf^{-1} denotes the inverse of the error function. Using the threshold γ determined by (5) in the likelihood ratio test (4) results in a false alarm probability $P_f = \alpha$. Therefore, the statistical inference made from the test can be determined by the choice of α.

The Generalized Likelihood Ratio Test for Unknown Parameters. If a hypothesis in a binary decision problem depends on an unknown parameter, the likelihood ratio test (1) is not directly applicable. This is due to the fact that the probability density function for that hypothesis, denoted as the likelihood function, also depends on the unknown parameter. Therefore, an estimate of the parameter is obtained under the assumption that the hypothesis which depends on this parameter is true. This estimate is then used in the formulation of a likelihood ratio test as if it was the correct value of the unknown parameter. A likelihood ratio test which is constructed with maximum likelihood estimates ([3, 13]) of some unknown parameters is called a *generalized likelihood ratio* test. Maximum likelihood estimates are obtained by minimizing the likelihood function using standard techniques of calculus.

Detection of a Cosine Waveform with Unknown Phase. In functional MRI observations of brain physiology are repeated many times in a single experiment. Since in these cycles the subject is switching from one condition to another, a periodic response in the time series of activated brain areas is expected. For this reason, in many functional MRI evaluation procedures a sinusoidal form of the hemodynamic response is proposed ([7, 8]). However, the phase of such sinusoidals which is associated with the delay of the hemodynamic response function is arbitrarily chosen or empirically assumed ([1, 10]). Therefore, we present a detection procedure for a cosine waveform time series with unknown phase. For this, we make the binary hypothesis

$$
\begin{aligned}
H_1 &: \quad Y_i = \cos(\omega t_i + \phi) + n_i, \quad i = 1, \cdots, N \\
H_0 &: \quad Y_i = \qquad\qquad\qquad n_i, \quad i = 1, \cdots, N
\end{aligned} \tag{6}
$$

Under H_1 the Y_i of the observed time series are assumed to be samples of a cosine function with known frequency ω at time instants t_i. However the phase ϕ is not known. Suppose that $\omega = 2k\pi/p$, where k is an integer number $\neq 0$ and p is an integer number > 0. Further, assume that $N \geq p$ and that N is a multiple of p. If we denote that $t_i = i$, then we have the conditions

$$
\sum_{i=1}^{N} \cos\left(\frac{2k\pi}{p}i + \phi\right) = 0 \quad \text{and} \quad \sum_{i=1}^{N} \cos^2\left(\frac{2k\pi}{p}i + \phi\right) = \frac{N}{2} \tag{7}
$$

for any possible value of ϕ. This means that the cosine function in (6) is sampled over an integer number of periods, and with the same number of samples per period. The observation under H_1 is assumed to be corrupted with Gaussian white noise of zero mean and variance σ_n^2. Under H_0 only pure noise of the same type is assumed.

After determining a maximum likelihood estimate for the unknown phase ϕ considering the conditions in (7) we can formulate the generalized likelihood ratio test

$$
\left(\sum_i y_i \cos \omega t_i\right)^2 + \left(\sum_i y_i \sin \omega t_i\right)^2 \underset{H_0}{\overset{H_1}{\gtrless}} \gamma \tag{8}
$$

The determination of the threshold γ is again based on the Neyman-Pearson criterion. Using equation (2) we obtain

$$\gamma = \frac{N}{2}\sigma_n^2 K_2(\alpha) \qquad (9)$$

where α is the constraint for false alarm probability P_f and $K_2(\cdot)$ denotes the χ^2-distribution with 2 degrees of freedom. Using the threshold γ determined by (9) in the likelihood ratio test (8) results in a false alarm probability $P_f = \alpha$. Therefore, the statistical inference made from the test can be determined by the choice of α.

2.2 Verification of the Gaussian Noise Model

The development of the likelihood ratio tests (8) and (4) was based on a Gaussian assumption about noise. Application of these tests on real data is legitimate only after verification of the Gaussian white noise model in real data. We have performed this verification empirically and with the help of the χ^2-distribution and the statistical χ^2-test. We have made use of a dummy data set acquired from a volunteer. The data set consists of 512 functional images with an image resolution of 128×128 pixels, acquired with EPI on a Bruker TOMIKON S200. Only pixels within brain tissue were incorporated in the verification process. The volunteer was not exposed to any specific sensory stimulation.

Equal Variance over Space and Time. A histogram of all pixel values within brain tissue in the time series of the dummy data set is shown in figure 1a. We see that this histogram is well approximated by a Gaussian distribution function with variance equal to the variance estimate over all pixels under investigation. The variance estimate has been obtained using the standard estimation calculus for the variance over all pixels, after subtracting the mean from each time series. This estimate, denoted as the overall variance, is assumed to be the true noise variance. Figure 1b shows a histogram of the normalized variance estimate from the time series within brain tissue (solid line). The computed histogram is well approximated by the theoretically expected χ^2-distribution (dotted line). The plot in figure 1b therefore supports our assumption that the measured overall variance is well the true noise variance, and that it is the same at any pixel location. To corroborate our assumption about equal variance over space we have performed the statistical χ^2-test for any two pairs of time series, to test if they are drawn from different distributions ([12], p. 489). 95% of the significance levels obtained from the χ^2-test were > 0.1. Therefore we can say that there are very insignificant differences in the distribution of practically any two time series in the dummy data set. This in turn is an indication that our assumption about the variance being the same in any time series, i.e. equal over space, holds.

To verify that the variance in the time series of the dummy data set is equal over time, we have observed the distribution of the normalized variance estimate in time series within a sliding time window. In the data set with 512 time samples, we have chosen a window width of 128 time instants. The computed mean and

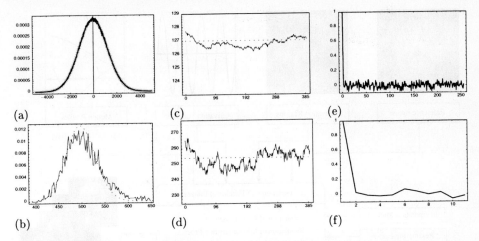

Fig. 1. Verification of the Gaussian white noise model in functional MRI data. (a), (b) Equal variance over space. (c), (d) Equal variance over time. (e) An example for independent time series samples. (f) An enlargement from the plot in (e).

standard deviation of the normalized variance estimate for any time section are shown in figure 1c and 1d (solid line), together with the mean and standard deviation of the theoretically expected χ^2-distribution (dotted line). We observe that the mean and the variance remain well the same over time. On the basis of the results in figure 1c and 1d it seems justifiable to conclude that the assumption of the equal variance over time is satisfied.

Gaussian Distribution of the Time Series Samples. The assumption we make, is that the time series data are drawn from a Gaussian distribution with zero mean and variance equal to the measured overall variance. Note that the mean of the assumed Gaussian distribution is zero, because the mean of each time series has been subtracted. To verify our assumption we have performed the statistical χ^2-test for the distribution of the samples of each time series and the assumed Gaussian distribution ([12], p. 488). 95% of the significance levels obtained from the χ^2-test were > 0.1. Therefore, we can say that there are very insignificant differences in the true distribution of the data and the Gaussian distribution. This in turn is an indication that our assumption about the time series data being Gaussian distributed holds.

Independent Time Series Samples. The assumption of the noise being white requires the verification that the samples in the time series are independent. For this verification we have made use of the Box-Pierce test for white noise ([6, 8]). The Box-Pierce test statistic calculates the sum of squared autocorrelation coefficients at lags $k = 1..K$. An example of autocorrelation coefficients calculated from a time series of the dummy data set are plotted in figure 1e,f. Under the null hypothesis that the time series in question is serially independent, or white noise, the Box-Pierce statistic is assumed to be χ^2-distributed with K degrees of freedom. Therefore, we can again use a χ^2-test for significant dependencies in

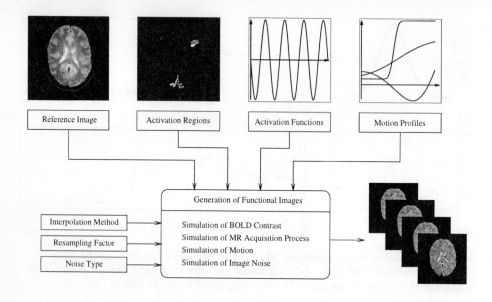

Fig. 2. Functional imaging simulation environment.

the time series samples. 90% of the significance levels obtained from the χ^2-test were > 0.1. This means that there are very insignificant dependencies in the time series samples. From this test result we can deduce that our assumption of the noise being independent holds.

2.3 Simulation of functional MRI Data

To fulfill the requirements for simulation a software environment for the generation of artificial functional images, as shown in figure 2, was designed and implemented using AVS as a development tool ([14, 9]. In the implementation the user determines different physiological and experimental parameters of a functional MRI measurement. This mainly consists of the outlining of brain activation regions on a reference image and of the assignment of a hemodynamic response to any of these regions. Further parameters, such as image resolution, number of images and the noise level in the images, can be determined. The software also supports the simulation of motion artifacts. For this, interpolation procedures for the spatial transformation of images are provided. In functional MRI the amplitude of the hemodynamic response may vary from experiment to experiment ([11, 2, 4]). Taking into account a constant noise level in the images, analysis methods for functional MRI data may therefore take advantage of high response amplitudes or may suffer from weak responses. For this reason, we have considered important to investigate the influence of the signal-to-noise ratio on the performance of methods applied to functional MRI data by the use of the simulation environment. For this investigation, the signal-to-noise ratio

SNR $\equiv \frac{\hat{A}}{\sigma_n}$ in artificial functional data sets was defined as the ratio of the amplitude $\hat{A}$ of the activation function and the standard deviation σ_n of the noise in the functional images.

3 Results

3.1 Comparison of Analysis Methods using Simulated Data

The performance of five different methods for functional MRI analysis with respect to the signal-to-noise ratio was investigated using simulated test data. These methods were:

- The averaged difference. This simple method averages the images taken under rest and stimulation conditions and calculates a difference image between these two averages.
- The correlation method [1]. This method calculates the linear correlation coefficient between each time series and a reference pattern.
- The Fourier method [5]. In the Fourier transform of the time series, the amplitude at the stimulation frequency is used as an index to responsiveness to the stimulation.
- Principle component analysis (PCA). This method identifies activated brain regions in the eigenimages obtained by singular value decomposition of the data.
- The likelihood ratio test (8) proposed herein.

In simulated functional images the amplitude $\hat{A}$ of a cosine waveform with phase $\phi = \pi/2$ used as an activation function was varied from a value of 40 to 1000 in 25 equidistant steps, and from a value of 1000 to 5000 in another 20 equidistant steps. Using a noise standard deviation σ_n of 1000, totally 45 image data sets were produced. Each data set contained 64 images of 128×128 pixels. The five different methods were used to produce activation maps from the generated image data sets with SNR increasing from 0.04 to 5. Statistical inference was automatically provided by the simulation environment by counting pixels inside and outside the simulated activation regions. For each method the false alarm probability P_f was constrained to a specified value while the detection probability P_d was evaluated for each SNR level. The plot in figure 3a shows the values of P_d for constrained $P_f = 0.05$. According to figure 3, the performance depending on the SNR shows more or less the same progression for different analysis methods. For SNR < 0.2 all the methods failed almost completely in detecting areas of activation, whereas for SNR > 3 all methods almost perfectly succeeded in the detection task, when the false alarm probability was constrained to 0.05. The correlation method is observed to be superior to the others. However, the improvement with respect to the other methods is not remarkable. The detection performance of the likelihood ratio test (8), the only method assuming the phase of the cosine waveform as unknown, is comparable to the other methods and justifies its application on real functional MRI data.

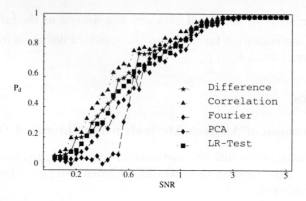

Fig. 3. Performance of different methods on simulated functional MRI data depending on the SNR. Detection probability P_d for constrained false alarm probability $P_f = 0.05$.

3.2 Detection and Inference of Brain Activation by Likelihood Ratio Tests

A functional image data set consisting of 64 images (128×128 pixels) was acquired from a volunteer with a Bruker TOMIKON S200 scanner (University Children's Hospital, Zurich) using a gradient echo imaging sequence. Goggles with a flicker display identical to those used in electrophysiological examinations were used to visually stimulate the volunteer. During the stimulation state the volunteer was exposed to flickering red light at 8 Hertz. This flickering light was switched off in the rest state. Both states had a duration of 30 seconds. The experiment started with one cycle of rest and activation state without data acquisition so that the volunteer became accustomed to the stimulation. Then 8 images under the rest state were acquired followed by 8 images acquired under stimulation conditions. This stimulus alternation was totally repeated for four cycles. We have chosen a cosine waveform with phase $\phi = \pi/2$ as a reference pattern for the hemodynamic response. Figures 4a-c show the results obtained by the correlation method and the two likelihood ratio tests at a significance level of 0.05. In the activation map in figure 4a, obtained by the correlation method, the result is not satisfactory because of many spurious pixels and regions all over the map. The map in figure 4b, obtained by the likelihood ratio test (4) gives a good visual impression about the extents of the activated brain areas. The spurious pixels in the background are reduced to a much greater degree than the result obtained by the correlation method. At the same time, there is no loss of pixels or regions within the head. In the activation map from figure 4c, obtained by the likelihood ratio test (8), almost no spurious pixels appear in the background. Although the phase of the cosine waveform was *assumed to be unknown*, the test still has succeeded to detect pixels forming activation regions similar to those in the map from figure 4b. Figures 4d-f show the results obtained by the correlation method and the two likelihood ratio tests at a significance level of 0.005. The activation map obtained with the correlation method still shows some residual spurious pixels in the background. The maps obtained with the likelihood ratio tests show practically no pixels in the background. Although the detected regions look quite similar, in detail we observe slight differences. A visual inspection of the detected time series can empirically give an impression about the fidelity of the results. Therefore we have plotted some time series which were detected by the three methods within brain tissue in figures 4g-j. These time series were all selected from within the detected activation regions in the occipital lobe. The plot in figure 4g shows a time series which was detected by all three methods. The plots in figure 4h and 4j show time series detected only by one of the two likelihood ratio tests (4) and (8). In figure 4g we see that the time series signal nicely follows the switching from the rest state to the activation state (indicated by the grey bars). This effect is visually not so impressive in figure 4h, but still observable. Figure 4j shows a time series which seems to be related to the stimulus in an opposite way. In fact a difference in phase of 180° with respect to the time series in figure 4k,l may be suspected. It is up to a neurophysiologist to relate time series as shown in figure 4j to a hemodynamic response evoked by neuronal activation due to the visual stimulus.

4 Conclusion

We have applied the likelihood ratio tests (4) and (8) also on data sets with a large number of images comprising visual stimulation. Thereby, we have obtained similar results as those presented in figure 4. Differences in location between detected pixels were only encountered in small detail. The example demonstrated is therefore representative for the results we obtained from all analyzed data sets. This may lead to the conclusion that activation signals evoked by a neuronal stimulus show no phase shift between onset of stimulation and hemodynamic response. From the time series example in figure 4j however, we see that the likelihood ratio test (8) has detected a signal which obviously represents a phase shift of 180° between stimulation onset and response. Although this effect was detected only at a few pixel positions, it shows that detection procedures like the test (8) may contribute to the elaboration of unclear behavior of hemodynamic effects. We conclude that the likelihood ratio tests perform well on real data. Providing coequal results as other methods their power lies in allowing for the assumption of unknown parameters. The derivation of the likelihood ratio statistic (and the subsequent test procedures) is based on the probabilistic model of the noise in the data and therefore provides a direct approach to the detection problem. Other methods are based on the probabilistic consideration about a chosen metric (averaged difference, correlation, etc.) and therefore address the detection problem indirectly. Consequently, in a signal detection task based on hypothesis testing with the likelihood ratio, the statistical inference is made about the assumed signal model, and not about a metric computed from the model. The design of a likelihood ratio test based on the Neyman-Pearson criterion does not require any knowledge about a priori probabilities or costs

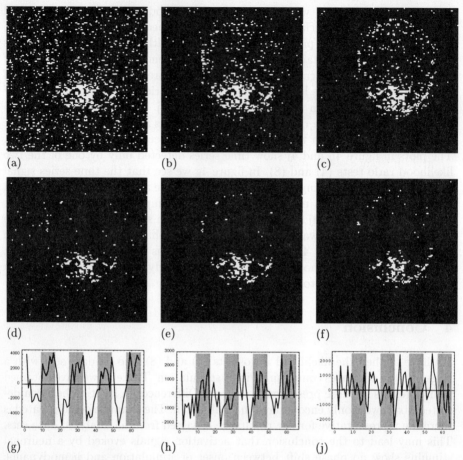

Fig. 4. Comparison between the activation map obtained by the correlation method and likelihood ratio tests (4) and (8), assuming a cosine waveform as a reference pattern. (a)-(c) Activation maps at a significance level of 0.05. (d)-(f) Activation maps at a significance level of 0.005. (g) Time series detected by all three methods, (h) only by the test (4), (j) only by the test (8).

and is therefore well suited for the detection of brain activation in functional MRI. Further, the statistical inference is completely determined by the design (i.e., the constraint for the false alarm probability). This allows a user who is not familiar with thresholds to decide himself about the inference made from test results by supplying a probability value. Taking a look at figure 4, the likelihood ratio tests are superior and more robust in making a statistical inference about detected regions compared with the correlation method [1]. The thresholds in our likelihood ratio tests all depend on the variance of the noise in the data. We have verified that the Gaussian white noise holds well in functional MRI data. We can therefore assume the value of the true noise variance from an estimate over a huge amount of pixels ($\approx 4 \cdot 10^6$) within brain tissue, and use this estimate for the determination of the threshold in the likelihood ratio tests. Therefore, statistical inference is made by accounting for the noise variance for time series within brain tissue. The correlation method relates the threshold for the calculated correlation coefficients to a Gaussian distribution with zero mean and variance $1/N$, N denoting the number of samples in the time series, which is an approximation to the true distribution of correlation coefficients. Consequently, the threshold for the correlation method does not account for the true noise variance. By comparing figure 4a and 4b it is seen that this can lead to an incorrect inference of the results.

References

1. P. A. Bandettini, A. Jesmanowicz, E. C. Wong, and J. S. Hyde. Processing strategies for time-course data sets in functional MRI of the human brain. *Magnetic Resonance in Medicine*, 30:161–173, 1993.
2. P. A. Bandettini, E. C. Wong, R. S. Hinks, et al. Time course EPI of human brain function during task activation. *Magnetic Resonance in Medicine*, 25:390–397, 1992.
3. M. Barkat. *Signal Detection & Estimation*. Artech House, Boston, 1991.
4. A. M. Blamire, S. Ogawa, K. Ugurbil, et al. Dynamic mapping of the human visual cortex by high-speed magnetic resonance imaging. In *Proc. Natl. Acad. Sci. USA*, volume 89, pages 11069–11073, 1992.
5. K. Boulanouar, I. Berry, J. F. Demonet, et al. A monofrequential approach to the detection of activated pixels in fMRI. In *NeuroImage, Second International Conference on Functional Mapping of the Human Brain, June 17-21, 1996, Boston, MA*, page 51, 1996.
6. G. E. P. Box, G. M. Jenkins, and G. C. Reinsel. *Time Series Analysis*. Prentice Hall, New Jersey, 3rd edition, 1994.
7. G. M. Boynton, S. A. Engel, G. H. Glover, and D. J. Heeger. Linear systems analysis of functional magnetic resonance imaging in human V1. *Journal of Neuroscience*, 16(13):4207–4221, 1996.
8. E. Bullmore, M. Brammer, S. C. R. Williams, et al. Statistical methods of estimation and inference for functional MR image analysis. *Magnetic Resonance in Medicine*, 35:261–277, 1996.
9. D. Ekatodramis, G. Székely, E. Martin, and G. Gerig. A simulation environment for validation and comparison of fMRI evaluation procedures. In *NeuroImage, Second International Conference on Functional Mapping of the Human Brain, June 17-21, 1996, Boston, MA*, page 57, 1996.
10. K. J. Friston, C. D. Frith, R. Turner, and R. S. Frackowiak. Characterizing evoked hemodynamics with fMRI. *NeuroImage*, 2:157–165, 1995.
11. K. K. Kwong, J. W. Belliveau, et al. Dynamic magnetic resonance imaging of human brain activity during primary sensory stimulation. In *Proc. Natl. Acad. Sci. USA*, volume 89, pages 5675–5679, 1992.
12. W. H. Press, B. P. Flannery, S. A. Teukolsky, and W. T. Vetterling. *Numerical Recipes in C*. Cambridge University Press, Cambridge, 1988.
13. H. L. Van Trees. *Detection, Estimation, and Modulation Theory*. John Wiley, New York, 1968.
14. AVS Developer's Guide. Advanced Visual Systems Inc.

A Fast Technique for Motion Correction in DSA Using a Feature-Based, Irregular Grid*

Erik H.W. Meijering, Karel J. Zuiderveld, Max A. Viergever

Image Sciences Institute, Utrecht University, Heidelberglaan 100, 3584 CX Utrecht, The Netherlands. http://www.isi.uu.nl; e-mail: erik@isi.uu.nl.

Abstract. In clinical practice, Digital Subtraction Angiography (DSA) is a powerful technique for the visualization of blood vessels in the human body. However, due to patient motion the diagnostic relevance of the images is often reduced by the introduction of artifacts. In this paper, we propose a new approach to the registration of DSA images, which is both effective, and very fast. The computational speed of our algorithm is achieved by applying a gradient based control point selection mechanism, which allows for a more efficient positioning of a reduced number of control points as compared to approaches based on regular grids. The results of preliminary experiments with several clinical data sets clearly show the applicability of the algorithm.

1 Introduction

In clinical practice, Digital Subtraction Angiography (DSA) is a powerful technique for the visualization of blood vessels in the human body. With this technique, a sequence of X-ray projection images is taken to show the passage of a bolus of injected contrast material through one or more vessels of interest. The background structures in these *contrast* images are largely removed by subtracting an image taken prior to the arrival of the contrast medium: the *mask* image. The subtraction technique is based on the assumption that during exposure, tissues do not change in position or density. Clinical evaluations following the introduction of DSA in the early eighties [1, 2] revealed that this assumption is not valid for a substantial number of examinations. Patient motion frequently occurs, which causes the subtraction images to show artifacts that may hamper proper diagnosis. In order to reduce motion artifacts, the misalignment of the successive images in the sequence needs to be determined and corrected for; operations often referred to as *registration* and *motion correction* [3, 4].

Although many studies have been carried out on this subject over the past two decades, they have not led to algorithms which are sufficiently fast so as to be acceptable for integration in a clinical setting. In this paper, we propose a new approach to the registration of digital angiographic image sequences which

---

* This work was done in cooperation with Philips Medical Systems, Department of X-Ray Diagnostics/Predevelopment, Best, The Netherlands and was supported by the Netherlands Ministry of Economic Affairs (IOP-project IBV96004).

is both effective, and computationally very efficient. The registration approach is described in Section 2. Results of preliminary experiments showing the performance of the algorithm are presented in Section 3, and discussed in Section 4. Concluding remarks are made in Section 5.

2 Registration Approach

Given a two-dimensional digital image sequence $I(x, y, t)$ of size $M \times M \times N$, the registration of one of the images with respect to a successive image in the sequence, involves two operations: (i) The computation of the correspondence between the pixels in the two images; (ii) The correction based on this correspondence. In this section, the proposed approach to perform these operations is described.

2.1 Control Point Selection

It is computationally very expensive to compute the correspondence separately for every pixel. To reduce the computation time to a clinically acceptable level (several seconds), assumptions have to be made concerning the nature of the underlying motion. From a physical point of view it is reasonable to assume a certain amount of coherence between the motion of neighboring pixels and to compute the correspondence only for a selected amount of *control points* $\mathbf{p}_i = (x_i, y_i)$. The overall correspondence can then be obtained by interpolation. Control points can be chosen manually by selecting a region of interest [5], or can be taken to lie on a regular grid [6–8]. More sophisticated algorithms use image features.

In the subtraction images, artifacts can only appear in those regions where strong object edges are present in the individual images. Moreover, edges can be matched better than more homogeneous regions. Therefore, the selection of control points should be based on an edge-detection scheme. Compared to algorithms where control points are chosen on a regular grid, this has three major advantages: (i) The control points are chosen at those positions where the artifacts can be expected to be largest; (ii) The reliability of the displacement estimates will be higher than in the case of arbitrarily selected points; (iii) The number of control points, and thus computation time, is reduced.

The location of edges can easily be computed by detecting local maxima of the grey-level gradient magnitude $\|\nabla I(x, y)\|$ of the mask image. In our algorithm, $\|\nabla I(x, y)\|$ is computed at a relatively small scale σ, using Gaussian regularization [9]. Since, in principle, the potential severeness of a motion artifact is directly related to the strength of the underlying edge, it is required to indicate which of the edges are sufficiently important to be considered further. The final selection of control points from $\|\nabla I(x, y)\|$ is carried out by dividing the image into blocks of size $D_{\max} \times D_{\max}$. In turn, these blocks are subdivided into smaller blocks of size $D_{\min} \times D_{\min}$. For every large block, every interior

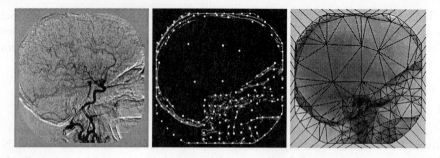

Fig. 1. An example of control point selection and mesh generation. **Left:** A cerebral DSA image showing motion artifacts. **Middle:** The thresholded gradient magnitude image of the mask, used as a prediction of the locations of motion artifacts, with the set of selected control points (white dots) superimposed. **Right:** The mask image with the resulting mesh (Delaunay triangulation) superimposed.

small block is scanned for pixels at which $\|\nabla I(x,y)\|$ is above a certain threshold Θ_e. From these pixels, the one with the largest value for $\|\nabla I(x,y)\|$ is taken as a candidate control point. If no edge-pixels are encountered, no candidate is selected. The candidate becomes a control point if it is positioned inside the exposure region $\mathcal{R}_E$ and at a distance of at least $D_{\exp}$ from the border $\partial \mathcal{R}_E$ of that region[1]. In order to enforce a minimum distance between control points, the gradient magnitude values in a $(2D_{\min} + 1) \times (2D_{\min} + 1)$ region around the selected point (that point being the center) are suppressed. If no point is selected after a large block has been scanned, the point with the largest gradient magnitude value in a small block around the center of the large block is taken as a control point so as to constrain the maximum distance between selected points.

2.2 Displacement Computation

For the computation of the actual displacements of the selected control points we use a template matching approach: for every control point, a small window $\mathcal{W}$ of $W \times W$ pixels is defined and the corresponding window in a successive image in the sequence is searched for by optimizing a predefined measure of match. In order for such a technique to be successful in angiographic images, the similarity measure is required to be insensitive to the inflow of contrast in some parts of the image. It has been demonstrated by Buzug *et al.* [10,11] that measures based on the histogram of difference are most suitable for this purpose. In order to find the optimal displacement in an efficient manner, we use a hill-climbing optimization approach.

---

[1] By $\mathcal{R}_E$ we denote the part of the image in which the grey-values were caused by the exposure of X-rays. Because of the shape of the image intensifier, it is more or less circular (see *e.g.* Fig. 1) and can be extracted quite easily.

As indicated by a clinical evaluation in the early eighties [2], even subpixel misalignments may produce significant artifacts in the subtraction image. In our algorithm, subpixel accuracy in the displacement computations is accomplished by local interpolation of the images and by determining the optimal measure of match at subpixel displacements around the optimum of integer displacements. An accuracy of 0.1 pixel is sufficient for angiographic images [7].

2.3 Displacement Interpolation

In order to be able to carry out the warping of the mask image with respect to the contrast image, it is required to have a complete description of the displacement vector field $\mathbf{d}: \mathbb{R}^2 \to \mathbb{R}^2$. In order to reduce the computation time to a minimum, the displacements at the remaining points in the image are linearly interpolated from the displacements at the control points. Therefore it is required that the set $P = \{\mathbf{p}_i\}$ of control points is properly tessellated. The only possible polygons that can be used for this purpose are triangles, so that the control points become the vertices of an irregular triangular mesh.

In our algorithm, the control points are tessellated into a Delaunay triangulation $\mathcal{D}(P)$ [12], since in this case it is guaranteed that the smallest of the three angles of every triangle will be as large as possible, thereby avoiding triangles with one or two highly acute interior vertex angles in which the displacement at certain points will become dependent on very distant control points (see Fig. 1). An important advantage of using such a tessellation is that the required operations for the final warping of the polygons can be carried out by graphics hardware, which will result in a very fast implementation.

3 Experimental Results

The algorithm as presented in the previous section was implemented in the C++ programming language, utilizing the Open Graphics Library. The experiments were carried out on a relatively low cost Silicon Graphics O2 workstation (one 180 MHz R5000 IP32 processor, 64MB/512kB main/cache memory), with graphics hardware for support of the OpenGL instructions. During the experiments, the parameters of the algorithm as described in the previous section were kept fixed at the values shown in Table 1. Clinical digital angiographic image sequences were acquired on a Philips Integris system. For all sequences, the first image was taken as the mask image.

The results of applying the proposed registration technique to a cerebral, peripheral and an abdominal image sequence are shown in Fig. 2. The left column shows the original subtraction images which contain motion artifacts. The middle column shows the registration results after applying a manual pixel-shifting technique[2], as provided on standard DSA imaging devices. With this technique, the regions for which corrections must be obtained have to be selected explicitly:

---

[2] That is, global translation only.

Param.	Value	Param.	Value
σ	1.0	$D_{\min}$	$0.04M$
Θ_e	15.0	$D_{\max}$	$0.20M$
W	51	$D_{\exp}$	$0.01M$

Table 1. The values of the parameters of the algorithm during the experiments. M denotes the x-y-dimension of the image sequence (either 1024 or 512 pixels in most DSA sequences). See further Section 2 for a description of these parameters.

In the cerebral image we corrected for artifacts in the middle-right part of the image; In the peripheral image, artifacts were corrected in the left part of the image; Finally, in the abdominal image, we attempted to correct for artifacts in the top-left part. Although some artifacts were eliminated by this procedure, in other parts of the images artifacts were reinforced or even introduced. That is to say, the artifacts could not be corrected for by means of 2D rigid transformations, even though the original 3D motion might have been rigid, e.g. in the case of the cerebral image. In general, the approach proposed in the present paper, based on a triangular mesh of irregularly spaced, edge-based control points yields better registrations and, consequently, better subtractions.

4 Discussion

It must be pointed out that angiographic images are in fact *two*-dimensional representations of a *three*-dimensional scene. It has been shown by Fitzpatrick [13] that, subject to a few conditions (which are easily met in X-ray projection imaging), given any two such images that are assumed to differ only as a result of the motion of particles *in* the three-dimensional scene, there *does* exist a one-to-one two-dimensional mapping that completely describes the changes in the images, caused by three-dimensional object motion. However, it should be stressed that it is not possible to uniquely and completely retrieve it from the two images only. There are three main reasons for this: (i) Since we are dealing with digital images, the retrieval of a displacement vector in a certain point in one image in a sequence inevitably requires neighborhood operations. If the neighborhood contains several objects that move independently of each other (which is very likely to occur in projection images), the computations can be expected to be unreliable and inaccurate; (ii) At points that lie on isophotes in the image, it is impossible to retrieve the tangential component of the displacement vector (generally known as the aperture problem); (iii) The assumption that the two images differ only as a result of the motion of particles *in* the three-dimensional scene, does not apply to angiography, since contrast material is introduced in certain parts of the scene. Although similarity measures can be designed to be relatively insensitive to inflow of contrast, the problems (i) and (ii) are more fundamental and cannot be solved without additional knowledge.

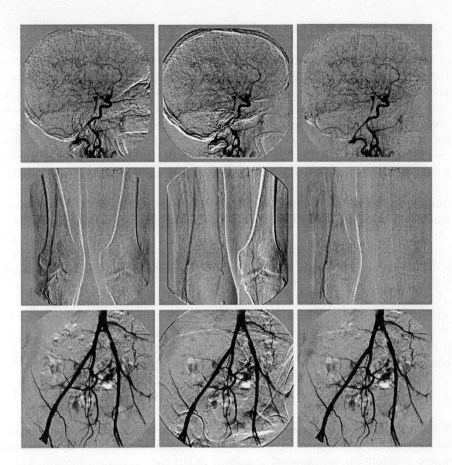

Fig. 2. Registration results for a cerebral, peripheral and an abdominal image sequence. **Left Column:** The original subtractions of one of the contrast images from the mask image. **Middle Column:** The subtractions after registration by global translation of the mask image (obtained by manual pixel-shifting; see Section 3 for a more detailed explanation). **Right Column:** The subtractions after registration using the proposed approach.

Therefore, successful application of our registration technique will be limited to regions where these problems are insignificant.

From the experimental results as shown in Fig. 2, it can be seen that there is a major difference between the registration results of the cerebral and peripheral sequences and the results of the abdominal sequence. In the first two sequences, the artifacts have been removed almost completely, *i.e.*, the algorithm gave near perfect registrations. In the abdominal data set, the motion artifacts have been removed partially, but the resulting subtraction still shows some major artifacts. We note that these artifacts could not be removed by adjusting one or more of the parameters of the algorithm so as to yield a larger density of control points. In fact, the artifacts could not even be removed by replacing the hill-climbing optimization by an exhaustive-search approach. The registration result of the abdominal sequence where manual pixel-shifting was applied reveals that there are parts in the image in which there are several important structures projected onto each other (in this case the spine, the pelvis and the bowels), as opposed to the cerebral and peripheral sequences, where the important structures resulted from the projection of only one object in the original three-dimensional scene, *viz.* bones. When multiple superimposed structures move independently, the displacement of only one of these structures can no longer be reconstructed from the resulting projections. This has been mentioned at the beginning of this section as the first limitation of any registration algorithm for X-ray projection images, and explains why even a full-search approach will not be able to retrieve the correspondence. In general, it was found that in most abdominal data sets the peristaltic motion locally causes severe changes in grey-values. In those cases, even when the correct local displacements are found, the final subtraction will still show serious artifacts. It is inherent to the nature of the current approach that these artifacts cannot be removed.

Finally, we note that the proposed approach is capable of registering at a speed of less than one second per image (on average). This is mainly due to the edge-based control point selection procedure which, in general, results in a reduction in the number of points for which the displacement needs to be computed explicitly.

5 Conclusions

We have presented a new approach for the registration of digital angiographic image sequences. The method involves the extraction of regions in the image where artifacts can be expected to appear in the case of patient motion. These regions are obtained by thresholding the gradient magnitude of the mask image. Based on assumptions about the coherence of motion of neighboring pixels, a selected set of control points is extracted, for which the displacement is computed explicitly by means of maximizing the energy of the histogram-of-differences and using a hill-climbing optimization approach. The complete displacement vector field is constructed from the displacements at these control points, using a Delaunay triangulation and linear interpolation. The final warping of the images is performed real-time by graphics hardware.

The algorithm is capable of registering complete sequences at a speed of less than one second per image. The results of a preliminary evaluation on various clinical image sequences show the viability of the method. We are currently undertaking a thorough clinical evaluation of the algorithm.

References

1. W.A. Chilcote, M.T. Modic, W.A. Pavlicek, J.R. Little, A.J. Furian, P.M. Duchesneau & M.A. Weinstein. Digital subtraction angiography of the carotid arteries: A comparitive study in 100 patients. *Radiology*, vol. 139, no. 2 (1981), pp. 287–295.

2. W.R. Brody, D.R. Enzmann, L.-S. Deutsch, A. Hall & N. Pelc. Intravenous carotid arteriography using line-scanned digital radiography. *Radiology*, vol. 139, no. 2 (1981), pp. 297–300.
3. L.G. Brown. A survey of image registration techniques. *ACM Computing Surveys*, vol. 24, no. 4 (1992), pp. 325–376.
4. J.B.A. Maintz & M.A. Viergever. A survey of medical image registration. *Medical Image Analysis*, vol. 2, no. 1 (1998), pp. 1–36.
5. A. Venot & V. Leclerc. Automated correction of patient motion and gray values prior to subtraction in digitized angiography. *IEEE Transactions on Medical Imaging*, vol. 3, no. 4 (1984), pp. 179–186.
6. K.J. Zuiderveld, B.M. ter Haar Romeny & M.A. Viergever. Fast rubber sheet masking for digital subtraction angiography. In *Science and Engineering of Medical Imaging*, M.A. Viergever (ed.), vol. 1137 of *Proceedings of SPIE*, The International Society for Optical Engineering, Bellingham, Washington, USA, 1989, pp. 22–30.
7. L. van Tran & J. Sklansky. Flexible mask subtraction for digital angiography. *IEEE Transactions on Medical Imaging*, vol. 11, no. 3 (1992), pp. 407–415.
8. G.S. Cox & G. de Jager. Automatic registration of temporal image pairs for digital subtraction angiography. In *Image Processing*, vol. 2167 of *Proceedings of SPIE*, The International Society for Optical Engineering, Bellingham, Washington, USA, 1994, pp. 188–199.
9. J.F. Canny. A computational approach to edge detection. *IEEE Transactions on Pattern Analysis and Machine Intelligence*, vol. 8, no. 6 (1986), pp. 679–698.
10. T.M. Buzug, J. Weese, C. Fassnacht & C. Lorenz. Image registration: Convex weighting functions for histogram-based similarity measures. In *CVRMed-MRCAS '97*, J. Troccaz, E. Grimson & R. Mösges (eds.), vol. 1205 of *Lecture Notes in Computer Science*, Springer-Verlag, Berlin, Germany, 1997, pp. 203–212.
11. T.M. Buzug, J. Weese, C. Lorenz & W. Beil. Histogram-based image registration for digital subtraction angiography. In *Image Analysis and Processing (ICIAP '97)*, A. Del Bimbo (ed.), vol. 1311 of *Lecture Notes in Computer Science*, Springer-Verlag, Berlin, Germany, 1997, pp. 380–387.
12. D.F. Watson. Computing the n-dimensional Delaunay tessellation with application to Voronoi polytopes. *The Computer Journal*, vol. 24, no. 2 (1981), pp. 167–172.
13. J.M. Fitzpatrick. The existence of geometrical density-image transformations corresponding to object motion. *Computer Vision, Graphics and Image Processing*, vol. 44, no. 2 (1988), pp. 155–174.

Autofocusing of Clinical Shoulder MR Images for Correction of Motion Artifacts

Armando Manduca, Kiaran P. McGee, E. Brian Welch, Joel P. Felmlee, and Richard L. Ehman

Mayo Clinic and Foundation, Rochester MN 55905

Abstract. A post-processing "autofocusing" algorithm for the reduction of motion artifacts in MR images has been developed and tested on a large clinical data set of high resolution shoulder images. The algorithm uses only the raw (complex) data from the MR scanner, and requires no knowledge of the patient motion during the scan, deducing that from the raw data itself. It operates by searching over the space of possible patient motions and optimizing the image quality. Evaluation of this technique on the clinical data set (for which navigator echo based measured motions and corrected images were available) show that the algorithm can correct for the effects of global translation during the scan almost as well as the navigator echo approach and is more robust.

1 Introduction

The most serious remaining limitation in many current MRI examinations is data corruption by patient motion. Such motion causes phase errors in the received signal in k-space, which leads to ghosting, blurring and other artifacts in the image. A wide variety of techniques have been developed to minimize or correct for such motion, with perhaps the most successful being the use of navigator echoes [1]. However, corruption due to global patient motion does not actually lose information - if the motion is known, and the appropriate phase corrections applied, the image can be perfectly restored. It is therefore possible in principle to correct for motion given only the raw data from the MR scanner by simply trying different possible motion corrections and searching for the highest quality resulting image with a suitable evaluation function. Such approaches are used in the autofocusing of synthetic aperture radar images and in certain problems in seismic data processing.

Atkinson et al. [2] recently described such an algorithm, which uses entropy minimization as a focus criterion. We have developed a similar algorithm which we term "autocorrection", detailed below, and applied it to a clinical problem - high-resolution shoulder imaging - in which the sharpness of the image is critical to the clinical evaluation of the supraspinatus tendon and rotator cuff. Navigator echoes have been shown to be effective on such images [3], and we used the data set from that study to directly compare autocorrection and navigator results.

2 Methods

Autocorrection does not attempt to track patient motion (as do navigator-based methods of motion correction), nor does it seek information about the motion explicitly in the k-space data, as do some phase retrieval techniques. Rather, autocorrection algorithms perform motion correction by defining a measure or metric of image quality, and evaluating many combinations of possible patient motions, searching for a set which optimizes this quantity after the appropriate corrections are made to the image. It is implicitly assumed that the metric has an optimal value if the object is stationary, and that any motion during the imaging sequence will corrupt the image and degrade this value. In other words, it is assumed that it is impossible to make an image better (in terms of the metric) than the stationary case. It is also assumed that the better the value of the metric, the better the image.

In mathematical terms, autofocusing casts motion correction as an optimization problem, with the metric as the cost function, in a very high-dimensional space (as many dimensions as there are views in the acquired data). While it is probably impossible in practice to find the true global minimum of such a cost function, it appears to be possible to search the space of possible solutions in a way which yields very good improvements in image quality in a reasonable amount of time, as described below. It should be noted that similar approaches are used in the processing of synthetic aperture data [4] and in problems concerning the inversion of seismic data [5].

Atkinson et al. [2] recently showed the feasability of autofocusing for the reduction of MR motion artifacts, presenting an algorithm which used entropy minimization as the focus criterion. They considered both 2-D translation and rotation, and presented good results for simple test images. The algorithm we describe here is fundamentally similar to theirs, with improvements and differences as noted below. We have evaluated this autocorrection technique on high-resolution shoulder images, a clinical application in which maximum image sharpness is critical. Although this is a demanding test of the algorithm's ability to sharpen the image, it is also known that motion in such images is primarily translational along the superior-inferior direction [3]. This greatly simplifies the operation of the algorithm, since we need only consider one degree of freedom (motion along the phase-encoding direction).

2.1 Optimization Algorithm

The algorithm begins with the acquired k-space data (384 lines of 256 points each), and initially groups frequencies in blocks of 64. A given block is temporarily "corrected for" a certain trial motion by applying the phase shifts that would correct for that motion, if the patient had in fact moved by that amount during the time corresponding to the acquisition of exactly those views. After these phase shifts, the data is transformed to image space and the metric is calculated. This metric is compared to the results for other trial motions, and, in this manner, the optimal motion correction for that block of frequencies can be determined. We use golden section optimization, and find the optimal motion to an accuracy of 0.1 pixel. This is done starting on one side of the center of k-space and working outward, then moving to the other side and working outward (although alternating sides while moving outward seems to work equally well). When corrections are complete for the blocks of 64, the process is begun again with blocks of 32, and so on until individual lines are considered one at a time. This procedure allows one to gradually approximate the motion record more and more accurately as one moves to smaller block sizes. It is not critical to start at a block size of 64 (any large number is fine), and, perhaps surprisingly, it does not seem to be necessary to go all the way to considering each line individually. If one stops at blocks of 2 or even 4 lines, the correction is essentially complete - one has already captured the major features of the motion record, and the finer details are not critical to the visual appearance.

The above paradigm of working with blocks of frequency space of gradually decreasing size has some similarities to the optimization strategy in [2]. Since they considered 2-D motions, however, they simply evaluated their metric on possible combinations of several discrete displacements in both x and y, rather than using a more sophisticated optimization scheme in 1-D as we do here.

2.2 Cost Function

The most important improvement we have made is the choice of a better cost function: we use the entropy of the gradient of the image, rather than the entropy of the image itself. Entropy from information theory is defined in terms of the probability of a quantity assuming various values, and is minimized when most values have probability zero and a few values have high probability. In terms of an image, the entropy of the image itself (the metric proposed by [2]) is maximized when the image is dark in as large an area as possible, and its brightness concentrated in as few pixels as possible. It is known, however, that entropy is most sensitive to how close the small values are to zero, and is less sensitive to the behavior of the large values. Thus, entropy as an autofocusing metric depends critically on the dark areas of the image (especially minimizing ghosts in the background), and is not using information from bright areas very well. This was noted by [2], and we have confirmed that a significant amount of dark area is necessary to the success of image entropy based autofocusing on test images [6]. In the shoulder data set, initial experiments using image entropy as the metric failed to produce good motion correction - typically, ghosting in the background areas was reduced somewhat, but the image did not appear to sharpen sufficiently. It was also observed that changes in entropy values did not correlate well with observer judgments of how much an image was improving.

The metric used here (the entropy of the gradient) is minimized when the image consists of areas of uniform brightness, separated by sharp edges - since in such a case, the gradient is zero everywhere except at the edges, where it has high values. This is a fairly good model for what is expected in MR images of the body in ideal situations. Any blurring or ghosting will increase the entropy, since the gradient will be non-zero at more points and will take on smaller values at the actual edge locations. This metric thus takes full advantage of both bright and dark areas of the image. In a separate study [7], we compared the values of 24 separate metrics on the set of shoulder images described below both before and after navigator corrections, and correlated how well the change in the metrics predicted the improvement in image quality as judged by the observers. Gradient entropy had the smallest variance and gave the highest correlation with the observer ratings ($R = 0.53$, where $R = 0.72$ was the inter-observer variability), and was much superior to image entropy ($R = 0.33$, with high variance).

2.3 Optimization on Selected Columns

The algorithm in [2] requires a long computation time (many hours for a 256x256 image), due to the need for an inverse 2-D FFT for every new set of trial motions to evaluate the image in real space. In our case, this time is much reduced due to the single degree of freedom. However, still faster processing is possible by considering only selected columns of an image, since evaluating their quality requires only 1-D FFTs. We proceed from the k-space data by performing an inverse FFT in x, transforming the data into hybrid space (spatial in x, frequency in y). Since the only motion we are considering is along y, which is the phase-encoding direction, the phase correction terms do not depend on x, and each column can be considered separately. We are therefore free to choose only columns of interest (in this case, those containing the humeral head), and need to inverse transform only those, greatly speeding up the calculations. We have to restrict the gradient used in the evaluation to consider only the y (phase encoding) direction, but it is in this direction that the ghosting occurs.

This approach also allows the calculations of corrections specific to a certain area of interest if the motion is not truly global. This is the case in the shoulder, since patient motion typically tends to be greater farther out towards the shoulder (the motion can be likened to a pump handle with the fulcrum along the central axis of the body) and the region of main clinical interest is relatively small. In synthetic test images, one can correct for induced motions with only a small number of columns [6]. In this clinical data set, we find a minimum of 32 to 64 columns seem to be necessary for stable motion correction, probably due to signal to noise considerations. We will report on this in more detail in the future.

3 Evaluation

The navigator study data set described in [3] comprises one hundred and forty four (144) high-resolution shoulder exams acquired under routine clinical conditions using an interleaved navigator pulse sequence. These were oblique coronal acquisitions with a double spin-echo sequence to provide proton-density and T2-weighted images. Further details of the acquisitions are provided in [3]. Raw k-space data representing a slice bisecting the rotator cuff was selected from each of the 144 exams for autocorrection. The original, autocorrected, and navigator-corrected images for the selected slices were printed onto film and evaluated by 4 observers experienced in reviewing shoulder images. For each case, they were asked to rank each image on the same scale of one through five (1 = non- diagnostic image quality, 2 = severe motion effect, 3 = moderate motion effect, 4 = mild motion effect, and 5 = no observable motion corruption) as used in [3]. The general results were that both correction techniques (autocorrection and navigator echoes) significantly improve the images, and while the navigator corrections are slightly better overall, the autocorrection corrections are nearly as effective.

Figure 1 shows the percentage of images which received each rating (from 1 to 5) for the original images and the two correction techniques. Both correction techniques significantly reduce the percentage of images with low ratings, increase the percentages with high ratings, and skew the distribution of ratings strongly towards the "excellent quality" side as compared to the original distribution. For the original images, only 23% were judged to be free of observable motion corruption. Autocorrection and navigator echoes both increased this value to 39%. Conversely, 48% of the original images showed moderate motion corruption or worse (ratings of 1-3). This number was reduced to 27% after navigator correction and 28% after autocorrection.

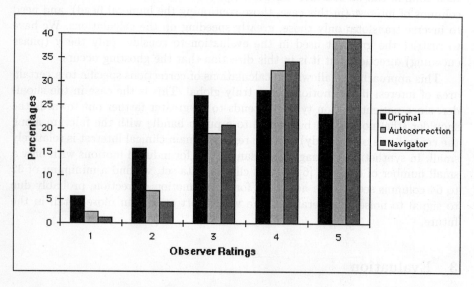

Fig. 1. Absolute observer ratings for images. Percentages of images receiving ratings of 1 (non-diagnostic image quality) through 5 (no observable motion corruption) are plotted for original images (black), autocorrected images (light gray), and navigator corrected images (dark gray). Both correction techniques significantly reduce the percentage of images with low ratings, increase the percentages with high ratings, and skew the distribution of ratings strongly towards the "excellent" side as compared to the original distribution.

Table 1 shows the changes in observer rating when the correction techniques were applied to the original images. Navigators were judged to have improved the image 307 times vs. 279 for the autocorrection (out of 576 total ratings). Autocorrection, however, was more robust: the navigator correction was judged to have degraded an image 6 times, while autocorrection was never judged to have degraded an image. Table 2 shows the average improvement in the observer ratings for an image for each technique. Images with an original rating of 5 were not considered in the averages, since they could not possibly be improved and were never degraded by either technique. The overall average improvement with autocorrection (0.71) is more than 90% of the average improvement achieved with navigator echoes (0.78). Figure 2 shows two examples of successful corrections for each technique.

Table 1. Changes in Observer Ratings for Correction Techniques

Change in score	Autocorrection	Navigator
-2	0	0
-1	0	6
0	297	263
+1	247	262
+2	32	45

Table 2. Average Improvement in Observer Ratings

Observer	Autocorrection	Navigator
Observer 1	0.69	0.70
Observer 2	0.58	0.76
Observer 3	0.89	0.92
Observer 4	0.66	0.75
Average	0.71	0.78

4 Discussion

It is clear that autocorrection performs well in this application to high resolution shoulder MRI, perhaps remarkably so when one considers that it has no knowledge of the actual patient motion. The effectiveness of the algorithm presented here is perhaps 90% that of navigator echo based correction, and (unlike navigators) autocorrection never degraded an image. It is possible that this performance will improve with future refinements of the algorithm.

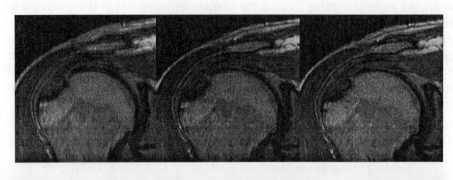

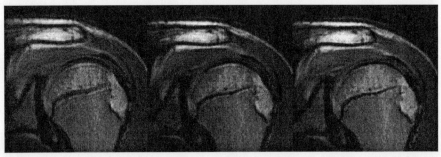

Fig. 2. Two sample images showing the original (left), autocorrected (middle), and navigator corrected versions (right). In these cases both techniques were judged to improve the image by +2 points.

We did not attempt to measure the effect of autocorrection on diagnostic accuracy, due to the difficulty of obtaining an independent test to establish the diagnosis. However, the improvements in image quality are readily apparent, and they are obtained without additional acquisition time, special pulse sequences, special hardware, or any sort of patient preparation. The autocorrection algorithm uses only the raw (complex) data from the scanner, and can be applied retrospectively to any data set from any scanner for which that information was saved, even data that is years old.

The computation times of the algorithm as used here are long, typically 15 minutes per slice on a Dec Alpha. We believe these times can be considerably shortened without affecting the quality of the result. Current experiments indicate that a time of 2-3 minutes per slice may suffice to give the level of performance achieved here. Future improvements in computing hardware and in the algorithm should further reduce computation time.

The autocorrection approach can be readily extended to more complicated motions. Atkinson et al. (21) demonstrated corrections for 2-D translations and rotation, although their work was on a few test images without pathology. We are presently extending the algorithm to include 3-D translations and rotations, and will report such results in the future. We are also researching similar approaches to correct other, non-motion types of artifacts, such as timing errors in EPI images or saturation effects in gated cardiac imaging.

5 Conclusion

Autocorrection has been shown to be a practical technique for the reduction of motion artifacts in a demanding clinical application. The algorithm presented here uses only the raw (complex) data from the scanner, requires 15 minutes of processing time per slice, and significantly reduces motion artifacts. It performs nearly as well as the navigator echo technique, which is remarkable considering that the navigator is explicitly tracking patient motion while autocorrection uses no motion information. The algorithm never degraded an image, while the navigator did so 1% of the time. The algorithm is flexible and should be easily extensible to other types of motion in other applications and, quite possibly, to other types of artifacts in MR images.

References

1. Ehman RL, Felmlee JP. Adaptive technique for high-definition MR imaging of moving structures. Radiology 1989; 173:225-263.
2. Atkinson D, Hill DL, Stoyle PN, Summers PE, Keevil SF. Automatic correection of motion artifacts in magnetic resonance images using an entropy focus criterion. IEEE Trans Med Img 1997; 16(6):903-910.
3. McGee KP, Grimm RC, Felmlee JP, Rydberg JR, Riederer SJ, Ehman RL. The shoulder: Adaptive motion correction of MR images. Radiology 1997; 205:341-354.
4. Bocker RP, Jones SA. ISAR motion compensation using the burst derivative measure as a focal quality indicator. Int J Imag Syst Technol 1992; 4:285-297.
5. Stoffa PL, Sen MK. Nonlinear multiparameter optimization using genetic algorithms: inversion of plane-wave seismograms. Geophysics 1991; 56:1794-1810.
6. Welch EB, Manduca A, Ehman RL. Fast autofocusing of motion-corrupted MR images using one-dimensional Fourier transforms. Proc SPIE Med Img 1998; 3338: 391-397.
7. McGee KP, Manduca A, Felmlee JP, Grimm RC, Riederer SJ, Ehman RL. Autocorrection of high resolution shoulder MR images: analysis of image metrics. Proc ISMRM 1998.

Reconstruction of Elasticity and Attenuation Maps in Shear Wave Imaging: An Inverse Approach

Armando Manduca[1], Vinayak Dutt[1], David T. Borup[2], Raja Muthupillai[1], Richard L. Ehman[1], and James F. Greenleaf[1]

[1] Mayo Clinic and Foundation, Rochester MN 55905
[2] University of Utah, Salt Lake City UT 84112

Abstract. Acoustic shear waves of low frequency can be detected and measured using a phase contrast based magnetic resonance imaging technique called MR Elastography or phase measurement based ultrasound techniques. Spatio-temporal variations of displacements caused by the propagating waves can be used to estimate local values of the elasticity of the object being imaged. The currently employed technique for estimating the elasticity from the wave displacement maps, the local frequency estimator (LFE), has fundamental resolution limits and also has problems with shadowing and other refraction-related artifacts. These problems can be overcome with an inverse approach using Green's function integrals which directly solve the wave equation problem for the propagating wave. The complete measurements of wave displacements as a function of space and time over the object of interest obtained by the above techniques permit an iterative approach to inversion of the wave equation to obtain elasticity and attenuation maps.

1 Introduction

New techniques that can directly visualize propagating acoustic strain waves in tissue-like materials subjected to harmonic mechanical excitation have recently been developed: a phase contrast based magnetic resonance imaging technique called MR Elastography [1, 2] and a related ultrasound technique based on the phase of quadrature echo signals [3]. These techniques present the opportunity of generating medical images that depict tissue elasticity or stiffness. This is significant because palpation, a physical examination that assesses the stiffness of tissue, can be an effective method of detecting tumors, but is restricted to parts of the body that are accessible to the physician's hand.

The spatio-temporal variations of wave displacements measured by these techniques allow the calculation of local mechanical properties. In particular, estimation of the local wavelength (or frequency) of the shear wave propagation pattern at each point in the image allows one to quantitatively calculate local values of shear modulus across the image and generate an image of tissue elasticity. We have previously described a local frequency estimation (LFE) algorithm based on log-normal quadrature wavelet filters [4, 5] and have used it to calculate such images for synthetic data, test phantoms, excised tissue specimens, and in vivo [4]. These "elastograms" or "stiffness images" clearly depict areas of different elastic moduli in these objects, and calculated values for test phantoms correlate well with moduli calculated independently by mechanical means [1, 4]. Although LFE is effective in reconstructing elasticity maps for simple objects, there are fundamental limits on the resolution it can achieve. The estimated values of the local frequency (and hence the shear modulus) are inaccurate within half a wavelength or so of a boundary with a different object. Also, LFE can produce artifacts in the presence of strong refraction and reflections. These limitations can be largely overcome by using an approach based directly on the wave equation, inverting the equation to estimate the mechanical properties of the object being imaged, as described below.

2 Inverse Approach

Any kind of wave propagation through an object has to satisfy the wave equation [6, 7],

$$\rho(\bar{x})\nabla \cdot \{\rho^{-1}(\bar{x})\nabla\phi(\bar{x})\} + k^2(\bar{x})\phi(\bar{x}) = 0 \tag{1}$$

where $\rho(\bar{x})$ is the medium density distribution, $k(\bar{x})$ is the complex wave number, $k^2(\bar{x}) = \omega^2(\kappa(\bar{x}) + j[\alpha(\bar{x})/\omega])$, where $\kappa(\bar{x})$ is medium compressibility and $\alpha(\bar{x})$ is the absorption factor, and $\phi(\bar{x})$ could be acoustic pressure or displacement. Since shear wave elastography provides information about $\phi(\bar{x})$ at every point $\bar{x}$ in the object, it should be possible to invert equation (1) to solve for the material properties $\rho(\bar{x})$, $\kappa(\bar{x})$ and $\alpha(\bar{x})$. This would provide the density, elasticity and attenuation maps for the object under investigation. We will normalize by density below and, from that point on, ignore density variations - in effect, assuming a uniform density of 1.0 everywhere (a fairly good approximation for soft tissues).

By a change of variable in equation (1), $\Phi = \phi/\sqrt{\rho}$, the equation can be written as the standard Helmholtz equation,

$$[\nabla^2 + \epsilon^2(\bar{x})]\Phi(\bar{x}) = 0 \tag{2}$$

where $\epsilon^2 = k^2 - \sqrt{\rho}\nabla^2 \frac{1}{\sqrt{\rho}}$. This can be solved if the incident energy into the object is known (i.e., the wave equation solution in the absence of the object). The solution in terms of the Green's function can be written as the volume integral [6, 7],

$$\Phi(\bar{x}) = \Phi_i(\bar{x}) - \epsilon_0^2 \iiint_V \gamma(\bar{x}')\Phi(\bar{x})g(\bar{x} - \bar{x}')d\bar{x}' \tag{3}$$

where ϵ_0 is the value of ϵ for the background medium, γ is relative value of ϵ^2 normalized by ϵ_0^2, $\gamma(\bar{x}) = \left(\frac{\epsilon(\bar{x})}{\epsilon_0}\right)^2 - 1$, $g(\bar{x})$ is the Green's function of the wave and

$\Phi_i(\bar{x})$ is the incident wave distribution. Equation (3) can be used to devise an iterative method to solve for γ (which we term the object function). The real part of γ contains the elasticity information and the imaginary part the attenuation information. Such an estimator based on wave equation inversion should robustly handle situations with interference and refraction, which cause problems for local frequency estimation techniques, and should also provide higher resolution estimates of the mechanical properties.

If the functions $g(\bar{x})$ and $\Phi(\bar{x})g(\bar{x})$ are written in terms of basis functions $\phi_j(\bar{x})$ which are shifted versions of each other, $\phi_j(\bar{x}) = \phi(\bar{x} - \bar{x}_j)$,

$$g(\bar{x}) = \sum_j g(\bar{x}_j)\phi(\bar{x} - \bar{x}_j), \tag{4}$$

and

$$\gamma(\bar{x})\Phi(\bar{x}) = \sum_j \gamma(\bar{x}_j)\Phi(\bar{x}_j)\phi(\bar{x} - \bar{x}_j), \tag{5}$$

then eq. (3) can be written as [6],

$$\Phi(\bar{x}) = \Phi_i(\bar{x}) + \sum_j \gamma(\bar{x}_j)\Phi(\bar{x}_j)C(\bar{x}, \bar{x}_j) \tag{6}$$

where

$$C(\bar{x}, \bar{x}_j) = -\epsilon_0^2 \iiint_V \phi(\bar{x}' - \bar{x}_j)g(\bar{x}' - \bar{x})d\bar{x}'. \tag{7}$$

The Green's function is a modified Bessel's function, $\frac{1}{4i}H_0^{(2)}(k_0 r)$, for the 2-D wave propagation problem and a complex sinusoid, $\frac{\exp(ik_0 r)}{r}$, for the 3-D wave propagation problem. For a given sampling function, the basis function, $\phi(x)$, is known (e.g., sinc function for uniform sampling) and thus the coefficients, $C_j(\bar{x}, \bar{x}_k)$, of equation (7) can be estimated numerically.

If the field is measured at a finite set of grid points $\bar{x}_k$, then eqn. (6) can be written as a linear transformation,

$$\Phi(\bar{x}_k) = \Phi_i(\bar{x}_k) + \sum_j \gamma(\bar{x}_j)\Phi(\bar{x}_j)C(\bar{x}_k, \bar{x}_j). \tag{8}$$

This equation can be iteratively solved for the total field, $\Phi(\bar{x})$, if the object function, $\gamma(\bar{x})$, and the incident field, $\Phi_i(\bar{x})$, are known. We have solved this forward problem by adapting a biconjugate gradient descent method previously shown to be useful for a related problem in diffraction tomography [8]. This allows the calculation of simulated data fields for known objects.

Conversely, if the total field, $\Phi(\bar{x})$, and the incident field, $\Phi_i(\bar{x})$, are known, then the inverse problem is to solve for the object function, $\gamma(\bar{x})$, obtaining the elasticity and attenuation values across the object. Equation (8) can be iteratively solved for $\gamma(\bar{x})$ using a conjugate gradient descent based pseudo inverse procedure based on modifications to the software described above [8].

Note that the total field at each point is a complex number, of which the measured displacement at a given moment is the real part. These complex displacements are measurable with both MR and ultrasound based shear wave elastography techniques by obtaining wave field images at different phases of the acoustic wave.

3 Validation

We first tested the efficacy of the inverse approach by simulating observed wave fields for given object functions using the forward scattering method described above. These wave fields were used to obtain estimates of the object function using the local frequency estimation algorithm. These estimates were then used as initial guesses in the iterative conjugate gradient inverse solutions for the object functions to evaluate the improvements in the reconstructed object functions over the LFE estimates. The inverse approach was also tested on in-vivo breast wave field images to verify the efficacy of the inverse approach for real data.

3.1 Simulations

Simple object functions with shear modulus and attenuation variations were used for simulating the wave field which would be measured in a shear wave imaging experiment, using the forward calculation method described above. The simulations used an image grid size of 128×128 with 1 mm pixel size. Simulations were performed for a shear wave frequency of 250 Hz with background wave speed of 2.56 m/s. Figure 1 shows the object function, the computed total field, and the reconstruction for one such experiment. This simulation does not have noise added.

The LFE was used to estimate the real part of the object function (LFE can not solve for the attenuation), using the real part of the field. The inverse approach then used this LFE estimate as its initial guess for the object function. From the figures it can be seen that the inverse approach shows improved edges and sharper object definitions than the LFE, as well as providing information on the attenuation (the imaginary component of the object function).

Simulations such as this show that the LFE has good reconstruction ability, but objects are blurry, edges are poorly defined, and some artifacts are obvious. The inverse approach significantly sharpens the reconstruction and reduces the artifacts. If the inverse approach is started from a random initial state instead of from the LFE estimate, the solutions are very similar, but more iterations are required. Typical computation speeds are 2-3 seconds for the LFE, 1 hour for the inverse approach starting from the LFE (200 iterations), and 75 minutes for the LFE from a random initial state (250 iterations).

3.2 Sensitivity to Incorrect Incident Field

The inverse algorithm requires an incident field to be defined everywhere in the image - essentially, what the field would be if the entire image had an object function of unity and zero attenuation. This may be difficult to estimate in a real experimental situation. To check the sensitivity of the reconstruction to variability in the incident field specification, reconstruction was attempted with the incident field incorrectly specified to be of twice the proper amplitude and wavelength. The results were that the shear modulus (real part) was correctly reconstructed, but with an offset to the object function - that is, the background was estimated to have an object function of 3.0 instead of 1.0, exactly what is needed to counter the effect of the incorrect input and yield the observed wavenumber. Similarly, the too-high amplitude specification was "corrected" by the algorithm by assigning a large attenuation to the pixels on the left edge of the image, which immediately brings the wave amplitude down to the proper value. This indicates that the algorithm is quite robust to inaccuracies in the amplitude and background wavenumber specification for the incident field.

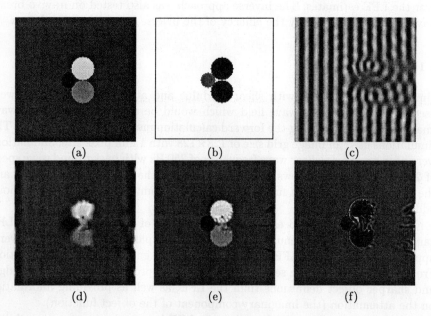

Fig. 1. Results for a simulated object function consisting of three circular objects with differing shear modulus and attenuation embedded in a uniform background. (a) and (b) show the real (shear modulus) and imaginary (attenuation) parts of the object function. (c) shows the real part of the complex total field, with the incident waves coming in from the left. (d) shows the LFE result. (e) and (f) show the real and imaginary parts of the object function using the inverse approach.

3.3 Sensitivity to Noise

The sensitivity of the algorithm to noise in the data was studied by adding Gaussian noise of varying amplitude to noise-free simulations such as those above. Fig. 2(a) shows a complicated psi-shaped object function, which (with no attenuation) yields the total field shown in Fig. 2(b). The LFE does a surprisingly good job of reconstructing the object (Fig. 2(c)), but artifacts and blurriness are evident. The inverse approach yields a much sharper and more accurate reconstruction (Fig. 2(d)) in the noise-free case, although some artifacts are present. Results when noise is added are shown in Figs. 2(e-f). At the 1% level, the noise has a substantial effect on the reconstruction, and at the 4% level, the reconstruction is seriously compromised. The LFE results at these noise levels (not shown) differ little from the noise-free case. It is evident that the inverse algorithm as currently formulated is quite sensitive to noise in the data, and reducing this sensitivity by regularizing the algorithm in some way is a priority for future research.

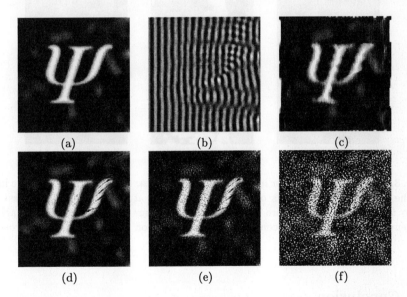

Fig. 2. Results for a simulation consisting of a psi-shaped object and smaller noise objects in a uniform background. (a) Object function: Real part of the object function. The imaginary part of the object function is zero (no attenuation). (b) The total field produced by such an object function (real part). (c) The LFE based reconstruction of the real part of the object function. (d) The real and part of the object function using the inverse approach. (e) The real and part of the object function using the inverse approach, after 1% Gaussian noise was added to the total field. (f) The real and part of the object function using the inverse approach, after 4% Gaussian noise was added to the total field.

4 Experimental Results

Fig. 3 shows the results for shear wave measurements for an in-vivo MRE breast exam on a volunteer. The data was acquired at a shear wave frequency of 100 Hz on a 16 cm field of view on a 256 × 256 grid. The LFE reconstruction (not shown) is unable to distinguish fatty tissue from the glandular tissue (as seen in the magnitude image). Some structure and distinction between the two tissues is seen with the inverse approach, in both the elasticity and attenuation images (Fig. 3(b-c)). The inverse approach is thus able to provide estimates of two distinct quantities, shear modulus and shear wave attenuation, which can provide complementary information on tissue properties.

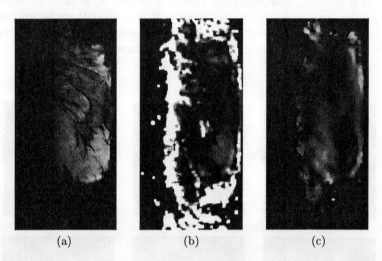

Fig. 3. Elasticity mapping for in-vivo breast MRE data. (a) The MR magnitude image of the scan. The breast rests on a vibrating surface at the right and the chest wall is to the left. (b) and (c) are the real (relative shear modulus) and the imaginary (attenuation) parts of the reconstructed object function using the inverse approach.

5 Conclusion

Acoustic shear wave elastography can provide the spatio-temporal distribution of shear wave propagation using either a phase contrast based MRI technique or an ultrasound based echo phase imaging technique. Such low frequency shear wave images can be utilized to reconstruct the elasticity and attenuation maps of the object imaged. The local frequency estimation (LFE) algorithm currently used provides useful reconstructions, but with limited resolution and some sensitivity to interference and refraction. The inverse approach to reconstruction described here provides sharper and more robust reconstructions, as demonstrated on simulations as well as on experiments with in-vivo breast images.

The inverse approach also provides the attenuation maps, which are not obtainable with LFE. The inverse approach does show more sensitivity to noise than the LFE (not discussed here). Reducing this sensitivity to noise and speeding up the algorithm are priorities for future research. The inverse approach developed here can also be extended to 3-D quite simply via the use of the 3-D Green's function, although the computation times may become prohibitive.

References

1. R. Muthupillai, D. J. Lomas, P. J. Rossman, J. F. Greenleaf, A. Manduca, and R. L. Ehman, "Magnetic resonance elastography by direct visualization of propagating acoustic strain waves," *Science*, vol. 269, pp. 1854–1857, Sept. 1995.
2. R. Muthupillai, P. J. Rossman, D. J. Lomas, J. F. Greenleaf, S. J. Riederer, and R. L. Ehman, "Magnetic resonance imaging of transverse acoustic strain waves," *Mag. Res. Med.*, vol. 36, pp. 266–274, 1996.
3. V. Dutt, R. R. Kinnick, and J. F. Greenleaf, "Shear wave displacement measurement using ultrasound," in *IEEE Ultrasonics Symp. Proc.*, (New York), pp. 1185–1188, IEEE, 1996.
4. A. Manduca, R. Muthupillai, P. J. Rossman, J. F. Greenleaf, and R. L. Ehman, "Image processing for magnetic resonance elastography," *Medical Imaging 1996: Image Processing*, SPIE vol. 2710, pp. 616–623, 1996.
5. H. Knutsson, C.-F. Westin, and G. Granlund, "Local multiscale frequency and bandwidth estimation," in *Proceedings of the 1994 IEEE International conference on Image Processing*, (Los Alamitos, CA), pp. 36–40, IEEE Computer Society Press, 1994.
6. S. A. Johnson and M. K. Tracy, "Inverse scattering solutions by a sinc basis, multiple source, moment method - part I: Theory," *Ultrasonic Imaging*, vol. 5, no. 4, pp. 361–375, 1984.
7. S.-Y. Kim, H.-C. Choi, J.-M. Lee, and J.-W. Ra, "Inverse scattering scheme based on the moment method in the spectral domain, part I: Theory," *Ultrasonic Imaging*, vol. 14, pp. 16–28, Jan. 1992.
8. D. T. Borup, S. A. Johnson, W. W. Kim, and M. J. Berggren, "Nonperturbative diffraction tomography via gauss-newton iteration applied to the scattering integral equation," *Ultrasonic Imaging*, vol. 14, no. 1, pp. 69–85, 1992.

Understanding Intensity Non-uniformity in MRI

John G. Sled and G. Bruce Pike

*McConnell Brain Imaging Centre, Montréal Neurological Institute,
McGill University, Montréal, Québec, Canada*

Abstract. Motivated by the observation that the diagonal pattern of intensity non-uniformity usually associated with linearly polarized radio-frequency (RF) coils is often present in neurological scans using circularly polarized coils, a theoretical analysis has been conducted of the intensity non-uniformity inherent in imaging an elliptically shaped object using 1.5 T magnets and circularly polarized RF coils. While an elliptic geometry is too simple to accurately predict the variations in individual anatomical scans, we use it to investigate a number of observations and hypotheses. (i) The widely made assumption that the data is corrupted by a smooth multiplicative field is accurate for proton density images. (ii) The pattern of intensity variation is highly dependent on the shape of the object being scanned. (iii) Elliptically shaped objects produce a diagonal pattern of variation when scanned using circularly polarized coils.

1 Introduction

Intensity non-uniformity is the smooth intensity variation often seen in MR images caused by such factors as RF excitation field inhomogeneity [1], non-uniform reception coil sensitivity, eddy currents driven by field gradients [2], as well as electrodynamic interactions with the object often described as RF penetration and standing wave effects [3]. In modern MRI scanners these variations are often subtle enough that they are difficult to detect by visual inspection, however, they do affect automated image analysis techniques [4], particularly segmentation techniques that assume homogeneity of intensity within each tissue class.

While initial efforts at correcting intensity non-uniformity were based on physical models or external measurements of the field variations [1,5], these methods are not sufficiently accurate to improve upon modern volumetric scans, such as those produced of the brain using a birdcage coil. Instead, recent efforts have focused on data driven strategies [6–9] based on statistical definitions of image uniformity. However, these methods are confounded by true anatomical variation that mimics the variations caused by intensity non-uniformity.

In this paper, we develop and validate, for a simple geometry, a physical model of intensity non-uniformity that has sufficient accuracy to predict the variations in a 1.5 T scanner using circularly polarized coils. While this geometry is too simple to accurately predict the variations in individual anatomical scans, it is sufficient to investigate a number of observations and hypotheses. (i) The widely made assumption that the data is corrupted by a smooth multiplicative field is accurate for proton density images. (ii) The pattern of intensity variation is highly dependent on the shape of the object being scanned. (iii) Elliptically shaped objects produce a diagonal pattern of variation when scanned using circularly polarized coils.

2 Methods

2.1 Modelling the RF excitation field and reception sensitivity

For simplicity, an analytic approach is used to investigate the effect of eccentric geometry on intensity non-uniformity. This treatment considers a long homogeneous dielectric cylinder with elliptic cross section excited by a circularly polarized field perpendicular to the cylinder axis. Interaction with the RF coil is neglected and far from the cylinder the excitation field (B_1) is assumed to be uniform. The propagation of electric and magnetic fields in dielectric media is governed by the equations:

$$\nabla^2 \mathbf{E} = \mu\epsilon \frac{\partial^2 \mathbf{E}}{\partial t^2} + \frac{\mu}{\rho} \frac{\partial \mathbf{E}}{\partial t} \qquad (1)$$

$$\nabla \times \mathbf{E} = -\frac{\partial \mathbf{B}}{\partial t}, \qquad (2)$$

where $\mathbf{E}$ and $\mathbf{B}$ are the electric and magnetic fields respectively, μ is the magnetic permeability, ϵ is the permittivity, and ρ is the resistivity of the media. The magnetic field B_1 is assumed to be oriented perpendicular to the cylinder axis while the electric field is oriented parallel. In addition, the solutions for the real vector fields $\mathbf{E}$ and $\mathbf{B}$ are assumed to vary sinusoidally in time at an angular frequency ω such that

$$\mathbf{E} = \text{Re}\left\{E_z \hat{z} e^{j\omega t}\right\} \qquad (3)$$

$$\mathbf{B} = \text{Re}\left\{(B_x \hat{x} - jB_y \hat{y}) e^{j\omega t}\right\}. \qquad (4)$$

Solutions to this problem for the cases of circular and elliptic cylinders are given in [10] and [11].

A so-called circularly polarized excitation field is created by driving two orthogonal linearly polarized coils 90° out of phase such that the field components that contribute to the MR signal add constructively. In general, the field produced by a linearly polarized coil will vary in magnitude and direction within the object such that the combined field from the two coils can have arbitrary elliptic polarization. This elliptically polarized field can be decomposed into a (+) rotating field, which causes the excitation, and a typically weaker (-) counter-rotating field that does not [12]. The orientation of this (+) rotating field with respect to the driving field can be interpreted as a phase shift, which we refer to as a geometric phase shift.

In general, the individual field components will be complex to reflect the phase delays caused by currents induced in the object. Geometric and inductive phase shifts combine to determine the local phase of the excitation field within the object as follows:

$$B^+ = B_{xx} + jB_{yx} - jB_{xy} + B_{yy}. \quad (5)$$

where the notation B_{yx} refers to the magnetic field in the y direction produced by a coil aligned along the x axis. While this derivation is based on two linearly polarized coils aligned with the x and y axes, the result is general for any combination of coils producing a circularly polarized field. Hence, it can used to predict the field pattern of a birdcage coil or a pair of linearly polarized coils not aligned with the x and y axes.

The same solutions for the field components apply when orthogonal coils are used for reception. However, the geometric phase shifts caused by reception cancel with those of the excitation field [1] whereas the phase shifts due to induced currents accumulate. Hence, the reception sensitivity is given by

$$R^+ = R_0(B_{xx} - jB_{yx} + jB_{xy} + B_{yy}), \quad (6)$$

where R_0 is a scale factor reflecting the sensitivity of the coil.

Images produced by a spin echo sequence are simulated using the derived excitation field and reception sensitivity. The signal measured for a spin echo pulse sequence is given by [10]

$$S = \rho R^+ S_{SE} \quad (7)$$

$$S_{SE} = \sin^3\left(\frac{\pi}{2}\frac{|B^+|}{B_m}\right)\exp(j\arg(B^+)), \quad (8)$$

where ρ is the spin density, S_{SE} is the emitted signal, S is the measured signal, and B_m is the nominal field strength needed to produce a 90° flip-angle. This derivation neglects relaxation and assumes complete recovery of the magnetization between repetitions.

2.2 Phantom studies

To validate our theoretical model of intensity non-uniformity, we constructed two 40cm long plastic cylindrical containers with elliptic and circular cross sections respectively. The circular cylinder has an inside diameter of 17.5cm, while the elliptic cylinder has major and minor diameters of 20cm and 15cm. Each cylinder was filled with various concentrations of NaCl solutions made from deionized water.

The conductivity and permittivity of each solution was computed based on the concentration of NaCl using data from [13]. The quantities of NaCl were 1.38g/L, 2.83g/L, and 58.2g/L, or roughly 24mM, 48mM, and 100mM, producing resistivities of $4.0\Omega m$, $2.0\Omega m$, and $1.0\Omega m$ respectively. These resistivities span the range typical of biological tissues [3] at frequencies around 64MHz. At this frequency, the relative permittivity of water is essentially unchanged from its D.C. value of $\epsilon_r = 80$, which is comparable to that of brain [14] at 64MHz.

In addition to NaCl, a small quantity of MnCl$_2$ was added to each solution to bring its concentration to 97μM so as to reduce T_1 relaxation times to approximately 910ms. Experiments using long repetition times (TR = 30s) showed no measurable change in intensity non-uniformity after addition of MnCl$_2$.

For the experiments, the cylinders were aligned axially with the isocenter of the body coil of a 1.5T Siemens Vision MRI scanner and scanned transversally using a B_1 field mapping sequence [15] as well as a standard spin echo sequence. All images were acquired at 2mm in-plane resolution and 6mm slice thickness. The spin echo sequence (TR/TE = 8s/14ms) had sufficiently short TE and long TR that relaxation can be neglected. The field mapping sequence is a stimulated echo technique ($90° - \tau_e/2 - 90° - \tau_1 - \alpha - \tau_2 - 90° - \tau_e/2 - acquire$ where $\tau_e/\tau_1/\tau_2/TR = 36\text{ms}/60\text{ms}/8\text{ms}/1\text{s}$) which yields a series of images whose intensities are related by

$$S_i = a \cos b\alpha_i. \tag{9}$$

The parameters a and b are computed at each voxel by a non-linear least squares fit to the flip angles α_i and complex image values S_i. Images were acquired at $\alpha = 0°, 40°, \ldots, 400°$. The resulting parameter map b is proportional to the excitation field strength, while the parameter map a is roughly proportional to spin density.

3 Results

3.1 Simulated spin echo images

Once the expressions for excitation field and reception sensitivity have been evaluated they can be used to simulate an imaging sequence. A simulated spin echo image for an elliptic geometry having $\mu = \mu_0$, $\epsilon_r = 80$, and $\rho = 2\,\Omega m$ is shown in Figure 1. Also shown are the corresponding excitation field and reception sensitivity.

It should be noted that the pattern of non-uniformity in the spin echo image resembles neither the excitation field nor the reception sensitivity. This is caused by the apparent reversal of the excitation field to produce the sensitivity map. However, close inspection of the phase images for the two cases reveals that the excitation field and reception sensitivity maps differ by more than a reversal. In particular the geometric phase in the two cases is opposite while the inductive phase lag, dominant in this medium, remains unchanged.

Due to the symmetry of the elliptic shape, the magnitude of the excitation and reception sensitivity maps differ only by a reversal of the y axis. However, the resulting spin echo image is not symmetric as reception sensitivity makes a stronger contribution to image non-uniformity than does excitation field variation.

3.2 Comparison with phantom studies

The experimental data admits two types of comparisons with the theoretical model: a direct comparison of the measured excitation field with that predicted,

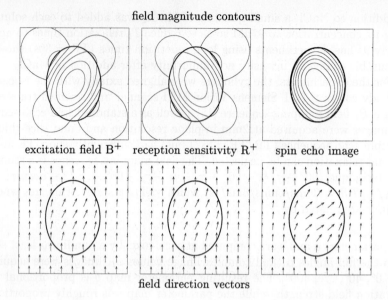

Fig. 1. Simulated spin echo images with nominal 90° and 180° flip-angles. Contours are at 5% of mean intensity. For the spin echo image the direction vectors can be interpreted as the phase of the complex image.

and a comparison of the measured spin echo image with that simulated from the predicted excitation field and reception sensitivity.

Before any comparisons were made all of the measured data was first automatically registered [16, 17] with the spin density map of the corresponding simulated image by linear transformation. A common mask was defined for each pair of images by automatically thresholding each image based on its histogram [18], taking the intersection of the two masks, and eroding it by 2mm. The RMS difference between two images was then computed within the common mask and expressed as a percentage of the mean intensity in the simulated image.

Figure 2 shows the excitation fields measured in the elliptic cylinder for each of the three NaCl solutions. Also shown are the predicted field patterns and the differences between the measured and predicted results. The prediction of a diagonal pattern of non-uniformity is confirmed by these experiments. When the gray scale of the difference image is expanded, it reveals spurious ghost images caused by the field mapping sequence as well as minor and largely random differences between the measured and predicted fields. The accuracy of the results for the circular cylinder is essentially the same.

The accuracy of the model at predicting the measured images was quantified by computing the root-mean-square (RMS) difference between the two. In all cases, the RMS difference was less than 2% and did not increase as the severity of the non-uniformity increased.

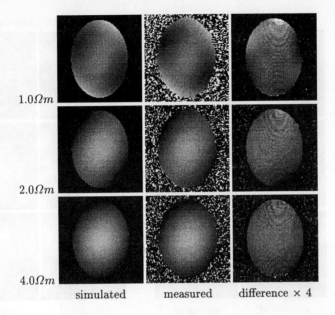

Fig. 2. Comparison of predicted and measured excitation fields B^+ in an elliptic phantom for three levels of resistivity. The normalized intensity scale for each image is 0.8 to 1.2 except for the difference images which are -0.05 to 0.05.

Figure 3 shows the measured and predicted spin echo images for the two geometries and three solutions. The pattern of variations in these images is more complicated and the variations are more severe owing to the contribution of the reception sensitivity. Note that the orientation of the diagonal pattern in the elliptic case is reversed with respect to the excitation field map. The RMS difference between measured and predicted images was 1%-2%.

4 Discussion

By modelling the electromagnetic interactions with the subject during excitation and reception from first principles, we are able to account for almost all of the intensity non-uniformity observed in volumetric scans at 1.5 T. This agreement is achieved in spite of making no explicit assumptions of a coil producing the fields. While this is reasonable for a head sized object in a body coil, one can expect that smaller coils such as a head coil would produce some variations caused by their interaction with the object. However, in either case electromagnetic interaction with the object is the primary cause of intensity non-uniformity. Hence, the use of equation (7) is justified, and verifies that non-uniformity is correctly modelled as a smooth multiplicative field for proton density imaging sequences. However, for other imaging sequences that depend on relaxation, the

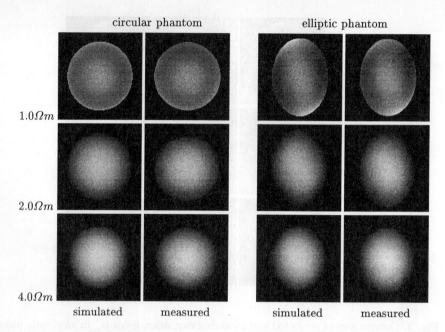

Fig. 3. Comparison of predicted and measured spin echo images for each level of resistivity. The normalized intensity scale for each image is 0.8 to 1.2.

term S_{SE} in equation (7) will depend on the relaxation rates and will not in general be spatially smooth for inhomogeneous media.

We have shown that an elliptic geometry imaged using a circularly polarized coil produces a diagonal intensity non-uniformity pattern qualitatively similar to the quadrapole artifact observed with a linearly polarized coil. Although, one would expect the circularly symmetric pattern seen for circular objects to generalize to an elliptically symmetric pattern for elliptic objects, in the elliptic case the two linear fields interact with the media differently, leading to asymmetric intensity variations that do not cancel in the combined field. Such asymmetry could be incorrectly attributed to right-left hemisphere differences in a sensitive statistical analysis of neurological scans. Furthermore, since the orientation of this diagonal pattern is determined by the orientation of the object and not the orientation of the coil, one can expect that non-uniformity patterns will, in general, be correlated with anatomy and hence will also be present in averages of multiple scans.

Inspection of the experimental results for the elliptic case would suggest that the reception sensitivity is the mirror image of the excitation field pattern. However, the theoretical results show a more subtle relationship. In particular, for conductive objects there is a distinction between the phase delays associated with induced currents and those inherent in imaging the object in the absence of conductivity. Accounting for excitation and reception, the latter phase terms cancel while the former do not, thereby leading to the non-uniformity pattern in the spin echo image being more complicated than either the excitation or receptions fields.

An important implication of this lack of cancellation is that for arbitrarily shaped conductive objects, measurement of the excitation field is not sufficient to predict the pattern of variations in the resulting image. In addition, since electrodynamic interaction significantly affects the reception sensitivity, neither measurement of the sensitivity in the absence of the subject nor scanning of a standard phantom is sufficient to predict the variations in a given subject. Furthermore, these variations will be present irrespective of the uniformity of the field produced by the unloaded coil. As we have shown, the variation can be predicted by an electrodynamic model provided it takes into account the pulse sequence, geometry, and resistive and permittive properties of the subject.

References

1. E. R. McVeigh, M. J. Bronskill, and R. M. Henkelman, "Phase and sensitivity of receiver coils in magnetic resonance imaging," *Med. Phys.*, vol. 13, pp. 806–814, Nov./Dec. 1986.
2. A. Simmons, P. S. Tofts, G. J. Barker, and S. R. Arridge, "Sources of intensity nonuniformity in spin echo images," *Magn. Reson. Med.*, vol. 32, pp. 121–128, 1994.
3. P. A. Bottomley and E. R. Andrew, "RF magnetic field penetration, phase shift and power dissipation in biological tissue: implications for NMR imaging," *Physics in Medicine and Biology*, vol. 23, pp. 630–43, Jul 1978.
4. J. G. Sled and A. C. E. Alex P. Zijdenbos, D. Louis Collins, "The impact of intensity non-uniformity on automated anatomical analysis of 3d mri images," in *Third International Conference on Functional Mapping of the Human Brain*, p. S399, 1997.
5. B. R. Condon, J. Patterson, D. Wyper, *et al.*, "Image non-uniformity in magnetic resonance imaging: its magnitude and methods for its correction," *Br. J. Radiology*, vol. 60, pp. 83–87, 1987.
6. B. M. Dawant, A. P. Zijdenbos, and R. A. Margolin, "Correction of intensity variations in MR images for computer-aided tissue classification," *IEEE Trans. Med. Imag.*, vol. 12, pp. 770–781, Dec. 1993.
7. C. R. Meyer, P. H. Bland, and J. Pipe, "Retrospective correction of intensity inhomogeneities in MRI," *IEEE Transactions on Medical Imaging*, vol. 14, pp. 36–41, Mar. 1995.
8. W. M. Wells III, W. E. L. Grimson, R. Kikinis, and F. A. Jolesz, "Adaptive segmentation of MRI data," *IEEE Trans. Med. Imag.*, vol. 15, no. 4, pp. 429–442, 1996.
9. J. G. Sled, A. P. Zijdenbos, and A. C. Evans, "A non-parametric method for automatic correction of intensity non-uniformity in MRI data," *IEEE Trans. Med. Imag.*, vol. 17, pp. 87–97, February 1998.
10. G. O. Glover, C. E. Hayes, N. J. Pelc, W. A. Edelstein, O.M.Mueller, H. R. Hart, C. J. Hardy, M. O'Donnel, and W. D. Barber, "Comparison of linear and circular polarization for magnetic resonance imaging," *J. Magn. Reson.*, vol. 64, pp. 255–270, 1985.

11. J. G. Sled and G. B. Pike, "Standing-wave and RF penetration artifacts caused by elliptic geometry: an electrodynamic analysis of MRI," *IEEE Trans. Med. Imag.*, 1997. (submitted).
12. P. S. Tofts, "Standing waves in uniform water phantoms," *J. Magn. Reson. B*, vol. 104, pp. 143–147, 1994.
13. P. S. Neelakanta, *Handbook of electromagnetic materials : monolithic and composite versions and their applications*, pp. 577–584. CRC Press, 1995.
14. D. Simunic, P. Wach, W. Renhart, and R. Stollberger, "Spatial distribution of high-frequency electromagnetic energy in human head during MRI: numerical results and measurements," *IEEE Transactions on Biomedical Engineering*, vol. 43, pp. 88–94, Jan 1996.
15. S. Topp, E. Adalsteinsson, and D. M. Spielman, "Fast multislice B_1-mapping," in *International Society for Magnetic Resonance in Medicine*, vol. 1, p. 281, 1997.
16. D. L. Collins, P. Neelin, T. M. Peters, and A. C. Evans, "Automatic 3D intersubject registration of MR volumetric data in standardized Talairach space," *J. Comput. Assist. Tomogr.*, vol. 18, no. 2, pp. 192–205, 1994.
17. MNI Automated Linear Registration Package, Version 0.98, 1997. Available by anonymous ftp at ftp://ftp.bic.mni.mcgill.ca/pub/mni_autoreg/
18. N. Otsu, "A threshold selection method from gray-level histograms," *IEEE Transactions on Biomedical Engineering*, vol. 9, pp. 63–66, 1979.

An Automatic Threshold-Based Scaling Method for Enhancing the Usefulness of Tc-HMPAO SPECT in the Diagnosis of Alzheimer's Disease

Pankaj Saxena[1], Dan G. Pavel[2], Juan Carlos Quintana[3] and Barry Horwitz[4]

[1] Biomedical Visualization Laboratory, Department of Neurosurgery, University of Illinois at Chicago, 912 S. Wood Street, Chicago, IL 60612
[2] Nuclear Medicine, Department of Radiology, University of Illinois at Chicago.
[3] Catholic University, Santiago, Chile
[4] Laboratory of Neurosciences, National Institute of Aging, NIH, Bethesda, MD 20892

Abstract. Functional imaging of the brain can aid in the diagnosis of Alzheimer's disease. Tc-HMPAO SPECT is widely available and relatively inexpensive to use. Combined with computer-based analysis of images, SPECT is a powerful tool in detecting decreases in brain perfusion caused by Alzheimer's disease. However, analysis can falsely elevate the perfusion of normal areas and diminish the perfusion of atrophic areas in the Alzheimer's brain when used with conventional scaling methods. In this paper, we present a technique for scaling images that overcomes the problems associated with conventional scaling methods. Our technique was successful in eliminating or attenuating the false increases in perfusion shown in probable Alzheimer's patients in over 90% of cases (n=17), and in enhancing the sensitivity of detection of degenerative changes by Statistical Parametric Mapping.

1 Introduction

Alzheimer's Disease (AD) is typically diagnosed through a process of exclusion [1]. A diagnosis of probable AD is made after excluding other possibilities in the differential diagnosis of dementia. Since the process of diagnosing AD is complex, and sometimes uncertain, there is a need for new tools and techniques that can aid in diagnosis, especially in its early stages, when the most benefit can be derived from drugs that may slow the progression of the disease.

Imaging is a relatively simple, non-invasive procedure that can provide useful structural and functional information about the brain. Anatomically, AD is characterized by the degeneration of cortical and subcortical structures. This is accompanied by a reduction in brain volume [2], which occurs globally, but is somewhat more marked in structures particularly affected by AD, such as the hippocampus, temporal and parietal lobes, and amygdala [2]. Functionally, AD is characterized by a reduction in cerebral metabolism, selectively targeting areas such as the posterior parietal, temporal and frontal cortex, while often sparing the primary sensorimotor and occipital cortex [3]. This reduction in metabolism is correlated with a decrease in blood supply to the affected areas of the brain, and usually appears before structural changes are observed [3].

Functional imaging techniques such as Positron Emission Tomography (PET) and Single Photon Emission Computed Tomography (SPECT) can detect changes in regional metabolism and blood flow. However, it is often difficult to distinguish the changes that accompany AD from normal aging, and from other causes of dementia and degeneration.

1.1 Functional Imaging in Alzheimer's Disease

PET has been used to study the reduction of cerebral metabolism in AD [8]. Because of the limited availability and high cost of PET, attention has focused on SPECT to provide a low cost alternative to PET. SPECT provides data on regional blood flow that correlates with the metabolic data provided by PET in patients with AD, such as decreases in blood flow to temporo-parietal areas [3], and is considered a useful tool to aid in the diagnosis of AD [9, 10]. Some investigators have found that the degree and extent of decreased cerebral blood flow correlates with severity [12] of AD. The synergistic use of SPECT with other imaging modalities adds a new dimension of anatomical-functional correlation, and is likely to further enhance the usefulness of SPECT in AD [11].

Computer-based techniques can extend the usefulness of SPECT. Statistical Parametric Mapping (SPM) [13] is a univariate approach based on the general linear model. A t-statistic is calculated in parallel for each voxel, and an image of this statistic is assembled (the SPM(t) map), which is transformed to a Gaussian Field (the SPM(Z) map). Regional variations of SPM(Z) can be used for statistical inference based on distributional approximations derived from the theory of Gaussian Fields. Corrected p-values can be calculated for clusters of voxels exceeding some given threshold [13, 14].

Although initially developed for PET and subsequently fMRI, SPM has been successfully adapted for SPECT [18]. We have previously used SPECT to evaluate motor activation, diamox and balloon occlusion tests, as well as paroxysmal psychiatric events.

Voxel intensities in SPECT images represent perfusion levels in the brain. There are several sources of variation among SPECT scans. Global variations may be caused by differences in the dose of radioactive tracer, scanner sensitivity, or the positioning of the head in the scanner. Local variations may occur normally as differences among patients, or within the same patient at different times, and/or as the result of brain pathology. These differences must be accounted for in order for statistical comparisons to be made, and is typically done by scaling the images to each other, or to some standard.

SPM provides several models to do the scaling. ANCOVA assumes a local linear model, for a small range of global values of CBF. It assumes that variance is constant, and that activations are additive. Therefore, ANCOVA best models the local non-linear relationship between regional CBF and global CBF, in the absence of sources of global variance and gross pathology. The proportional model (followed by ANOVA) assumes that there is a proportional relationship between global and regional changes, that is, activations are proportional to the underlying global blood flow, and that the variance increases with global CBF. If global counts vary greatly due to scanner sensitivity or dosage, and noise increases proportionally with the signal, the proportional scaling model is appropriate.

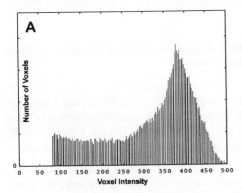
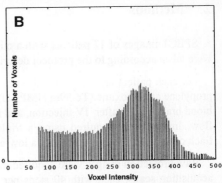

Figure 1: Histograms showing the global distribution of voxel intensities in (A) control image, and (B) image from an AD patient. Both images are normalized to Talairach space (see Methods section below) and represent approximately identical volumes. The images were thresholded at a number proportional to their global means in order to remove extra-cerebral voxels and the highest voxels were scaled to a value of 500. The marked flattening of the peak in the AD image indicates a reduced blood supply to cortical areas.

We use SPECT to diagnose Alzheimer's patients by comparing their scans to those of a control group. The decrease in blood flow in AD is large enough to depress the global mean of voxel intensities (rCBF equivalent) significantly below the control group, making ANCOVA a poor choice for scaling, since it assumes that there is little or no global variance. The proportional scaling model is also inappropriate, because it scales the global means of the images to each other. Since the global mean of the AD images is depressed, these images are scaled up to match the global means of the controls. This scaling-induced elevation of counts in the AD images has unfortunate effects. First, areas which had normal counts before the scaling (areas that are generally spared by AD, such as the primary sensorimotor cortex) are scaled up to an extent that they appear as "better than normal perfusion" areas in the SPM results. Second, the scaling-induced global elevation of counts in AD also affects areas that show atrophy from the disease. Scaling up these areas produces a loss of sensitivity seen when the AD images are subtracted from the controls.

It has been suggested that in PET images [19], the problems of these scaling methods can be avoided by choosing areas unaffected by the disease to do a proportional scaling. An average calculated from such unaffected areas should be resistant to the false hyperperfusion and loss of sensitivity seen with SPM-based proportional scaling. Since selecting "normal" areas manually is a time-intensive and subjective process, we developed a method to automatically scale the images based on normal areas for the routine evaluation of SPECT images from AD patients.

2   Methods

SPECT images of 17 patients with a clinical diagnosis of probable AD, and 17 controls were taken according to the protocol described below:

For each patient or control, rCBF was assessed with technetium-99m-D L-hexamethyl-propylene amine oxime (Tc-99m HMPAO), a lipophilic radiotracer that readily crosses the blood brain barrier after IV injection, and is trapped inside the brain in proportion to blood flow. Images were acquired using a triple-head camera system (Picker Prism 3000XP). Each camera head is equipped with a low-energy ultra-high-resolution fan beam collimator.

Raw projection images were acquired in a 128x128 matrix using a protocol with 5 rapid acquisition scans; each with 40 steps per camera head at 7 seconds per step, for a total acquisition time of 23.3 minutes. The summed data was reconstructed using a Parzen filter, and the resulting transverse slices post-filtered using a low-pass (order=6, cutoff=0.26) filter. An attenuation correction map was applied to the filtered data sets, and orthogonal slices were obtained in preparation for SPM-based analysis.

After doing a roll-yaw correction on a single scan, all other scans were aligned to it using the Automated Image Registration (AIR) program [15]. A subsequent alignment was repeated in SPM95 [16], following which the images were edited to remove the skull and extra-cerebral tissues. This is necessary in SPECT Tc-HMPAO images since scalp/skull are prominent, and will affect the subsequent normalization unless they are removed.

In order to compare images from different subjects, all images were then normalized in SPM95 to the standard anatomical space described by Talairach and Tournoux [17]. A smoothing kernel (FWHM 20×20×12) was applied to the normalized images (which had anisotropic voxels, larger along the z-axis. These images were scaled as described below:

1. The average of the top 1% (in terms of intensity) voxels for each image was calculated in our control and AD groups. Our assumption was that the voxels with the highest intensities (denoting highest levels of perfusion) would be in those areas that are relatively unaffected by AD.
2. Every voxel in each image was divided by the top 1% average for that image.
3. In order to retain more significant digits, we multiplied all voxels by a factor of 100.

4. These scaled images were provided to SPM95 for analysis using a single-subject-replication-of-conditions design. SPM(Z) statistics were calculated using different thresholds and a p-value of 0.05 was chosen as statistically significant.

We experimented with other levels of averaging, ranging from the top 30% average to the top 0.25% average. Results continued to improve on both contrasts (in terms of attenuating the false increase in contrast A and sensitizing contrast B) as we progressed from 30% towards 0.25%. The 0.5% and 0.25% averaging did not consistently improve results compared to the 1% averaging. Because of this, and because we suspected that outliers might exert a substantial effect on averages taken from a small number of voxels, we picked 1% as the standard.

We plotted frequency histograms of the voxel intensities for each image (Figure 1). We were able to distinguish between a normal and an AD-type frequency distribution of voxel values. The AD histogram is characterized by a flattening of the peak in the upper-middle range, which represents degenerated cortical areas. Of our 17 probable AD patients, 4 did not show this characteristic flattening of the peak. The numbers for kurtosis and skewness showed that of these 4 probable AD patients, 3 were intermediate between the control and probable AD group, while one was indistinguishable from the control group.

3 Results

We compared results of processing a clinically diagnosed probable AD patient with and without our scaling procedure. Figure 2 illustrates the different types of scalings.

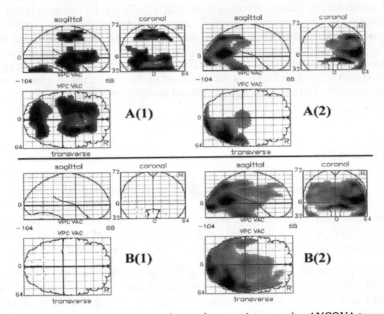

Figure 2: SPM(Z) maps comparing an AD patient to the control group using ANCOVA type scaling (A) & top 1% averaging (B). Contrast 1 shows areas that are better perfused in the AD patient than the controls. Contrast 2 shows areas with reduced perfusion in AD compared to the control group.

We fused the SPM image maps to a Talairach-normalized, co-registered MR image in order to better locate the affected areas (Figure 3). Visual inspection of the SPECT images, which shows no significant increase in perfusion on the left side in the areas corresponding to the hot spots in Figure 3 (A(1)), supports the conclusion that the areas eliminated by our top 1% average scaling method were false positives. The second contrast (areas that are less perfused in the AD patient compared to the control group) underestimates, in most cases, the extent and significance of the affected areas.

Of the 17 patients in the Alzheimer's group, 9 showed elimination, and 5 an average 80% attenuation of the false positive effect in Contrast A. These patients also showed an average 70% increased sensitivity in Contrast B when using our top 1% average scaling. Three patients showed a minor improvement in contrast A, but no gain in sensitivity in contrast B.

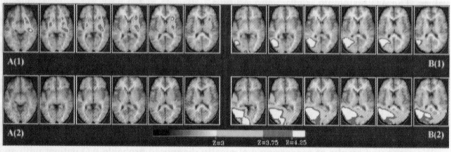

Figure 3: SPM processing results superimposed on patient's MRI. The slices are displayed in the Radiological Convention (Left is Right). Images on the left (Contrast A) show areas better perfused in the patient than the controls, according to ANCOVA [A(1)] and 1% averaging [A(2)]. The areas found in the ANCOVA processing are mainly located in the subcortical region, sensorimotor areas, and cerebellum. While these areas are indeed least affected in AD, they are unlikely to be better in the AD patient than the control group. Images on the right (Contrast B) show areas with less perfusion in the patient than in the controls, according to ANCOVA [B(1)] and 1% averaging [B(2)]. The areas most affected are located in the right parieto-temporal area and, to a lesser extent, in the left parietal region. These areas are typically affected by Alzheimer's disease.

4 Discussion

Our scaling method appears to be effective in countering the effects of globally decreased counts seen in AD patients processed with SPM. In the majority of cases, it attenuated or eliminated the false positive effect of better-than-control perfusion in AD patients, and significantly increased the sensitivity in terms of number of voxels affected and/or their associated Z-value in detecting the perfusion deficits in AD patients.

In cases where the top 1% averaging method failed to produce any improvement over the ANCOVA processing results in contrast B, we found that the histograms of the AD patient's data resembled our control group more than they resembled the other AD patients. The arithmetic of scaling indicates that there is no advantage to scaling to the top 1% average rather than the global average in these cases. In other words, the patient's image is scaled up approximately equally in both cases. This indicates that either (1) the global average for these patients is not as depressed as it is for the other AD patients, and/or (2) the top 1% average for these patients is more depressed for these patients than for the other AD patients, relative to the control group. Since the top 1% pixels represent the areas that are generally spared by AD, (1) above is the more likely explanation. This is further supported by the fact that histograms of their image data resemble the control group more than they resemble other Alzheimer's patients, and by the actual values of the global averages, which are unusually high. It is possible that these patients represent an atypical presentation of AD, or misdiagnosis.

In principle, this type of scaling should be useful for any pathological state which involves a substantial decrease in perfusion, such as other types of cerebral degeneration and large focal deficits caused by infarction or trauma. We are presently evaluating the utility of this technique in such cases. The differential diagnosis of probable AD requires an extension of this method to a large group, and further correlation with definite cases of AD.

References

1. Murden, R.A.: The diagnosis of Alzheimer's Disease. Adv. Exp. Med. Biol. **282** (1990) 59-64
2. Fox, N.C., Freeborough, P.A., and Rossor, M.N.: Visualization and quantification of rates of atrophy in Alzheimer's Disease. Lancet. **348** (1996) 94-97
3. Mayberg, H.S.: Clinical correlates of PET- and SPECT-identified defects in dementia. J. Clin. Psychiatry. 55 (1994) Supplement 12-21
4. Freeborough, P.A., Woods, R.P. and Fox, N.C.: Accurate registration of serial 3D MR brain images and its application to visualizing change in neurodegenerative disorders. J. Comp. Assisted Tomography. **20(6)** (1996) 1012-1022
5. Freeborough, P.A., and Fox, N.C.: The boundary shift integral: An accurate and robust measure of cerebral volume changes from registered repeat MRI. IEEE Trans. Med. Imag. **16(5)** (1997) 623-629
6. Fox, N.C. and Freeborough, P.A.: Brain atrophy progression measured from registered serial MRI: validation and application to Alzheimer's Disease. J. Magn. Reson. Imag. **7(6)** (1997) 1069-1075
7. Aylward, E.H., Rasmusson, D.X., Brandt, J., Raimundo, L., Folstein, M., and Pearlson, G.D.: CT measurement of suprasellar cistern predicts rate of cognitive decline in Alzheimer's Disease. J. Int. Neuropsychol. Soc. **2(2)** (1996) 89-95
8. Azari, N.P., Pettigrew, K.D., Schapiro, M.B., Haxby, J.V., Grady, C.L., Pietrini, P., Salerno, J.A., Heston, L.L., Rapoport, S.I., and Horwitz, B.: Early detection of Alzheimer's Disease: a statistical approach using Positron Emission Tomographic data. J. Cereb. Blood Flow and Metab. **13** (1993) 438-447
9. McMurdo, M.E., Grant, D.J., Kennedy, N.S., Gilchrist, J., Findlay, D., and McLennan, J.M.: The value of HMPAO SPECT scanning in the diagnosis of early Alzheimer's Disease in patients attending a memory clinic. Nucl. Med. Commun. **15(6)** (1994) 405-9
10. Golan, H., Kremer, J., Freedman, M., and Ichise, M.: Usefulness of follow-up regional cerebral blood flow measurements by Single Photon Emission Computed Tomography in the differential diagnosis of dementia. J. Neuroimaging. **6(1)** (1996) 23-28
11. D'Asseler, Y.M., Koole, M., Lemahieu, I., Achten, E., Boon, P., De Deyn, P.P., and Dierckx, R.A.: Recent and future evolutions in neuroSPECT with particular emphasis on the synergistic use and fusion of imaging modalities. Acta Neurol. Belg. **97(3)** (1997) 154-62

12. Eagger, S., Syed, G.M.S., Burns, A., Barette, J.J., and Levy, R.: Morphological (CT) and functional (rCBF SPECT) correlates in Alzheimer's Disease. Nucl. Med. Commun. **13** (1992) 644-647
13. Friston, K.J., Holmes, A.P., Worsley, K.J., Poline, J.P., Frith. C.D., and Frackowiak R.S.J.: Statistical Parametric Maps in Functional Imaging: A General Linear Approach. Human Br. Mapping. **2** (1995) 189-210
14. Friston, K.J.: Statistical Parametric Mapping: Ontology and Current Issues. J. Cerebral. Blood Flow. **15** (1995) 361-370
15. Woods, R.P.: Automated Image Registration software for Unix, version 3.0. Available through the Internet at the URL: http://bishopw.loni.ucla.edu/AIR3/index.html. (1995–98)
16. Friston, K., Ashburner, J., Heather, J., Holmes, A., Poline, J-B., et al.: SPM Software. Wellcome Department of Cognitive Neurology. URL: http://www.fil.ion.ucl.ac.uk/spm/. (1994-1998)
17. Talairach, P. and Tournoux, J.: A stereotactic coplanar atlas of the human brain. Thieme, Stuttgart, Germany. (1988)
18. Pavel, D.G., Thompson, D., Patel, B., Lin, Q., Brint, S., Dujovny, M., and Ibanez, V.: Evaluation of brain SPECT changes using Statistical Parametric Mapping following diamox challenge. J. Nucl. Med. **38** (1997) 280
19. Pavel, D.G., Horwitz, B., Saxena, P., Schapiro, M.B., Pietrini, P., and Ibanez, V.: Quantification of Alzheimer's PET Images using a special scaling method and Statistic Parametric Mapping. Soc. For Neurosci. Ann. Meeting. New Orleans. Vol **23** (1997), 563

Automatic Computation of Average Brain Models

Alexandre Guimond[1,2], Jean Meunier[2], and Jean-Philippe Thirion[1]*

[1] INRIA Sophia Antipolis, Epidaure Project 2004, France
{guimond,thirion}@sophia.inria.fr
http://www.inria.fr/Equipes/EPIDAURE-eng.html
[2] Université de Montréal, Département d'informatique et de recherche opérationnelle,
Montréal, Canada.
meunier@iro.umontreal.ca
http://www.IRO.UMontreal.CA/labs/vision

Abstract. We present a completely automatic method to build average anatomical models of the human brain using a set of MR images. The models computed present two important characteristics: an average intensity and an average shape. We provide results showing convergence toward the barycenter of the image set used for the computation of the model.

1 Introduction

Someone suffering from a neurological disorder such as epilepsy or schizophrenia will usually undergo a series of tests to assess the anatomy and the functional activity of his or her brain. The results of these tests are then analyzed to identify if abnormal variations are present, providing valuable information for future medical treatment.

An important tool used to diagnose abnormal anatomical variations are medical atlases. Traditional ones [14, 12] are presented in textbooks, but computerized atlases comprising information in a more practical and quantitative manner are becoming available [10]. They also usually include information obtained from a set of subjects [8] instead of a single individual, making them more representative of a population and enabling the calculation of normal variations [17].

The following work aims to develop and validate the concepts introduced in a previous paper [9] to build an average model of the human brain using a set of magnetic resonance (MR) images obtained from normal subjects. We intend to fabricate an image with two important characteristics: average tissue intensity and average tissue shape up to an affine transformation.

As depicted in Fig. 1, our method can be summarized in the following manner. Affine registration between all the images of the set and a reference image corrects for differences due to translations, rotations, scalings and shearings. These are morphometrical variations that are not of concern for our study. Elastic registration is then used to evaluate residual variations due to pure morphological

---
* Now in Focus Imaging, Sophia Antipolis, France

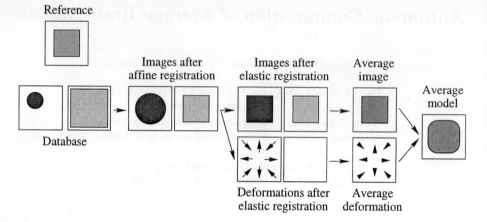

Fig. 1. Average model construction method.

differences and produce images having the same shape as the reference. The images and the residual deformations are averaged and the average deformation applied to the average image to produce the model. It presents an average intensity and an average shape modulo an affine transformation corresponding to the affine characteristics of the reference image.

The main contribution of this paper is the description of a fully automatic technique to obtain an *average intensity* image combined with an *average shape* image, producing the *average model M*.

The most similar work regarding average intensity atlases is that of [3] who created from nine MR scans a two-dimensional image representing the average intensity of the mid-sagittal plane. Thirteen manually identified landmarks in the mid-sagittal plane of each scan where matched with a reference image using the thin-plate spline interpolant [2]. The nine resampled images where then averaged to result into a morphometric average atlas. Our method differs mainly by two aspects. First, as suggested by [3], we make full use of the three-dimensionality of the scans to compute a three-dimensional average image. Second, our registration method is automatic and computes a dense deformation field instead of an interpolated function based on thirteen landmarks. This deformation identifies for each voxel of the reference the corresponding positions in the other scans. Within this process, every voxel of the reference can be though of as a landmark automatically determined in the other scans.

The work of [8], where three hundred and five (305) three-dimensional MR scans were registered using translations, rotations and scalings, and averaged to build a statistical neuroanatomical model, also relates to our work. We follow the same idea but proceed further by using a less constrained type of deformation.

As will be shown, compared to these previous efforts, our method provides clearer images with higher contrasts and more sharp definitions of tissue boundaries.

The average shape concept is most similar to the work of [13], [4] and [11] who compute average shapes modulo similarity or affine transformations. We have not tried to strictly follow the theory developed in their works. Our intention was to conform to the idea of making abstraction of differences between images due to first order transformations, and analyze residual variations. Our main contribution resides in the characteristics used to build the average shape, that is the image intensities instead of landmarks or crestlines. Again, this enables the computation of dense deformations fields representing variations everywhere is the MR scan, as opposed to interpolating transformations found using landmarks, lines or surfaces. We believe this technique may find less accurate matches in the close surroundings of the landmarks, but provides better overall registration.

The remaining sections of this paper are organized in the following manner. First, we detail the method used to construct the average model. We then present results showing the convergence of the method towards an average intensity and an average shape, and show the effect of the choice of reference image. We conclude by a discussion on future research tracks.

2 Methodology

2.1 Registration

The work that follows assumes each point in one image has a corresponding equivalent in the others. It also assumes available a matching method able to find these correspondences and capable of providing a vector field representing those relationships. In theory, neither of these conditions is realized. That is, at a microscopic scale, there is not a one to one relationship between the brain cells of two individuals, and assuming there was, to this day, no algorithm is able to find it. In practice however, deforming one brain so its shape matches the one of another is conceivable and many algorithms realizing this process have been developed [2, 1, 6, 7, 16].

The procedure used in the following work is the demons method [15] which is a fully automated intensity-based registration method. It provides results qualitatively similar to [1] and [6] but with an implementation one or two orders of magnitude faster. From a practical point of view, it is worth mentioning that although the algorithm matches intensities and that a *global* intensity correction is made over the whole image, the transformed image of I_1 is not an exact duplicate of I_2. This is due to the smoothness constraint applied to the displacement field which establishes a compromise between intensity resemblance and uniform local deformations.

2.2 Average Model Construction

The average model construction (See Fig. 2) needs as input a reference image I_R and a set of N images $I_1, \ldots, I_N$ representing the group of subjects under consideration. The method can be divided in six steps as follows:

1. The first step regards the evaluation of shape differences between the reference and each image of the set. Elastic registration between I_R and I_i provides vector fields D_i giving for each voxel x_R of I_R the analogous anatomical location x_i in I_i.

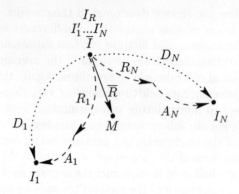

Fig. 2. Average model construction. First step (dotted arrows): the D_i are obtained. Second step: I_i are resampled into I'_i. Third step: $\overline{I}$ is computed. Fourth step (dashed arrows): D_i are decomposed in A_i and R_i. Fifth step: $\overline{R}$ is computed. Sixth step (full line): Combination of average intensity and shape to obtain the average model M.

2. These correspondences found, the second step resamples the I_i using trilinear interpolation to provide I'_i presenting the same shape as I_R with the intensities of I_i.
3. In the third step, the I'_i are averaged pixelwise, producing a mean intensity image $\overline{I}$ with the shape of I_R.
4. The fourth step concerns the decomposition of D_i into affine (A_i) and residual (R_i) components. Since we want correspondences between anatomical points of the I_i and I_R that have the form $x_i = D_i(x_R) = A_i(R_i(x_R))$, we compute the A_i by minimizing the distance $\sum_x ||x - A_i^{-1}(D_i(x))||^2$, where the summation is performed on the voxels positions in I_R corresponding to cerebral tissues[1]. The residual components are obtained by computing $R_i(x) = A_i^{-1}(D(x))$.
5. The fifth step aims to produce the deformation presenting the shape variations between I_R and the average shape of the set elements after correction of affine differences. Since the residual deformations R_i are all defined in the same anatomical space, that of I_R, calculating their vectorwise average $\overline{R}(x) = 1/N \sum_i^N R_i(x)$ will provide the desired deformation.
6. The sixth and final step consists of applying this average residual deformation to the average intensity image to obtain an average intensity and average shape image representing the anatomical average model M.

Considering numerical errors due the fact that automatic registration methods usually perform better when images are closer to each other, all these steps may be repeated by replacing I_R with M, thus constructing a model with a reference image closer to the barycenter of our set. Intuitively, this should reduce the mean registration error and provide a new model M' closer to the theoretical solution.

---

[1] These positions are obtained using an automatic method for brain segmentation similar to that of [5]. From hereon, all summations over x are assumed to be on the voxel positions obtained using this algorithm.

3 Results

The method is tested by computing four models using two reference images I_{R_1} and I_{R_2} (See Figs. 5(a) and 5(b)) and two image sets S_1 and S_2, each composed of five images (See Table 1).

Model	Reference	Image Set
M_{11}	I_{R_1}	S_1
M_{21}	I_{R_2}	S_1
M_{12}	I_{R_1}	S_2
M_{22}	I_{R_2}	S_2

Table 1. References and image sets used to build the different models.

The 3D MR protocol provides coronal images obtained using a 1.5 Tesla SIGNA (General Electric, Milwaukee, U.S.A.) whole body MR imaging system. One hundred and twenty four (124) coronal T1-weighted images were obtained using a spoiled gradient echo (SPGR) pulse sequence (TE=9 seconds, TR=34 seconds, flip angle=45°). Two NEX acquisitions took 27 minutes and 52 seconds. The Field of View (FOV) of the images was 20 cm and each image refers to a contiguous section of tissue of 1.6 mm thickness. The $256 \times 256 \times 124$ voxels of size 0.78mm $\times$ 0.78mm $\times$ 1.6mm were trilinearly interpolated to $200 \times 200 \times 198$ to give cubic voxels of 1mm side.

We analyze our results with regards to two factors. First, the iteration process is investigated to see if convergence is achieved, and if so how fast is the convergence rate. Second, we study the effect of changing the reference image. If the model is a veritable average of the image set, changing the reference should produce an identical model up to an affine transformation defined by the affine difference between references.

In our evaluation procedure, three metrics are used. The first determines the average distance from an image I to the elements of a set S_j, $\text{AD}(I, S_j) = \sqrt{\frac{1}{n}\sum_x \frac{1}{N}\sum_{i=1}^N ||x - R_i(x)||^2}$, where R_i is the residual deformation from I to the ith element of S_j, n is the number of voxels characterizing cerebral tissues and N represents the number of elements in S_j. The second is the root mean square (RMS) norm which supplies information regarding the shape variation expressed by a deformation field D, $\text{RMSn}(D) = \sqrt{\frac{1}{n}\sum_x ||x - D(x)||^2}$. The third provides a measure of brightness disparity between two images I_i and I_j. It is the RMS difference of the images intensities at corresponding locations, $\text{RMSd}(I_i, I_j) = \sqrt{\frac{1}{n}\sum_x (I_i(x) - I_j(x))^2}$.

3.1 Effect of Iterating

To evaluate the effect of iterating, we construct the four models repeating the process five times and using the result of the previous iteration as the reference image. We will designate the model M_{jk} computed at the ith iteration by $M_{jk}^{(i)}$. For convenience, $M_{jk}^{(0)}$ will be identified to the average intensity image having the shape of I_j.

Four measures were computed:

AD$(M_{jk}^{(i)}, S_k)$ The average distance from the reference of the current iteration to all the elements of the set.

RMSn$(\overline{R}_{jk}^{(i)})$ The shape variation expressed by the residual deformation field $\overline{R}_{jk}^{(i)}$ when $M_{jk}^{(i)}$ is used as the reference.

RMSn$(D_{jk}^{(i)})$ The shape difference between models computed at successive iterations. $D_{jk}^{(i)}$ is the deformation obtained by registering $M_{jk}^{(i)}$ with $M_{jk}^{(i+1)}$.

RMSd$(M_{jk}^{(i)}, M_{jk}^{(i+1)})$ The brightness disparity between models obtained at successive iterations.

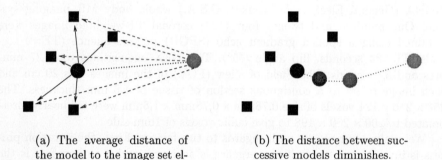

(a) The average distance of the model to the image set elements decreases.

(b) The distance between successive models diminishes.

Fig. 3. Evolution of the model (circles) toward the center of the image set (squares).

If the models computed tend towards the barycenter of the image set, the first measure should diminish. This process is depicted in Fig. 3(a): as the model evolves towards the center (dotted line), the average distance to the image set elements decreases. The second and third measures, representing the shape evolution of the model (See Fig. 3(b)), should tend towards zero. Finally, the fourth value should also decrease to zero since it represents the brightness differences between successive models.

The results of these calculations on the four models are presented in Fig. 4. Note that the iterations range up to 4 and not 5 since we compare models computed at iterations i and $i+1$. We remind the reader that "models" $M_{jk}^{(0)}$, that is models before the first iteration, characterize only average intensities and not average shapes.

From Fig. 4(a), we know the average distance from the references to the image set elements is close to 4.0mm and reduces to about 2.5mm when the model gets to the center of the image set, that is when the average shape is obtained. Compared to these values, the variation between successive models (See Figs. 4(b) and 4(c)), which is about 0.5mm, seems minor. Figure 4(d) presents numbers showing the brightness difference between successive models diminishes rapidly, increasing our belief that models do not evolve significantly after the first iteration.

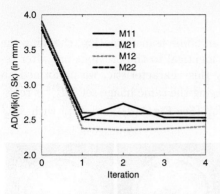

(a) Average distance to the reference of the current iteration.

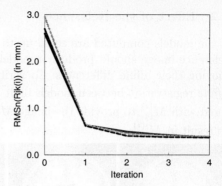

(b) Shape variation of the reference for the current iteration.

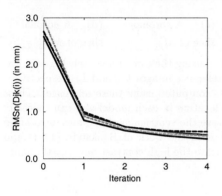

(c) Shape difference between models computed at successive iterations.

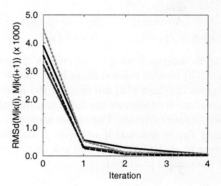

(d) Brightness disparity between models computed at successive iterations. Values are multiplied by 1000.

Fig. 4. Impact of the iteration process when computing the models. Note that the iterations range up to 4 and not 5 since we compare models computed at iterations i and $i+1$. We remind the reader that "models" $M_{jk}^{(0)}$, that is models before the first iteration, characterize only average intensities and not average shapes.

3.2 Effect of the Reference

If the models computed are equal up to an affine transformation, changing the reference image should produce a model identical to the previous one after removing their affine differences. To verify this characteristic, we performed an *affine* registration between models built using the same image set. $M_{21}^{(i)}$ is registered with $M_{11}^{(i)}$ to provide the image $M'^{(i)}_{21}$ (See Fig. 5(d)) and $M_{22}^{(i)}$ with $M_{12}^{(i)}$ to result in $M'^{(i)}_{22}$.

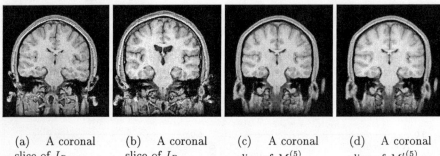

(a) A coronal slice of I_{R_1}. (b) A coronal slice of I_{R_2}. (c) A coronal slice of $M_{11}^{(5)}$. (d) A coronal slice of $M'^{(5)}_{21}$.

Fig. 5. Reference images and models computed using the same image set. Figures 5(a) and 5(b) present coronal slices from the two reference images I_{R_1} and I_{R_2} respectively. Figures 5(c) and 5(d) are slices of the models computed using these references. These two slices are taken at the same anatomical location in each model and can therefore be compared directly. The reader should observe the ventricular shape bias introduced using I_{R_2} is minimal if not null. If familiar with the work of Bookstein (1991) and Evans et al. (1993), he or she will also appreciate the high contrast and visual quality of the images produced.

Two measure were used:

RMSn($D_k^{(i)}$) The shape variation from $M_{2k}^{(i)}$ to $M'^{(i)}_{1k}$. $D_k^{(i)}$ is the deformation obtained by registering the two images.

RMSd($M_{1k}^{(i)}$, $M'^{(i)}_{2k}$) The brightness disparity between the two models.

Results are show in Figs. 6(a) and 6(b) respectively. We notice that shape variation between the models reduces from 3.0mm to 1.0mm. This last value is close to the difference between successive models which we know from Figs. 4(b) and 4(c) to be approximately 0.5mm. The brightness disparity also diminishes rapidly and does not change drastically after the first iterations.

4 Discussion

Figure 4 presents numbers showing that our method constructs average models well representing the average intensity and shape of our image sets. In particular, Fig. 4(a) shows that the average distance from one image to the set elements is about 4.0mm. This distance reduces and stays at approximately 2.5mm after the first iteration. Figures 4(b) and 4(c) illustrate a minor shape evolution of

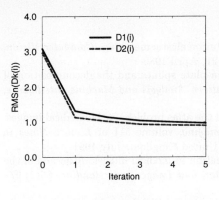 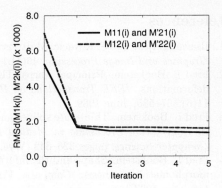

(a) Shape variation between $M_{1k}^{(i)}$ and $M'^{(i)}_{2k}$.

(b) Brightness disparity between $M_{1k}^{(i)}$ and $M'^{(i)}_{2k}$. Values are multiplied by 1000.

Fig. 6. Influence of the reference on the model computed.

the models at each iteration, we believe due to numerical errors. Furthermore, Fig. 4(d) allows us to claim the visual aspect of the models changes only minimally. This leads us to the conclusion that models constructed are different, but equivalent from a practical point of view. Their intensity difference is practically null, and their shapes, although different, all have the same average distance to the other elements of the set. Hence, we believe one iterations is sufficient to build representative average models.

Concerning the invariance of the models to the reference images used in the method, Fig. 6 shows that the models built using different references seem to converge towards the same solution. Their shape difference presented in Fig. 6(a) of about 1.0mm is low compared to the average distance of 2.5mm between the models and the set elements, and just over the distance of 0.5mm between successive average models. Figure 6(b) also presents a low disparity between the different models intensities.

5 Conclusion

We have presented a completely automatic method to build average anatomical models of the human brain using a set of MR images. To this end, brain shape variations between subjects were identified. Differences due to linear transformations were excluded, resulting in the quantification of pure morphological differences. The result is an average intensity and average shape image representative of the characteristics of the image set elements used for the construction. The coupling of such a high quality model with statistical information regarding normal deformations, such as the work of [17], could enrich the significance of statistical tests by adding intensity information, useful for example in detecting gliosis in T2 MR images, and would supply an important tool in the analysis of normal anatomy.

References

1. Ruzena Bajcsy and S. Kovacic. Multiresolution elastic matching. *Computer Vision, Graphics and Image Processing*, 46(1):1–21, April 1989.
2. Fred L. Bookstein. Principal warps: Thin-plate splines and the decomposition of deformations. *IEEE Transactions on Pattern Analysis and Machine Intelligence*, 11(6):567–585, June 1989.
3. Fred L. Bookstein. Thin-plate splines and the atlas problem for biomedical images. In *Information Processing in Medical Imaging*, volume 511 of *Lecture Notes in Computer Science*, pages 326–342, Wye, United Kingdom, July 1991.
4. Fred L. Bookstein. Shape and the information in medical images: A decade of the morphometric synthesis. *Computer Vision and Image Understanding*, 66(2):97–118, may 1997.
5. M.E. Brummer, R.M. Mersereau, R.L. Eisner, and R.R.J. Lewine. Automatic detection of brain contours in MRI data sets. *IEEE Transactions in Medical Imaging*, 12(2):153–166, June 1993.
6. Gary Christensen, Richard D. Rabbitt, and Michael I. Miller. 3D brain mapping using a deformable neuroanatomy. *Physics in Medecine and Biology*, 39:608–618, March 1994.
7. D. Louis Collins, Terry M. Peters, and Alan C. Evans. An automated 3D non-linear image deformation procedure for determination of gross morphometric variability in human brain. In *Visualisation in Biomedical Computing*, volume 2359 of *SPIE Proceedings*, pages 180–190, Rochester, October 1994.
8. Alan C. Evans, D. Louis Collins, S. R. Mills, E. D. Brown, R. LO. Kelly, and Terry M. Peters. 3D statistical neuroanatomical models from 305 MRI volumes. In *IEEE Nuclear Science Symposium/Medical Imaging Conference*, pages 1813–1817, 1993.
9. Alexandre Guimond, Gérard Subsol, and Jean-Philippe Thirion. Automatic MRI database exploration and applications. *International Journal of Pattern Recognition and Artificial Intelligence*, 11(8):1345–1365, December 1997.
10. Karl Heinz Höhne, Michael Bomans, Martin Riemer, Rainer Schubert, Ulf Tiede, and Werner Lierse. A volume-based anatomical atlas. *IEEE Computer Graphics and Applications*, pages 72–78, July 1992.
11. David G. Kendall. A survey of the statistical theory of shape. *Statistical Science*, 4(2):87–120, 1989.
12. Eduard Pernkopf. *Atlas d'anatomie humaine*. Piccin, 1983.
13. Gérard Subsol, Jean-Philippe Thirion, and Nicholas Ayache. A general scheme for automatically building 3D morphometric anatomical atlases: applications to a skull atlas. In *Medical Robotics and Computer Aided Surgery*, pages 373–382, Baltimore, November 1995.
14. Jean Talairach and Pierre Tournoux. *Co-Planar Stereotaxic Atlas of the Human Brain*. Thieme Medical Publishers, New York, United-States, 1988.
15. Jean-Philippe Thirion. Fast non-rigid matching of 3D medical images. In *Medical Robotics and Computer Aided Surgery*, pages 47–54, Baltimore, November 1995.
16. P. Thompson and A. W. Toga. A surface-based technique for warping 3-dimensional images of the brain. *IEEE Transactions in Medical Imaging*, 15:1–16, 1996.
17. Paul M. Thompson and Arthur W. Toga. Detection, visualization and animation of abnormal anatomic structure with a deformable probabilistic brain atlas based on random vector field transformations. *Medical Image Analysis*, 1(4):271–294, September 1997.

Brain Shift Modeling for Use in Neurosurgery

Oskar Škrinjar[1], Dennis Spencer[2] and James Duncan[1]

[1] Departments of Diagnostic Radiology and Electrical Engineering
[2] Department of Neurosurgery
Yale University, New Haven, CT 06520, USA

Abstract. Surgical navigation systems are used intraoperatively to help the surgeon to ascertain her or his position and to guide tools within the patient frame with respect to registered structures of interest in the preoperative images. However, these systems are subject to inaccuracy caused by intraoperative brain movement (brain shift) since they assume that the intracranial structures are rigid. Experiments show brain shifts of up to several millimeters, making it the cause of the dominant error in those systems. We propose a method for reducing this error based on a dynamic brain model. The initial model state is obtained from pre-operative data. The brain tissue is modeled as a homogeneous linear visco-elastic material, although the model allows for setting the tissue properties locally. Gravity draws the brain downwards which in turn interacts with the skull and other surrounding structures. The simulation results are presented both for a 2D model (the mid-sagittal slice) and a 3D model. The results show the time evolution of the brain deformation. The complete 3D validation of the simulated brain deformation is a rather complicated task and is currently in progress within our laboratory, but a procedure is proposed for updating the model in time by one or more of several intraoperative measurements.

1 Introduction

The use of surgical navigation systems is a standard way to assist the neurosurgeon in navigating within the intraoperative environment, allowing her or him to "see" through the body and relate the position of the surgical instruments to the features in preoperative images. It is important that these systems be as precise as possible. Ideally, they should provide a 3D display of the neuroanatomical structures of interest and include visualization of surgical instruments within the same frame. Furthermore, if 3D acquisition systems were fast enough, brain shift would not cause an error. Thus, the ideal goal would be to sense 3D intraoperative volumetric information in real time. Since the brain deforms rather slowly even a slower acquisition rate would be acceptable. However, hardware for obtaining true 3D data is limited probably to MR or CT and is typically bulky and expensive, restricting surgical access and therefore is not currently widely used in the OR[1].

---

[1] There exists a system using intraoperative MRI (see [5] and [6]) but it does not provide a complete 3D dataset of the head at a fast enough rate, but rather single slices at lower fields.

Alternatively, one may improve the hardware of the current systems or develop new ones that would be fast and practical enough to work as described above. Another way is to obtain the 3D data preoperatively and then to register it to estimates of portions of 3D structure via video or other intraoperative sensors. Most of current systems use the latter approach (see [12], [13] and [14]). However, they assume that the brain and other intracranial structures are rigid and fixed relative to the skull. The brain or its structures of interest are registered to the image of the patient at the beginning of the surgery. While this can be done with a precision within 1 mm at the initial moment (see [13]), since the brain deforms in time, the accuracy of the system deteriorates. The median brain shift of points on the brain surface was estimated to range from 0.3 mm to 7.4 mm (see [1]). It is clear that the system based on the rigid brain assumption cannot achieve a precision better than a few millimeters at the outer structures. Since the deeper brain structures deform less than the outer ones the error is the largest at the cortical surface. The brain deforms even more after interventions, e.g. post-resections. Furthermore, the average brain shift for cases in which hematoma or tumors were removed was reported to be 9.5 mm and 7.9 mm, respectively (see [2]). In such cases the error is even larger.

For the above reasons we propose a method that treats the brain as a dynamic deformable structure. The model initialization is based on preoperative data. The model deforms in time and will ultimately be guided by intraoperative information. Then the structures of interest can be displayed using the current model state rather than the rigid brain model obtained preoperatively. By doing this one reduces the error due to brain shift. Eventually the system will receive data about brain deformation intraoperatively using it to update the model. Possible sources of the deformation data are sets of points on the open brain surface obtained by stereo video imaging and 2D slices normal to the brain surface acquired by intraoperative ultrasound.

As we move in these directions, we note relevant work in soft tissue modeling related to recovering image-derived information, including: an attempt to intraoperatively reduce the brain shift error (see [2]), a paper on brain tissue modeling (see [9]), a computationally efficient tissue modeling for knee surgery (see [10]) and cardiac motion modeling (see [7] and [8]). It is also worth mentioning an algorithm for 3D finite element mesh generation (see [15]).

2 Model

2.1 Brain Tissue Modeling

The fact that the brain shift is a relatively small deformation facilitates the brain tissue modeling. A linear stress-strain relation is a good approximation for small tissue displacements. The model consists of a set of discrete interconnected nodes each representing a small part of the brain tissue. Nodes have masses depending on the size of the volume they represent and on the local tissue density. Each connection is modeled as a parallel connection of a linear spring and dashpot, known as the Kelvin solid model (see [3]). Like for the nodes, the connection parameters can depend on their position in the brain. The Kelvin solid model is a model for a visco-elastic material subject to slow and small deformations, which is exactly the case with brain shift. It is also a rather simple approach, which is a desirable property since the model deformation should be computed in real time, i.e. faster or at least at the speed of the brain deformation, since it must be displayed during the surgery. The constitutive relation for the Kelvin solid model is

$$\sigma = q_0 \epsilon + q_1 \dot{\epsilon}, \qquad (1)$$

where σ is stress and ϵ strain, while q_0 and q_1 are local parameters.

If two nodes are at positions r_1 and r_2, have velocities v_1 and v_2, and are connected in the above fashion, then the force acting on the first node is

$$f_{inner}(r_1, r_2, v_1, v_2) = [k_s(\|r_2 - r_1\| - r_{12}) - k_d(v_2 - v_1)n_{21}] n_{21}, \qquad (2)$$

where k_s is the stiffness coefficient, k_d is the damping coefficient and r_{12} is the rest length of the spring connecting the two nodes. In a general case they can vary from connection to connection depending on the local material properties. n_{21} is the unit vector from r_1 to r_2. Note that the same force acts on the other node but in the opposite direction.

While a continuum mechanics approach, implemented using finite elements, such as the one employed by our group for cardiac motion modeling (see [7] and [8]), better physically models the tissue, the discrete modeling approach, in addition to having reasonable results, is computationally faster. This is very important for our application, since the ultimate goal is to run the simulation in real time or close to real time.

2.2 Modeling the Brain - Skull Interaction

If a point mass is far enough away from a rigid body there is no interaction between them. When the point mass is closer than a "critical distance" to the rigid body there is an interaction, and the closer they are the greater the interaction, becoming very large if the point mass is very close to the body. Furthermore, this interaction is in the direction of the surface normal of the body. Based on the above intuitive reasoning, the following model of the interaction between a point mass and rigid body is proposed

$$f_{outer}(r) = \begin{cases} C \left(\frac{1}{r^2} - \frac{1}{r_0^2} \right) n &, 0 \leq r \leq r_0 \\ 0 &, r > r_0 \end{cases}, \qquad (3)$$

where f is the force vector, r is the minimal distance between the rigid body and point mass, r_0 is the "critical distance", C is a proportionality constant and n is the body surface normal. This force acts on both the rigid body and point mass but in the opposite directions.

If a brain model node comes closer than r_0 to the skull it interacts with the skull in the above way. In small deformation situations, such as the brain shift case, only the outer brain surface nodes will interact with the skull, which reduces the simulation time. Since the skull is assumed to be fixed, the skull - brain interaction in the simulation is applied only to the brain nodes.

2.3 The Model Equations

Newton's Second Law for node j gives

$$m^j a^j = m^j g + f_{outer}{}^j + \sum_{i=1}^{n^j} f_{inner}{}^j_{s^j_i}, \qquad (4)$$

where m^j is the node's mass, a^j is its acceleration, $f_{outer}{}^j$ is its interaction with the skull defined by (3), $f_{inner}{}^j_{s^j_i}$ is the interaction between nodes j and s^j_i defined by (2) and g is the gravity acceleration, while $\{s^j_1, s^j_2, \ldots, s^j_{n^j}\}$ is the set of the neighboring nodes of the node j. Equation (4) represents a system of second order nonlinear ordinary differential equations.

One can define the state variables to be $x_{2j-1} = r^j$ and $x_{2j} = v^j$ for $j = 1, \ldots, N$, where N is the number of the brain model nodes. Obviously, $\dot{x}_{2j-1} = x_{2j}$. The expression for $\dot{x}_{2j}$ follows directly from (4). It depends only on state variables but not on their time derivatives. Now it is clear that (4) can be rewritten in the compact state-space form

$$\dot{\mathcal{X}} = f(\mathcal{X}), \qquad (5)$$

where $\mathcal{X}$ is the vector of the state variables. It is assumed that the brain starts deforming from a rest position, i.e. $v^j(t = 0) = 0$ for all j. The initial node positions $r^j(t = 0)$ were obtained from the preoperative images, as discussed in the next section.

The system defined by (5) is suitable for numerical integration (see [4]). In this case the fourth order Runge-Kutta method with adaptive stepsize was employed.

3 Results

3.1 2D Results

The mid-sagittal slice of a MRI data set is chosen for testing the 2D model. We developed a tool in MATLAB for preprocessing the slice and setting the initial model state. A part of the skull is artificially erased to simulate the craniotomy. The tool allows one to set the tissue properties, which affect the node masses and connection parameters, to define the initial node positions as well as the orientation of the head. It also offers an initial level of automation. Figure 1 shows the head in a certain orientation and the corresponding 2D mesh.

As the model deforms in time, the nodes change positions and the image of the brain deforms. Since the deformation is rather small one can assume that the interior of each triangle in the model deforms in an affine manner, as dictated by the following equations. Let (x^i_1, y^i_1), (x^i_2, y^i_2) and (x^i_3, y^i_3) be the node coordinates of a triangle in the initial state and (x^c_1, y^c_1), (x^c_2, y^c_2) and (x^c_3, y^c_3)

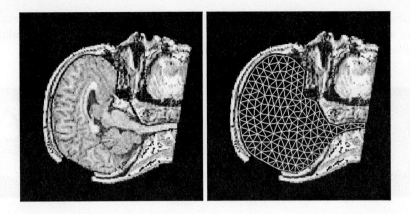

Fig. 1. The initial node positions as well as the connection properties are set by a special purpose tool developed in MATLAB.

their corresponding coordinates in the current state. One can define local triangle coordinates α and β through the following equation

$$\begin{bmatrix} x^i \\ y^i \end{bmatrix} = \begin{bmatrix} x_1^i \\ y_1^i \end{bmatrix} + \alpha \begin{bmatrix} x_2^i - x_1^i \\ y_2^i - y_1^i \end{bmatrix} + \beta \begin{bmatrix} x_3^i - x_1^i \\ y_3^i - y_1^i \end{bmatrix} \quad (6)$$

where $0 \leq \alpha \leq 1$, $0 \leq \beta \leq 1 - \alpha$ and (x^i, y^i) is a point inside or at the boundary of the initial triangle. The affine transformation is defined by

$$\begin{bmatrix} x^c \\ y^c \end{bmatrix} = \begin{bmatrix} x_1^c \\ y_1^c \end{bmatrix} + \alpha \begin{bmatrix} x_2^c - x_1^c \\ y_2^c - y_1^c \end{bmatrix} + \beta \begin{bmatrix} x_3^c - x_1^c \\ y_3^c - y_1^c \end{bmatrix} \quad (7)$$

where (x^c, y^c) is the point in the current triangle corresponding to (x^i, y^i). One can eliminate α and β from (6) and (7) obtaining the direct affine transformation between the two triangles. The transformation is invertable as long as both triangles have non-zero areas. This is true since the deformation is small and triangles do not change shape significantly, preserving non-zero areas. Equations (6) and (7) are used to calculate the image deformation knowing the node positions in time.

Although the tissue properties could be set locally, at this point the brain is assumed to be homogeneous. A time sequence of a deforming brain is shown in Fig. 2. Figures 3 and 4 show the difference in the brain deformation if the tissue is made stiffer[2], but still homogeneous. The final (rest) state is the state after which there is no noticeable change in the model. For a 2D brain model with 176 brain nodes, 57 skull (rigid) nodes and 469 connections it takes approximately ten minutes to simulate the brain deformation to the rest state on a Hewlett Packard 9000 (C110) machine. However, the code was not optimized for an

---

[2] The "stiffer" case has 10 times greater the stiffness coefficient (k_s in (2)) than the "softer case".

efficient computation. The primary goal was to test the model but certainly there are many ways to go about reducing the simulation time. More simulation results can be found at http://pantheon.yale.edu/~os28/.

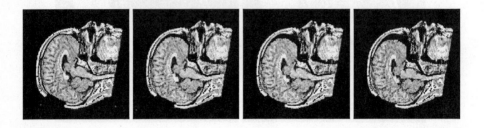

Fig. 2. A time sequence showing the brain model deformation. From left to right are the initial state, two middle states and the final (rest) state after equal intervals. As the brain settles down due to gravity, there are not only posterior movements, but also slight extensions in superior and inferior directions.

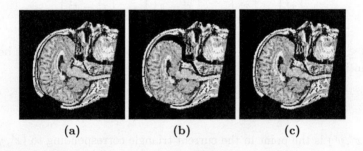

(a)   (b)   (c)

Fig. 3. Deformation comparison of the models with different tissue properties. (a) initial state, (b) final (rest) state for a "softer" case, (c) final (rest) state for a "stiffer" case. Note the difference in the curvature of the brain boundary at the position of the skull opening for the two cases. The largest deformation is at the anterior part of the brain.

3.2   3D Results

The initial state geometry of the 3D model is based on a MRI dataset of a patient's head. The aforementioned tool allows one to create an artificial craniotomy, set tissue properties and the model orientation and automatically set the model connections and initial node positions. The equations driving the model are completely analogous to the ones in the 2D case, the only difference being the number of nodes and connections. Figure 5 represents a time sequence of

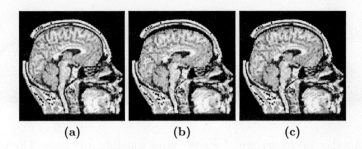

Fig. 4. Deformation comparison of the models with different tissue properties (another angle). (a) Initial state, (b) final (rest) state for a "softer" case, (c) final (rest) state for a "stiffer" case. Note the deformation at the top of the superior part of the brain.

states of the model in a certain orientation. The sequence shows how the brain settles down, supported by the skull and other surrounding structures. Figure 6 shows a time sequence of states for the model in another orientation.

The 3D model has 1093 nodes and 4855 connections. It takes approximately four hours for the simulation to reach the final state. At the other hand a real brain typically deforms for 30 minutes, which is about 8 times smaller than the simulation time. However, we believe that computational time can be reduced to or close to 30 minutes for the following reasons. We employed the fourth order Runge-Kutta method for numerical integration which is not the fastest method (see [4]). Also, we imposed rather strict conditions on the precision (required for the adaptive stepsize control part). By relaxing them one can increase the computational efficiency. Moreover, one can optimize the data organization for the specific application further reducing the simulation time. Finally, the computational time can be reduced by using a faster computer.

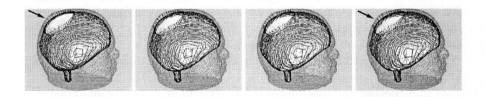

Fig. 5. A time sequence of model states equidistant in time. The left image represents the initial state while the right one shows the final (rest) model state. The brain slightly settles down due to gravity. One can notice through the artificially made craniotomy the increase in the gap between the skull and the brain over time (the black gap under the arrow). For larger images refer to http://pantheon.yale.edu/∼os28/.

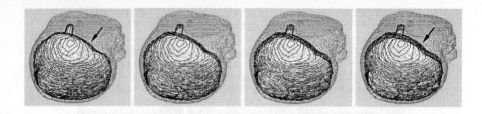

Fig. 6. Another time sequence of model states equidistant in time. The left image represents the initial state while the right one shows the final (rest) model state. Note how the brain settles down (the increase in the top black gap under the arrow). As opposed to Fig. 5 in this case the gap between the brain and the skull at the craniotomy decreases over time.

4 Discussion

The two main problems with this modeling are how to reliably estimate the model parameters and how to validate the model deformation. Research is being conducted in our laboratory addressing both problems. Since the physical brain tissue properties in humans and animals are very similar one can perform tissue property measurements on an animal brain. Those results can be used to initialize the model parameters. However, brain tissue properties might change during the surgery due to reducing intracranial pressure, by controlling CO_2 concentration in the blood and reducing the water content of the brain by administering an osmotically active drug. Cerebrospinal fluid also leaks from the subarachnoid space at a variable rate. We are working on including these effects both directly in the model as well as through intraoperative information that will guide the model. Currently our model incorporates the visco-elastic brain tissue properties, initially set homogeneously within the brain, and the effect of gravity. In addition, our current research includes cerebrospinal fluid modeling motivated by interaction between fluid particles given by Lennard-Jones model (see [11], Chapter 15). Since the grey and white matter do not have the same visco-elastic properties the geometry of the sulci affects the brain deformation. This is also a problem we are working on.

We believe that our model, with appropriately set tissue parameters and intraoperatively guided, can significantly reduce the error introduced by the brain shift, making the surgical navigation system more precise and reliable.

5 Acknowledgements

We are grateful to prof. Turan Onat from Department of Mechanical Engineering, Yale University, for useful discussions as well as to graduate students Sudhakar Chelikani and Aleksandar Milošević from the Departments of Applied Physics and Physics, Yale University, respectively.

References

1. Hill, D., Maurer, C., Wang, M., Maciunas, R., Barwise, J., Fitzpatrick, M.: Estimation of Intraoperative Brain Surface Movement. *CVRMed-MRCAS'97*, Grenoble, France, March (1997) 449–458
2. Bucholz, R., Yeh, D., Trobaugh, J., McDurmont, L., Sturm, C., Baumann, C., Henderson, J., Levy, A., Kessman, P.: The Correction of Stereotactic Inaccuracy Caused by Brain Shift Using an Intraoperative Ultrasound Device. *CVRMed-MRCAS'97*, Grenoble, France, March (1997) 459–466
3. Pamidi, M. R., Advani, S. H.: Nonlinear Constitutive Relations for Human Brain Tissue. *Journal of Bio-Mechanical Engineering*, February (1978), Vol. 100, 44–48
4. Press, W. H., Teukolsky, S. A., Vettrling, W. T., Flannery, B. P.: *Numerical Recipes in C*, 2nd Edition, Camridge University Press, 1992.
5. Ferenc, A. J.: Image-guided Procedures and the Operating Room of the Future. *Radiology*, September (1997), Volume 204, 601–612
6. Revolution in the O.R., Brigham and Women's Hospital, *BWH* Fall 1997, 10–16
7. Shi, P., Sinusas, A. J., Constable, R. T., Duncan, J. S.: Volumetric Deformation Analysis Using Mechanics-Based Data Fusion: Applications in Cardiac Motion Recovery. *International Journal of Computer Vision*, Kluwer, submitted.
8. Duncan, J., Shi, P., Constable, R.T., Sinusas, A.: Physical and Geometrical Modeling for Image-Based Recovery of Left Ventricular Deformation. *Progress in Biophysics and Molecular Biology*, in press.
9. Edwards, P. J., Hill D. L. G., Little, J. A., Hawkes, D. J.: Deformation for Image Guided Interventions Using a Three Component Tissue Model. *15th International Conference, IPMI'97, Proceedings*, (1997) 218–231
10. Gibson, S., Samosky, J., Mor, A., Fyock, C., Grimson, E., Kanade, T., Kikinis, R., Lauer, H, McKenzie, N., Nakajima, S., Ohkami, H., Osborne, R. Sawada, A.: Simulating Arthroscopic Knee Surgery Using Volumetric Object Representations, Real-Time Volume Rendering and Haptic Feedback. *CVRMed-MRCAS'97*, Grenoble, France, March (1997) 369–378
11. Fosdick, L. D., Jessup, E. R., Schauble, C. J. C., Domik, G.: *An Introduction to High-Performance Scientific Computing*, The MIT Press, 1995.
12. Grimson, W. E. L., Ettinger, G. J., White, S. J., Gleason, P. L., Lozano-Perez, T., Wells III, W. M., Kikinis, R.: Evaluating and Validating an Automated Registration System for Enhanced Reality Visualization in Surgery.
13. Grimson, W. E. L., Ettinger, G. J., White, S. J., Gleason, P. L., Lozano-Perez, T., Wells III, W. M., Kikinis, R.: An Automatic Registration Method for Frameless Stereotaxy, Image Guided Surgery, and Enhanced Reality Visualization. *IEEE Transactions on Medical Imaging*, Vol. 15, No. 2, April (1996) 129–140
14. Peters, T., Davey, B., Munger, P., Comeau, R., Evans, A., Olivier, A.: Three-Dimensional Multimodal Image-Guidance for Neurosurgery. *IEEE Transactions on Medical Imaging*, Vol. 15, No. 2, April (1996), 121–128
15. Hartmann U., Kruggel F.: A Fast Algorithm for Generating Large Tetrahedral 3D Finite Element Meshes from Magnetic Resonance Tomograms. *Workshop on Biomedical Image Analysis, Proceedings*, Santa Barbara, CA, June (1998) 184–191

Proximity Constraints in Deformable Models for Cortical Surface Identification

David MacDonald, David Avis, and Alan C. Evans

McConnell Brain Imaging Centre, Montréal Neurological Institute,
McGill University, Montréal, Canada
david@bic.mni.mcgill.ca
http://www.bic.mni.mcgill.ca

Abstract. Automatic computer processing of large multi-dimensional images such as those produced by magnetic resonance imaging (MRI) is greatly aided by deformable models. A general method of deforming polyhedra is presented here, with two novel features. Firstly, explicit prevention of non-simple (self-intersecting) surface geometries is provided, unlike conventional deformable models which merely discourage such behaviour. Secondly, simultaneous deformation of multiple surfaces with inter-surface proximity constraints provides a greater facility for incorporating model-based constraints into the process of image recognition. These two features are used advantageously to automatically identify the total surface of the cerebral cortical gray matter from normal human MR images, accurately locating the depths of the sulci even where under-sampling in the image obscures the visibility of sulci. A large number of individual surfaces (N=151) are created and a spatial map of the mean and standard deviation of the cerebral cortex and the thickness of cortical gray matter are generated. Ideas for further work are outlined.

Contact: David MacDonald
Address: McConnell Brain Imaging Centre, Webster 2B,
Montréal Neurological Institute,
3801 University, Montréal, Québec, H3A 2B4
Fax: 514-398-8948

Keywords: Image Segmentation, Surface Deformation, Cerebral Cortex

1 Introduction

Digitally acquired information is increasingly being used in medical fields for surgery planning and intra-operative navigation, diagnosis and monitoring of disease, as well as in investigations of normal and pathological anatomy. In the realm of computational neuroanatomy, large amounts of three- and four-dimensional anatomical and functional information are available in the form of such modalities as magnetic resonance imaging (MRI), positron emission tomography (PET), and computed tomography (CT). The diverse nature of the image data, in addition to the large size of individual images, motivates researchers to explore automated methods of processing the data into forms more useful for subsequent analysis. Deformable models provide a promising technique for registration, segmentation, and matching tasks in computational neuroanatomy, by combining the bottom-up approach of edge detection with the top-down approach of model-based geometric constraints. The active contour method of Kass et al. [1], commonly referred to as "SNAKES", has been the foundation upon which deformation methods have been based. Essentially, a two or three dimensional spline is assigned an energy function which consists of a stretching and smoothing term based on first and second derivatives, and an image term which decreases in energy as the spline moves closer to image boundaries. Numerical integration techniques deform the spline from a starting position to a minimum energy configuration, which represents a compromise between the shape constraints and the image edge features. Many adaptations of deformable models in medical imaging have since been presented [2–6], and a survey of these methods is presented in [7]. Here we address two of the limitations of conventional methods. Firstly, deformable surfaces typically use stretching and bending constraints for a regularization effect which penalizes but does not prevent non-simple (self-intersecting) surface geometries. Secondly, single surface deformation methods are sensitive to partial volume effects in images due to under-sampling. Some existing methods ([8,9]) attempt to disambiguate the location of cerebral cortical surfaces in human MR images by combining information from both gray and white matter image boundaries. This idea is extended here to present a novel formulation of deformable polyhedra which incorporates a variety of proximity constraints in order to identify the entire cortical surface of the human brain from MR images of normal volunteers. The use of inter- and intra-surface intersection avoidance as well as a two-surface model of the inner and outer boundaries of the cortical gray mantle results in a fully automatic identification of the entire surface, even in deep, narrow sulci which may be confounded by partial volume effects. Surfaces are guaranteed not to intersect themselves or each other. The formulation of this method as a minimization problem is described in the next section. Application to a population of datasets, inter-subject averaging, and mapping of cortical surfaces to simpler parameter spaces is described. Finally, ideas for further application are presented.

2 Method

The essence of the method is the formulation of an objective function which when minimized provides a solution to an image recognition problem. The domain of the function is the set of vertex coordinates describing one or more polyhedra to be deformed, and the range is a scalar value representing a goodness of fit of the polyhedra to the target data. The objective function and its terms are described, followed by the method of minimization.

2.1 Objective Function

The objective function, $O(S)$, may be defined generally as a weighted sum of N_t terms, each of which may be thought of as a data or model term, depending on whether it constrains the deforming polyhedra to match image data or some model-based *a priori* information:

$$O(S) = \sum_{k=1}^{N_t} w_k T_k,$$

where w_k is a weighting factor, S is a set of N_s deforming polyhedral surfaces,

$$S = \{S_i \ : \ S_i \text{ is a polyhedral surface}, \ 1 \leq i \leq N_s\},$$

and $\hat{S}$ is a set of N_s model polyhedral surfaces where each $\hat{S}_i$ has the same topology as S_i. Each term, T_k, is formulated as:

$$T_k(S) = W(D_k(S)),$$

where $D_k(S)$ is a signed scalar measure of deviation from some ideal, and $W(x)$ is a general weighting function. Usually this is just a squaring function, $W(x) = x^2$, but the function $W(x)$ can be also be used as an attenuation function by increasing the cost sharply when the measure of deviation passes a certain threshold. Each objective term is described here for the simple case where $W(x)$ is a squaring function. As a prolog, some definitions are presented:

$\bar{x}_v = (x_v, y_v, z_v)$, the 3D position of vertex v in a deforming polyhedral mesh,

$\hat{\bar{x}}_v = (\hat{x}_v, \hat{y}_v, \hat{z}_v)$, the 3D position of vertex v in a static model polyhedral mesh,

n_v, the number of vertices in a polyhedral mesh.

n_e, the number of edges in a polyhedral mesh.

n_p, the number of polygons in a polyhedral mesh. and

m_v, the number of neighbours of vertex v,

$d(\bar{x}, \bar{y})$, the Euclidean distance between two three dimensional points,

$n_{v,j}$, the j'th neighbour of vertex v, and

$\bar{N}_v$, the surface normal at vertex v, defined as the unit normal to the polygon consisting of the counterclockwise ordered neighbours of the vertex.

Image Term The image term is based on the distance from each vertex to the nearest image boundary in the direction of the local surface normal, and is expressed as

$$T_{boundary\_dist} = \sum_{v=1}^{n_v} d_B(\bar{x}_v, \bar{N}_v, t)^2$$

where $d_B(\bar{x}_v, \bar{N}_v, t)$ is the distance to the nearest image contour of the threshold, t, from the vertex, v, along the line defined by the surface normal, $\bar{N}_v$. The explicit search in both directions along the surface normal increases the power of locating image boundaries that are relatively far from the current surface position. This term may be modified to use first and second derivative information, or improved by over-sampling between vertices.

Stretching Term The stretch term increases as lengths between vertices are stretched or compressed relative to a user-defined model surface representing the ideal lengths,

$$T_{stretch} = \sum_{v=1}^{n_v} \sum_{j=1}^{m_v} \left(\frac{d(\bar{x}_v, \bar{x}_{n_{v,j}}) - L_{v,j}}{L_{v,j}} \right)^2,$$

where $L_{v,j}$, the ideal length of an edge, is defined as the corresponding length in the model polyhedron:

$$L_{v,j} = d(\hat{x}_v, \hat{x}_{n_{v,j}}).$$

The intended effect of this term is to make distances between corresponding pairs of vertices on the model and deformed surface roughly equivalent, and is analogous to the term involving the magnitude of the first derivative of the spline in the original Snakes formulation.

Bending Term The bending term provides a measure of deviation from a model shape based on an estimate of local curvature, and is analogous to the second derivative term in the Snakes formulation,

$$T_{bend} = \sum_{e=1}^{n_e} \left(a(S, e) - a(\hat{S}, e) \right)^2,$$

where $a(S, e)$ is the signed angle between the two polygons adjacent to the edge, e. This term is intended to be used for shape-based matching and segmentation.

Self-Proximity Term and Inter-Surface Proximity Term The previous three terms are found in some form in most conventional deformable models. Here we introduce the self-proximity term, which measures the proximity of pairs of non-adjacent polygons in a surface,

$$T_{self-proximity} = \sum_{i=1}^{n_p-1} \sum_{j=i+1}^{n_p} \begin{cases} (\hat{d}(P_i, P_j) - d_{i,j})^2, & \text{if } \hat{d}(P_i, P_j) < d_{i,j} \\ 0, & \text{otherwise,} \end{cases}$$

where $\hat{d}(T_i, T_j)$ is the smallest Euclidean distance between the i'th polygon, P_i, and the j'th polygon, P_j, and $d_{i,j}$ is a distance threshold. In practice, pairs of adjacent polygons are not included in the above equation, as their $\hat{d}(P_i, P_j)$ is a constant zero value for any deformation of the polyhedra. The self-proximity term is used to explicitly prevent non-simple topologies by assigning a prohibitively high cost to self-intersecting topologies. The inter-surface proximity term, $T_{surface-surface}$, is formulated in a similar fashion, and is used to prevent two surfaces from coming within a certain distance of each other.

Vertex-Vertex Proximity Constraints Two surfaces may be designated to prefer to stay a certain distance apart by defining a term constraining the desired distance between specific points on the two surfaces:

$$T_{vertex-vertex} = (d(\bar{x}_v, \bar{x}_w) - d_B)^2$$

where d_B is the preferred distance between vertex v on one surface and vertex w on a second surface. This term keeps specific points of two surfaces a fixed distance apart, but does not explicitly prevent inter-surface intersection, which is achieved by the inter-surface proximity term defined previously.

2.2 Minimization of Objective Function

Deformation of polyhedra is achieved by minimization of the objective function using a conjugate gradient method, which involves iteratively computing a derivative direction and a line minimization along a direction computed from successive derivatives. In order to increase the chances of finding the global minimum, a multi-scale approach is employed. Deformation begins with a low-resolution initial guess for each of the polyhedral surfaces being deformed, which may be a hand-crafted model or statistically generated approximation to the surfaces being identified. The low-resolution surfaces are deformed to fit blurred image data, then resampled to contain more triangles. The resampled surfaces are then deformed to fit a less blurred version of the image data, and the process repeated until the desired resolution is achieved. Typically, triangles with lengths of one millimetre are sufficient to capture the surfaces in the MR data being segmented.

3 Solving Partial Volume Effects with a Double Surface Model

One of the most interesting applications of this general deformation framework is the identification of deep, narrow sulci that are obscured by partial volume effects. Figure 1a illustrates a cross section through a three dimensional simulated brain phantom. Conventional deformable methods find the sulcus in the white matter (Fig. 1c), but fail to find a sulcus in the gray matter (Fig. 1b) due to partial volume effects in the image. The new deformation method successfully locates a reasonable approximation to the gray matter sulcus (shown in three dimensions in Fig. 1d), using a double surface formulation. The gray-cerebrospinal fluid (CSF) (Fig. 1e) and the gray-white (Fig. 1f) surfaces are simultaneously deformed to fit the image, with the constraint that the two surfaces prefer to be a specific distance apart. While neuroanatomical estimates of gray matter thickness vary from three to seven or more millimetres, it was felt that for a preliminary evaluation of this method, five millimetres was a reasonable constraint on the thickness, with a range of plus or minus two millimetres. The gray-CSF surface follows gray-white surface deep into the sulci, and self-proximity constraints prevent it from intersecting itself as the two boundaries of the sulcus are pushed together.

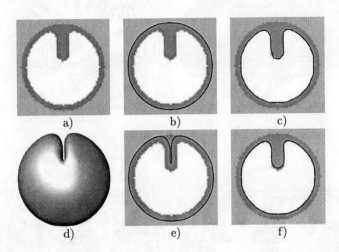

Fig. 1. a) Cross section of image representing sulcus obscured by partial volume. b) Cross section of apparent gray-CSF boundary. c) Cross section of apparent gray-white boundary. d) Results of dual-model deformation. e) Dual-model gray-CSF surface. f) Dual-model gray-CSF surface.

4 Application to Cortical Surface Segmentation

The deformation method presented is applied to a large number of normal human MR images to automatically identify the total surface of the cerebral cortical gray matter. T1-weighted, T2-weighted, and PD-weighted images are acquired at a isotropic sampling of one millimetre. The images are corrected for RF inhomogeneity artifacts [10], linearly transformed into a stereotaxic coordinate system [11], and classified into gray matter, white matter, and CSF. The identification of the cortical surface is accomplished with two steps. The first step is use high stretching and bending weights to rigidly deform a coarse cortex mask to fit the classified volume, to remove non-cerebral white matter from the volume. Then the dual-surface deformation described previously is performed on the masked volume, in a multi-scale fashion. The initial surfaces contain 320 triangles, and after several iterations of deformation and sub-sampling the surfaces, the resulting surfaces contain about 90 000 triangles. The segmentation for a single subject takes about 100 hours of time on a Silicon Graphics Origin 200 R10000 processor running at 180 megahertz. Figure 2 shows the right view of the outer surface of a cerebral cortex, as well as cross sections of the surface superimposed on the classified volume.

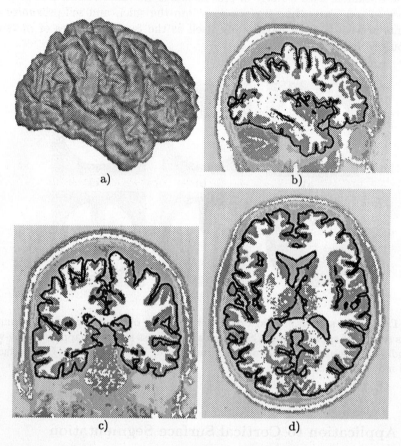

Fig. 2. a) Gray-CSF boundary automatically extracted. b) Sagittal section. c) Coronal section. d) Transverse section.

Choice of Weights A drawback of most deformable methods is the necessity to balance the various objective terms by carefully choosing weights. Most deformable methods use some sort of constraint on stretching and/or bending as regularization terms to avoid degenerate deformation configurations. In the experiments with the current formulation, it has been found that the self-proximity term provides an alternative to the conventional regularization by preventing self intersections, and therefore, it is possible that the stretching and bending terms may be discarded when shape constraints are not needed. This reduces the number of arbitrary weights that must be chosen, and a method of assigning the remaining weights has been devises. The image term is arbitrarily assigned a value of one, and the weighting functions for the surface proximity terms are constructed in such a way that geometric measures are specified, rather than weights. For instance, the self-proximity term is constructed so that above 0.25 millimetres the term is 0, and below .25 millimetres, the weight increases from 10^{-10} at 0.25 millimetres to 10^{10} at .01 millimetres. This large range of weights works for almost any application, and only the millimetre thresholds for proximity constraints must be chosen.

4.1 Averaging and Mapping to Two Dimensions

The surfaces deformed have a topology based on a triangulation of a sphere, and there exists a one-to-one mapping between points on any two deformed surfaces or between a deformed surface and a sphere. The result is that the convoluted cortical surface can be mapped onto a sphere, and sets of deformed surfaces may be averaged into a mean surface. Figure 3a shows the average of 151 individual cerebral cortical surfaces automatically identified by the deformation method. The average curvature of the surfaces is mapped onto the average surface where black areas correspond to sulci, and brighter areas are gyri. Figure 3b shows the same curvature information mapped onto a unit sphere. Aside from the visual simplification aspect, it is possible that some types of analysis may be more easily performed in the two dimensional parameter space of the sphere or on the average surface. Depending on the specific analysis requirements, it may be necessary to perform a further step of warping within the two dimensional space, for instance, in order to make the mapping preserve distances, angles, or areas.

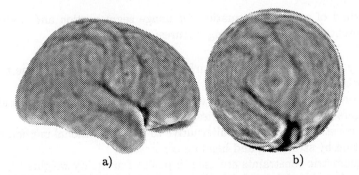

Fig. 3. Curvature of cortex from Fig. 2a mapped onto a) the average surface, and b) a sphere.

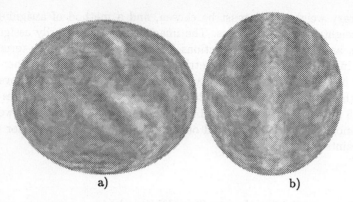

Fig. 4. a) Right view, and b) Top View of thickness of cortex from Fig. 2a mapped onto an ellipsoid,(range: 3 mm to 7 mm).

4.2 Cortical Thickness Map

The thickness of the gray matter can be measured at any point on an individual cortical surface, using the two deformed surfaces, and averaged over the entire set of surfaces, shown on an ellipsoid in Fig. 4. However, the resulting thickness is biased towards the original proximity constraints defined in the dual-surface model. In order to minimize this bias, the current estimate of local cortical thickness should be used to define a second-generation model and the surface deformation process repeated for all 151 surfaces. Such refinement of the cortical thickness map may be repeated until a convergence is achieved. More work is required to determine to what extent the *a priori* constraints and the deformation algorithm itself control the perceived thickness of the cortex.

5 Summary

A novel method of surface deformation for image segmentation and matching has been presented, with the following features:

- a boundary search along the local surface normal is used to increase the range of attraction of edges,
- the use of proximity constraints with appropriate weights guarantees avoidance of intersecting surface geometries,
- proximity constraints provide an alternative to the conventional method of regularization by stretching and bending constraints,
- intuitive geometric constraints are used in place of arbitrary weights,
- multiple surfaces, models, and datasets may be combined into a single objective function,
- and finally, the application of this surface deformation method to the identification of the total cerebral cortical surface from MR images is achieved with improved insensitivity to partial volume effects.

The ability to automatically generate surface represenations from images provides opportunities for sophisticated analysis of large populations of neuroanatomical data. Generation of average surface models which incorporate descriptions of mean position, shape, and thickness is in progress. Future directions include improving the mapping of cortical surface between subjects, as well as sulcal recognition, and application to identification of cerebellum, brainstem, and other neuroanatomic structures.

References

1. M. Kass, A. Witkin, and D. Terzopoulos, "Snakes: Active contour models," *International Journal of Computer Vision*, pp. 321–331, 1988.
2. D. Collins, T. Peters, W. Dai, and A. Evans, "Model-based segmentation of individual brain structures from mri data," in *Proceedings Visualization in Biomedical Computing 1992*, pp. 10–23, 1992.
3. C. Davatzikos and R. N. Bryan, "Using a deformable surface model to obtain a shape representation of the cortex," *Proceedings of the IEEE International Conference on Computer Vision 1995*, pp. 212–217, 1995.
4. S. Sandor and R. Leahy, "Surface-based labeling of cortical anatomy using a deformable atlas," *IEEE Transactions on Medical Imaging*, vol. 16, pp. 41–54, Feb 1997.
5. L. D. Cohen and I. Cohen, "Finite-element methods for active contour models and balloons for 2-d and 3-d images," *IEEE Transactions on Pattern Analysis and Machine Intelligence*, vol. 15, pp. 1131–1147, Nov 1993.
6. L. Staib and J. Duncan, "Deformable fourier models for surface finding in 3d images," in *Proceedings Visualization in Biomedical Computing 1992*, pp. 90–104, 1992.
7. T. McInerney and D. Terzopoulos, "Deformable models in medical image analysis: a survey," *Medical Image Analysis*, vol. 1, no. 2, 1996.
8. M. Vaillant, C. Davatzikos, and N. R. Bryan, "Finding 3d parametric representations of the deep cortical folds," *Proceedings of the Workshop on Mathematical Methods in Biomedical Image Analysis 1996*, pp. 151–159.
9. A. M. Dale and M. I. Sereno, "Improved localization of cortical activity by combining eeg and meg with mri cortical surface reconstruction: a linear approach," *Journal of Cognitive Neuroscience*, vol. 5, pp. 162–176, 1993.
10. J. G. Sled, A. P. Zijdenbos, and A. C. Evans, "A comparison of retrospective intensity non-uniformity correction methods for MRI," in *Information Processing in Medical Imaging*, 1997. in press.
11. D. Collins, P. Neelin, T. Peters, and A. Evans, "Automatic 3d intersubject registration of mr volumetric data in standardized talairach space," *Journal of Computer Assisted Tomography*, vol. 18, pp. 192–205, Mar. 1994.
12. R. Bajcsy and K. cič, "Multiresolution elastic matching," *Computer Vision, Graphics, and Image Processing*, vol. 46, pp. 1–21, 1989.
13. C. Nastar and N. Ayache, "Non-rigid motion analysis in medical images: a physically based approach," in *Proceedings of Information Processing in Medical Imaging*, (Flagstaff, Arizona), pp. 17–32, June 1993.

Fast Analysis of Intracranical Aneurysms Based on Interactive Direct Volume Rendering and CTA

P. Hastreiter[1], Ch. Rezk–Salama[1], B. Tomandl[2], K.E.W. Eberhardt[2], T. Ertl[1]

[1] Computer Graphics Group, University of Erlangen–Nuremberg,
Department of Computer Science, Am Weichselgarten 9, 91058 Erlangen, Germany
{hastreiter|ertl}@informatik.uni-erlangen.de
[2] Division of Neuroradiology, University of Erlangen–Nuremberg,
Department of Neurosurgery, Schwabachanlage 6, 91054 Erlangen, Germany

Abstract. The diagnosis of intracranial aneurysms and the planning of related interventions is effectively assisted by spiral CT-angiography and interactive direct volume rendering. Based on 3D texture mapping, we suggest a hardware accelerated approach which provides fast and meaningful visualization without time–consuming pre–processing. Interactive tools provide reliable measurement of distance and volume allowing to calculate the size of vessels and aneurysms directly within the 3D viewer. Thereby, the expensive material required for coiling procedures is estimated more precisely. Interactively calculated shaded iso–surfaces, presented in [1] were evaluated in respect of enhanced perception of depth. Based on the integration into OpenInventor, global overview and simultaneous detail information is provided by communicating windows allowing for intuitive and user–guided navigation. Due to an average of 15–20 minutes required for the complete medical analysis, our approach is expected to be useful for clinical routine. Additional registration and simultaneous visualization of MR and CT-angiography gives further anatomical orientation. Several examples demonstrate the potential of our approach.

1 Introduction

Current clinical routine is supported by different imaging modalities which allow to perform angiographic procedures. They provide important information for the diagnosis of a diversity of vessel pathologies. DSA *(Digital Subtraction Angiography)* is the most established imaging technique for cerebral blood vessels and their malformations. Although there is a certain risk of complications due to its invasive nature, DSA is the method of choice for cerebral aneurysms providing optimal spatial and temporal resolution. However, in case of complex topology the superposition of vessels makes the analysis difficult since the resulting projection images contain little depth information (see Fig. 1). Therefore, tomographic imaging techniques like CTA *(Computed Tomography Angiography)* and MRA *(Magnetic Resonance Angiography)* gain growing attention since they provide three–dimensional *(3D)* information.

Intracranial aneurysms are berry–like blisters of the cerebral arteries which are caused by a weakness of all vessel wall layers. They incidentally occur in 1 to 5 out of 100 individuals [2] as congenital lesion or after a disease of the vessel wall. As a major risk, hemorrhage may cause serious damage to the brain, if the rupture of an aneurysm occurs. In preparation of interventional procedures or surgery a clear understanding of the surrounding vessel situation is required. The location and size of the neck which is the connection between the aneurysm and the feeding vessel, strongly influences the further strategy. In general, there are two methods of treatment, with surgery performed in most cases. More recently, an alternative procedure allows to direct a platinum coil into the aneurysm using an intra-vascular access. In order to perform a fast and precise analysis the choice of the imaging modality combined with an appropriate visualization approach are of great importance.

Aiming at 3D imaging modalities, aneurysms with a diameter of 3 − 11 mm are reproduced with similar quality. However, in case of MRA it is still difficult to delineate the neck and small arterial branches due to the nature of the resulting images. Above all, a meaningful visualization requires several hours of pre-processing, as presented in [3]. Therefore, as proposed in [4], we use CTA which provides the highest sensitivity for lesions of arbitrary size including small ($>$ 3 mm) and large ($>$ 11 mm) aneurysms.

Since it is difficult to integrate the information of tomographic slice images to a correct 3D model, reconstruction is efficiently assisted by techniques of volume rendering. For the analysis of angiographic data sets maximum intensity projection has positioned itself as one of the most popular visualization techniques. However, using only the highest gray value along every ray of sight, it prohibits to distinguish overlapping vessels clearly and to see intra-vascular abnormalities. Alternatively, techniques of surface rendering became very popular [3, 5] which allow to compute images interactively based on an intermediate geometric model. However, its calculation requires time-intensive segmentation which must be repeated for every correction of the result.

In order to overcome these limitations, we suggest direct volume rendering which uses the entire data volume, giving insight to interior and superimposed information. In order to provide interactive manipulation of the visualization parameters which is essential for the analysis in practice [6], we propose to use hardware accelerated 3D texture mapping [7] which we expect to be commonly available on PCs in the near future. After a short survey of our visualization approach in section 2, we briefly review the interactive calculation of iso-value representations in section 3 which has been previously published in [1]. Their integration was evaluated for the diagnosis of cerebral aneurysms in respect of enhanced perception of depth. Subsequently, in section 4, we suggest intuitive manipulation based on the integration into OpenInventor. In sections 5 and 6 tools are presented which consider convenient measurement of aneurysms and the registration of MR and CT based on a hardware accelerated approach, which was introduced in [8]. Finally, the strategy of the medical diagnosis is presented in section 7 with several examples demonstrating the value of our approach.

2 Direct Volume Rendering

For the visualization of tomographic image data, direct volume rendering proved to be very suitable. It allows to apply user-defined transfer functions which assign a specific color and opacity to all voxels of a certain scalar value. According to [9], all known approaches of direct volume rendering can be reduced to the transport theory model which describes the propagation of light in materials. Approximations of the underlying equation of light transfer have been developed and differ considerably in the physical phenomena they account for and in the way the emerging numerical models are solved.

The large amount of data of a typical tomographic scan makes the interactive manipulation of the volume object difficult which is essential for the ease of interpretation and the convenient analysis in medical practice. Therefore, based on ray–casting different optimization techniques were proposed [10, 11] which allow to traverse the volume data more efficiently. Alternatively, the time–intensive re–sampling of the original data is circumvented by voxel based projection methods [12]. More recently, considerable acceleration was achieved by expressing the rotation of a volume object by a 2D shear and a consecutive image warp [13]. However, most impressive frame rates are obtained with special purpose hardware [14, 15].

The 3D texture mapping hardware of high–end graphics computers provides a huge amount of trilinear interpolation operations and thereby allows to perform direct volume rendering at high image quality and interactive frame rates [7]. After converting the volume data set to a 3D texture, it is loaded to the respective memory. In a first step equidistant planes parallel to the viewport are clipped against the bounding box of the volume data set. Subsequently, the resulting polygons are projected onto the image plane. During rasterization they are textured with their corresponding image information directly obtained from the 3D texture by trilinear interpolation. Finally, the 3D representation is produced by successive blending of the textured polygons back-to-front onto the viewing plane. Since this process uses the blending and interpolation capabilities of the underlying hardware, the time consumed for the generation of an image is negligible compared to software based approaches. Interactive frame rates can be achieved even when applied to data sets of high resolution.

3 Fast Iso–Surfaces

Semi–transparent representations produced with direct volume rendering techniques allow to see superimposed structures. However, for some directions of view the spatial relation is evaluated much easier if lighting effects are integrated (see Fig. 2). If interactive navigation through complex vessel structures is envisaged, shaded surfaces assist to improve the users sense of orientation.

Different approaches like the Marching Cubes algorithm [16] provide iso–value representations of structures contained in volume data sets. However, as a major drawback, time–intensive calculations are required for every change of the iso–value prohibiting interactive manipulation. In addition, the complexity of the intermediate geometric model rapidly exceeds the available rendering capacity.

As presented in [1], interactive manipulation of iso–value surfaces and realistic lighting effects are possible if hardware assisted 3D texture mapping and two frame buffer operations are applied. This requires to define a cut plane for every scan line of the resulting image which has an orientation orthogonal to the viewing plane. Applying the rendering procedure, described in section 2, the corresponding image information of every cut plane is interpolated within the 3D texture memory and written to the frame buffer. After accessing its contents, all data values required for a complete scan line are simultaneously available in real–time. Using a standard ray–casting procedure they have to be calculated separately for every pixel of the current scan line along rays in the direction of view. After checking the obtained cut plane for the current iso–value the identified 2D locations are re–projected to their 3D positions within the volume data. Interpolation of the neighboring voxel gradients finally provides the surface normals required for the shading procedure.

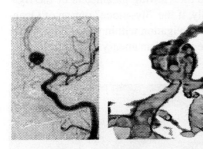

Fig. 1. Intracranial aneurysm: DSA *(left)* and direct volume rendering of CTA *(right)*.

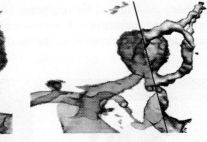

Fig. 2. Comparison of semi–transparent *(left)* and shaded iso–surface *(right)* representation.

4 Manipulation and Navigation

The presented approach builds on top of a frame work based on OpenInventor which was previously presented in [1]. Thereby, a variety of functionality is available which ensures intuitive manipulation. As a basis, a standardized interface is offered which provides a selection of sophisticated 3D viewers including various editors, light sources and other features. Additionally, several built–in manipulators are available which are attached to an object after selection. They considerably support a convenient navigation within 3D space if a 2D input device is applied. Consequently, the user–guided interactive inspection and analysis of an angiographic volume data set is accelerated.

In order to inspect interior structures , independent clip planes provide an intuitive way to virtually cut off parts of the volume data set. As can be seen in Fig. 4, the wall of the aneurysm was partly removed in order to view the connection to a related vessel from inside. Alternatively, choosing normal rendering mode and full opacity for the whole data set, clip planes assist the clinician to inspect the local gray value information at slices with arbitrary orientation.

In many situations during the analysis of an angiographic data set it is necessary to inspect detail information by approaching the structures very closely. However, at the same time, it is desirable to view the lesion from a more distant eye–point. Therefore, two communicating 3D displays are provided (see Fig. 3) which allow for an individual adjustment of the camera position. Within the right window typically local information is focused while a more distant view point gives global overview of the vessel situation within the left window. In order to provide improved orientation a geometric representation of the viewing frustum of the right window is integrated into the left display. Thereby, the small arrow connected to a sphere indicates the direction of view and the eye–point. Optionally, if the camera parameters of the right window change, the position of the camera of the left window remains unchanged, either relative to the arrow–sphere model or to the volume object. Thereby, the user gets the impression of a passing volume object in the first case, or of an arrow which flies through the fixed data set. Alternatively, if the arrow–sphere model is selected in the left window different manipulators are attached which allow to change the viewing parameters of the right window from a more distant viewing point. Finally, if the "fly–mode" option of Open-Inventor is applied interactive and user–controlled navigation within vessels is possible which provides endoscopic views of the sac or the neck of an aneurysm.

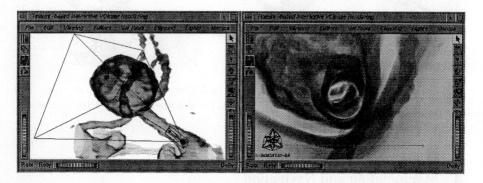

Fig. 3. Navigation inside a vessel approaching the aneurysm. The arrow within the left window indicates the direction of view of the right window

5 Measurements

For the preparation of interventions it is helpful to have information about the size of the aneurysm, the size of vessels or the distance between adjacent structures. Therefore, simple interactive tools are provided which allow for measurements directly within the 3D viewer (see Fig. 5). Thereby, the calculation of the distance between two points is performed on–the–fly, after placing the corresponding markers in 3D space. Finding the right position is assisted by appropriate manipulators inherited from the OpenInventor toolkit. But, more efficiently the correct location can be identified, if additional clip planes are used to reduce the degrees of freedom.

If treatment with a platinum coil is envisaged, additional knowledge about the volume of the aneurysm allows better estimation of the required expensive material. Using simple geometric objects the actual shape of an aneurysm or vessel is approximated. During an iterative procedure the shape of the selected object is distorted with an appropriate manipulator of OpenInventor while the quality of the fit is visually inspected by rotating the whole scene.

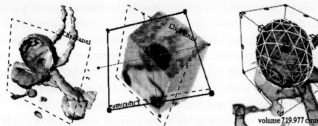 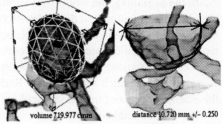

Fig. 4. Clip planes: inspect interior structures *(left)* and gray value information *(right)*.

Fig. 5. On–the–fly measurement of volume *(left)* and distance *(right)*.

6 Registration

In order to provide further anatomical orientation an additional tool is provided which allows for fast registration of the angiographic CT data with MR. As presented just recently [17], voxel based approaches gained more attention since they allow to perform retrospective and accurate alignment. Taking into account the entire gray value information at geometrically corresponding grid positions, the similarity of the involved data sets is optimized using a functional which evaluates the quality of alignment. Having introduced mutual information [18, 19], a very general functional is available which proved to provide very robust registration. However, the optimization procedure which is required to re–sample the volume data, typically consumes a huge amount of trilinear interpolation operations. Ensuring fast performance which is fundamental for medical applications, an approach is provided which integrates registration into the process of visualization, as suggested in [8]. Similar to the technique used for direct volume rendering the method uses the imaging and texture mapping subsystem of graphics computers. Thereby, all trilinear interpolation operations are completely performed with hardware assisted 3D texture mapping. The histograms of the data sets which are necessary for the calculation of mutual information are obtained with different hardware accelerated imaging operations. Using similar hardware supported procedures, as applied to visualization, the process of registration is considerably accelerated.

7 Strategy of Data Analysis

The visualization and inspection of CTA data sets is performed according to a specific protocol in order to ensure a fast and consistent analysis. After transferring the data from the scanner to a graphics workstation the range of gray values which describes the vessel information is transformed linearly to a new representation while data values below are suppressed and those above are mapped to maximum value. Due to the stretching of the histogram in the area of interest, subsequent manipulation of transfer functions for color and opacity values is performed in a more convenient way. Applying pre–defined lookup tables, a fast and meaningful initial visualization is obtained. Subsequently, the transfer functions are adjusted interactively to the individual data set by simple manipulation operations while the result is reviewed by a skilled user.

In the beginning, the whole data volume is loaded in order to detect all aneurysms. Pre–defined eye points and directions of view allow for a fast access of the most important areas for the medical analysis. Subsequently, the user may rotate, translate or zoom the 3D representation interactively in order to inspect detail information. Following the step of identification, bounding boxes are applied which define a sub-volume around every aneurysm which was detected. Reducing the amount of data allows to focus on the essential details of the vessel topology and ensures real–time manipulation.

For the documentation of every case, snap shots of the current visualization can be taken at any time of the analysis. Additionally, short movie sequences are recorded in order to provide an enhanced perception of depth.

8 Results and Discussion

All image data was obtained with a *Siemens Somaton Plus 4* spiral–CT scanner. For the angiography 100 ml of non–ionic contrast agent were injected with a delay time dependent on the circulation time and a flow rate of 3 ml/sec. With the lowest possible table–feed and a slice thickness of 1 mm, volume data sets with a resolution of 0.2 x 0.2 x 0.5 mm were reconstructed. The applied imaging technique proved to be optimal for small vessels and aneurysms including those of the basilar artery. All visualization was performed on a *SGI Indigo^2 Maximum Impact* and a *SGI Onyx Reality Engine II* which provide 4 Mbytes and 16 Mbytes of 3D texture memory respectively. Concerning the amount of available trilinear interpolation operations the underlying hardware has the same order of magnitude.

Subsequently, image data of three patients is presented which was obtained with the proposed approach. The overview image of Fig. 6 shows the location of a large basilar bifurcation aneurysm relative to the surrounding vessel situation. Choosing a closer semi–transparent representation the connections to the basilar artery and both posterior cerebral arteries are clearly conveyed. Within Fig. 7 an aneurysm of the right anterior communicating artery (ACoA) is delineated. Intra-operative views *(before and after applying a clip for treatment)* demonstrate the similarity between real and virtual presentation. Finally, Fig. 8 shows an aneurysm of the middle cerebral artery (MCA) bifurcation. The close semi–transparent visualization of the aneurysm clearly depicts the connected vessels and their location relative to the lesion. (see the color page at: **http://www9.informatik.uni-erlangen.de/eng/gallery/vis/med/miccai.html**)

Our experiments have shown that the visualization method is of major importance for the diagnostic value of the obtained images. In comparison to exclusively using shaded surface representations, direct volume rendering has proved to be an optimal visualization approach in order to delineate the sac and the neck of intracranial aneurysms including the surrounding vessels. Besides the ability to show opaque vessel structures, the semi–transparent representation is most informative since it conveys important information about the relation between the vessels and the lesion. Above all, the ability of real–time image generation and intuitive manipulation based on the functionality of OpenInventor is most important for a convenient analysis. Since motion enhances the perception of depth, the understanding of complex vessel situations is thereby improved considerably.

Additionally, integrating shaded vessels obtained by interactive extraction of iso–value surfaces proved to make the understanding of the spatial relation of neighboring objects much easier. Especially, if a fixed direction of view is chosen superimposed structures are inspected more conveniently. Selecting hybrid visualization consisting of a semi–transparent and a iso–surface representation, improved ease of orientation is provided inside cavities or during a user–controlled flight through vessels.

In comparison to other approaches which perform extensive segmentation, the proposed method only provides relative information about the actual vessel wall due to the soft delineation based on transfer functions for color and opacity values. However, the interactivity of the whole visualization process allows a skilled user to change parameters immediately and to evaluate the results by direct visual feedback. As further source of information which ensures the quality of the 3D visualization, clip planes of arbitrary orientation are optionally integrated which provide the original gray values of the data set. As a major advantage of our approach all visualization procedures and the medical diagnosis are performed in less than 15 – 20.

The interactive tools which allow to measure distance and volume information directly within the 3D viewer provide valuable information about the size and the distance of structures. Since clip planes of arbitrary orientation are used for the placement of markers, either the 3D visualization of objects or the original gray value information, optionally shown on every plane, is used to find the correct location. Measurements performed with a phantom data set confirmed the precision of the obtained results.

9 Conclusion

A fast and interactive approach was presented for the visualization and analysis of intracranial aneurysms. Using direct volume rendering based on 3D texture mapping and spiral CT angiography, the neck of the aneurysm and the surrounding vessels are optimally conveyed including small aneurysms and complex vessel topology. Improving the perception of depth iso–surface representations are integrated. Based on OpenInventor and communicating windows intuitive manipulation and convenient user–guided navigation are ensured. Further functionality comprises tools for hardware accelerated registration and for volume and distance measurement. The presented results demonstrate the value of our approach which proved to effectively assist pre–operative planning due to the short amount of time required for the complete medical analysis.

References

1. O. Sommer, A. Dietz, R. Westermann, and T. Ertl. An Interactive Visualization and Navigation Tool for Medical Volume Data. In V. Skala, editor, *WSCG'98 Conf. Proc.*, Feb. 1998.
2. J.L.D. Atkinson, T.M. Sundt, and O.W. Houser. Angiographic frequency of anterior circulation intracranial aneurysms. *Neurosurg.*, 70:551–555, 1989.
3. S. Nakajima, H. Atsumi, A. Bhalerao, F. Jolesz, R. Kikinis, T. Yoshimine, T. Moriarty, and P. Stieg. Computer-assisted Surgical Planning for Cerebrovascular Neurosurgery. *Neurosurgery*, 41:403–409, 1997.

4. K.E.W. Eberhardt, B. Tomandl, W.J. Huk, R. Laumer, and R. Fahlbusch. Value of CT–angiography (CTA) in patients with intracranial aneurysms. Comparison with MR–angiography (MRA and digital subtraction angiography (DSA)). In *Proc. of 11th Int. Congr. of Neurolog. Surg.*, pages 1963–1967, Bologna, 1997.
5. A. Puig, D. Tost, and I. Navazo. An Interactive Cerebral Blood Vessel Exploration System. In *Proc. Visualization*, pages 433–436, Phoenix, AZ, 1997. IEEE Comp. Soc. Press.
6. K.J. Zuiderveld, P.M. van Ooijen, J.W. Chin-A-Woeng, P.C. Buijs, M. Olree, and F.H. Post. Clinical Evaluation of Interactive Volume Visualization. In *Proc. Visualization*, pages 367–370, San Francisco, Calif., 1996. IEEE Comp. Soc. Press.
7. B. Cabral, N. Cam, and J. Foran. Accelerated Volume Rendering and Tomographic Reconstruction Using Texture Mapping Hardware. *ACM Symp. on Vol. Vis.*, pages 91–98, 1994.
8. P. Hastreiter and T. Ertl. Integrated Registration and Visualization of Medical Image Data. In *Proc. CGI*, pages 78–85, Hannover, Germany, 1998.
9. W. Krüger. The Application of Transport Theory to the Visualization of 3D Scalar Data Fields. In *Proc. Visualization*, pages 273–280. IEEE Comp. Soc. Press, 1990.
10. J. Danskin and P. Hanrahan. Fast Algorithms for Volume Ray Tracing. In *Worksh. of Vol. Vis.*, pages 91–98. ACM, 1992.
11. R. Yagel and Z. Shi. Accelerating Volume Animation by Space Leaping. In *Proc. Visualization*, pages 62–69, Los Alamitos, 1993. IEEE Comp. Soc. Press.
12. D. Laur and P. Hanrahan. Hierarchical Splatting: A Progressive Refinement Algorithm for Volume Rendering. *Computer Graphics*, 25(4):285–288, July 1991.
13. P. Lacroute and M. Levoy. Fast Volume Rendering Using a Shear–Warp Factorization of the Viewing Transform . *Computer Graphics*, 28(4):451–458, 1994.
14. G. Knittel and W. Straßer. A Compact Volume Rendering Accelerator. In A. Kaufman and W. Krüger, editors, *Symp. on Vol. Vis.*, pages 67–74. ACM SIGGRAPH, 1994.
15. H. Pfister and A. Kaufman. Cube–4 — A Scalable Architecture for Real–Time Volume Rendering. In R. Crawfis and Ch. Hansen, editors, *Symp. on Vol. Vis.*, pages 47–54. ACM SIGGRAPH, 1996.
16. W.E. Lorensen and H.E. Cline. Marching Cubes: A High Resolution 3D Surface Construction Algorithm. *Computer Graphics*, 21(4):163–169, 1987.
17. J. West and J.M. Fitzpatrick and M.Y. Wang and B.M. Dawant and C.R. Maurer Jr. and R.M. Kessler and R.J. Maciunas. Retrospective Intermodality Registration Techniques: Surface–Based Versus Volume Based. In *Proc. CVRMed–MRCAS*, pages 151–160, 1997.
18. A. Collignon, D. Vandermeulen, P. Suetens, and G. Marchal. Automated Multi-Modality Image Registration Based on Information Theory. *Kluwen Acad. Publ's: Computational Imaging and Vision*, 3:263–274, 1995.
19. W.M. Wells, P. Viola, H. Atsumi, S. Nakajima, and R. Kikinis. Multi-modal Volume Registration by Maximization of Mutual Information. *Medical Image Analysis, Oxford University Press*, 1(1), March 1996.

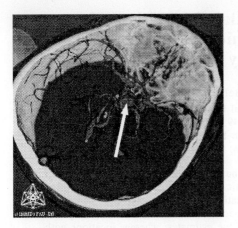 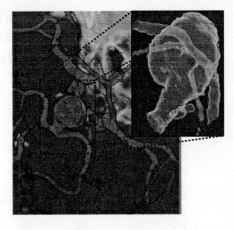

Fig. 6. Basilar bifurcation aneurysm with closer view showing the connected vessels.

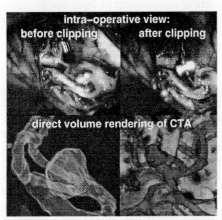 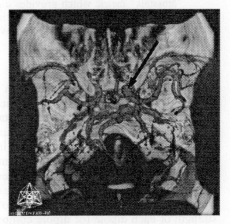

Fig. 7. Aneurysm of anterior communicating artery and comparison with intra-operative views.

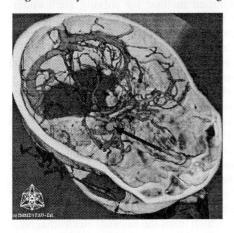 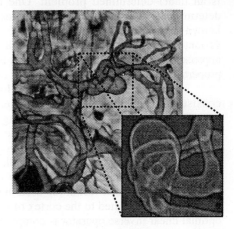

Fig. 8. Aneurysm of middle cerebral artery bifurcation and related vessels.

Visualizing Spatial Resolution of Linear Estimation Techniques of Electromagnetic Brain Activity Localization

Arthur K. Liu[1], John W. Belliveau[1], Anders M. Dale[1]

[1]Massachusetts General Hospital NMR Center
Bldg. 149, #2301
13th St.
Charlestown, MA 02129

Abstract. Various linear methods have been proposed to localize brain activity from external electromagnetic measurements. When interpreting the estimated spatiotemporal localizations, one must consider the spatial resolution of the particular approach. Locations with high spatial resolution increase the confidence of the estimates, whereas locations with poor resolution provide less useful localization estimates. We describe a "crosstalk" metric which provides a quanitative measurement of distortion at a given location from other locations within the brain. Crosstalk maps over the entire cortical surface provide a useful visualization of the spatial resolution of the inverse method.

1 Introduction

Localization of neuronal activity within the brain, based upon external measurement of the electric potential (EEG) and/or the magnetic field (MEG), is fundamentally ill-posed [12]. That is, for any set of instantaneous EEG and/or MEG measurements, there are infinitely many current source distributions within the head that are consistent with those recordings. Thus, in order to solve the electromagnetic "inverse problem" one must place some constraints on the otherwise infinite solution space.

A number of linear approaches have been proposed to overcome the ill-posedness of the inverse problem. These methods take advantage of the fact that if the locations of all possible sources are known *a priori*, the problem of determining the strength of each dipole (or dipole component) is a linear one. Since the number of possible source locations is, in general, much larger than the number of sensors, this is an under-determined problem. One common method for solving such under-determined linear problems is to choose the solution with the least power, also known as the minimum-norm (Moore-Penrose pseudo-inverse) solution [10, 24]. A variant of this method is to solve for the "smoothest" solution, as in the LORETA approach [19]. These linear approaches have certain advantages, including statistical properties that are well-known and easily characterized.

Given the ill-posedness of the localization problem, numerous solutions are consistent with any given set of external electromagnetic measurements. An important consideration in interpreting any localization approach is the spatial resolution of the method. Here, we describe a "crosstalk" metric that provides a quantitative measurement of the resolution inherent in the linear estimation approach. In addition, the mapping of the crosstalk metric onto the cortical surface provides a representation of resolution that is easily visualized.

The particular technique used in these studies is an anatomically constrained (all activity is restricted to the cortex of the brain) linear estimation approach [4]. An optimal linear inverse operator is computed, which maps the external electromagnetic field measurements into an estimated distribution of dipole strength across the cortical surface.

2 Methods

2.1 Forward solution

The "forward problem" of calculating the electric potential and magnetic field outside the head, given the conductive current source distribution within the head and the individual conductive properties of the tissues, is a well-defined problem, governed by the quasi-static limit of Maxwell's equations [9, 17, 20]. As has been noted previously by numerous authors, this results in a simple linear relationship between the electric and magnetic recordings, and the components of dipole moment at any location in the brain. This allows us to express the forward solution in simple vector notation:

$$\mathbf{x} = \mathbf{As} + \mathbf{n} \qquad (1)$$

where **x** is the vector of instantaneous electric and/or magnetic recordings, **A** is the so-called *gain matrix* (with each column specifying the electric and/or magnetic forward solution for a given dipole component), **s** is a vector of dipole component strengths, and **n** is a vector specifying the noise at each electrode/sensor. The elements of **A** are complicated non-linear functions of the sensor locations, and the geometry and electric properties of the head. Historically, the gain matrix has been calculated assuming an idealized head-shape, typically multiple concentric spheres of different conductivities. However, recent advances in numerical techniques and computer technology have made it practical to compute the forward solution for a more realistic non-spherical head. Furthermore, the advent of high-resolution 3-D MRI scans has made it possible to customize such realistic models to each individual subject's anatomy.

In this demonstration, we used conductivity boundaries and cortical surfaces determined from the MRI anatomy of a normal volunteer. The gain matrix calculations assumed the standard sensor geometry of the 122-channel Neuromag, Inc. MEG system [14]. We have adapted a realistic boundary element method (BEM) for calculating the forward solutions [5, 18].

The EEG forward solution computation requires the specification of boundaries between brain and skull, skull and scalp, and scalp and air, and the relative conductivities of each of those regions. The MEG forward solution, on the other hand, has been shown to require only the inner skull boundary to achieve an accurate solution [11, 13].

The surfaces required for computation of the magnetic forward solution (cortical surface and inner skull) are automatically reconstructed from high-resolution T1-weighted 3-D anatomical MRI data using the technique described by Dale and Sereno [4]. Briefly, the skull is first automatically stripped off the 3-D anatomical data set by inflating a stiff deformable spherical template of 642 triangles from a starting position in the white matter. The surface expands outward until it settles exactly at the outer edge of the brain. Since bone appears dark on MR images, this outer brain surface is then used to estimate the inner skull surface. The gray/white matter boundary for each cortical hemisphere is then estimated with a region-growing method, starting from a seed point in the white matter. The boundary between filled and unfilled 1 x 1 x 1 mm voxels is tessellated to generate a surface that typically consists of about 150,000 vertices for each hemisphere. The resulting surface is smoothed using a deformable template algorithm. Each vertex is moved according to the vector sum of a curvature-minimizing force and an MRI force that works to prevent each vertex from penetrating the white matter. The resulting refined surface settles approximately near layer 4. For calculation of the forward solution, the cortical surface is tiled with approximately 5600 vertices.

Here we evaluated the results only for the MEG case. The biomagnetic sources were constrained to be within the cortical gray matter. Each possible source location was represented either by three orthogonal current dipoles placed at that location.

2.2 Inverse Solution

Minimization of expected error [3], Bayesian estimation [7], Tichonov regularization [22], and the generalized Wiener filter [6] all result in an equivalent inverse operator (**W**):

$$\mathbf{W} = \mathbf{R}\mathbf{A}^T\left(\mathbf{A}\mathbf{R}\mathbf{A}^T + \mathbf{C}\right)^{-1} \quad (2)$$

where **C** is the covariance matrix of **n**, and **R** is the *a priori* covariance matrix estimate for **s** from Eq. 1 [4]. **W** is a linear operator that maps a recording vector **x** into an estimated solution vector $\hat{\mathbf{s}}$. Note that if both **C** and **R** are set to a scalar multiple of the identity matrix then this approach reduces to the well-known minimum-norm solution [9, 10]. Two derivations, based on the minimization of expected error and Bayesian estimation, which arrive at different, but equivalent, inverse operators are shown below.

The minimization of expected error [3, 4, 7], begins with a set of measurements specified by Equation 1. One would like to calculate a linear inverse operator **W** that minimizes the expected difference between the estimated and the correct source solution. The expected error can be defined as:

$$Err_W = \left\langle \|\mathbf{Wx} - \mathbf{s}\|^2 \right\rangle \quad (3)$$

Assuming both **n** and **s** are normally distributed with zero mean and covariance matrices **C** and **R**, respectively, the expected error can be rewritten as:

$$Err_W = \left\langle \|\mathbf{W}(\mathbf{As} + \mathbf{n}) - \mathbf{s}\|^2 \right\rangle \quad (4)$$

$$= \left\langle \|(\mathbf{WA} - \mathbf{I})\mathbf{s} + \mathbf{Wn})\|^2 \right\rangle \quad (5)$$

$$= \left\langle \|\mathbf{Ms} + \mathbf{Wn}\|^2 \right\rangle \quad (6)$$

where
$$\mathbf{M} = \mathbf{WA} - \mathbf{I}$$

$$= \left\langle \|\mathbf{Ms}\|^2 \right\rangle + \left\langle \|\mathbf{Wn}\|^2 \right\rangle \quad (7)$$

$$= tr(\mathbf{MRM}^T) + tr(\mathbf{WCW}^T) \quad (8)$$

where tr(**A**) is the trace of **A** and is defined as the sum of the diagonal entries

Re-expanding the expression gives

$$= \text{tr}(\mathbf{WARA}^T\mathbf{W}^T - \mathbf{RA}^T\mathbf{W}^T - \mathbf{WAR} + \mathbf{R}) + \text{tr}(\mathbf{WCW}^T) \qquad (9)$$

This last expression can be explicitly minimized by taking the gradient with respect to $\mathbf{W}$, setting it to zero and solving for $\mathbf{W}$.

$$0 = 2\mathbf{WARA}^T - 2\mathbf{RA}^T + 2\mathbf{WC} \qquad (10)$$
$$\mathbf{WARA}^T + \mathbf{WC} = \mathbf{RA}^T \qquad (11)$$
$$\mathbf{W}(\mathbf{ARA}^T + \mathbf{C}) = \mathbf{RA}^T \qquad (12)$$

This yields the expression for the linear inverse operator:

$$\mathbf{W} = \mathbf{RA}^T(\mathbf{ARA}^T + \mathbf{C})^{-1} \qquad (13)$$

The Bayesian linear inverse operator [7] derivation begins with the expression for conditional probability:

$$\Pr(\mathbf{s}|\mathbf{x}) = \frac{\Pr(\mathbf{x}|\mathbf{s})\Pr(\mathbf{s})}{\Pr(\mathbf{x})} \qquad (14)$$

which one would like to maximize. Again, beginning with a measurement vector $\mathbf{x}$: specified in Equation 1, and assuming both $\mathbf{n}$ and $\mathbf{s}$ are normally distributed with zero mean and covariance matrices $\mathbf{C}$ and $\mathbf{R}$, respectively, rewrite $\Pr(\mathbf{x}|\mathbf{s})$ and $\Pr(\mathbf{s})$:

$$\Pr(\mathbf{x}|\mathbf{s}) = e^{-(\mathbf{As}-\mathbf{x})^T\mathbf{C}^{-1}(\mathbf{As}-\mathbf{x})} \qquad (15)$$
$$\Pr(\mathbf{s}) = e^{-\mathbf{s}^T\mathbf{R}^{-1}\mathbf{s}} \qquad (16)$$

This gives a simplified Bayesian expression:

$$\max[\Pr(\mathbf{s}|\mathbf{x})] = \max\left[\frac{\left(e^{-(\mathbf{As}-\mathbf{x})^T\mathbf{C}^{-1}(\mathbf{As}-\mathbf{x})}\right)\left(e^{-\mathbf{s}^T\mathbf{R}^{-1}\mathbf{s}}\right)}{\Pr(\mathbf{x})}\right] \qquad (17)$$

$$= \max\left[-(\mathbf{As}-\mathbf{x})^T\mathbf{C}^{-1}(\mathbf{As}-\mathbf{x}) - \mathbf{s}^T\mathbf{R}^{-1}\mathbf{s}\right] \qquad (18)$$
$$= \min\left[(\mathbf{As}-\mathbf{x})^T\mathbf{C}^{-1}(\mathbf{As}-\mathbf{x}) + \mathbf{s}^T\mathbf{R}^{-1}\mathbf{s}\right] \qquad (19)$$

Taking the derivative with respect to $\mathbf{s}$ and setting it to zero:

$$2\mathbf{A}^T\mathbf{C}^{-1}\mathbf{As} - 2\mathbf{A}^T\mathbf{C}^{-1}\mathbf{x} + 2\mathbf{R}^{-1}\mathbf{s} = 0 \qquad (20)$$
$$\mathbf{s} = \left(\mathbf{A}^T\mathbf{C}^{-1}\mathbf{A} + \mathbf{R}^{-1}\right)^{-1}\mathbf{A}^T\mathbf{C}^{-1}\mathbf{x} = \mathbf{Wx} \qquad (21)$$

which yields the expression for the Bayesian linear operator

$$\mathbf{W} = \left(\mathbf{A}^T\mathbf{C}^{-1}\mathbf{A} + \mathbf{R}^{-1}\right)^{-1}\mathbf{A}^T\mathbf{C}^{-1} \tag{22}$$

Finally, it is possible to show that the linear operators given by Equations 13 and 22 are equivalent (assuming that both $\left(\mathbf{A}\mathbf{R}\mathbf{A}^T + \mathbf{C}\right)$ and $\left(\mathbf{A}^T\mathbf{C}^{-1}\mathbf{A} + \mathbf{R}^{-1}\right)$ are invertible).

$$\mathbf{R}\mathbf{A}^T\left(\mathbf{A}\mathbf{R}\mathbf{A}^T + \mathbf{C}\right)^{-1} = \tag{23}$$

$$\left(\mathbf{A}^T\mathbf{C}^{-1}\mathbf{A} + \mathbf{R}^{-1}\right)^{-1}\left(\mathbf{A}^T\mathbf{C}^{-1}\mathbf{A} + \mathbf{R}^{-1}\right)\mathbf{R}\mathbf{A}^T\left(\mathbf{A}\mathbf{R}\mathbf{A}^T + \mathbf{C}\right)^{-1}$$

$$= \left(\mathbf{A}^T\mathbf{C}^{-1}\mathbf{A} + \mathbf{R}^{-1}\right)^{-1}\left(\mathbf{A}^T\mathbf{C}^{-1}\mathbf{A}\mathbf{R}\mathbf{A}^T + \mathbf{A}^T\right)\left(\mathbf{A}\mathbf{R}\mathbf{A}^T + \mathbf{C}\right)^{-1} \tag{24}$$

$$= \left(\mathbf{A}^T\mathbf{C}^{-1}\mathbf{A} + \mathbf{R}^{-1}\right)^{-1}\left(\mathbf{A}^T\mathbf{C}^{-1}\right)\left(\mathbf{A}\mathbf{R}\mathbf{A}^T + \mathbf{C}\right)\left(\mathbf{A}\mathbf{R}\mathbf{A}^T + \mathbf{C}\right)^{-1} \tag{25}$$

$$= \left(\mathbf{A}^T\mathbf{C}^{-1}\mathbf{A} + \mathbf{R}^{-1}\right)^{-1}\mathbf{A}^T\mathbf{C}^{-1} \tag{26}$$

Although these two operators are equivalent, it is computationally more efficient to use the inverse operator given by Equation 13 (based on the minimization of expected error) since it only requires the inversion of a matrix that is square in the number of sensors, compared to square in the number of dipoles. Typically, the number of sensors is on the order of 200, whereas the number of dipoles can easily be in the thousands.

Once the optimal linear inverse estimator $\mathbf{W}$ is calculated for a given anatomy (cortical surface), and sensor placement, the estimated spatiotemporal pattern of electric/magnetic activity (dipole strength) can be calculated using the simple expression:

$$\hat{\mathbf{s}}(t) = \mathbf{W}\mathbf{x}(t) \tag{27}$$

where $\hat{\mathbf{s}}(t)$ and $\mathbf{x}(t)$ are the estimated dipole strength and recording vectors as a function of time, respectively.

2.3 Crosstalk Metric

The estimated source strength ($\hat{s}_i$) at each location i can be written as a weighted sum of the actual source strengths at <u>all</u> locations, plus a noise contribution. This is due to the linearity of both the forward solution and our inverse operator. More formally,

$$\hat{s}_i = \mathbf{w}_i \mathbf{x} \tag{28}$$
$$= \mathbf{w}_i (\mathbf{A}\mathbf{s} + \mathbf{n}) \tag{29}$$
$$= \mathbf{w}_i \left(\sum_j \mathbf{a}_j s_j + \mathbf{n} \right) \tag{30}$$
$$= \sum_j (\mathbf{w}_i \mathbf{a}_j) s_j + \mathbf{w}_i \mathbf{n} \tag{31}$$

where $\mathbf{w}_j$ is the *i*th *row* of $\mathbf{W}$, and $\mathbf{a}_j$ is the *j*th *column* of $\mathbf{A}$ (i.e., the lead field including orientation information at location *j*). Note that the first term in Equation 31 is the sum of the activity (S_j) at every location *j*, weighted by the scalar $\mathbf{w}_i \mathbf{a}_j$. The second term reflects the noise contribution to the estimated activity at location *i*.

We would like an explicit expression for the relative sensitivity of our estimate at a given location to activity coming from other locations. We define a "crosstalk" metric (ξ_{ij}), similar to the averaging kernel of the Backus-Gilbert method [1, 2] as follows:

$$\xi_{ij}^2 = \frac{|(\mathbf{WA})_{ij}|^2}{|(\mathbf{WA})_{ii}|^2} = \frac{|\mathbf{w}_i \mathbf{a}_j|^2}{|\mathbf{w}_i \mathbf{a}_i|^2} \tag{32}$$

where $\mathbf{WA}$ is the resolution matrix [8, 16] or resolution field [15].

By comparing Equations 31 and 32, we see that the crosstalk metric x_{ij} describes the sensitivity (or weighting) of the estimate at location *i* to activity at location *j*, relative to activity at location *i*, and provides a measurement of the distortion due to location *j* . A crosstalk value of 0% means that the estimated activity at location *i* is completely insensitive to activity at location *j*. A crosstalk value of 100% means that the estimated activity at location *i* is equally sensitive to activity at locations *i* and *j*.

Two locations, one on the top of a gyrus and one in the bottom of a neighboring sulcus, were selected for display. For each location, the crosstalk from all other locations was calculated. This computation shows the spatial spread of the estimate at each location.

3 Results

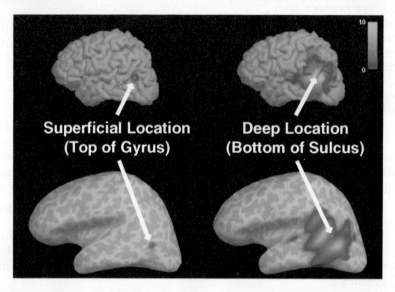

Fig. 1. Maps of the crosstalk metric (x_{ij}) for two different locations i (see arrows) were computed for all locations j, shown in folded (top) and inflated (bottom) cortical surface views. Surface curvature is represented in grayscale (light and dark gray corresponding to gyri and sulci, respectively). The crosstalk represents the relative sensitivity of the dipole strength estimate at a given location to activity at other locations (shown in color, ranging from 0 (gray), to 10 (yellow)). Note the greater spread of the crosstalk for the deep location (right) relative to the superficial location (left), reflecting different intrinsic spatial resolution for these locations.

All cortical locations may potentially contribute to the estimated activity at any given location (see Equation 31). The computed crosstalk for two locations is shown in Figure 1 on the normal and inflated cortical surfaces. The cortical inflation process allows for visualization of the entire cortical surface, including areas buried within deep sulci [4, 21, 23]. The maps indicate the relative weighting of activity at each and every location (j) contributing to the estimated activity at the indicated locations (i, white arrow). The superficial location on top of the gyrus (left figures) clearly shows much less sensitivity to activity at other locations, and consequently intrinsically higher spatial resolution, than the deeper location at the bottom of the nearby sulcus (right figures).

4 Discussion

The estimate of activity at a given location is potentially affected by activity at other locations. The crosstalk metric, as described here, provides a quantitative measurement of the sensitivity of the estimate at a location to the activity at other locations. Spatial maps of crosstalk can be generated by combining the crosstalk metric with an explicit representation of the cortical surface. The interpretation of brain activity localized based on external electromagnetic measurements is greatly enhanced by the additional computation of crosstalk maps. This type of spatial information can show which regions of the brain are intrinsically less sensitive to localization error.

Such crosstalk maps can directly address the issue of mis-localized activity between two or more areas of activation. If there is little overlap between the crosstalk maps of those areas, one can be confident that the localization at one area is unaffected by activity at the other area. Conversely, if the spatial crosstalk map of one region of activity encompasses another region of activity, the particular inverse method examined would not be able to accurately separate the activity from those two areas. Using the spatial crosstalk map potentially provides a principled argument for determining which brain regions can be well localized, allowing confident analysis of estimated activity using the linear estimation approach.

References

1. Backus, G.E., F. Gilbert: Geophysical Journal of the Royal Astonomical Society. **16** (1968) 169-205
2. Backus, G.E., F. Gilbert: Philosophical Transactions of the Royal Society of London A. **266** (1970) 123-192
3. Dale, A.M.: Source Localization and Spatial Discriminant Analysis of Event-Related Potentials: Linear Approaches. Ph.D. Thesis UCSD (1994).
4. Dale, A.M., M.I. Sereno: Improved localization of cortical activity by combining EEG and MEG with MRI cortical surface reconstruction: A linear approach. J. Cog. Neurosci. **5** (1993) 162-176
5. de Munck, J.C.: A linear discretization of the volume conductor boundary integral equation using analytically integrated elements. IEEE Trans. Biomed. Eng. **39** (1992) 986-990
6. Deutsch, R.: Estimation Theory. Prentice Hall Englewood Cliffs, NJ (1965)
7. Gelb, A.: Applied Optimal Estimation. MIT Press, Cambridge (1974).
8. Grave de Peralta Menendez, R., S. Gonzalez Andino, B. Lutkenhoner: Figures of merit to compare linear distributed inverse solutions. Brain Topography. **9** (1996) 117-124
9. Hamalainen, M., R. Hari, R.J. Ilmoniemi, J. Knuutila, O.V. Lounasmaa: Magnetoencephalography - theory, instrumentation, and application to noninvasive studies of the working human brain. Review of Modern Physics. **65** (1993) 413-497
10. Hamalainen, M.S., R.J. Ilmoniemi: Interpreting measured magnetic fields of the brain: estimates of current distributions. Helsinki Univ. of Technology Helsinki, Finland (1984)
11. Hamalainen, M.S., J. Sarvas: Realistic conductivity geometry model of the human head for interpretation of neuromagnetic data. IEEE Trans. Biomed. Eng. **36** (1989) 165-171
12. Helmholtz, H.: Ueber einige Gesetze der Vertheilung elektrischer Strome in korperlichen Leitern, mit Anwendung auf die thierisch-elektrischen Versuche. Ann. Phys. Chem. **89** (1853) 211-233, 353-377
13. Ilmoniemi, R.J.: Magnetoencephalography-A tool for studies of information processing in the human brain. In: Lubbig, H. (ed.): The Inverse Problem. Akademie Verlag, Berlin (1995) 89-106
14. Knuutila, J.E.T., A.I. Ahonen, M.S. Hamalainen, M.J. Kajola, P.O. Laine, O.V. Lounasmaa, L.T. Parkkonen, J.T.A. Simola, C.D. Tesche: A 122-channel whole-cortex squid system for measuring the brains magnetic fields. IEEE Trans. Magn. **29** (1993) 3315-3320

15. Lutkenhoner, B., R. Grave de Peralta Menendez: The resolution-field concept. EEG and Clin. Neurophysiol. **102** (1997) 326-334
16. Menke, W.: Geophysical Data Analysis: Discrete Inverse Theory. Academic Press San Diego, CA (1989)
17. Nunez, P.L.: Electric fields of the brain. Oxford University Press New York (1981)
18. Oostendorp, T.F., A. van Oosterom. "Source parameter estimation using realistic geometry in bioelectricity and biomagnetism." Biomagnetic Localization and 3D Modeling, Report TKK-F-A689. Nenonen, Rajala and Katila ed. Helsinki University of Technology. Helsinki. (1992)
19. Pascual-Marqui, R.D., C.M. Michel, D. Lehmann: Low resolution electromagnetic tomography: a new method for localizing electrical activity in the brain. Inter J Psychophysiology. **18** (1994) 49-65
20. Plonsey, R.: Bioelectric Phenomena. McGraw-Hill, New York (1969)
21. Sereno, M.I., A.M. Dale, J.B. Reppas, K.K. Kwong, J.W. Belliveau, T.J. Brady, B.R. Rosen, R.B.H. Tootell: Borders of multiple visual areas in humans revealed by functional magnetic resonance imaging. Science. **268** (1995) 889-893
22. Tichonov, A.N., V.Y. Arsenin: Solutions of ill-posed problems. Winston, English translation by F. John Washington D.C. (1977)
23. Tootell, R.B.H., J.D. Mendola, N.K. Hadjikhani, P.J. Ledden, A.K. Liu, J.B. Reppas, M.I. Sereno, A.M. Dale: Functional analysis of V3A and related areas in human visual cortex. J Neuroscience. **17** (1997) 7060-7078
24. Wang, J.-Z., S.J. Williamson, L. Kaufman: Magnetic source images determined by a lead-field analysis: the unique minimum-norm least-squares estimation. IEEE Trans.Biomed.Eng. **39** (1992) 665-675

Biomechanical Simulation of the Vitreous Humor in the Eye Using an Enhanced ChainMail Algorithm

Markus A. Schill[1,2,3], Sarah F. F. Gibson[1], H.-J. Bender[3], and R. Männer[2]

[1] MERL – A Mitsubishi Electric Research Laboratory, 201 Broadway, Cambridge, MA, 02139, USA, http://www.merl.com
[2] Lehrstuhl für Informatik V, Universität Mannheim, B6, D-68131 Mannheim, Germany, http://www-mp.informatik.uni-mannheim.de
[3] Institut für Anästhesiologie und Operative Intensivmedizin, Fakultät für klinische Medizin Mannheim der Universität Heidelberg, D-68135 Mannheim, Germany
markus.schill@ti.uni-mannheim.de gibson@merl.com

Abstract The focus of this paper is the newly developed Enhanced ChainMail Algorithm that will be used for modeling the vitreous humor in the eye during surgical simulation. The simulator incorporates both visualization and biomechanical modeling of a vitrectomy, an intraocular surgical procedure for removing the vitreous humor. The Enhanced ChainMail algorithm extends the capabilities of an existing algorithm for modeling deformable tissue, 3D ChainMail, by enabling the modeling of inhomogeneous material. In this paper, we present the enhanced algorithm and demonstrate its capabilities in 2D.

Introduction

A vitrectomy removes the vitreous humor, a gelatinous substance filling the eyeball (see Figure 1). This procedure is performed under numerous pathological conditions, including an opaque vitreous body or traction ablatio, where thin pathological membranes and tissue fibers on the retina contract and start to lift the retina from the sclera. In the case of an opaque vitreous body, the vitreous humor is removed and replaced with a clear fluid. To address traction ablatio, the vitreous humor is first removed to allow access to the pathological membranes.

During the vitrectomy, two narrow instruments are inserted into the eye – a vitrector and a cold light lamp. The vitrector has a hole at the side of its tip through which material is sucked in and extracted with an internal oscillating knife. The extracted material is then pumped out through the handle of the vitrector. The cold light lamp is used to generate reflections on the surface of the otherwise highly transparent vitreous humor, helping the surgeon to visualize remaining material. The lamp also casts a strong shadow of the instrument onto the retina. This shadow provides depth cues to the surgeon, an important means for estimating the distance between the instrument and the highly sensitive retina.

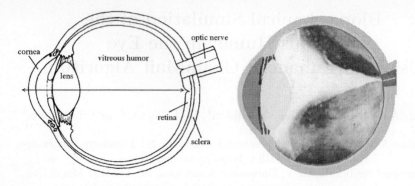

Figure1. The EyeSi project will simulate removal of the vitreous humor from the eyeball. (Left) A diagram of the eye. (Right) Pathological vitreous humor. For this picture a photography and a 2D model were superposed.

A collision between the vitrector and the retina can result in loss of eye sight. Unfortunately, because vitrectomies are performed using a stereo microscope, hand-eye coordination can be extremely difficult within the small volume of the eye (the eye's diameter is 2.6 cm). These constraints, in addition to a lack of well-defined mechanical feedback from motion of the instruments, mean that vitrectomies are challenging both to perform and to teach. To address the need for better teaching tools, the University of Mannheim has begun the EyeSi project, a computer-based simulator for intra-ocular surgery.

The EyeSi Project

The EyeSi project aims to develop a computer-based training workstation for the simulation of a vitrectomy, the removal of the vitreous humor from the eyeball. The simulator is designed to augment the training and rehearsal of intra-ocular surgery. The project addresses both navigation inside the eye and the removal of the vitreous humor with a vitrector. During the simulation, the user manipulates a vitrector and a cold light lamp. The positions of these two instruments are tracked by an optical tracking system[1] and monitored by a PC-based workstation. The instrument positions are used to render the instruments in a graphical representation of the computer eye model and to detect possible interactions with the vitreous humor. Because the vitreous humor is an inhomogeneous, semi-transparent, highly deformable gel, the system uses a volumetric representation (rather than a surface-based representation) for modeling and visualization of this substance.

---

[1] The tracking system uses i-cam, an intelligent camera system developed by the Fachhochschule für Technik, Mannheim. Each CCD camera is equipped with a digital signal processor (DSP) which can be programmed to perform simple image processing tasks and position tracking. Using the DSPs for motion prediction is planed for the future.

EyeSi will use a volume rendering system developed at the Lehrstuhl für Informatik V, Universität Mannheim[2] which provides combined visualization of volume and surface objects and shadow casting [4], [7]. As described above, rendering shadows is particularly important for providing depth cues to the surgeon to help avoid damaging the retina with the vitrector tip. The system will combine surface-based object representations for the surgical instrument and the outer geometry of the eyeball with a volumetric representation of the vitreous humor (Figure 1 (right) shows a 2D model). The biomechanical behavior of the volumetric vitreous humor will be simulated with the Enhanced ChainMail Algorithm presented in this paper. The enhancement allows the modeling and deformation of inhomogeneous volumetric material at interactive rates.

Recent Work on Eye Surgery Simulation

The structure and function of the human eye are well understood. This together with its spherically symmetric shape and its relatively simple structure on one hand, and its high sensitivity and fragility on the other hand make it a good candidate for surgical simulation.

A number of others have developed computer based simulations of the eye for education and training. For example, the Biomedical Visualization laboratory at the University of Illinois have developed an anatomical atlas of the eye [1]. Most systems that have been developed for simulating eye surgery deal with structures, such as cataracts, that are on or near the surface of the eye Hence, these systems use surface-based object representations and surface rendering (e.g. [6], [5]). In these systems, interactions with surgical instruments have been modeled using Finite Element Methods, where either on-line computation limits the rates of interactions with the object models [6] or off-line calculations or the incorporation of previously measured interaction forces limit the flexibility of the system [5].

The Enhanced ChainMail Algorithm

Because of the highly deformable nature of the vitreous humor and the mechanical complexity of the extraction process, the surgical procedure is not well modeled with conventional deformation techniques such as mass-spring systems or Finite Element Methods. Solving Navier Stokes based 3D computational fluid dynamics for this problem can not be performed at the required update rates. While particle systems provide a possible solution [2], the lack of direct interparticle communication can also make these systems too slow for an interactive simulation when a relatively large number of particles are used. In contrast, the 3D ChainMail algorithm, introduced by Gibson in 1997 [3], provides fast interactions with highly deformable materials containing 10's of thousands of elements.

---

[2] http://www-mp.informatik.uni-mannheim.de/research/VIRIM

This capability provides the potential for addressing the highly demanding requirements of the EyeSi project. However, 3D ChainMail has a number of limitations. In the rest of this paper, we outline the capabilities and limitations of 3D ChainMail and introduce an Enhanced ChainMail Algorithm that addresses some of these limitations. The features of this new algorithm are defined and illustrated in 2D.

3D Chainmail: 3D ChainMail is the first step in an iterative process that models shape changes in deformable objects. Its function is to approximate the new shape of a deformed object by minimally adjusting element positions to satisfy geometric constraints between the elements in the volumetric object. The second step in the deformation process, Elastic Relaxation, relaxes the approximate shape of a deformed object to reduce an elastic energy measure in the object.

3D ChainMail is physically-based in the sense that the information of a deformation process is propagated through the object by passing it from one volume element to another. As information travels through the object, each element reacts by adjusting its own position within certain material constraints. By adjusting its position, an element changes the information (the amount of deformation still to be performed) that is propagated to neighboring elements. Once this deformation information is reduced to zero or there are no more neighbors to propagate the information to, the process ends. Fig. 2 illustrates the ChainMail process in one dimension.

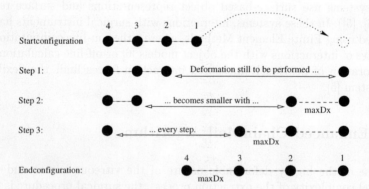

Figure2. The deformation is initiated by moving element #1. In the next step, element #2 implicitly changes the information that is passed on to element #3 by adjusting its position according to the material constraint, maxDx, where maxDx is the maximum allowed distance between two elements. When the original elements are separated by a distance less than maxDx, the amount of deformation that remains to be performed decreases with every step

The ChainMail algorithm enables fast propagation of the deformation information because connections to neighboring elements are explicitly stored in the object data structure. The algorithm described in [3] uses 4-connected neighborhoods in 2D and 6-connected neighborhoods in 3D. The relative positions between neighboring elements are governed by a set of deformation and shear constraints. Figure 3 shows the six constraints that determine the material properties in 2D. Different constraints controlling vertical, horizontal, and front-to-

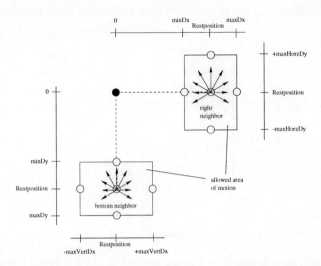

Figure 3. The geometric constraints between an element (black) and its right and bottom neighbors are illustrated In 2D, six material constraints are used to model different material properties with ChainMail: maxDx, minDx, maxDy, and minDy govern the compression or stretch of the material, while maxVertDx and maxHorzDy govern the possible shear between neighbors.

back deformation and shear allow anisotropic material properties. However, the algorithm is particularly fast because it assumes that these constraints are constant throughout the volumetric object. Because the vitreous humor is not homogeneous, especially in pathological cases, it is important that we expand the algorithm presented in [3] to address inhomogeneous tissues.

Enhanced ChainMail: For inhomogeneous materials, the first-moved-first-processed element processing order that was used in 3D ChainMail is no longer appropriate. As expected, a straightforward application of ChainMail using this processing order gave inconsistent deformations for inhomogeneous materials that resulted in holes and tears. The Enhanced ChainMail algorithm addresses this problem with a new element processing order.

Refining the ChainMail algorithm for inhomogeneous materials required thinking about deformation as a physical process in which deformation information travels through the material as a sound wave. In general, the speed of sound is higher in denser material because the "connection" between elements is stiffer. In

ChainMail the "stiffness" of a connection between two neighbors is determined by the material constraints of the two elements. In inhomogeneous materials, when neighboring elements have different material constraints, the constraints for the link between the two neighbors are calculated using contributions from both elements. Fig. 4 shows the constraints that are assigned to a single element in the enhanced ChainMail algorithm and Fig. 5 illustrates how the two neighbors contribute to the constraints that determine their relative behavior.

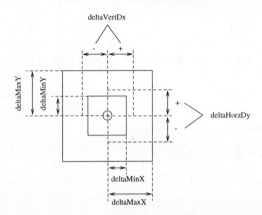

Figure4. Constraints assigned to a single element in the Enhanced ChainMail Algorithm. deltaMaxX, deltaMinX, deltaMaxY, and deltaMinY, correspond to maximum allowed stretch and compression in the horizontal and vertical directions respectively. +/-deltaVertX and +/-deltaHorzY correspond to the maximum allowed shear to vertical and horizontal neighbors respectively.

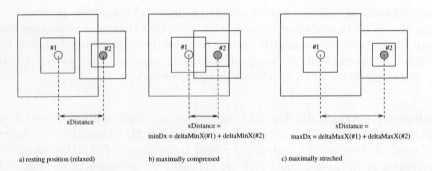

Figure5. The contributions of both neighbors combine to give the constraints that govern the link between them.

The order in which neighbors of a moved element are processed determines where the deformation information is propagated first. Hence, the processing order can be used to model material and direction-dependent propagation speeds in the object. The Enhanced ChainMail Algorithm uses this observation to order the processing of elements in the object so that the deformation travels most quickly through stiff materials. The ordering is determined by comparing the constraint violations between neighboring elements and processing elements with the largest constraint violations first. For example, the constraint violations for element #2 in step 1 of Fig. 2 is determined as follows:

$$amount\ of\ constraint\ violation = distance_{\#1,\#2} - maxDx$$

After moving an element, its neighbors are examined to determine whether any constraint has been violated. If so, the neighbor with the largest constraint violation is processed first. This is equivalent to processing neighbors in the order in which their constraints were violated, guarenteeing that the deformation information is propagated fastest through stiff materials.

Algorithm outline

The Enhanced ChainMail Algorithm maintains an ordered list of elements that must be considered for a movement. The ordering criteria for the list is the size of the constraint violation. The process starts when an initial sponsoring element in the object is moved to a new position. After this, neighboring elements are inserted into the list, whereby the previous ordering principle is maintained, according to which the element with the largest constraint violation is always at the head of the list. Next the first element is popped from the list and moved to satisfy the constraint against its sponsor. (The sponsor is the element by whose movement the current element was added to the list.) The process ends when the list is exhausted. The following is pseudo code for the Enhanced ChainMail Algorithm:

```
initialSponsor.position = newPosition ;
insertNeighborsToList(initialSponsor) ;
while (elements in lists)
   popFirstElementFromList ;
   if(checkVsSponsor demands move)
      thisElement.updatePosition ;
      addNeighborsToList(thisElement) ;
```

The candidate list can be sorted easily if new elements are inserted into the correct position when they are added to the list. Currently the list is implemented as a binary tree, making it relatively fast and easy to insert and find elements. However element insertion is the most time-consuming process in the current implementation.

Results

To model inhomogeneous material with ChainMail the first-moved-first-processed criteria used for homogeneous materials is no longer valid. It must be replaced by the mode general princible first-"vioalation of constraint"-first-processed. The Enhanced ChainMail Algorithm was implemented and tested in 2D for a number of test objects and integrated into a general system which enables a 2D gray-scale image to be read into the system, material constraints to be set using a lookup table on gray-scale values, and the resultant 2D model to be interactively manipulated. The sequence in Figure 6 shows the deformation of a gray-scale picture using this system. The gray values in the original picture (top, left) were mapped to material constraints that were a linear function of the gray scale value, where black pixels became rigid elements and white pixels became highly deformable elements. The sequence shows the deformation of the image when an element on the right side of the image is grabbed and moved to the right. Notice how the more rigid hair on the left border of the picture affects the softer surrounding material during the deformation.

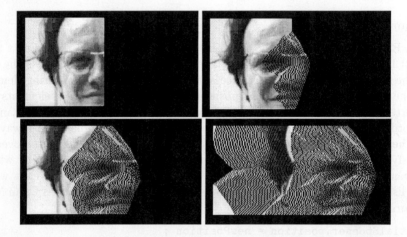

Figure6. The gray values of the original picture (top left) are interpreted as material constraints. White is soft and black is rigid material.

Because of the sorting required for determining the processing order of object elements, the Enhanced ChainMail algorithm is slower than the original 3D ChainMail algorithm. However, we were able to achieve interactive rates for deforming a 100 × 100 inhomogeneous image. The system was implemented in C++ on a PC with a Pentium 200 MHz processor.

Discussion

The Enhanced ChainMail algorithm addresses the need for modeling complex, inhomogeneous materials at interactive rates in simulations such as modeling the vitreous humor in the EyeSi project. The algorithm will be used in the EyeSi

Project but is also well suited for other tissue modeling applications. While the results and analysis presented here were limited to 2D, extension to 3D is straightforward.

While this work has demonstrated that the algorithm presented here will make simulation of the vitreous humor feasible, there are a number of important areas of future work. First, speed of the algorithm must be improved. For this reason, we have begun investigating parallelizing the Enchanced ChainMail algorithm. Because the algorithm considers x, y, and z displacements independently and the resultant deformation is a superposition of the solutions along these three axes, the system can easily be parallelized by calculating deformations along the x, y, and z axes on different processors.

Two additional limitations of the current Enhanced ChainMail Algorithm are that it does not model volume conservation, an important characteristic of many tissues in the human body, and that, because of the axis-aligned material constraints, it does not model inter-element rotation. There are at least two ways to impose volume conservation on the deforming volume. The first is to incorporate volume conservation into the Elastic Relaxation step of the two-process deformation system described above. The second is to change material constraints along the axes perpendicular to the deformation axis according to constraint violations in the direction of deformation. We have implemented this second approach in a test system with promising results. We have also begun investigating the addition of a new degree of freedom to indicate element orientation so that inter-element rotation can be modeled.

References

1. Biomedical Visualization Laboratory at University of Illinois. Model of the Eye. http://www.bvl.uic.edu/bvl/eye/.
2. M. Desbrun and M-P. Gascuel. Animating Soft Substances with Implicit Surfaces. In *SIGGRAPH '95*, pages 287 – 290, Los Angeles, CA, USA, 1995.
3. S. Gibson. 3D ChainMail: A Fast Algorithm for Deforming Volumetric Objects. In *1997 Symposium on Interactive 3D Graphics*, pages 149 – 154, Providence, RI, USA, April 1997.
4. A. Gröpl, T. Günther, J. Hesser, J. Kröll, R. Männer, C. Poliwoda, and C. Reinhart. Interactive Operation Planning and Control with VIRIM. In *Proc. Medicine Meets Virtual Reality 4*, pages 121–133, San Diego, CA, January 1996.
5. Medical College of Georgia & IMTC at GeorgiaTech. Simulation of a Catheract Surgery. http://www.oip.gatech.edu/MMTLPROJ/eye.html.
6. Mark A. Sagar, David Bullivant, Gordon D. Mallinson, and Peter J. Hunter. A Virtual Environment and Model of the Eye for Surgical Simulation. In *SIGGRAPH '94*, Anual Conference Series, pages 205–212, July 1994.
7. M. Schill, Ch. Reinhart, T. Günther, Ch. Poliwoda, J. Hesser, M. Schinkmann, H.-J. Bender, and R. Männer. Biomechanical Simulation of Brain Tissue and Real-time Volume Visualisation. Integrating Biomechanical Simulations into the VIRIM System. In *Proceedings of the international Symposium on Computer and Communication Systems for Imageguided Diagnosis and Therapy, Computer Assisted Radiology*, pages 283–288, Berlin, Germany, June 1997.

A Biomechanical Model of the Human Tongue and Its Clinical Implications

Yohan Payan[1], Georges Bettega[1,2], and Bernard Raphaël[2]

[1] Laboratoire TIMC/IMAG – UMR CNRS 5525 – Faculté de Médecine
Domaine de la Merci, La Tronche - France - Yohan.Payan@imag.fr
[2] Service de Chirurgie Plastique et Maxillo-Faciale
Centre Hospitalier Universitaire de Grenoble – France

Abstract. Many surgical technics act on the upper airway in general, and on the tongue in particular. For example, tongue is one of the anatomical structures involved in the case of Pierre Robin syndrome, mandibular prognathism, or sleep apnoea syndrome.
This paper presents the biomechanical and dynamical model of the human tongue we have developed, and the method we have used to fit this model to the anatomical and physical properties of a given patient's tongue. Each step of the modeling process is precisely described: the soft tissues modeling through the Finite Element Method (geometrical design of the FE structure within the upper airway and representation of lingual musculature), and the motor control of the model with the corresponding dynamical simulations. Finally, the syndromes listed above are presented, with some focus on the clinical implications of the model.

INTRODUCTION

Tongue is one of the anatomical structures implicated in the collapse of the upper airway, in obstructive sleep apnoea ([13]). Its muscular structure is also affected in the neonate troubles known as the syndrome of Pierre Robin ([15], [17]), or in the mandibular prognathism ([1], [4]). The development of a biomechanical model of tongue structure seems thus interesting, to understand the role played by human tongue tissues in the case of those syndromes. It may also be useful to evaluate and simulate some of the implications of surgical acts. This paper will present the biomechanical model of the human tongue, originally developed in the framework of an articulatory speech synthetiser ([12]). We will insist here on the way we have fit this model to the physical properties of a given patient. Finally, some syndromes involving tongue structure will be presented, and the usefulness of our model, in relation to those syndromes, will be discussed.

1 TONGUE ANATOMY

Tongue arrangement consists of a complex interweaving of active structures, the muscular fibers, and passive ones, mainly formed by glands and mucosa. The fantastic dexterity of this articulator is due to its structure, which contains a large amount of muscles, each of them being highly innervated. Indeed, ten muscles or so are able to shape precisely tongue structure in its sagittal, transverse and coronal planes. One particularity of those muscles is that most of them are internal to the structure, and are then responsible for their own deformation. Among all muscles which act on tongue structure, seven have an important influence on its shaping: the *genioglossus*, the *styloglossus*, the *hyoglossus*, the *verticalis*, the *transverse*, and the superior and inferior parts of the *longitudinalis* (figure 1).

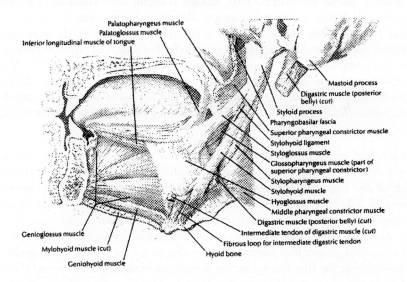

Fig. 1. Sagittal view of the human tongue musculature (from [11])

2 THE TONGUE MODEL

Perkell ([14]), with his 2D mass-spring model, has for the first time shown the interest of a physiological model of the tongue, to understand the respective contribution of each muscle in tongue's shaping. Following this concept, other biomechanical tongue models have been developed ([9], [18]). All of them have proposed a better analytical description of the continuous elastic structure of the tongue by the Finite Element Method. However, those models have not been evaluated and compared to measured tongue movements, as they were developed without any reference to the real measured properties of a given biological human tongue. To evaluate the ability of our model to precisely replicate the deformations observed on human tongue, we have decided to build a patient-specific model, i.e. the copy of the biological tongue of a human subject.

2.1 Definition of the model

Our modeling approach was first dedicated to the choice of a mathematical tool able to describe the lingual deformations. Then, the structure was designed to fit the external shape of the reference patient's upper airways, and inserted into their corresponding contours. Finally, internal and external muscular fibers were defined, in order to give to the tongue structure its ability to move.

The Finite Element Method to model tongue soft tissues. The mathematical tool chosen to describe tongue deformation was the Finite Element Method (FEM). This method allows a precise description of the continuous, elastic and uncompressible properties of a body. For this, the physical properties of the body are taken into account through two elastic constants : the Young modulus E, which measures its stiffness, and the Poisson's ratio ν, related to its compressibility. Moreover, it permits, via the notion of element, to attribute specific biomechanical properties to individual regions of the structure.

Geometrical shaping of the FE structure within the upper airways. Our aim was to develop a biomechanical model as close as possible to the morphological and physical characteristics of a given patient. That is the reason why the patient PB, who had already been subject to a large amount of articulatory data recordings (X-Ray, electropalatographies, electromagnetic recordings, MRI), was retained as our reference patient. Tongue description was limited to the midsagittal plane, in accordance with the fact that the main articulatory data available in the literature describe tongue movements in this sagittal plane. The first stage of tongue shaping was then to collect a given X-ray picture of PB's tongue, associated to a rest position of his lingual articulator. The corresponding radiography gives, in the midsagittal plane, the upper airways contours (hard palate, velar regions, pharynx and larynx), the shape and position of the mandible, the lips, the hyoid bone, and the external contour of the tongue, as a reference for the rest shaping of our model (figure 2.a). An isoparametric mesh, composed of 48 elements, was then defined and distributed inside the tongue structure. The FE tongue model was finally inserted into PB's upper airways contours (figure 2.b). Tongue insertions on jaw and hyoid bone were modeled by imposing no displacements of the corresponding nodes.

Tongue muscles modeling. The great majority of tongue muscles are left/right muscle pairs, i.e. muscles composed of two symmetrical parts along the sagittal plane. Our modeling approach has considered the two symmetrical parts of each tongue muscle as a unique entity, acting in the sagittal plane. Furthermore, we have only modeled muscles whose action has significant influence on tongue shaping in the sagittal plane, namely the posterior and anterior parts of the genioglossus, the hyoglossus, the styloglossus, the inferior and superior longitudinalis, and the verticalis.

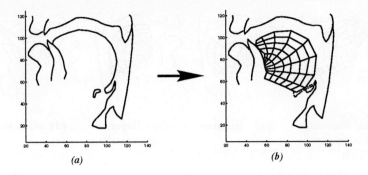

Fig. 2. The 48 elements (63 nodes) building the model are shaped (b) to give the model the rest configuration of the patient's tongue (a).

Choice for the FE elastic parameters. Young modulus E and Poisson's ratio ν values have to be carefully chosen, as they directly influence the way the FE structure will be deformed under muscular actions. The choice for the ν value was the simplest one, because of the specific tongue physiological structure. Indeed, tongue tissues are mainly composed of water (see for example the density of $1040 kg/m^3$ reported by Duck ([6]) for human muscle tissues). In order to model this quasi-incompressibility, a 0.49 ν value was chosen. As concerns the Young modulus, its value is directly related to the stiffness of tongue body. If no data, from our knowledge, are available in the literature about E value for tongue tissues, some measurements are reported for other soft part of human body ([10], [6]). Moreover, some measurements of forces developed by each tongue muscle during speech production were provided by Bunton and Weismer ([2]). Those levels of forces were used to act on tongue muscles, in order to compare the FE deformations with the lingual deformations measured on PB during some speech sequences. This helped us in tuning the Young modulus value, which was finally fixed to 15 kPa. Once the elastic parameters have been chosen, the lingual deformations induced by each modeled muscle can be computed. Figure 3 plots the actions of four muscles, namely the posterior part of the genioglossus, the hyoglossus, the superior longitudinalis, and the styloglossus. Each muscle is composed of one to three macro-fibers, on which global muscle force is distributed.

Dynamics in the model. The biomechanical model of the tongue is now able to be animated under the coordination of all the modeled muscles. For this, we have retained, for the control of tongue movements, the concepts developed by feldman ([7]), and proposed more generally for the control of human limb movements. Those propositions are based on a *functional* model of force generation, for which the level of force depends on muscle length and rate of length from one hand, and on a central command, called the "λ command", on the other hand (see [12] for more details about this neurophysiological model for force generation). Following this hypothesis, it is assumed that the Central Nervous System

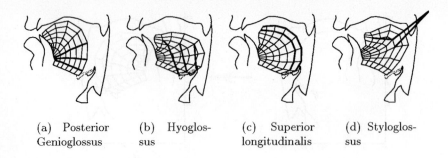

(a) Posterior Genioglossus (b) Hyoglossus (c) Superior longitudinalis (d) Styloglossus

Fig. 3. Contribution of some tongue muscles to the global tongue shaping. The macrofibers, modeling the muscles forces, are shown by the bold lines.

controls the temporal evolution of each muscular λ command. The corresponding movements of the FE tongue structure has then to be computed. For this, the temporal evolution of U, $\dot{U}$ and $\ddot{U}$, respectively the displacement, velocity and acceleration vectors (dimension: 63 x 2) of the structure's nodes, is computed by solving the equation of motion via the adaptive Runge Kutta method :

$$M\ddot{U} + f\dot{U} + K(U,\dot{U},\lambda)U = F(U,\dot{U},\lambda) + P \qquad (1)$$

M is the global mass matrix (100 g for the whole tongue);
f is the global passive damping matrix (viscosity coefficient = 15 N s/m) ;
K is the stiffness matrix, modeling the passive elastic behaviour of the tongue and computed by means of the FE technique ; this matrix depends on central commands, muscle length and rate of muscle length change, since some elements have a Young modulus modified by muscle activation ;
F is a vector of forces exerted by muscles, and concentrated on specific nodes ;
P is the vector of all external forces acting on each node : gravity and contact forces (tongue against the teeth or the palate).

Figure 4 shows the successive tongue shapes obtained with a linear shift of the hyoglossus and posterior genioglossus central commands (patterns used to move the tongue from a front and high position towards a back and low one).

3 CLINICAL IMPLICATIONS OF THE MODEL

Some implications could be drawn concerning the usefulness of a biomechanical modeling, at the clinical level. In particular, it is interesting to focus on syndromes involving tongue structure, namely the Pierre Robin syndrome ([15], [17]), mandibular prognathism ([1], [4]), or sleep apnoea syndrome ([13]).

3.1 Pierre Robin Syndrome

The combination of micro-retromandibulism, glossoptosis, palatal clefting and respiratory troubles observed in the neonate is known as the syndrome of Pierre

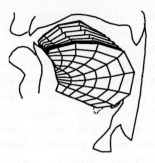

Fig. 4. Dynamical tongue deformations under the coordinated action of posterior genioglossus and hyoglossus muscles.

Robin ([15]). The pathogenesis is a disturbance of muscular maturation of nervous origin and the syndrome belongs to the category of muscular dysmaturations which affects the masticatory muscles, the tongue and the pharyngeal slings. Swallowing is disturbed and airway obstructed, resulting in the aspiration of secretion and foods. The respiratory difficulties are further increased by the low and posterior position of the tongue. A lateral radiographic soft tissue view shows the ptotic tongue to be positioned below the mandibular angle, pressing on the epiglottis. Clinical inspection shows three crests: mandibular, sublingual and lingual. The malformation is characterised by a functional disturbance of the tongue which may be associated with a palatal cleft. The degree of lingual protrusion is a criterion of the evolution of the syndrome. Various treatments are possible. Skilled nursing care with the child in prone position, maintained by a frame, is the treatment most commonly used ([3]). Application of a palatal plate to hold the tongue in forward position and lingual rehabilitation by stimulation of suction are complementary methods of treatment. Some cases are surgically treated, either by mandibulohyoid fixation or better by a submental myoplasty ([5]) ; the tracheotomy is exceptionally used.

The biomechanical model of the tongue could be useful to obtain a prognostic factor of the neuro-muscular dysmaturation. This would help to precise the therapeutic strategy and should give objective elements for the follow-up.

3.2 Mandibular prognathism

Dentofacial deformity of the lower third of the face resulting from excess mandibular growth is not as common as mandibular deficiency. However the frequency of class III malocclusion (anterior placement of mandibular teeth compared with maxillary teeth) is approximately 1 to 3 % of the population, depending on age and geographic variation. The deformity is related to an excess of mandibular development or to a retrusion of maxilla, but the majority of patients associate both abnormalities. The etiology of mandibular excess has been studied extensively, but the primary determinant is still controversial. However, tongue position and tongue function seem to be an important factor in the etio-pathogeny of the problem, and seem to be one of the major causes of relapse of the dysmorphosis after treatment (either orthodontic or surgical). Very often, the tongue of those patients is flat and anteriorly displaced, this causes a widened mandibular arch and a narrow maxillary arch with high palate. The goal of treatment is to correct the occlusion (dental position) either with an isolated orthodontic work or with an association of orthodontics and orthognathic surgery. But the therapeutic plan must include the correction of tongue position and function to avoid relapse. Usually this part is assumed by the orthophonist, but in some cases surgical tongue reduction (glossectomy) should be discussed, even if controversial. In the framework of the mandibular prognathism, the implications of a biomechanical model of the human tongue are numerous :

- To identify and appreciate the participation of tongue malposition or of tongue dysfunction in the etiology of mandibular prognathism.
- To identify the patients who present a risk of relapse after treatment (orthodontic or surgical treatment) in a way to prevent this by activation of the re-education by the orthophonist.
- To prove the uselessness of glossectomy in the treatment of prognathism.
- The same protocol should be extended to the dysmorphosis with an open bite anomaly. In this case the problem seem to be, very often, the interposition of the tongue between dental arches.

3.3 Sleep apnoea syndrome

Airway closure during sleep apnoea syndrome (SAS) comes from the interaction between inspiratory flow and the upper airway that is formed by the succession of anatomical and physiological singularities with their own geometrical and mechanical properties ([13]). The tongue is one of the anatomical structures implicated in the collapse. Some of the surgical techniques associated to the SAS reduce the volume of the tongue, while others try to have a more global and progressive action on the entire upper airway. In order to fully understand the metamorphosis in inspiratory flow pattern that has been reported during SAS, some mechanical models of the upper airway have been developed, assuming that upper airways can be represented by a single compliant segment ([16]), or by series of individual segments representing singularities ([8]).

In this framework, a complete biomechanical model of the tongue appears thus to be interesting, to describe and explain, at the mechanical point of view, the upper airway obstruction.

CONCLUSION

The biomechanical model of the tongue we have developed was presented in details, with specific focuses on its relation to the physical properties of a given patient. Special emphasis was put onto the shaping of the FE tongue structure, the definition of muscular fibers, as well as the choice of FE elastic parameters. Some points supporting an anthropomorphic modeling and its use for clinical applications were given and discussed.

ACKNOWLEDGEMENTS

The biomechanical work was carried out with Pascal Perrier, from the ICP (Grenoble, France), and supported by the grant INSERM PARMPSTRC 9607.

References

1. H. Bell. *Modern practice in orthognathic and reconstructive surgery*, volume 3. WB Saunders company, Philadelphia, 1992.
2. K. Bunton and G. Weismer. Evaluation of a reiterant force-impulse task in the tongue. *Journal of Speech and Hearing Research*, 37:1020–1031, 1994.
3. W.R Burston. *Neonatal surgery*, chapter Mandibular retrognathia. Rickham P.P. and Johnston J.H. eds, London, 1969.
4. J. Delaire. *la langue et dysmorphie*, chapter la langue et dysmorphie, page 81. Masson, Paris, 1996.
5. R.P Delorme, Y. Laroque, and L. Caouette-Laberge. Innovative surgical approach for the pierre robin anomalad : subperiostal release of the floor of the mouth musculature. *Plast. Reconstr. Surg.*, 83:960–64, 1989.
6. F.A. Duck. *Physical properties of tissues: a comprehensive reference book*. Academic Press, London, 1990.
7. A.G. Feldman. Once more on the equilibrium-point hypothesis (λ model) for motor control. *Journal of Motor Behavior*, 18(1):17–54, 1986.
8. R. Fodil, C. Ribreau, B. Louis, F. Lofaso, and D. Isabey. Interaction between steady flow and individualised compliant segments: application to upper airways. *Medical & Biological Engineering & Computing*, November 1997.
9. K. Honda. Organization of tongue articulation for vowels. *Journal of Phonetics*, 24:39–52, 1996.
10. Y. Min, I. Titze, and F. Alipour. Stress-strain response of the human vocal ligament. *NCVS Status and Progress*, 7:131–137, 1994.
11. F.H Netter. Atlas of human anatomy. Technical report, CIBA-GEIGY Corporation editor, 1989.
12. Y. Payan and P. Perrier. Synthesis of v-v sequences with a 2d biomechanical tongue model controlled by the equilibrium point hypothesis. *Speech Communication*, 22(2–3):185–205, 1997.
13. J.L Pépin, D. Veale, and G. Ferreti. Evaluation of the upper airway in sleep apnea syndrome. *Sleep*, 15:s50–s55, 1992.
14. J.S Perkell. *A physiologically-oriented model of tongue activity in speech production*. PhD thesis, Massachusetts Institute of Technology, Boston, 1974.
15. P. Robin. La glossoptose. Un grave danger pour nos enfants. Doin ed., Paris, 1929.
16. P.L. Smith, R.A. Wise, A.R. Gold, A.R. Schwarts, and S. Permutt. Upper airway pressure-flow relationship in obstructive slepp apnea. *J. Appl. physiol*, 64:789–795, 1998.
17. M. Stricker, J. Van Der Meulen, B. Raphael, and R. Mazzola. *Craniofacial malformations*. Churchill Linvingstone ed., Edingburgh, 1990.
18. R. Wilhelms-Tricarico. Physiological modeling of speech production: Methods for modeling soft-tissues articulators. *J. Acoust. Soc. of Am.*, 97(5):3085–3098, 1995.

Three-Dimensional Joit Kinematics Using Bone Surface Registration: A Computer Assisted Approach with an Application to the Wrist Joint *in vivo*

*[†]Joseph J. Crisco, *Robert D. McGovern, [‡]Scott W. Wolfe

*Department of Orthopaedics, Rhode Island Hospital, Providence, RI;
[†]Division of Engineering, Brown University, Providence, RI;
[‡]Department of Orthopaedics, Yale University School of Medicine, New Haven, CT

Please address correspondence to:
Joseph J. Crisco, Ph D
Bioengineering Lab SWP-3
Rhode Island Hospital
593 Eddy Street
Providence, RI 02903
phone: 401-444-4231
fax: 401-444-4559
email: joseph_crisco_iii@brown.edu

Abstract. The majority of the present knowledge of the three-dimensional kinematic behavior of skeletal joints has been acquired in studies employing cadaveric models using invasive procedures. In the wrist, the small size and complex motion of the carpal bones present a difficult challenge for an invasive kinematic analysis or external marker system. This paper describes an approach to quantify the three-dimensional kinematics of the wrist and carpal bones *in vivo*, using non-invasive computed tomographic (CT) imaging. The applications of this method include quantification of normal wrist motion, analysis of pathomechanics, and evaluation of surgical intervention. The approach is also applicable to other joints and imaging modalities.

INTRODUCTION

Kinematic analysis has been widely used to study normal joints, and the effects of pathology, acute trauma, and reconstructive procedures on joint motion. Most of the studies on human joints have been performed in cadaveric specimens. Previous *in vivo* joint motion studies have been limited to a two-dimensional kinematic analysis with plane radiography or to invasive procedures such as transcutaneous bone pins[7] or implantable bone markers[5]. Such invasive procedures are not well accepted by volunteers and the utility of bone pins is further compromised by mechanical impingement and tethering of soft tissues. The advantages of analyzing joint motion *in vivo* include the incorporation of true muscular forces, which are either neglected or simulated in cadaveric studies, and the ability to evaluate the long term effects of healing and surgical intervention. Recently, researchers have successfully measured the three-dimensional *in vivo* kinematics of the long bones of the knee joint using non-invasive techniques[1]. Due to the complexity, shape and small size of the carpal bones, the existing techniques for measuring three-dimensional kinematics are not applicable to the wrist.

Our aim was to develop a noninvasive method to measure 3D *in vivo* motion of the carpal bones. The purpose of this paper is to briefly present our approach and interactive computer method for quantification and visualization of complex 3D *in vivo* kinematics. This method may be used to evaluate surgical treatments, study kinematics of joint replacement, generate quantified diagnostic information on aberrant kinematics, and provide 3D animation for professional and patient education.

METHODS

For the purposes of illustrating the method, the *in vivo* kinematics of selected carpal bones were quantified in a single uninjured subject. The steps described in the method are image acquisition, segmentation of bone surfaces, kinematic analysis, and visualization.

Image acquisition was performed while the left wrist was positioned in three different positions: radial deviation, neutral, and ulnar deviation. Volume images of a 60 mm segment of the wrist extending from the radioulnar metaphysis to the proximal metacarpals were acquired using a HiSpeed Advantage CT scanner (GE Medical Systems, Milwaukee, WI) and exposure parameters of 80 mA, 80 kVp and 1 second. Volume images were collected in axial format with voxel dimensions of 0.187 x 0.187 x 1 mm^3. The images were transferred to a Silicon Graphics workstation (Indigo^2 XZ, SGI, Mountain View, CA) on which all image processing was done using a 3D biomedical imaging software system (*Analyze*, Biomedical Imaging Resource, Rochester, MN).

Segmentation was defined as the process of extracting bone contours and associating each contour with the individual carpal bones. Defining the outer surfaces of the eight carpal bones presents a challenging segmentation problem because of the narrow articular spaces and highly curved shapes. Segmentation was performed in several steps: thresholding, extraction, and association. The CT volumes were thresholded to emphasize the outer cortical shell. In each image slice, bone contour coordinates were extracted after each bone cross-section was closed and filled[10]. This resulted in multiple contours for each cross-section. To associate each contour with its respective carpal bone, we developed an interactive approach using custom software (Open Inventor, C++, Silicon Graphics, Inc.; MATLAB, Mathworks, Natick, MA). The software generated 3D images of the contours and created an interactive handle at each contour's centroid. The interactive handles enabled the user to manipulate the view and manually associate each contour with its proper bone. Segmentation was completed by exporting the 3D surface coordinates for the contours of each bone.

Kinematic analysis was performed under the assumption that each bone moved independently as a rigid body in 3D. The kinematic variables were calculated by registering the bone, described by its surface points obtained from segmentation, from one position to another position. Registering the bone's centroid and principal axes of inertia provided an initial estimate of the kinematic variables[3]. Final registration and the resulting kinematic variables were obtained by minimizing the mean distance between the bone's surfaces using an algorithm developed by Pelizzari et al[9]. The helical axis of motion (HAM) was chosen to uniquely describe the 3D kinematics with a rotation about and translation along an axis in space. The motions of each of the capitate, scaphoid, and lunate bones were calculated relative to the radius.

Visualization of bone position and orientation was helpful to ensure successful reconstruction of the images. The segmented contours were rendered as solid bone cross-sections using specifically written code in C++ and Open Inventor. Better visualization and an improved estimate of the bone's true surface was obtained by generating a triangular surface mesh (B. Geiger, Nuages, INRIA, France). Animations using the kinematic data and reconstructed bones can also be created to provide dynamic viewing of the results.

RESULTS

The simple motion of wrist radial and ulnar deviation resulted in complex coupled motions of the carpal bones that were visualized by rendering the bone surfaces. These renderings are three dimensional models that can be viewed from any orientation (Fig. 1).

For the single subject in radial deviation, the motions of the scaphoid and lunate were notably distinct from those of the capitate (Fig. 2A). The helical rotation angle of the capitate (33.9°) was nearly twice that of both the scaphoid (18.4°) and lunate (14.7°). The helical translation of the capitate (0.7 mm) was similar to that of the scaphoid (0.6 mm), while there was no measurable helical translation of the lunate (<0.01 mm). Each helical axis passed through the proximal portion of the capitate. The orientation of the helical axis of the capitate was approximately dorsal-ventral, while the helical axes of the scaphoid and lunate were roughly orthogonal in a medial-lateral orientation. These relative orientations of the helical axis demonstrate that the scaphoid and lunate exhibited coupled flexion as the capitate rotated with the wrist in radial deviation.

In ulnar deviation, the motions of scaphoid and lunate were more similar to those of the capitate (Fig. 2B). The helical rotation of the capitate (25.9°) was similar to both the scaphoid (25.2°) and lunate (24.8°). In contrast to radial deviation, the helical translations of each carpal bone were notable and similar (each approximately 2.5 mm). While the helical axes passed through the proximal capitate, as in radial deviation, there was less of a difference in their orientation.

DISCUSSION

We have demonstrated a method to accurately and noninvasively measure 3D joint kinematics *in vivo*. The method was illustrated using CT volume images of a single wrist, however it can be applied to the study of all skeletal joints with any medical imaging modality from which 3D surfaces can be accurately segmented. Despite the small size, complex shape and motion patterns of the carpal bones, the present method was shown to be capable of tracking *in vivo* 3D motions. The motions reported here were similar to those reported previously using cadaveric specimens implanted with radio-opaque markers[6]. A more detailed comparison can be accomplished once this methodology has been a applied to a larger number of subjects.

A detailed analysis of accuracy is an extensive study because of the numerous contributing factors such as bone size and shape, voxel size, image quality, scanning orientation, and the particular registration method. Accuracy varies for each bone within the same the wrist image because of differences in bone size and shape. A preliminary study of kinematic accuracy found that the HAM angle and translation errors were typically less than 0.6 degrees and 0.5 mm, although the lunate errors were slightly larger[4]. When the method is employed to study pathokinematics, the most crucial issue will become the level of accuracy required to detect clinically significant differences, and this will be determined in part by the specific clinical disease to be studied. Each of these factors requires further study.

Application of segmentation techniques to medical imaging has developed rapidly and several investigators have developed protocols for use in studying the carpus[2, 8, 11]. A detailed comparison of the efficacy of the various approaches to segmenting the bone surface is difficult because of the lack of a common data base, however, any segmentation method may be used with the kinematic analysis presented here. One limitation of our method is that the calculated kinematics are quasi-static; motion is calculated between two fixed positions. This limitation is not inherent in the method, but is due to the time required to acquire multiple CT volume images. Decreasing the interval between fixed positions will improve the ability of this technique to simulate true motion, however radiation exposure will increase. Future advances in real time scanning techniques may eliminate this limitation. While radiation exposure is always a concern, the recent generation CT scanner used in this study produced exposure levels for nine complete volume images that totaled well below governmental guidelines.

The complexity and the number of wrist bones results in a voluminous amount of kinematic data. Our approach includes a method for visualizing these complex motions which should help in understanding joint kinematics and aid in research and educational applications. Future studies should also generate a database with which *in vitro* and computer models can be validated. The application of this 3D kinematic method to pathological conditions and to evaluation of surgical interventions may assist in diagnosis and treatment of complex disorders of the carpus.

ACKNOWLEDGMENTS.

We would like to thank Lee Katz, M.D. for his assistance in acquiring the CT images. This work was supported in part by NIH AR44005.

REFERENCES

1. Banks SA, Markovitch GD, Hodge WA. In vivo kinematics of the cruciate retaining and substituting knee replacements. *J Arthroplasty*, 12(3): 297-304, 1997.
2. Belsole RJ, Hilbelink DR, Llewellyn JA, Dale M, Ogden JA. Carpal orientation from computed reference axes. *J Hand Surg*. 16A(1): 82-90, 1991.
3. Crisco JJ, McGovern RD. Efficient calculation of mass moments of inertia for segmented homogeneous 3D objects. *J Biomech*, 31(1):97-101, 1998.
4. Crisco JJ, McGovern RD, Wolfe SW. Three dimensional kinematics of carpal bones: an in vitro error analysis. *Am Soc Biomech Conference*, Clemson, SC, Sept 22-24, 1997.
5. de Lange A, Kauer JMG, Huiskes R. Kinematic Behavior of the Human Wrist Joint: A Roentgen-Stereophotogrammetric Analysis. *J Orthop Res*, 3:56-64, 1985.
6. Horii E, Garcia-Elias M, An KN, Linscheid RL, Bishop AT, Cooney WP, Chao EYS. A kinematic study of lunotriquetral dissociations. *J Hand Surgery*, 16(2):355-362, 1991.
7. Lafortune MA, Cavanagh PR, Sommer HJ, Kalenak A. Three-dimensional kinematics of the human knee during walking. *J Biomech*, 25(4):347-358, 1992.
8. Patterson RM, Elder KW, Viegas SF, Buford WL. Carpal bone anatomy measured by computer analysis of three-dimensional reconstructions of computed tomography images. *J Hand Surgery*, 20(6):923-929, 1995.
9. Pelizzari CA, Chen GT, Spelbring DR, Weichselbaum RR, Chen CT. Accurate three-dimensional registration of CT, PET, and/or MR images of the brain. *J Comput Assist Tomogr*, 13(1):20-26, 1989.
10. Robb RA. Three-dimensional Biomedical Imaging: Principles and Practice. VCH, N.Y., N.Y., 1995.
11. Viegas SF, Hillman GR, Elder K, Stoner D, Patterson RM. Measurement of carpal bone geometry by computer analysis of three-dimensional CT images. *J Hand Surg*, 18A(2):341-349, 1993.

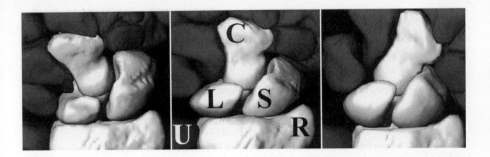

Fig. 1. Three-dimensional dorsal view of the left wrist of a healthy subject. The CT volume images were collected in ulnar deviation (left), neutral (middle) and radial deviation (right) of the wrist. The long axis of the capitate (C) follows wrist motion which is occurring in the plane of the paper. These renderings illustrate the complex 3D motion of the scaphoid (S) and lunate (L): in ulnar deviation the lunate and the scaphoid also extend (rotate out of the paper) and in radial deviation they also flex (rotate into the paper), relative to their neutral orientations. For reference and clarity the ulna (U) and radius (R) are labeled and the other bones have been darkened.

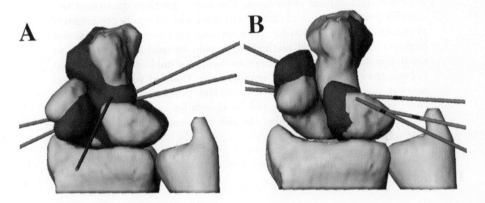

Fig. 2. The location and orientation of the helical axes are rendered here for the motion of the scaphoid, lunate and capitate from the neutral position to radial deviation (A) and ulnar deviation (B) relative to the radius (palmer view).

Range of Motion After Total Hip Arthroplasty: Simulation of Non-axisymmetric Implants

Constantinos Nikou[1], Branislav Jaramaz[1,2], and Anthony M. DiGioia[1,2]

[1] Center for Medical Robotics and Computer Assisted Surgery,
Carnegie Mellon University, Pittsburgh, PA
costa@ri.cmu.edu   http://www.mrcas.ri.cmu.edu
[2] Center for Orthopaedic Research, UPMC Shadyside Hospital, Pittsburgh, PA
{branko, digioia}@cs.cmu.edu   http://www.cor.ssh.edu

Abstract. Dislocation following total hip replacement surgery represents a significant cause of early failure, incurring additional medical costs and patient distress. One major cause of dislocation is implant impingement. The most important factor in preventing implant impingement is correct implant orientation. This paper describes the newest version of a prosthetic range of motion simulator which permits prediction of prosthetic range of motion for non-axisymmetric femoral and acetabular implants. This analytical methodology could be used as a preoperative simulation tool that can help surgeons decide the implant placement that reduces the chance of implant impingement. Coupled with a computer-assisted clinical system for precise implant positioning, this approach could significantly reduce the risk of dislocation, maximize the "safe" range of motion, and minimize the risk for complications arising from impingement.

1 Introduction

The incidence of implant dislocation following total hip replacement (THR) surgery ranges between 2 and 6% [3, 12] and represents a significant cause of early implant failure, incurring additional costs to the total surgery expenses. The causes of dislocation are related to factors such as surgical approach, soft tissue tension, prosthetic design, and most importantly, orientation of components. One possible dislocation mechanism is the impingement of prosthetic components, in which the implant neck hits the rim of the acetabular liner and levers the head out of the socket [2]. In addition to dislocation, implant impingement causes excessive wear of the cup liner and creation of debris. Proper alignment of implant components, which is patient and implant specific, reduces the incidence of impingement and reduces the risk of associated complications.

Previously, we have developed and experimentally verified a preoperative analytical simulator that takes into account implant design, placement and orientation, and predicts the range of motion (ROM) and impingement limits [5, 6]. The simulator enabled surgeons to preoperatively optimize the parameters in the placement of axisymmetric implants in order to reduce the probability of implant impingement and dislocation during normal patient motion. However, non-axisymmetric cup liners and femoral implant necks, provided as part of commercial pre-designed implant systems and as custom implants, are in wide use. Recognizing this, we have extended the prosthetic range of motion (PROM) simulator to include models of non-axisymmetric implants.

Coupled with CT-based three-dimensional preoperative planning and image-guided positioning of implant components, this methodology has the potential of precise implementation, ensuring optimal outcomes with respect to risk of dislocation.

2 Background

The most common cause of dislocation after THR is implant impingement caused by malposition of components [12]. A number of researchers and clinicians have examined this phenomenon, in an effort to explain mechanisms of dislocation. Amstutz and Markolf [2] described three modes of dislocation: 1) due to poor tissue tension, the prosthetic head climbs the socket wall and slips over the rim of the socket, 2) the neck impinges on the socket wall and levers the head from the socket, and 3) the neck impinges on a bony prominence.

Some researchers have tried to identify the range of cup orientations that are less prone to dislocations, based on the geometric similarity of human anatomies. Lewinnek et al. [10] demonstrated that the cases falling in the zone of 15±10 degrees of anteversion and 40±10 degrees of abduction have an instability rate of 1.5%, compared with a 6% instability rate for the cases falling outside this zone. No attention was paid, however, to the design of either the cup, the design of the femoral component, or the femoral component orientation.

Although the mechanism of implant impingement is well understood, the attempts to model the phenomenon were until recently limited mainly to experimental procedures, in which a physical model is created to simulate the range of motion. Most investigators [2, 12] realized that the head-to-neck ratio of the femoral component is the key factor of the implant impingement. However, few have attempted to quantify the relationship between the implant design and orientation and the incidence of dislocation. Some experimental studies examined how specific implant design influences the prosthetic range of motion. Amstutz et al. [1] and Krushell et al. [8] examined experimentally the influence of different prosthetic designs and the influence of prosthetic orientation. However, general quantitative results based on constant head-neck ratios cannot be readily applied to use of non-axisymmetric implants because the head-neck ratio for an implant pair changes as a function of implant and position.

Other researchers have examined the effect of acetabular cup design. Krushell et al. [9] evaluated the ROM of two types of elevated-rim liners compared with standard liners. They concluded that an optimally oriented elevated-rim liner may improve the joint stability with respect to implant impingement. Cobb et al. [3] have demonstrated a statistically significant reduction of dislocations in the case of elevated-rim liners, compared to standard liners. The two-year probability of dislocation was 2.19% for the elevated liner, compared with 3.85% for the standard liner. They raised the concern, however, of possible long-term effects of the elevated liner on wear and loosening. Initial results of a finite element study by Maxian et al. [11] indicate that the contact stresses and therefore the polyethylene wear are not significantly increased in the extended lip case.

Analytical modeling of range of motion has only recently become a subject of interest for researchers. Maxian et al. [11] have looked at the dislocation propensity for different liner designs, although dislocation was not considered in the context of range of motion. Jaramaz et al. developed an analytical model (along with experimental validation) for calculating range of motion for a given size and orientation of only axisymmetric implant components [5,6].

3 Methods

3.1 Coordinate systems and transformations

In order to establish appropriate relationships between the leg motion, position of the pelvis in the body, and relative orientations of implant components, we have to define relevant coordinate systems. We define the body coordinate system as follows: the Y axis points superiorly, parallel to the coronal and midsagittal planes; the X axis points to the patient's left, parallel to the coronal and transversal body planes; the Z axis is perpendicular to both X and Y and points to the anterior (Figure 1).

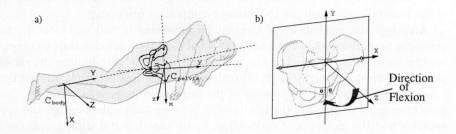

Fig. 1. a) Body and pelvic coordinate systems. b) Definition of the pelvic coordinate system as defined by landmark points on the pelvis

To define the pelvic coordinate system we use the pelvic anterior plane, defined by the anterior superior iliac spine and pubis symphisis points, and the symmetry plane of the pelvis (Figure 1). The pelvic X and Y axes lie parallel to this plane, with X to the patient's left, and Y pointed toward the patients head. Position of the pelvis is expressed as a flexion value. We define flexion as rotation about the body X axis. Neutral pelvic position (where the pelvis has zero degrees flexion) is defined as being aligned with the body coordinate system. The orientation of the pelvis relative to the body can be expressed as a 3x3 rotation matrix $^{body}\text{R}_{pelvis}$. This transform, along with its inverse, $^{pelvis}\text{R}_{body}$, can be easily derived from the flexion value.

Furthermore, we define a femoral coordinate system so that one axis (Y) corresponds to the mechanical axis of the femur, i.e., connects the center of the femoral head and the center of the condyles. The other axes are parallel with corresponding body axes in neutral standing position. Following common definitions, flexion/extension is then defined as rotation around the body X axis, ab/adduction as rotation around the body Z axis, and internal/external rotation as rotation around the femoral Y axis. Ab/adduction in flexion is rotation around the body Y axis subsequent to flexion. Any motion and position of the leg can be described as a result of a sequence of these basic motion components. We can establish a 3D rotation matrix $^{body}\text{R}_{femur}$ which describes the position of the femur relative to the body frame. Femoral neutral position is attained when the femoral coordinate frame is aligned rotationally with the body frame.

Both the femoral implant neck and the acetabular cup have associated coordinate systems as well. The orientation of the femoral implant neck is described as an ordered pair of abduction and anteversion rotations relative to the femoral coordinate frame. Neck abduction is defined as rotation about the femoral Z (the coordinate axis pointing to the anterior) and neck anteversion is rotation about the femoral Y. Again, these rotations are sequential, with abduction occurring first. The rotations from the neutral position define a 3D rotation matrix $^{femur}\text{R}_{neck}$.

The coordinate frame of the cup is defined as follows: the origin lies at the center of femoral rotation; the Z axis (also referred to as the cup axis) is normal to the opening of the cup; the other axes are normal to the Z axis. Normally, cup placement is described as a pair of rotations. DiGioia et al. described three systems for describing cup placement [4]. Their studies, however, assumed an axisymmetric cup, so only two parameters were required to describe cup orientation. The current PROM simulator supports these three description systems appending a rotation about the cup Z axis (a cup "twist") to each. Any of these systems is sufficient to define a full 3D rotation in the pelvic frame $^{pelvis}\text{R}_{cup}$, along with its inverse $^{cup}\text{R}_{pelvis}$. By the rules of transform arithmetic, we can calculate the position of the implant neck in the cup coordinate frame by the equation:

$$^{cup}\text{R}_{pelvis} * {}^{pelvis}\text{R}_{body} * {}^{body}\text{R}_{femur} * {}^{cup}\text{R}_{neck} = {}^{cup}\text{R}_{neck} \ . \quad (1)$$

3.2 Displaying range of motion

The parameters necessary to evaluate PROM limited by neck-liner impingement are the geometries of both the implant neck and the cup liner, and the orientation of the neck relative to the cup implant liner. Leg motion is defined as motion relative to the body coordinate system. It is important to define leg motion to be relative to the body and independent of pelvic position because studies have shown significant differences in pelvic orientation for various patient positions (e.g., sitting vs. standing positions) [7].

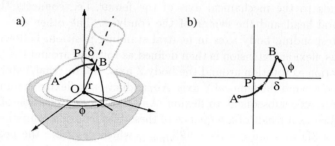

Fig. 2. Definition of angles ϕ and δ and their corresponding value on the PROM plot. Movement of the neck axis from point A to point B (diagram "a") corresponds to curve AB on the PROM plot (diagram "b")

The knowledge of these parameters allows us to analyze the motion of the femoral implant neck in the coordinate frame of the acetabular cup. In a special case of the axisymmetric femoral neck, the problem can be reduced to tracking the axis of the neck liner and detecting whether it is within a domain defined by the cup liner geometry. For any position of the leg during motion one can track the position of the femoral neck in the spherical coordinate system placed in the center of the femoral head. These positions can be simply displayed on a two-dimensional polar coordinate plot as a function of two angles, ϕ and δ (Figure 2). The permissible ROM domain of the cup for a given neck geometry can then be defined by an "impingement circle" (this object is not necessarily circular, but a closed curve in (ϕ, δ) space) where the limits of motion are plotted in the same (ϕ, δ) space as the neck trajectory [5].

For more general implant geometries, such a simplification is not possible. In the non-axisymmetric case, the safe PROM will change for a given cup/femoral implant pair depending on femoral orientation. The safe ROM envelope is therefore not independent of neck orientation as in the axisymmetric case because the limits in any direction are dependent on the point of the neck where impingement will occur (Figure 3). In order to keep analysis simple, however, a two-dimensional ROM plot is still desired.

The rim of the cup liner is represented on the plot as a closed curve in (ϕ, δ) space. This curve also represents the envelope of safe (non-impinging) PROM. The trajectory of the implant neck can be displayed as the path of its axis in (ϕ, δ) cup space. Any trajectory that maintains safe PROM will lie within the cup liner curve. The neck trajectory curve represents only the path of the neck axis, however. We need to represent the surface of the neck because that is what will collide with the cup liner.

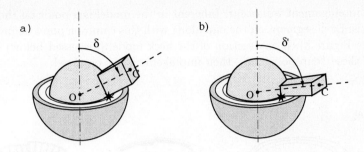

Fig. 3. Dependency of maximum δ angle on rotation orientation of the femoral implant neck. PROM is much greater in certain directions for case "a" than case "b"

When the neck of the implant impinges, it most likely impinges at one point only. This point lies on the cup liner as well as the neck. This point lies on a sphere centered at the origin O. The intersection of this sphere with the femoral neck surface is a closed curve which can be plotted on the PROM plot in (ϕ, δ) coordinates. The impingement point lies on the plot at the intersection of the cup liner curve and the neck outline (Figure 4).

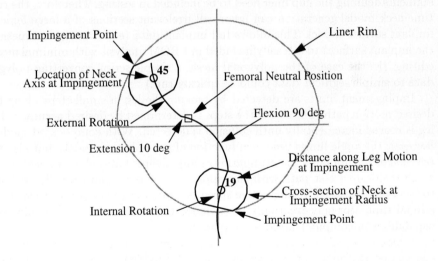

Fig. 4. PROM Plot example

3.3 Modeling and collision detection

The cup liner model is defined by a collection of ordered segments. These segments are a discretization of a continuous curve on the edge of the cup liner where impingement will occur. Inherent in the model is a point on the negative cup axis. Each segment on the cup along with this common point defines a triangle (see Figure 5). If any section of the neck model (discussed below) intersects one of these "cup polygons", then impingement has occurred.

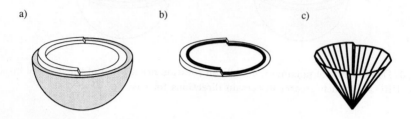

Fig. 5. Diagrams showing a) the cup with liner, b) the liner with highlighted rim, and c) the generated model of the cup

The femoral neck is modeled as a set of segments that is a discretization of the surface of the implant neck. During collision detection, only the neck segments that lie in the same range of distance from the center of rotation as the segments defining the cup liner need to be included in testing. Therefore, the runtime neck model generation can ignore all irrelevant sections of a large femoral implant surface model. This allows full implant data (e.g. a polygonal mesh of the implant surface) to be easily included in PROM analysis with minimal model editing. (In the case of the polygonal mesh, a simple script converting polygon data to simple segment data could be quickly run.)

Impingement limits are detected by moving the leg in small steps along the desired motion path. The size of the steps is determined by desired accuracy. The leg is moved incrementally until collision is detected. With complicated models, however, the angle limits become a function of not only the models, but also the position of the implants. Determination of impingement at each incremental step along the desired test path with this approach is too computationally intensive to be done interactively. Interactive speed is desired in the long run because the PROM simulator may eventually be extended to provide intra-surgical planning capabilities in computer-aided hip replacement.

In order to gain speed while retaining accuracy, a binary searching method can be implemented. For each leg motion path (divided into independent movements of flexion, abduction, extension, etc.), the full movement is first tried. If no impingement occurs during the movement, then the next movement is considered. Full movements are attempted until there are no more movements to try, or until impingement is detected. For the movement in which impingement is detected, movements of decreasing distance along the path are attempted until impingement occurs. The incremental distance attempted is halved each time, hence the term "binary search". When the incremental distance needed for impingement falls below a pre-set threshold, the position of the leg at this impingement point can be recorded. Below is pseudocode for the impingement detection algorithm:

```
D = {angular distance entered for final impinging movement};
e = {desired accuracy};
R = {current leg position};
t = 0;

do {
   R' = {leg position after moving D from R};
   if({no impingement is detected at R'}) {
      R = R';
      t = t+D;
   }
   D = D/2;
} while (D > e);
```

At this point, t is the distance travelled along the movement path before impingement.

4 Results

Various simulations were performed with combinations of the Trilogy line of acetabular cup implants and VerSys femoral stem implants (both by Zimmer Inc.). A head size of 28 mm was assumed for all tests as well as a stem size of 17. Work is currently being done to develop a database of implant data. Unless otherwise noted, all examples used an identical cup orientation (45° abduction, 15° flexion, and 135° clockwise twist), an identical neck orientation (40° abduction, 15° anteversion) and no pelvic flexion.

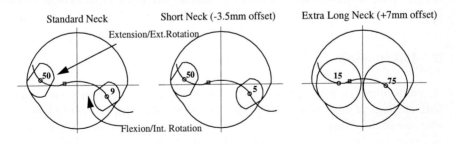

Fig. 6. PROM Plots for identical leg motions, but for different neck lengths

The first example illustrates the effect of neck length on PROM for the VerSys 20 degree elevated cup liner. In Figure 6, we see two sets of motions: 1) 90° leg flexion followed by maximum internal rotation and 2) 10° extension followed by maximum external rotation. The PROM is least limited by use of the standard neck length, though use of a shorter neck does not shrink the envelope of possible motion by much. However, use of the +7mm neck extension results in a loss of 35° possible external rotation. Flexion is limited to 75° with no possible internal rotation. Notice the dramatically increased cross-sectional area of the effective neck for the extra long neck case, resulting from the "flange" on the long neck.

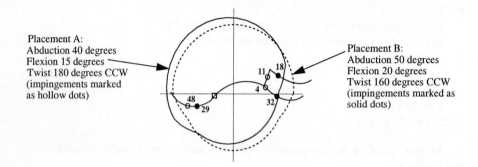

Fig. 7. PROM Plots for different placements of the cup and liner

The second example of the PROM simulator reiterates the importance of proper placement of the cup during THR. Figure 7 shows a set of motions (the previous two motions along with 90° flexion followed by 20° adduction and maximum internal rotation) for two different cup placements. The PROM simulator allows the surgeon to superimpose two cup placements for comparative purposes. (The neck outlines have been removed to aid reading of the plots.) Although both cup orientations are within a commonly accepted "safe" range [10], Placement A will allow 6° more external rotation, while Placement B provides a greater range of motion in the direction of forward leg motion, providing 11 to 14 degrees more internal rotation.

5 Discussion

Non-axisymmetric implants are used to increase implant stability and improve patient range of motion without compromising the strength of the implant. However, use of these implants increases the need for both proper selection and proper placement of the implant. Use of analytical simulators for implant design can allow suppliers to perform "trial runs" on their implants in order to fine tune their designs. They can allow surgeons to provide better care for their patients by placing the implants in order to optimize ROM on a per patient basis. Our studies along with others have shown that even within a widely-accepted "safe" zone, patient range of motion limited by impingement is affected significantly by cup placement. With the growing variety of available implant designs, some method of accurately performing optimally planned implant placement is increasingly important.

Though the current PROM simulator may predict impingement for various fixed positions of the pelvis, our results do not take into account motion of the pelvis during leg motion. Pelvic motion during movement will allow range of motion greater than the limits predicted by our system, although the extent of the allowance has yet to be determined. This system currently does not address dislocation via bone impingement. However, the complications that arise from implant impingement may be avoided with the proper combination of preoperative planning and technologically enhanced surgical procedures.

References

1. Amstutz, H. C., Lodwig, R. M., Schurman, D. J. and Hodgson, A. G.: Range of motion studies for total hip replacements. Clinical Orthopaedics and Related Research (111), September 1975, 124-130.
2. Amstutz, H. C. and Markolf, K. L.: Design features in total hip replacement. In Harris W.H. (ed.): Proceedings of the Second Open Scientific Meeting of the Hip Society, New York, C.V. Mosby, 1974.
3. Cobb, T. K., Morrey B. F., Ilstrup D. M.: The elevated-rim acetabular liner in total hip arthroplasty: Relationship to postoperative dislocation. The Journal of Bone and Joint Surgery, Vol 78-A, No. 1, January 1996, 80-86.
4. DiGioia III, A. M. et al.: An image guided surgical navigation system for the accurate measurement and alignment of acetabular implants. Accepted for publication: Clinical Orthopaedics and Related Research, 1998.
5. Jaramaz, B., Nikou, C., DiGioia III, A. M.: Effect of cup orientation and neck length in range of motion simulation. 43rd Annual Meeting, Orthopaedic Research Society, February 9-13, 1997, San Francisco, California, 286-48.
6. Jaramaz, B., Nikou, C., Simon D. A., DiGioia III, A. M.: Range of motion after total hip arthroplasty: Experimental verification of the analytical simulator. In Troccaz, J., Grimson, E., Mosges, R. (eds.): Proceedings of CVRMed-MRCAS97, Grenoble, France, March 1997: 573-582.
7. Johnson, R. C., and Smidt, G. L: Hip motion measurements for selected activities of daily living. Clinical Orthopaedics and Related Research 1970 Sept-Oct (72): 205-215.
8. Krushell, R. J., Burke, D. W., and Harris, W. H.: Range of motion in contemporary total hip arthroplasy (the impact of modular head-neck components). The Journal of Arthroplasty Vol. 6 (2 1991): 97-101.
9. Krushell, R. J., Burke, D. W., and Harris, W. H.: Elevated-rim acetabular components: Effect on range of motion and stability in total hip arthroplasty. The Journal of Arthroplasty 6, Supplement October 1991: 1-6.
10. Lewinnek, G. E., Lewis, J. L., Tarr R., Compere, C. L., Zimmerman, J. R.: Dislocation after total hip-replacement arthroplasties. J. Bone Joint Surg.: 217-220, Vol 60-A, No. 2, March 1978.
11. Maxian, T. A., Brown, T. D., Pedersen, D. R. and Callaghan, J. J.: Finite element modeling of dislocation propensity in total hip arthroplasty. 42nd Annual meeting, Orthopaedic Research Society, February 19-22, 1996, Atlanta, Georgia, 259-44.
12. McCollum, D. E. and Gray, W. J.: Dislocation after total hip arthroplasty (causes and prevention). Clinical Orthopaedics and Related Research 261 (1990): 159-170.

4D Shape-Preserving Modelling of Bone Growth*

Per Rønsholt Andresen[1,2], Mads Nielsen[2], and Sven Kreiborg[2]

[1] Department of Mathematical Modelling,
Technical University of Denmark, Denmark
pra@imm.dtu.dk   http://www.imm.dtu.dk/~pra

[2] 3D-Lab, School of Dentistry, University of Copenhagen, Denmark
http://www.lab3d.odont.ku.dk

Abstract. From a set of temporally separated scannings of the same anatomical structure we wish to identify and analyze the growth in terms of a metamorphosis. That is, we study the temporal change of shape which may provide an understanding of the biological processes which govern the growth process. We subdivide the growth analysis into growth simulation, growth modelling, and finally the growth analysis. In this paper, we present results of growth simulation of the mandible from 3 scannings of the same patient in the age of 9 months, 21 months, and 7 years. We also present the first growth models and growth analyzes. The ultimative goal is to predict/simulate human growth which would be extremely useful in many surgical procedures.

1 Introduction

This paper presents a non-linear growth model which to a very good approximation interpolates the growth as seen on the human mandible (the lower jaw). The results comply with the existing 2D theory on mandibular growth [1]. These experiments use a unique 4D data set containing three Computerized Tomography (CT) scans[1] of the same patient with Apert syndrom, but with normal mandibular development, taken at three ages (9 months, 21 months, and 7 years old). In many situations, surgeons need information about the growth of the jaws, particularly when performing pediatric cranio-facial surgery. After surgery, the bones continue to grow, and therefore in order to optimize the intervention, there is a need to predict/simulate growth. Also for basic understanding and teaching, we have a need for these models. We subdivide the growth study into growth simulation, growth modelling, and finally the growth analysis. Growth simulation is the data driven analysis, where we try to fit an (almost) arbitrary model to the data. In growth modelling, we have a model and wish to evaluate if the data fits the model. When we are doing growth analysis, the process is

---

* This work is partly supported by the Danish Technical Research Council, registration number 9600452

[1] The scans were performed for diagnostic and treatment planning purposes.

reversed, and we try to extract information from the models, such as active areas, spatial correlations, predicted changes, etc. In contrast to normal biological tissue growth, bone grows only on the surface. The interior is rigid and does not change shape [1]. The growth of a bone can be subdivided into *deposition* (adding bone) and *resorption* (removal of bone). Because the deposition and resorption happen all over the surface of the bone at different speeds, this results in non-linear growth [1]. For the mandible the condyles are the most active areas, and are therefore important to be followed over time. Homologous[2] points followed over time, define a spatio-temporal vector field (the *growth vector field* or just *vector field* or *flow field*). The goal of *growth simulation* is the identification of the spatio-temporal vector field. Many different vector fields will satisfy the constraints given by the data and the definitions of homologous points. Thus a *growth model* (or interpolation model) must be used for the determination of a unique vector field.

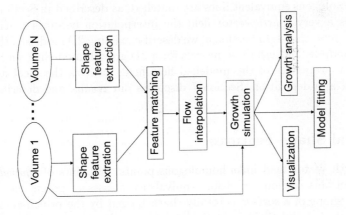

Fig. 1. *Flow chart of the algorithms involved in the growth analysis.*

We distinguish between models having the same number of degrees of freedom as the data and over-constrained models. We will use the first in the process of growth simulations, while over-constrained models are used for growth modelling. The simulation is a mere data interpolation, whereas the modelling will test whether data comply to a given model. In Figure 1 the information flow is shown.

Finally, in the *growth analysis*, we will extract information from the simulated or modelled vector field in order to identify local biological processes and/or physical conditions that govern the remodelling of the bone. In this paper, we estimate the resorption and deposition on the surface of the mandibular bone.

In earlier work on simulating the growth of the mandibular bone [2] the interpolation has been performed directly on the surface position. But the time steps are large, and a direct surface position interpolation as carried out in

---

[2] Homologous = having the same relative position, value, or structure.

that work will not preserve the overall shape. Thus, intermediate steps will not necessarily look like mandibles. See figure 2.

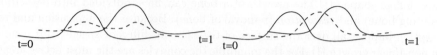

Fig. 2. *Surface interpolation illustration to the left is a linear interpolation in position of closest point. The top at t = 0 will disappear and at the same time a new top will appear. To the right is a linear interpolation of shape feature positions such as maximally curved points on the surface. Here, the top moves to the right over time.*

In Section 2, we will give one definition of homologous points in terms of the extremal mesh [15] (which are lines) and the different types of ridge lines. These homologous equivalent lines are matched, as described in Section 3. Since this yields a very sparse vector field the interpolation becomes crucial and is described in Section 4. In Section 5, we describe existing 2D models of the growth of the mandible, and use these models for a 3D growth modelling. In Section 6, we extract properties of the modelled flow fields such as the local amount of resorption and deposition. Section 7 discusses our results and describes future work.

2 Local Shape Features

The growth vector field links homologous points, or points of *equivalent morphology*. In this section, we define equivalence classes of points on a surface. The local shape of a surface is totally characterized by the principal curvatures k_1, k_2 ($k_1 > k_2$) and their derivatives in the coordinate system defined by the principal directions (t_1, t_2) [6]. Since the bone topology is not changing in our

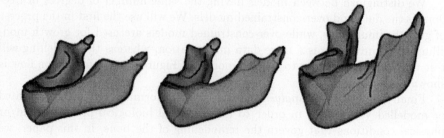

Fig. 3. *The crest lines on the three smoothed mandibles at 9 months (left), 21 months (middle), and 7 years old (right). The surfaces are translucent.*

studies, we may model the growth process by a 3D diffeomorphism (a one-to-one differential mapping). This corresponds to D'Arcy Thompson classical methods of transformations [5]. The principal curvatures and directions will in general change when exposed to this non-linear diffeomorphism, and cannot directly be used for registration. However, certain *shape singularities* are stable in the sense that they cannot be removed by an infinitesimal perturbation [3]. Here, we give a list of some stable shape features.

Shape feature	Definition	Dimensionality
Umbilic point	$k_1 = k_2$	0
Critical curvedness [11]	$\partial_{t_1} C = 0 \wedge \partial_{t_2} C = 0$, def: $C = k_1^2 + k_2^2$	0
Extremal points	$\partial_{t_1} k_1 = 0 \wedge \partial_{t_2} k_2 = 0$	0
Parabolic line	$k_1 = 0 \vee k_2 = 0$	1
Ridge line (or extremal mesh)	$\partial_{t_1} k_1 = 0 \vee \partial_{t_2} k_2 = 0$	1
Crest line	$\partial_{t_1} k_1 = 0 \wedge \partial_{t_1}^2 k_1 < 0$, def: $|k_1| > |k_2|$	1
Sub-parabolic line [3]	$\partial_{t_2} k_1 = 0 \vee \partial_{t_1} k_2 = 0$	1

Shape features with dimension ≥ 2 will not be discussed in this paper.

The ridge lines (or extremal mesh) can be partitioned into four types corresponding to respectively maximum or minimum in k_1 and k_2. We use the maxima in (the absolute value of) both k_1 and k_2.

The above mentioned shape features are all *structurally stable*, but even though they can not be removed by infinitesimal perturbations, they will in general change topology under finite perturbations.

We work with the extraction and matching of ridge lines in a scale-space setting [10] (see the following section). Also the scale-space evolution of ridge lines is not totally understod even though some aspects are covered in the literature [4,7,8]. Thus, theoretical issues are still to be clarified. However, by making a matching which only accepts good matches (see the following section), we obtain satisfying results. The crest lines of the mandibles can be seen in Figure 3.

3 Feature Matching

As features we will only consider the lines with maximally k_1 (crest-lines) and maximally k_2 (here, called k_2-max lines) in the extremal mesh. The overall framework follows the ideas of [14]. First we extract the crest lines and k_2-max lines for each dataset at scale 3.0 (matching scale) and 1.0 (localization scale). The crest lines at scale 3.0 are registered pairwise (here, it means only the temporally neighboring datavolumes), and initial vector fields are calculated. The k_2-max lines are then deformed according the initial vector fields and registered. From the two sets of matches (one from the crest-lines, the other from the k_2-max lines) final vector fields are calculated. This procedure is repeated for scale 1.0, but the lines are initially deformed according to the the final vector fields for scale 3.0.

The steps in the registration are always the same. First moment-registration, then two first order polynomial deformations, followed by two second order polynomial deformations. Lastly a totally non-rigid deformation is applied (all points on the lines move freely). For all the registration methods (including the non-rigid) they must satisfy the restriction that the deformation must be a 3D diffeomorphism. See Figure 6 for an example of matches between two set of crest lines at scale 3.0.

4 Flow Interpolation

The matching provides us with a very sparse set of vectors. This vector field must be interpolated such as to yield a differentiable spatially dense field of spatio-temporal deformation vectors: A diffeomorphism (that its, spatial the Jacobian is nowhere vanishing).

We wish the interpolation to satisfy the following constraints: (i) approximation, (ii) regularity, (iii) shadowing, (iv) maximum principle. (i) The interpolated vector field must approximate the data values well since localization of the features are assumed relatively precise. (ii) In regions of missing features a smooth solution must be created. We do assume a regular growth. (iii) The data must be able of shadowing each other. That is, in a given direction only the nearest data must be weighted. In this way, we avoid that features from the "other side" of a thin structure influence the local solution. (iv) The solution must not extend the solution to values larger than the largest data value or smaller than the smallest data value. We assume that the ridge lines also correspond to lines of extreme growth.

We address this as a statistical inference problem. Assume that the covariance function $C(x, x')$ is known. The covariance function expresses the covariance of the vector field values in two points x and x'. Typically, the closer the points are, the more correlated their data values are assumed to be. An interesting aspect is that if this covariance defines a distribution of functions, and if $C(x, x') = exp(-(|x - x'|/\lambda)^\alpha)$, some well-known function classes appear with probability 1, for different choices of α: $\alpha = 0$ yields white noise, $\alpha \in]0; 2[$ yields fractional Brownian motions with $\alpha = 1$ as the classical Brownian motion [12], while $\alpha = 2$ (the Gaussian) yields C^∞ functions. Given the covariance function $C(x, x')$ and an expression of the belief in data as the assumed variance of data values r^2, we can make a maximum likelihood estimation of $f(x)$ as [16]

$$f(x) = \frac{w(x, \boldsymbol{x})Q^{-1}g(\boldsymbol{x})}{w(x, \boldsymbol{x})Q^{-1}\mathbf{1}} \tag{1}$$

where $w(x, \boldsymbol{x})$ is a vector containing $w_i = C(x, x_i)$, and Q is a matrix containing $Q_{ij} = C(x_1, x_2) + r^2 \delta_{ij}$. The intuitive interpretation of the introduction of Q^{-1} is that, prior to the regularizations based on the covariance function, an inverse filtering is performed to make the samples uncorrelated. In terms of scale-space, we might say that we have data given at some scale λ. To interpolate, we first perform a deblurring to scale zero, then interpolate and then blur back to the current scale.

This method satisfies all criteria when $\alpha = 1$ and $r = 0$ [13]. λ can be chosen freely, so as to adjust the smoothness of the interpolated vector field. In

Figure 4, the deformation of the mandible is shown as it is transported along the deformation vector field.

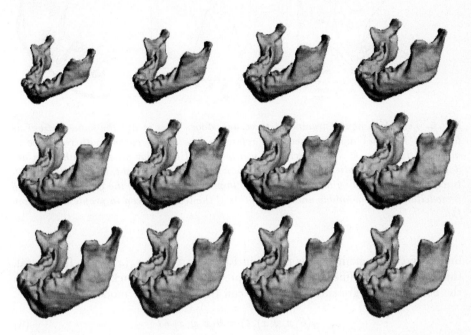

Fig. 4. *Result of deformations on the 7 years mandible using a second order polynomial model (see section 5). The top left and right images are the deformation at 9 months and 21 months, respectively. The bottom right image is the original 7 years old mandible.*

5 Growth Modelling

We have the general model $g(\theta(x,y,z),t)$, $g : \mathcal{R}^3 \mapsto \mathcal{R}^3$ (for fixed t), and the 3D volumes $v_i(x,y,z)$, where $\theta(x,y,z)$ is the parameters for g, and (x,y,z) defines a point in $\mathcal{R}^3$. t is the time. $i = \{1,\ldots,n\}$. n is the total number of volumes. t_i is the time at the ith scan. We need to pick a reference volume, let's say v_n. All deformations will then be applied to this set, i.e. a simulated volume at time t is given by $\tilde{v}_n(g(\theta(x,y,z),t),v_n(x,y,z))$ or $\tilde{v}_n(x,y,z,t)$ for short. We want to solve the problem

$$\hat{\theta} = \arg\min_{\theta} \sum_{i=1}^{n} \left[\sum_{x,y,z} \{\tilde{v}_n(x,y,z,t_i) - v_i(x,y,z,t_i)\}^2 \right] \quad (2)$$

Note, when having $g(\theta(x,y,z),t)$, the actual deformation on the volume v_n from time t_n to t, can always be made by a linear deformation (we just pick the straight

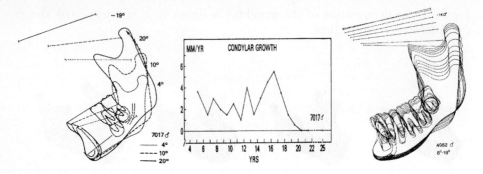

Fig. 5. *Left: Mandibular tracing at three age stages (this is not the same patient as for the CT scans) superimposed in a reference line in the corpus with reference to natural structures. Middle: Curve for yearly rate of condylar growth. Both plots are data from the same patient with a normal mandibular growth. Right: Mandibular growth tracing superimposed by means of metallic implants, illustrating the yearly growth and remodelling of the mandible and the eruption if the teeth, as seen in profile view. From [1].*

line between two homologous points in $\tilde{v}_n(x,y,z,t)$ and $v_n(x,y,z)$). In general, this leads to a non-linear optimization problem, but if we pick models, linear in the parameters, regression analysis [9] can be used. Linear models

$$g(\theta(x,y,z),t) = \theta(x,y,z) * t \tag{3}$$

have been used in previous work [2]. This model has the drawback that a point, p, can only grow in the direction of the vector $\theta(p)$. From Figure 5, it is obvious that the growth of the mandible is not linear. The simplest non-linear model is a polynomial model (with $k \leq 2$)

$$g(\theta(x,y,z),t) = t^k\theta_k + \cdots + t^2\theta_2 + t\theta_1 + \theta_0, \ \theta = [\theta_k \cdots \theta_2\ \theta_1\ \theta_0] \tag{4}$$

As seen from Figure 5, the growth speed is not constant, but this can be handled by the model by re-parametrizing the time variable, t.

Because we only have three scans of the same patient, we can not go above the second order model[3] (k=2). A second order polynomial model is estimated using the matches between scan one and two, and scan two and three. Interpolation of the volumes is carried out by deforming the last scan (see Figure 4). Because the calculation of the deformation field from one scan to the next scan is not perfect, we have some model errors (even though the model itself doesn't have any error) which are seen in Figure 7. Other possible models include logarithmic spirals and power functions, known from the theory of growth [5] or spatially constrained models.

---

[3] This leads to a model error equal zero, because the number of parameters equals the number of volumes.

6 Growth Analysis

The growth modelling is on its own also a growth analysis since residuals to an over-constrained model may be used for validating the model. The growth simulations, as we obtain it in Figure 4, can be used for a local characterization of the growth. The model errors at 9 months are shown in Figure 7. Using anatomical structures which are also spatially stable, a rigid registration of the different time instances of the bone can be obtained. In the mandible, the nerve canal is known to be spatially stable, and can serve as an anchor for a rigid registration. In this coordinate system, the spatio-temporal growth simulation vector field can be used directly for estimation of the amount of surface resorption and deposition. In Figure 8 we show the surface remodelling in terms of a color coding of the mandible as respectively the remodelling (the local velocity vector projected to the surface normal) and the speed of the homologous points. The remodelling is consistent with earlier 2D studies on larger statistical material [1]. Especially we see the expected large movement of the condyle.

7 Summary

We have simulated the growth of the mandible from 3 CT scans of the same patient at ages 9 months, 21 months, and 7 years. The intermediate interpolated time instances also exhibit shapes that clearly are "mandible shaped". This is due to the strategy of interpolating in shape feature position instead of a simple surface position interpolation [2]. The major errors in the simulations are found in the region where teeth are appearing. In principle, they should a priori have been removed from the mandible surfaces, as they are not part of the mandible but separate objects, and the shape change can not be contributed to a surface remodelling. The shape modelling in this paper has used simple second order polynomial temporal models. They exhibit some inexpedient features inherent for polynomial approximations. An example is a tendency to a contraction of the two condyles towards each other if a time extrapolation is attempted. Since the ultimate goal of a growth analysis and modelling is a prediction of the shape of the craniofacial complex. Future work will be devoted to examination of superior temporal models and validation on more datasets. Extension of the feature matching from ridge lines to iso-surfaces, as mentioned in Figure 7, may reduce errors. Also development of a skeletal growth atlas, which contains growth models for all bones would be interesting.

References

1. A. Björk and V. Skieller. Normal and abnormal growth of the mandible. A synthesis of longitudinal cephalometric implant studies over a period of 25 years. *European Journal of Orthodontics*, 5:1–46, 1983.
2. M. Bro-Nielsen, C. Gramkow, and S. Kreiborg. Non-rigid image registration using bone growth model. In *CVRMed-MRCAS'97*, Lecture Notes in Computer Science, pages 3–12. Springer Verlag, 1997.

3. J. W. Bruce and P. J. Giblin. *Curves and Singularities*. Cambridge University Press, Cambridge, 1984.
4. J. Damon. Local Morse theory for solutions to the heat equation and Gaussian blurring. *Jour. Diff. Eqtns.*, 1993.
5. D'Arcy Thomsen. *On Growth and Form*. Cambridge Unversity Press, 1971.
6. M. P. Do Carmo. *Differential Geometry of Curves and Surfaces*. Prentice Hall, Inc., New Jersey, 1976.
7. D. Eberly, R. Gardner, B. Morse, S. Pizer, and C. Scharlach. Ridges for image analysis. *Journal of Mathematical Imaging and Vision*, 4(4):353–373, 1994.
8. M. Fidrich. Following feature lines across scale. In *ScaleSpace97*, 1997.
9. D. Kazakos and P. Papantoni-Kazakos. *Detection and Estimation*. Computer Science Press, W. H. Freemann and Company, New York, 1990.
10. J. J. Koenderink. The structure of images. *Biological Cybernetics*, 50:363–370, 1984.
11. J. J. Koenderink. *Solid Shape*. MIT Press, Cambridge, Massachusetts, 1990.
12. B. B. Mandelbrot and J. W. van Ness. Fractional Brownian motions, fractional noises, and applications. *SIAM Review*, 10(4):422–437, 1968.
13. M. Nielsen and P. R. Andresen. Feature displacement interpolation. In *IEEE 1998 International Conference on Image Processing*, Chicago, Illinois, USA, 1998. To appear.
14. G. Subsol, J.-P. Thirion, and N. Ayache. A general scheme for automatically building 3D morphometric anatomical atlases: application to a skull atlas. *Medical Image Analysis*, 2(1):37-60, 1998.
15. J.-P. Thirion. The extremal mesh and the understanding of 3D surfaces. *International Journal of Computer Vision*, 6(58):503–509, November 1996.
16. C. K. I. Williams and C. E. Rasmussen. Gaussian processes for regression. *Advances in Neural Information Processing Systems*, 8, 1996.

Comments on color images. **Fig. 6**: The final matches (lines in black) between two sets of crest lines. The crest lines on the 21 months and 7 years mandible are red and green, respectively. It is seen that the condyles on the two mandibles are matched together. For visual clarity only every eighth match is shown. **Fig. 7**: The plots in the middle and right shows the frequency and accumulated distribution of the distance errors (the distance errors are measured as the minimal distances from the deformed surface to the original surface) between the 9 months old mandible and the 7 years old mandible deformed to 9 months. The mean error is 0.57mm, and 95% of the errors are less than 1.46mm. The maximal error is 2.79mm. This should be compared to the size of the 7 years old mandible whice is approximately $(X, Y, Z) = (80mm, 100mm, 40mm)$. The left surface is colored red when the error $> 1.46mm$, else white. When the surface changes a lot the matching algorithm does not match with lines in the "holes" of the surface, but are more likely to match with a line on the "top", therefor we see the errors located at places with a lot of changes in the shape. If we applied a surface to surface registration afterwards, the errors would be minimal. **Fig. 8**: First row: The 7 years mandible colored with the local velocity vector projected to the surface normal (left) and the length of the velocity vector (right). The next row shows X (first two images), Y (next two images), and Z (last two images) components of the velocity vector (projection and length, respectively). Read text in "Growth Analysis" for further explanation.

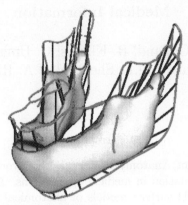

Fig. 6. *See "Comments on color images".*

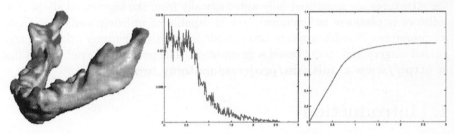

Fig. 7. *See "Comments on color images".*

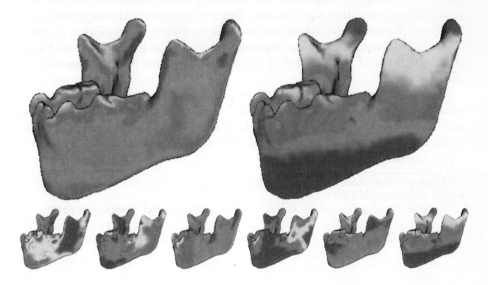

Fig. 8. *See "Comments on color images".*

AnatomyBrowser: A Framework for Integration of Medical Information

P. Golland,[*] R. Kikinis,[†] C. Umans[†],
M. Halle[†], M.E. Shenton[†], J.A. Richolt[†]

Abstract

In this paper we present AnatomyBrowser, a framework for integration of images and textual information in medical applications. AnatomyBrowser allows the user to combine 3D surface models of anatomical structures, their cross-sectional slices, and the text available on the structures, while providing a rich set of cross-referencing and annotation capabilities. The 3D models of the structures are generated fully automatically from the segmented slices. The software is platform independent, yet is capable of utilizing available graphics resources. Possible applications include interactive anatomy atlases, image guided surgery and model based segmentation. The program is available on-line at **http://www.ai.mit.edu/projects/anatomy_browser**.

1 Introduction

With recent developments in MRI technology it has become possible to obtain high quality medical images that are extremely useful for clinical studies, surgical planning and other applications. This has spurred rapid development of a family of information extraction and analysis algorithms using medical imagery. These include segmentation and registration, shape and deformation modeling, etc. Importance of visualization of the results, especially 3D data, became apparent as well.

This paper presents AnatomyBrowser, a visualization and integration framework for medical applications. It provides visualization capabilities for slice sets and 3D surface models of anatomical structures, as well as a useful set of cross-referencing and annotation features. It can also be used as an aid tool for the model driven segmentation.

---

[*]Corresponding author. Artificial Intelligence Laboratory, Massachusetts Institute of Technology, Cambridge, MA 02139
[†]Surgical Planning Laboratory, Brigham and Women's Hospital, Boston, MA 02115

The system is written as a Java applet, which makes it platform independent. It can be readily run using any web browser that supports Java. In fact, the system is available on-line [1].

Although no special hardware or software is required to run AnatomyBrowser in its basic setup, it is capable of utilizing specialized graphics resources (hardware/software). For this purpose, an additional 3D viewer was created that generates dynamic renderings of the 3D surface models using rendering capabilities of the graphics software available.

This paper is organized as follows. The next section reviews the differences between AnatomyBrowser and other systems available in the field. Then AnatomyBrowser is discussed in detail and its interface is described. After that, uses of AnatomyBrowser in various application areas are reported. It is followed by a discussion of possible extensions to the system, which include merging the dynamic and the static versions of the 3D rendering components of the system.

2 Related Work

Interactive anatomy atlases are one important example of possible applications for the visualization and integration system we propose. In fact, it was an original inspiration for this work.

The work on digital atlases has been pioneered by Höhne et al. [4]. A digital brain atlas integrating several image modalities with the information on anatomy hierarchy was proposed in [6]. The goal of the work presented in this paper was to develop a system for visualization of segmentation results (both in 2D and 3D) and their integration with original scans and text information available on the structures. We do not restrict the application of the system to atlas generation. It can be used on any data set, including clinical cases.

In addition to anatomy studies, digital atlases are used for model driven segmentation. The atlas data is treated by the algorithm as a reference template, to which the input data set is registered. Several registration algorithms (using both rigid and elastic matching) have been developed by different groups [2, 3, 10]. Another approach is to extract anatomical knowledge from the atlas and use it to build a prior model of the input data [5]. In both cases, AnatomyBrowser can serve as an aid tool in the model based segmentation 'loop': segmented images are used to accumulate knowledge of anatomy, which is used, in turn, for segmentation of the new data sets.

In the visualization field, there are several packages available for rendering of 3D surface models (Inventor by SGI, VTK by GE, and many others), but to the authors' best knowledge, AnatomyBrowser is the only integration environment that provides extensive referencing and annotation capabilities. This is extremely important in clinical applications, when a user wants to establish a clear correspondence between all types of pictorial information available. Another significant difference between AnatomyBrowser and other visualization

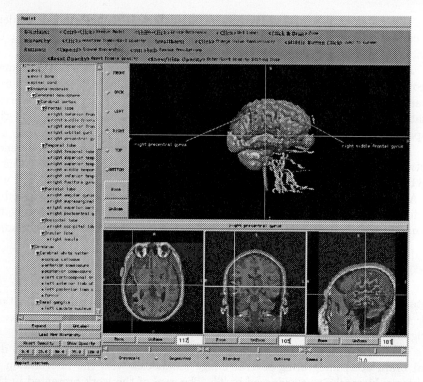

Figure 1: An example of AnatomyBrowser for a brain data set. The crosshair positions correspond to the same 3D point. Some of the structures are annotated on the 3D display. The sagittal slice is slightly zoomed in.

packages is its portability. It can be a great advantage, considering the target applications and the user community.

3 AnatomyBrowser

In this section the user interface of AnatomyBrowser is described, and the design considerations are introduced and discussed.

AnatomyBrowser integrates three main types of information: the slice sets, the 3D models and the text information on the structures (structure names and general text notes on some structures). Accordingly, its interface consists of three main components, namely, the slice displays, the 3D display and the hierarchy panel (Fig.1). In addition to visualization capabilities, AnatomyBrowser provides cross-referencing among all types of displayed information. The cross-referencing among the images is different in its nature from the correspondence between image and text information. While the former can be established au-

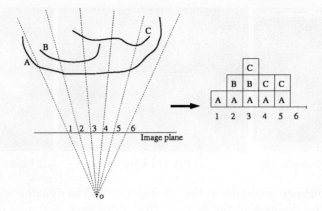

Figure 2: A multi-layer image. The 3D scene consists of three surfaces (A,B and C). The view rays and the stacks in the multi-layer image are shown for six different pixels.

tomatically, the latter requires some user input.

The sections below discuss each interface component, the information it provides to the user and its interaction with other components of the system.

3.1 3D Model Generation

We used the traditional approach of polygon (triangle) meshes for representation of 3D surface models. We use the Marching Cubes algorithm [7] to construct a triangle approximation of a surface from a set of segmented slices. We assume the segmentation to be available. Section 4 discusses connections between AnatomyBrowser and segmentation algorithms used for the medical applications.

To build a surface model, the algorithm first considers each border voxel of the segmented structure independently of its neighbors. In this phase, a planar patch of a surface is built for every border voxel. Next, patches from neighboring voxels are merged to form a single mesh that approximates the surface of the structure. In order to decrease the number of polygons (triangles) in the representation and improve the surface appearance, some amount of decimation and smoothing is performed on the mesh under constraints on the accuracy of the representation.

The model construction process uses a coordinate system naturally defined by the input slice set, and therefore the models can be straightforwardly registered to the pixels in the original slices. This greatly simplifies implementation of cross-referencing between the 3D models and the cross-sectional views.

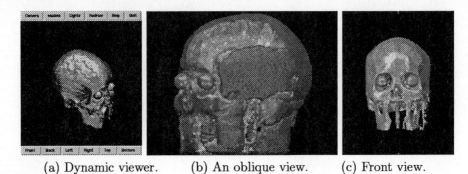

(a) Dynamic viewer. (b) An oblique view. (c) Front view.

Figure 3: Different examples of the 3D display. (a) The dynamic viewer allows one to render any view of the models. (b,c) Additional examples of the static views. Skin was made fully transparent, skull was made partially transparent, and in (c) muscles were removed.

3.2 3D Model Visualization

The viewer program for visualization of 3D surface models was created using the Visualization Toolkit (VTK) [8], a software package that uses available GL libraries (e.g. openGl, xGl, Mesa, etc.) to take advantage of graphics resources of a particular machine. Any other visualization library that provides dynamic rendering (such as Inventor by SGI) could be used for implementation of the viewer.

The viewer provides controls for the scene's global parameters, such as the observer's position relative to the scene and the light locations and intensities, as well as the surface properties of the models (color, transparency and reflectivity). Fig.3a shows the viewer interface with the surface models for the brain data set.

Since the goal of this work was to produce an easily portable, platform independent system, a static version of the viewer was implemented as well. The static viewer does not require any special graphics hardware or software, but it is restricted to a set of static views rather than allowing the user to choose a view dynamically. In the current implementation, a user specifies several views of the 3D models, which are rendered off-line and then displayed by AnatomyBrowser. The user still has control over the surface properties of the model (color and transparency), but the properties that would require re-rendering the entire scene (for example, lighting) are kept constant. The AnatomyBrowser interface shown in Fig.1 uses the static version of the viewer.

We use so-called *multi-layer images* [9] to save the information necessary for rendering and depth recovery for the static viewer. The idea of the multi-layer image is the following. For each pixel in the image, a view ray is constructed (Fig.2).

This ray might intersect several surfaces in the scene. For each surface that

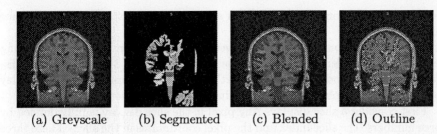

(a) Greyscale   (b) Segmented   (c) Blended   (d) Outline

Figure 4: Slice display. The same coronal slice from the brain data set is displayed using four different ways of combining greyscale and segmented images.

is intersected by the view ray, a tuple of the surface index, the intensity and the depth of the intersection point is saved. Thus each pixel in the multi-layer image is represented by a (possibly empty) stack of <index,intensity,depth> tuples, which are used later for rendering and establishing relative location of the structures.

Note that in a proper representation the multi-layer images are almost as easily compressed as the segmented images. Since most of the models are smooth, each of the tuple channels contains (hopefully large) uniform patches. If the channels are compressed separately, high compression rates can be achieved.

Since the pixel value is computed at rendering time by composing the surface points that project onto that pixel, surface transparency and color can be easily handled by the static version of the viewer. Fig.3c shows the brain data set with the skin made fully transparent and the skull being only partially transparent.

3.3 Cross-Sectional Slices

Axial, coronal and sagittal[1] cross-sections are displayed on the three slice displays. The cross-sectional slices are computed from the original scan by resampling it along the three orthogonal directions.

Each slice display has a set of original greyscale images and a set of segmented slices associated with it. AnatomyBrowser provides four different ways to view the slices. The user can choose to view just the greyscale images, or just the segmented set, or blend them together, or view the greyscale images with the outlines of the segmentation. Fig.4 demonstrates all four choices for one slice from the brain data set.

3.4 Cross-Reference Among the Displays

An important capability provided by AnatomyBrowser is cross-referencing among the displays. If a user clicks on one of the display areas (<Shift-Click>), a

---

[1]These are the standard orthogonal cross-sections used in the medical community. They correspond to bottom-to-top, front-to-back, left-to-right cross-sections respectively.

cross-hair appears on all four displays at locations corresponding to the same 3D point.

Even though all four displays exhibit very similar behavior, the cross-referencing definition and implementation must be different for the 3D and the slice displays. To understand why this is so, let's consider a mapping from the display coordinates to the physical volume defined by the input set of slices.

First consider a slice display. Any pixel in the slice display is fully defined by three numbers: the slice index and the pixel coordinates in the slice. These three numbers are also sufficient to compute the 3D coordinates of the corresponding point in the volume defined by the slice set. Therefore, the mapping between pixels in the slice set and physical points in the 3D volume is one-to-one and can be readily computed from the physical dimensions of the voxel.

This is not true for the 3D display. Each pixel in the 3D display is described by only two coordinates. The user has no means to specify nor to obtain depth values from the 3D display, and therefore the depth dimension is lost for the images on the 3D display. The natural one-to-one correspondence between the pixels of the 3D display and the entities in the 3D space is the one from pixels to view rays and *vice versa*. This construction provides us with a useful interpretation of the cross-referencing for the 3D display.

If a cross-reference is initiated from the slice display, the corresponding 3D point can be uniquely computed. For the 3D display, we place the cross-hair on the pixel corresponding to the selected 3D point, but we might not see the point itself on the display. Instead, we will see a surface that occludes the selected 3D point. The cross-hair on the 3D display should be interpreted as a view ray along which the selected 3D point lies.

In a similar way, by clicking on the 3D display, a user may specify a view ray rather than a single 3D point. We use the depth information available to AnatomyBrowser to disambiguate this problem. We assume that the point of interest lies on the intersection of the view ray with the closest visible surface. This decision is justified by a natural notion of pointing[2]: when interpreting one's pointing, an observer follows the imaginary ray defined by the pointer until it meets an object. This object is assumed to be the answer.

3.5 Model Hierarchy

Textual information is a third important component of AnatomyBrowser. This includes names of anatomical structures and text notes associated with some of the structures.

AnatomyBrowser uses a directed acyclic graph (DAG) to model the anatomical hierarchy. The text file that defines the hierarchy is essentially a list of internal nodes that represent groups of structures, and their children, each of

---

[2]One can argue that this is a very simplistic interpretation of the human interaction by pointing, and the authors would fully agree with that.

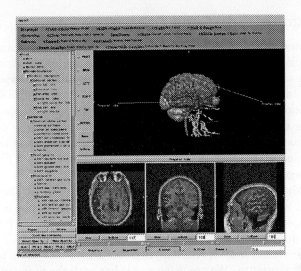

Figure 5: AnatomyBrowser for the brain data set with the frontal lobe collapsed into one node. Compare to Fig.1 for the differences in the hierarchy panel, the colors of the structures and annotation labels.

which can be either another group or a single structure. The hierarchy file is parsed by AnatomyBrowser and displayed in the hierarchy panel.

We use a tree model to display the hierarchy, because it is more suitable than a DAG for visualization purposes. If a particular group (or structure) is shared by several parents, several instances of the corresponding subgraph (or leaf) are generated and displayed under each of the parents. Since the internal representation uses a DAG, and all the instances of a group or a structure point back to the same element in the representation, the element properties can be changed using any of the instances. This implies that the changes will affect all the instances. For example, after a certain instance of a structure in the hierarchy panel was used to change the structure transparency, all the instances of this structure will report the new value for transparency.

A hierarchy tree (graph) is a natural, systematic way to classify and present anatomical structures. It also allows the user to set a desirable level of details for the 3D models and segmented slices. Any subtree in the hierarchy panel can be collapsed into a single node (leaf). This causes all the structures in the sub-tree to be re-rendered using the color of the new collapsed node and to be treated as one structure that point forward (Fig.5).

This feature can be very useful for studying anatomy with the help of AnatomyBrowser. A user can start with a very coarse hierarchy tree and expand the group nodes gradually, rather than try to learn the whole tree at once.

3.6 Integrating Text and Images

AnatomyBrowser also provides annotation capabilities, which can be viewed as cross-referencing between text and images. Annotation of the structures can be invoked from any of the main components of the AnatomyBrowser interface.

Implementation of the annotation using the hierarchy panel is fairly straightforward. Clicking on a node name in the hierarchy tree causes this name to appear on the title bar below the 3D display. If this structure – which can be a group that was collapsed into a single structure – can be seen on the 3D display, it is also labeled with a pointer and the structure name (Fig. 5,6).

Using images for annotation requires additional effort. We use segmented slices for the slice displays and multi-layer images for the 3D display to determine for each pixel what structure, if any, contains this pixel. When a user clicks on any of the displays, the corresponding structure is located in the hierarchy graph and used for annotation.

As was mentioned before, AnatomyBrowser allows text notes to be attached to a particular structure. We are using a title bar with the name of the structure as a 'hypertext' link to a collection of text notes. Clicking on it brings up a text window with all the text information available on the structure.

It is worth mentioning that both annotation and text documentation can be used for all leaves in the hierarchy panel, whether they represent real structures or groups collapsed into a single node.

4 Applications

AnatomyBrowser provides a framework for visualization of medical image information and integrating it with text available on the structures in the images. Anatomy studies are the most obvious application for such a system. AnatomyBrowser can effectively replace a conventional anatomical atlas book, as it provides at least as much information as the book. Students can see anatomical structures, view an MR or CT scan of those structures, read attached description and study the hierarchy of the structures. Visualization and full cross-referencing make AnatomyBrowser a very useful interactive teaching tool.

We have generated several atlases using AnatomyBrowser. They include brain (Fig. 1), knee, abdominal and inner ear data sets. They are available on-line [1].

The atlas can also be used for model driven segmentation. We can view the process of model based segmentation as a loop, in which the results of the segmentation of the previous scans are used in segmentation of the new data sets. And the digital atlas is an intermediate step in this loop, where the knowledge about anatomy is accumulated in a particular representation, visualized for the user, and possibly processed for the future use by the segmentation algorithm. In a way, its purpose is to 'close the loop' from one stage of the segmentation

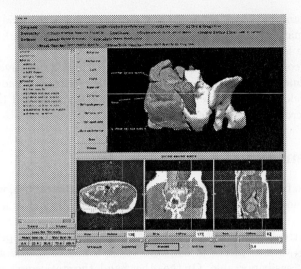

Figure 6: Clinical case example. AnatomyBrowser for the pelvic tumor data set demonstrating cross-reference and label correspondence.

to the next one, which uses the result of the first stage.

We want to point out that there is a significant difference between AnatomyBrowser and a standard anatomy atlas, and it is in the data. An atlas is usually one data set – real or phantom – that is used as a 'normal' reference. AnatomyBrowser, however, is a software package that takes images and text as input and produces a user-friendly interface for viewing and cross-referencing all the pieces of data. It can be used on any data set, and not necessarily on the reference case that would be used for an atlas. This naturally brings up another application for AnatomyBrowser. It can be used as a visualization and annotation tool for clinical cases, when the analysis has to be performed on a per-case basis.

We tested AnatomyBrowser on several tumor cases in different anatomical areas: pelvis (Fig. 6), sacrum, brain, and kidney. Again, all of the cases are available on-line [1]. The tool was tested for both surgical planning and image guided surgery. During the planning stage, the surgeons used AnatomyBrowser to familiarize themselves with the 3D structure of the tumor and structures around it and to plan the directions of the cuts. Then AnatomyBrowser, with the set of views specified by the surgeon, was used as a reference tool during the surgery.

We would like to mention that in two of those cases AnatomyBrowser allowed the surgeons to significantly improve their performance. In case of the sacral tumor, the visualization system made it obvious that certain vertebra were covered by the tumor on the right side, but not on the left side of the sacrum, which was of a great help in planning the surgery. For the pelvic tumor case, the initial plan made by the surgeon, was changed after the analysis of the 3D models in AnatomyBrowser had demonstrated that the originally planned cut would not be feasible.

The surgeons' response to the system was extremely positive. It provided them with much greater visualization capabilities than they had before, while establishing clear correspondences between the 3D models and the more commonly used cross-sectional slice sets.

5 Extensions

In addition to further testing of AnatomyBrowser for clinical use, we are working on merging the dynamic and the static versions of the 3D viewer under the same framework.

In the current implementation, the dynamic viewer is a separate program that requires various pieces of software to be available in the system. It is, therefore, not easily portable. On the other hand, the static version of the viewer is an integral part of the Java applet that implements the AnatomyBrowser interface. It can be viewed using any web browser that supports Java.

We are currently working on an implementation of the dynamic viewer in Java using Java3D, a package that provides an interface between Java and the GL libraries. The dynamic version of AnatomyBrowser will still depend on the graphics hardware and GL support, but this will eliminate its dependency on intermediate 'layers' of software (VTK, tcl/tk) used for visualization of the 3D models. The users with graphics support will be able to run AnatomyBrowser with no extra effort, while the users of the low-end machines with no graphics capabilities will still use the static version of the system.

6 Conclusions

We have presented a framework for generating and combining different modalities of medical imaging data. 3D models generated from the segmented slices provide the user with useful visualization capabilities, while the full cross-reference among all the sources of information allows flexibility in viewing modes with the possibility of bringing the displays in correspondence.

The software is easily portable to various platforms and doesn't require special resources. However, if the fast graphics hardware is available, the system can take advantage of it in a straightforward way.

AnatomyBrowser has been used to generate an interactive atlas for several data sets. The digital atlas can be used as an interactive teaching tool, as well as for model based segmentation. Surgical planning and image guided surgery are another example of the applications that can greatly benefit from using AnatomyBrowser. Different applications proved certain subsets of features to be useful. While hierarchical representation of the textual information and annotation capabilities were very important for the teaching tool, 3D visualization combined with cross-referencing were valuable for the clinical applications. The system as a whole combined a set of capabilities rich enough for both purposes.

References

[1] AnatomyBrowser URL.
http://www.ai.mit.edu/projects/anatomy_browser.

[2] R. Bajcsy and S. Kovacic. Multiresolution elastic matching. *Comp. Vision, Graphic and Image Processing*, 46:1–21, 1989.

[3] D.L. Collins, C.J. Holmes, T.M. Peters, and A.C. Evans. Automatic 3D model-based neuroanatomical segmentation. *Human Brain Mapping*, 3:190–208, 1995.

[4] K.H. Höhne et al. A 3D anatomical atlas based on a volume model. *IEEE Computer Graphics Applications*, 2:72–78, 1992.

[5] M. Kamber et al. Model-based 3D segmentation of multiple sclerosis lesions in dual-echo mri data. *SPIE Visualization in Biomed. Computing*, 1808:590–600, 1992.

[6] R. Kikinis et al. A digital brain atlas for surgical planning, model driven segmentation and teaching. *IEEE Transactions on Visualization and Computer Graphics*, 2(3), 1996.

[7] W.E. Lorensen and H.E. Cline. Marching cubes: A high resolution 3d surface construction algorithm. *Computer Graphics*, 21:163–169, 1987.

[8] W. Schroeder, K. Martin, and B. Lorensen. *The visualization toolkit : an object-oriented approach to 3D graphics*. Prentice-Hall, NJ, 1996.

[9] C. Umans, M. Halle, and R. Kikinis. Multilayer images for interactive 3d visualization on the world wide web. Technical Report 51, Surgical Planning Lab, Brigham and Women's Hospital, Boston, MA, September, 1997.

[10] S. Warfield et al. Automatic identification of gray matter structures from mri to improve the segmentation of white matter lesions. In *Proceedings of Medical Robotics and Computer Assisted Surgery (MRCAS)*, pages 55–62, 1995.

Automatic, Accurate Surface Model Inference for Dental CAD/CAM

Chi-Keung Tang[1], Gérard Medioni[1], and François Duret[2]

[1] Inst. Rob. Intell. Sys., University of Southern California, Los Angeles, CA 90089-0273.
{chitang, medioni}@iris.usc.edu
[2] School of Dentistry, University of Southern California, Los Angeles, CA 90089-0641.
duret@hsc.usc.edu

Abstract. Dental CAD/CAM offers the prospects of drastically reducing the time to provide service to patients, with no compromise on quality. Given the state-of-the-art in sensing, design, and machining, an attractive approach is to have a technician generate a restorative design in wax, which can then be milled by a machine in porcelain or titanium. The difficulty stems from the inherent outlier noise in the measurement phase. Traditional techniques remove noise at the cost of smoothing, degrading discontinuities such as anatomical lines which require accuracy up to 5 to 10 μm to avoid artifacts. This paper presents an efficient method for the automatic and accurate data validation and 3-D shape inference from noisy digital dental measurements. The input consists of 3-D points with spurious samples, as obtained from a variety of sources such as a laser scanner or a stylus probe. The system produces faithful smooth surface approximations while preserving critical curve features such as grooves and preparation lines. To this end, we introduce the *Tensor Voting* technique, which efficiently ignores noise, infers smooth structures, and preserves underlying discontinuities. This method is non-iterative, does not require initial guess, and degrades gracefully with spurious noise, missing and erroneous data. We show results on real and complex data.

1 Introduction and overall approach

Dental CAD/CAM has been revolutionizing dentistry for the past ten years, and is ubiquitous in every major dental group and laboratory today. Its main components are data acquisition, modeling, and milling systems. The only system widely used commercially is the CEREC system, produced by Siemens Inc. It is a self-contained unit with an imaging camera, a monitor, and an electrically controlled machine to mill inlay and onlay restorations from ceramic blocks. The accuracy is not good, and significant manual processing is required. Another system of interest, developed by Duret *et al.*, was able to produce crowns with an average gap of 35 μm. The system is no longer commercially available, and suffered from lack of speed and a cumbersome interface.

An alternative approach, followed here, is to perform the restoration design manually, in a laboratory, by using a conventional medium such as wax; then to transfer this physical design into a digital model. This information can be directly used to control a CAM machine to mill the restoration from a ceramic (or other) block. Typically, digital measurements are sampled from a wax model, using palpation or optical sensing [4].

Figure 1 shows the set up of one such commercial, multiple-view registration system, from which our data was obtained. As we shall see, though mostly accurate, the point sets obtained also contain many erroneous outlier readings. Given such noisy measurements, the challenge is to derive an accurate shape description automatically. Otherwise, even slight errors may result in artifacts which need to be corrected manually, or worse, may make the restoration unusable.

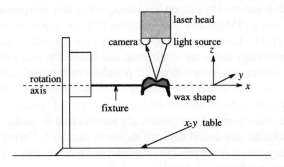

Fig. 1. Data acquisition by a laser digitizer (courtesy of GC Corporation, Tokyo, Japan).

While filter-based techniques such as discrete Fourier transform [10] are effective in suppressing spurious samples, they often "oversmooth", degrading sharp discontinuities and distinct features that correspond to important anatomical (preparation) lines and features. At present, unless intensive human intervention is used, it is impossible to construct an accurate representation that respects both medical and dental criteria requiring accuracy of up to 5 to 10 μm [5]. Recently, much progress has been made in computer vision for robust surface inference from clouds of points. Their application should result in better 3-D dental model descriptions. This paper presents an integrated approach for inferring dental models in the form of surfaces (for capturing smoothness) and 3-D curves (for preserving shape discontinuities) from noisy dental data.

Much work has been done in surface fitting to clouds of points. The majority of the approaches use the deformable model approach (first proposed by Kass *et al.* in [9] and then in [19]) which attempts to deform an initial shape for fitting the input, using energy minimization. The work by Boult and Kender [2], Poggio and Girosi [13], Blake and Zisserman [3], Fua and Sander [6], Szeliski *et al.* [14], and many others belong to this category. Physics-based approaches proposed by Terzopoulos *et al.* [17, 18] model the problem as a multi-particle system governed by physics laws and equations. The initial surface (or model), originally in equilibrium, is subject to external forces exerted at each data point. Such forces make the system converge to another equilibrium. Hoppe *et al.* [8] and Boissonnat [1] use computational geometry techniques, treating the data as graph vertices and constructing edges using local properties.

Most methods above are computationally expensive as an iterative process is taking place. Also, they have limited potential in inferring faithful 3-D models from dental data: most do not work in the presence of spurious noise; and surface discontinuities are usually smoothed out. Our method attacks these problems by applying [7, 15, 16], in which a non-linear voting process is used to achieve efficient feature segmentation and discontinuity detection. Our method is robust to outlier noise since its effect is reduced by accumulating a large number of tensor votes.

Our overall approach is depicted in Figure 2. Each input point is first quantized in a 3-D voxel array. A preprocessing step is then applied to estimate the normal to the surface. This step, as well as the surface and curve inference processes, is realized by *tensor voting*, which is outlined in section 2. Consequently, two independent 3-D *saliency maps*, one for surface (SMap) and one for curve (CMap), are produced. More details can be found in [7, 11]. Local extrema in these maps are extracted, resulting in a triangulation mesh (surfaces) and a set of directed and connected 3-D poly-line segments (curves). These features are then refined (if possible) to localize detected discontinuities and remove inconsistent surface patches (such as the spurious patches labeled in Figure 2). Finally, the surfaces and curves inferred in the 3-D model are coherently integrated. Feature extraction and integration are summarized in section 3 (also detailed in [15, 16]). Results on real dental data are shown in section 4. Owing to space limitation, we omit many details in the present coverage, and refer readers to [7, 11, 15, 16] for more technical and mathematical details.

2 Tensor voting and saliency maps

The noisy dental data is in fact a scalar field, for which a preprocessing step for normal estimation at each point, or "vectorization", is required. Having produced a vector field, then, a "densification" step is needed for surface and curve extraction. Both processes are realized by *tensor voting* [11], in which data are represented by *tensors*, and data communication is achieved by *voting*.

Tensor representation. A point in the 3-D space can assume either one of the three roles: surface patch, discontinuity (curve or point junctions), or outlier. Consider the two extremes, in which a point on a smooth surface is very certain about its surface (normal) orientation, whereas a point on a (curve or point) junction has absolute orientation uncertainty. This whole continuum is thus abstracted as a general, second-order symmetric 3-D *tensor*, which can be visualized geometrically as a 3-D **ellipsoid** (Figure 3). Such an ellipsoid can be fully described by the corresponding eigensystem with its three eigenvectors $\hat{V}_{max}, \hat{V}_{mid}$, and $\hat{V}_{min}$ and the three corresponding eigenvalues $\lambda_{max} \geq \lambda_{mid} \geq \lambda_{min}$. Rearranging the eigensystem, the 3-D ellipsoid is given by: $(\lambda_{max} - \lambda_{mid})\mathbf{S} + (\lambda_{mid} - \lambda_{min})\mathbf{P} + \lambda_{min}\mathbf{B}$, where $\mathbf{S} = \hat{V}_{max}\hat{V}_{max}^T$ defines a *stick tensor*, $\mathbf{P} = \hat{V}_{max}\hat{V}_{max}^T + \hat{V}_{mid}\hat{V}_{mid}^T$ defines a *plate tensor*, and $\mathbf{B} = \hat{V}_{max}\hat{V}_{max}^T + \hat{V}_{mid}\hat{V}_{mid}^T + \hat{V}_{min}\hat{V}_{min}^T$ gives a *ball tensor*. These tensors define the three *basis* tensors for any 3-D ellipsoid.

Geometric Interpretation. The *eigenvectors* encode *orientation (un)certainties*: surface orientation (normal) is described by the *stick* tensor, which indicates *certainty* in a single direction. *Uncertainties* are abstracted by two other tensors: *curve* junction results from two intersecting surfaces, where the uncertainty in orientation only spans a single *plane* perpendicular to the tangent of the junction curve, and thus described by a *plate* tensor. At *point* junctions where more than two intersecting surfaces are present, a *ball* tensor

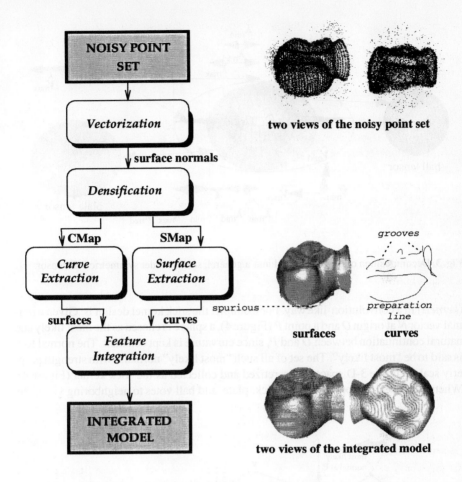

Fig. 2. Overall strategy of our method, using *Crown-24* as illustration.

is used since all orientations are equally probable. The *eigenvalues* encode the *magnitudes* of orientation (un)certainties, since they indicate the size of the corresponding 3-D ellipsoid. We define three *dense vector maps*, in which each voxel of these maps has a 2-tuple $(s, \bar{v})$, where s is a scalar indicating *saliency* and $\bar{v}$ is a unit vector:

- *Surface map (SMap)*: $s = \lambda_{max} - \lambda_{mid}$, and $\bar{v} = \hat{V}_{max}$ indicates the normal direction.
- *Curve map (CMap)*: $s = \lambda_{mid} - \lambda_{min}$, and $\bar{v} = \hat{V}_{min}$ indicates the tangent direction.
- *Junction map (JMap)*: $s = \lambda_{min}$, $\bar{v}$ is arbitrary.

Tensor voting. Having outlined the tensor formalism, we now describe the *voting* algorithm for obtaining the tensor representation at *each* voxel and the above dense vector maps, thus achieving field densification. Suppose that we already have a vector field for densification (vectorization will be described shortly). First, each input vector is encoded as a general tensor, which is actually a very thin and elongated ellipsoid. Then, these input tensors are made to align with predefined, discrete versions of the three basis tensors

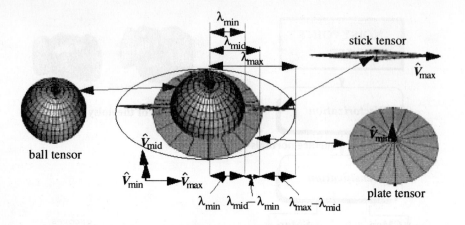

Fig. 3. Decomposition of a 3-D ellipsoid into a general, second-order symmetric 3-D tensor.

(*kernels*) in a convolution-like way. For example, the stick kernel design is: Given a normal vector N at origin O and a point P (Figure 4), a sphere is chosen as the most likely and natural continuation between O and P, since curvature is kept constant. The normal to P is said to be "most likely". The set of all such "most likely" normals (with strength properly scaled) in the 3-D space is discretized and collected as the stick kernel (Figure 4). When each input tensor has cast its stick, plate, and ball votes to neighboring voxels by

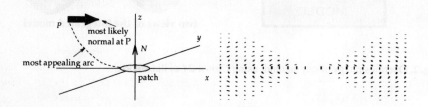

Fig. 4. The design, and one projection view of Stick kernel.

aligning with the respective *dense* basis kernels, each voxel in the volume receives a set of directed votes. These directed votes are collected, using tensor addition, as a 3x3 covariance matrix. Then, we diagonalize this matrix into the corresponding eigensystem and the above tensor formalism is applied.

Vectorizing scalar fields. Vectorizing a scalar field into a dense vector field is implemented *exactly* as the densification described above, except that each scalar input site is encoded as *ball* tensor, since no orientation information is given. After the voting step, the original input "balls" are replaced by true ellipsoids, which encode surface normal and curve tangent information.

3 Feature extraction and integration

Local extrema in CMap (resp. SMap) are extracted by our extremal curve (resp. surface) algorithms [16]. The extracted features are integrated to produce a coherent surface and curve description, whenever possible. These processes are outlined in the following:

Extremal curve extraction. Each voxel in the CMap holds a 2-tuple $(s,\bar{t})$, where s is curve saliency and $\bar{t}$ indicates tangent direction. Suppose the CMap is continuous in which $(s,\bar{t})$ is defined for every point p in 3-D space. A point p with $(s,\bar{t})$ is on an extremal curve if any displacement from p *on the plane normal to* $\bar{t}$ will result in a lower s value, i.e. $\frac{\partial s}{\partial u} = \frac{\partial s}{\partial v} = 0$, where u and v define the plane normal to $\bar{t}$ at the voxel center. This definition therefore involves the detection of zero crossing in the u-v plane normal to $\bar{t}$. To do this, we compute the saliency gradient $\bar{g}$ as, $\bar{g} = \nabla s = \left[\frac{\partial s}{\partial x} \; \frac{\partial s}{\partial y} \; \frac{\partial s}{\partial z}\right]^T$. Define $\bar{q} = \mathbf{R}(\bar{t} \times \bar{g})$ where $\mathbf{R}$ defines a frame aligned with the u-v plane. By construction, $\bar{q}$ is the projection of $\bar{g}$ onto the plane normal to $\bar{t}$. Therefore, an extremal curve is the locus of points for which $\bar{q} = \bar{0}$. The corresponding discrete $\bar{q}$ can be similarly defined, from which a tracing algorithm can be readily defined. The output is a set of connected and oriented poly-line segments representing the extremal curves.

Extremal surface extraction. Each voxel in the SMap holds a 2-tuple $(s,\bar{n})$ where s indicates surface saliency and $\bar{n}$ denotes normal direction. As before, suppose the SMap is continuous in which $(s,\bar{n})$ is defined for every point p in 3-D space. A point is on an extremal surface if its saliency s is locally extremal along the direction of the normal, i.e., $\frac{ds}{d\bar{n}} = 0$. This definition involves the detection of zero crossing on the line aligned with $\bar{n}$, which is computed by defining a scalar $q = \bar{n} \cdot \bar{g}$, where $\bar{g}$ was defined earlier. Therefore, an extremal surface is the locus of points for which $q = 0$. We define the corresponding discrete q, which can be processed directly by the Marching Cubes algorithm [12]: A polygonal mesh is thus produced.

Feature integration. The final phase integrates surfaces, curves and junctions to produce an unified 3-D model description. While tensor voting produces good results on smooth structures, it only detects discontinuities but does not properly localize them. This is because the SMap and CMap are independently interpreted. To integrate them, a curve detected in CMap is first treated as *surface inhibitor* in SMap so that when a smooth surface is traced, it is forbidden to enter region close to any detected discontinuities. With such a "trimmed" surface, the same curve is then treated as *surface exciter* for computing precise and natural surface junction. A set of "extended" surfaces are produced, which will undergo subsequent refinement.

4 Results

We tested our system on a variety of crowns and inlays. An inlay is a cast filling that is used to replace part of a tooth, while a crown is a larger restoration. The data is acquired using the set-up shown in Figure 1. The wax shape, obtained from the dental laboratory, is rotated about the x-axis in 15° (or 90°) increment so that 24 (or 4) successive views are visible to the sensor. The following tabulates the running times (in min) on a Sun Ultra 2 (Model 1300 with 256 MB RAM).

Data	No. of points	Voting	Feature extraction	Feature integration	Total
Mod-4	5217	4	2	-	6
Inlay-4	2447	3	1	-	4
Crown-4	8844	6	2	-	8
Crown-24	60095	35	5	5	45

Table 1. Processing times (in min) on Sun Ultra 2 (Model 1300 with 256 MB RAM).

Mod-4. We first demonstrate in this and the next two examples the graceful degradation of tensor voting in the presence of spurious and missing samples. Because of this, feature integration is skipped (as outlined in section 3). A set of only 4 views of a *Mod* are digitized and quantized in 100x100x100 array, which contains 5217 points. This data set is difficult because it has a complicated shape, and has many missing and misleading data resulting from fewer registered views and self occlusion. Using the inferred surface and curve model, we can perform **data validation** (Figure 5(a)): after voting, we validate each input point by simple thresholding of its associated surface or curve saliency. This shows a simple application of spurious noise elimination with the availability of a faithful model. The extracted extremal surfaces and curves are depicted in Figure 6(a). Note that surfaces are only correct from the discontinuity curves, for which they have low surface saliencies. However, these discontinuities are detected and marked since they are characterized by high curve saliencies. These detected junction curves allow further refinement or intervention to take place.

Inlay-4. A set of 4 views of an *Inlay* are digitized, having 2447 data points quantized in a 70x50x70 array. This is a very complicated surface, and the data set is noisy, and contains many missing and erroneous readings. Result of data validation is shown in Figure 5(b). The extremal surfaces and curves extracted are shown in Figure 6(b).

Crown-4. A sparse set of only 4 views of a *Crown* are digitized and quantized, using a 100x100x100 voxel array. This data set contains 8844 points. We can recover the underlying surface model, which is automatically marked with curves representing grooves and preparation lines. With a faithfully inferred model, we can perform data validation (Figure 5(c)). Figure 7(a) shows the resultant extremal surfaces and curves.

Crown-24. A set of 24 views of a *Crown* are registered. The data set contains 60095 points, quantized in a 100x100x100 array. We can detect the upper and lower surfaces of the *Crown*. The detected preparation line and the grooves are in turn used to produce a coherently integrated surface and curve description. Result of data validation is shown in Figure 5(d). Figure 7(b) shows the extracted extremal surfaces and curves.

5 Conclusion

We have presented an efficient and robust method, *tensor voting*, to automatically generate faithful dental models, consisting of surfaces and 3-D curves, from very noisy measurements. As shown by our results, while further improvement can still be made (or simply provide us with more views of data), our working prototype indeed demonstrates a very promising potential on significantly improving current dental CAD/CAM technology, as our system produces faithful results despite that some sample data are noisy, missing and confusing. We not only interpolate smooth structures, but also respect important anatomical lines, and filter out spurious outlier points as well, and hence offer the prospects for reducing time in providing necessary service. We expect to perform more quantitative error analysis, investigate the right level of details (e.g. data quantization), and compare our results on same complex data with outputs from other sites.

References

1. J.D. Boissonnat, "Representation of Objects by Triangulating Points in 3-D space", in *Proc. Intl. Conf. Patt. Recogn.*, pp.830–832, 1982.
2. T.E. Boult and J.R. Kender, "Visual Surface Reconstruction Using Sparse Depth Data", in *Proc. IEEE Comput. Vision Patt. Recogn.* (Miami Beach, FL), pp.68–76, 1986.
3. A. Blake and A. Zisserman, "Invariant Surface Reconstruction Using Weak Continuity Constraints", in *Proc. IEEE Comput. Vision Patt. Recogn.* (Miami Beach, FL), pp.62–67, 1986.
4. F. Duret, The Dental Robotic: "State of the Science Dental CAD/CAM", Clark's Clinic. Den. Ency, Philadelphia, Lincholl ed.
5. F. Duret, "Functionality and accuracy of Sopha CAD/CAM system today", in *Proc. Intl. Conf. Comput.*, vol. 1, p.500.
6. P. Fua and P. Sander, "Segmenting Unstructured 3D Points into Surfaces", in *Proc. Euro. Conf. Comput. Vision* (Santa Margherita Ligure, Italy), pp.676–680, 1992.
7. G. Guy and G. Medioni, "Inference of Surfaces, 3-D Curves, and Junctions from Sparse, Noisy 3-D Data", *IEEE Trans. on Patt. Anal. and Machine Intell.*, vol.19, no.11, pp.1265–1277, 1997.
8. H.Hoppe, T.DeRose, T.Duchamp, J.McDonald, W.Stuetzle, "Surface Reconstruction from Unorganized Points", *Computer Graphics*, 26, pp.71–78, 1992.
9. M. Kass, A. Witkin, and D. Terzopoulos, "Snakes: Active Contour Models", *Int. J. Comput. Vision*, pp.321–331, 1988.
10. H.Kimura, H.Sohmura, et al., "Three Dimensional Shape Measurement of Teeth (part 3)", *J. Osaka Uni. Dent Sch.*
11. M.-S. Lee and G. Medioni, "Inferring Segmented Surface Description from Stereo Data", in *Proc. IEEE Comput. Vision Patt. Recogn.*, (Santa Barbara, CA), pp.346–352, 1998.
12. W.E. Lorensen and H.E. Cline, "Marching Cubes: A High Resolution 3D Surface Reconstruction Algorithm", *Computer Graphics*, 21(4), 1987.
13. T. Poggio and F. Girosi, "A theory of networks for learning", *Science*, pp.978–982, 1990.
14. R. Szeliski, D. Tonnesen, and D. Terzopoulos, "Modeling Surfaces of Arbitrary Topology with Dynamic Particles", in *Proc. IEEE Comput. Vision Patt. Recogn.*, pp.82–85, Jun 1993.
15. C.-K. Tang and G. Medioni, "Integrated Surface, Curve and Junction Inference from Sparse 3-D Data Sets", in *Proc. IEEE Intl. Conf. Comput. Vision*, pp.818–824, Jan 1998.
16. C.-K. Tang and G. Medioni, "Extremal Feature Extraction from Noisy 3-D Vector and Scalar Fields", to appear in *Proc. IEEE Visualization Conf.*, Oct 1998.
17. D. Terzopoulos and D. Metaxas, "Dynamic 3D models with local and global deformations: deformable superquadratics", *IEEE Trans. on Patt. Anal. and Machine Intell.*, vol. 13, no. 7, pp.91–123, 1991.
18. D. Terzopoulos and M. Vasilescu, "Sampling and reconstruction with adaptive meshes", in *Proc. IEEE Comput. Vision Patt. Recogn.*, (Lahaina, Maui, HI), pp.70–75, 1991.
19. M. Vasilescu and D. Terzopoulos, "Adaptive Meshes and Shells: Irregular Triangulation, Discontinuities, and Heretical Subdivision", in *Proc. IEEE Comput. Vision Patt. Recogn.*, pp.829-832, 1992.

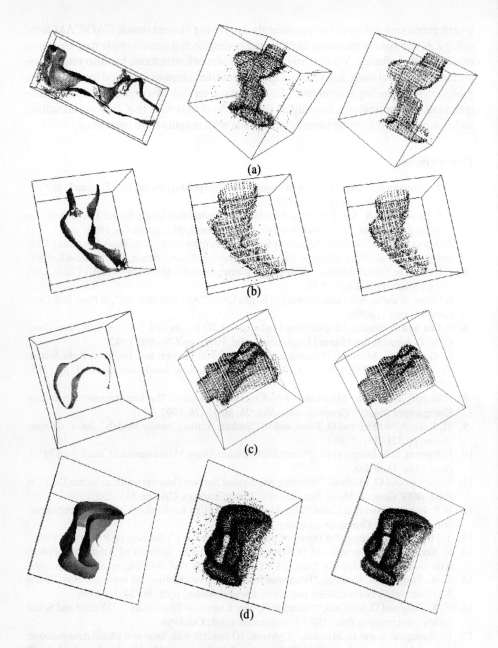

Fig. 5. A middle slice of extremal surfaces, the original noisy data, and the validated data set, for (a) *Mod-4*, (b) *Inlay-4*, (c) *Crown-4*, and (d) *Crown-24*

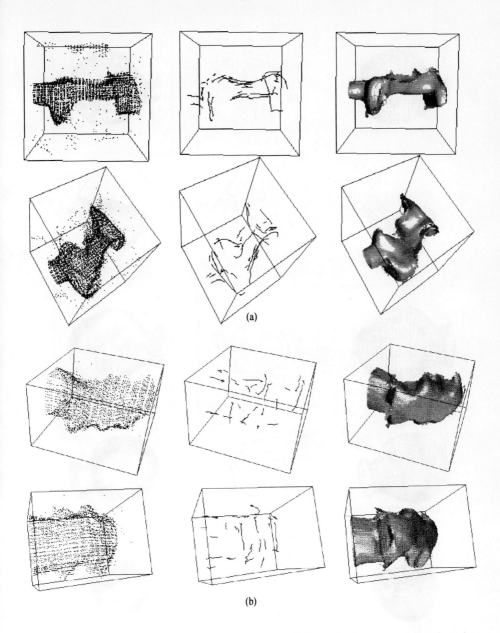

Fig. 6. Two views of the original noisy data, the extremal discontinuity curves and surfaces inferred for (a) *Mod-4* and (b) *Inlay-4*.

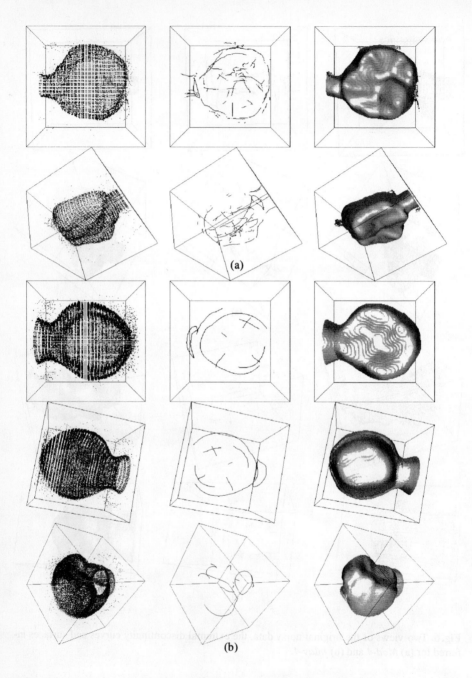

Fig. 7. Different views of the original noisy data, the extremal discontinuity curves and surfaces inferred for (a) *Crown-4* and (b) *Crown-24*.

Initial In-Vivo Analysis of 3D Heterogeneous Brain Computations for Model-Updated Image-Guided Neurosurgery

Michael Miga[1], Keith Paulsen[1,2,3], Francis Kennedy[1], Jack Hoopes[1,2,3], Alex Hartov[1,2], and David Roberts[2,3]

[1] Dartmouth College, Thayer School of Engineering, HB8000, Hanover, NH 03755
{michael.miga, keith.paulsen, francis.kennedy, p.jack.hoopes, alex.hartov, david.w.roberts}@dartmouth.edu
http://www.thayer.dartmouth.edu/thayer/
[2] Dartmouth Hitchcock Medical Center, Lebanon, NH 03756
[3] Norris Cotton Cancer Center, Lebanon, NH, 03756

Abstract. Registration error resulting from intraoperative brain shift due to applied surgical loads has long been recognized as one of the most challenging problems in the field of frameless stereotactic neurosurgery. To address this problem, we have developed a 3-dimensional finite element model of the brain and have begun to quantify its predictive capability in an *in vivo* porcine model. Previous studies have shown that we can predict the average total displacement within 15% and 6.6% error using intraparenchymal and temporal deformation sources, respectively, under relatively simple model assumptions. In this paper, we present preliminary results using a heterogeneous model with an expanding temporally located mass and show that we are capable of predicting an average total displacement to 5.7% under similar model initial and boundary conditions. We also demonstrate that our approach can be viewed as having the capability of recapturing approximately 75% of the registration inaccuracy that may be generated by preoperative-based image-guided neurosurgery.

1 Introduction

Current state-of-the-art image-guided surgery involves coregistration of the patient, the operating room coordinate space, patient-specific images generated by CT (computed tomographic) or MR (magnetic resonance), and surgical instrument location [1], [2]. This capability has dramatically impacted the field of frameless stereotactic neurosurgery by allowing detailed navigational information to be monitored in real-time during surgery. However, often during a neurosurgical procedure, tissue is purposely retracted/resected which causes a subsequent shift of the cortical surface as well as subsurface structures. Roberts et. al. performed a detailed study tracking cortical surface shift over 28 surgeries involving a variety of neurosurgical procedures and found on average a 1cm shift of the surface with a definite predisposition in the direction of gravity [3]. Hill et. al. performed a comparable study on 5 cases and evaluated overlays of the deformed surface on the original MR to understand the nature of the intraoperative brain shift. They found surface shifts that ranged from 0.3-7.4mm and that the surface tended to sink in the direction of gravity[4]. Dickhaus et. al. performed a 10 patient study with only tumor resections but used intraoperative MR which allowed quantification of subsurface movement. They found that surface shift was on the order of 2 cm, while subsurface movement was 6 to 7 mm for positions located at the interhemispheric fissure and the lateral ventricles [5].

This data suggests that coregistered image studies performed preoperatively cannot accurately account for such shift which in turn could lead to surgical error when relied upon for navigational information. To date, the only solutions to account for this shift have come in the form of intraoperative CT/MR which is costly and cumbersome and intraoperative ultrasound which provides a limited database with significantly lower contrast resolution. We have elected to pursue a physics-based modeling approach to account for intraoperative tissue deformation. Using the finite element method (FEM), we have modeled the brain using porous-media physics and have begun to quantify computational model accuracy using an *in vivo* porcine system in which we impart simulated surgical loads [6]. Previous studies have shown we can produce an average total displacement with errors less than 15% for an intraparenchymal placement of the deformation source [7], and less than 6.6% for a temporally located source under assumptions of homogeneous tissue properties [8]. In this paper, we have modeled the temporal mass expansion with added tissue heterogeneity, specifically gray/white matter delineation, in order to investigate the extent to which this increase in model complexity improves the data-model match.

2 Model

The theory used to model the brain originates from the soil mechanics literature and has been used in the context of soil consolidation. Deformation by consolidation theory [9] is characterized by an instantaneous deformation at the load contact area followed by subsequent additional displacement over time as the interstitial fluid drains in the direction of strain-induced pressure gradients (i.e. from high to low pressure). This theory characterizes brain tissue as a biphasic system consisting of a solid matrix and an interstitial fluid. The solid matrix is isotropic and follows the laws of linear elasticity. The fluid component represented by a pressure distribution flows in accordance with Darcy's law and is usually considered incompressible. The governing equation describing mechanical equilibrium is,

$$\nabla \cdot G\nabla \mathbf{u} + \frac{G}{1-2\nu}\nabla\varepsilon - \alpha\nabla p = 0. \quad (1)$$

where G is the shear modulus ($G = \frac{E}{2(1+\nu)}$), ν is Poisson's ratio, α is the ratio of fluid volume extracted to volume change of tissue under compression, ϵ is the volumetric strain ($\epsilon = \nabla \cdot \mathbf{u}$), $\mathbf{u}$ is the displacement vector, and p is the interstitial pressure. In order to complete the description, a constitutive equation relating volumetric strain to fluid drainage is represented as

$$\nabla \cdot k \nabla p - \alpha \frac{\partial \varepsilon}{\partial t} - \frac{1}{S} \frac{\partial p}{\partial t} = 0, \qquad (2)$$

where k is the hydraulic conductivity, and $1\backslash S$ is a void compressibility constant. In the literature, the fluid component of the model is typically considered incompressible for brain tissue, which we have also adopted (i.e. $\frac{1}{S} = 0$, $\alpha = 1$). The weighted residual form of the above equations along with a stability analysis has been presented previously [7], [10]. The method of solution used is a fully implicit Galerkin finite element scheme.

Unfortunately, only a modest amount of data on brain tissue mechanical properties has been reported in the literature. Early studies used mechanical devices to measure properties *in vivo* but were semi-quantitative at best [11]. A new and exciting area of research has emerged using MR and ultrasound to image transverse strain waves thereby allowing the calculation of regional mechanical properties based on strain measurements [12]. While more quantitative tissue property information can be anticipated in the future based on these newer techniques, the current uncertainty in brain tissue mechanical properties has led us to investigate the effect of varying Young's modulus and Poisson's ratio in our simplified homogenous model as well as the pressure gradient which acts as a distributed body force with respect to elastic deformation [13]. The results indicate that an optimal Young's modulus exists which varies with Poisson's ratio. The calculations also indicate that an optimal pressure gradient for a given Young's modulus and Poisson's ratio exists as well.

Based on previous results and the few literature citations on brain tissue properties which exist, we have performed a set of six calculations with different combinations of tissue properties as reported in Section 4. For comparison purposes three of these simulations use our homogeneous model with the elastic properties taken from our previous experience [13]. In addition, two different values of hydraulic conductivity have been assumed which span the maximum and minimum values in [14], [15]. In the three heterogeneous calculations, tissue property parameters have been taken from Nagashima et. al. [14] and Basser [15]. The Nagashima data is based on the feline brain for moduli whereas Basser performed analytical work to deduce his property values.

3 Methods

In conjunction with the realization of a numerical model, we have developed a method of quantification using an *in vivo* porcine experimental protocol. Prior to surgical procedures, a detailed MR series is taken of the pig cranium. These scans guide the FEM discretization process. Using **ANALYZE Version 7.5 - Biomedical Imaging Resource** (Mayo Foundation, Rochester, M.N.), we segment the 3D volume of interest and execute a discrete marching cubes algorithm to render a discretized description of the surface [16]. We then produce a tetrahedral grid on the interior of the domain defined by this boundary using customized mesh generation software [17]. Following the generation of the volumetric grid, we proceed to derive element tissue types by examining the average intensity value over an element based on the original MR image voxels thus creating a heterogeneous model. In this paper, we used thresholding to classify the tissue type but we also have the ability to determine tissue moduli using a functional interpolant description of the MR intensity values.

During the surgical procedure, the pig brain is implanted with 1 mm stainless steel beads in a grid-like fashion which serve as tissue markers. A balloon catheter (filled with contrast agent) is positioned temporally. All implants are easily observable in the CT images. Following the procedure, incremental inflations of the balloon catheter are performed and the beads are tracked in the CT yielding 3-dimensional deformation maps. Following the experiment, similar boundary conditions are applied to the model producing the predicted bead displacements which are subsequently compared to the deformation maps.

4 Results

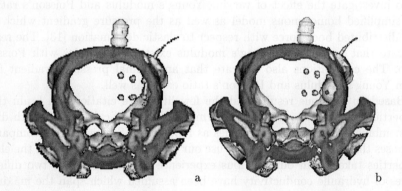

Fig. 1. Experimental model (a) baseline (b) 1 cc inflation.

The results from our *in vivo* porcine model can be seen in Figure 1a-b. Figure 1a-b illustrates the pig cranium with parenchymal tissue eliminated which enhances the visibility of the implants. Figure 1a represents the baseline position of the bead implants and the uninflated balloon catheter. The comparison figure shows movement by some beads resulting from the expanding temporally located balloon catheter. The expanded balloon surface can also be observed. The maximum displacement associated with balloon diameter for the 1cc inflation level is approximately 9.3 mm. The average bead displacement over 15 beads is 1.52 mm with a maximum of 5.61 mm.

Figures 2a illustrates a typical coronal MR slice from the pig cranium. Figure 2b shows the corresponding heterogeneous slice in the discretized volume mesh.

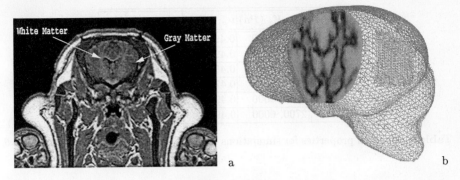

Fig. 2. Representation of heterogeneity in model with MRI slice (left) and respective heterogeneous model slice (right): (a) MRI coronal slice of pig cranium with white matter and gray matter designated (notice that white matter has a slightly higher image intensity value), (b) Volume grid boundary with equivalent rendered coronal heterogeneous slice where the dark border and its contents represent the complex material pattern of white matter surrounded by the lighter area corresponding to gray matter.

In this preliminary heterogeneous model, we have classified the continuum as one of two tissue types, white matter shown in the right image as the material enclosed by (boundary between materials is an interpolated color mapped to greyscale) the dark border and gray matter shown as the lighter material outside the border.

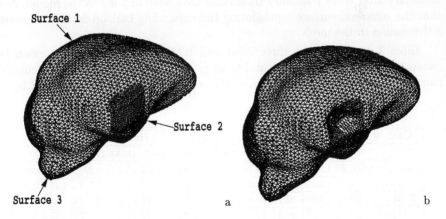

Fig. 3. (a) Boundary representation of tetrahedral grid with boundary condition surfaces designated (b) Deformed mesh from applied boundary conditions

Figure 3a displays the volumetric mesh generated by our mesh generation software with three surfaces designated where different boundary conditions are applied [17]. Surface 1 is the larger cortical surface and its boundary condition

Calc. #	E_w, E_g (Pa)	ν_w, ν_g	k_w, k_g ($\frac{m^3 s}{kg}$)
1	2100, 2100	0.49, 0.49	1e-7, 1e-7
2	2100, 2100	0.49, 0.49	7.5e-12, 7.5e-12
3	2100, 2100	0.45, 0.45	1e-7, 1e-7
4	4000, 8000	0.47, 0.47	1e-7, 1e-10
5	2700, 6000	0.49, 0.49	7.5e-12, 5e-12
6	2700, 6000	0.49, 0.49	1e-7, 1e-10

Table 1. Material properties for simulations with $dt = 180$ sec, # steps=3, $\mathbf{u}=0$, $p=0$.

represents a fixed, impermeable (to the fluid) surface. Surface 2 marked by the refined mesh is the location for balloon inflation. Displacement values correspond to the net balloon expansion (as measured from the CT scans) and are specified over this temporal area with an interstitial pressure of 5mmHg. Just outside the expansion area, the surface can move freely but is impermeable to flow. Surface 3 corresponds to the brain stem and was allowed to move freely (allowing the brain to herniate) and fixed with a pressure of 0 mmHg (gradient is formed from application area to brain stem). Under brain loading, strain-induced pressure gradients form and drainage occurs preferentially at the spinal column as the tissue is allowed to herniate. The field equations were solved on a mesh consisting of 21,732 nodes and 116,341 elements. The material properties (subscript 'g' and 'w' refer to gray and white matter, respectively) defining each calculation and the initial conditions are shown in Table 1. Figure 3b displays the mesh boundary after these boundary conditions have been applied to the model. Note that the temporal surface representing the expanding balloon front has created a depression in the mesh.

Table 2 quantifies the directional and total displacement comparison between calculated and experimental bead positions. The background calculation can be viewed as a representation of the errors that would be generated by us-

Calc. #	dx (mm) avg. (max.)	dy (mm) avg. (max.)	dz (mm) avg. (max.)	D (mm) avg. (max.)	D (%) avg. (max.)
background	0.39 (1.17)	0.26 (0.78)	1.35 (5.47)	1.52 (5.61)	27.2% (100.0%)
1 (Hom.)	0.53 (2.75)	0.32 (0.94)	0.39 (1.68)	0.33 (1.75)	5.9% (31.1%)
2 (Hom.)	0.57 (2.86)	0.29 (0.67)	0.54 (1.02)	0.51 (1.07)	9.2% (19.1%)
3 (Hom.)	0.53 (2.59)	0.31 (0.87)	0.40 (1.87)	0.32 (1.83)	5.7% (32.6%)
4 (Het.)	0.52 (2.53)	0.34 (1.07)	0.43 (1.86)	0.36 (1.86)	6.4% (33.2%)
5 (Het.)	0.57 (2.70)	0.31 (0.85)	0.48 (1.08)	0.42 (1.27)	7.5% (22.6%)
6 (Het.)	0.54 (2.61)	0.35 (1.09)	0.42 (1.70)	0.38 (1.77)	6.8% (31.6%)

Table 2. Comparison over several homogeneous (Hom.) and heterogeneous (Het.) calculations showing average (maximum) directional and total displacement error in absolute terms and the total displacement error as a percentage of the maximum bead displacement (background calculation assumes no bead movement).

ing preoperative-based image-guided neurosurgery (i.e. assumes no movement during surgery). The first column lists the respective calculation followed by 4 columns reflecting the mean and maximum of the absolute error between experimental and calculated displacements followed by the last column relating total displacement error to the maximum experimental bead displacement as a percentage. Column 4 shows a substantial recovery of error in the 'dz' component which is the direction of greatest motion for all calculations when compared to the background. Looking at the last two columns, the model-based method demonstrates an average improvement over the complete set of six different calculations of 75% (worst/best = 66%/79%) and 72% (worst/best = 67%/81%) with respect to the mean and maximum total displacement relative to a surgical technique which employs no updating.

Figure 4 is representative of the physical mapping of the deformation of each bead for each directional component as well the total displacement. Each subfigure plots the displacement component versus bead number. The complete directional trajectory of a particular bead can be determined from the top two subfigures (x and y directions) and the bottom left subfigure (z direction) while the total displacement can be found in the bottom right subfigure. In each subfigure, the measured (x) and calculated (o) bead displacement is compared where the line segment between the two symbols represents error between predicted and actual bead movement.

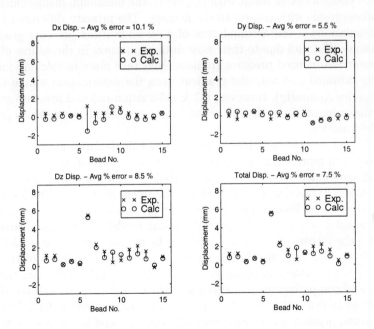

Fig. 4. Calculation #5 (heterogeneous) comparison between measured and calculated data for directional and total displacements for 1 cc inflation of the balloon catheter (Avg. % error is the average error relative to the maximum bead displacement).

5 Discussion

From Table 2, we see a dramatic improvement in total bead displacement for (homogeneous) calculation #1 over the background marked by the change in absolute error from 1.52 mm to 0.33 mm in column 5. Interestingly, we observe a slightly greater decrease in error in (homogeneous) calculation #3 to 0.32 mm. These simulations differ only with respect to Poisson's ratio. Calculations #1 & #4 as well as #2 & #5 are similar in hydraulic conductivity but substantively different in Young's modulus with #1 & #2 being homogeneous and #4 & #5 being heterogeneous. The nominal change in total displacement between calculations #1 & #4 (0.03mm) and between calculations #2 & #5 (0.09 mm) suggests the impact of heterogeneity on the model may be small. However, it is important to recognize that the homogeneous property values were based on the optimal data-model match [13] whereas no such optimization has been performed with heterogeneous properties rather the values were taken from the literature.

In a similar manner we can compare these simulations by grouping them according to hydraulic conductivity. Using this criterion, we could compare homogenous calculations #1 & #2 as well as heterogeneous calculations #5 & #6. In the first comparison we find that calculation #1 provides a better data-model match with respect to average total displacement whereas caclulation #2 is the better with respect to the maximum displacement. Comparing calculations #5 & #6 we find a similar trend where the simulation with smaller hydraulic conductivity yields a better result with respect to the maximum displacement error but a worse result with respect to the average. The primary difference between these simulations is the accumulation of a strain-induced pressure gradient in calculations #2 & #5 due to their slow draining nature. In the course of 9 minutes, the strain-induced pressure gradients that take place in calculations #1 & #6 have subsided and only the gradient from the deformation source to brain stem remains (5 mmHg). However, #2 & #5's strain-induced pressure gradients are on the order of 35 mmHg and act as a distributed body force which produces more deformation.

In Table 2, we have provided a background calculation. This calculation can be viewed as a representation of the loss in accuracy due to using preoperative-based image-guided surgery; it assumes that no movement has occurred from the initial image baseline which is exactly the same assumption which underpins preoperative-based image-guided neurosurgery. Using this measure as a background against which to compare subsequent model calculations provides insight into the recovery of accuracy that can be attained using our model-guided approach. It also suggests the degree to which each component of the model influences the accuracy outcome. Examining the averages in the last column of Table 2 and comparing the percentages to the background, we can see that our calculations indicate that elasticity accounts for approximately 63%-79% of the deformation, pressure gradients account for 5%-12% and heterogeneity accounts for 0.5%-2%. This breakdown ranks the importance of each component of the model and the approximate recovery of accuracy that might be expected using our approach.

Analyzing Figure 4 yields an indication of how well the model can track bead displacement. The majority of displacement in this case occurs along the z axis which is the direction approximately normal to the expanding balloon front. Overall, we can see that the directional trends are quantitatively captured and there is excellent agreement between experimental and calculated total displacement. Given the simplicity and approximate nature of the boundary conditions, the results presented here are very encouraging for the future of model-updated image-guided stereotactic neurosurgery.

6 Conclusions

In previous results, we have shown that a 3D consolidation model is capable of predicting the total average displacement to within 15% of measured values for an intraparenchymally located expanding mass [7], [13] and 6.6% for a temporally located mass [8] within a porcine brain. In this paper, we have demonstrated that we are able to predict a total average displacement within 5.7% for a temporally expanding mass using a more complex model which includes pressure gradients, tissue property heterogeneity and better mesh resolution. In the analysis of several calculations, we have found that the effects of heterogeneity are relatively minor, accounting for a 0.5%-2% change in results, while effects from elasticity and pressure gradients account for 63%-79% and 5%-12%, respectively. However, it is important to recognize that we have not explored the full range of possible combinations of heterogeneous tissue properties in order to best fit the experimental data. Further, there is no consensus on the exact values for these properties in gray versus white matter. Hence, we may have underestimated the importance of tissue heterogeneity at this point and further study is warranted. Nonetheless, our approach has shown an ability to capture nearly 75% of the tissue registration inaccuracy generated by the equivalent of preoperative-based image-guided neurosurgery. The remaining 25% has likely been lost for several reasons of which the most significant may be the inability to adequately describe the expanding balloon front creating error associated with bead directionality. We are presently in the process of designing a piston-like delivery system for more controlled applications of deformation. Undoubtedly, there is additional accuracy loss due to large deformation, non-linearities and experimental error (i.e. coregistration and bead fixation problems); but, overall the results shown here, as well as previously, are very encouraging for this model-updating approach.

Acknowledgments: This work was supported by National Institutes of Health grant R01-NS33900 awarded by the National Institute of Neurological Disorders and Stroke. ANALYZE software was provided in collaboration with the Mayo Foundation.

References

1. D. W. Roberts, J. W. Strohbehn, J. F. Hatch, W. Murray, and H. Kettenberger, ' A frameless stereotactic integration of computerized tomographic imaging and the operating microscope', *J. Neurosurg.*, vol. 65, pp. 545-549, 1986.

2. T. Peters, B. Davey, P. Munger, R. Comeau, A. Evans, and A. Olivier, 'Three-dimensional multimodal image-guidance for neurosurgery', *IEEE Trans. Med. Imaging*, vol. 15, pp. 121-128, 1996.
3. D. W. Roberts, A. Hartov, F.E. Kennedy, M. I. Miga, K. D. Paulsen, 'Intraoperative brain shift and deformation: a quantitative clinical analysis of cortical displacements in 28 cases', *Neurosurgery*, (in press), 1998.
4. D. L. G. Hill, C. R. Maurer, M. Y. Wang, R. J. Maciunas, J. A. Barwise, J. M. Fitzpatrick, 'Estimation of intraoperative brain surface movement', *Proc. CVRMed-MRCAS'97*, ed. J. Troccaz, E. Grimson, R. Mosges, Springer Lecture Notes in Computer Science, vol. 1205, pp. 449-458, 1997.
5. H. Dickhaus, K. Ganser, A. Staubert, M. M. Bonsanto, C. R. Wirtz, V. M. Tronnier, and S. Kunze, 'Quantification of brain shift effects by mr-imaging', *Proc. An. Int. Conf. IEEE Eng. Med. Biology Soc.*, 1997.
6. M. I. Miga, K. D. Paulsen, F. E. Kennedy, P. J. Hoopes, A. Hartov, and D. W. Roberts, 'A 3D brain deformation model experiencing comparable surgical loads', *Proc. 19th An. Int. Conf. IEEE Eng. Med. Biology Soc.*, 773-776, 1997.
7. K. D. Paulsen, M. I. Miga, F. E. Kennedy, P. J. Hoopes, A. Hartov, and D. W. Roberts, 'A computational model for tracking subsurface tissue deformation during stereotactic neurosurgery', *IEEE Transactions on Biomedical Engineering*, (in press), (1998).
8. M. I. Miga, K. D. Paulsen, F. E. Kennedy, P. J. Hoopes, A. Hartov, and D. W. Roberts, 'Quantification of a 3D brain deformation model experiencing a temporal mass expansion', *Proceedings of the 24th IEEE Northeast Bioengineering Conference*, pp. 68-71, 1998.
9. M. Biot, 'General theory of three dimensional consolidation', *J. Appl. Phys.*, vol. 12, pp. 155-164, 1941.
10. M. I. Miga, K. D. Paulsen, F. E. Kennedy, 'Von Neumann stability analysis of Biot's general two-dimensional theory of consolidation', *Int. J. of Num. Methods in Eng.*, (in press), 1998.
11. E. K. Walsh, and A. Schettini, 'Calculation of brain elastic parameters in vivo', *Am. J. Physiol.*, 247, R693-R700, 1984.
12. R. Mathupillai, P. J. Rossman, D. J. Lomas, J. F. Greenleaf, S. J. Riederer, and R. L. Ehman, 'Magnetic resonance elastography by direct visualization of propagating acoustic strain waves', *Science*, vol. 269, pp. 1854-1857, 1995.
13. M. I. Miga, K. D. Paulsen, F. E. Kennedy, P. J. Hoopes, A. Hartov, and D. W. Roberts, 'Modeling Surgical Loads to Account for Subsurface Tissue Deformation During Stereotactic Neurosurgery', *IEEE SPIE Proceedings of Laser-Tissue Interaction IX, Part B: Soft-tissue Modeling*, vol. 3254, pp. 501-511, 1998.
14. T. Nagashima, T. Shirakuni, and SI. Rapoport, 'A two-dimensional, finite element analysis of vasogenic brain edema,' *Neurol. Med. Chir.*, vol. 30, pp. 1-9, 1990.
15. P. J. Basser, 'Interstitial pressure, volume, and flow during infusion into brain tissue', *Microvasc. Res.*, vol. 44, pp. 143-165, 1992.
16. C. Montani, R. Scateni, and R. Scopigno, 'Discretized Marching Cubes Visualization 1994', *Conf. Proc.*, Washington, 1994.
17. J. M. Sullivan Jr., G. Charron, and K. D. Paulsen, 'A three dimensional mesh generator for arbitrary multiple material domains, *Finite Element Analysis and Design*, vol. 25, pp. 219-241, 1997.

A New Dynamic FEM-Based Subdivision Surface Model for Shape Recovery and Tracking in Medical Images

Chhandomay Mandal[1], Baba C. Vemuri[1], and Hong Qin[2]

[1] Dept. of CISE, University of Florida, Gainesville
[2] Dept. of CS, SUNY at Stony Brook

Abstract. A new dynamic FEM-based subdivision surface model is proposed to reconstruct and track shapes of interest from multi-dimensional medical images. The model is based on the butterfly subdivision scheme, a popular subdivision technique for generating smooth C^1 (first derivative continuous) surfaces of *arbitrary topology*, and is embedded in a physics-based modeling paradigm. This hierarchical model needs *very few* degrees of freedom (control vertices) to accurately recover and track complex smooth shapes of arbitrary topology. A novel technique for locally parameterizing the smooth surface of arbitrary topology generated by the butterfly scheme is described; physical quantities required to develop the dynamic model are introduced, and the governing dynamic differential equation is derived using Lagrangian mechanics and the finite element method. Our experiments demonstrate the efficacy of the modeling technique for efficient shape recovery and tracking in multi-dimensional medical images.

1 Introduction

Advances in the medical imaging technology over the last few decades have given us an opportunity to obtain a detailed view of the internal anatomical structures using state-of-the-art high resolution imagery. However, efficient recovery and tracking of the embedded complex shapes from large volume data sets is still an open area of research. Accurate shape recovery requires distributed parameter models which typically possess a large number of degrees of freedom. On the other hand, efficient shape representation imposes the requirement of geometry compression, i.e., models with fewer degrees of freedom. These requirements are conflicting and numerous researchers have been seeking to strike a balance between these requirements [1–6]. A physics-based model best satisfying both the criteria is a good candidate for a solution to the shape recovery problem for obvious reasons. Deformable models, which come in many varieties, have been used to solve this problem in the physics-based modeling paradigm. These models involve either fixed size [1, 6] or adaptive size [2, 5] grids. The models with fixed grid size generally use less number of degrees of freedom for representation, but the accuracy of the recovered shape is lacking in most cases. On the other hand, models using adaptive grids typically use large number of degrees of freedom to recover the shapes accurately. In most medical imaging applications, the anatomical shapes being recovered from image data are smooth in spite of the complex details inherent in the shapes. Under these circumstances, the finite element approaches as in [1, 5] need a *large* number of degrees of freedom for deriving a smooth and accurate representation. In addition, they can not represent shapes with known arbitrary topology.

Subdivision surfaces, widely used in computer graphics for modeling shapes of arbitrary topology, offer a compact representation of smooth complex shapes. In a typical subdivision scheme, a simple polygonal mesh a.k.a. the control mesh is refined recursively using a fixed set of refinement rules to generate a smooth C^1 or C^2 (second derivative continuous) limit surface. *This smooth limit surface is described by the degrees of freedom of the initial mesh*, thereby offering a very compact representation of a potentially complicated shape. If these purely geometric subdivision models were to be set in a physics-based paradigm, they will offer an elegant solution to the problem of reconstructing arbitrarily complex shapes. However, the problem lies in the fact that the limit surface obtained via subdivision process does not have a closed-form analytic expression. Dynamic subdivision surfaces were first introduced by Mandal et al. [4] to address the aforementioned shape recovery problem. The technique however was limited to a very specific subdivision scheme. The approach taken in this paper is much more general in the sense that it can be used with any type of subdivision schemes. However, we choose the butterfly scheme [7] to demonstrate the concept. A detailed discussion on the advantages of the proposed model can be found in [8]. Once we embed the chosen subdivision surface model into physics-based paradigm, the initialized model deforms under the influence of synthesized forces to fit the underlying shape in the data set via the principle of energy minimization. Recalling the fact that the smooth limit surface in any subdivision scheme is a function of the degrees of freedom of the initial mesh, once an approximate shape is recovered from the data, the model adopts a new initial mesh which is obtained via a subdivision of the original initial mesh. Note that this new initial mesh and the original initial mesh have the same limit surface, but the new initial mesh has more degrees of freedom thereby assisting in the recovery of the local features of the underlying shape. This process is continued till a prescribed error criteria for fitting the data points is achieved. This model can also be used in the context of tracking dynamic shapes via a straight-forward extension – once the shape is recovered from a data set in a time sequence, the recovered shape can be used as the initialization for the next data set in the sequence. The experimental results show that the proposed method outperforms the existing methods, including the technique in [4], in terms of the number of degrees of freedom to represent a given shape. We also demonstrate better performance of this model in compactness of shape representation in comparison with the now popular balloon (FEM-based) model in the context of tracking an underlying shape in a time sequence of CT images.

2 Formulation

The butterfly subdivision scheme [7] starts with an initial triangular mesh which is also known as control mesh. The vertices of the control mesh are known as control points. In each step of subdivision, the initial (control) mesh is refined through the transformation of each triangular face into a patch with four triangular faces. After one step of refinement, the new mesh in the finer level retains the vertices of each triangular face in the previous level and hence, "interpolates" the coarser mesh in the previous level. In addition, every edge in each triangular face is spilt by adding a new vertex whose position is obtained by an affine combination of the neighboring vertex positions in the coarser level as shown in Fig.1(a). The name, butterfly subdivision, originated from the "butterfly"-like configuration of the contributing vertices. The weighting factors for different contributing vertex positions are shown in Fig.1(b). The vertex $\mathbf{e}_{12}^{j+1}$ in the $j+1$-th

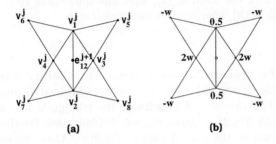

Fig. 1. (a) The contributing vertices in the j-th level for the vertex in the j+1-th level corresponding to the edge between $\mathbf{v}_1^j$ and $\mathbf{v}_2^j$; (b) the weighing factors for different vertices.

level of subdivision, corresponding to the edge connecting vertices $\mathbf{v}_1^j$ and $\mathbf{v}_2^j$ at level j, is obtained by $\mathbf{e}_{12}^{j+1} = 0.5(\mathbf{v}_1^j + \mathbf{v}_2^j) + 2w(\mathbf{v}_3^j + \mathbf{v}_4^j) - w(\mathbf{v}_5^j + \mathbf{v}_6^j + \mathbf{v}_7^j + \mathbf{v}_8^j)$, where $0 \leq w \leq 1$, and $\mathbf{v}_i^j$ denotes the position of the i-th vertex at the j-th level.

The butterfly subdivision scheme produces a smooth C^1 surface of an arbitrary topology in the limit (except possibly at very few degenerate points) whose global parameterization may not be possible. However, we can locally parameterize the limit surface over the domain defined by the initial mesh. The idea is to track any arbitrary point on the initial mesh across the meshes obtained via the subdivision process, so that a correspondence can be established between the point being tracked in the initial mesh and its image on the limit surface. We note that the smooth limit surface has as many smooth triangular patches as the triangular faces in the initial mesh. Therefore, the limit surface s can be expressed as $\mathbf{s} = \sum_{k=1}^{n} \mathbf{s}_k$, where n is the number of triangular faces in the initial mesh and $\mathbf{s}_k$ is the smooth triangular patch in the limit surface corresponding to the k-th triangular face in the initial mesh.

We now briefly describe the parameterization of the limit surface over the initial mesh, the details of which can be found in [8]. We choose a simple planar

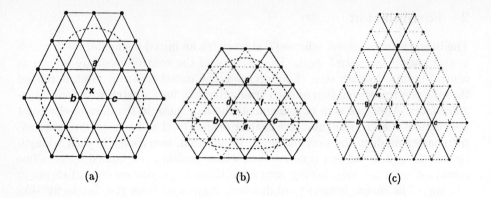

Fig. 2. Tracking a point x through various levels of subdivision : (a) initial mesh, (b) the selected section of the mesh in (a), after one subdivision step, (c) the selected section of the mesh in (b), after another subdivision step.

mesh shown in Fig.2(a) as the initial mesh. An arbitrary point **x** inside the triangular face abc is tracked over the meshes obtained through subdivision. After one level of subdivision, it falls inside the triangular face dbe as shown in Fig.2(b). Note that Fig.2(b) shows the subdivided mesh for the portion of the initial mesh selected by the dotted lines in Fig.2(a). After one more subdivision step, the tracked point **x** is inside the triangular face dgi. We have developed a systematic tracking strategy and it can be shown that *any point inside the smooth triangular patch in the limit surface corresponding to the face abc in the initial mesh depends only on the vertices in the initial mesh which are within the 2-neighborhood of the vertices* **a**, **b** *and* **c** *due to the local nature of the subdivision process* [8]. Let $\mathbf{v}^0_{abc}$ be the collection of vertices in the initial mesh which are within the 2-neighborhood of the vertices **a**, **b** and **c** in the initial mesh (Fig.2(a)). Now, the smooth triangular patch in the limit surface corresponding to the triangular face abc in the initial mesh can be written as $\mathbf{s}_{abc}(\mathbf{x}) = \mathbf{B}_{abc}(\mathbf{x})\mathbf{v}^0_{abc}$, where $\mathbf{B}_{abc}$ is the collection of basis functions at the vertices of $\mathbf{v}^0_{abc}$. In [8], we describe the details of the construction of an approximation to these basis functions generated by the butterfly subdivision which do not have any closed-form expression. Finally, we can collect all the triangular patches in the limit surface together, and the expression for the smooth limit surface can be written as $\mathbf{s}(\mathbf{x}) = \mathbf{J}(\mathbf{x})\mathbf{p}$, where **J** is the collection of basis functions for the corresponding vertices in the initial mesh. The vector **p** is also known as the degrees of freedom vector of the smooth limit surface **s**.

We now treat the vertex positions in the initial mesh defining the smooth limit surface **s** as a function of time in order to develop the new dynamic butterfly subdivision model. The velocity of the surface model can be expressed as

$\dot{\mathbf{s}}(\mathbf{x}, \mathbf{p}) = \mathbf{J}(\mathbf{x})\dot{\mathbf{p}}$, where an overstruck dot denotes a time derivative and $\mathbf{x} \in S^0$, S^0 being the domain defined by the initial mesh.

3 Finite Element Implementation

We have already pointed out in Section 2 that the smooth limit surface obtained by the recursive application of the butterfly subdivision rules can be represented by smooth triangular patches. We consider each patch in the limit surface as an element. The number of such patches is equal to the number of triangular faces in the initial mesh as mentioned earlier. The governing motion equation of the dynamic model is given by $\mathbf{M}\ddot{\mathbf{p}} + \mathbf{D}\dot{\mathbf{p}} + \mathbf{K}\mathbf{p} = \mathbf{f}_p$, where $\mathbf{f}_p$ is the generalized force vector and $\mathbf{M}$, $\mathbf{D}$, and $\mathbf{K}$ are the mass, damping and stiffness matrices of the model. We now provide an outline on how to derive the mass, damping and stiffness matrices for these elements so that a numerical solution to the governing second-order differential equation can be obtained using finite element analysis techniques. We use the same example as in Section 2 (refer Fig.2) to develop the related concepts.

The mass matrix for the element $\mathbf{s}_{abc}$, corresponding to the triangular face abc, can be written as $\mathbf{M}_{abc} = \int_{\mathbf{x} \in \mathbf{s}_{abc}} \mu(\mathbf{x}) \mathbf{B}_{abc}^T(\mathbf{x}) \mathbf{B}_{abc}(\mathbf{x}) d\mathbf{x}$. However, the basis functions (stored as entries in $\mathbf{B}_{abc}$) do not have any analytic form, hence computing this integral is a difficult proposition. We solve the problem by approximating the smooth triangular patch in the limit surface corresponding to the face abc in the initial mesh by a triangular mesh with 4^j faces obtained after j levels of subdivision of the original triangular face abc (each subdivision step splits one triangular face into 4 triangular faces). In addition, we choose a discrete mass density function which has non-zero values only at the vertex positions of the j-th subdivision level mesh. Then the mass matrix can be expressed as $\mathbf{M}_{abc} = \sum_{i=1}^{k} \mu(\mathbf{v}_i^j) \{\mathbf{B}_{abc}^j(\mathbf{v}_i^j)\}^T \{\mathbf{B}_{abc}^j(\mathbf{v}_i^j)\}$, where k is the number of vertices in the triangular mesh with 4^j faces. This approximation has been found to be very effective and efficient for implementation purposes. The elemental damping matrix can be obtained in an exactly similar fashion.

We assign internal energy to each element in the limit surface, thereby defining the internal energy of the smooth subdivision surface model. We take a similar approach as in the derivation of the elemental mass and damping matrix and assign the internal energy to a j-th level approximation of the element. In this paper, we assign spring energy to the discretized model as its internal energy. For the example used throughout the paper, this energy at the j-th level of approximation can be written as

$$E_{abc} \approx E_{abc}^j = \frac{1}{2} \sum_{\Omega} \frac{k_{lm}(|\mathbf{v}_l^j - \mathbf{v}_m^j| - \ell_{lm})}{|\mathbf{v}_l^j - \mathbf{v}_m^j|} (\mathbf{v}_l^j - \mathbf{v}_m^j)$$

$$= \frac{1}{2} \{\mathbf{v}_{abc}^j\}^T (\mathbf{K}_{abc}^j) \{\mathbf{v}_{abc}^j\},$$

where k_{lm} is the spring constant, $\mathbf{v}_l^j$ and $\mathbf{v}_m^j$, the l-th and m-th vertex in the j-th level mesh, are in the 1-neighborhood of each other, Ω is the domain defined by all such vertex pairs, ℓ_{lm} is the natural length of the spring connected between $\mathbf{v}_l^j$ and $\mathbf{v}_m^j$, and $\mathbf{v}_{abc}^j$ is the concatenation of the (x,y,z) positions of all the vertices in the j-th subdivision level of the triangular face abc in the initial mesh. Now, the vertex positions in $\mathbf{v}_{abc}^j$ are obtained by a linear combination of the vertex positions in $\mathbf{v}_{abc}^0$, and hence we can write $\mathbf{v}_{abc}^j = (\mathbf{A}_{abc}^j) \mathbf{v}_{abc}^0$ where $(\mathbf{A}_{abc}^j)$ is the transformation (subdivision) matrix. Therefore, the expression for the elemental stiffness matrix is given by $\mathbf{K}_{abc} = (\mathbf{A}_{abc}^j)^T (\mathbf{K}_{abc}^j)(\mathbf{A}_{abc}^j)$.

The generalized force vector $\mathbf{f}_p$ represents the net effect of all externally applied forces. The current implementation supports spring, inflation as well as image-based forces. However, other types of forces like repulsion forces, gravitational forces etc. can easily be implemented.

Model Subdivision. The initialized model grows dynamically according to the equation of motion and when an equilibrium is achieved, the number of control vertices can be increased by replacing the original initial mesh by a new initial mesh obtained through one step of butterfly subdivision. This increases the number of degrees of freedom to represent the same smooth limit surface and a new equilibrium position for the model with a better fit to the given data set can be achieved. The error of fit criteria for the discrete data is based on distance between the data points and the points on the limit surface where the corresponding springs are attached. In the context of image-based forces, if the model energy does not change between successive iterations indicating an equilibrium for the given resolution, the degrees of freedom for the model can be increased by the above-mentioned replacement scheme until the model energy is sufficiently small and the change in energy between successive iterations becomes less than a pre-specified tolerance.

4 Results

In the first experiment, we present the shape extraction of a caudate nucleus from 64 MRI slices, each of size 256×256. Fig.3(a) depicts a slice from this MRI scan along with the points placed by an expert neuroscientist on the boundary of the shape of interest. Fig.3(b) depicts the data points (placed in each of the slices depicting the boundary of the shape of interest) in 3D along with the initialized model. Note that points had to be placed on the boundary of the caudate nucleus due to lack of image gradients delineating the caudate from the surrounding tissue in parts of the image. The control mesh of the smooth initialized model has only 14 vertices (degrees of freedom). Continuous image based forces as well as spring forces are applied to the model and the model deforms under the influence of these forces until maximal conformation to the data is achieved. The final fitted model, which has a control mesh comprising 194 vertices, is shown in Fig.3(c). We like to point out the fact that the recovered shape in [4] for the same data set has 386 degrees of freedom and therefore, we achieve a factor of 2 improvement in the number of degrees of freedom required to represent the model in this particular example.

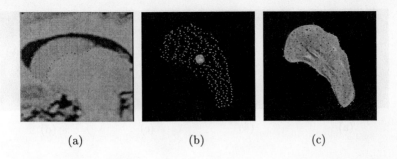

Fig. 3. (a) Data points identifying the boundary of the caudate nucleus on a MRI slice of human brain, (b) data points (from all slices) in 3D along with the initialized model, and (c) the fitted dynamic butterfly subdivision model.

In the second experiment, we recover and track the left-ventricular chamber of a canine heart over a complete cardiac cycle. The data set comprised of eight 3D CT images, with each volume image having 118 slices each of 128 × 128 pixels. First, we recover the shape from one data set using image-based (gradient) as well as point-based forces. After achieving this, the fitted model is used as the initialization for the next data set to track the shape of interest. The tracking results are shown in Fig.4 for the eight volume data sets. It may be noted that the control mesh describing the smooth surfaces shown in Fig.4 has only 384 triangular faces with a total of 194 vertices. This is an improvement by a factor of approximately 15 over the results reported in [5] for representing the same data set.

5 Conclusions

In this paper, we have presented a finite element method based dynamic butterfly subdivision surface model which is very useful for shape recovery and tracking. We have presented a local parameterization of the subdivision scheme, incorporated the advantages of free-form deformable models in the butterfly subdivision scheme and introduced hierarchical dynamic control. Our experiments show that the model outperforms the existing shape recovery schemes in terms of the compactness in the representation of the smooth recovered shape, and can also be used successfully in tracking applications.

6 Acknowledgments

This research was supported in part by the NSF grant ECS-9210648 and the NIH grant RO1-LM05944 to BCV, the NSF CAREER award CCR-9702103 and DMI-9700129 to HQ. We wish to acknowledge Dr. T. McInerney, Dr. G. Malandain, Dr. D. Goldgof, and Dr. C.M. Leonard for the data sets.

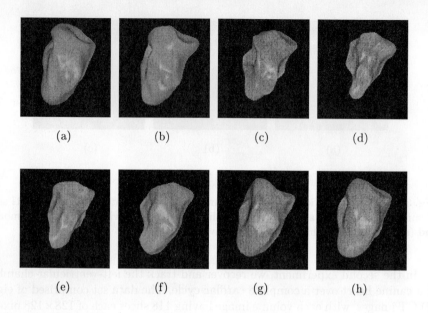

(a) (b) (c) (d)

(e) (f) (g) (h)

Fig. 4. Tracking of the LV chamber of a canine heart over a cardiac cycle using the dynamic butterfly subdivision model.

References

1. L.D. Cohen, and I. Cohen, "Finite-element methods for active contour models and balloons for 2D and 3D images," *PAMI*, vol. 15, no. 11, pp. 1131 – 1147, November 1993.
2. E. Koh, D. Metaxas and N. Badler, "Hierarchical shape representation using locally adaptive finite elements," in *ECCV'94*, Springer-Verlag, vol. 800, pp. 441 – 446.
3. F. Leitner and P. Cinquin, "Complex topology 3D objects segmentation," in *Model-based Vision Development and Tools*, SPIE, vol. 1609, pp. 16 – 26, 1991.
4. C. Mandal, B.C. Vemuri and H. Qin, "Shape recovery using dynamic subdivision surfaces," in *ICCV'98*, pp. 805 – 810.
5. T. McInerney and D. Terzopoulos, "A dynamic finite element surface model for segmentation and tracking in multidimensional medical images with application to cardiac 4D image analysis," *CMIG*, vol. 19, no. 1, pp. 69 – 83, 1995.
6. D. Terzopoulos and D. Metaxas, "Dynamic 3D models with local and global deformations: Deformable superquadrics," *PAMI*, vol. 13, no. 7, pp. 703 – 714, July 1991.
7. N. Dyn, D. Levin and J.A. Gregory, "A butterfly subdivision scheme for surface interpolation with tension control," *TOG*, vol. 9, no. 2, pp. 160 – 169, April 1990.
8. C. Mandal, H. Qin and B.C. Vemuri. "Direct manipulation of butterfly subdivision surfaces : A physics-based approach," Technical Report CISE-TR-98-009, University of Florida, 1998.

Automatic Quantification of Changes in the Volume of Brain Structures

Guillaume Calmon[1], Neil Roberts[1], Paul Eldridge[2], and Jean-Philippe Thirion[3]

[1] Magnetic Resonance and Image Analysis Research Centre (MARIARC),
University of Liverpool, UK
{gcalmon, neil}@liv.ac.uk
[2] Walton Centre for Neurology and Neurosurgery, Liverpool, UK
eldrid-p@wcnn.co.uk
[3] Épidaure Project, Institut National de Recherche en Informatique
et en Automatique (INRIA), Sophia Antipolis, France
thirion@epidaure.inria.fr

Abstract. We present an automatic technique to quantify changes in the volume of cerebral structures. The only manual step is a segmentation of the structure of interest in the first image. The image analysis comprises: *i)* a precise rigid co-registration of the time series of images, *ii)* the computation of residual deformations betweens pairs of images. Automatic quantification can be obtained either by propagation of the segmentation or by integration of the deformation field. These approaches have been applied to monitor brain atrophy in one patient and to investigate a 'mass effect' in tissue surrounding a brain tumour in four patients undergoing radiotherapy. Segmentation propagation gave good results for quantifying contrasted structures such as ventricles or well-circumscribed tumours; however, integration of the deformations may be more appropriate to quantify diffusive tumours.

1 Introduction

The combination of Magnetic Resonance (MR) imaging and computer-based image analysis offers the opportunity for non-invasive measurement of changes in brain compartment volumes associated with a variety of diseases. Images obtained on successive occasions may be analysed separately, thanks to point-counting technique [1], or repeated segmentations of the structure of interest. Alternatively, an increasingly popular approach involves first co-registering all the images obtained in the time series. Changes may be visualised by subtracting consecutive co-registered images in the time series [2], [3]. Quantification may be achieved by integrating small intensity changes within the boundary region [4].

Furthermore, pathologies can be studied by comparison to a reference patient or model, thanks to non-rigid inter-patient registration. Several methods have been put forward, including the use of anatomical landmarks [5], [6] or differential features (e.g. edges, crest-lines or ridges). The possible output transformations include linear deformations [7], splines [8],[9], elastic models [10], [11], and viscous fluid models [12].

In this work, after an automatic rigid co-registration of succesive magnetic resonance (MR) images of a patient, a 3-D deformation field resulting from an intra-patient non-rigid registration is used to propagate an initial segmentation to each image in the time series. An alternative approach is to integrate the deformation field over a family of surfaces equidistant from the initial segmentation. The difference in the volume variation obtained by integration and by segmentation propagation may be accounted for by a mass effect in the surrounding tissue. A detailed description of the methods of segmentation propagation and deformation field integration are given in Sect. 2 below. In Sect. 3, we describe the application of segmentation propagation to a patient with primary progressive aphasia (PPA). In Sect. 4 we describe the application of both approaches to four patients with brain tumours undergoing radiotherapy.

2 Quantification of Volume Variation

2.1 Overview of the Technique

The technique comprises: *i)* a rigid co-registration of all the images in the series with the image acquired first, using an automatic detection of crest-lines in the images and a matching of their maxima of curvature [13]; *ii)* a non-rigid matching used to compute the residual deformations between successive pairs of images. Our implementation utilises the 'demons' algorithm [14], close to viscous-fluid models [15]. It outputs a 3-D vector field called **f**. The only manual step of the technique is a (semi-automatic) segmentation of the structure of interest in the first image of the series. Automatic quantification can then be obtained either by propagation of the segmentation (see Sect. 2.2) or by integration of the deformation field **f** (see Sect. 2.3).

2.2 Segmentation Propagation

Given two images, I_1 and I_2, a segmentation S_1 in I_1, and assuming a regular grid G lying in I_1, (see Fig. 1, left), the number of nodes of G within S_1, times the volume associated with a single node, is an approximation of the total volume $V(S_1)$. The number of nodes of G within the deformed surface $\mathbf{f}(S_1)$ gives an approximation of $V(S_2)$, volume of the segmentation in the second image (Fig. 1, right). $V(S_1)$ is also the number of nodes of $\mathbf{f}(G)$ within $S_2 = \mathbf{f}(S_1)$ (Fig. 1, centre), or, conversely, $V(S_2)$ is the number of nodes of $\mathbf{f}^{-1}(G)$ within S_1. This shows how we can efficiently compute $\Delta V_{propag} = V(S_2) - V(S_1)$ and resample S_1 into S_2 in a single pass over I_1, using the *inverse* deformation field $\mathbf{f}^{-1}$.

2.3 Integration of the Deformation Field

Motivations. Precise segmentation of a structure of interest is not always possible. A physical boundary to the tumour may not exist, due to the infiltration

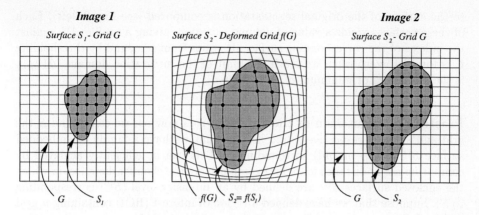

Fig. 1. Segmentation propagation: the volume variation is equal to the number of nodes (55) of the grid G inside the segmentation S_2 in the second image minus the number of nodes (25) of G inside the segmentation S_1 in the first image (which is the same as the number of nodes of the deformed grid $\mathbf{f}(G)$ inside the segmentation S_2). In this case, $\Delta V_{propag} = 55 - 25$ voxels.

of tumourous cells through the healthy tissue. To quantify the pathological evolution of the tumour and its effects on the surrounding tissue more reliably, we have developped the following model (see also [16]):

Model for the Integration. The brain is divided into three components: tumour, healthy tissue, surrounding tissue. The 'tumour' is a (sometimes arbitrarily) delineated region in which we assume no brain function. The 'healthy tissue', is normal-looking tissue away from the tumour. Between these two, tissue surrounding the tumour can be a mix of tumourous cells, edema, brain tissue... To monitor volume variation in surrounding tissue, a family of surfaces parallel

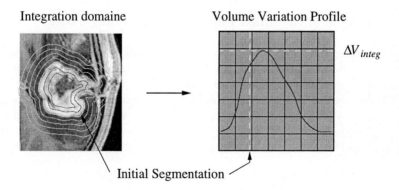

Fig. 2. Integration of the deformation over embedded surfaces yields a profile of the volume variation.

to the surface of the original segmentation is computed (see Fig. 2, left). Each of these surfaces yields a value of volume variation, giving a profile ΔV against the index i of the corresponding surface. It starts from zero, and by thresholding **f**, is forced to zero when we reach the limit of the integration domain. ΔV_{integ} is the maximum or minimum of the profile.

Practical Computation of the Profile. From now on, we call G and S the grid and surface, respectively, and assume that we have a family of embedded surface $S^{(i)} (i \in [-m...m])$ surrounding S. This can be efficiently achieved by computing a 3-D distance map, for example using the chamfer distance, in which the enclosed surfaces $S^{(i)}$ are defined by an intensity level ($S^{(0)}$ corresponding to S). Suppose that we have defined a region of interest (ROI) containing n grid nodes of G:

- We define two arrays of numbers $\{M_i^G\}$ and $\{M_i^{\mathbf{f}(G)}\}$, $i \in [-m...m]$.
- For the n nodes of G, $P_j(x, y, z)$ ($j \in [0..n]$), we determine the index i of the shell delimited by the surfaces $S^{(i)}$ and $S^{(i+1)}$ which contains P_j (resp. $\mathbf{f}(P_j)$). The index i can be obtained in constant time with the distance map described above For each P_j, we increment the corresponding bucket M_i^G (resp. $M_i^{\mathbf{f}(G)}$).
- Next, we compute incrementally the arrays

$$N_i^G = \sum_{k=0}^{i-1} M_k^G \text{ and } N_i^{\mathbf{f}(G)} = \sum_{k=0}^{i-1} M_k^{\mathbf{f}(G)}.$$

N_i^G (resp. $N_i^{\mathbf{f}(G)}$) represents the total number of nodes of G (resp. $\mathbf{f}(G)$) within $S^{(i)}$.
- Finally, the volume variation profile is $\Delta V_i = (N_i^G - N_i^{\mathbf{f}(G)}) \times V(voxel)$ against i, $i \in [-m...m]$.

2.4 Definition of the 'Mass Effect' in Surrounding Tissue

Segmentation propagation and deformation field integration represent two different ways of automatically quantifying the variations in the volume of a structure of interest. If we call V_1 (resp. V_2) the volume of the tumour in the initial (resp. final) image, and $V_1 + v_1$ (resp. $V_2 + v_2$) the volume of tumour plus surrounding tissue, then ΔV_{propag} is a quantification of $V_2 - V_1$, whereas ΔV_{integ} is a (more imprecise) estimation of $(V_2 + v_2) - (V_1 + v_1)$. To monitor brain response to the treatment and/or to tumour evolution, we introduce the 'mass effect' as

$$\frac{v_2 - v_1}{\Delta t} = \frac{\Delta V_{integ} - \Delta V_{propag}}{\Delta t},$$

where Δt is the time gap between the two acquisitions.

3 Quantification of Ventricular Enlargement in Primary Progressive Aphasia

The application of segmentation propagation to monitor the increase in the volume of the lateral ventricles in a patient with primary progressive aphasia (PPA) is examined. We compared the rate of ventricular enlargement to the estimation of the rate of whole brain atrophy obtained by stereology.

3.1 Subject and MRI

A 65 year old male with a diagnosis of PPA was scanned using 1.5 T SIGNA whole body MR imaging system (General Electric, Milwaukee, USA). High resolution T1-weighted SPGR images were obtained on four separate occasions approximately one year apart. The images, of an initial resolution of $0.78 \times 0.78 \times 1.6$ mm^3 for $256 \times 256 \times 124$ voxels were sinc-interpolated to an array of $200 \times 200 \times 199$ isotropic (i.e. cubic) voxels of side 1.0 mm.

3.2 Segmentation of Left and Right Ventricles

Segmentation of the left and right lateral ventricles (LV and RV) was achieved by interactively thresholding the image and classifying connected components

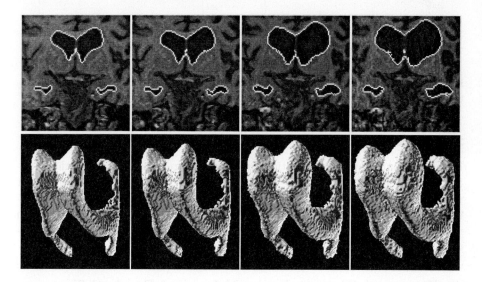

Fig. 3. Segmentation of the lateral ventricles in 4 MR images of a patient with brain atrophy, approximately one year appart. Top, from left to right: coronal sections in successive time points. Bottom: 3-D rendering of the lateral ventricles (images have been flipped to reflect upper coronal sections).

of the eroded binary image. Minimal manual editing was necessary to cut the lateral ventricles from the third and fourth ventricles. We manually partitioned the left and right ventricles to separately compare volume variations in the left and right hemisphere.

3.3 Results

The rate of increase of volume of the left (resp. right) ventricle as measured by image analysis was 33.0 mm^3 per day (resp. 17.3 mm^3 per day) compared with the findings of stereology: 31.3 mm^3 per day (resp. 15.5 mm^3 per day); linear regression relationship $R > 0.952$ in all cases (see Fig. 4). Corresponding values for the rate of decrease of left (resp. right) cerebral hemisphere volume obtained using stereology was -137.9 mm^3 per day (resp. -124.2 mm^3 per day); linear regression relationship $R > 0.88$.

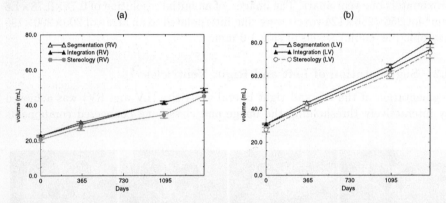

Fig. 4. Patient with brain atrophy. Variation of volume of (a) right and (b) left ventricles over a period of four years

3.4 Discussion

Results of automatic segmentation propagation are consistent with those obtained by stereology. The larger rate of increase of volume observed for the left ventricle is consistent with a preferential decrease in the volume of the left cerebral hemisphere associated with the loss of language. Segmentation propagation represents a reliable and sensitive technique for monitoring and quantifying ventricular enlargement.

4 Temporal Changes in the Volume of Cerebral Tumours Following Radiotherapy

We investigated changes in brain tumours and lateral cerebral ventricles in four patients undergoing radiotherapy (RT). We computed the variation in the volume of the tumour and ventricles over time, and tried to quantify the 'mass effect' in the brain tissue surrounding the tumour.

4.1 Subjects and MRI

Four patients with surgically confirmed high grade astrocytoma were imaged on an average of 5 occasions. The patients gave informed written consent of their willingness to participate in the study, which was approved by the local Ethics Committee. For each patient, prior to and approximately monthly after RT (and brachytherapy in the case of patient C), T1-weighted 3-D MR IRPREP images have been obtained following intravenous injection of the contrast agent Gd-DTPA. The resolution of the $256 \times 256 \times 124$ acquired voxels is $0.78 \times 0.78 \times 1.6$ mm^3.

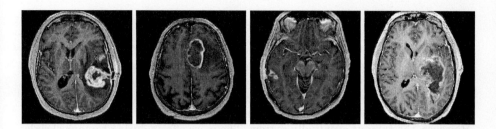

Fig. 5. Glioma study: from left to right, patient A, B, C, D.

4.2 Segmentation of Structures of Interest

We used the same approach to segment the lateral ventricles as described in Sect. 3.2. In patients A, the disruption of the blood-brain barrier produced a conspicuous ring of enhancement around the tumour, so that segmentation could be achieved by thresholding followed by minimal manual editing. Patient C had a small, well contrasted tumour, for which the same procedure applied. In patient B and D, the tumour margins were more diffuse and more approximate segmentations were obtained. Nevertheless, for all patients, the effect of therapy could be quantified.

4.3 Results and discussion

Segmentation propagation proved useful for the monitoring of volume changes in the lateral ventricles following administration of RT to cerebral tumours (see Table 1). The approach also proved appropriate for studying changes in volume of tumours with enhanced boundaries (patients A and C). However, integration of the deformation field represented a useful approach for quantifying changes in volume of tumours in patients B and D. In addition, it enabled quantification of changes in tissue surrounding the tumour.

In patients A and B, renewed growth of the tumour approximately 100 days after RT corresponded to a to a decrease in the rate of ventricular enlargement. The brain tissue surrounding the tumour expanded by between 60 mm^3 per day

Table 1. Ventricles and tumours volumes and surrounding tissue mass effect in four patients with brain tumour.

Patients		A	B	C	D
Ventricles (ml)	before RT	26.3	13.6	25.3	15.7
	after RT	30.3	15.1	31.9	27.5
Tumour (ml)	before RT	23.6	36.4	1.4	62.3
	after RT	19.2	32.1	0.85	50.8
	regrowth	33.3	36.3	n/a	62.1
Mass effect	after RT	+20	-80	-40	-200
(mm^3 per day)	regrowth	+60	+80	n/a	+130

in patient A, and 80 mm^3 per day in patient B. In patient C, brachytherapy at day 49 induces an enlargement of the tumour, followed by a shrinkage between days 70 and 130. Negative mass effect occurs after brachytherapy (-30 mm^3 per day). In patient D, the tumour decreased in volume over a period of at least 100 days following radiotherapy, during which time the lateral ventricles enlarged. However, the tumour eventually regrew. The mass effects during tumour shrinkage (-200 mm^3 per day) and renewed growth (120 mm^3 per day) are larger than in all the other patients.

5 Conclusion

Non-rigid registration of 3-D MR images obtained on successive occasions is a reliable and sensitive technique for monitoring and quantifying changes in volume in brain structures. Results are consistent with those obtained by stereology. Furthermore, analysis of the deformation field may give an estimation of tissue expansion or compaction in a region of interest. In the case where the region of interest is the exact segmentation of a structure of interest (e.g. the lateral ventricles), accurate changes in volume can be automatically quantified by segmentation propagation.

Acknowledgments

We gratefully acknowledge the support of our partners, Dr. M. Doran and Dr. A. Brodbelt from the Walton Centre for Neurology and Neurosurgery, Liverpool, UK, and Dr. B. Jones from the Clatterbridge Centre for Oncology, Wirral, UK. We also wish to thank Ms. J. Webb and Mr. Q. Gong, from MARIARC, who performed the stereological measurements, and performed the scanning of the patients.

References

1. N. Roberts, A. S. Garden, L. M. Cruz-Orive, G. H. Whitehouse, and R. H. T. Edwards. Estimation of fetal volume by MR imaging and stereology. *Bristish Journal of Radiology (BJR)*, 67:1067–1077, 1994.
2. Joseph V. Hajnal, Nadeem Saeed, Angela Oatridge, Elaime J. Williams, Ian R. Young, and Graeme M. Bydder. Detection of subtle brain changes using subvoxel registration and subtraction of serial MR images. *Journal of Computer Assisted Tomography (JCAT)*, 19(5):677–691, 1995.
3. Louis Lemieux. The segmentation and estimation of noise in difference images of co-registered MRI scan pairs. In *Medical Image Understanding and Analysis (MIUA'97)*, Oxford, UK, July 1997.
4. Peter A. Freeborough, Roger P. Woods, and Nick C. Fox. Accurate registration of serial 3D MR brain images and its application to visualizing change in neurodegenerative disorders. *Journal of Computer Assisted Tomography (JCAT)*, 20(6):1012–1022, 1996.
5. D. Lemoine, C. Barillot, B. Gibaud, and E. Pasqualini. An anatomical-based 3D registration system of multimodality and atlas data in neurosurgery. In *Lecture Notes in Computer Science*, volume 511, pages 154–164, 1991.
6. Jean Talairach and Pierre Tournoux. *Referentially oriented cerebral MRI anatomy*. Thieme Medical Publishers, New York, United-States, 1993.
7. D. Louis Collins, Peter Neelin, Terrence M. Peters, and Allan C. Evans. Automatic 3D intersubject registration of MR volumetric data in standardized Talairach space. *Journal of Computer Assisted Tomography (JCAT)*, 18(2):192–205, 1994.
8. Fred L. Bookstein. Principal warps: Thin-plate splines and the decomposition of deformations. *IEEE Transactions in Pattern Analysis and Machine Intelligence (PAMI)*, 11(6):567–585, June 1989.
9. J. Declerck, G. Subsol, Jean-Philippe Thirion, and N. Ayache. Automatic retrieval of anatomical structures in 3D medical images. In *Computer Vision, Virtual Reality and Robotics in Medicine, CVRMed '95*, pages 153–162, Nice, France, April 1995.
10. R. Bajcsy and S. Kovačič. Multiresolution Elastic Matching. *Computer Vision, Graphics and Image Processing*, 46:1–21, 1989.
11. Jim C. Gee, Martin Reivich, and Ruzena Bajcsy. Elastically deforming 3D atlas to match anatomical brain images. *Journal of Computer Assisted Tomography (JCAT)*, 17(2):225–236, 1993.
12. G. E. Christensen, R. D. Rabbitt, and M. I. Miller. 3D brain mapping using a deformable neuroanatomy. *Physics in Medicine and Biology*, 39:609–618, 1994.
13. Jean-Philippe Thirion. New feature points based on geometric invariants for 3D image registration. *International Journal of Computer Vision*, 18(2):121–137, 1996.
14. Jean-Philippe Thirion. Non-rigid matching using demons. In *Computer Vision and Pattern Recognition*, San Francisco, California USA, June 1996.
15. Morten Bro-Nielsen and Claus Gramkow. Fast fluid registration of medical images. In *Visualization in Biomedical Computing (VBC'96)*, pages 267–276, Hamburg, Germany, September 1996.
16. Jean-Philippe Thirion and Guillaume Calmon. Measuring lesion growth from 3D medical images. In *IEEE Non Rigid and Articulated Motion Workshop in conjunction with CVPR'97*, pages 112–119, Puerto Rico, USA, June 1997. also available as technical report RR-3101 at ftp.inria.fr/INRIA/tech-reports/RR.

Automatic Analysis of Normal Brain Dissymmetry of Males and Females in MR Images

Sylvain Prima[1], Jean-Philippe Thirion[2], Gérard Subsol[1], and Neil Roberts[3]

[1] INRIA Sophia Antipolis, EPIDAURE Project, France
Sylvain.Prima@sophia.inria.fr
[2] Focus Imaging SA, Sophia Antipolis, France
[3] MARIARC, University of Liverpool, U.K.

Abstract. In this paper, we present a statistical analysis of the normal dissymmetry in brain MR images. Our method consists in: computing a dense 3D field characterizing the dissymmetry of a subject, analysing it with an operator (*relative volume variation*), computing 3D statistical maps from populations of subjects (*learning series*) and extracting interesting regions. The results are then tested on an independent *validation series*. We use a database of 36 normal young subjects, 18 males and 18 females, strongly right-handed. We show that the brain hemispheres can be reliably discriminated thanks to a consistent size difference in the white matter of the temporal and frontal lobes, with a very high level of confidence (36/36, α-value=0.000001). We also exhibit a difference of brain dissymmetry with respect to sex.

1 Introduction

In [10], we presented a general method to study the dissymmetry of anatomical structures such as the human brain. This work was initially motivated by clinical studies assuming a connection between diseases such as schizophrenia and abnormalities in brain symmetry [1]. In this work, we computed at each voxel of a 3D MR brain image a vector characteristic of the dissymmetry and we obtained a dense 3D vector field F called the "dissymmetry field" of the image. This was then analysed with the operator $||F||div(F)$ that gives a "dissymmetry image" enhancing the differences between "symmetric" anatomical structures in the hemispheres, such as ventricles, temporal lobes, etc. From images computed using several subjects, we deduced 3D statistical maps to detect significantly dissymmetrical locations in a given population, or to compare the dissymmetry between 2 populations, or between one subject and a population.

In this paper, we present a more detailed statistical analysis of the dissymmetry field and we apply the whole method to large databases of subjects. In section 2, we recall the general scheme of the method and introduce a new 3D vector field operator, the *relative volume variation* measure. In section 3, we propose a further step in the statistical analysis to validate the results: after computing statistical maps from a *learning series* of subjects, we automatically extract interesting areas that we investigate in a different *validation series*. In section

4, we present new experiments on a large database of subjects: after analysing the "normal" dissymmetry in one population (normal right-handed young males, normal right-handed young males plus females) we compare brain dissymmetry between males and females.

2 Description of the general scheme

2.1 General presentation

The gross symmetry of the human brain is very well known by clinicians. The cortical surface of the brain, as well as the substructures such as the ventricles, the hippocampi, the white and grey matters, etc., are mainly symmetrical. Some subtle differences can be noted with a closer visual inspection, showing morphometrical (e.g., the size of the ventricles) and morphological (e.g., the number of white matter tracks) differences between homologous structures in both hemispheres. Our goal is to quantify and localise those differences in human brain MR images. Assuming the existence of a symmetry plane in the brain, the basic idea is to compare the initial image with its symmetrical counterpart with respect to this plane. By matching homologous voxels in both hemispheres, a non-rigid registration algorithm gives a 3D field characterizing the dissymmetry at each voxel; e.g., a perfectly symmetrical brain leads to a null field.

2.2 Computation of the mid-sagittal plane

The first step of the algorithm consists in computing the "symmetry plane". The position of the patient's head during the scanning process is variable, and taking the "geometrical" mid-plane of an MR image is only a rough approximation of the sought after "anatomical" mid-plane. The medical description of this plane, usually called the "mid-sagittal plane", relies on an anatomical landmark: the inter-hemispheric fissure of the brain. In [4], the hemisphere boundaries defining this fissure in an MR image are segmented using snakes, and the plane is fitted to a set of control points taken on inter-hemispheric curves. In [3], the plane is estimated from each "mid-sagittal symmetry axis" in all axial (or coronal) slices of an MR or CT image. Each axis maximizes the similarity between the slice and its 2D symmetric reflexion in relation to this axis; the similarity criterion is the 2D cross-correlation. Some other techniques have been developed for centering functional brain images [5], however the generalization to anatomical modalities seems difficult. Our method, developed in [10] and briefly described in Figure 1, does not require any preprocessing such as segmentation and relies on the whole volume of the MR image, without any anatomical knowledge; it computes directly the 3D plane minimizing a least-squares criterion. Moreover, it can be generalized to realign any approximately symmetrical object.

In the second step, we compute the rigid transform that realigns automatically the mid-sagittal plane with the mid-plane of the MR image.

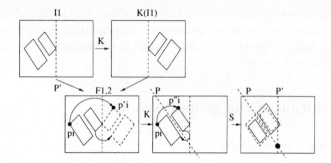

Fig. 1. Overview of the mid-sagittal plane determination: the image I_1 is transformed into a symmetrical image $K(I_1)$ with respect to any given plane P' (in general, the midplane of the image). Then a point to point correspondance $F_{1,2}$ is computed between both images, leading to pairs (p_i, p'_i). Applying K to the p'_i points gives couples (p_i, p''_i) of corresponding points with respect to the mid-sagittal plane P, which are used to compute the final symmetry S or equivalently the mid-plane P itself, by minimization of $C = \sum_i (S(p''_i) - p_i)^2 = \sum_i (S \circ K(p'_i) - p_i)^2$.

2.3 Computation of the 3D dissymmetry image

Computation of the 3D dissymmetry field. Once the the mid-plane of the MRI is aligned with the mid-sagittal plane, the 3D deformation field obtained by non-rigid registration between the image and its symmetric is called the "dissymmetry field" of the brain. This 3D field is costly: it is difficult to visualize, to analyse statistically (it requires multivariate analysis tools) and requires a lot of memory. An intuitive idea to extract the most relevant information provided by this field F is to reduce it to a 3D scalar image, by applying an operator. In [10], we proposed to use the operator $||F||div(F)$, introduced in [9], which gives good results, but whose "physical" meaning is difficult to interpret. Here, we introduce a new operator, dv/v, more quantitative and intuitive, that computes the relative volume variation of a set of *cells* submitted to a deformation field.

Volume variation of a cell. The non-rigid registration provides a 3D deformation vector for each voxel of the MRI of size $X \times Y \times Z$. We assume that these vectors are applied to the centers of the voxels. Considering the voxel of coordinates (i, j, k), the centers of the voxels (i, j, k), $(i, j + 1, k)$, $(i, j, k + 1)$, $(i, j+1, k+1)$, $(i+1, j, k)$, $(i+1, j+1, k)$, $(i+1, j, k+1)$, and $(i+1, j+1, k+1)$ define unambiguously the vertices of a cube that we call the *cell* (i, j, k). We want to compute the volume variation of each cell under the action of the deformation applied to its eight vertices, to build the 3D image of size $(X-1) \times (Y-1) \times (Z-1)$ where the value of the voxel (i, j, k) is the volume variation of the cell (i, j, k). This first "dissymmetry image", associated with the original MRI, enhances the local differences of size between the hemispheres of the brain.

A priori, each deformed cell is a non-regular hexahedron; we partition each cell into 6 tetrahedra. If (u, v, w) defines a positively oriented tetrahedron, its volume is $\frac{1}{6}Det(u, v, w)$. The deformation field, F, transforms u, v, w into $F(u)$, $F(v)$, $F(w)$ respectively; we define the volume of the deformed tetrahedron as

$\frac{1}{6}Det(F(u), F(v), F(w))$. If $(F(u), F(v), F(w))$ is no longer direct, the volume of the "transformed tetrahedron" is negative. We define the volume variation of the cell by summing the volume variation of the 6 tetrahedra.

The partition is the same for all cells, so that 2 adjacent cells have a common triangle partition on their common face. We define the volume variation of a whole region of (non-necessarily connected) cells as the sum of each cell volume variation. The result is the actual volume variation of the whole region deformed by the field, which depends only on its boundary displacement. In particular, if the region boudary remains the same, the integration of volume variation over the cells composing this region is null.

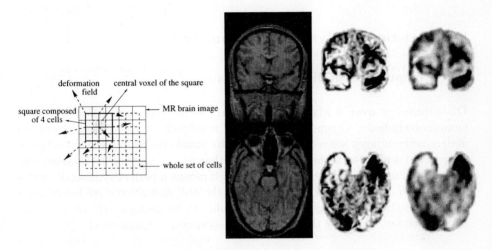

Fig. 2. Left: Integration on a larger cube: here, we present an illustration in the 2D case with $N = 1$. From the original MRI and its associated 2D deformation field, we compute the area variation of all cells, that we integrate on the squares of $(2N)^2 = 4$ cells and set the normalised value (i.e., area variation divided by 4) to the center voxel in the MR image. **Right:** Comparison between the first dissymmetry image and the smoothed one (coronal and axial views). From left to right: reference subject; first dissymmetry image (white means that the voxel is larger than its correspondent in the other hemisphere); smoothed dissymmetry image, with $N = 3$. In accordance with the medical convention, the right side of the subject is shown on the left in the MRI.

Computation of the dv/v image. To compare all the database subjects, we align their dissymmetry images in the same frame (i.e., with respect to a reference subject), with a non-rigid registration algorithm.

This is the third use of this algorithm in the scheme: the method is based on the "demons" algorithm [8], relying on grey values, entirely automatic, and relatively fast: the time computation of the 3D deformation field is about 20 minutes for two $256 \times 256 \times 128$ MRI on a DEC Alpha workstation of 400 MHz.

Experimentally, we can obtain a rough idea of the accuracy of this registration method: the comparison with other methods gives mutually coherent results with an average difference of about 3 voxels [11]. Consequently, it seems inconsistent to perform a voxel-by-voxel statistical analysis on these aligned images. Thus, we perform a linear filtering of these images by taking into account the neighbourhood of each cell. Given an integer N, we sum the volume variation of the $(2N)^3$ cells belonging to the cube centered in each voxel (see Figure 2). After division by $(2N)^3$, we obtain a relative volume variation that takes into account the neighbouring values and the new "dissymmetry" (dv/v) image is a smoother version of the first dissymmetry image (see Figure 2). The smoothing of high frequency variations in this one reduces the effects of misregistration, but as N increases, some anatomical details are lost and we get more global dissymmetry measures. Given the estimated accuracy of the registration, we chose $N = 3$.

3 Statistical analysis of dissymmetry

3.1 Computation of dissymmetry maps

Dissymmetry over a given population. We use basic univariate statistical analysis techniques. Given a population of n subjects, their aligned, smoothed dissymmetry images are comparable voxel by voxel. We denote the value of the subject i at a given voxel as x_i. We assume that $x_1, ..., x_n$ follow a Gaussian law, of unknown mean μ_0 and variance σ_0^2. $\mu_0 = 0$ means a perfect symmetry at this voxel. Let $H_0 : \mu_0 = 0$ and $H_1 : \mu_0 \neq 0$ be the null and alternative hypotheses. We compute the α-value, giving the probability to be wrong in rejecting the null hypothesis, i.e., in saying that there is a dissymmetry at this voxel:

$$\alpha = F^{-1}_{1,n-1}(T^2), \qquad (F_{1,n-1} \text{ is a Fisher's law})$$

where: $T^2 = \frac{n\mu^2}{\sigma}$, $\mu = \frac{1}{n}\sum_{i=1}^{n} x_i$, and $\sigma = \frac{1}{n-1}\sum_{i=1}^{n}(x_i - \mu)^2$. Computing this α-value for each voxel gives a dense 3D statistical map.

Dissymmetry between 2 given populations. Given two populations of n_1 and n_2 subjects, whose dissymmetry images are computed and aligned, we denote the intensity of a given voxel for the first (resp. second) population as x_i^1 (resp., x_i^2). We assume that $(x_1^1, ..., x_{n_1}^1)$ (resp., $(x_1^2, ..., x_{n_2}^2)$) follow a Gaussian law, of unknown mean μ_1 (resp., μ_2) and unknown variance σ_1^2 (resp., σ_2^2). $\mu_1 = \mu_2$ means that the dissymmetry of the two populations is the same at this voxel. Let $H_0 : \mu_1 = \mu_2$ and $H_1 : \mu_1 \neq \mu_2$ be the null and alternative hypotheses. The probability to be wrong in saying that there is a difference of dissymmetry is:

$$\alpha = F^{-1}_{1,n_1+n_2-2}(T^2), \qquad (F_{1,n_1+n_2-2} \text{ is a Fisher's law})$$

where: $T^2 = \frac{n_1 n_2}{(n_1+n_2)} \frac{(\bar{x}_2 - \bar{x}_1)^2}{S}$, $\bar{x}_1 = \frac{1}{n_1}\sum_{i=1}^{n_1} x_i^1$, $\bar{x}_2 = \frac{1}{n_2}\sum_{i=1}^{n_2} x_i^2$,

and $S = \frac{1}{n_1+n_2-2}[\sum_{i=1}^{n_1}(x_i^1 - \bar{x}_1)^2 + \sum_{i=1}^{n_2}(x_i^2 - \bar{x}_2)^2]$.

3.2 Interpretation of the dissymmetry maps

The first idea is to set a significance level l and to focus on the significant voxels using this level, which is equivalent to computing a two-tailed *t-test*: we keep voxels whose $\alpha < l$. The dense 3D map is then reduced to a binary image. A typical level for clinical studies is 0.001, which means, for each voxel there is one-in-a-thousand chance to reject wrongly the null hypothesis. However, the interpretation of these tests can be strongly misleading. Let us suppose that the voxels are uncorrelated; then, the tests are independent, and the probability of wrongly rejecting the null hypothesis for at least one of the n voxels in the image is equal to $1 - (1 - l)^n$. For $l = 0.001$, with an image of $n = 128^3 \simeq 2 \times 10^6$ voxels, this probability is very close to 1: we are nearly sure to have *false positives* between significant voxels, that is voxels for which $\alpha < l$ "by chance".

However, we notice that isolated significant voxels are very rare in this binary map and most of them compose connected clusters of several voxels. This can be partially explained by the spatial correlation between the voxel values of the dissymmetry images; thus, the n *t-tests* we compute (as many as there are voxels in the MR images) are not independent. This correlation can be explained by:

- The anatomical consistency of the dissymmetry: the dissymmetry in substructures, such as the ventricles or the hippocampi, results in a non-null dissymmetry field over their whole volume.
- The iterative Gaussian filtering applied on the deformation field by the *demons* non-rigid registration algorithm. The smoothing parameter σ is constant along iterations and is set to 2.0.
- The linear filtering of the dissymmetry image, controlled by N.

It is then natural to focus on clusters more than on individual voxels in binary maps, and to identify the most "significant" clusters. Such a method is proposed in the software *SPM* [7], in the field of functional image statistical analysis. A spatially limited cluster is usually considered less "significant" than larger ones, and a further quantitative analysis, with computation of exact probabilities for sets of voxels, can be found in [2]. We propose a simplified method to validate our results. First, we divide the whole database into a *learning series* and a *validation series*, and we compute the first dissymmetry image and its smoothed version for each subject. Second, we follow the scheme (see also Figure 3):

- First step: the 3D dense statistical maps are computed on the *learning series*. Then a significant level is arbitrarily fixed, and the clusters of connected significant voxels are extracted. The 2 hemispheres contain the same information of dissymmetry, and we choose to study one of them only. We identify the k most significant clusters as the k largest ones in this hemisphere.
- Second step: we associate to each of these voxel clusters the corresponding cluster of cells (i.e., the cell (i, j, k) to the voxel (i, j, k)), whose relative volume variation is computed on the *validation series*, independently of the *learning series*. This leads to a series of values that we statistically analyse according to the formulae of section 3.1.

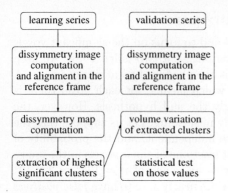

Fig. 3. General scheme of the method. Note: it is also possible to define other clusters as "interesting" ones, relying on clinical knowledge: for example, if the largest sized clusters are inside an anatomical (temporal, frontal, occipital lobes, ventricles, etc.) or functional (Broca's, Wernicke's, etc.) area, it is natural to apply the dissymmetry analysis to the whole region, and then to choose this area as a cluster for further statistical studies.

4 Results

4.1 Materials

Our database is composed of 19 MR brain images of healthy young males and 18 of healthy young females, provided by the MARIARC, University of Liverpool. All of them are strongly right-handed to restrict the possible influence of the laterality on dissymmetry results. One of the males is chosen as the reference subject for all our experiments (perfectly right-handed: laterality coefficient of 100). This leaves 36 subjects, divided into the *learning series* (10 males and 10 females, chosen with the highest laterality coefficient), and the *validation series* (8 males and 8 females). In the following, we perform several experiments.

4.2 The dissymmetry over the male population

Figure 4 shows the average dissymmetry and the dissymmetry map for $l = 0.001$, computed on the 10 males of the *learning series*. We reaffirm the preliminary results presented in [10] with a different operator. Two main areas appear in the map: one in the white matter of the temporal lobe, the other in the frontal lobe. Both seem to be significantly larger in the right hemisphere. We focus on these two areas in the left hemisphere (at right on the images, according to the medical convention), and compute their relative volume variation for the 8 males of the *validation series*. From those values, we deduce the probabilities to be wrong in saying that those areas are dissymmetrical: 0.00041 (temporal lobe) and 0.00044 (frontal lobe). Those values are largely lower than usual significance levels (typically, $l = 0.001$): this is very conclusive.

One must note another interesting result: in the average dissymmetry image, we recover the *torque* effect, very well known by clinicians. There is an "inversion" of dissymmetry between the front and the back of the brain. This does not appear in the map: it is not significant over the whole population for $l = 0.001$.

4.3 Comparison males/females

The comparison of dissymmetry between males and females has been largely studied by biologists. It is widely assumed that language functions are likely to

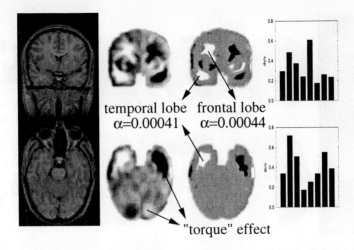

Fig. 4. From left to right: reference subject; average of the dv/v images of the male *learning series*; statistical map for this series (each voxel is displayed with its α-value bearing the sign of the average dissymmetry at this point, $l = 0.001$); dv/v measure on the *validation series* for the 2 most significant clusters in the left hemisphere, located in the frontal (top) and temporal (bottom) lobes.

be more lateralized in males [6]. Males also seem to show greater anatomical dissymmetry than females, e.g., for the Sylvian fissure [12]. Figure 5 shows the average dissymmetry for the 10 males and the 10 females of the *learning series* and the statistical map for $l = 0.001$ comparing these 2 populations. We kept the area in the top of the left hemisphere. The computation of the relative volume variation of this area for the *validation series* gives 2 series of 8 values. The α-value is equal to 0.11. The area seems to be smaller in the left hemisphere than in the right for the males, and larger for the females. Further experiments on a larger dataset is probably needed to lead to definitive conclusions.

4.4 The dissymmetry over the whole population

The comparison between males and females does not lead to a significant difference in the temporal and frontal lobes, which correspond to the largest natural dissymmetry in the male population. The computation of the dissymmetry map for the whole *learning series* allows one to enhance a "normal dissymmetry" on a wider population. The map, shown in Figure 6, reveals a large set of voxels, in the same area as for the male only population, but wider, i.e., intuitively more significant. The largest "significant" volume is a "V" shape in the white matter of the cortex, spreading from the frontal to the temporal lobe. Computing the relative volume variation of this "V" shape in the left hemisphere for the whole database of males and females gives a series of 36 values all superior to 0, which means that for all subjects, this volume is larger in the right hemisphere than in the left: for our database, we have a criterion allowing to discriminate consistently the left hemisphere from the right one. The computed α-value on the *validation series* is equal to 0.000001, which confirm these results.

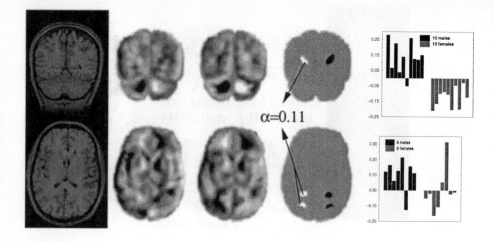

Fig. 5. From left to right: reference subject; average of dv/v im the female *learning series*; statistical map comparing the 2 populations (coronal and axial views, $l = 0.001$); dv/v measure on the *learning* (top) and the *validation* (bottom) *series* for the most significant cluster in the left hemisphere.

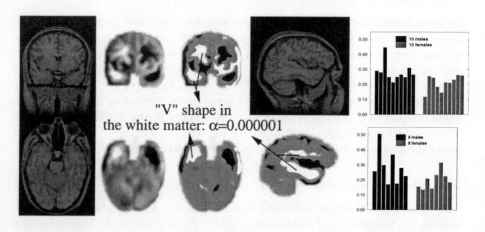

Fig. 6. From left to right: reference subject; average of dv/v images for the whole learning series; statistical map (coronal and axial views, $l = 0.001$); sagittal view of the reference subject and the map; dv/v measure on the *learning* (top) and the *validation* (bottom) *series* for the most significant cluster in the left hemisphere: the "V-shape".

5 Conclusion

We have presented a method to study the dissymmetry of roughly symmetrical objects such as brains. We have shown the usefulness of this method to assess firmly essential results for brain normal anatomy. It was long known that brains in normal subjects were dissymmetrical with always the same laterality, i.e., with the right temporal lobe generally larger than the left one. We have shown on a population of 36 normals (18 males and 18 females) that this phenomenon is consistent (36 out of 36), with a high level of confidence (p=0.000001). Furthermore, we have been able to refine the shape of this dissymmetric region, which defines a kind of "V" shape, mainly located in the white matter of the brain, with one branch extending in the frontal lobe and the other one in the temporal lobe. The comparison between males and females has lead to the definition of a discriminant area that should be validated on a larger database. We are currently applying the same method on a database of 40 schizophrenic patients and 40 controls within the EC Biomed II BIOMORPH Project.

References

1. T.J. Crow. Schizophrenia as an anomaly of cerebral asymmetry. In K. Maurer, editor, *Imaging of the Brain in Psychiatry and Related Fields*, pages 1–17. Springer-Verlag, Berlin Heidelberg, 1993.
2. K.J. Friston, K.J. Worsley, R.S.J. Frackowiak, J.C. Mazziotta, and A.C. Evans. Assessing the Significance of Focal Activations Using their Spatial Extent. *Human Brain Mapping*, 1:214–220, 1994.
3. Y. Liu, R.T. Collins, and W.E. Rothfus. Automatic bilateral symmetry (midsagittal) plane extraction from pathological 3D neuroradiological images. In *SPIE, International Symposium on Medical Imaging*, San-Diego, CA, February 1998.
4. P. Marais, R. Guillemaud, M. Sakuma, A. Zisserman, and M. Brady. Visualising Cerebral Asymmetry. In Höhne, K.H. and Kikinis, R., editor, *Visualization in Biomedical Computing*, volume 1131 of *Lecture Notes in Computer Science*, pages 411–416, Hamburg (Germany), September 1996. Springer.
5. S. Minoshima, K.L. Berger, K.S. Lee, and M.A. Mintun. An automated method for rotational correction and centering of three-dimensional brain images. *J Nucl Med*, 33(8):1579–1585, August 1992.
6. B.A. Shaywitz, S.E. Shaywitz, K.R. Pugh, R.T. Constable, P. Skudlarski, R.K. Fulbright, R.A. Bronen, J.M. Fletcher, D.P. Shankweller, L. Katz, and J.C. Gore. Sex differences in the functional organization of the brain for language. *Nature*, 373:607–609, February 1995.
7. SPM96. http://www.fil.ion.bpmf.ac.uk/spm/.
8. J-P Thirion. Fast non-rigid matching of 3D medical images. In *Medical Robotics and Computer Aided Surgery (MRCAS'95)*, pages 47–54, Baltimore, November 1995. Electronic version: http://www.inria.fr/RRRT/RR-2547.html.
9. J-P Thirion and G. Calmon. Measuring lesion growth from 3D medical images. In *Nonrigid and Articulated Motion Workshop (NAM'97)*, Puerto Rico, June 1997. IEEE. Electronic version : http://www.inria.fr/RRRT/RR-3101.html.
10. J.-P. Thirion, S. Prima, G. Subsol, and N. Roberts. Statistical Analysis of Normal and Abnormal Dissymmetry in Volumetric Medical Images. In *IEEE Workshop on Biomedical Image Analysis, WBIA'98*, Santa Barbara, USA, June 1998. Electronic version : http://www.inria.fr/RRRT/RR-3178.html.
11. J-P Thirion, G. Subsol, and D. Dean. Cross validation of three inter-patients matching methods. In *VBC*, volume 1131 of *Lecture Notes in Computer Science*, pages 327–336, Hamburg, Germany, September 1996.
12. S.F. Witelson and D.L. Kigar. Sylvian fissure morphology and asymmetry in men and women: Bilateral differences in relation to handedness in men. *The Journal of Comparative Neurology*, 323:326–340, 1992.

Marching Optimal-Parameter Ridges: An Algorithm to Extract Shape Loci in 3D Images

Jacob D. Furst, Stephen M. Pizer

Medical Image Display and Analysis Group
University of North Carolina, Chapel Hill, NC 27599
furst@cs.unc.edu
fax: 1 (919) 962-1799

Abstract. This paper presents a method for identifying image loci that can be used as a basis for object segmentation and image registration. The focus is on 1D and 2D shape loci in 3D images. This method, called *marching ridges*, uses generalized height ridges, oriented medialness measures and a marching cubes like algorithm to extract optimal scale-orientation cores. This algorithm can can also be used for other image processing tasks such as finding intensity skeletons of objects and identifying object boundaries.

Keywords: marching ridges, scale-space, orientation, medialness

1 Introduction

There are a variety of problems in medical imaging for which height ridges are generally useful. For example, height ridges of intensity can be used to track the centers of blood vessels. Ridges of boundariness can also be used to identify edges using the Canny definition. Of particular interest to this paper are height ridges of medialness (called cores) that can be used as the basis for a figural shape model, the deformable shape locus, described by Pizer [15].

In this paper, we will concentrate on height ridges as they are defined in [8]. In particular, we will use the definition of optimal parameter ridges, in which certain parameters of the space in which we are finding ridges are distinguished. These ideas can be used for identifying boundaries, in which the boundary normal provides a distinguished orientation or in seaching for ridges (cores) in a scale-orientation space of medialness, in which we will distinguish scale and orientation.

This paper describes an algorithm for finding cores of 3D images, similar in structure to Lorensen's marching cubes [11] and Bloomenthals' tracked partitioning [1] (when finding 2D cores) and Thirion's [16] marching lines (when finding 1D cores). This paper presents algorithms and results for 2D cores. 1D cores in 3D images are the subject of current work.

2 Methods

The methods used in this paper combine much of the work described in Section 1 into a common algorithm called marching ridges. We measure an image using oriented medialness kernels and then find ridges within the marching framework using the optimal scale-orientation definition of height ridges.

2.1 Height ridges

Maximum convexity height ridges The maximum convexity height ridge is dealt with extensively in Eberly's fine book [3]. Here we will only repeat the definition of the maximum convexity height ridge:

Definition 21 *(Maximum Convexity Height Ridge) An m-dimensional (mD) maximum convexity height ridge of a function $M : \mathcal{X} \to \mathbb{R}$, or m-ridge of M, is an mD locus in the (nD, $n > m$) domain of M. In general, the definition of this locus involves*

1. *given the Hessian matrix of second derivatives $\mathcal{H}(M)$, order the Hessian's eigenvalues λ_i according to $\lambda_i < \lambda_{i+1}$. Let the vector $\boldsymbol{v}^i$ be the eigenvector associated with λ_i. The first $n - m$ such $\boldsymbol{v}^i$ are transverse directions.*
2. *require that M have a relative maximum in each of the transverse directions; that is,*
   (a) $\boldsymbol{v}^i \cdot \nabla(M)(\bar{x}) = 0$ for $i = 1, \ldots, n - m$, where $\nabla(M)$ is the gradient of M, and
   (b) $\lambda_{n-m} < 0$ at $\bar{x}$

Generalized height ridges We have expanded upon Eberly's definition to create a more generalized definition of height ridge, one that includes many definitions and algorithms already existing in the image processing literature (See [9, 10, 5]).

Definition 22 *(Height Ridge) An m-dimensional (mD) height ridge of a function $M : \mathcal{X} \to \mathbb{R}$, or m-ridge of M, is an mD locus in the (nD, $n > m$) domain of M. In general, the definition of this locus involves*

1. *a rule for choosing $n - m$ linearly independent directions, $\boldsymbol{v}^i$, transverse to the putative ridge at a location x, and*
2. *requiring that M have a relative maximum in each of the (1D) $\boldsymbol{v}^i$ directions; that is,*
   (a) $\boldsymbol{v}^i \cdot \nabla(M)(\bar{x}) = 0$ for $i = 1, \ldots, n - m$, and
   (b) $(\boldsymbol{v}^i)^t \mathcal{H}(M)(\bar{x}) \boldsymbol{v}^i < 0$ for $i = 1, \ldots, n - m$.

Note that the maximum convexity height ridges are a specific example of the generalized height ridge in which the rule for choosing transverse directions involves an eigen analysis of the Hessian matrix. Also, the generalized definition provides a mechanism for computing Canny edges [2], for example, by choosing one direction transverse to the ridge as the gradient direction, and maximizing gradient magnitude in that direction.

Optimal parameter height ridges There are a number of tasks in image processing, to include finding skeletons [9] and edges [10], that require a choice of directions different than that of the maximal convexity definition. One way to do this is the optimal parameter height ridge. In this work, we choose to calculate optimal parameter ridges for three major reasons:

1. Distinguishing certain parameters seems a natural and intuitive choice when dealing with certain functions. Pizer [15] has described how position, radius, and orientation are natural parameters to separate for modeling shape. The maximum convexity height ridge does not guarantee such separation.
2. The incommensurability of position, radius and orientation can provide for non-Euclidean geometries in the domain of M. In the case of position and scale alone, Eberly [3] has shown a hyperbolic geometry in the domain of M. However, even then, there is a parameter involved relating derivatives in space to derivatives of radius. The optimal parameter hight ridge avoids this notion and guarantees Euclidean derivatives.
3. Algorithmically, the problems of discontinuity in eigensystems becomes unmanageable in higher dimensions. Morse [12] was able to show success in 2D, Eberly [4] in 3D, and Furst [7] some success in 4D, but both Eberly and Furst have failed to robustly generate maximum convexity height ridges for medical images using a 4D domain of position and scale.

Working from our definition of generalized height ridges, we can define an optimal parameter ridge as follows:

Definition 23 *(Optimal Parameter Height Ridge) An m-dimensional (mD) optimal parameter height ridge of a function $M : \mathcal{X} \times \mathcal{S} \to \mathbb{R}$, or m-ridge of M, is an mD locus in the (nD, n > m) domain of M. Define it as follows*

1. *given the Hessian matrix of M restricted to the subspace $\mathcal{S}$, $\mathcal{H}|_\mathcal{S}(M)$, let each of the eigenvectors of $\mathcal{H}|_\mathcal{S}(M)$ be a transverse direction, and have a rule for choosing the remaining transverse directions from $\mathcal{X}$ in a way possible dependent on the eigenvectors of $\mathcal{H}|_\mathcal{S}(M)$.*
2. *requiring that M have a relative maximum in each of the (1D) v^i directions; that is,*
   (a) *the gradient of M restricted to the subsace $\mathcal{S}$, $\nabla|_\mathcal{S}(M)$, vanishes, and $v^i \cdot \nabla(M)(\bar{x}) = 0$ for each $v^i \in \mathcal{X}$, and*
   (b) *$\mathcal{H}|_\mathcal{S}(M)$ is negative definite at $\bar{x}$ and $(v^i)^t \mathcal{H}(M)(\bar{x}) v^i < 0$ for each $v^i \in \mathcal{X}$.*

Let $M(\bar{x}; \bar{s}) : \mathcal{X} \times \mathcal{S} \to \mathbb{R}$. Let $\mathcal{X}$ be called the underlying image space (typically $\mathbb{R}^2$ or $\mathbb{R}^3$; this paper uses $\mathbb{R}^3$) and let $\mathcal{S}$ be called the distinguished space whose spanning parameters will be optimized. We have identified distinguished spaces containing from one to five dimensions; this paper uses three. We can view these three as a radius and an angular orientation: $\mathbb{R}_+ \times S^2$ (spherical coordinates) or we can view them as a vector: $\mathbb{R}^3$ (Cartesian coordinates). The spherical coordinates provide an intuitive idea of the optimized parameters, while the Cartesian coordinates provide a computational advantage. When looking for a 2D ridge in a 6D space ($\mathbb{R}^3 \times \mathbb{R}^3$) we need four transverse directions. Requiring a maximum of M in the distinguished space $\mathcal{S}$ identifies three transverse directions. As required by Definition 23, these directions are eigenvectors of $\mathcal{H}|_\mathcal{S}(M)$. The last transverse direction is taken from the underlying image space $\mathcal{X}$. This direction can be chosen using the maximum convexity rule as given in Definition 21. However, given that one of our distinguished parameters is orientation, we can use the particular orientation that produces a maximum of M in $\mathcal{S}$ to determine the final transverse direction in $\mathcal{X}$. That is, if $\bar{s} \in \mathcal{S}$ is the point at which $M(\bar{x}; \bar{s})$ is maximal for a particular $x \in \mathcal{X}$, then $v^4 = \frac{\bar{s}}{\|\bar{s}\|}$ in the Cartesian formulation of $\bar{s}$ or $v^4 = [\cos s_2 \cos s_3, \sin s_2 \cos s_3, \sin s_3]$ in the spherical formulation of $\bar{s}$.

Once having determined this direction, we must satisfy the derivative conditions to label it a ridge point. We do this by assuming that the locus of points $\{(\bar{x}; \bar{s}) | (\bar{x}; \bar{s}) \in \mathcal{X} \times \mathcal{S}\}$ for which $M(\bar{x}; \bar{s})$ is maximal in $\mathcal{S}$ creates a well-defined manifold $\mathcal{M}$. Except for non-generic situations, this assumption holds. (See [8] for failure of genericity).

We then define a coordinate chart $\bar{i} : \mathcal{X} \to \mathcal{M}$. This coordinate chart is well defined except at folds of $\mathcal{M}$ with respect to its projection onto $\mathcal{X}$. These folds, however, occur only where one of the eigenvalues of $\mathcal{H}|_\mathcal{S}(M)$ vanishes. Since a ridge point is possible only where $\mathcal{H}|_\mathcal{S}(M)$ is negative definite, the coordinate chart will be well defined at all ridge points.

We then define $\hat{M} : \mathcal{X} \to \mathcal{S} = f \circ i$. We must then satisfy the following two conditions to establish a ridge point at x

1. the first derivative of $\hat{M}$ in the v^4 direction ($\hat{M}_{v^4}$) vanishes, and
2. the second derivative of $\hat{M}$ in the v^4 direction ($\hat{M}_{v^4 v^4}$) is less than 0.

See Section 2.3 for a the mathematical implementation of these conditions.

Any point $(\bar{x}; \bar{s})$ that satisfies these two conditions and for which $M|_\mathcal{S}(\bar{x}; \bar{s})$ is maximal is an optimal scale-orientation ridge point of M. The collection of all such points forms the optimal scale-orientation ridge.

Subdimensional maxima Given the definition of a generalized height ridge, there is no guarantee that a point satisfying the derivative conditions in some subset of transverse directions will be a local maximum of the function restricted to the space spanned by those transverse directions. This concern was detailed in [8]. However, we have proved that for optimal parameter ridges, each ridge point is a maximum of the functions M restricted to the space spanned by the directions transverse to the ridge.

2.2 Marching ridges

Both marching cubes and marching lines share the common characteristic of finding implicitly defined manifolds by finding intersections of the manifold with line segments of the space. Marching cubes does this with a characteristic functions and line segments whose endpoints are sample points of the original image. Marching lines does this with zero-trapping along line segments whose endpoints are image sample points and then zero-trapping along line segments whose endpoints are the previously defined zeroes. Marching ridges incorporates both these strategies for finding both curve and surface ridges in 3D images. However, the ridge definition requires more than just that we identify zero-crossings of first derivatives. It also requires that second derivatives are less than zero. This condition produces boundaries of the ridge, a situation not encountered in marching cubes or marching lines, in which the surfaces and curves, respectively, are closed.

Marching ridges is a general purpose algorithm for finding height ridges; we have used it to calculate skeletons, edges, and cores using a variety of ridge definitions. This paper uses a specific implementation of the algorithm for finding optimal parameter ridges of medialness, which I will hereafter refer to as marching cores.

The marching cores algorithm consists of the following steps:

1. **Initialization** Using a mouse to specify a spatial location in a target image and sliders to specify distinguished parameters, the user identifies a starting point in $\mathcal{X} \times \mathcal{S}$ for the marching.
2. **Search** Given the starting spatial point, the algorithm constructs a cube containing the initial point and the seven points whose coordinate values are 1 greater than the initial point for some subset of coordinates. This cube serves as the structure for the rest of the algorithm. E.g., starting at image coordinate (34,123,12) produces the cube with vertices at (34,123,12), (35,123,12), (35,124,12), (34,124,12), (34,124,13), (35,124,13), (35,123,13) and (34,123,13).
3. **Maximization** Each vertex of the cube maximizes the medialness M with respect to the distinguished parameters, producing values for each spatial point.
4. **First derivative calculation** As described in Section 2.1, each vertex of the cube calculates first derivatives of $\hat{M}$. This is done using weighting functions as described in Section 2.3.
5. **Trap zeroes** If the value of $\hat{M}_{v^4}$ at any two vertices joined by an edge of the cube differ in sign, we use a linear approximation of $\hat{M}_{v^4}$ to interpolate the location along the edge where $\hat{M}_{v^4} = 0$.
6. **Second derivative calculation** Each such zero-crossing of $\hat{M}_{v^4}$ then performs an optimization of distinguished parameters and a subsequent calculation of second derivatives of $\hat{M}$. If $\hat{M}_{v^4 v^4} < 0$, then the point is a ridge point and is labeled appropriately in the image.
7. **Expansion** Each face of the original cube that contains any ridge points among its edges identifies an adjacent cube to be searched for ridge points. Each such cube is entered into a list.
8. **Marching** The algorithm explores each cube in the list in a breadth-first pattern in a manner similar to the initial cube with the exception that initial values for the optimization of distinguished parameters is the average of the optimal values already determined among its vertices.

The marching cores algorithm continues this loop until there are no more cubes to process. This occurs as the ridges ends, closes or exits the image.

2.3 Oriented medialness

Pizer [13, 15] describes a variety of options for producing medialness in 3D images. The medialness used to produce the examples in this paper is the semilinear, central medialness described in [13]. It is designed to reduce the effects of interfigural interference on the calculation of cores, as well as to give a more accurate width estimation of objects. More importantly, the orientation component of the medialness kernel can be used in an optimal parameter ridge to determine the final transverse direction as described in Section 2.1.

The underlying medialness is thus $M(\bar{x}; n) = L_{nn}(\bar{x}; \|n\|)$, where $L(\bar{x}; r) = I(\bar{x}) * G(\bar{x}; r)$, the original image convolved with a Gaussian of standard deviation r. The algorithm does not, however, calculate medialness, since only derivatives of medialness are required for ridge identification. Since the medialness is a function of image derivatives, the derivatives of medialness are also derivatives of the original image intensity. First derivatives of medialness require third derivatives of image intensity, while second derivatives of medialness require fourth derivatives of image intensity.

Given that $\hat{M}(\bar{x}) = M(\bar{x}, \bar{i}(\bar{x}))$ and that M can be defined in terms of derivatives of the original image, the derivatives necessary for ridge calculation are as follows:

$$\hat{M}_n = M_{\bar{i}(n)}$$
$$= L_{nnn}$$
$$\hat{M}_{nn} = M_{\bar{i}(n)\bar{i}(n)} - (\nabla|_S(M_{\bar{i}(n)}))^t \, (\mathcal{H}^{-1}|_S(M)) \, (\nabla|_S(M_{\bar{i}(n)}))$$
$$= L_{nnnn} - (\nabla|_S(L_{nnn}))^t \, (\mathcal{H}^{-1}|_S(L_{nn})) \, (\nabla|_S(L_{nnn}))$$

Where $\bar{i}$ is the coordinate chart described in Section 2.1. Each of these derivatives is implemented as a spherical weighting function applied to the original image intensities.

3 Results

Figure 1 shows the result of using the marching ridges algorithm on a human brain ventricle in an MR image. Only four slices of the head are shown; the core extends further in the ventricle on higher and lower slices.

4 Discussion

4.1 Skeletons and object edges by marching ridges

The marching ridges algorithm has been used to produce intensity ridges (skeletons) of objects in 2D images. It has also been used in 3D images to find curvilinear skeletons of tube-like objects and surface skeletons for more general objects.

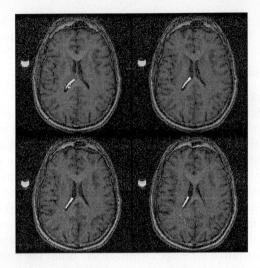

Fig. 1. Optimal scale-orientation core of brain ventricle in 4 adjacent MR image slices.

The marching ridges algorithm has also been used to produce edges of objects in both 2D and 3D images using the Canny definition.

4.2 1D cores in 3D images

This paper presents a method for calculating cores of general objects in 3D images, objects whose cores will generally be surface manifolds. There are, however, structures in the human body which are better described by curvilinear cores, e.g., blood vessels and bronchial tubes. We have modified the marching cores algorithm to calculate cores for these structures; space limitations prevent the inclusion of our results here.

4.3 Medialness with two orientations

The medialness we are currently using is a weighting function of spatial position, radius, and a single orientation. We have begun using Blum-like medialness measures that are functions of spatial position, radius, and two orientations.

5 Acknowledgements

The work presented here was accomplished partially under the support of NIH grants P01 CA47982, R01 CA67812 and R01 LM05508. The UNC Department of Computer Science also provided important support. We gratefully acknowledge the ideas of James Damon, Jason Miller and Rob Keller which have contributed to the mathematical aspects of this work.

References

1. J. Bloomenthal. Polygonization of implicit surfaces. *Computer Aided Geometric Design*, pages 341–355, 1988.
2. J. Canny. A computational approach to edge detection. *IEEE Transactions on Pattern Analysis and Machine Intelligence*, PAMI-8(6):679–698, November 1986.
3. D. Eberly. *Ridges in Image and Data Analysis*. Computational Imaging and Vision Series. Kluwer Academic Publishers, Dordrecht, NL, 1996.
4. D. Eberly and S. Pizer. Ridge flow models for image segmentation. In *SPIE Proceedings on Mathematical Methods in Medical Imaging II*, pages 54–64, 1994.
5. M. Fidrich. Iso-sruface extraction in 4d with applications related to scale space. Technical Report 2833, Institut National de Recherche en Informatique et en Automatique, March 1996.
6. D. S. Fritsch, S. M. Pizer, L. Yu, V. Johnson, and E. L. Chaney. Localization and segmentation of medical image objects using deformable shape loci. In H. H. Barrett and A. F. Gmitro, editors, *Information Processing in Medical Imaging*, Lecture Notes in Computer Science, pages 127–140. Springer-Verlag, 1997.
7. J. Furst, S. Pizer, and D. Eberly. Marching cores: a mehtod for extracting cores from 3d medical images. In *Proceedings of the workshop on Mathematical Methods in Biomedical Image Analysis*, pages 124–130. IEEE Computer Society Technical Committee on Pattern Analysis and Machine Intelligence, June 1996.
8. Jacob D. Furst, Robert S. Keller, Jason E. Miller, and Stephen M. Pizer. Image loci are ridges in geometric spaces. In Bart ter Haar Romeny, Luc Florack, Jan Koenderink, and Max Viergever, editors, *Scale Space Theory in Computer Vision*, Lecture Notes in Computer Science, pages 176–187. Springer-Verlag, 1997.
9. R. M. Haralick. Ridges and valleys on digital images. *Computer Vision, Graphics, and Image Processing*, 22:28–38, 1983.
10. T. Lindeberg. Edge detection and ridge detection with automatic scale selection. Technical Report ISRN KTH/NA/P-96/06-SE, KTH (Royal Institute of Technology), 1996.
11. W. E. Lorensen and H. E. Cline. Marching cubes: a high resolution 3d surface construction algorithm. *Computer Graphics*, 21(4):163–169, July 1987.
12. B. S. Morse, S. M. Pizer, and A. Liu. Multiscale medial analysis of medical images. *Proceedings on Information Processing in Medical Images*, 687:112–131, 1993.
13. S. M. Pizer, D. Eberly, B. S. Morse, and D. S. Fritsch. Zoom-invariant vision of figural shape: The mathematics of cores. *Computer Vision and Image Understanding*, 1998. to appear.
14. S. M. Pizer, D. S. Fritsch, V. Johnson, and E. Chaney. Segmentation, registration and measurement of shape variation via image object shape, 1996. tutorial notes *Visualization in Biomedical Computing*.
15. Stephen M. Pizer, Daniel S. Fritsch, Kah-Chan Low, and Jacob D. Furst. 2d & 3d figural models of anatomic objects from medical images. In *Proceedings of ISMM98*, 1988. to appear.
16. J. Thirion and A. Gourdon. The marching lines algorithm: new results and proofs. Technical Report 1881, Institut National de Recherche en Informatique et en Automatique, April 1993.
17. Paul Yushkevich, Daniel Fritsch, Stephen Pizer, and Edward Chaney. Towards automatic, model-driven determination of 3d patient setup errors in conformal radiotherapy, 1998. Submitted to MICCAI98.

Singularities as Features of Deformation Grids

Fred L. Bookstein

University of Michigan, Ann Arbor, Michigan 48109 USA

Abstract. Biological shape differences often are represented as diffeomorphisms of a Cartesian coordinate grid. This paper suggests that their spatially discrete, localized features, for instance the details that suggest underlying developmental or pathological processes, can often be identified with variants of the singularity $(x, y) \to (x, x^2y + y^3)$. This is an unfamiliar singularity, generic of codimension 1, at which a pair of cusps appears as a function of a parameter for "extrapolation." I introduce canonical coordinates for such singularities and show how they may be used to produce objective reports of grids encountered in an empirical context. An example is shown involving the corpus callosum in Fetal Alcohol Syndrome. These features appear to be robust under relaxation of bending energy against Euclidean distance, the analogue to multiscale analysis for discrete punctate data.

1 Introduction

In the rapidly growing literature of image analysis of the whole human brain, two principal methodological themes are *object detection* and *visualization by deformation grid*. The "objects" may be segmented regions (ventricle, hippocampus, tumor) from an anatomical image, or perhaps "hot spots" of metabolism exceeding baseline in a contrast of functional images. Deformations may be from atlas to patient, between different images of the same patient (pre- to intraoperative, or MR to PET), or, as will be the case in this paper, between averages of classes of patients whose contrast is important for scientific understanding of the causes and concomitants of anatomical anomalies. Yet our literature has not paid much attention to the interrelation of these two themes. Displacement and deformation grids have typically not been searched for focal features in the same way that the raw anatomical or functional images have been, and reports of features of deformation, whether focal or global, are typically not filtered through the multiscale machinery so fruitful in the contemporary methodologies of object detection for structural images and functional contrasts.

The present paper suggests a technique for bridging this gap: a method for finding focal features of deformation or displacement grids that is consistent with a multiscale approach and also with the existing biometric machinery for causes and effects of shape. Section 2 introduces a parametric template for such features, the *crease* singularity, and Section 3 shows how it is produced when empirical deformations are extrapolated to high multiples. Section 4 applies the method to an instructive example from the neuroanatomy of Fetal Alcohol Syndrome, an irreversible but somewhat cryptic structural-behavioral disorder, and Section

5 shows a multiscale extension that supports a useful statistical significance test for findings like these.

2 The basic singularity

Consider the deformation function at right in Figure 1. (Note that the scales of the axes here are unequal.) This figure is a transformation of originally square Cartesian axes according to the composition of three functions. Two are uninteresting: the map $(x,y) \to (x - 2y^2, y)$, which bends lines $x = c$ into parabolas of vertical vertex tangent, and the map $(x,y) \to (x + 8y, y)$, which imposes a shear along the x-axis. The core of the transform, however, is quite interesting: the map $(x,y) \to (x, x^2 y + y^3)$, at the left in the figure, with that curious singularity at $(0,0)$. The generic singularities of maps $R^2 \to R^2$ are folds and cusps (Whitney's theorem [1]) having canonical forms $(x,y) \to (x, y^2)$ and $(x,y) \to (x, xy + y^3)$, respectively. Clearly the singularity here is neither of these. Lines $y = c$ are transformed here into a nested family of parabolas $cx^2 + c^3$ whose spacing shrinks faster than curvatures as they approach the real axis. In both panels of the figure, the heavy line is the image of the original locus $x = 0$. Its singularity is concealed on the left—it falls to speed zero as it traverses the axis—but, unfolded on the right, we can see how when symmetry is broken this meridian can change direction there.

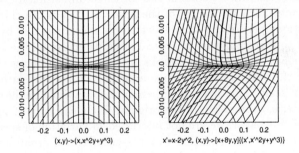

Figure 1. The basic singularity and a generalization.

Nongeneric singularities can be usefully approached as limiting cases of generic ones. In the present instance, the map $(x,y) \to (x, x^2 y + y^3)$ can be viewed as the limit as $a \to 0$ of maps $(x,y) \to (x, (x^2 - a)y + y^3)$, Figure 2. For $a > 0$, each of these has two ordinary cusps at $\pm\sqrt{a}$. The Jacobian of the map is negative in the lip-shaped region between the cusps. As a passes through 0, the two cusps momentarily fuse in our higher-order singularity, then vanish.

3 How these arise in data

The manner in which singularities like these arise as descriptors of biological shape phenomena is, needless to say, not as the limit of the parametrized mappings in Figure 2. Realistic maps of one biological form onto another do not have cusps or folds. Instead, our singularity is encountered when realistic deformations are extrapolated to arbitrarily high multiples.

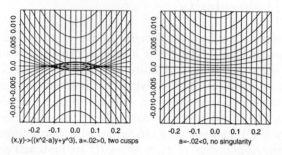

Figure 2. Limit of paired cusps: $(x, y) \to ((x^2 - a)y + y^3, y)$ for a near 0.

The maps we are exploring arise as expressions of statistical contrasts corresponding to a variety of applied biometric questions, such as dimensions of greatest natural variations in shape or aspects of shape that optimally covary with exogenous causes or effects of shape. (The example here illustrates the simplest such context, the visualization of the difference between two group average shapes.) In this version of morphometrics, shape data are formalized via ordered n-tuples of *landmark points* in two- or three-dimensional Cartesian space. Landmark points, such as "bridge of the nose" or "tip of the chin," have operational definitions permitting their location on specimens one by one but also are presumed to correspond on biological grounds across all the specimens of a sample. The shape of a set of landmarks is the equivalence class of their configuration under the ordinary Euclidean similarity group of translations, rotations, and changes of scale. This space is a Riemannian manifold under the celebrated *Procrustes metric*, submersion of the original Euclidean sum-of-squares [2]. For the purpose of this paper, we are not interested in variation of specimens within samples, but restrict our attention to representations of group average shapes, where the "average" is the form of least summed squared Procrustes distance to all the forms of the subsample. The computational geometry of the Procrustes methods has been reviewed elsewhere [3]; its details are not important for the analysis of singularities to follow.

Rather more important is the algebra of the thin-plate splines that we use for smooth interpolation between different shapes, such as averages of different subgroups of one data set. This formalism has appeared many times previously [3,4]. For the equations to follow we borrow the standard notations: L is the bordered kernel matrix, H is the vector of target landmark coordinates with three zeroes appended, $L^{-1}H$ is the vector of spline coefficients, and L_k^{-1} is the quadratic form for bending energy.

The spline helps visualize statistical summaries based in these Procrustes coordinates in a remarkably effective manner. Any vector computed in the course of a multivariate analysis—a mean difference, for example—can be visualized as a deformation in this way. That the double integral of second derivatives is minimized means that the spline fits shape changes with the smallest possible variation of affine derivative (shapes of the little grid cells in these figures). If a given change of affine derivative can be managed over a larger interval, its contribution to the integral of squares is lower; hence the spline tries to represent deformations "as globally as possible." Global features of such changes are plainly visible in the grids without further parameterization. Furthermore, because the spline's coefficients $L^{-1}H$ are linear in H, the deformed configuration, we can unambiguously construct an α-fold extrapolation (magnification) of the map $S_1 \to S_2$ as the map $S_1 \to S_1 + \alpha(S_2 - S_1)$.

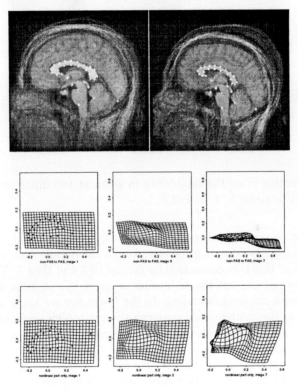

Figure 3. A two-group contrast (FAS average at top right) with ordinary (middle row) and affine-free (bottom row) extrapolates. α, left to right: 1,3,7.

4 An instructive example

Figure 3 shows, in the upper row, landmark-registered mean images from midsagittal brain MR for 4 adults with Fetal Alcohol Syndrome (FAS) and 8 persons not so affected. (Fetal Alcohol Syndrome is an irreversible process of prenatal brain damage discovered in 1973 and known to be caused by exposure to very high levels of alcohol early in fetal life.) At center left in the figure is the deformation grid from left to right mean landmark configuration. In the bright white curving arch (center of the raster images, from left to top of the punctate diagrams) is the *corpus callosum*, the principal conduit of information between the cerebral hemispheres; cerebellum is at the lower right. The left part of the callosum is called "genu"; the bulb at the right, "splenium"; the narrowing just to its left, "isthmus."

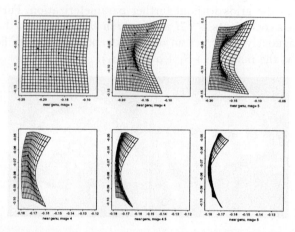

Figure 4. Zooming in on the singularity in genu, at two different scales. α, top to bottom, left to right: 1, 4, 5, 4, 4.5, 5.

The grid at center left in Figure 3 is obviously not affine, but it is difficult to put into words exactly what it is instead. Across the middle row of the figure are extrapolations of this transformation by factors of 3 and then 7. The bending is becoming more patent, but the collapsing of the shape at large extrapolations is interfering with our understanding. In the lower row we apply an elementary stratagem from the contemporary morphometric toolkit, removing the affine term by linear projection in the Procrustes geometry [3,5]. Now it is clear that there is an extended extremum of hypoplasia (compression) across the entire length of the corpus callosum. Somewhere between the threefold extrapolation and the sevenfold, the deformation goes singular in two different regions.

Figure 4 enlarges regions around genu near the extrapolation at which the singularity appears. In the top row are shown the actual deformation of the region in question and also multiples of the original transformation by four and by five; the singularity appears somewhere in between. In the lower row, a further enlargement localizes the singularity quite near the multiple of 4.5. The higher extrapolation at lower right shows the expected paired-cusp structure.

Something here is not yet as symmetrical as it might be. In the lower left panel of Figure 4, count down about eight grid lines on the left and the right margins of the little grid cell. You will find that their images are not aligned—none of the grid lines drawn appear to be transversals of the singularity. We can make this a bit clearer, Figure 5, by rotating the data through a range of orientations with respect to the starting grid. At some orientations, lines slew upward along the singularity; at others, they slew downward. There is thus some orientation along which they do not slew at all, the orientation exploited at right in the figure. Here grid lines approximate a proper corner where they cross the tangent to the singularity just upstream or just downstream.

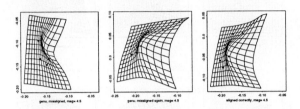

Figure 5. Rotating the starting grid through the singularity ($\alpha = 4.5$).

What is the meaning of such a finding? I suggest that it constitutes a *finite feature*, a salient organizing focus for description of the map in the large. Figure 3, lower right, shows this interpretation quite clearly. We have located the center of horizontal compression of a vertically organized dysmorphogenic field that, extended, generates the cusp visible there right up to the boundaries of the next such structure (to be encountered in Figure 6). That the singularity appears at extrapolation 4.5 means that the largest compression in any direction is by 1/4.5=22% of the original length, and the field of compression extends for a considerable distance upward from this feature.

These grids look remarkably like the prototype I led you to expect (recall Figure 1). The parameters of one of these features total eight: location (two), direction of the axis of the singularity, angles between the tangent to the singular locus and the principal transversal at its "corner" (two), first derivative of the map in the tangent direction, second derivative in the transversal direction, and extrapolation α at which all this goes singular.

This decomposition contrasts considerably with the existing methods for feature extraction from deformations. The method of biorthogonal grids, for instance [7], computes principal strains of the affine derivative at every point, but its singularities are umbilics. It offers no formalism for finding the local extrema of strain rate analogous to the analysis here. And studies that compare areas or that search for sources, sinks, or peaks (cf. [6]) have hitherto been scalar-based, lacking the very important directional features of this parameterization.

Returning to the full transformation, Figure 3 (lower right), let us track down the structure of the other salient compression, at its upper center. As Figure 6 shows, this is a composite of two singularities at about the same maximal compression ($\frac{1}{5}$ to $\frac{1}{6}$) but different principal axes. In the rightmost of the two singularities, the corner of the transversal makes rather different angles with the tangent to the singularity on its two sides, as Figure 1 already prototyped (by shear along the tangent line). All along this arc of tissue (a histological locus, not a mathematical one), the average FAS case falls short of normal by about 1/5.5=18% in callosal thickness—that's a lot of neural tissue missing. The pair

of findings here owe to the same alcohol-induced dysmorphogenesis that leads
to the characteristic facial features by which FAS is diagnosed [8].

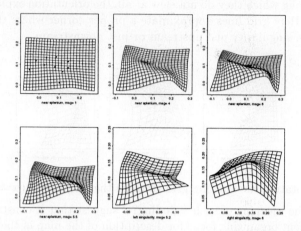

Figure 6. Near splenium, there are two more singularities, nearly collinear. α, top to bottom, left to right: 1, 4, 6, 5.5, 5.2, 6.

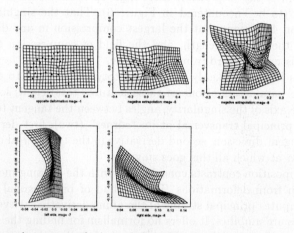

Figure 7. Negative extrapolation of the affine-free FAS grid shows two foci of expansion. α, top to bottom, left to right: $-1, -5, -8, -7, -6$.

To complete the analysis of this transformation, we need to look at the singularities of the opposite transformation (negative extrapolations of the same map). Figure 7 shows that this transformation has two singularities of its own, rather close together, both of the same familiar structure. Because these are creases of the opposite map, they are local extrema of expansion, not compression, of the original comparison; together they account for the great whitened area at the lower right in Figure 3. These loci of greatest expansion are both within the fluid compartment of this brain section, so the expansion does the victim of the syndrome no good at all. For other empirical examples, dealing with schizophrenia, see [9].

5 Relaxation preserves creases as features

As an exact interpolant, the thin-plate spline here tracks variation in a mapping function at all pertinent scales. This is not necessarily a virtue in a world where data incorporate noise right alongside signal. By trading imprecision for bending energy, the spline can be made more similar in spirit to other energy-based methods, regularized from the outset, that compromise a pictorial mismatch energy against a complexity cost. The following approach, for instance, has been developed twice before [10,11].

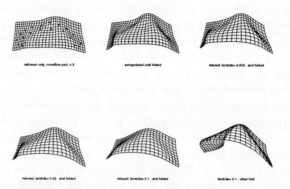

Figure 8. The relaxation that smooths the grids does not alter the creases as features. Values of λ: upper right, .005; lower row, .02, .01, .01. The analysis is of the nonaffine signal only.

In the notation introduced earlier, reorder the Cartesian coordinates of a set of k landmarks (X_i, Y_i) as the $2k$-vector $V = (X_1, X_2, \ldots, X_k, Y_1, \ldots, Y_k)^t$. To relax a perturbed configuration V_p onto a standard configuration V_s, seek the configuration V_r that minimizes the weighted sum of two energies. One term is the bending $(V_r - V_s)^t BE(V_r - V_s)$ of V_r considered as a deformation of the standard form. (Here BE is the duplication $\text{diag}(L_k^{-1}, L_k^{-1})$ of the bending-energy matrix corresponding to V_s.) The other term is "pictorial" energy, the sum-of-squares $(V_r - V_p)^t(V_r - V_p)$ that corresponds to squared Procrustes distance between the relaxed landmark configuration V_r and the data vector V_p actually encountered. In the references cited, there was also introduced a *log-likelihood* $\frac{1}{2}(V_r - V_s)^t \Sigma^-(V_r - V_s)$, where Σ is a sample variance-covariance matrix, but we shall not need that third term here.

For any relative weight λ, we seek the relaxed configuration V_r that minimizes the weighted sum $(V_r - V_p)^t(V_r - V_p) + \lambda(V_r - V_s)^t BE(V_r - V_s)$ of the two energies. Setting the gradient of this expression to zero straightforwardly leads to

$$V_r \equiv V_r(\lambda) = (I_{2k} + \lambda BE)^{-1}(V_p + \lambda BE \, V_s) \,.$$

As λ varies, $V_r(\lambda)$ traverses a smooth curve in the space of landmark configurations, the charmingly named *curve décolletage* [10]. Note that $V_r(0) = V_p$—in the absence of any penalty for deviation from the standard V_s, the best fit to any data is the selfsame data. In the other limit $\lambda \to \infty$, V_r tends to the configuration of zero bending having the least Euclidean cost: the best fit to the data by an affine transform of the standard. Because BE is a function of V_s, this formulation is not symmetric in V_p and V_s.

As λ increases, naturally the transformation $V_s \to V_r(\lambda)$ moves closer to a uniform map. Its features, in the sense of this paper, may be restored by enhancing the extrapolation of maps $V_s \to V_r$ to compensate. (In effect we are following a curve in the two-dimensional "control space" parameterized by λ and $\alpha(\lambda)$.) From the sequence of just-creased maps that results I have extracted the examples in Figure 8 for your consideration. Clearly these comparisons are becoming steadily smoother as the value of λ increases; but also, just as clearly, the creases that we found in Figure 3 are fairly stable against energy-driven smoothing as operationalized by the relaxation here.

The last two frames of this figure suggest an appropriate statistical significance test for the effect claimed here. Over a range of spatial scales the deformation appears to have two creases (at two different values of α) which together span nearly all of the callosal arc. Features like these are susceptible to permutation-based methods of statistical inference analogous to those now securely in place for global features [3]. Without the need for any parametric modeling, we can test the claim of a significant difference between the FAS subset and the others by examining the distribution of analogous features, at values of α that are no greater, when cases are permuted over group [12]. There are $\binom{12}{4} = 495$ permuted subsettings of this data set. In addition to the one given by the actual diagnosis, 19 others show creasing along the callosum as extensive as we see here. Hence the significance level of the crease report here is 4%, precisely.

6 Future work

The visualizations and the computational geometry associated with the search for creases are at very early stages of development. The representations here were produced slowly and interactively by hand; we need very fast algorithms for locating these structures in real data so that permutation-based statistical tests for reliability of these features can go forward in practical time. (The data set here is at the upper limit of size for which the enumeration of creased permutations is feasible by eye.) In addition to the crease singularity there are limiting cases of higher degeneracy [9] that need parametric models. In three dimensions [13] the equivalent of the catastrophe here is the emergence of a pair of the equivalently isolated singularities, *swallowtails*, from a diffeomorphism. We have such a finding in 3D already (see the projected images in [14]), but the parametric template for the mapping is still obscure, and the interactive search for its features is a good deal more difficult than the equivalent in two dimensions.

Acknowledgements. The work reported here was supported in part by NIH grants DA-09009 and GM-37251 to Fred L. Bookstein. I am grateful to Hemant Tagare (Yale) for the tip about Whitney's theorem, and to my longtime collaborator Bill Green for his `ewsh` package permitting free play with extrapolation and grid placement in two and three dimensions. The FAS data set was gathered under NIH grant AA-10836 to Ann P. Streissguth.

7 Literature Cited

1. Bruce, J. W., and P. J. Giblin. *Curves and Singularities*, second edition. Cambridge University Press, 1992.
2. Kendall, D. G. Shape-manifolds, procrustean metrics, and complex projective spaces. *Bulletin of the London Mathematical Society* 16:81–121, 1984.
3. Bookstein, F. L. Shape and the information in medical images. *Computer Vision and Image Understanding* 66:97–118, 1997a.
4. Bookstein, F. L. *Morphometric Tools for Landmark Data*. New York: Cambridge University Press, 1991.
5. Bookstein, F. L. Biometrics and brain maps: the promise of the Morphometric Synthesis. Pp. 203–254 in S. Koslow and M. Huerta, eds., *Neuroinformatics*. Hillsdale, NJ: Lawrence Erlbaum, 1997b.
6. Thompson, P. M., and A. W. Toga. Detection, visualization, and animation of abnormal anatomic structure with a deformable probabilistic brain atlas. *Medical Image Analysis* 1:271–294, 1997.
7. Bookstein, F. L. *The Measurement of Biological Shape and Shape Change*. Lecture Notes in Biomathematics, vol. 24. Springer-Verlag, 1978.
8. Bookstein, F. L., A. P. Streissguth, P. Sampson, P. Connor, and H. Barr. Does the face predict the brain? The corpus callosum in Fetal Alcohol Syndrome. *NeuroImage*, submitted for publication, 1998.
9. Bookstein, F. L. Singularities and the features of deformation grids. Pp. 46–55 in B. Vemuri, ed., *Proc. Workshop on Biomedical Image Analysis*, IEEE Computer Society, 1998.
10. Bookstein, F. L. Four metrics for image variation. Pp. 227–240 in D. Ortendahl and J. Llacer, eds., *Proceedings of the XI International Conference on Information Processing in Medical Imaging*. Progress in Clinical and Biological Research, vol. 363. New York: Wiley-Liss, Inc., 1990 [1991].
11. Rohr, K., H. Stiehl, R. Sprengel et al. Point-based elastic registration of medical image data using approximating thin-plate splines. Pp. 297–306 in K. Höhne and R. Kikinis, eds., *Visualization in Biomedical Computing. Lecture Notes in Computer Science*, vol. 1131. Springer-Verlag, 1996.
12. Good, P. *Permutation Tests*. Springer, 1994.
13. Whitney, H. Singularities of mappings of Euclidean spaces. In his *Collected Papers*, Birkhäuser, 1992, vol. 1, pp. 436–452.
14. Buckley, P. F., D. Dean, F. Bookstein et al. Three-dimensional MR-based morphometrics and ventricular dysmorphology in schizophrenia. *Biological Psychiatry*, in press, 1998.

Morphological Analysis of Terminal Air Spaces by Means of Micro-CT and Confocal Microscopy and Simulation within a Functional Model of Lung

Andres Kriete[1], Henrik Watz[2], Wigbert Rau[2], Hans-Rainer Duncker[1]

[1]Institute of Anatomy and Cell Biology
Image Processing Laboratory
Aulweg 123, 35385 Giessen, Germany
[2]Department of Diagnostic Radiology
University Clinic Giessen
Klinikstr. 36, 35385 Giessen, Germany

Abstract. We devise a new methodology to investigate terminal air spaces of lung. Micro-CT imaging and a computer guided technique for scanning and image fusion in confocal microscopy enable the acquisition of extended and highly resolved data volumes exhibiting respiratory units. Segmentation and the analysis of the topography of respiratory airways leads to a finite volume model suitable for computational physics within a computer lung model.

1 Introduction

Terminal air spaces such as alveoli, alveolar ducts and acini, also called respiratory units, are responsible for the gas exchange and herewith represent the important functional part of lung. There are up to 150000 acini or respiratory units in mammalian lungs, each containing 300-2000 alveoli. The fundamental knowledge about the spatial and functional relationships of terminal air spaces need to be obtained before a structural and functional model can be constructed suitable for a computer simulation.

There is a long history of experimental difficulties in the quantitative investigation of terminal air spaces. Due to the lack of appropiate imaging techniques most studies were based on casts,e.g. [1], which do not permit any insight into the structural organization of the dense and undifferentiated lung tissue (see Fig. 1). This paper explores a new set of methodologies to image, quantify and model terminal air spaces of mammalian species including micro-CT and a complementary confocal microscopic imaging technique.

2 Material and Methods

2.1 Micro-CT

Micro-CT investigations require structures of high density to give sufficient contrast. Applications reported so far are limited to the analysis of bones or applications in material sciences [2]. To give highly resolved images at sufficient contrast of the lung parenchyma, we introduce histological staining techniques not very much unlike to those known in light and electron microscopy. Exstirpated human lungs were inflated and fixed with hot formalin vapor via the main bronchus. Respiratory movements were simulated over a period of 8 hours to get a sufficient amount of fresh formalin vapor into the alveoli, which were inflated to nearly full inspiratory volume. Cylindric specimens of the fixed lungs of 10 mm in diameter were taken perpendicular to the lung surface. In order to augment the contrast between alveolar walls and air, the lung tissue was impregnated with 0.8 molar $AgNO_3$. Subsequently the specimens were mounted in the micro-CT. An X-ray tube with a microfocus of 10 microns diameter was used as a source, a CCD-array as a detector, the peak of the X-ray spectrum was at 25 keV. The images acquired by this device have a spatial isotropic resolution of 14 microns at a matrix of 1024^2 pixels in an isotropic volume data set.

Visualization of lung parenchyma is a difficult task. Because of an undifferentiated appearance, no prominent structures can be outlined. Visualizations of surfaces without preprocessing don't give any insight, but deliver a sponge like appearence. An interesting feature to visualize the lumen is that of virtual endoscopy, as illustrated in Fig. 2. However, for a morphological analysis a carefull segmentation technique, such as the one described in Chapter 3, has to be applied.

2.2 Confocal microscopy

The confocal microscope is used in the sense of an optical tomograph to acquire image sequences with precise registration at thick specimen. The axial resolution of such an device is improved with lenses of high numerical aperture, but unfortunatly the today available lens designs bring along a narrow field of view at the same time. Certain studies like that of the lung parenchyma however require both a good axial resolution and in particular a wide field of view. This conflict is resolved here by an image fusion technique which combines a series of histological thick sections, each of these sections is confocally resolved and scanned in an array-like fashion and all the resulting subvolumes are digitally combined. The distinct advantage of using this

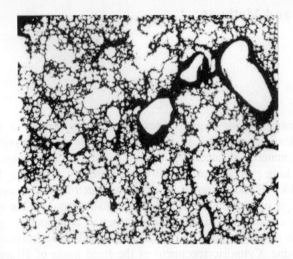

Fig.1 A section of lung tissue (rat) imaged with a confocal microscope. This image illustrates the undifferentiated appeerance of the densely packed structures, only some prominent bronchioli can be easily identified. Size is about 2x2 mm

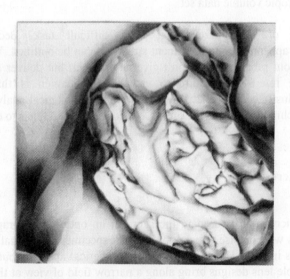

Fig.2 Endoscopic view of the acinar pathways at a human respiratory unit. The data set stems from micro-CT imaging, size of the pathway is about 0.05 mm in diameter

imaging technique is that it is scalable for resolution and is also usefull for other than human lungs when higher resolutions are required, such as rat or mouse.

Histological sections of 50-80 micron thickness of a rat lung stained with HE are the material for this example. For imaging, an upright Zeiss confocal laser scan microscope was used (Zeiss LSM 410) equipped with a HeNe laser emitting at 535 nm. Fluorescence was detected with one photomultiplier above 545 nm from the lung parenchyma.

To increase the accessible volume in confocal microscopic imaging, a framework for a computer guided imaging technique was developed. First the sections were imaged with a low magnifying lens of 5x (imaged area was 2000x2000 microns). These images were aligned for linear shift and rotation. Transfered back to the confocal microscope, these preprocessed images serve for alignement of the histological sections. Variation of the scanning offset, i.e. shifting the scanning beam electronically away from the center in all 8 possible directions at a lateral distance of 600 microns, gave 9 reference images and at a zoom factor of 4 they construct a frame of 1800 μm side length (see Fig. 1). Switching to a 20x magnifying lens, the field of view at zoom factor 1 fits exactly to that of the 9 individual reference images, so that non-overlapping subvolumes can be acquired by optical sectioning. Typically, some hundred images have to be fused, the example given in Fig. 3 is based on 819 fused images of 768x768x91 voxels each, equivalent to a volume of 1800x1800x910 microns. Such a volume may enclose a complete acinus, but exhibits as well all structural details like the alveoli.

3 Segmentation and 3-D Analysis of Terminal Air Spaces

The segmentation and labeling of structures within lung parenchyma is a step to prepare measurements and structural attributes for 3-D visualizations. Segmentation often requires interaction by the user, since automatic algorithms almost rely on the intensities of the voxels only. Here, the threshold selected was interactively controlled, which is used as a demarcation between lung parenchyma and background.

Once binary images had been obtained, it was necessary to identify structures out of the images like the outer boundary of the acinus, ductus, bronchi and alveoli. During the labeling the black and white pixel are replaced by user selected gray levels. To differentiate ductus and alveolar sacs completely from the alveoli, binary morphological operations using structuring elements for erosion and dilatation were performed. This procedure, if performed several times, removed all structures lying beyond a given size. Here, the filter size and the number of operations were selected in a way that mostly all alveoli, many of them in a sponge like open form, could be differentiated from the ducts. By this procedure, about 80% of all structural details were identified. Since the exact boundary of the acinus is difficult to define, in particular in the outer areas some of the structures remain questionable and had to be identified interactively.

The overwhelming structural detail of the data sets make the above described labeling method very time-consuming, since all the procedures have to be applied anew for the sections following until the whole data set is processed. What was tested instead was a still more automated seeding procedure. First, one representative image out of the middle of the data stack was selected as a starting point. At this image, an interactive guided labeling of structures as described above was performed. Next, this identified image was used as an marker or reference for the following one. If combined with one selected label of the reference image, this label was transferred to those objects which overlap by at least one pixel of the area with the reference object. Due to changes from section to section not all the structures were identified correctly, and some interactive correction was always necessary. Fig. 3 depicts an completely segmented data set with opaque rendered bronchioli. Alveolar ducts and aveoli have a high transparency.

For a morphological analysis of the branching pattern of airways within an acinus, a topological skeleton was extracted. We used our software package 3D-TOP, explained in detail elsewhere [3]. This skeleton may be embedded in a volume rendering, such as in Figure 3. The topological skeleton starts with the bronchiolus terminalis, splits into two short segments, which are devided up further into two daughter ducts each. Assuming a circular form of the ducts, the cross-sectional area was calculated. The sum of cross-sectional areas along the distance from the origin of the acinus reveals a normal, Gaussian distribution. The maximum of the distribution occurs around the 5-6 th order of branching.

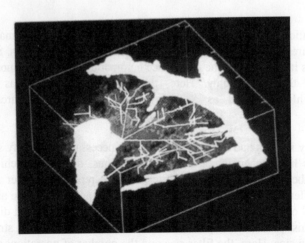

Fig.3 A volume rendered view of a complete respiratory unit with bright bronchioli. Embedded lines indicate the branching pattern of the airspaces. Size is about 2x2x1 mm

4 Simulation of Gas Transport within a Computer Lung Model

A computer modeling is often complicated by the structural complexity at the various levels [4]. As an example, the mammalian lung requires an investigation of some thousand air conducting bronchial segments and, in addition, the investigation of respiratory units (acini) at microscopic resolution as discussed here. The use of models for substructures is essential to realize a computer aided functional simulation of complex biological systems like that of a lung. As an initial step, a hierarchical model was reported previously which concerns the structure of the bronchial, air conducting part of the rat lung. This model features about 4000 bronchial segments [5,6], to which a dynamical model of the respiratory units has to be attached.

The Gaussian shape of the diameter distribution of airways at respiratory units allows to develop a model being composed of individual volumetric segments or subsections. This procedure is a typical approach in computational fluid dynamics [7]. Based on the analytical findings reported above, a Gaussian volume distribution can be modeled consisting of individual segments. From here the number of alveoli and the volume-to-surface ratio can be calculated. Depending on the breathing amplitude typical variations in volume size of all segments within the acini occur (Fig. 4).

To model gas distribution, each segment gains mass from the distal segment or losses mass due to transport into the daughter segments or gas uptake. Parameters necessary to perform such calculations include diffusion coefficient, difference of concentration across segment and gradient, way of flow partitioning and dispersion coefficient [6,8].

For each of the segments, such an equation describing conservation of mass can be postulated. A solution of the complete bronchial tree can not be found analytically, instead an iterative method was used, where the breathing cycle is devided up into many time-steps. The number of steps necessary depends on the mathematics used to yield a stable solution, typically 10000 time steps are necessary. For each of the segments at each time step the mass transport equation which is a differential equation is solved by Gauss-Seidel iteration. The calculation proceeds from the first order branches to more distal branches down to the respiratory units, and the resulting concentrations are stored along with the segments. The actual concentration values may be visualized.

Calculations can be performed for various amplitudes of the breathing cycle within the complete model of the organ of a rat lung. It was found that mass transport is about equal for convection and diffusion when entering the acinus, but the fast decrease in flow velocity quickly drops the rate of convectional mass transport. Diffusion however, dependent on the cross-sectional areas of the individual segments, increases towards the center of the acinus. Diffusional mass transport drops at a higher rate towards the periphery of respiratory units because of oxygen absorption.

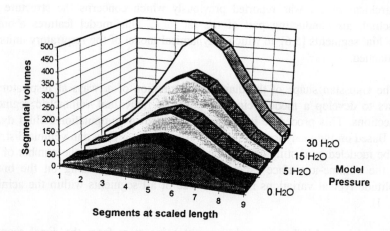

Fig. 4. Variation of segment sizes of modeled acini at different tidal volumes

5 Conclusions

For the investigation of terminal air spaces at the respiratory part of lung two novel imaging techniques are explored, which close a gap between the field of view obtainable with high resolution clinical imaging devices and the resolution of microscopical imaging. Complementary to micro-CT of stained lungs a novel 3-D image compositing technique at precise registration is described, which increases the accessible volume imaged with a confocal laser scanning microscope. The latter method is scalable and can also be applied to smaller mammalien lungs. Both methods allow to image complete respiratory units with all structural details.

The problems involved in the segmentation and visualization of the undifferentiated lung parenchyma is discussed, as well as the topological quantification of the acinar pathways. Subsequently a model of respiratory units is developed based on finite volumes to be used within a functional model of lung incorporating dynamics at breathing. Mass transport equations are solved iteratively describing convection, diffusion and gas uptake. Depending on the size and location of these units, a different amount of gas concentration and uptake is predicted .

Research addressing the microstructure of lung can now benefit of digital image processing by using advanced imaging techniques. Overall, new roads are opened to develop precise functional computer lung models usefull in clinical investigations, research and teaching.

Acknowledgements

We would like to thank K-P.Valerius, Giessen for loaning corrosion casts and histological sections. Special thanks go to T.Hildebrand and P.Rügsegger from the ETH Zürich for support in micro-CT imaging.

References

[1] Haefeli-Bleuer,B.; Weibel,E.R.(1988): Morphometry of the humal pulmonary acinus. Anat.Record, 220, pp. 401-414
[2] Rügsegger,P.,Koller, B., Müller, R.(1996) A microtomographic system for the nondestructive evaluation of bone architecture. Calcif.Tissue Res., 58, pp 24-29
[3] Kriete,A., Schwebel,T.(1996) : 3-D Top - a software package for the topological analysis of image sequences. J. of Structural Biology 116 , Academic Press (1996), pp 150-154
[4] Hersh,J.S.(1990): A survey of modeling representations and their application to biomedical visualization and simulation. in: Proc. of the Conf. on Visualization in Biomedical Computing. Atlanta, IEEE Comp.Soc.Press, pp 432-440
[5] Kriete,A.(1969): Hierarchical data representation of lung to model morphology and function. in: (Eds. Höhne,K.-H., Kikinis, R).: Visualization in Biomedical Computing. Springer, NY, pp 399-404
[6] Kriete,A.(1998): Form and function of mammalian lung: analysis by scientific computing. in press for: Advances in Anatomy, Embryology and Cell Biology, Vol. 145, Springer - Verlag, Berlin
[7] Davidson,L., Nielsen,P.(1995): Calculation of two-dimensional airflow in facial regions and nasal cavities using an unstructured finite volume solver. Conference on Finite Volume Methods, ISSN 1395-7953 R9539, Dec.1995
[8] Mercer,R.R.,Anjilvel,S.,Miller,F.J.,Crapo,J.D.(1991): Inhomogenity of ventilatory unit volume and its effects on reactive gas uptake. J.Appl.Physiol. 70,5, pp 2193-220

2D+T Acoustic Boundary Detection in Echocardiography

Miguel Mulet-Parada and J. Alison Noble
{miguel,noble}@robots.ox.ac.uk

Department of Engineering Science. University of Oxford, Oxford OX1 3PJ, UK

Abstract. In this paper we address the problem of spatio-temporal acoustic boundary detection in echocardiography. We propose a phase-based feature detection method to be used as the front end to higher-level 2D+T/3D+T reconstruction algorithms. We develop a 2D+T version of this algorithm and illustrate its performance on some typical echocardiogram sequences. We show how our temporal-based algorithm helps to reduce the number of spurious feature responses due to speckle and provides feature velocity estimates. Further, our approach is intensity-amplitude invariant. This makes it particularly attractive for echocardiographic segmentation, where choosing a single global intensity-based edge threshold is problematic.

1 Introduction

This paper develops a novel technique for finding acoustic boundaries in 2D and 2D+T echogram sequences. Most prior work has involved the development of 2D spatial processing methods, based on, for example, template mask feature detection [1]; 'snakes' [2], or integrated backscatter (IBS) boundary detection [3]. However, spatial methods ignore temporal continuity, which can potentially be used to improve the reliability of feature detection. Herlin and Ayache investigated this idea [4]. They proposed tracking cardiac boundaries using a method that employed a spatio-temporal based version of the Deriche edge detector [5] and assumed a Gaussian noise model. However, their approach was not fully developed or validated on clinical data.

Acoustic image feature detection needs to be robust to speckle noise and attenuation imaging artefacts. Speckle noise corrupts the data by introducing sharp changes in the image intensity profile, while attenuation artefacts alter the intensity of equally significant cardiac structures depending on their orientation with respect to the ultrasound beam. This suggests that measures based on phase information rather than intensity derivatives may be more appropriate for acoustic feature detection.

In previous work we have discussed the application of phase-based feature extraction methods to echocardiographic data [7]. We used a local-phase measure to selectively detect step edges associated with cardiac boundaries in 1D echocardiographic profiles. Local phase was computed via the convolution of the image with a quadrature pair of filters [6]. A scalogram was used to show that local phase signatures of cardiac boundaries are detectable and well localised at large scales. This is not the case for small scale speckle noise. Further, we showed that step-like cardiac boundaries can be selectively extracted according to the value of their local-phase signature which is different from that of the ridge-like structures associated with speckle. We applied this approach to 1D acoustic boundary detection in a Kalman-filter based tracking algorithm, and showed that this method gives better tracking performance than using simple gradient-based edge detection.

Unfortunately, the technique used in [7] cannot be readily extended to two or more dimensions. Building on the work of Kovesi [8], in the rest of this paper we present a new phase-based measure that shares the good localisation and selectivity properties of local phase but which can be extended to 2D and 2D+T. We also show how the 2D+T version of this algorithm provides an estimate of feature velocity. We are currently investigating how this idea can provide input to a higher level algorithm.

The outline of the paper is as follows. Section 2 presents the 2D acoustic feature detection algorithm and motivates the need for spatio-temporal analysis. This leads us to propose a 2D+T measure in Section 3 and to show how feature velocity can be estimated. Section 4 presents preliminary experimental segmentation results on real 2D cardiac sequences. We conclude with a summary and a discussion of current and future work in Section 5.

2 The 2D feature asymmetry algorithm

Kovesi proposed a 2D multi-scale, intensity-invariant, feature detection measure for finding step features in visual images [8]. In [7] we showed that a simplified version of this algorithm, using a single large scale, gives well localised segmentation results. We call this measure 2D feature asymmetry, $FA_{2D}(x,y)$, which we define as,

$$FA_{2D}(x,y) = \sum_m \frac{\lfloor [|o_m(x,y)| - |e_m(x,y)|] - T_m \rfloor}{A_m(x,y) + \epsilon}. \quad (1)$$

Here $o_m(x,y)$ ($e_m(x,y)$) is the output of a convolution of an image with an orientable odd (even) symmetric log-Gabor wavelet filter, and the summation is taken over m filter orientations. A_m is the local energy amplitude of the mth filter response given by $A_m(x,y) = \sqrt{e_m(x,y)^2 + o_m(x,y)^2}$, $\lfloor \rfloor$ denotes zeroing of negative values and ϵ avoids division by zero. The orientable 2D filters are defined by "spreading" a log-Gabor function into two dimensions. Namely, an orientable filter tuned to a particular orientation ϕ_0 is constructed in the frequency domain by masking a radial log-Gabor function with an angular Gaussian tuned to ϕ_0,

$$G(\omega_r, \phi) = \exp-\left(\frac{(log(\omega_r/\omega_{r_0}))^2}{2(log(\kappa/\omega_0))^2} + \frac{(\phi - \phi_0)^2}{2\sigma_\phi^2}\right). \quad (2)$$

Here ϕ_0 is the orientation of the filter and σ_ϕ defines the extent of the spreading function as a scaling s of the separation between filters $\Delta\phi$ i.e. $\sigma_\phi = s \times \Delta\phi$. The value κ/ω determines the wavelength of the filters. In our experience we have found that $\Delta\phi = 30°, s = 0.6, \kappa/\omega = 0.55$ (2 octaves), provides a good compromise between even spectral coverage, orientation resolution and computation time for a six filter bank. The orientation-dependent noise threshold, T_m, and the zeroing operation make each filter respond to only those features in its orientation range. In Equation 1, amplitude normalisation provides invariance to contrast. Thus, the response of each feature is normalised according to the local energy measure around its neighbourhood. In this way local feature significance prevails over general feature strength.

The result of computing 2D feature asymmetry on a short-axis ultrasound image with no pre-filtering is shown in Figure 2(B). In our images a filter wavelength of 20 pixels has been found to give good feature localisation while avoiding the detection of speckle. The results show good detection of the chamber boundaries. However, the limitation of using a 2D feature asymmetry measure is highlighted if the 2D (spatially) processed images are displayed as a movie sequence. In this case, a number of small flickering spurious features are observed. In any given frame, there will always be a number of spurious features, due to noise and artefacts, that share similar intensity, shape and scale characteristics as responses from chamber boundaries. However, and unlike cardiac chamber boundaries, most of these features are not persistent from one frame to the next. In fact, most are due to speckle patterns that decorrelate with tissue movement. To remove the flickering noise, we now extend the 2D analysis into the temporal domain.

3 The 2D+T algorithm and feature velocity estimation

The extension of the feature asymmetry measure to 2D+T involves the design of a set of filters oriented in a number of spatio-temporal directions. This is achieved by re-defining the 2D filters in 3D spherical co-ordinates,

$$G(\omega_r, \phi, \theta) = \exp - \frac{(log(\omega_r/\omega_{r_0}))^2}{2(log(\kappa/\omega_0))^2} \exp - \left(\frac{(\phi - \phi_0)^2}{2\sigma_\phi^2} + \frac{(\theta - \theta_0)^2}{2\sigma_\theta^2} \right). \quad (3)$$

The velocities to which each filter responds are encoded in terms of ϕ_0 the spatial orientation, and θ_0 the temporal orientation. Figure 1 shows a diagrammatic representation of the filter orientations. Twenty-one filters are located on a spatio-temporal hemisphere at the vertices of an 80 faceted tesselation of the unit sphere obtained from the subdivision of a regular icosahedron. This provides an approximately even distribution of filters over the spatio-temporal space. Note that for $\theta = 0$ (*time* = 0 plane) only orientations in the $\phi = [0°, 180°)$ interval are required. The spread parameters are chosen to be the same, making the filters isotropic in the spatial and temporal dimensions ($\sigma_\phi = \sigma_\phi$). The value of the spatio-temporal spread is set to a fraction (0.6) of the average angular spacing between filters to ensure even spectral coverage.

In order to improve the contrast of a segmented image, the maximum filter output over all orientations is taken rather than the sum. The 2D+T feature asymmetry measure then becomes,

$$\text{FA}_{2D+T}(x,y) = \max_{v,m} \frac{\lfloor [|o_{m,v}(x,y)| - |e_{m,v}(x,y)|] - T_{m,v} \rfloor}{A_{m,v}(x,y) + \epsilon}, \quad (4)$$

where the indices v, m respectively indicate the temporal and spatial orientation of each filter.

Note that we do not choose particular velocities but sample over all the spatio-temporal space. The current implementation does not optimise filter design to a velocity range because cardiac motion varies during the cardiac cycle, depends on position on the heart surface, and image velocities ultimately depend on the temporal resolution of the data. In practice, provided that the spatio-temporal filters have sufficient resolution and tile the spatio-temporal volume evenly, any velocity will be detected by at least one filter. The $\theta = 90°$ filter detects very fast changes that persist over time, i.e. pure temporal steps due to occlusions.

Note further that by recording which of the filters gives the strongest response an estimate of feature velocity is obtained. Given the sparse sampling of the 2D+T space the estimate can be improved by interpolating the responses around the maximum to approximate the true feature velocity.

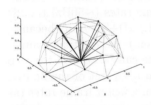

Fig. 1. *The 21 2D+T filter orientations.*

The current implementation performs filter convolutions by multiplication in the frequency domain using Temperton's FFT algorithm [9]. The filters are built in the frequency domain using Equation 3. The separability of the 3D FFT operation allows us to resample the filter's spectrum according to the relative data lengths of each axis in space-time. We treat the 2D+T volume to be isotropically sampled. In the results presented in Section 4 the data dimensions are 256×256 pixels in space by 32 frames in time.

4 Results

In this section we present the results of applying our 2D+T acoustic boundary detection algorithm to a number of echogram sequences. We illustrate some of the distinguishing features of this type of approach to acoustic feature detection and highlight some potential areas of application of the technique. We encourage the reader to visit http://www.robots.ox.ac.uk/~miguel/MICCAI98.html where the movies referred to in this section and further examples can be seen.

4.1 Comparing 2D and 2D+T filters: The purpose of the first experiment is to highlight some of the differences between 2D and 2D+T boundary detection. A 2D+T filter bank, consisting of 21 filters, was designed as described in Section 3. The wavelength of the Log-Gabor component was 20 pixels for all the filters, their bandwidth was 2 octaves, $\kappa/\omega_0 = 0.55$, and $s = 0.6$.

Three consecutive frames (11, 12 and 13 in the movie sequences) of the 2D+T segmentation are shown in Figure 2(C). For comparison we have included the original data and the results of a 2D segmentation using the same scale, Figures 2(A) and 2(B) respectively.

Note the absence of small scale flicker features in the 2D+T measure when compared with the 2D result. The significant features in the 2D+T results can be easily traced across the three frames and they all correspond to relevant cardiac structure. In the 2D segmentation this is not the case. Many inconsistent blob-like features are detected as well as a number of short-lived small-scale line features corresponding to speckle. Furthermore, in the 2D+T result the left wall of the ventricle is visible as a faint arc. This structure is not detected by 2D segmentation. The results illustrate how the 2D+T segmentation weighs the importance of spatial features according to their temporal significance.

With larger filter scales, smoother contours are obtained and less noise is detected, but this is at the price of less accurate localisation and detail. Obviously, increasing the scale of the 2D filters does not remove flicker noise, (see the web page for an illustration of this). In Figure 3(A) we show 2D and 2D+T results on a very cluttered long axis image. This is the other standard view used to quantify left ventricle dynamics by cardiologists. The results show very clearly the removal of the flickering speckle features and the enhancement given to the main cardiac structures by 2D+T filtering.

A limitation of our current 2D+T algorithm is that it cannot detect fast cardiac motions that have similar temporal characteristics to speckle; for example the mitral valve leaflets. At typical diagnostic frame rates (∼50Hz) the 2D segmentation of the mitral valve appears superior to the 2D+T results because, during opening, the leaflets cannot be tracked consistently across time frames. This is illustrated in Figure 3(B). The whole sequences can be seen in the web page. Note that this is not a problem of the algorithm itself but of the limited sampling rate of the data. This can be overcome by using faster frame rates (as available on new commercial machines) or interpolating the sequence prior to detection.

4.2 Gradient vs. phase-based filtering: The full spatio-temporal character of our method and its invariance to contrast, are illustrated in this section by comparison with a gradient-based spatio-temporal algorithm developed by Herlin and Ayache [4].

Herlin and Ayache used a modification of Deriche's edge detector in 3D based on smooth derivatives [5]. They estimated the two spatial components of the gradient vector N_x and N_y from the convolution of the 2D+T intensity function $I(x, y, t)$ with two spatial derivative kernels (D_x, D_y) and a temporal smoothing filter (L_t) so that $N_x = (D_x, L_y, L_t) \otimes I(x, y, t)$, and, $N_y = (L_x, D_y, L_t) \otimes I(x, y, t)$. Edges were obtained from the local maxima of the norm of the gradient given by, $N(x, y, t) = \sqrt{N_x^2 + N_y^2}$.

The result of applying the Deriche method to our short axis sequence is shown in Figure 3(C). The same parameters as in [4] were used. The Deriche method is contrast dependent and features are detected based on the size of intensity derivatives rather than on their spatio-temporal significance and shape. The result is a cluttered edge strength image where relevant and irrelevant features are detected with similar strength. Further, the Deriche method is not truly spatio-temporal. The derivation is only performed in the spatial domain and the temporal filtering only contributes by smoothing the image over time, not by detecting temporal features.

4.3 Velocity measurements: Finally, we present results of feature velocity estimation. Velocity is estimated from the inclination of the filter exhibiting the strongest response. As the cardiac muscle gains speed during systole, wall features in the spatio-temporal domain are detected by faster moving filters (larger θ_0). At end-systole the muscle velocity decreases to zero before diastolic relaxation and the features are detected by static filters in the spatial plane ($\theta_0 = 0$). Colour coded response maps for a series of views can be seen at our web page. Figure 3(D) shows two frames during systole and diastole. Arrows have been marked on the detected features after non-maximal suppression of the feature asymmetry image. In this case the orientation and magnitude of these arrows corresponds to the velocity vector estimated from the interpolated filter responses around the maximum. We are currently investigating how these measurements can provide input to an active-contour based tracker. Current research is also comparing this approach to velocity estimation using Doppler Tissue Imaging [11].

5 Discussion

We have presented a new approach to spatio-temporal acoustic boundary detection based on phase-based methods. The main contributions of this work are (1) to propose a new phase-based scheme for detecting acoustic boundaries in echocardiographic image sequences and (2) to develop a 2D+T version of this algorithm that is resistant to temporally inconsistent speckle and that can provide a measure of feature velocity. A key advantage of this approach is that it is intensity-amplitude invariant. This makes it especially attractive for echocardiographic 3D+T reconstruction where choosing a single global intensity-based edge threshold is problematic due to position dependent attenuation.

We are currently using our phase based segmentation and velocity estimation as the front end to a higher level interpretation system based on a snake framework similar to our work in [10, 7], and also plan to extend our ideas to volumetric spatio-temporal data. We also plan to perform a more detailed study of filter design and filter response interpolation in order to improve the accuracy of feature velocity estimation. Quantitative assessment and evaluation against related measurement protocols, particularly Doppler Tissue Imaging will also be performed. Finally, an interesting variant of this work might be to investigate the use of a *symmetry* measure for speckle tracking.

References

1. D.C. Wilson, E.A. Geiser, and J-H. Li. Feature extraction in two-dimensional short-axis echocardiographic images. *J. of Math. Imag. and Vis.*, 3:285–298, 1993.
2. V. Chalana, et al. A multiple active contour model for cardiac boundary detection on echocardiographic sequences. *IEEE Trans. Med. Imag.*, 15(3):290–298, 1996.
3. A. Lange, et al. The variation in integrated backscatter in human hearts in differing ultrasonic transthoracic views. *JASE*, pages 830–838, Nov-Dec 1995.

4. I. Herlin and Ayache.N. Feature extraction and analysis methods for sequences of ultrasound images. In *ECCV92*, pages 43–57, 1992.
5. R. Deriche. Fast algorithms for low-level vision. PAMI-12(1):78–87, January 1990.
6. S. Venkatesh and R.A. Owens. An energy feature detection scheme. In *ICIP98*, pages 553–557, Singapore, 1989.
7. G. Jacob, A. Noble, M. Mulet-Parada, and A. Blake. Evaluating a robust contour tracker on echocardiographic sequences. *MedIA Journal*, to appear 1998.
8. P. Kovesi. *Invariant measures of image features from phase information*. PhD thesis, University of Western Australia., 1996.
9. C. Temperton. A generalised prime factor FFT algorithm for any $n = 2^p \times 3^q \times 5^r$. *SIAM J. Sci. Stat. Comp.*, May 1992.
10. G. Jacob, A. Noble, and A. Blake. Robust contour tracking in echocardiographic sequences. In *ICCV98*, Bombay, India, pages 408-413, January 1998.
11. M.A. Garcia Fernandez et al.. Doppler Tissue Imaging Echocardiography. McGraw-Hill, Madrid 1998.

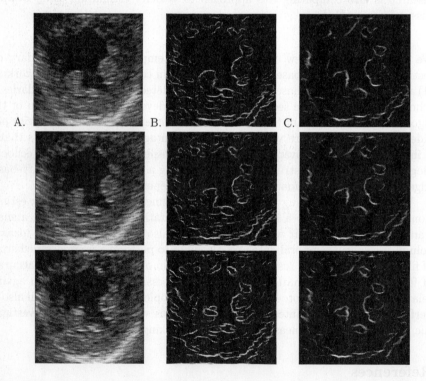

Fig. 2. *Comparison of (A) input frames, (B) 2D feature asymmetry results, (C) 2D+T feature asymmetry results.*

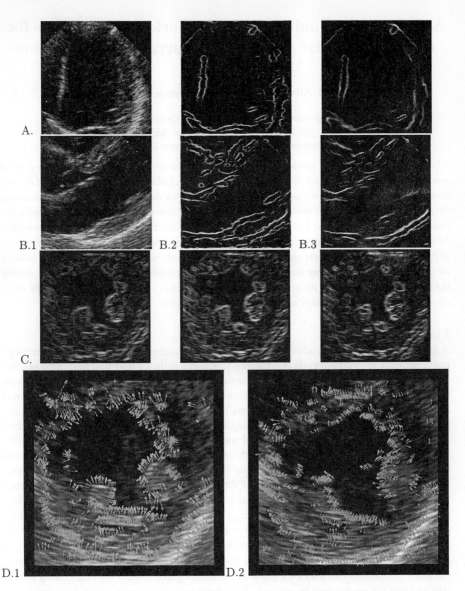

Fig. 3. (A) *Long axis frame, 2D and 2D+T feature asymmetry results.* (B) *Valve Results. (1) View of the Mitral and Aortic Valves at opening. (2) 2D and (3) 2D+T feature asymmetry results* (C) *Results of running Herlin and Ayache's method on our data.* (D) *Interpolated filter response velocity estimates, (1) systole: arrows point inwards, (2) diastole: arrows point outwards.*

Automatically Finding Optimal Working Projections for the Endovascular Coiling of Intracranical Aneurysms

Dale Wilson[1], J. Alison Noble[1], Duncan Royston[2], and James Byrne[2]

[1] Dept. of Engineering Science, University of Oxford, Oxford, OX1 3PJ
{dale,noble}@robots.ox.ac.uk
[2] Dept. of Neuroradiology, Radcliffe Infirmary, Oxford OX2 6HE

Abstract *The endovascular coil embolisation of intracranial saccular aneurysms requires a set of specific X-ray images with which to view the aneurysm during coiling. These two-dimensional images, known as* **working projections** *should be optimal for measuring the aneurysm sac diameter, inserting the first coil, and checking coil overhang into the surrounding vessels. At present the gantry angle that produces these images is found by the radiologist by trial and error. In this paper we present a method for automatically finding the angles that will produce the desired X-ray projections. Our method consists of four steps: (1) segmenting the vasculature from three-dimensional angiographic data; (2) locating the aneurysm neck; (3) labelling the aneurysm sac; and (4) determining the optimal angle for viewing the aneurysm during coiling. We discuss details of the algorithm steps and present the results of the algorithm applied to one synthetic and two pathological examples.*

1 Introduction

A novel technique for the endovascular treatment of intracranial aneurysms with electrolytically detachable platinum coils (Guglielmi detachable coils, GDCs) was described in 1991 [1]. Since then endovascular occlusion of aneurysms with GDCs has become a widely practised technique. Total occlusion of the aneurysm sac can be achieved in up to 90% of small (< 10 mm) and large (10-25 mm) aneurysms, but in only 50% of giant aneurysms (> 25 mm) [2]. Mid-term clinical outcomes are encouraging, with an excellent or good outcome reported in 86% of patients where the GDC method was the definitive treatment of the aneurysm [3].

Aneurysm coiling is carried out in an X-ray angiography suite where catheters and coils are positioned using two-dimensional X-ray fluoroscopy, road-mapping and digital subtraction angiography (DSA). A clear view of the aneurysm sac and neck and of the adjacent vessels in the image is required to accurately place the coils. However, it may be difficult from visual assessment to determine the best X-ray images to use, and even if the optimal projections are found it may still be hard to define the relationship of the aneurysm to the adjacent vessels with 2D projection information alone.

There are standard projections that are used for the diagnosis of intracranial aneurysms, but these projections can only be a guide to the radiologist choosing the best coiling projection and will not necessarily be optimal. The gantry angles that produce the best projections are generally found using a combination of information from DSA images acquired immediately prior to coiling, the clinical experience of the radiologist, and trial and error. It is not uncommon for up to seven DSA images to be acquired before the radiologist is satisfied with the working projection.

In this paper we propose a protocol for automatically predicting the optimal projections, known as *working projections*, using 3D angiographic data acquired prior to treatment, and a simulated geometric set-up of an X-ray machine.

The automatic technique presented in this paper is aimed specifically at coiling procedures. However, it is a technique that may well be applied to other areas, such as radiation therapy planning. If, for example, a tumour is identified, the optimal gantry angles could be determined based on the geometry of the tumour and surrounding tissues.

The authors know of only one group [4] who have previously worked on a GDC angle prediction method. Building on their method we have added several new features: firstly, once our input data has been selected, our algorithm is fully automatic; we treat different aneurysm sites specifically; we include the application specific X-ray machine geometry to improve algorithm accuracy; and finally, we incorporate a sac labelling step into our algorithm, which allows for sac volume estimation.

There are four main steps to our algorithm: (1) segmenting the relevant vasculature from 3D (volumetric) angiography data; (2) determining the location and orientation of the aneurysm neck; (3) labelling all voxels in the segmentation that belong to the aneurysm sac; and (4) combining the information found in the previous steps to predict the angle that produces the best working projection. In this paper we discuss each step of the prediction method, concluding with a discussion of the completed algorithm applied to one synthetically modified data set and two pathological data sets. Details of a study on a larger number of data sets are forthcoming [5].

2 Segmenting the 3D angiographic data

Currently there are two clinically available techniques for producing 3D angiographic data: computed tomography angiography and magnetic resonance angiography (MRA). A segmentation of the cerebral vasculature from either data source is suitable input for our viewing angle optimisation algorithm. We use a 3D segmentation from time-of-flight MRA data, because of availability. Details of an early version of the segmentation algorithm are presented elsewhere [6]. The segmentation algorithm must output a 3D binary volume consisting of the arteries that would appear in a DSA image where contrast agent was injected to allow visibility of the aneurysm. Hence the segmentation must be of either the left or right carotid circulation, or the vertebro-basilar circulation, depending on the aneurysm site.

3 Determining the neck location and orientation

For our angle prediction algorithm we need to know the neck location to aid in the labelling of the sac, and the neck orientation to initialise the search for the optimal working projection angle. We obtain the geometry of the neck (location and orientation) by analysing spherical projection images computed from voxels inside the parent artery and the aneurysm neck and sac. In the following sections we describe how to choose these voxels and create the spherical projection images, and how these images are used to find the neck position and orientation.

3.1 Setting up the spline and its local axes   To create a spherical projection image we need a point in 3D and a set of orthogonal coordinate axes originating at that point to parameterise the vectors about the sphere. To define the points we skeletonise a 3D segmentation of the vessels using Euclidean Homotopic Thinning [7] and then fit an approximating open cubic B-spline [8] to the section of the skeleton that passes from the parent artery into the sac. The definition of the coordinate axes is then fairly straightforward, as the spline has intrinsically defined local coordinate axes, the tangent and two normals, at every point along its length. We adjust the two normal vectors so that they vary continuously along the curve, not flipping at inflection points, so that the spherical projection images also vary continuously. It is possible to create spherical projection images at each point on the skeleton if, say, we define each spherical projection image with respect to a global set of 3D axes. However, this would result in the images having no direct relationship to the local geometry of the surrounding vessels, which is a feature we use later.

The spline gives a very good approximation to the medially situated skeleton, with spline points lying within a voxel's distance of the skeleton. In Fig. 1(a) we show a 3D spline fitted to a skeleton, and in Fig. 1(b) show the spline as it is located inside the corresponding segmentation of a posterior communicating artery aneurysm.

3.2 Creating spherical projection images   Each pixel position in a spherical projection image references a direction (ϕ, θ) in spherical coordinates that is defined with respect to the local coordinate frame centred at a given point along the spline. We can think of the parameter ϕ as longitude and θ as latitude, where $\phi \in [0, 360)$ and $\theta \in [-90, 90)$. The two parameters represent the respective indices of the x and y axes of the spherical projection images. The unit vector in 3D Cartesian coordinates with longitude ϕ and latitude θ is $\mathbf{u}(\phi, \theta) = (\cos\theta \sin\phi, \cos\theta \cos\phi, \sin\theta)^T$.

The intensity of a pixel in a spherical projection image represents the Euclidean distance from the spline point to the vessel lumen in the direction $\mathbf{u}(\phi, \theta)$. Thus, low intensities in the image indicate directions where the lumen is close to the spline, and higher intensities indicate directions where there is a greater distance between the spline and lumen.

Two typical spherical projection images, one from inside the internal carotid artery, and one from inside a posterior communicating artery aneurysm, are shown in Figs 1(c) and (d) respectively. Note that Fig. 1(c) has high intensity regions at the top and bottom of the images. These regions correspond to θ close to $-90°$ and $90°$, where the vectors point up and down the internal carotid artery, and hence there is a large distance to the lumen. In Fig. 1(d) there is only one high intensity region at the bottom of the image, which corresponds to the vectors pointing out through the aneurysm neck. This region will be smaller for small diameter necks, and larger for large necks. Here the neck is quite small.

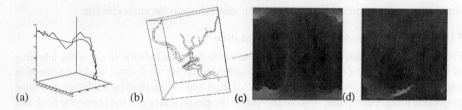

Fig. 1. *In (a) a cubic B-spline fitted to a selected part of the segmentation skeleton is shown. In (b) the spline and (a transparent) segmentation of a posterior communicating artery aneurysm are displayed. Two spherical projection images are shown in (c) and (d): (c) is from inside the internal carotid artery, and (d) is from inside the sac of a posterior communicating artery aneurysm.*

3.3 Defining the neck parameters   Given a sequence of spherical projection images acquired at equal steps along a spline, we want to use them to find the point on the spline that passes through the neck, and the angle of the plane that slices through the least area of the neck. We term this plane the *neck plane*, and use it later to initialise the optimisation of the working projection angle.

In spherical coordinates, if a plane intersecting the origin is defined by its normal $(\phi_n, \theta_n)^T$, then all the vectors through the origin that lie parallel to the plane are defined by $\theta = \theta' \cos\phi'$

for all $\phi \in [0, 360)$, where $\theta' = \theta_n + 90$, and

$$\phi' = \begin{cases} \phi - \phi_n & \text{if } \phi \geq \phi_n, \\ (\phi + 360) - \phi_n & \text{otherwise.} \end{cases}$$

As ϕ varies from 0 to 360, the (ϕ, θ) pairs around the plane describe points along a sinusoid in a spherical projection image. It is one of these curves that corresponds to the *neck plane*.

The area of a region in a plane can be approximated by polygonal integration. Referring to the illustration in Fig. 2(a), the area within the triangle **pqr** is defined as $\frac{1}{2}a.b.\sin(\varphi)$. The distances a and b correspond to intensity values at adjacent positions along one of the sinusoids within a spherical projection image. The area of a plane within the vessel is the sum of all the triangular regions around the plane. To find the plane most likely to be the neck plane, we seek the minimal area over all images and all plane normals (ϕ_n, θ_n).

Minimising over the area is not accurate enough to define the neck location and orientation. We must add two normalised weighting functions, one, ω^m, over the set of images corresponding to spline points along the skeleton section, and the other, ω^t, over the plane normal latitude parameter θ_n. These two sets of weights incorporate our prior knowledge of the aneurysm neck in our search for a minimum.

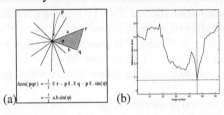

Fig. 2. *(a) An illustration of the vectors circumscribing a region of a plane. The definition of the area of one of the triangular regions is also shown. (b) A plot of the weighted minimum plane areas for each image in the sequence for a posterior communicating aneurysm.*

The weightings ω^m for the images (and hence spline points) are included because there is no guarantee that the neck diameter will be smaller than the parent artery diameter, so it is possible that the minimum plane area will be found somewhere along the artery before the neck. We avoid this by weighting the images closer to the sac end of the spline with greater likelihood.[1]

The weightings ω^t on the plane normal parameter θ_n simply give greater likelihood to planes with normals closer to the spline tangents. This is because the spline is directed straight up into the sac, and one would expect the neck plane to be close to perpendicular to the spline as it enters the sac. Choosing the two weighting functions is a non-trivial problem and is discussed in more detail in related work [5].

The cost function that is minimised is

$$C = \min_{i \in [0, M)} \min_{\phi_n, \theta_n} \omega_i^m \omega_{\theta_n}^t A(\phi_n, \theta_n),$$

where M is the number of images (spline points) in the sequence, and A is the area of the region of the plane with normal $(\phi_n, \theta_n)^T$ that is within the vessel lumen. A plot of the minimum plane areas for images in the sequence for a posterior communicating aneurysm is shown in Fig. 2(b). The minimum of the image sequence occurs at image 46, and is shown by the crossed lines.

4 Labelling the sac

There is one step remaining before we can compute the working projection angles, and that is to identify the 3D segmentation voxels that belong to the aneurysm sac. We need to do this

---
[1] Note that this does not cause a problem in mislabelling the neck for bilobal sacs, as the neck is always much smaller than the waist-line of the bilobal sac.

because one of our criteria for determining the optimal working projections is to minimise the vessel and sac overlap, so the two structures must be distinctly defined. A feature of spherical projection images computed from points inside the sac is the discontinuity between the lengths of vectors pointing out through the neck, which are large, and the lengths of vectors pointing to the sac walls, which are small [4]. We use this characteristic for labelling the sac.

We use the discrete version of the graduated non-convexity algorithm [9], a method for smoothing an image which allows the smoothing function to break at discontinuities, to identify and exclude the regions of high intensities in a spherical projection image (corresponding to vectors pointing out through the neck) and then interpolate between the neighbouring low intensity regions. Using the interpolated, or 'smoothed' image we can label all voxels that lie within the 'smoothed' distances of the centre voxel (that was used to compute the spherical projection image) as being part of the aneurysm sac.

More specifically, we firstly find the pixels in a spherical projection image P that correspond to the long vectors, pointing out through the aneurysm neck. These pixels are the ones that differ significantly from the rest of the image, based on an estimate of the noise, σ, in the image. We can estimate the noise in P by comparing P to an image that is a lightly smoothed version of P, where breaks in the smoothing function are allowed. Then by creating a heavily smoothed version of P, S, where breaks are *not* allowed, the high intensities in P can be labelled as those pixels that deviate more that 3σ from S. Finally, P is smoothed, not allowing for breaks, with the exclusion of the labelled high intensity pixels. To label the aneurysm sac we simply identify all voxels along each of the vectors around the sphere that are within the distance specified in the final smoothed image.

We perform this entire process for every spherical projection image from the end of the spline (within the sac) to the image corresponding to the point a quarter of the way along the spline towards the aneurysm neck. We use more than one point (and therefore image) for the labelling process, so as to ensure complete labelling of all lobes of the sac. Often some of the larger aneurysms can be distinctly bilobal. An example of a spherical projection image and its 'smoothed' version, for a middle cerebral artery aneurysm, are shown in Fig. 3(a) and (b). A rendered picture of the final segmented aneurysm sac is shown in Fig. 3(c).

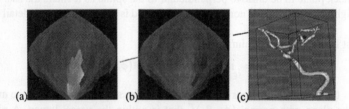

Fig. 3. *A spherical projection image (a) computed from a point within the sac of a middle cerebral artery aneurysm, next to (b) the 'smoothed' version of the image. The final segmentation of the aneurysm is shown in (c). Note that the spherical projection images have been corrected for the distortion caused when spherical coordinates are mapped onto a rectangular grid.*

5 Predicting the working projection angles

We now have all of the information required to find the optimal working projections. We have based our method for predicting the working projection angles on the same criteria that radiologists use for manual predictions. We have divided the six most common intracranial saccular aneurysm sites into two groups, based on the aneurysm geometry. Within each group we quantitatively optimise features of the X-ray projections that are particular to that group. The two groups are illustrated in Fig. 4.

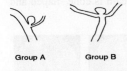

Fig. 4. *Aneurysm types.*

The group A sites are side-wall aneurysms that arise adjacent to the origin of a vessel that is relatively small with respect to the parent artery. Included in this group are posterior communicating and carotid ophthalmic artery aneurysms. The second set of sites, group B, consists of termination aneurysms, where the parent artery divides into two or more branches. Basilar termination, terminal internal carotid, middle cerebral and anterior communicating artery aneurysms are included in group B. The anatomy at the anterior communicating artery level is complicated, with 80% of aneurysms occuring at this site being associated with hypoplasia of one of the proximal cerebral arteries (A1) [10]. Hence most aneurysms at this site occur at the junction of the hyperplastic A1, the A2 and the anterior communicator, and we therefore class them as being similar to the other bifurcation aneurysms in group B.

The projection criteria for group A are (1) to minimise the overlap of the vessels and the sac in the X-ray image, and (2) to minimise the foreshortening of the parent artery. For group B the criteria are (1) to minimise the overlap of the sac by the left T-junction branch, and (2) to minimise overlap by the right branch. These two optimisations for group B result in two working projections.

Overlap of the sac is measured by fixing the gantry angle and computing the average proportion of X-rays that are attenuated by the sac, compared to the attenuation by the surrounding arteries. If the average normalised proportion is α, then values of $1 - \alpha$ close to 0 represent little sac overlap, and values closer to 1 indicate more overlap of the sac by arteries.

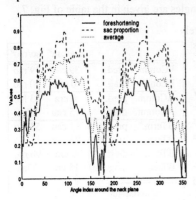

Fig. 5. *Plot of the sac overlap and parent artery foreshortening measures, along with their average for the neck plane angles for an anterior communicating artery aneurysm.*

Parent artery foreshortening is measured by analysing the section of the parent artery immediately below the aneurysm neck. This arterial section is separated using a method described in previous work [11]. The quantitative value of interest here is the average attenuation of the X-rays passing through the parent artery. When normalised, the average value is minimised at the gantry angle for the X-ray image showing the least foreshortening of the parent artery.

Thus, the optimisation procedure for the aneurysm sites in group A is to take the average between the normalised foreshortening measure and the normalised sac overlap measure, and search for the minimum. We firstly find the minimum over all the gantry angles parallel to the neck plane (see Section 3). Then from this initial angle we do a brute force search through the neighbouring angles, updating the current angle if a better projection under the described criteria is found. If none of the neighbouring angles, up to a radius of 20 degrees, is found to produce a better projection then the search is stopped. Note that we do not consider any angles outside the limits of the X-ray machine gantry. The entire (non-optimised) minimisation procedure takes less than six minutes on a Silicon Graphics 200 MHz workstation.

The sac overlap and foreshortening measures, along with their average for all angles parallel to the neck plane for an anterior communicating artery aneurysm are shown in Fig. 5. The minimum is marked with the crossed lines. In the plot the measures are almost, but not quite symmetric at 180° intervals. This asymmetry is because the beam is cone shaped and not parallel.

The optimisation for the group B sites follows a very similar procedure to that of the group A sites, except that two final angles are found, one for the minimisation of sac overlap from the left, and one for overlap from the right. X-ray images for some of the final prediction angles for a posterior communicating and an anterior communicating artery aneurysm (pathological examples), and a synthetically composed basilar termination artery aneurysm are shown in Fig. 6(a). The standard projections for the diagnosis (not coiling) of these three aneurysm sites are shown in Fig. 6(b). The angles for each of the coiling prediction angles and the standard diagnosis angles are given in the table of Fig. 7.

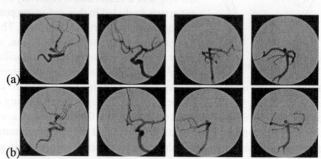

Fig. 6. *Left to right in (a) are some of the final prediction results for a posterior communicating and an anterior communicating artery aneurysm (both pathological cases), and a synthetically constructed basilar termination artery aneurysm. The standard views used for angiographic diagnosis screening of the same aneurysm sites are shown in (b). The gantry angles for all of these images are given in the table of Fig. 7.*

Although the standard diagnosis projections are rarely used as working projections, they are often used as starting points in the manual search for a good working projection. We use them as comparisons to our predicted working projections because it would currently be invalid to compare our results with the actual working projections used during the coilings, as we have not performed a registration between the 3D MRA data and the 2D data acquired during coiling. We are currently carrying out experiments on a method for computing the change in orientation of the patient's head between their position in the MR screening and their position during coiling. When we have this registration information along with the working projection information we will be able to correctly assess our results.

		cra/cau[a]	lao/rao[b]
PComm.[c]	pred.	39 cau	99 rao
PComm.	diag.	0 cra	90 rao
AComm.[d]	pred.	0 cra	43 lao
AComm.	diag.	15 cau	0 lao
BTerm.[e]	pred. (A)	11 cau	53 lao
BTerm.	pred. (B)	25 cau	36 rao
BTerm.	diag. (A)	0 cra	90 rao
BTerm.	diag. (B)	15 cra	0 lao

[a] cranio/caudal
[b] left/right anterior oblique
[c] posterior communicating
[d] anterior communicating
[e] basilar termination

Fig. 7. *Gantry angles for the predicted working projections and the standard diagnosis projections.*

6 Conclusions

We have outlined a pre-treatment algorithm for determining the best X-ray gantry angle for viewing intracranial saccular aneurysms during endovascular coiling procedures. There is clearly a necessity for such predictions to reduce the time, radiation and contrast dose associated with GDC treatments, and to provide the radiologist with maximal information regarding the state of the aneurysm.

The results from each step of our optimisation algorithm can be used independently to provide both qualitative and quantitative information to the radiologist prior to coiling. The first step, the segmentation of the vessels, if rendered to show a fully 3D representation of the vessel structure, can provide important qualitative information about the geometric structure of the arteries and aneurysm. The orientation of the neck, which is often difficult to ascertain by eye, even from 3D data, can be a guide to the radiologist for precise adjustments when inserting the coil. The third step in our algorithm, labelling the sac voxels, can result in an estimate of the aneurysm volume, a measure previously unattainable except by extrapolation from 2D measurements. Finally, the prediction of the working projection angles can avoid repeated injections of contrast agent while the radiologist searches for the best projection, and may provide more information than the projection found by the radiologists' trial and error method.

In conjunction with the work described in this paper we have also developed a planning tool for simulating DSA images, that allows the radiologist to view synthetic X-ray images from any angle prior to coiling. The geometric set-up of the simulations is the same as for the X-ray machine that is used during coiling. This leaves the finer adjustments on the working projection gantry angle up to the radiologist, who would use our predictions as a guide. Analysis of our predictions in clinical use, incorporating the registration procedure, along with the clinical application of the planning tool will be forthcoming [12, 5].

Acknowledgements Thanks are given to Paul Hayton who provided code for the graduated nonconvexity algorithm. DW is supported by the Assoc. Comm. Universities and the AFUW-QLD.

References

1. G. Guglielmi, F. Vinuela, I. Septka, and V. Macellar. Electrothrombosis of saccular aneuryms via endovascular approach. Part 1. *J. Neurosurg.*, 75:4–7, 1991.
2. J.V. Byrne. Interventional neuroradiology: an emerging subspeciality. *Clinical Radiology*, 52(12):891–902, 1997.
3. T.W. Malisch, G. Guglielmi, and F. Vinuela *et al.* Intracranial aneurysms treated with the Guglielmi detachable coil. *J. Neurosurg.*, 87(2):176–183, 1997.
4. R. van der Weide, K.J. Zuigerveld, W.P.Th.M. Mali, and M.A. Viergever. Calculating optimal angiographic angles of cerebral aneurysms. In H. U. Lemke, M. W. Vannier, and K. Inamura, editors, *Comp. Assist. Radiol.*, pages 289–294. Elsevier Science, Amsterdam, June 1997.
5. D.L. Wilson. Planning For Endovascular Treatments of Cerebral Aneurysms. DPhil. thesis, University of Oxford. In preparation, 1998.
6. D.L. Wilson and J.A. Noble. Segmentation of cerebral vessels and aneurysms from MR angiography data. In *Proc. IPMI'97*, pages 423–428, Poultney, June 1997.
7. C.J. Pudney. Distance-ordered homotopic thinning: A skeletonization algorithm for 3D digital images. *Int. J. of Comp. Vis.* To appear, 1998.
8. B.A. Barsky. *Computer graphics and geometric modeling using beta-splines.* Springer-Verlag, London, 1988.
9. A. Blake and A. Zisserman. *Visual Reconstruction.* MIT Press, Cambridge, Mass, 1987.
10. M.G. Yasargil. *Microneurosurgery. Vol II: Clinical Considerations, Surgery of The Intracranial Aneurysms and Results.* Georg Thieme Verlag, Stuttgart, 1984.
11. D.L. Wilson, J.A. Noble, and C.J. Pudney. From MR angiography to X-ray angiography. In *Proc. of Med. Im. Understanding and Anal. '97*, pages 161–164, Oxford, U.K., July 1997.
12. D.D. Royston. Endovascular Treatment of Intracranial Aneurysms - Preoperative Evaluation and Treatment Planning Using Magnetic Resonance Angiography. MSc. thesis, University of Oxford., 1998.

Computer Assisted Quantitative Analysis of Deformities of the Human Spine

B. Verdonck[1], R. Nijlunsing[1], F. A. Gerritsen[1], J. Cheung[2], D. J. Wever[2],
A. Veldhuizen[2], S. Devillers[3], S. Makram-Ebeid[3]

[1] Philips Medical Systems Nederland B.V., P.O.Box 10.000, NL-5680 DA Best,
The Netherlands, Bert.Verdonck@best.ms.philips.com
http://www.medical.philips.com
[2] Academic Hospital Groningen, P.O. Box 30.001,
NL-9700 RB Groningen, The Netherlands
[3] Laboratoires d'Electronique Philips S.A.S., P.O. Box 15,
F-94453 Limeil-Brevannes cedex, France

Abstract. Nowadays, conventional X-ray radiographs are still the images of choice for evaluating spinal deformaties such as scoliosis. However, digital translation reconstruction gives easy access to high quality, digital overview images of the entire spine. This work aims at improving the description of the scoliotic deformity by developing semi-automated tools to assist the extraction of anatomical landmarks (on vertebral bodies and pedicles) and the calculation of deformity quantifying parameters. These tools are currently validated in a clinical setting.

1 Introduction

The interest in three dimensional (3D) analyses of spinal deformities is increasing over the last decades. This evolution is partially due to the progress of digital imaging technology and automated image processing. The description and quantification of the geometry of scoliosis, a complex 3D deformity of the spine, is essential and will assist the clinician in the accurate and reliable follow up of natural history, brace and operative treatment.

Computer Tomography (CT) imaging could give immediate access to 3D information. However, it does not allow the patient to be in a natural standing posture and it would expose him to higher X-ray dose. Optical and opto-electronic image capture is without any risk for the patient but yields limited accuracy and gives only indirect information about the deformity of the vertebral column. Large focus, long film X-ray radiographs are still the images of choice for evaluating deformities of the entire spine in general and scoliosis more specifically.

We have developed a digital method for creating complete overview images of the human vertebral column [1]. The image is reconstructed from a series of overlapping X-ray images acquired with a dedicated protocol on a conventional image intensifier based digital X-ray system (with constant translation speed and frame acquisition rate). Successive images are matched and merged into one overview image. These overviews have demonstrated improved image quality for equivalent X-ray dose as compared to conventional film-based techniques (figure 1). This reconstruction technique is commercially available as one of the software modules of the EasyVision product line of Philips Medical Systems.

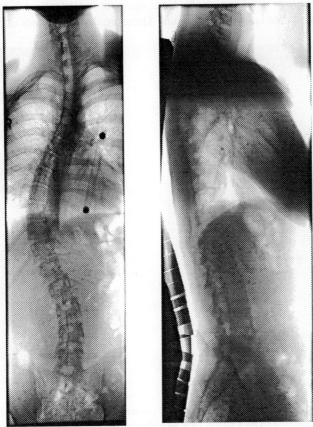

Fig. 1. Digital overview image of the spine, constructed from a translated series of digital images with optimized exposure and contrast. Fontal and lateral acquisitions.

The EasyVision Spine software includes utilities for the measurement of Cobb's angle, vertical alignment and femur height difference. At the end of a previous paper [1] some attention was drawn to the accuracy of measurements on translation reconstructed images and to the limited precision of the conventionally used Cobb's angle.

We now further develop the appropriate functionality to assist the diagnosis of spinal deformities based on one or more overview images, according to the clinical specifications of the orthopaedic department of the Academic Hospital Groningen, The Netherlands. In a prototype environment, we are developing more advanced measuring functions based on a set of anatomical landmarks of vertebral bodies and pedicles. The localization of these landmarks on a frontal projection image gives access to a set of interesting deformity parameters such as axial rotation, wedge and tilt angles. Similar analyses can be performed using a lateral projection image. Two projections can be combined to approximate a three-dimensional vertebrae model.

The access to digital images and the development of a dedicated user interface are meant to replace the time-consuming and unpractical film-based procedures using digitizer tablets. In order to further limit time-consuming and tedious user interaction and to reduce the variability of human observers, some automated processing techniques are explored to assist the landmark extraction. These are the main topics of this paper.

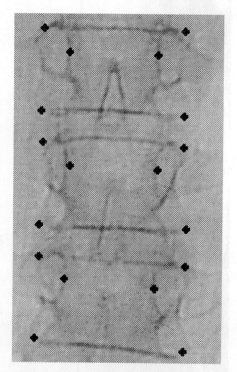
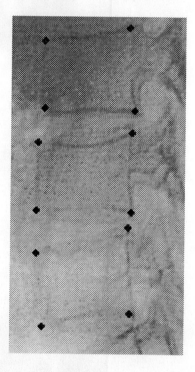

Fig. 2. Vertebral landmarks on a frontal view (4 corner points of the vertebral body and 2 inner edges of the pedicles) and on a lateral view (4 corner points of the vertebral body).

Vertebral body segmentation was also addressed by D'Amico et al. [2] using manual indication of end-plates on gradient direction encoded images. In Kauffman et al. [3] a vertebral body template is first rigidly matched using the generalized Hough transform. These templates are then deformed while optimizing a generalized active contour model energy. We try to develop semi-automated methods that closely cooperate with user interactions and that benefit from the improved image quality of our digital images.

Several authors have described the estimation of 3D models of the human spine, a.o. Stokes [4], Godillon et al. [7] and Dansereau et al. [6] using biplanar orthogonal radiography and André et al. [5] using two vertical stereo radiographs. All of these methods depend on landmark localization on X-ray films using a digitizer tablet or on digitally scanned X-ray films. We have access to digital images directly which simplifies the indication of landmarks considerably thanks to optimal zooming, contrast/brightness correction, edge enhancement, etc.

2 Methods

2.1 Vertebral landmarks

Literature uses a blend of different anatomical landmarks on vertebral bodies to capture the geometry of individual vertebrae and of the vertebral column. A frequently used set of landmarks consists of the four corners of the vertebral body in frontal and/or lateral projections and some characteristic points of the pedicles, e.g. the inner edge point (i.e. the most interior point of the pedicle contour) (figure 2). This makes 6 landmarks on a frontal projection and 4 points on a lateral projection.

These landmarks have to be well visible and easily identifiable in the projection images. We therefore avoid the centers of both superior and inferior endplates and the (overall) center of the vertebral body since they cannot be deduced directly from image features. Moreover, these centers can be deduced from the four corner points that are more clearly correlated to image features. In places where the corner points are badly visible, they can sometimes be determined better as the result of the intersection of two line segments: top/bottom plate intersecting with left/right vertebral body sides. If the pedicle contours are entirely delineated, the most interior point can be determined automatically. We do not indicate the spinous process since it is not always clearly visible and its position is not proportionally related to the degree of scoliosis.

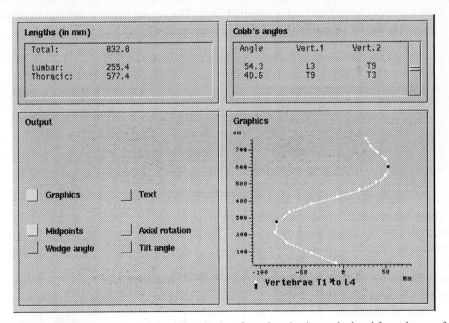

Fig. 3. Analytical parameters of the deformity in a frontal projection, calculated from the set of vertebral landmarks of all vertebrae of the patient in figure 1. The graph can show different parameters. In this example it represents the coordinates of the midpoints of the vertebral body as projected in the frontal (x,z) plane (the z (vertical) and x (horizontal) coordinates are represented with different scales in the graph).

We have developed a user interface for indicating these landmarks manually. For each vertebra, the user selects its name (thoracic 1-12, lumbar 1-5) and locates the landmarks in a random order. An algorithm automatically sorts out the meaning of all points using some heuristics on the relative positions of each pair of points.

2.2 Analytic parameters

Literature defines all kinds of parameters that assist the orthopaedic surgeon in evaluating the scoliotic deformity. Stokes [8] gives a summary of clear and detailed definitions.

We selected the most significant parameters, calculated them using the vertebral landmarks and summarized them as a set of numbers and charts. An example for the patient on the right of figure 1 is shown in figure 3.

The output includes both global and local parameters: length of the vertebral axis (total, thoracic and lumbar length), Cobb's angles (with automatic determination of the most inclined vertebrae), coordinates of the midpoints of vertebral bodies (with automatic determination of the apex vertebrae (i.e. the most horizontally displaced vertebrae)) and three vertebral body angles (axial rotation, wedge and tilt angle). The center of the vertebral body is calculated as the intersection of the line connecting the centers of the superior and inferior endplates with the line connecting the centers of the left and right body sides. Axial rotation is the intrinsic rotation of the vertebral body around its vertical axis and is approximated using Stokes' method [9]. The wedge angle is the angle between the endplates of a vertebral body. The tilt angle is the average angle of both endplates with respect to the horizontal direction.

2.3 Semi-automatic extraction of vertebral landmarks

We are currently experimenting with several techniques to speed up and automate the landmark selection process.

Interpolation. After the user has localized landmarks on some key vertebrae, interpolation can be used to estimate the landmark positions on the intermediate vertebrae. Since the user labels the vertebra for which he is entering landmarks, the number of missing vertebrae between each two given vertebrae is known.

This is illustrated in figure 6a where user-indicated points are shown in white. Automatically interpolated landmarks are shown in black. Another example is shown in figure 4 for the entire spine where only 6 out of

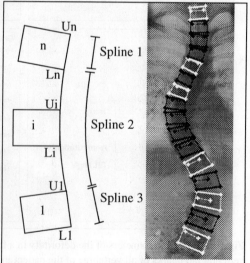

Fig. 4. Automatic interpolation of vertebral landmarks: manually specified landmarks in white, interpolated landmarks in black.

16 vertebrae where localized manually. In this image the corner and pedicle points are connected with a set of lines in order to clarify their meaning.

This interpolation links the corresponding sides of two manually specified vertebrae with a natural cubic spline, formed by three spline segments that have first and second order continuity on connecting points. The positions of the end plates on this spline are defined using the following hypotheses (U_i and L_i are curvilinear coordinates):
- the height of successive vertebrae follows a geometrical law, i.e. $U_i - L_i = r \cdot (U_{i-1} - L_{i-1})$ where $r^n = (U_n - L_n)/(U_1 - L_1)$;
- the ratio between the height of the vertebrae and the distance between vertebrae is the same.

Vertebral axis. As initialization for further automation, we need to have a global idea of the position and course of the vertebral axis (defined as the line connecting the centers of all vertebral bodies). Since this task is difficult for a computer algorithm but rather easy for a human being, we ask the user to indicate a limited number of points on the spinal axis. These points are interpolated on the fly with a poly-Bezier curve that can be edited interactively (figure 6b).

Automated global outline detection. Starting from the vertebral axis we extract the global outline of all vertebral bodies as two curves that are more or less parallel to this axis (figure 6c). We calculate an oriented edge map (on an appropriate scale) and search for an optimal almost-vertical path using dynamic programming.

The edge detection algorithm chains low-pass recursive filtering of the image with gradient calculation: gradient magnitude and orientation (quantised into 16 directions). An edgeness map is then calculated: only those points for which the projected gradient intensity is a local maximum along the direction of the gradient are given a non-zero edgeness equal to the gradient magnitude.

A path through the edge map is determined which optimizes a cost function that combines constraints on the edge feature strength (edgeness), orientation (gradient orientation with respect to vertebral axis tangent orientation) and path continuity (local path curvature). The path is forced to link strong edge features while remaining approximately parallel to the global vertebral axis.

Automated end plate detection. The edge map also allows to search for a set of lines approximately orthogonal to the global vertebral axis: the vertebral body end-plates. Originally all points on the axis are end-plate candidates. They are qualified according to the quality of an edge path growing out from each of them, orthogonally to the axis.

For this task the gradient image is thresholded with a low threshold in order to capture as many faint edges as possible, resulting in a binary feature image. This image is grey level dilated with a small isotropic structuring element to increase the number of edge point candidates.

For each point on the vertebral axis, one can calculate the cost for linking the current point to the rightmost spine outline and another cost for linking it to the leftmost spine outline. Loosely speaking, each of these costs is the shortest path length linking the current vertebral axis point to one of the spine outlines and going through high gradient edge-points. Two paths can thus be determined: one with preferred upward directed gradients, one with downward directed gradients.

Each path is determined in an angular sector as illustrated in figure 5. Length and slope constraints are imposed to each discretized path representing an endplate candidate. The maximal length is limited to half the approximated width of the vertebrae. The slope angle is forced to remain within +/- 45 degrees. The cost for having an end-plate going through a vertebral axis point is then defined as the sum of the costs for the left and right paths. This defines the end-plate's "length".

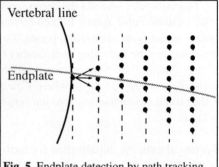

Fig. 5. Endplate detection by path tracking.

This leads to two functions of end plate quality with respect to vertebral axis coordinate: one for end plates with upward gradients, one with downward gradients. Each local minimum of these functions is a candidate end plate position. The user has to indicate the height of the first and the last vertebra and to label them: this allows to determine the number of endplates between both vertebrae and to estimate the approximative height of each vertebra (using a geometric law as described before).

The optimal set of end-plates is then selected with dynamic programming using a cost function that combines the end-plate "length" with the deviation from the expected vertebral body heights. This can be seen as an optimal labeling of all vertebra axis minima to an appropriate vertebra end-plate. End-plates that appear to be missing because they are too far off an expected position, can be filled in by interpolating well detected end-plates. A result of this procedure is illustrated in figure 6d.

The vertebral body corner points can then be located automatically at the intersection of the endplates with the global vertebral column outlines.

2.4 3D modeling

A simplified 3D model of the vertebral column can be fitted to two sets of landmarks on frontal and lateral views. The translation reconstructed images closely approximate the orthogonal projections geometry. Therefore these views are only calibrated for differences in scaling and vertical alignment.

A 3D ellipse is fitted to the four landmarks of each vertebral body end-plate while making use of the axial rotation as estimated from the pedicle positions. Top and bottom ellipses are filled with a triangulated surface and the intrinsic orientation is visualized by two tetrahedra that represent the pedicles. This generates a model as illustrated in the three surface rendered views of figure 7. One of the vertebrae is missing since it was not possible to trace some of the landmarks on the lateral projection image.

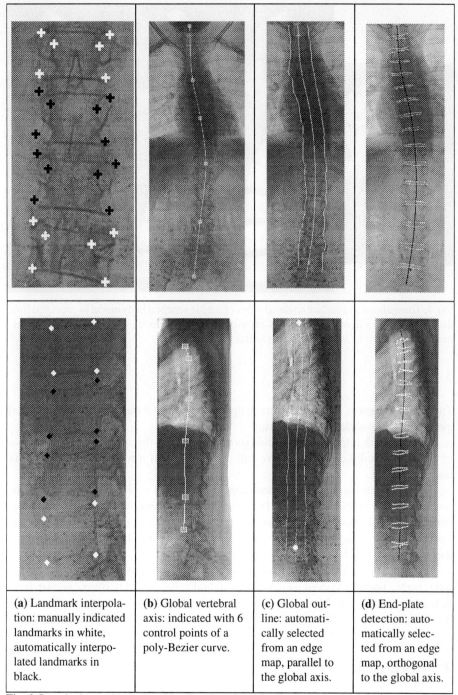

Fig. 6. Steps in the semi-automated localization of vertebra landmarks on frontal (top) and lateral (bottom) views.

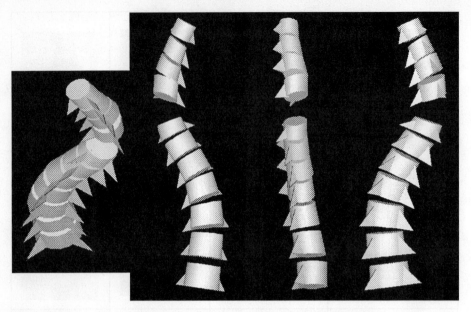

Fig. 7. Triangulated and surface rendered views of the 3D vertebral body model as estimated from the landmarks on a frontal and lateral X-ray projection. One vertebra is missing because it was impossible to trace its landmarks on the lateral view.

3 Results

The previous figures illustrated some preliminary results of the analysis and modeling methods that are under development.

The landmark interpolation method shows to facilitate the approximative indication of landmarks in difficult regions. We still need to prove if it really decreases the total interaction time.

The other semi-automated methods appear to perform well but tend to be sensitive to the vertebral axis initialization. Therefore they are currently improved by allowing simple user interactions to correct erroneous results (e.g. small corrections of the global vertebra outline of figure 6c). They will then be added to the clinical prototype for further validation.

Image quality of lateral projections is dependent on the degree of the scoliotic deformity: highly laterally curved parts of the vertebral column lead to overprojected vertebrae in the lateral view. Moreover, as the direction of the X-rays is much less parallel to the end plates than in the frontal view, these become poorly visible. The detection of landmarks on lateral projections of high-degree scolioses is thus often problematic.

4 Discussion

The overall purpose of this work is to facilitate the analysis of the 3D deformity of the vertebral column of scoliotic patients. A practical and interactive user interface has been developed to indicate vertebral anatomical landmarks easily and to calculate a set of clinically useful parameters. Attempts to locate those landmarks automatically look promising but they remain to be incorporated in an interactive landmark setting procedure and to be extended for pedicle contour extraction.

The reproducibility of manual semi-automated landmark indication is currently investigated by a panel of clinical experts. Additionally, they compare measurements on digital images using the prototype graphical user interface with measurements from digitized landmarks on conventional X-ray films. These studies should establish the accuracy and reliability of the proposed methods.

Due to the inherent problems of lateral acquisitions we are looking for other imaging protocols that are dedicated to 3D modeling and that could result in more clearly identifiable landmarks.

Acknowledgments

The authors thank N. Pivet and P. Lacour for their wonderful trainee-work. We acknowledge the inspiration of A. van Eeuwijk and S. Lobregt during the start up phase of this research project.

References

1. A. H. W. van Eeuwijk, S. Lobregt and F.A. Gerritsen: A novel method for digital X-ray imaging of the complete spine", Proceedings of CVRMed-MRCAS'97, Lecture Notes in Computer Science vol. 1205, pp. 521-530, 1997.
2. M. D'Amico, S. Dell'era, P. Roncoletta: New procedure for computation and automatic classification of spinal clinical parameters by image processing of digitised radiography, Three dimensional analysis of spinal deformities, M. D'Amico et al. (Eds.), pp. 39-43, 1995.
3. C. Kauffman, J.A. de Guise: Digital radiography segmentation of scoliotic vertebral body using deformable models, SPIE, vol. 3034, pp.243-251, 1997.
4. I.A.F. Stokes: Biplanar radiography for measurement of spinal shape and motion, Automedica, Vol. 5, pp. 37-49, 1985.
5. B. André, J. Dansereau, H. Labelle: Optimized vertical stereo base radiographic setup for the clinical three-dimensional reconstruction of the human spine, J. Biomechanics, vol. 27:8, pp. 1023-1035, 1994.
6. J. Dansereau, A. Chabot, N.T. Huynh, H. Labelle, J. de Guise: 3-D reconstruction of vertebral endplate wedging, Three dimensional analysis of spinal deformities, M. D'Amico et al. (Eds.), pp. 69-73, 1995.
7. A.P. Godillon, F.X. Lepoutre, D. Chopin: Evaluation of a 3D geometrical spinal model, Three dimensional analysis of spinal deformities, M. D'Amico et al. (Eds.), pp. 191-195, 1995.
8. I. A. F. Stokes: Three-dimensional terminology of spinal deformity, SPINE, vol. 19:2, pp. 236-248, 1994.
9. I.A.F. Stokes, L.C. Bigalow and M.S. Moreland: Measurement of axial rotation of vertebrae in scoliosis, Spine, Vol. 11:3, pp. 213-218, 1986. And a correction in a "letter to the editor" in Spine, Vol. 16:5, 1991.

Motion Measurements in Low-Contrast X-ray Imagery

Martin Berger and Guido Gerig

Swiss Federal Institute of Technology
Communication Technology Lab, Image Science
8092 Zürich, Switzerland
{berger,gerig}@vision.ee.ethz.ch

Abstract. Measuring motion in medical imagery becomes more and more important, in particular for object tracking, image registration, and local displacement measurements. Such measurements are especially difficult in megavoltage X-ray images (*portal images*), which are used to control the position of patients in high precision radiotherapy. Low contrast, blur, and noise render accurate measurements difficult.

In this work we review the framework of a generic matching algorithm only based on the image signal and not on binary image features. Thus, the often unreliable step of feature extraction in such imagery is circumvented. Another major advantage is the possibility of self-diagnosis, which is used for restricting the transformation in motion measurements if the image quality is not sufficient.

The method of digitally reconstructed radiographs (DRR) allow for the computation of error free reference images, avoiding the additional step of therapy simulation. The multi-modal match between such DRRs and portal images lead to an estimate of the patient position during radiotherapy treatment. Results of generated data with known ground truth as well as results of a multi-modal match are presented.

1 Introduction

Accurate motion measurements in images are essential to solve numerous problems in computer vision. For medical imagery in particular, precise position measurements and registration of image series represent two important applications. Wherever feature extraction is difficult or high precision is required, the least squares template matching algorithm (LSM) reviewed in this paper has many advantages over other methods. LSM is a generic matching algorithm suitable for many applications including motion estimation in low-contrast megavoltage X-ray images, also called *portal images*.

The specific goal in this work is the exact positioning of patients during radiotherapy, which is essential for high precision treatment. This involves automatically measuring patient setup deviation between or even during treatment sessions. One possible sensor is an electronic portal imaging device (EPID), which delivers images of the exit dose distribution during treatment. Unfortunately, the contrast of these megavoltage X-ray images is very low due to the high energy beam, and, since we are dealing with projected images, parts of a rigid 3D motion must be estimated by evaluating projected 2D images.

Because portal images are inherently noisy and low in contrast, it is difficult to robustly extract features like edges, ridges or cores. This is the weakness of feature-based methods applied to portal images like chamfer matching [Gilhuijs and van Herk 1993] and core-based image registration [Fritsch et al. 1995]. Previous area-based methods include the greyvalue correlation techniques described in [Dong and Boyer 1996, Moseley and Munro 1994]. Their limitations lie in the restriction to a translation or in a coarse search grid for computational reasons.

In [Berger and Danuser 1997] we proposed the area-based LSM algorithm to find displacements between two portal images. The method of LSM with deformable templates meets the requirements of being an area-based approach with the possibility of self-diagnosis. Early work in this field was presented by [Lucas and Kanade 1981], who published an iterative image registration scheme base on LSM. Among the first papers that discussed the concept of exploiting the full information of the statistical models for robust template matching are [Grün 1985] and [Förstner 1987]. Following and extending the work of Grün, [Danuser and Mazza 1996] achieved highly accurate results at the resolution limit of a light microscope. Compared to these previous applications of LSM, additional problems arise in portal images from the higher complexity of the image scene and the out-of-plane rotations.

A similar technique for the registration of medical image series is reported by [Unser et al. 1995], where each image is matched to the reference image based on a global greyvalue difference measure. In contrast to their work, our framework does not rely on one global template, but on several small templates each containing a significant image structure. Thus, the inclusion of distinct but insignificant image features which vary between the data of one sequence is avoided and the impact of global greyvalue errors such as intensity inhomogeneity is reduced.

Extending the approach in [Berger and Danuser 1997], we further exploit the self-diagnosis capabilities. The variation of image quality of portal images inhibits the estimation of a 2D affine transformation for all cases. An adaptive scheme based on self-diagnostic measures allows for an automatic reduction of the parameter set where the full parameter set is not determinable. Furthermore we include the multi-modal matching of portal images against digitally reconstructed radiographs (DRR) computed from the CT volume data.

2 Least squares template matching

LSM is an area-based matching algorithm, thus does not depend on the extraction of binary image features. This is a very important advantage in low-contrast and blurred imagery, where feature extraction is mostly unreliable. Furthermore, unlike in most correlation methods, the optimum transformation is not searched on a discrete grid, but approached using an optimization scheme. Assuming that a fair initial guess can be supplied, this is not only faster but also more accurate.

The following sections give a short review over the LSM framework. Further information can be found in [Berger 1998, Berger and Danuser 1997].

2.1 Unconstrained LSM

The LSM includes two observations, the template image $f[.]$ and the search image $g[.]$, called patch. The geometric relation between the original template and the matched area is defined by an arbitrary transformation. Depending on the type of the chosen transformation, this allows for displacement, rotation and/or deformation of the template.

In addition to the geometric transformation, the observations must be adjusted radiometrically. The simultaneous estimation of both types of transformations would lead to an overdetermined system, since it is not possible to distinguish them locally. In order to overcome this problem, the parameters of the radiometric transformation are estimated based on a global measure within the template region apart from the actual least squares optimization. The resulting radiometrically adjusted patch $\bar{g}[.]$ is then used for the next optimization step. We use a linear transformation which can be written as $\bar{g}[u] = \alpha + \beta\, g[u]$, where u stands for the discrete image coordinates.

The general geometric transformation is denoted by $x = \psi(\boldsymbol{\xi}, u)$, transforming the image coordinates u using the parameter vector $\boldsymbol{\xi}$. Applying the least squares framework, this leads to the observation equation

$$f[u] + e[u] = \bar{g}(x) \,. \tag{1}$$

Equation (1) represents a relation between each greyvalue within the template and its corresponding image intensity in the search image.[1] Interpolating the greyvalues for a given $\boldsymbol{\xi}$ we substitute $\tilde{g}_\xi[u] := \bar{g}(\psi(\boldsymbol{\xi}, u))$. Based on a coordinate list $u[k]$, equation (1) is reordered into a vector notation

$$\boldsymbol{f} + \boldsymbol{e} = \tilde{\boldsymbol{g}} \,, \tag{2}$$

building a series of n equations, where n is the number of pixels included in the template and $k = 1 \ldots n$. Together with the least squares objective function $e^T P e$, with P as optional weight matrix, this defines an unconstrained nonlinear least squares (NLS) problem. This nonlinear problem is iteratively solved using a Newton-Raphson scheme. A new estimate $\hat{\boldsymbol{\xi}} = \boldsymbol{\xi}° + \boldsymbol{\Delta\xi}$ is computed linearizing the observation equations (1) around the current estimate $\boldsymbol{\xi}°$

$$\boldsymbol{f} + \boldsymbol{e} = \tilde{\boldsymbol{g}}° + \boldsymbol{A} \cdot \boldsymbol{\Delta\xi} \,. \tag{3}$$

Matrix $\boldsymbol{A}$ is the $n \times r$ Jacobian matrix $\nabla_\xi\, \bar{g}(x°)$ with respect to the parameter vector $\boldsymbol{\xi}$ and r denotes the number of parameters. The linear problem (3) is

---

[1] Notice that square brackets denote functions defined on a discrete grid. The functions $g(.)$ and $\bar{g}(.)$ simply represent the continuous versions of $g[.]$ and $\bar{g}[.]$, respectively.

solved analytically setting the first derivative of the least squares goal function $e^T P e$ to zero, which yields the normal equation system

$$A^T P A \cdot \Delta \xi = -A^T P (\tilde{g}^\circ - f) . \qquad (4)$$

This linear equation system is then solved using Cholesky decomposition. After each iteration step, matrix A must be recomputed using the updated set of parameters $\xi^{t+1} = \xi^t + \Delta \xi$. When the parameter change $\Delta \xi$ falls below a specified numerical resolution the iteration process is stopped.

2.2 Error propagation and parameter determinability

Parameter estimation in linear least squares problems are extensively discussed in standard literature on parameter estimation theory, for instance in [Koch 1988]. The iterative solution of equation (1) is an unbiased estimate for the unknowns with a stochastic variance expressed by the diagonal elements of the covariance matrix $\Sigma_{\xi\xi} = \hat{\sigma}_0 \cdot Q_{\xi\xi}$. The value $\hat{\sigma}_0$ denotes the a posteriori noise estimate and $Q_{\xi\xi} = (A^T P A)^{-1}$ is the cofactor matrix.

The determinability of a parameter i is tested using its relative contribution δ_i to the trace of the cofactor matrix $Q_{\xi\xi}$

$$\delta_i = \frac{|\text{tr}[Q_{\xi\xi}] - \text{tr}[Q^i_{\xi\xi}]|}{\text{tr}[Q_{\xi\xi}]} = \frac{\sum_j q_{ij}^2}{q_{ii} \sum_j q_{jj}^2} , \qquad (5)$$

where $Q^i_{\xi\xi}$ is the cofactor matrix with parameter i excluded and q_{ij} denote the elements of the full cofactor matrix $Q_{\xi\xi}$. The efficient implementation on the right hand side is achieved employing the Kalman-Bucy filter technique (cf. [Koch 1988]), computing the partial cofactor matrix $Q^i_{\xi\xi}$ directly from $Q_{\xi\xi}$.

If a contribution δ_i of the parameter i is high, this parameter strongly correlates to one or more parameters. One should either exclude parameter i or combine it with the correlating parameters by applying parameter constraints as described in section 2.5.

2.3 Multi template extension

Using multiples template instead of one large template allows significant and stable regions to be selected without including regions unsuitable for matching. There are several ways to extend the standard LSM to multiple templates. For all of them, the equation (1) has to be adapted to include multiple templates and their corresponding patches.

The most straightforward extension is to keep one single transformation for all patches with the same parameter set shown in equation (7), leading to

$$f[u^K] + e[u^K] = \bar{g}^K (x^K) , \qquad (6)$$

where $\bar{g}[.] = \alpha^K + \beta^K g[.]$ and $x^K = \psi(\xi, u^K)$. Formally, this procedure is similar to defining one large template with several scattered regions of interest. However, since the radiometric parameters α^K and β^K may vary between the templates, it is possible to compensate for global greyvalue differences like bias fields.

2.4 Affine transformation as geometric transformation

So far no assumptions have been made on the dimensionality of the problem and on what type of transformation is used. In the following, the case of a two dimensional affine transformation is presented. The corresponding parameter vector consists of six variables $\boldsymbol{\xi} = [t_1, t_2, m_1, s_1, s_2, m_2]^T$ and the coordinate transformation is written as

$$x = \begin{bmatrix} t_1 \\ t_2 \end{bmatrix} + \begin{bmatrix} m_1 & s_1 \\ s_2 & m_2 \end{bmatrix} u. \qquad (7)$$

The derivative $\nabla_{\boldsymbol{\xi}} \bar{g}(\boldsymbol{x})$ is then calculated explicitly using the chain rule. In vector notation, this leads to the $n \times 6$ Jacobian matrix $\boldsymbol{A}$ (cf. equation (3)), each line $\boldsymbol{A}_k$ representing the derivatives at $\boldsymbol{x}_k = \boldsymbol{\psi}(\boldsymbol{\xi}, \boldsymbol{u}[k])$.

2.5 Employing constraints

The least squares formalism allows one to introduce additional constraints in a simple and intuitive way. In addition to the observation equations, zero observations are included in the framework using large weights in the weight matrix $\boldsymbol{P}$. In this section, we will apply this technique to LSM. As an examples serves the reduction of an affine to a similarity transformation. Instead of reparametrization we still employ equation (7) as transformation equation and add the following constraints to the parameter vector $\boldsymbol{\xi}$:

$$m_1 - m_2 + e_m = 0 \qquad \boldsymbol{A}_m = [0, 0, 1, 0, 0, -1]$$
$$s_1 + s_2 + e_s = 0 \qquad \boldsymbol{A}_s = [0, 0, 0, 1, 1, 0] \ .$$

Analogous to the observation equations (1), the constraints are linearized around the current estimates m_i° and s_i°. Thus, the matrix $\boldsymbol{A}$ is augmented by the constraint vectors $\boldsymbol{A}_m$ and $\boldsymbol{A}_s$.

Employing constraints instead of reparametrization is easier to implement and more versatile. On the one hand, constraints can easily be changed during the iteration, quickly switching from a similarity to an affine transformation. On the other hand, only a few types of constraints can actually be expressed by reparametrization, which makes constraints more flexible to use.

3 Controlling patient position in radiotherapy

The steps before high precision conformal therapy include the acquisition of a CT, then a 3D planning of beam directions, field shape and dose distribution and finally the positioning of the patient using a simulator with the same geometry as the linear accelerator (figure 1). During radiotherapy treatment, either portal films or electronic portal images are acquired for quality control.

The portal images in this work were acquired at the University Hospital of Zürich using a Varian accelerator and their electronic portal imaging device

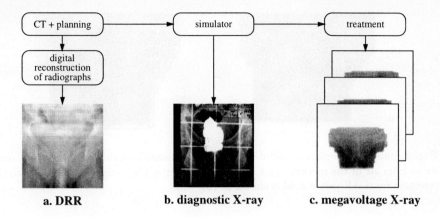

Fig. 1. Overview of the different steps of radiotherapy treatment.

(EPID). This device delivers a distortion free image with a resolution of 256×256 pixel on an area of 32×32 cm² [van Herk and Meertens 1988].

The diagnostic X-ray images from the simulator are often used as a reference image for measuring the patient motion in subsequent portal images. Besides the fact that simulator images are not suitable for automated area-based matching due to their different greyvalue characteristics, they also represent an additional source of error with respect to the original planning data. Hence, one goal of this project is to eliminate the need for simulator X-ray images for motion measurements by direct comparison with a megavoltage DRR (figure 1a).

DRRs are computed simulating the therapy setup by a ray-tracing based algorithm, also correcting for the different absorption coefficients at different beam energies. Thus, a DRR representing the correct patient position serves as reference image. Subsequent portal images are compared to this reference image and the estimate of a 2D affine transformation leads to a correction of the patient position. However, in order to compute DRRs with sufficient quality, the CT slice thickness should be no larger than 5 mm.

3.1 Selecting suitable templates

In the particular problem of portal images, two displacements must be computed. Since the EPID is in general not in a fixed position, a common coordinate system must be established using the edges of the radiation field. These edges are very distinct features and pose no problems to the matching algorithm. We refer to [Berger and Danuser 1997] for a more detailed description of the fieldedge match.

In the following, we will concentrate on the anatomy match. The selection of the template regions follows the previous work. Due to artifacts and the presence of distinct but unstable features (for instance originating from air in the rectum), a fully automated template selection is beyond the possibilities of computer vision. Thus, the physician has to position predefined standard templates onto the significant structures in the reference image (figure 2).

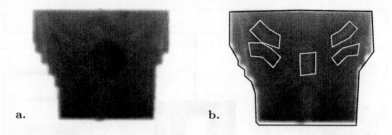

Fig. 2. Image (a) depicts a portal image with a common unstable features that originates from air in the rectum (dark blur in the center of the image). A typical template selection for a AP pelvis field is shown in (b).

3.2 Self-diagnosis within LSM

The statistics behind the self-diagnosis outlined in section 2.2 is only valid in the adjusted state. Therefore, this measure can not be applied directly to the initial system. However, an upper bound for the determinability is computed matching the templates onto themselves. Based on this upper bound, a coarse result is computed using a restricted parameter set which still approximates the final parameter set sufficiently, usually a congruent transformation.

At this first estimate, the full affine parameter set is tested for determinability. If none of the parameters show large contributions δ_i, the optimization is continued with the full parameter set. A general flowchart is depicted in figure 3.

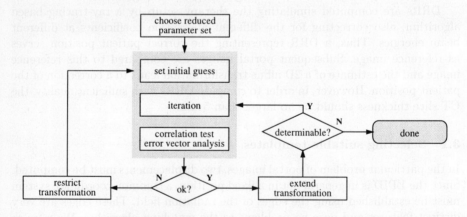

Fig. 3. Flowchart of the diagnostic measures.

The cross-correlation between the template $f[.]$ and the patch $\tilde{g}[.]$—which is interpolated from the search image using the final parameter set ξ—should be very close to 1.0. For multiple templates, the correlation value is computed for each template. Since a low correlation value indicates a mismatch for this

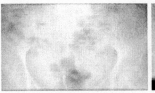 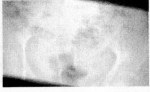 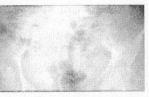

a. reference image   b. 35 images translated and rotated in-plane   c. 200 images rotated around x and z axis

Fig. 4. Example DRR images from the in-plane (b) and out-of-plane (c) test series computed from CT volume.

region, excluding such a template and reoptimizing the geometric transformation usually results in a better parameter set.

4 Results

The high precision capabilities of LSM are extensively shown in [Berger and Danuser 1997, Danuser and Mazza 1996]. In the following sections, the emphasis is on the estimation of the in-plane part of the 3D patient motion based on the evaluation of projected 2D images. We first apply the algorithm to generated datasets to test the potential of LSM. In the last section, we present results of the multi-modal match.

In all examples, an affine transformation was used for matching and the initial position was set to the fieldedge position. The typical run time including Gauss filtering of the search image, matching the fieldedge and matching the anatomy templates is about 4 seconds on a Sun Ultra 1 (167 Mhz UltraSPARC CPU).

4.1 In-plane translation and rotations

The following test series consisted of 35 simulated portal images with a maximum patient displacement of 20 mm in x and y direction and a maximum rotation of 10° (figure 4b). The standard deviations of the translation measurements were 0.25 pixel (0.23 mm) in x direction and 0.37 pixel (0.33 mm) in y direction. These systematic errors are caused by the unknown y position in the CT coordinate system of the template features. Within the rotation measurement, these systematic error do not occur and the standard deviations are below 0.01°.

4.2 Including out-of-plane rotation

In order to test under more realistic conditions, a test series of 200 images with small out-of-plane rotations is generated (figure 4c). The LSM still found the corresponding regions with a correlation well above 0.9. The systematic errors already encountered in the example above, which are an inherent problem of using projected images, were of course higher in this example. But the total point errors of 1.24 mm for 2° rotation and 3 mm for 5° still are promising results.

4.3 Multi-modal match with portal images

Figure 5a shows a DRR and the chosen templates including four validation lines, which are not used for matching. The DRR was computed from a CT volume with a voxel size of $2\times2\times3\,\text{mm}^3$. The corresponding portal image series contained 22 images, two of which are depicted in 5b and c. The results were visually validated and all but one were accepted to be correct, which indicates a success rate of well over 90 %.

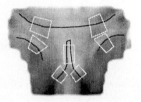
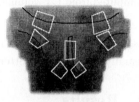

a. reference image (DRR)   b. translation (0,-4) mm   c. translation (3,-3) mm
                               rotation 1.5°   rotation 2.6°

Fig. 5. Multi-modal match between a DRR image computed from CT data (a) and a portal image series (b,c). The match is based on an affine transformation model. White polygons outline the template regions and patches respectively, black lines represent validation lines which are not used for matching.

5 Conclusion and Outlook

The LSM method with deformable templates is a versatile matching algorithm. Since it is an area-based method, the often unreliable step of feature extraction is circumvented. Especially in low-contrast imagery like megavoltage X-ray images (portal images), this is an important feature.

In earlier work, LSM has been successfully applied to matching megavoltage X-ray images of the same modality. The results presented in this paper show the suitability for a multi-modal match between digitally reconstructed radiographs as reference images and the portal images acquired during radiotherapy. The area-based method LSM proved robustness even when matching slightly distorted patterns.

In two test series with generated data, the systematic error caused by estimating a 3D motion from projected 2D images is examined. Furthermore, tests with a DRR matched to real portal images show promising results which will be validated more thoroughly in the near future. Another goal is to combine multiple 2D measurements from different directions to better estimate the 3D motion and to reduce the influence of the systematic error occurring in the 2D measurements.

The presented methods are a step further in the direction of automatically controlling the patient position in radiotherapy. Applied in daily hospital routine, this should lead to an improved quality assurance in radiotherapy.

Acknowledgments. We would like to thank Dr. U. R. Meier and Prof. Dr. U. M. Lütolf for providing the portal images and useful information concerning medical topics. This work was granted by the Swiss Cancer League and the Walter Honegger Foundation.

References

[Berger and Danuser 1997] Martin Berger and Gaudenz Danuser. Deformable multi template matching with application to portal images. In *Proc. CVPR '97*, pages 374–379. IEEE Computer Society Press, 1997.

[Berger 1998] Martin Berger. The framework of least squares template matching. Technical Report 180, Image Science Lab, ETH Zürich, 1998. Available at http://www.vision.ee.ethz.ch/.

[Danuser and Mazza 1996] G. Danuser and E. Mazza. Observing deformations of 20 nanometer with a low numerical aperture light microscope. In *Optical Inspection and Micromeasurements*, volume 2782, pages 180–191. SPIE, 1996.

[Dong and Boyer 1996] L. Dong and A. L. Boyer. A portal image alignment and patient setup verification procedure using moments and correlation techniques. *Phys. Med. Biol.*, 41(4):697–723, 1996.

[Förstner 1987] W. Förstner. Reliability analysis of parameter estimation in linear models with applications to mensuration problems in computer vision. *Computer Vision, Graphics, and Image Processing*, 40:273–310, 1987.

[Fritsch et al. 1995] D. S. Fritsch, E. L. Chaney, A. Boxwala, M. McAuliffe, S. Raghavan, A. Thall, and J. R. D. Earnhart. Core-based portal image registration for automatic radiotherapy treatment verification. *Int. J. Rad. Onc. Biol. Phys.*, 33(5):1287–1300, 1995.

[Gilhuijs and van Herk 1993] K. G. A. Gilhuijs and M. van Herk. Automatic on-line inspection of patient setup in radiation therapy using digital portal images. *Med. Phys.*, 20(3):667–677, 1993.

[Grün 1985] A. Grün. Adaptive least squares correlation: A powerful image matching technique. *South African J. of Photogrammetry*, 14(3):175–187, 1985.

[Koch 1988] K. R. Koch. *Parameter estimation and hypothesis testing in linear models*. Springer, 1988.

[Lucas and Kanade 1981] Bruce D. Lucas and Takeo Kanade. An iterative image registration technique with an application to stereo vision. In *International joint conference on artificial intelligence*, pages 674–679, 1981.

[Moseley and Munro 1994] J. Moseley and P. Munro. A semiautomatic method for registration of portal images. *Med. Phys.*, 21(4):551–558, 1994.

[Unser et al. 1995] M. Unser, P. Thévenaz, L. Chulhee, and U. Ruttimann. Registration and statistical analysis of pet images using the wavelet transform. *IEEE Engineering in Medicine and Biology*, Sep./Oct. 1995.

[van Herk and Meertens 1988] M. van Herk and H. Meertens. A matrix ionisation chamber imaging device for on-line patient setup verification during radiotherapy. *Radiother. Oncol.*, 11(4):369–378, April 1988.

Pitfalls in Comparing Functional Magnetic Resonance Imaging and Invasive Electrophysiology Recordings

DLG Hill[1], A Simmons[2,3], AD Castellano Smith[1], CR Maurer, Jr.[1], TCS Cox[1,2], R Elwes[2], MJ Brammer[3], DJ Hawkes[1], CE Polkey[2]

[1]Radiological Sciences & Medical Engineering, [2]Clinical Neurosciences and [3]Institute of Psychiatry, King's College London, UK. <D.Hill@umds.ac.uk>

Abstract. Several authors have recently compared the results of fMRI studies on neurosurgery patients with invasive electrophysiology. These studies aim to validate fMRI against an accepted gold standard, and ascertain whether fMRI could replace invasive electrophysiology in neurosurgical patients. We have identified and quantified two characteristics of these data that make such comparisons problematic. Firstly, the epilepsy surgery patients (n=8) studied move significantly more during fMRI experiments than normal volunteers (n=6) performing the same task. This motion has a particularly large out-of-plane component, and is significantly more correlated with the stimulus than for the normal volunteers. This motion is especially large when performing a task on the side affected by the lesion. This additional motion is hard to correct and substantially degrades the quality of the resulting fMRI images, making it a much less reliable technique on these surgical patients than on other subjects. Secondly, we have found that, following electrode implantation, the brain surface can shift by more than 10 mm relative to the skull compared to its preoperative location, substantially degrading the accuracy of the comparison of electrophysiology measurements made on the deformed brain and fMRI studies carried out preoperatively. Taken together, these findings suggest that studies of this sort are currently of limited use for validating fMRI, and further image analysis research is necessary to solve the problems caused by subject motion and brain deformation.

1 Introduction

Several authors have recently compared the results of functional Magnetic Resonance imaging (fMRI) studies on neurosurgery patients with subsequent electrophysiology studies carried out using chronically implanted sub-dural electrodes or intraoperative evoked potentials and stimulation [1–5]. These studies, which are reviewed below, contribute to an understanding of the relationship between functional regions localised using fMRI and the same regions localised using invasive electrophysiology. They do not, however, demonstrate that fMRI is sufficiently accurate and sensitive to replace invasive cortical mapping in surgery planning. Neither do they accurately validate fMRI against the established alternative technique of invasive cortical mapping. The results described in the literature tend to be qualitative, for example concluding that there is "good agreement" between the techniques, without stating what constitutes good agreement. Where quantitative data is provided, the accuracy of the measurements (eg: from aligning preoperative images with intraoperative photographs) is unclear.

We have carried out a similar study of epilepsy surgery patients, and noticed several features of our data that have important consequences for studies of this type. In particular, during fMRI, the neurosurgical epilepsy patients move more than volunteers and other patients studied at our institution, which affects the quality of the fMRI results. Furthermore, there is a clear shift in the position of the brain surface between preoperative MR panel and post-implantation CT scans. This brain deformation has implications for the position of sites in the brain identified during the two measurements, and any comparison of their location. We have quantified both the subject motion and brain deformation on a series of eight patients.

1.1 Review of literature

Jack's paper [1] states two benefits of this sort of study: to assess the suitability of fMRI as a tool for "localization of functional areas relative to the surgical target", and "validation of the physiologic truth of functional localization with MR imaging... with the accepted criterion standard of invasive cortical mapping". Two epilepsy surgery cases were studied. Both had fMRI and intraoperative electrode recordings (evoked potentials and median nerve stimulation). The first patient additionally had measurements taken using chronically implanted subdural electrode strips. For patient 1, two volume renderings of the brain surface were generated. The first shows the relationship between the brain surface, the tumour boundary and the orientation of the single fMRI slice. The second showed the position of the electrodes and tumour overlaid on the rendered MR brain surface. The electrodes were localised using a post-implantation CT scan registered to the preoperative MR. Visual comparison of the two renderings "confirmed the impression formed from the functional MR study that the tumour straddled the functional sensorimotor strip". The results from the second patient were more problematic due to motion during fMRI imaging, but once again, the electrode measurements "confirmed the impression formed at functional MR imaging".

Yousry et al [2] share the objectives of Jack et al. They studied six patients and four volunteers. All the patients had space occupying lesions close to the pre-central gyrus, and one had a slight palsy. All patients and volunteers underwent an fMRI examination while carrying out a motor task. Electrophysiological measurements were made on the patients using intraoperative stimulation under local or balanced anaesthesia. The patients were administered corticosteroids and diuretics before craniotomy, so "there was no detectable brain displacement after opening the dura." Functional regions identified during stimulation were marked with small numbered labels placed on the brain surface, and the positions of the labels was recorded using an intraoperative photograph and sketch. In order to compare the fMRI and electrophysiology results, they first defined the motor hand area from the fMRI as the parenchymal area where the motor task resulted in a temporally correlated statistically significant regional signal increase. The corresponding functional region was defined intraoperatively as the area where electrical cortical stimulation of the central region elicited compound muscle action potentials from the contralateral hypothenar or thenar muscle, or a tonic opening or closing of the contralateral hand. Comparison of the locations of the functional region identified in these ways was achieved by measuring the distance between the target point and each of four anatomical landmarks (lines) visible in both the MR image and intraoperatively. The precise nature of the coordinate systems defined by these landmarks is unclear from the paper. The discrepancy in the measurements varied from -3 to 10 mm. A Wilcoxon test was used to assess the significance of these discrepancies. The resulting P value was greater than 0.5, from which the authors appear to have concluded that the two sets of measurements agreed. No study of the reproducibility of the measurements was reported. Yousry et al additionally found that the activated region in the fMRI was more diffuse in the patients than for the normal volunteers.

Puce et al [3] studied 4 patients (3 with focal epilepsy, 1 with intractable post-traumatic seizures) and six normal volunteers. For both groups, fMRI images were acquired using both dual slice conventional gradient echo and three-slice gradient-echo EPI, with motor and sensory hand activation tasks. For all patients, electrophysiological measurements were made using intraoperative cortical stimulation. For one patient, measurements were also made using chronically implanted subdural electrodes. Intraoperative photographs were taken using a camera mounted above the surgical field. A photograph was first taken of the bare brain, then with a recording grid in place, and also of the brain together with numerical labels placed on the brain surface to indicate sites of positive cortical stimulation. The coordinates of these sites were transferred onto an image of the rendered brain surface obtained from a segmented gradient echo MR volume. There is no consideration of errors introduced by the perspective geometry of the photograph compared to the rendering. For the patient who underwent chronic recordings, a post implantation MR volume was acquired to localize the electrodes. The fMRI was aligned with the anatomical gradient echo MR volume using an unspecified registration algorithm. Inspection of the renderings and comparison with the photographs lead them to report that "the delineation of hand sensorimotor cortex using functional MR imaging and two electrophysiological methods revealed good agreement on the location of sensory and motor areas". They conclude that "the correspondence of the functional MR imaging and electrophysiological maps, however, argues strongly for the accurate localization of the hand sensorimotor cortex by our MR imaging methods". No quantitative assessment of the discrepancy between the location of functional regions by the two methods is given.

Yetkin et al [4] study a relatively large series of 28 patients (22 with chronic epilepsy, 5 with a cerebral tumour, and one with an AVM). Their primary aim is to validate fMRI. These subjects carried out two tasks during fMRI imaging, word generation and finger tapping. Seven 1 cm thick sagittal EPI slices were acquired at a rate of 1 per second during the activation paradigm. All subjects underwent intraoperative stimulation mapping under local anesthesia. Each subject's hand, fingers, face and tongue were monitored during the stimulation and that subject counted or recited sentences while the surgeon searched for a region which, when stimulated, resulted in reproducible interruption of speech. Labels were placed on the brain at each stimulation site, and the marker placement was recorded photographically using a camera "positioned so as to minimize parallax and distortion". The fMRI and electrophysiological location of the functional regions were compared by aligning the most superficial slice of the fMRI showing activation with the digitized intraoperative photograph using Adobe Photoshop to scale, rotate and translate the images. Anatomical landmarks in the region were used as cues in performing this alignment. The discrepancies in the location of the corresponding functional regions in the two modalities were quantified by measuring the in-plane distance between the centre of the cortical stimulation site and the centre of the corresponding region activated in fMRI. Where there was no continuous region activated in fMRI, the distance between the centre of the cortical stimulation site and the closest activated pixel in the fMRI was measured instead. In all cases, the in-plane discrepancy was less than 20mm, and for 86% of measurement it was within 10mm. There is no estimate of out-of-plane discrepancy in location, or of errors in the registration of a single slice of fMRI to the photograph. They estimated the distortion in the EPI to reach one pixel and the precision of the fMRI to be 5mm from reproducibility studies. They conclude that, despite the significant methodological problems, functional MR imaging represents a non-invasive means of anticipating the results of cortical mapping.

Fitzgerald et al [5] studied 11 patients with a lesion in the presumed dominant hemisphere, 8 with tumours, 1 with a cyst, 1 with epilepsy and one with a cavernous angioma. Their aim was to evaluate fMRI as a predictive technique for locating eloquent areas in the dominant hemisphere, and in particular, its accuracy at locating language areas for planning surgical resection. They also stated that the study had implications for validating fMRI on normal volunteers. All subjects underwent fMRI examinations using multi-slice spin-echo EPI, while performing one or more language tasks. Cortical stimulation was carried out intraoperatively with the patient under local anesthesia. Tags were placed on the brain surface to mark language areas, and an intraoperative photograph was used to record the location of the tags. A volumetric gradient echo MR image from each patient was registered to an MR angiogram using Analyze, and a rendering produced showing the brain surface and blood vessel landmarks. The statistical fMRI map was registered to the rendering in an unspecified way, and cortical activity could then be projected onto the surface of the brain. The lateral projection of the rendering was aligned with the intraoperative photograph using Adobe Photoshop to scale, translate and rotate the images until the user considered the position of the landmarks in the photo and in the rendering to be in "good agreement". The authors estimated the error in this process to be less than 7mm for all patients, with 1 mm matching accuracy achieved for four patients. Agreement between the modalities was assessed by counting the number of activation areas in fMRI that contacted, overlapped or surrounded a language tags in the photograph. They additionally measured the distance between the centre of the region of activation in the fMRI and the language tags (it is not clear whether these measurements were carried out in the plane of the overlay, or in three dimensions). Sensitivity was considered to be the percentage of matches between fMRI regions and language tags, and specificity was the percentage of regions activated in fMRI that matched with a non-language tag. Depending on the stringency of the match criterion, the sensitivity across all subjects varied from 81% with a specificity of 51% to 92%, with a specificity of 0%.

2 Method

2.1 Data Acquisition

Eight patients with intractable epilepsy (4 of whom were judged clinically to have a motor deficit), were studied. Preoperatively, each patient was imaged using a 3D spoiled GRASS sequence and functional MRI on a 1.5T GE Signa MR system retrofitted with Advanced NMR hardware and software. For each study, 100 T2* weighted multi-slice datasets (TE=40ms, TR=3s, 128x64 acquisition matrix, 3.1x3.1x5mm voxels, 0.5mm slice gap, 10 slices) were acquired using gradient echo EPI. We refer to each multi-slice dataset as a frame. Rest and activation epochs are alternated for 30 second periods over a total imaging time of five minutes. Activation experiments were performed for both hands using a finger opposition task. Head movement was limited by foam padding within the head coil and a restraining band across the forehead. Daily quality assurance was carried out to ensure high signal to ghost ratio, high signal to noise ratio and excellent temporal stability using an automated quality control procedure [6]. Each patient subsequently had surgery to implant one or more subdural electrode mats, varying in size from 8 to 64 electrodes per mat, on a 1cm grid. All patients in this study had at least 32 electrodes implanted. During the days following implantation, electrophysiological measurements were carried out to localize the epileptogenic zone, and eloquent regions of the cortex in the vicinity of the site of surgery. Immediately after implantation of the mat, or immediately prior to removal, the patient had a neuro-CT scan. Subsequent resection was planned in the normal way, without taking into account the fMRI data. Six normal volunteers under-went the same fMRI paradigm.

2.2 Data Processing

For each fMRI study, all 100 frames were registered to the first frame using an algorithm that minimises the mean square difference between voxel intensities [7]. This algorithm produces a motion trajectory for each subject showing movement during the scan for six degrees of freedom (three translations and three rotations). Subject motion was quantified using two indices for each degree of freedom: the range of motion; and the value of the power spectrum of the motion at the stimulation frequency. The second index measures how correlated the motion is with the stimulus. The indices were used to compare the patients with the volunteers, and also to compare the amount of subject motion when a patient was carrying out a task using the side of the brain affected by the lesion with the contralateral side. Subsequent fMRI processing was carried out using the algorithm of Bullmore et al [8].

Each patient's gradient echo MR volume was registered to the post-implantation CT scan using an algorithm that optimises the mutual information of the joint probability distribution of the two images [9]. This algorithm was found in an international multi-centre trial to have a median registration error of less than 2mm for retrospective MR-CT registration [10]. The MR and CT images being registered in the current study are different from those in the multi-centre study (eg: the CT scans contain high contrast structures such as electrodes and air within the head that were not present in the MR), but this did not cause the algorithm to fail, and visual assessment of the results suggested the accuracy was similar [11]. For all patients in this study, the electrode mat is clearly visible in the post-implantation CT scan lying some distance medial to the inner table of the skull. The region between the mat and the skull is filled with air and fluid. If the CT scan is thresholded to show only bone and electrodes and overlaid on the registered MR volume, the electrodes are seen to lie several mm inside the MR brain surface. We believe that this shift in position is due to deformation of the brain tissue caused by the surgical procedure to open the dura and implant the electrodes. We quantified the magnitude of this brain deformation in two ways: by measuring the displacement between each electrode on the mat and nearest point on the inner table of the skull, and secondly by measuring the distance between each electrode on the mat and the envelope of the brain surface. We identified the 3D coordinates of the electrodes in the mat using a cursor in surface renderings of the CT scans. The rendering is a parallel projection in the sagittal plane with a z-buffer that stores the distance to the first voxel with an intensity over a specified threshold. The two dimensional coordinates of the cursor on the rendering can therefore be converted to three dimensional coordinates in the post-implantation CT scan using the z-buffer depth information. By rendering both sides of the brain, it is possible to identify the inner and outer surfaces of the electrodes (which are about 1mm thick). The Analyze software package (Biomedical Imaging Resource, Mayo Clinic, Rochester MN) was used to automatically trace the inner table of the skull from the CT scan, and also to manually trace the envelope of the brain surface from the MR volume. The brain envelope is an estimate of where the electrode mat might lie in MR coordinates in the absence of brain deformation. The envelope does not follow the convoluted surface of the cortex, as the electrode mat is relatively stiff, and cannot, therefore penetrate sulci. Also, the envelope is not the same as the dura surface, as in some of our patients, there was atrophy in the region where the mat was placed, so the tops of the gyri are separated from the dura by CSF. The rigid body transformation found by registering the MR and CT images was then used to transform the brain envelope surfaces into the same coordinate frame as the CT electrodes and inner surface of the skull. The skull and brain surfaces were then triangulated using the Nuages software package [12]. The Euclidean distance between each electrode and the closest facet in the two surfaces was calculated.

3 Results

In our neuroimaging unit, we regularly produce high quality fMRI images from normal volunteers and non-surgical patients (eg: [13–15]). The fMRI images from the epilepsy surgery patients presented in this paper were, however, visually judged to be of much lower quality, probably because of motion.

degree of freedom	volunteer	patient
x translate (mm) †	0.18	0.35
y translate (mm) †	0.19	0.39
z translate (mm) †	0.31	0.91
x rotate (deg.) †	0.20	0.71
y rotate (deg.) †	0.20	0.48
z rotate (deg.) †	0.18	0.42

(a)

degree of feedom	volunteer	patient
x translate †	24	120
y translate †	39	134
z translate †	42	2350
x rotate †	85	175
y rotate †	13	467
z rotate	10	257

(b)

Table 1. Median values of (a) range of translational and rotational motion and (b) value of the power spectrum at the stimulation frequency in each degree of freedom for six normal volunteers and eight epileptic patients. †represents significant difference between groups at 95% level.

The median range of motion and value of the power spectrum for the patient and volunteer groups are compared in table 1. For both indices and all degrees of freedom, the median motion of the patients is greater than for volunteers. The distributions fail a normality test, so the Mann-Whitney non-parametric test was used to test the significance of the difference in these median values. For the range of motion index, the null hypothesis that both groups come from the same population was rejected for all degrees

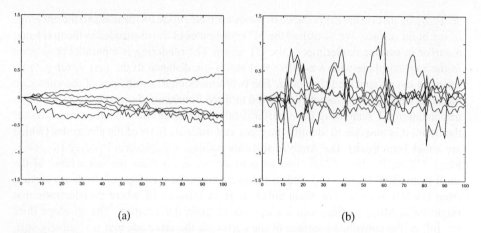

Fig. 1. Example motion trajectories for a normal volunteer (a) and patient (b). All six degrees of freedom are plotted for each subject. Frame number is along the horizontal axis, and motion amplitude (mm for translation and degrees for rotation) on the vertical axes. Note the large amplitude, and more periodic nature of the patient motion.

of freedom at the 95% level. For the power spectrum measure, the same hypothesis was rejected at the 95% level for all three translational degrees of freedom and the two rotational degrees of freedom with through-plane component, and at the 90% level for the in-plane rotational degree of freedom. The degree of freedom of motion that was most significantly greater for the patient group than for the normal group corresponded to through-slice translational motion (99.9% level). The median patient motion when carrying out tasks using the side of the brain affected by the lesion was greater than for the contralateral side for both indices and all degrees of freedom. This data is paired, so the significance of these differences was tested using the paired t-test if a normality test was passed, or Wilcoxon test if the normality test failed. We initially tested for significant difference in motion for each degree of freedom separately. For both motion indices, the motion was significantly greater (at the 95% level) in the anterio-posterior translation direction (in plane), and for both rotational degrees of freedom with an out-of-plane component. The lack of significant difference for the remaining degrees of freedom may be due to lack of statistical power. We therefore also concatenated the results for all degrees of freedom and carried out a single paired test between the two groups. In this case, for both indices, subject motion when undertaking a motor task on the normal side was significantly less (99.9% level) than when carrying out the same task on the side affected by the lesion.

Figure 2 shows axial and coronal slices through a pre-operative MR scan from patient 2. The CT scan has been thresholded so that only the bone and electrodes are visible and overlaid on the MRI. It is clear that the electrodes lie several millimetres inside the MR brain surface, and this can only be due to brain deformation. The right panel shows combined fMRI and post-implantation CT images from patient 7, with the significant voxels from the fMRI overlaid as white squares. The electrodes are visible as a row of grey elipses, which, because of brain deformation, lie several mm inside

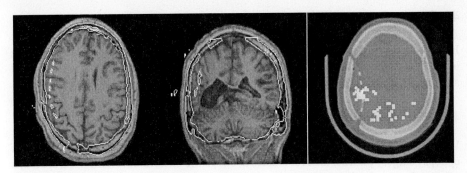

Fig. 2. Thresholded post-implantation CT images overlaid on registered MR image for patient 2 (left panel axial, centre panel coronal). The white lines show the outline of the bone, and the electrodes. Right panel: slice from post-implantation CT scan of patient 7 with significant activated fMRI voxels overlaid in white. The electodes are visible as grey rectangles in the CT. For all patients, there is a considerable gap between the electrodes and inner surface of the skull as a result of brain deformation similar to that shown here.

the surface of the activated cortex. Brain surface deformation has been quantified for the eight patients, and is summarised using the median, 10 percentile and 90 percentile displacements in table 2.

Patient	median displacement		90 percentile displacement		10 percentile displacement	
	MR brain	CT skull	MR brain	CT skull	MR brain	CT skull
1	3.6	4.5	7.5	7.0	1.4	0.2
2	4.9	5.2	9.3	9.3	2.5	2.4
3	3.5	3.8	7.8	6.8	-2.0	1.4
4	4.4	5.9	10.1	10.4	0.7	1.3
5	10.3	7.4	13.4	11.9	6.2	1.1
6	6.8	5.8	10.2	10.9	2.9	4.0
7	3.5	5.6	9.2	13.1	0.7	2.3
8	5.4	7.5	11.2	12.0	0.4	1.7
mean (stdev)	5.3 (2.3)	5.7 (1.3)	9.8 (1.9)	10.2 (2.3)	1.6 (2.4)	1.8 (1.1)

Table 2. Median, 90 percentile and 10 percentile displacement between the position of the electrodes located in the post-implantation CT scan and the closest point on the brain envelope delineated from the registered pre-operative MR scan (MR brain), and the position of the same electrodes and the closest point on the inner table of the skull (CT skull). Distances are in mm inside the brain envelope and inner table of the skull respectively.

There is good agreement between the values of the displacements calculated in these two ways. The displacements are all in the same direction, with the electrodes lying inside the brain boundary, as illustrated by figure 2. The largest shifts, which are more than 1 cm for most patients, were observed near the centre of the craniotomy, which in many cases is the brain region of greatest interest. These measurements do not provide any estimate of the lateral shift of the brain surface, but provide a lower bound on the deformation of points on the brain surface between the pre-operative MRI and post-implantation CT images.

4 Discussion

In carrying out this study we have identified several sources of error that make it difficult to determine how accurate fMRI is at localizing functional regions, or how well fMRI agrees with invasive electrophysiology measurements.

4.1 Patient motion during fMRI

We have found that fMRI is much more unreliable when applied to this group of epilepsy surgery patients than for studies at our centre on normal volunteers. Our results suggest that this is likely to be due to the greater magnitude of motion during scanning of the patient group, and especially the greater magnitude of motion correlated with the stimulus and motion with a large through-plane component.

During fMRI studies, it is necessary to detect changes in image intensity of a few percent [16]. Small amounts of motion can lead to changes of at least this magnitude. For example, consider an imaging sequence in which CSF is 100% brighter than grey matter. If, between two serial studies, the patient moves laterally by 0.1 of a sampling interval, voxels on the boundary between grey matter and CSF will experience a resulting change in partial volume effect. If the amount of CSF in the voxel increases by 10%, then the intensity of that voxel will increase by 5%. Such changes in partial volume effect at tissue boundaries can either mask signal changes resulting from blood oxygenation effects, or lead to "artefactual activations": signal changes that might be mistakenly interpreted as resulting from functional changes. For properly sampled data, these partial volume changes can be corrected using suitable interpolation kernels. Patient motion within a non-uniform B_0 or B_1 field can introduce further artefacts, as tissue moving relative to the magnetic field and RF coils will produce signal changes that cannot be corrected for simply by interpolation.

Patient motion that has a component through the slice plane can cause additional problems in multi-slice image sequences. Such through-slice motion can lead to tissue entering the slice that has not previously been excited in the same way as tissue in the slice plane (ie, the tissue has experienced a different "spin excitation history") [17]. Small volumes of particular tissues (eg: grey matter, white matter, CSF) moving into the slice in this way may contribute a different amount of signal to the identical volume of tissue they displace.

If the subject moves with a frequency unrelated to the frequency of the applied stimulus, then this motion can be separated from "true" activation because the period of the activation is known. The patient motion we measured, however, is strongly correlated with the applied stimulus, so its effects cannot be separated from functional effects by their period [18].

4.2 Brain deformation

There are numerous sources of error in making the comparison between electrode positions and corresponding positions in the functional MR data. The deformation in the brain surface we have observed for these patients can introduce errors of more than 10 mm in comparing the location of electrodes to structures and functional regions in the pre-operative images. Photographic methods for aligning the location of intraoperatively identified regions or electrodes have been used by other investigators [4,5]. These methods are potentially capable of correcting for any rigid body displacement or scale change in the position of the brain. The methods described are, however, unable to correct for deformations of the sort we have observed because they are not simply translational shifts, and the perspective geometry of the intraoperative photographs will introduce further errors that are hard to quantify.

There will be further difficulties in aligning pre-operative functional information from EPI MR images with either intra-operative or post-operative image coordinates because of distortion in the EPI images, which we have not quantified in this study. All these errors taken together make it hard to quantify the degree of agreements between modalities.

5 Conclusions

Using current processing techniques, we have found fMRI to be unsatisfactory for localisation of eloquent regions of the cortex in epilepsy neurosurgical patients who have lesions in the vicinity of their sensorimotor cortex. We believe this to be because these patients move more while carrying out motor tasks than other subjects investigated at our centre, and also because this motion tends to have a large component with the stimulus frequency. This is especially true when the subject is carrying out a task using the side of their brain ipsilateral to the lesion. We found substantial deformation in brain surface position between pre-operative MR imaging and post-implantation CT imaging. These brain shifts are of a similar magnitude to the intraoperative shifts recorded by other surgical centres in conventional neurosurgery [19–21]. This, together with possible EPI distortion, suggests that comparisons of the position of regions of activation seen on the fMRI study and the location of electrodes associated with the same functional task are subject to errors that can be in excess of 10mm. Errors of this magnitude are likely to be clinically significant for many types of surgical procedures, and makes it very difficult to accurately compare the location of electrophysiological measurements with the location of the corresponding blood flow changes measured by fMRI. Methods of comparison involving either post-operative CT, an intraoperative localiser, or intraoperative photographs will all be affected by these errors. Such measurements should, therefore, be interpreted with care, and, using current analysis techniques, are likely to be of limited use in the validation of fMRI protocols. We believe that substantial additional image analysis methodology needs to be developed and applied to these data before accurate comparison of fMRI and invasive electrophysiology can be performed.

References

1. C. R. Jack, R. Thompson, R. K. Butts, F. W. Sharbrough, P. Kelly, D. P. Hanson, S. J. Riederer, R. Ehman, N. J. Hangiandreou, and G. D. Cascino, "Sensory motor cortex: correlation of presurgical mapping with functional mr imaging and invasive cortical mapping," *Radiology*, vol. 190, pp. 85–92, 1994.
2. T. A. Yousry, U. D. Schmid, A. G. Jassoy, D. Schmidt, W. E. Eisner, H.-J. Reulen, M. F. Feiser, and L. J., "Topography of the cortical motor hand area: prospective study with functional mr imaging and direct motor mapping at surgery," *Radiology*, vol. 195, pp. 23–28, 1995.

3. A. Puce, R. T. Constable, M. L. Luby, G. McCarthy, A. C. Nobre, D. D. Spencer, J. Gore, and T. Allison, "Functional magnetic resonance imaging of sensory and motor cortex: comparison with electrophysiological localization," *J. Neurosurg.*, vol. 83, pp. 262–270, 1995.
4. F. Z. Yetkin, W. M. Mueller, G. L. Morris, T. L. McAuliffe, J. L. Ulmer, R. W. Cox, D. L. Daniels, and V. M. Haughton, "Functional mr activation correlated with intraoperative cortical mapping," *Am. J. Neuroradiol.*, vol. 18, pp. 1311–1315, 1997.
5. D. B. FitzGerald, G. R. Cosgrove, S. Ronner, H. Jiang, B. R. Buchbinder, J. W. Belliveau, B. R. Rosen, and R. R. Benson, "Location of language in the cortex: a comparison between functional mr imaging and electrocortical stimulation," *Am. J. Neuroradiol.*, vol. 18, pp. 1529–1539, 1997.
6. A. Simmons, E. Moore, and S. C. R. Williams, "Automated quality control for functional MRI studies," *Neuroimage*, vol. 5, p. S466, 1997.
7. D. L. G. Hill, D. J. Hawkes, C. Studholme, P. E. Summers, and M. G. Taylor, "Accurate registration and transformation of temporal image sequences," *Proc. Soc. Magn. Reson. 2nd Annual meeting*, p. 820, 1994.
8. E. Bullmore, M. Brammer, S. C. Williams, S. Rabe-Hesketh, N. Janot, A. David, J. Mellers, R. Howard, and P. Sham, "Statistical methods of estimation and inference for functional mr image analysis," *Magn. Reson. Med.*, pp. 261–277, 1996.
9. C. Studholme, D. L. G. Hill, and D. J. Hawkes, "Automated 3D registration of MR and CT images of the head," *Med. Image Anal.*, vol. 1, pp. 163–175, 1996.
10. J. West, J. M. Fitzpatrick, M. Y. Wang, B. M. Dawant, C. R. Maurer, Jr., R. M. Kessler, R. J. Maciunas, C. Barillot, D. Lemoine, A. Collignon, F. Maes, et al., "Comparison and evaluation of retrospective intermodality image registration techniques," *J. Comput. Assist. Tomogr.*, vol. 21, pp. 554–566, 1997.
11. J. M. Fitzpatrick, D. L. G. Hill, Y. Shyr, J. West, C. Studholme, and C. R. Maurer, Jr., "Visual assessment of the accuracy of retrospective registration of brain images," *IEEE Trans. Med. Imaging*, 1998 (in press).
12. J.-D. Boissonnat, "Shape reconstruction from planar cross-sections," *Comput. Vision Graph. Image Processing*, vol. 44, pp. 1–29, 1988.
13. A. Sahraie, L. Weiskrantz, J. L. Barbur, A. Simmons, S. C. Williams, and M. J. Brammer, "Pattern of neuronal activity associated with conscious and unconscious processing of visual signals," *Proceedings of the National Academy of Sciences of the United States of America*, vol. 94, pp. 9406–9411, 1997.
14. M. L. Phillips, A. W. Young, C. Senior, M. Brammer, C. Andrew, A. J. Calder, E. T. Bullmore, D. I. Perrett, D. Rowland, S. C. Williams, J. A. Gray, and A. S. David, "A specific neural substrate for perceiving facial expressions of disgust," *Nature*, vol. 389(6650), pp. 495–498, 1997.
15. G. A. Calvert, E. T. Bullmore, M. J. Brammer, R. Campell, S. C. Williams, P. K. McGuire, P. W. Woodruff, S. D. Iversen, and A. S. David, "Activation of auditory cortex during silent lipreading," *Science*, vol. 276(5312), pp. 593–596, 1997.
16. S. Ogawa, R. S. Menon, D. W. Tank, S. G. Kim, H. Merkle, J. M. Ellermann, and K. Ugurbil, "Functional brain mapping by blood oxygenation level-dependent contrast magnetic resonance imaging. a comparison of signal characteristics with a biophysical model," *Biophysical Journal*, vol. 64, pp. 803–812, 1993.
17. K. J. Friston, S. Williams, R. Howard, R. S. Frackowiak, and R. Turner, "Movement-related effects in fmri time-series," *Magn. Reson. Med.*, vol. 33, pp. 346–366, 1996.
18. J. V. Hajnal, R. Myers, A. Oatridge, J. E. Schwieso, I. R. Young, and G. M. Bydder, "Artifacts due to stimulus correlated motion in functional imaging of the brain," *Magn. Reson. Med.*, vol. 31, pp. 283–291, 1994.
19. D. L. G. Hill, C. R. Maurer, Jr., R. J. Maciunas, J. A. Barwise, J. M. Fitzpatrick, and M. Y. Wang, "Measurement of intraoperative brain surface deformation under a craniotomy," *Neurosurgery*, 1998 (in press).
20. N. L. Dorward, O. Alberti, B. Velani, F. A. Gerritsen, W. F. J. Harkness, N. D. Kitchen, and D. G. T. Thomas, "Postimaging brain distortion: Magnitude, correlates, and impact on neuronavigation," *J. Neurosurg.*, vol. 88, pp. 656–662, 1998.
21. R. D. Bucholz, D. D. Yeh, J. Trobaugh, L. L. McDurmont, C. D. Sturm, C. Baumann, J. M. Henderson, A. Levy, and P. Kessman, "The correction of stereotactic inaccuracy caused by brain shift using an intraoperative ultrasound device," in *CVRMed-MRCAS '97* (J. Troccaz, E. Grimson, and R. Mösges, eds.), pp. 459–466, Berlin: Springer-Verlag, 1997.

Specification, Modelling and Visualization of Arbitrarily Shaped Cut Surfaces in the Volume Model

B. Pflesser and U. Tiede and K.H. Höhne

Institute of Mathematics and Computer Science in Medicine (IMDM)
University-Hospital Eppendorf
Martinistraße 52, 20246 Hamburg, Germany
pflesser@uke.uni-hamburg.de

Abstract. So far, exploration of volume models is limited to cut planes or addition/removal of segmented objects. More capable exploration techniques are needed in order to allow a 'look and feel' close to a real dissection. This is especially important for applications like the simulation of osteotomy surgery. Therefore, we have developed methods for free-form volume-sculpting operations which allow the interactive specification, representation and high-quality rendering of free form regions. The novelty of this approach is that these regions are represented within the generalized-voxel-model, together with a simulation of the partial-volume-effect, which allows a sub-voxel localization of cut surfaces. These techniques are implemented in our VOXEL-MAN visualization system, thus enhancing the exploration techniques for volume data. Furthermore, we developed an extended ray-casting algorithm for 3D-visualization of object motion with detection and visualization of interpenetrating volumes. These methods together provide a powerful tool for volume exploration and applications like the rehearsal of surgical interventions.

1 Introduction

Systems for rehearsal and planning of surgical interventions are mostly based on traditional computer graphics methods where an object is represented by its surface only [4, 5, 9]. Often, these approaches concentrate on deformation techniques rather than cutting operations. For the specification of cuts, it is necessary to generate a new polygonal representation of cut regions. Therefore interactive specification tools are limited to basic techniques like cut planes and can not provide the 'look and feel' close to a real dissection. Furthermore, these approaches suffer from the lack of information about the interior of an object.

Several applications for object manipulation have been suggested that are based on the binary-voxel-model [16], which certainly does not overcome the limitation of surface based methods. The specification of arbitrarily shaped objects within the gray-level-volume model is a less developed subject. Some approaches have been presented by [1, 17]. However, these applications do not provide flexible dissection tools or proper visualization methods for cut surfaces. In a first approach [7], we have developed a method for free form cutting based on gray level modification. This method provided a fairly good visualization of cut surfaces but proved to be not flexible enough for complex interactive cutting operations.

Therefore, we wanted to establish free form operations in the VOXEL-MAN volume visualization system [11, 13] which already provides a set of tools for object manipulation in a volume representation. For example, objects defined in a previous segmentation step may be removed or added like in an assembly kit, or arbitrary cut planes may be specified.

In order to enhance the potential of these techniques, the following qualitites are required for methods of specification, representation and visualization of free-form cut regions:

- Representation of cut regions with preservation of object information.
- Sub-voxel modelling of cut surfaces (position, shape and surface normals)
- Interactive and flexible cutting tools.
- High-quality visualization of cut regions with preservation of object surfaces.

2 Method

2.1 Modelling of Cut Regions

Attribute Level. Within the VOXEL-MAN system anatomical objects are described using a two level data structure [3]. The lower level is a discrete data volume, as obtained from a medical imaging system. In addition, a set of attributes is assigned to every voxel, indicating its membership to anatomical regions under various aspects (e.g. morphology, functional anatomy). This level is equivalent to the previously described generalized voxel model [2]. On the upper level, objects and their relations are described symbolically [8].

For achieving the new functionality of representing arbitrarily formed cut-out regions within the generalized voxel model, we are using an additional voxel attribute. In contrast to other attributes, this kind of information is not static but subject to changes during the interactive specification process. By computing a table of all possible occurences of attribute combinations, it is possible to represent cut out regions without an additional label volume, thus minimizing memory requirements. This way, the original object information is available at any point of a cut-out region, and all operations can easily be reversed.

Data Level. Apparently, voxel attributes are limited to the resolution of the underlying data volume and do not provide means for a proper visualization of cut surfaces. An accurate estimation of surface normals is needed to visualize 3D-objects. For rendering surfaces in tomographic volume data the gray-level-gradient method has proven to be accurate. Therefore, we model cut surfaces within a data volume where the partial-volume-effect, which is the prerequisite for the gray-level-gradient method, is calculated as it would be generated by an imaging system. This way, the gray-level-gradient method which provides an accurate determination of the surface shape can be applied for visualization of arbitrarily shaped cut surfaces. Furthermore, the determination of the position of a surface point can be achieved within sub-voxel resolution, so that the decision of whether an object has been cut or not is very accurate.

2.2 Specification

Interactive Tools. The specification of 3D-areas within a data volume in the context of perspective 2D-images is not achieved easily. By utilizing the known image transformation an interactive tool can be moved arbitrarily in 3D-space (position and direction) and can be projected to image-space. The tip of such a tool can be defined in many ways, allowing the imitation of different instruments like a scalpel or a laser beam:

- Shape:
    - Geometrical representations, e.g. cuboid, ellipsoid, cylinder.
    - Polygonal models.
- Size and direction (relatively to direction of tool).
- "Sensibility": Which objects can be affected by an instrument?
- "Roughness": The modelling of the cut surface can be parameterized.

This tool kit provides very flexible methods for the specification of free-form regions within the volume model:

- Larger regions for the "in depth" exploration of the model.
- Gradual cutting with smaller instruments ("scalpel").
- Section anatomical parts.

Modelling of Cut Surfaces. Once shape and position of a tool have been specified, the voxel inside the tool can easily be determined and therefore be labeled. For an accurate representation of the tool shape in the data volume, it is necessary to estimate the partial-volume-effects on the surface very accurately. This can be achieved by calculating the percentage of a given sample region, which is covered by the tool tip. Since the tool tip is geometrically or polygonally represented, it can easily be determined whether a sample point lies inside the tool or not (Fig. 1, left). Whenever this sampling process results in a gray value which satifies the threshold definition of the cut region, the voxel has to be labeled.

Especially for gradual cutting with a "scalpel"-like tool, it is important to preserve existing cut surfaces. Therefore, it is not sufficient to resample only the tool. Also the amount of an existing cut region which is unaffected by the new cutting has to be determined (Fig. 1, right). Since the geometry and position of the tool which generated these cut surfaces are no longer known, the region has to be resampled by gray-level interpolation. The decision of whether a sample point is inside the cut region or not, is then made by the threshold definition specified for the cut region.

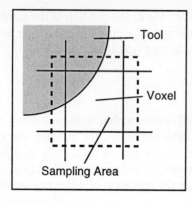 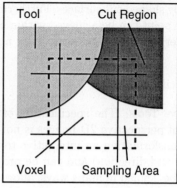

Fig. 1. Resampling of tool geometry for partial-volume-effect estimation (left). Resampling with preservation of existing cut surfaces (right).

2.3 Visualization

For rendering surfaces in tomographic volume data the gray-level-gradient method [14] has proven to be accurate. However, when visualizing a surface where a cut region has been removed, this method can not be used directly, because gray-level differences inside an object are not related to a surface. On the other hand the cut region itself is represented as an "artificial" object and the visualization of its surface would e.g. lack the morphological information. Therefore we extended the visualization algorithm in such a way that the morphological information and the information about cut surfaces are combined. Obviously it is not sufficient to make this combination with label information only. Rather, for each sample point during the ray casting process, the surfaces of morphological objects as well as cut surfaces have to be determined at subvoxel resolution. Both the morphological objects and cut-out regions are represented in the generalized-voxel-model with partial-volume-effects. Hence the position of the surfaces can be determined precisely with gray-level-interpolation using thresholding, and the surface normal estimation at this position can be calculated using the gray-level-gradient method [15].

The key point here is to detect if a cut surface really truncates an object or if the object has not been affected by a cutting operation. The situation is clear when only a cut surface has been detected. In this case the object should be visualized using the cut surface information. When multiple surfaces have been found between successive sample points we must determine which surface should be used.

The situation of multiple surfaces can occur when:

- an object has been cut close to its surface
- an object has been uncovered by a selective cutting operation

In both cases the information about the location of the surfaces is not sufficient to determine which surface should be visualized. Therefore we developed a method of adaptive sampling: Fig. 2, left, shows an example of this situation. At the sample position $s2$ an object which has been truncated by a cut region has been found. Between the successive sample points $s1$ and $s2$ we calculate the surface boundaries of the object and the cut region. Without the information which object is located between these surfaces the decision which surface (or any surface at all) should be visualized can not be made. Therefore we generate an additional sample point ($s3$) between the surface boundaries. In this case, the object is located at $s3$, so it is visualized using its "original" surface.

Fig. 2, right, shows the situation where an object has been uncovered partly by a selective cutting operation. Clearly this part of the object should be visualized with its "original" surface. This situation can not be solved by adaptive sampling only because the cut region produces an "artificial" surface which should not be used for visualization. Hence the information about the objects to which a cutting operation is restricted is used during the ray casting process and a cut surface which affects a "forbidden" object is ignored.

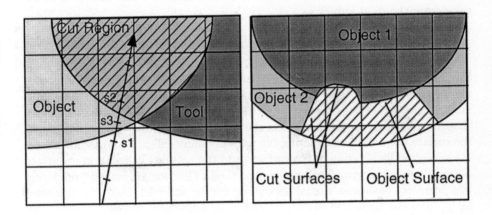

Fig. 2. Situation with multiple surfaces.
Left: an object has been cut close to its surface. With the method of adaptive sampling (sample point $s3$ between the surfaces) it can be decided that the object is to be visualized with its "original" surface. Right: an object has been uncovered partly by a selective cutting operation. Since the cut operation has been restricted to object 2 the "artifical" cut surface close to object 1 is ignored and the object surface is used for visualization.

For applications like the simulation of osteotomy surgery the visualization of object motion is needed. Therefore we developed an extension of our ray casting algorithm (ray compositing) which allows the movement of objects in the volume model. A detailed description of this algorithm can be found in [6].

3 Results

Figure 3 demonstrates some of the capabilities of the described method. In the upper left image parts of soft tissue and bone have been resected and an interactively specified ellipsoid-shaped region has been removed. It can be seen that the surface normal estimation on the "artifical" cut surfaces is very accurate. The upper right image shows the simulation of an osteotomy. The blue lines indicate the planning of the osteotomy and show the principle of the "scalpel"-like specification method. A part of the frontal bone (a region which is limited by a closed contour) has been resected and moved forward.

Since modelling and representation of cut surfaces is independent from the representation of the anatomical objects, our method can be applied identically to the data of the Visible Human Project^{TM} [12]. Figure 3, lower left, shows how the anatomy of the visual system can be explored within the context of surrounding structures by specifying a cut region where the eyes, optic tracts and optic muscles have been excluded from the operation. The lower right image demonstrates the simulation of an anatomical dissection. The abdomen have been opened and parts of the large and small bowels have been removed in order to uncover the right kidney.

4 Conclusion

The novel approach presented in this paper provides powerful exploration techniques as well as the basis for simulation of surgical interventions in the voxel-model which could not be achieved with any surface-based method. Arbitrarily shaped cut regions are represented in the volume model with proper modelling of the surface normals via simulating the partial-volume-effect. This method allows the sub-voxel localization of cut surfaces and the accurate calculation of surface normals using the gray-level-gradient method. This way, a realistic rendering which greatly facilitates spatial perception can be achieved. Since the representation of a cut surface is iteratively modified, arbitrarily complex surfaces can be modelled, which can not be achieved by surface based representations. We have implemented a wide range of flexible and interactive specification tools, as needed for surgical simulation. In combination with the technique for simulation of object movement, these methods create a capable tool kit for applications in the field of planning and rehearsal of surgical interventions.

For the future, one exciting field will be the combination of this approach with methods for elastic object deformation, also implemented in the VOXEL-MAN environment [10]. This way, applications may be extended to a more realistic handling of soft tissue as well.

References

1. Arridge, S. R.: Manipulation of Volume Data for Surgical Simulation. In Höhne, K. H. et al. (Eds.): 3D-Imaging in Medicine: Algorithms, Systems, Applications, NATO ASI Series F 60, Springer-Verlag, Berlin, 1990, 289–300.

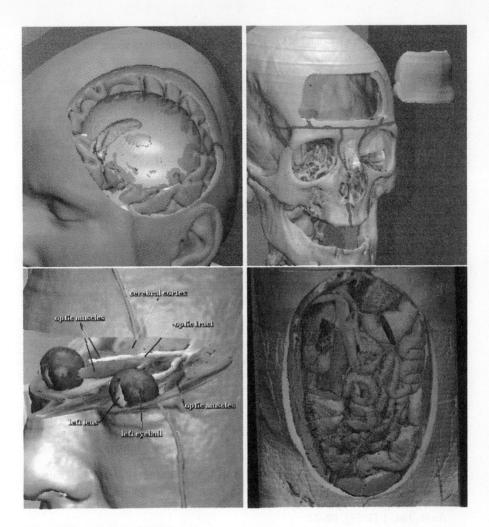

Fig. 3. Visualization of Cut Surfaces:
Upper left: Parts of soft tissue and bone have been resected and the model have been further explored "in depth" by removal of an ellipsoid shape.
Upper right: Simulation of craniofacial surgery. The blue lines represent the planning of the operation and a part of the frontal bone has been removed using a "scalpel".
Lower left: The extended exploration possibilities are demonstrated with data from the Visible Human Project. The eyes, optic tract and optic muscles have been uncovered by removal of an ellipsoidal region.
Lower right: This image demonstrates the simulation of an anatomical dissection. The abdomen have been opened and parts of the large and small bowel have been removed in order to uncover the right kidney.
Note: The smooth appearance of the cut surfaces is achieved by our new method which simulates the partial-volume-effect.

2. Höhne, K. H., Bomans, M., Pommert, A., Riemer, M., Schiers, C., Tiede, U., Wiebecke, G.: 3D-visualization of tomographic volume data using the generalized voxel-model. Visual Comput. 6, 1 (1990), 28–36.
3. Höhne, K. H., Bomans, M., Riemer, M., Schubert, R., Tiede, U., Lierse, W.: A 3D anatomical atlas based on a volume model. IEEE Comput. Graphics Appl. 12, 4 (1992), 72–78.
4. Keeve, E., Girod, S., Girod, B.: Craniofacial Surgery Simulation. In Höhne, K. H., Kikinis, R. (Eds.): Visualization in Biomedical Computing, Proc. VBC '96, Lecture Notes in Computer Science 1131, Springer-Verlag, Berlin, 1996, 541–546.
5. Koch, R. M., Gross, M. H., Carls, F. R., von Büren, D. F., Fankhauser, G., Parish, Y. I. H.: Simulating facial surgery using finite element models. In Proc. SIGGRAPH 96. New Orleans, LA, 1996, 421–428.
6. Pflesser, B., Tiede, U., Höhne, K. H.: Simulating motion of anatomical objects with volume-based 3D-visualization. In Robb, R. A. (Ed.): Visualization in Biomedical Computing 1994, Proc. SPIE 2359. Rochester, MN, 1994, 291–300.
7. Pflesser, B., Tiede, U., Höhne, K. H.: Towards realistic visualization for surgery rehearsal. In Ayache, N. (Ed.): Computer Vision, Virtual Reality and Robotics in Medicine, Proc. CVRMed '95, Lecture Notes in Computer Science 905, Springer-Verlag, Berlin, 1995, 487–491.
8. Pommert, A., Schubert, R., Riemer, M., Schiemann, T., Tiede, U., Höhne, K. H.: Symbolic modeling of human anatomy for visualization and simulation. In Robb, R. A. (Ed.): Visualization in Biomedical Computing 1994, Proc. SPIE 2359. Rochester, MN, 1994, 412–423.
9. Reinig, K., Spitzer, V., Pelster, H., Johnson, T., Mahalik, T.: More Real-Time Visual and Haptic Interaction with Anatomical Data. In Morgan, K. et al. (Eds.): Medicine Meets Virtual Reality: Global Healthcare Grid, MMVR'97, Studies in Health Technology and Informatics 39, IOS Press, Amsterdam, 1997, 155–158.
10. Schiemann, T., Höhne, K. H.: Definition of volume transformations for volume interaction. In Duncan, J., Gindi, G. (Eds.): Information Processing in Medical Imaging, Proc. IPMI '97, Lecture Notes in Computer Science 1230, Springer-Verlag, Berlin, 1997, 245–258.
11. Schubert, R., Höhne, K. H., Pommert, A., Riemer, M., Schiemann, T., Tiede, U., Lierse, W.: A new method for practicing exploration, dissection, and simulation with a complete computerized three-dimensional model of the brain and skull. Acta Anat. 150, 1 (1994), 69–74.
12. Spitzer, V., Ackerman, M. J., Scherzinger, A. L., Whitlock, D.: The Visible Human male: A technical report. J. Am. Med. Inf. Ass. 3, 2 (1996), 118–130.
13. Tiede, U., Bomans, M., Höhne, K. H., Pommert, A., Riemer, M., Schiemann, T., Schubert, R., Lierse, W.: A computerized three-dimensional atlas of the human skull and brain. Am. J. Neuroradiology 14, 3 (1993), 551–559.
14. Tiede, U., Höhne, K. H., Bomans, M., Pommert, A., Riemer, M., Wiebecke, G.: Investigation of medical 3D-rendering algorithms. IEEE Comput. Graphics Appl. 10, 2 (1990), 41–53.
15. Tiede, U., Schiemann, T., Höhne, K. H.: High quality rendering of attributed volume data. In Proc. IEEE Visualization '98, IEEE Computer Society Press, 1998. (accepted for publication).
16. Udupa, J. K., Odhner, D.: Fast visualization, manipulation and analysis of binary volumetric objects. IEEE Comput. Graphics Appl. 11, 6 (1991), 53–62.
17. Yasuda, T., Hashimoto, Y., Yokoi, S., Toriwaki, J.-I.: Computer system for craniofacial surgical planning based on CT images. IEEE Trans. Med. Imaging MI-9, 3 (1990), 270–280.

An Object-Based Volumetric Deformable Atlas for the Improved Localization of Neuroanatomy in MR Images

Tim McInerney[1,2] and Ron Kikinis[3]

[1] University of Toronto, Toronto, ON, Canada M5S 3H5
[2] Massachusetts Institute of Technology, Cambridge, MA 02139, USA
[3] Harvard Medical School, Boston MA 02115, USA

Abstract. We present a hierarchical object–based deformable atlas, a promising new approach for the automatic localization and quantitative analysis of neuroanatomy in MR images. The 3D finite element-based elastic atlas combines the advantages of both volumetric– and surface–based deformable atlases in one single unifying framework. This multi-resolution framework is not only capable of deforming entire volumes or subvolumes but can deform individual atlas objects, allowing greater and more effective use of object shape and local image feature information. Object surface representations are embedded in the volumetric deformable atlas and image-feature-derived forces acting on these surfaces are automatically transferred to the containing 3D finite element lattice. Consequently, spatial relationship constraints of the atlas objects are maintained via the elastic lattice while an object is deformed to match a target boundary. Atlas objects are deformed in a hierarchical fashion, begining with objects exhibiting well-defined image features in the target scan and proceeding to objects with slightly less well-defined features. Experiments involving several subcortical atlas objects are presented.

1 Introduction

The automatic localization of neuroanatomy in MR images and the subsequent quantitative analysis using 3D elastically deformable atlases is gaining increased attention in medical imaging research [10, 11, 6, 3, 12, 5, 8, 13, 7]. These model-based techniques can dramatically decrease the time required for the localization task over interactive methods as well as improve the objectivity, reproducibility, and, potentially, the accuracy of the localization. A fitted anatomical atlas can then be used as a fundamental component for the assessment of structural brain abnormalities, for mapping functional activation of the brain onto the corresponding anatomy, and for computer-assisted neurosurgery.

There are essentially two approaches to deformable atlas matching: volumetric–based and surface–based. While both approaches offer a powerful strategy for efficient localization and analysis, they suffer from several well-known deficiencies affecting the accuracy of the localization. Volumetric approaches maintain the spatial relationships of the atlas objects implicitly via the elastic medium in which they are embedded. However, these methods are sensitive to their initial placement – if the initial rigid alignment is off by too much, parts of the atlas may incorrectly warp onto the boundaries of neighboring features. This problem is exacerbated by the fact that volumetric methods discard the shape information of each atlas object and use only local intensity variations between the atlas and the target scan to drive the matching process.

Surface-based methods typically manually initialize several parametrically defined deformable surfaces – each representing a different neuroanatomical structure – and subsequently elastically deform the surfaces to extract the shapes of the target object boundaries. Each atlas object surface and its corresponding deformed surface in the target scan are then matched to produce surface warping functions. Using this surface warping information, a volumetric warp can be calculated via interpolation to deform the atlas material between the surfaces and register it with the target scan. One problem with this approach is that the surfaces are warped independently - the spatial relationship constraints provided by the elastic medium in the volumetric approach are initially discarded. Furthermore, if generic deformable surfaces are used — that do not make use of the known atlas object shape— then pieces of the object in the target scan could be missed by the deformable surface due to poor resolution or noise.

In this paper, we describe a new hierarchical object-based deformable atlas that combines the advantages of both the volumetric and surface based models in one unifying framework. The multi-resolution framework is not only capable of deforming entire volumes or subvolumes but can deform individual atlas objects and make use of image feature knowledge of an object. By embedding smooth surface representations of atlas objects into the finite element-based volumetric deformable atlas, image-feature-derived forces acting on these surfaces are automatically transferred to the surrounding volumetric finite elements. The subsequent deformation of the elements automatically deforms the embedded surfaces. Consequently, we maintain the spatial relationship constraints of the atlas objects via the elastic "medium" while also making use of shape and intensity information of each object. The atlas is deformed in a hierarchical fashion, beginning with an initial rigid alignment and elastic match over the entire volume. We then warp individual atlas objects and the surrounding volume in a specified neighborhood, starting with objects exhibiting well-defined image features in the target scan (such as the lateral ventricles), and then proceeding to objects with slightly less well-defined image features, and so on.

The motivation behind our approach is that while the standard volumetric deformable atlas approach can provide an automatic, efficient and good "overall" match of the atlas, there are still mismatches in individual atlas objects that can only be corrected by adjusting the object itself. At the same time, this "fine–tuning" should maintain and use the correct spatial relationships of neighboring objects. In the remainder of the paper, we will first describe an initial implementation of our model and then present some preliminary results using several subcortical structures to demonstrate the potential of this promising new approach.

2 Deformable Atlases

The idea behind a deformable anatomical atlas is to take the information contained in the atlas (typically a set of labeled voxels where the labels correspond to anatomical structures) and transfer this information onto the target dataset via a nonlinear warping function. To perform the warp, the atlas is typically modeled as a physical object and is given elastic properties. After an initial global alignment, the atlas deforms and matches itself onto corresponding regions in the brain image volume in response to forces derived from image features such as voxel similarity or image edges. To maintain the atlas topology and connectivity, the elastic properties of the atlas give rise to internal forces which regularize the deformation. The assumption underlying this approach is that at some representational level, normal brains have the same topological structure and differ only in shape details.

The idea of modeling the atlas as an elastic object was originated by Broit [4]. Bajcsy and Kovacic [1] subsequently implemented a multiresolution version of Broit's system where the deformation of the atlas proceeds step-by-step in a coarse to fine strategy, improving the robustness of the technique. The elastically deformable volume approach has become a very active area of research [10, 11, 6, 3, 7], and has recently been extended to a viscous fluid deformable volume [6] in an attempt to overcome the small deformation assumptions inherent in the linear elastic formulations. Although surface based deformable models have been widely used to segment medical images, surface-based deformable brain atlases are a more recent development [12, 5, 8, 13].

3 Hierarchical Object-based Deformable Atlas

Our model combines the advantages of the volumetric and surface based methods by integrating both approaches into one framework. This hybrid model embeds the surface of atlas objects into the solid deformable finite element mesh or lattice representing the elastic atlas. The result is that the deformation of atlas objects can be controlled individually or in combination while automatically maintaining the spatial relationships of each object via the elastic lattice. The model also has other distinct advantages:

- Multiple object-based image features can be used to attract an atlas object towards its boundary in the image. For example, known image intensity statistics of individual objects and *neighboring objects* can be used to weight a pressure force, driving the model towards salient boundary edges.
- Computing forces on the object surface and distributing these forces to the volumetric finite elements results in an accurate deformation of the object without discarding the contextual knowledge of the neighboring objects. The displacements of the deformed object are automatically passed on to the neighbors through the surrounding elastic lattice, resulting in improved localization of these objects. In addition, several neighboring objects can be

deformed concurrently in which case each object "competes" for the ownership of image features.
- The atlas is initially deformed over its entire volume to provide a good initialization of each atlas object. Atlas objects can be then deformed in a hierarchical fashion - from objects exhibiting very well-defined image features to objects with weaker features. After an object has been deformed we compute forces on it to maintain its equilibrium position. This acts to constrain the deformation of neighboring objects with adjacent boundaries (and less well-defined image features).
- The material properties of the 3D finite elements can be controlled on an object basis. Each object can use predefined elastic properties based on knowledge of the amount of deformation that typically will take place. If very large deformations are required an object can be deformed in phases, using coarse and rigid finite element meshes in initial phases and using finer, more flexible meshes in subsequent phases.

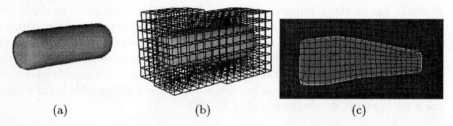

(a) (b) (c)

Fig. 1. (a) Synthetic object surface, (b) surface embedded in elastic 3D lattice, (c) cross-sectional view of deformed lattice and surface (surface: white, lattice: black, target data: gray).

3.1 Model Structure

We construct our object-based elastic atlas using a deformable 3D lattice or grid consisting of cubical finite elements. Each finite element corresponds to a labeled atlas voxel (or group of voxels). To deform a specified atlas object, we reconstruct a smooth triangulated surface of the object from the atlas using a modified marching cubes algorithm (Figure 1(a)). For each surface vertex, we compute its containing cubical element (Figure 1(b)) and the relative position of the vertex within the element. Image feature forces are calculated for each vertex and are then distributed to the nodes of the containing finite elements using the element basis (interpolation) functions. The elastic elements are then deformed and the nodal displacements calculated (Figure 1(c)). The new positions of the surface vertices are then computed based on their relative positions within their containing cubical element and the displacement of the element nodes. This process is repeated for a specified number of iterations.

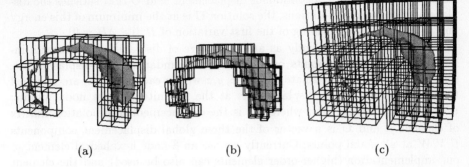

(a) (b) (c)

Fig. 2. Surface of caudate nucleus embedded in finite element mesh, (a) element *size*: 8 voxels, *e*lement *l*ayers: 1, (b) es: 4, el: 1, (c) es: 8, el: 2.

The lattice of cubical elements surrounding an atlas object can be controlled in a number of ways (Figure 2) by varying the element size, the number of element layers surrounding the object, and the element material properties.

3.2 Finite Element Implementation

The elastically deformable lattice model is implemented using the displacement-based finite element method. A brief description of this method for linear elastic bodies is provided below. Readers are referred to [2] for complete details.

In the displacement-based finite element method, a three dimensional body is located in a fixed coordinate system $\mathbf{X} = [X, Y, Z]^\mathsf{T}$. The body is subjected to externally applied forces:

$$\mathbf{f}^B = [f^B_x \; f^B_y \; f^B_y]^\mathsf{T}, \; \mathbf{f}^S = [f^S_x \; f^S_y \; f^S_z]^\mathsf{T}, \; \mathbf{F}^i = [F_{x_i} \; F_{y_i} \; F_{z_i}]^\mathsf{T} \quad (1)$$

where $\mathbf{f}^B$ are the body forces (force per unit volume), $\mathbf{f}^S$ are the surface traction forces (force per unit area), and $\mathbf{F}^i$ are the concentrated forces (i denotes the point of force application) due to attachments. The displacements of the body from the unloaded configuration are measured in the coordinate system $\mathbf{X}$ and are denoted by $\mathbf{U}(X, Y, Z) = [UVW]^\mathsf{T}$. The strains corresponding to $\mathbf{U}$ are:

$$\boldsymbol{\epsilon}^\mathsf{T} = \left[\frac{\partial U}{\partial X}, \frac{\partial V}{\partial Y}, \frac{\partial W}{\partial Z}, \frac{\partial U}{\partial Y} + \frac{\partial V}{\partial X}, \frac{\partial V}{\partial Z} + \frac{\partial W}{\partial Y}, \frac{\partial W}{\partial X} + \frac{\partial U}{\partial Z} \right]^\mathsf{T}, \quad (2)$$

the corresponding stresses are denoted $\boldsymbol{\tau}^\mathsf{T} = [\tau_{XX} \; \tau_{YY} \; \tau_{ZZ} \; \tau_{XY} \; \tau_{YZ} \; \tau_{ZX}]$, and finally the stress-strain relationship for a linear elastic body is given by $\boldsymbol{\tau} = \mathbf{D}\boldsymbol{\epsilon}$, where $\mathbf{D}$ is the stress-strain material matrix (the elastic coefficients).

Assuming a linear elastic continuum with zero initial stresses, the total potential energy of the body can be written as

$$\Pi(\mathbf{U}) = \frac{1}{2} \iint_V \boldsymbol{\epsilon}^\mathsf{T} \mathbf{D} \boldsymbol{\epsilon} \, dV - \iint_V \mathbf{U}^\mathsf{T} \mathbf{f}^B \, dV - \iint_S \mathbf{U}^{S\mathsf{T}} \mathbf{f}^S \, dS - \sum_i \mathbf{U}^{i\mathsf{T}} \mathbf{F}^i. \quad (3)$$

Assuming, furthermore, a continuous displacement field $\mathbf{U}$ that satisfies the displacement boundary conditions, the solution $\mathbf{U}$ is at the minimum of this energy and is found at the vanishing of the first variation of Π (i.e. $\delta \Pi = 0$).

We approximate the body as an assemblage of discrete finite elements interconnected at nodal points on the element boundaries. The displacements, measured in a local coordinate system x, y, z within each element, are assumed to be a function of the displacements at the N finite element nodal points: $\mathbf{u}^j(x, y, z) = \mathbf{H}^j(x, y, z)\hat{\mathbf{U}}$, where $\mathbf{H}^j$ is the displacement interpolation matrix of element j, and $\hat{\mathbf{U}}$ is a vector of the three global displacement components U, V, W at all nodal points. Currently we use an 8-node hexahedral element in our implementation (higher-order elements can also be used) and the element interpolation functions are specified in [2].

One typically calculates all element matrices using only element nodal displacements and the corresponding nonzero components of $\mathbf{H}^j$ for element j so that: $\mathbf{u}^j = \mathbf{N}^j \hat{\mathbf{u}}^j$, where $\hat{\mathbf{u}}^j$ and $\mathbf{N}^j$ are the element nodal displacements and basis functions, respectively. Using equations (2) and the stress-strain relationship, we can then evaluate the element strains as, $\epsilon^j = \mathbf{B}^j \hat{\mathbf{u}}^j$, where $\mathbf{B}^j$ is obtained by differentiating the components of $\mathbf{N}^j$. Using these two equations, the potential energy (3) can be rewritten in terms of its elemental contributions and subsequently minimized on an element-by-element basis:

$$\Pi = \sum_j \Pi^j(\mathbf{u}) = \sum_j \left\{ \frac{1}{2} \iint_{V^j} \hat{\mathbf{u}}^{j\mathsf{T}} \mathbf{B}^{j\mathsf{T}} \mathbf{D}^j \mathbf{B}^j \hat{\mathbf{u}}^j \, dV \right. \\ \left. - \iint_{V^j} \hat{\mathbf{u}}^{j\mathsf{T}} \mathbf{N}^j \mathbf{f}^{B(j)} \, dV - \iint_{S^j} \hat{\mathbf{u}}^{j\mathsf{T}} \mathbf{N}^j \mathbf{f}^{S(j)} \, dS - \sum_i \hat{\mathbf{u}}_i^{j\mathsf{T}} \mathbf{N}^j \mathbf{F}_i^j \right\}. \quad (4)$$

Solving for the first variation of Π leads to the equilbrium equation $\frac{\partial \Pi^j}{\partial \hat{\mathbf{u}}^j} = \mathbf{K}^j \hat{\mathbf{u}}^j - \mathbf{f}^j$, where $\mathbf{K}^j$ and $\mathbf{f}^j$ are the element stiffnes and load matrices, respectively. We introduce a simple velocity-proportional damping force and rewrite the equibrium equations as $\mathbf{C}^j \frac{d\hat{\mathbf{u}}^j}{dt} + \mathbf{K}^j \hat{\mathbf{u}}^j = \mathbf{f}^j$, where $\mathbf{C}^j$ is a diagonalized damping matrix with velocity damping coeficients γ along the main diagonal. We currently integrate this equation forward through time using an explicit first-order Euler method on an element-by-element basis, making the model fitting process efficient and easily parallelizable.

An isotropic linear elastic material is characterized by the Lamé constants, λ and μ. These constants are also related to Young's modulus of elasticity E and Poisson's ratio ν:

$$E = \frac{\mu(2\mu + 3\lambda)}{\mu + \lambda}, \quad \nu = \frac{\lambda}{2(\mu + \lambda)}, \quad (5)$$

where E relates tension of the object and its stretch in the longitudinal direction and ν is the ratio of lateral contraction to longitudinal stretch. We typically set λ to zero and allow E to range from 0.25 to 0.75, producing a range of stable elastic behavior from relatively stretchy to relatively rigid.

3.3 Applied Forces

As mentioned earlier, forces are computed for each of the surface vertices and are then distributed to the 8 nodes of the containing element using the element shape functions $\mathbf{N}^j$. We use a weighted pressure force, where the weights are derived from precomputed atlas object intensity statistics, to deform the object surface:

$$F(I(\mathbf{x}_i)) = +1, \ |I(\mathbf{x}_i) - \mu| \leq k\sigma, \quad F(I(\mathbf{x}_i)) = -1, \ |I(\mathbf{x}_i) - \mu| > k\sigma, \quad (6)$$

where μ is the mean image intensity of the target object, σ the standard deviation of the object intensity and k is a user defined constant.

We also use a functional F based on intensity gradients computed along a surface vertex normal. It is often the case that the intensity of an object varys considerably over its extent, limiting the usefulness of functionals based on absolute image statistics. However, the intensity gradients between an object and its neighbors is often fairly consistent when computed over a large enough surface region surrounding a surface vertex:

$$F(I(\mathbf{x}_i)) = -1, \ |\nabla I(\mathbf{x}_i) \cdot \mathbf{n}_i| >= C, \quad F(I(\mathbf{x}_i)) = +1, \ |\nabla I(\mathbf{x}_i) \cdot \mathbf{n}_i| < C, \quad (7)$$

where C is the known average difference in intensity between two objects. The signs are reversed in the functional if C is negative.

4 Experiments

The deformable atlas is based on an MR brain atlas developed in our laboratory [9]. To match the atlas to the target MRI scan, we first apply a rigid registration to the atlas followed by a generic volumetric elastic match [7] to initially deform the atlas and provide good initial positions of atlas objects [1]. We then use the deformed atlas to generate smooth surfaces of objects and apply our model to deform the objects.

We have used our technique in a set of preliminary experiments to deform several subcortical structures and match them onto a target MRI scan. Although the technique has not yet been validated with a large number of datasets, the results of our experiments are extremely promising - the model appears robust to noise and in regions containing sufficient image feature information, generates visually accurate results. In these preliminary experiments, we use a merged left and right lateral ventricle, the left and right caudate nucleus, the corpus callosum, and the left and right putamen. Two deformation phases were used with 30 steps in the first phase and an element size of 4 voxels and 30 steps in the second with an element size of 2 voxels. This unoptimized version of our system is still quite efficient and each deformation step takes from 1 to 10 seconds (depending on the number of objects deformed concurrently and the number of elements). In the first experiment we deform the merged lateral ventricles, the

---

[1] Although a separate elastic matching program is currently used to initially deform the atlas, we will eventually incorporate this stage into our model framework.

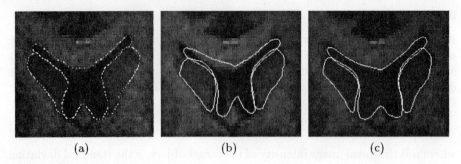

Fig. 3. (a) Manual tracing of left and right caudate nucleus and merged left and right lateral ventricle for slice 72, (b), (c) cross-section of initial and deformed surfaces.

left and right caudate nucleus and the surrounding volume (4 element layers are used). A significant segmentation improvement is obtained (figure 3(b, c)). In the second example, we deform the right putamen (Figure 4(a)(b)). The image intensity of the putamen varys considerably over its extent and its boundary is very noisy. For this reason, we integrate image feature information over a surface region centered at each surface vertex and then average this information to compute more reliable applied forces. In the final experiment we deform the corpus callosum (Figure 4(c)(d)). The strong edge features of this object results in a very accurate localization near the center of the object.

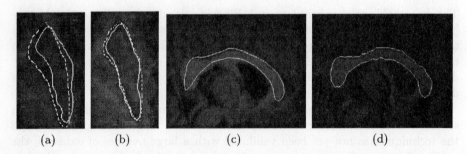

Fig. 4. Cross-section of initial and deformed surface of (a)(b) right putamen, (c) (d) corpus callosum. The dashed line in (a)(b) is a manual tracing.

5 Conclusion

We have created a 3D finite element-based object-oriented model to control the elastic deformation of a neuroanatomical atlas. The model framework provides us with the ability to deform not only the entire atlas or subvolumes of the atlas, but individual objects, separately or in combination. This ability allows us to accurately localize neuroanatomical structures in a target scan. The model has demonstrated considerable potential in preliminary experiments. We are currently applying our model to a large number of datasets to validate its effectiveness. We are also exploring several model improvements with the goal of creating a single unified framework for the precise control of atlas deformation, ranging from the elastic deformation of deep subcortical structures, to a constrained viscoelastic deformation of the cortical surface. In particular, we intend to replace the cubical mesh lattice with a 3D finite element mesh that conforms to the geometry of each atlas object. The goal is to generate an axial-based or skeleton-based object parameterization so that the shape of an object can be constrained to maintain a feasible shape and its deformation can be controlled in a scheduled, global-to-local manner. This will allow us to make optimal use of object shape, symmetry, and image feature information.

References

1. R. Bajcsy and S. Kovacic. Multiresolution elastic matching. *Computer Vision, Graphics, and Image Processing*, 46:1–21, 1989.
2. K.J. Bathe. *Finite Element Procedures*. Prentice Hall, 1996.
3. F.L. Bookstein. Thin-plate splines and the atlas problem for biomedical images. In *Information Processing in Medical Imaging: Proc. 12th Int. Conf. (IPMI'91), Wye, UK, July*, pages 326–342, 1991.
4. C. Broit. *Optimal Registration of Deformed Images*. PhD thesis, Computer and Information Science Dept., University of Pennsylvania, Philadelphia, PA, 1981.
5. C.A. Davatzikos, J.L. Prince, and R.N. Bryan. Image registration based on boundary mapping. *IEEE Trans. on Medical Imaging*, 15(1):112–115, Feb. 1996.
6. G. Christensen et al. Deformable templates using large deformation kinematics. *IEEE Transactions on Image Processing*, Sept. 1996.
7. Iosifescu et al. An automated measurement of subcortical brain mr structures in schizophrenia. *Neuroimage*, 6:13–25, 1997.
8. J.W. Snell et al. Model-based boundary estimation of complex objects using hierarchical active surface templates. *Pattern Recognition*, 28(10):1599–1609, 1995.
9. R. Kikinis et al. A digital brain atlas for surgical planning, model driven segmentation, and teaching. *IEEE: Visualization and Computer Graphics*, 2(3):232–241, 1996.
10. A.C. Evans, W. Dai, L. Collins, P. Neelin, and S. Marrett. Warping of a computerized 3D atlas to match brain image volumes for quantitative neuroanatomical and functional analysis. In *Medical Imaging V: Image Processing*, volume 1445 of *SPIE Proc.*, pages 236–246, 1991.
11. J. Gee, M. Reivich, and R. Bajcsy. Elastically deforming 3D atlas to match anatomical brain images. *Journal of Computer Assisted Tomography*, 17(2):225–236, March-April 1993.
12. D. McDonald, D. Avis, and A. Evans. Multiple surface identification and matching in magnetic resonance images. In *Proc. Third Conf. on Visualization in Biomedical Computing (VBC'94), Rochester, MN, October, 1994*, pages 160–169, 1994.
13. P. Thompson and A.W. Toga. A surface-based technique for warping three-dimensional images of the brain. *IEEE Trans. on Medical Imaging*, 15(4):402–417, August 1996.

Automated Labeling of Bronchial Branches in Virtual Bronchoscopy System

Kensaku MORI[1], Jun-ichi HASEGAWA[2], Yasuhito SUENAGA[1],
Jun-ichiro TORIWAKI[3], Hirofumi ANNO[4], and Kazuhiro KATADA[4]

[1] Dept. of Computational Science and Engineering, Graduate School of Engineering,
Nagoya University, Furo-cho, Chikusa-ku, Nagoya, Aichi, 464-8603 JAPAN
{mori,suenaga}@nuie.nagoya-u.ac.jp,
WWW home page: http://www.toriwaki.nuie.nagoya-u.ac.jp/~ mori
[2] School of Computer and Cognitive Sciences, Chukyo University,
101, Tokodachi, Kaizu-cho, Toyota, Aichi, 470-0348 JAPAN
hasegawa@sccs.chukyo-u.ac.jp
[3] Dept. of Information Engineering, Graduate School of Engineering,
Nagoya University, Furo-cho, Chikusa-ku, Nagoya, Aichi, 464-8603 JAPAN
toriwaki@nuie.nagoya-u.ac.jp
[4] School of Health Sciences, Fujita Health University,
Dengakugakubo, Kutsukake-cho, Toyoake, Aichi, 470-1192 JAPAN
{hanno, kkatada}@fujita-hu.ac.jp

Abstract. This paper proposes a method for automated labeling of bronchial branches in virtual bronchoscopy system. Anatomical names of bronchial branches are assigned basing upon a set of rules. If it is possible to assign the anatomical names to bronchial branches extracted from CT images by the computer and is possible to display the name of the currently observed branch on a virtual bronchoscopy image, it will help us to understand the current observing position. The proposed method constructs the knowledge base of anatomical names of bronchial branches. Tree structure of bronchus region is extracted from CT image. Labeling is performed by comparing tree structure information of the extracted bronchus with information of the branches described in the knowledge base. We implemented the proposed method with the virtual bronchoscopy system and obtained satisfactorily result.

1 Introduction

Rapid progress of three dimensional imaging equipment enables us to acquire very precise 3-D images of human body. However the doctors' load of diagnosing them is increasing. Therefore useful observation methods for those 3-D image are strongly expected. Virtualized endoscope system (virtual endoscopy system) has been developed as one of new observation tools of 3-D images. This system enables us to fly through inside and outside the human body in real time. If it is possible to display the anatomical name of the organ in a view of virtualized endoscope system corresponding to changing viewpoints and view directions, this will help us to know the current observation point.

Many researchers have reported a various kind of automated extraction methods of the organ from 3-D medical images. However there was no report about automated assignment of anatomical names to the organs extracted from a 3-D image. While some researchers including authors have reported about virtual endoscopy system, no paper has been published for automated display of the anatomical name of the organ in virtual endoscopy system [1–7]. Hoehne and colleagues have constructed the atlas of human body on computer. Anatomical names which are labeled manually are displayed on the rendered image of organ as the atlas [8]. Our method automatically assigns the anatomical name of the bronchus by using the knowledge base of the anatomical name of the bronchus and display the assigned result on the virtual bronchoscopy image corresponding to the viewpoint and view direction for helping the user to understand the current observation point.

This paper describes about a method for automated assignment of anatomical names of bronchial branches which were extracted from 3-D chest X-ray CT images and its application to virtual bronchoscopy system [9] for displaying branch names in the system. In section 2, the outline of the knowledge base of anatomical names of bronchial branches is briefly described. Section 3 shows the whole procedure of automated assignment and the method for displaying the branch name in the virtual bronchoscopy system. Experimental results are shown in Section 4 and brief discussion is added to the results.

2 Knowledge Base of Anatomical Names of Bronchial Branch

Bronchus is the organ which has the tree structure. The anatomical name of each branch is assigned basing upon a set of rules. We implement this assignment rule of anatomical name as knowledge base. Assignment of branch names is performed by comparing this knowledge base and the branching structure of bronchus which was extracted from a given CT image.

The algorithm of this name assignment accompanies the knowledge base of anatomical name of bronchial branch described by the frame representation which is one of the well-known methods for knowledge representation (Fig.1). Each frame keeps the knowledge of each branch consisting of the information of tag name, anatomical name, parent branch name, position and direction of branch, and weighted value for each evaluation item.

3 Processing Procedure

3.1 Automated Labeling of The Anatomical Name of Bronchial Branches

Fig.2 shows the processing procedure of automated labeling of bronchial branches. In the procedure, the bronchus region is extracted from 3-D CT images. Tree structure of bronchus is obtained from the extracted region. Automated labeling is performed, being based on the extracted tree structure of bronchus.

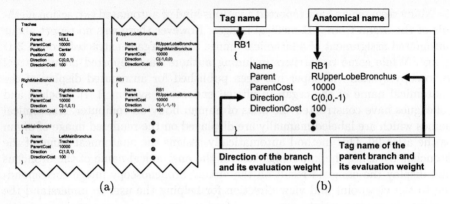

Fig. 1. An example of the knowledge base represented by frame description method. (a) overview of knowledge base, and (b) knowledge of one branch of the bronchus

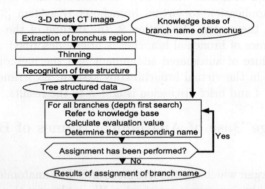

Fig. 2. Automated labeling procedure (automated assignment of anatomical name for bronchial branches)

1) Extraction of Branching Structure of Bronchus (Fig. 3) The bronchus region is extracted from 3-D chest X-ray CT image automatically by employing the method shown in [9]. This method segments the bronchus region by thresholding for CT numbers. The threshold value is automatically adjusted. The medial axis of the bronchus is calculated by using the thinning method [10]. Branching structure of bronchus is extracted from the thinned image [11]. The graph representation is generated also from the thinned result. In the graph, trachea is the root and each branches and branching points of bronchus are represented by arcs and nodes of the graph, respectively. Each arc (branch) has the following information : connecting branching point, direction of the arc, and the pointers to the parent arc and the child arc.

2) Labeling of Anatomical Name for Each Branch This procedure assigns the anatomical name to the bronchial branch by comparing the knowledge base with the structure information extracted in 1). The assignment procedure starts from the trachea and is performed sequentially from the center to the peripheral by the depth first search. The method selects the most appropriate name of a bronchial branch, which is described in the knowledge base, for each branch of the bronchial tree. Selection is performed by finding the branches of the knowledge base which has the highest evaluation value. Evaluation value is calculated from the information (such as running direction, parent branch) of each branch which is extracted from a CT image and the information described in the knowledge base. The following shows the detail of the procedure.

step1) The tree structure information of the extracted bronchus and the knowledge base are inputted.

step2) One branch B_i (B_i means the branch i of the bronchus extracted from a given CT image. $B_i \in$ {all branches of the bronchus extracted from CT image}) is selected from tree structure. This selection is performed sequentially for all branches of the bronchus extracted from CT image by the depth search from trachea.

step3) Evaluation values E_{ij} for B_i and K_j are calculated (K_j means the branch j described in the j-th item of the knowledge base. $K_j \in$ {all branches described in the knowledge base}) for all j. The evaluation value E_{ij} is calculated by

$$E_{ij} = w_d \frac{\mathbf{d}_{B_i} \bullet \mathbf{d}_{K_j}}{|\mathbf{d}_{B_i}||\mathbf{d}_{K_j}|} + w_p V \quad (1)$$

where $\mathbf{d}_{B_i}$ represents the running direction of the branch B_i, $\mathbf{d}_{K_j}$ the running direction of the branch K_j. w_d and w_p are weighted values. V takes V_p if the anatomical name of the parent branch of B_i is equal to the name of the parent branch of K_j, or 0 if the name is not equal.

step4) The branch K_{jmax}, which has the highest evaluation value for B_i and its evaluation value is greater than a given threshold value, is selected from a set of branches described in the knowledge base. Then we assign the anatomical name of K_{jmax} to the branch B_i. If we could not find the branch K_{jmax} which satisfies the above stating condition, assignment is not performed for B_i. If K_{jmax} was already assigned to another branch B_l, we compare two evaluation values E_{ijmax} (evaluation value for B_i and K_{jmax}) and E_{ljmax} (evaluation value for B_l and K_{jmax}). If $E_{ijmax} > E_{ljmax}$, the branch name of K_{jmax} is assigned to B_i and assignment to B_l and its child branches are canceled. Otherwise the assignment is not performed.

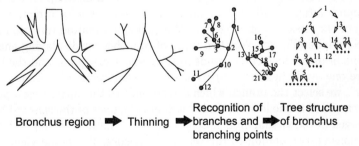

Fig. 3. Extraction of the tree structure of bronchus from a 3-D CT image

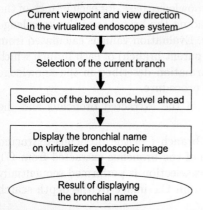
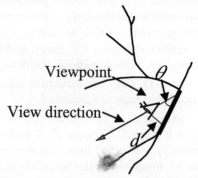

Fig. 4. Processing procedure for automated display of anatomical names of bronchial branches

Fig. 5. Selection of the branch corresponding to the current view point

step5) If all branches have been processed, go to step6). Otherwise, go to step2).

step6) If new assignment is performed in the iteration of step2)-step6), go to step2) and start from trachea again. Otherwise, labeling is terminated.

3.2 Display of The Branch Name in Virtual Bronchoscopy System

Anatomical names of bronchial branches are displayed in the virtual bronchoscopy system (Fig.4) which we have developed [4, 6]. In the virtual bronchoscopy system, bronchus region is extracted from a 3-D chest X-ray CT image. The shape of bronchus is represented by triangle patches. Marching Cubes method [12] was employed here for patch generation and the triangle patches are rendered by gouraud shading, perspective projection and spot light model. The user can specify the viewpoint and the view direction by mouse interactively and the corresponding image is rendered in real time.

The branch corresponding to the current viewpoint is found from the branching structure of the bronchus extracted in 3.1 1). The current branch is determined by calculating the closest branch from the current viewpoint. The current observation direction ("from center to peripheral" or "from peripheral to center") is also found automatically by the angle of the current view direction and the direction of the closest branch (Fig.5). When the observation direction is "from center to peripheral", we select two types of branches for displaying anatomical names, the branch which corresponds to the current viewpoint and the branches which are one level ahead (Fig.6). When the view direction is "from peripheral to center", we select the branch which corresponds to the current view point and the branch which is one level behind. Anatomical names of the selected branches are displayed in the virtual bronchoscopy image by character string in English at the positions corresponding to the selected branches. When the viewpoint and the view direction are changed, the name of branch and its displaying position are also changed.

4 Experimental Result and Discussion

4.1 Automated Labeling of Bronchial Branches

We applied the proposed method to eleven cases of real 3-D chest X-ray CT images which were taken by helical CT scanner. Image specifications are follows : image size is 512 (pixels) x 512 (pixels), the number of slices is 60 - 118 (slices), pixel size is 0.63mm, reconstruction pitch is 1mm or 2mm, width of X-ray beam is 2mm or 5mm. Knowledge base was created manually from textbook of anatomy. As the evaluation items for assignment, we used the parent name and the direction of the branch. Fig. 7(a) displays the outside view of bronchus extracted from CT image. Fig.7 (b) is the thinned results of the extracted bronchus region. Fig.7 (c) shows the tree structure and assignment results of anatomical names. Table 1 shows the results of assignments. The experimental result showed that this methods can assign correct anatomical names to about 90% of the extracted branches. This methods is considered as one of the method which uses knowledge based processing for medical image processing. This method will be very useful for automated description by anatomical name of the lung cancer extracted automatically [13].

4.2 Automated Display of Anatomical Name in The Virtual Bronchoscopy System

Fig.8 shows the scene of displaying the branch name in the virtual bronchoscopy system. Anatomical names are appropriately selected and automatically displayed on the images rendered by the virtual bronchoscopy system. Frame rate was about 6 frames / second. The computer was Silicon Graphics Octane MXI (cpu :R10000 195MHz, main memory: 512MByte). We confirmed that automatic display of branch name is very useful for understanding the current observation location.

The proposed method enables to display anatomical name on the endoscopic image rendered by the virtual bronchoscopy system. This is one of new diagnosis systems of medical images, which combines the observation method of 3-D medical images and the implementation of the knowledge based processing. Furthermore it is especially useful for education of medical students who are learning branching structure of the bronchus. Authors are collaborating with medical doc-

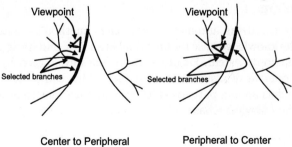

Fig. 6. Selection of the bronchial branches for displaying anatomical name

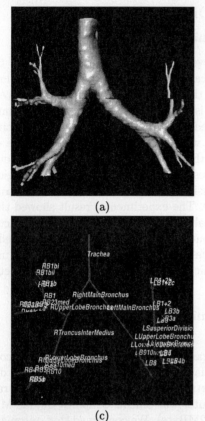

Fig. 7. Results of automated assignment of the bronchial names. (a) the extracted region of the bronchus, (b) the thinned result, (c) automated assignment result of the branch names

Table 1. Results of automated assignments of the anatomical name of bronchial branches

Data No.	The number of branches extracted from CT images	The number of branches assigned by proposed method successfully
001	28	24
002	27	23
005	9	9
006	9	9
007	19	19
010	19	15
014	9	9
018	11	11
019	11	11
021	43	43
024	23	7

tors for application of the proposed method to the education at medical college (Fig.9).

5 Conclusion

This paper presented the automated assignment method of anatomical names basing upon the knowledge base for bronchial branches, and its application to the virtual bronchoscopy system. Future work includes evaluation by large number of cases, development of assignment algorithm which can treat variation in the shapes of bronchus among patients efficiently, applications to other organs, and extension of the knowledge base.

Acknowledgment

Authors thank to Dr. Hiroshi Natori of Sapporo Medical University and Dr. Hirotsugu Takabatake of Hokkaido Keiai-kai Minami Ichi-jyo Hospital for providing CT images, useful comments and clinical validation of our system. Also authors thank to our colleagues for useful suggestion and discussion. Parts of this research was supported by the Grant-In-Aid for Scientific Research from the Ministry of Education, the Grant-In-Aid for Cancer Research from the Ministry of Health and Welfare of Japanese Government and Hori Information Promotion Foundation.

References

1. Vining, D.J., Shitrin, R.Y., Haponik, E.F., et. al. : Virtual Bronchoscopy. Radiology **193** (P, Supplement to Radiology (RSNA Scientific Program)) (1994), 261
2. Mori, K., Hasegawa, J., Toriwaki, J., Anno, H., Katada, K. : A method to extract pipe structured components in three dimensional medical images and simulation of bronchus endoscope image. Proc. of 3-D Image Conf.94 (1994) 269-274
3. Mori, K., Hasegawa, J., Toriwaki, J., Anno, H., Katada, K.: Automated extraction and visualization of bronchus from 3-D CT images of Lung. In: Ayache, N. (ed.) : Computer Vision, Virtual reality and Robotics in Medicine. Lecture Notes in Computer Science, Vol. 905. Springer-Verlag, Berlin Heidelberg New York (1995) 542-548
4. Mori, K., Hasegawa, J., Toriwaki, J., Anno, H., Katada, K. : Bronchus endoscope simulation system based on three dimensional X-ray CT images (Virtualized Bronchus Endoscope System). Japanese Journal of Medical Electronics and Biological Engineering **33** (1995) 343-351
5. Geiger, B., Kikinis, R. : Simulation of Endoscopy. In: Ayache, N. (ed.) : Computer Vision, Virtual reality and Robotics in Medicine. Lecture Notes in Computer Science, Vol. 905. Springer-Verlag, Berlin Heidelberg New York (1995) 542-548
6. Mori, K., Urano, A., Hasegawa, J., Toriwaki, J., Anno, H., Katada, K. : Virtualized Endoscope System - An Application of Virtual Reality Technology to Diagnostic Aid -. IEICE Transaction of Information and System **E79-D** (1996) 809-819
7. Ge, Y., Stelts, D.R., Vining, D.J. : 3D Skeleton for Virtual Colonoscopy. In: Hoehne, K.H., Kikinis, R. (eds.) : Visualization in Biomedical Computing. Lecture Notes in Computer Science, Vol. 1131. Springer-Verlag, Berlin Heidelberg New York (1996) 449-454
8. Hoehne, K.H., Pflesser, B., Pommert, A., Riemer, M., Schiemann, T., Schubert, R., Tiede, U. : A 'virtual body' model for surgical education and rehearsal. : IEEE computer **29** (1996) 25-31
9. Mori, K., Urano, A., Hasegawa, J., Toriwaki, J., Anno, H., Katada, K. : Recognition of bronchus in three dimensional X-ray CT images with application to virtualized bronchoscopy system. Proc. of 13th ICPR. Vol.III (1996) 528-532
10. Saito, T., Toriwaki, J., : A sequential thinning algorithm for three dimensional digital pictures using the euclidean distance transformation, Proc. of the 8th Scandinavian Conf. on Image Analysis (1995) 507-516
11. Mori, K., Urano, A., Hasegawa, J., Toriwaki, J., Anno, H., Katada, K. : A fast rendering method using the tree structure of objects in virtualized bronchus endoscope system. In: Hoehne, K.H., Kikinis, R. (eds.) : Visualization in Biomedical Computing. Lecture Notes in Computer Science, Vol. 1131. Springer-Verlag, Berlin Heidelberg New York (1996) 33-42
12. Lorensen, W., Cline, H.E. : Marching Cubes - a high resolution 3D surface construction algorithm. Computer graphics 21 (1987) 163-169
13. Kanazawa, K., Kubo, M., Niki, N., et. al. : Computer aided diagnosis for lung cancer based on helical CT image. Proc. of 13th ICPR. Vol.III (1996) 381-385

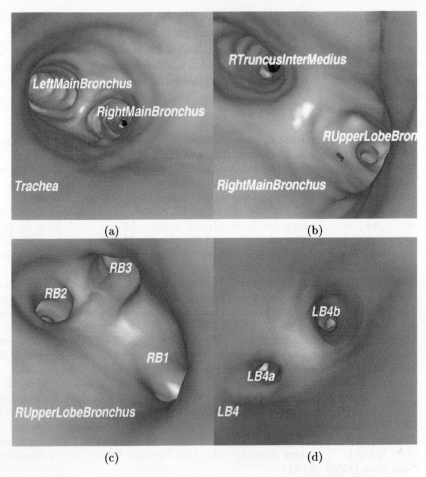

Fig. 8. An example of the images of automated display of anatomical names in the virtual bronchoscopy system. (a)-(d) are rendered at different viewpoints and from different view directions.

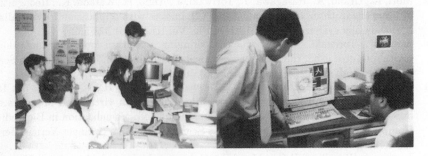

Fig. 9. Scenes of using the proposed system for education of medical students (at Sapporo Medical University, Japan)

Building a Complete Surface Model from Sparse Data Using Statistical Shape Models: Application to Computer Assisted Knee Surgery

Markus Fleute and Stéphane Lavallée, PhD

TIMC - IAB, Faculté de Médecine de Grenoble, 38 706 La Tronche Cedex FRANCE
markus.fleute@imag.fr

Abstract. This paper addresses the problem of extrapolating very few range data to obtain a complete surface representation of an antomical structure. A new method that uses statistical shape models is proposed and its application to modeling a few points manually digitized on the femoral surface is detailed, in order to improve visualization of a system developped by TIMC laboratory for computer assisted anterior cruciate ligament (ACL) reconstruction. The model is built from a population of 11 femur specimen digitized manually. Data sets are registered together using an elastic registration method of Szeliski and Lavallée based on octree-splines. Principal Components Analysis (PCA) is performed on a field of surface deformation vectors. Fitting this statistical model to a few points is performed by non-linear optimisation. Results are presented for both simulated and real data. The method is very flexible and can be applied to any structures for which the shape is stable.

1 Introduction

A system for computer assisted anterior cruciate ligament (ACL) reconstruction has been developped by TIMC laboratory since 1993. Details about the technique and its clinical validation can be found in [DLO+95,DLJ+95,JLD98].

The system uses only intra operative data obtained with an optical localizer (Optotrak, Northern Digital, Toronto), without requiring additional images such as x-rays, CT or MRI. The system enables the surgeon to digitize 3D points interactively, to track relative bone motion, and to locate the pose of surgical tools in real time. Rigid bodies made of infra-red LEDs are attached to the bones, the pointers, and the tools (Fig.1(a)). In the current version of the system, clouds of digitized points are approximated by spline patches. Those data enable the surgeon to navigate in the computer screen in real-time with any surgical tool equipped with an optical rigid body, and to compare the position of the tool with an optimal position of a graft defined by 2 points F and T on the femoral and tibial surfaces. Currently, the system enables the surgeon to minimize the anisometry of the graft by displaying anisometry maps [DLO+95], whilst avoiding impingement between the graft and the femoral notch [JLD98].

Fig.2(a) shows the Graphical User Interface of the current system for Computer Assisted ACL surgery including anisometry maps, a 3D view with spline

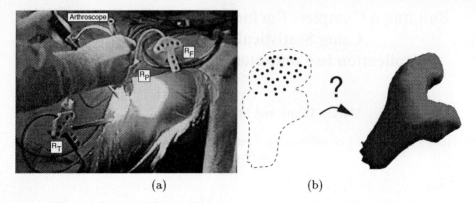

Fig. 1. (a) Surface digitizing during surgery. (b) Problem: How to extrapolate a few data points to a complete femur?

surfaces and a model of the graft envelope. Since only a small surface area has been digitized, it is very difficult to recognize the actual pose of the tibia and the femur only from the small surfaces patches generated by the bicubic splines. In order to provide the surgeon with a more complete and realistic view of the scene it is desirable to have a visualization of the whole femur (respectively tibia) as shown in Fig.2(b) (only the femur is visualized).

As illustrated in Fig.1(b), the problem addressed in this paper is to recover the complete shape of the bones from the few available data points. The objectives of this work are quadruple:

- Visualization of a complete anatomical model, including anatomical landmarks, for better orientation.
- Post-operative referencing of clinical results in the model coordinate system
- Shape-based interpolation in the area of digitized points
- Extrapolation coherent with the anatomy in the areas far from the digitized points

2 Related Work

The literature of computer vision and deformable models proposes a large variety of methods for building a surface model from range data. Overviews can be found in [BV91,MT96]. However, most of methods use only local constraints such as smoothness or they fit global shapes such as planes, cylinders or superquadrics which are not apropriate for our purpose, since the resulting shapes are not coherent with the anatomy if only a few data points locally distributed are used. It is therefore necessary to incorporate global a priori knowledge contained in statistical models, using Fourier representations [SkBG96], modal analysis performed directly [PS91] or based on features such as crest lines [STA96], or

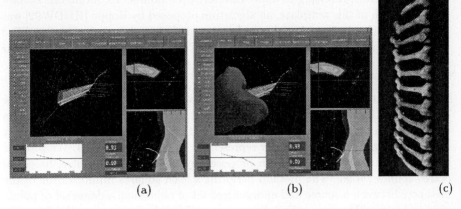

Fig. 2. (a) GUI for computer assisted ACL reconstruction (b) GUI using a complete model of the femur instead of a bicubic spline in the 3D view window : the global orientation and anatomy of the knee can be understood. (c) 11 right femurs of specimen used to build the model

Point distribution Models (PDM) proposed by Cootes and Taylor [CTCG95]. Our method is based on the latter approach.

A PDM is a deformable model built from the statistical analysis of examples of the object being modelled. Given a collection of N 3D training shapes of an object, the Cartesian coordinates of M landmark points are recorded for each image. Each training example is represented by a vector $\mathbf{m} = (x_1, y_1, z_1, ..., x_M, y_M, z_M)$. After aligning of the training shapes the pointwise mean shape $\bar{\mathbf{m}} = \frac{1}{N} \sum_{i=1}^{N} \mathbf{m}_i$ is then calculated. Modes of variation are found using Principal Component Analysis (PCA) on the deviations of examples from the mean. These modes are represented by $3M$ orthonormal eigenvectors $\mathbf{e}_i$. A new instance of the shape is generated by adding linear combinations of the t most significant variation vectors to the mean shape: $\mathbf{m} = \bar{\mathbf{m}} + \sum_{i=1}^{t} w_i \mathbf{e}_i$ where w_i is the weighting for the ith variation vector. By ensuring $t < 3M$, only the important deformations are extracted, discarding training data noise, and thus object shape and variation can be captured compactly. A key requirement for building such a model is the collection of several sets with corresponding landmarks from training images. This is presented in the following section.

3 Building a statistical shape model

Acquiring the Training Shapes: A set of 11 dry femurs of specimen (Fig.2(c)) was digitized manually using a 3-D optical localizer, resulting in 11 non-organized point sets. Ten of the femurs have been digitized with approximately 1500 points randomly distributed on the bone surface. The eleventh case was considered separately as a template and was digitized with a superior density in a larger area of the femur, resulting in approximately 6000 points. To obtain one surface representation of this template, an algorithm proposed by Hoppe [HDDW92] was used to build facets from the cloud of points, and then the result was simplified using the decimation method proposed in [CCMS97]. The result is a triangular mesh TM_{ref} of approximative 1500 vertices.

Aligning and matching the training shapes using Octree Splines: Now each of the 10 point sets has to be matched to the template mesh in such a way that each vertex of the template mesh TM_{ref} is mapped to its anatomically corresponding point on the femur represented by the set of points. We propose to use a multiresolution approach proposed by Szeliski and Lavallée, based on octree-splines [SL96]. The method performs a least squares minimization of the distances between a sparse and unorganized set of points and a dense set of points used to build a 3D octree-spline distance map [LSB91]. In our case, the dense set of points is obtained by resampling each facet of the template triangular mesh TM_{ref} up to 10,000 points. Fig.3(a) shows the octree containing the two shapes to be registered after rigid registration (top) and after non rigid registration (bottom).

The result of the octree-spline based registration technique is a smooth volumetric transform T that maps every point P of the data space to a point $M = T(P)$ of the model space. Reciprocally, it is possible to inverse this transformation. Given a point M of the template mesh, an iterative search is performed to find the point $P = T^{-1}(M)$ such that $||M - T(P)|| < \epsilon$. By this process, each point M_i of the template mesh is assigned to a data point P_i for each data set j of the N data spaces. Note that the points P_i were not in the data sets initially, but they were implicitly interpolated using the octree-spline deformation.

To avoid having the template mesh as the reference while registering the training shapes, all objects have to be registered to the *final* mean shape. This is done using an iterative algorithm: At first all training shapes are matched to the template mesh as described above. After calculating the mean shape, now all training shapes are matched to this current mean. This process is repeated until convergence occurs. The displacement vectors $\mathbf{d}_{m_i} = \mathbf{m}_i - \bar{\mathbf{m}}$ describe the mapping between the mean shape and each of the training objects.

Principal Component Analysis: Hence one can apply a Principal Component Analysis to the data which results in finding the eigenvectors of the covariance matrix $\mathbf{C} = \frac{1}{N} \sum_{i=1}^{N} \mathbf{d}_{m_i} \mathbf{d}_{m_i}^T$, of dimension $3M \times 3M$ which can be calculated from the displacement vectors. If $N \geq 3M$ one obtains $3M - 1$ nonzero eigenvectors. If $N < 3M$ it can be shown that the eigenvectors of the covariance matrix can be calculated from a smaller $N \times N$ matrix derived from the same data [CTCG95]. In this case there are only $N - 1$ nonzero eigenvectors. Because the eigenvector calculation time goes as the cube of the size of the matrix, this can give substantial time savings, as $3M$ may be in the range of several thousands, while N normally is much smaller. As $\mathbf{C}$ is real and symmetric effective Jacobi transformations can be applied to obtain the eigenvectors [PFTV92].

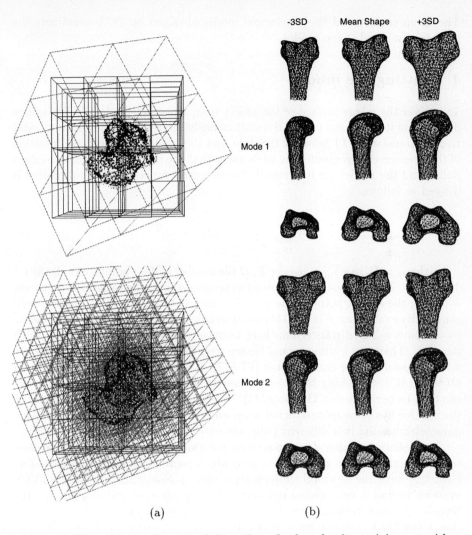

Fig. 3. (a) Hierarchical volumetric deformation of a low density training set with a high density template mesh, using Octree Splines. Up: after rigid alignment. Bottom: after elastic registration. (b) Applying 3 standard deviations of the first and second deformation modes on the mean shape

The mean surface and the t principal modes obtained by PCA constitute the statistically-based shape model.

4 Fitting the model

To recover the whole surface of the object from a new set made of a few sparse data points it is necessary to find simultaneously the rigid transformation (rotation $\mathbf{R}$, translation $\mathbf{T}$) between the data and the model and the decomposition of the t preserved eigenvectors in such a way that the distances between the data points and the model are minimized. The objective function to be minimized is defined as follows:

$$f = \sum_{i=1}^{D} \min_{1 \leq j \leq M} \|\mathbf{d}_i - \mathbf{m}_j\|^2 \tag{1}$$

with $\mathbf{m}_j = \mathbf{R}(\bar{\mathbf{m}} + \sum_{i=1}^{t} w_i \mathbf{e}_i) + \mathbf{T}$, D the number of data points, and $\mathbf{d}_i$ the ith data point. The computationally most expensive step in the registration process is finding the closest point in the model to each data point. The computational complexity evaluating f is $\mathbf{O}(DM)$ using exhaustive search. It is not interesting to compute a 3-D distance map here because the model is deformed at each iteration. Therefore k-dimensional binary trees (k-d trees, in this case k=3) are used to speed up the computation [FBF77]. A k-d tree can be constructed in $\mathbf{O}(M \log(M))$. Searching the closest point in the tree to the given data points can then be performed in $\mathbf{O}(D \log(M))$. Notice that for each function evaluation the k-d tree has to be reconstructed since using different weights w_i for the shape parameters results in a different point distribution.

The defined function f is a nonlinear function depending on $6 + t$ parameters. To minimize f an algorithm is used which combines a simulated annealing technique with the downhill simplex algorithm by Nelder and Mead [PFTV92] in order to find a near global minimum. This requires an initial guess for the rigid-body transformation, which is obtained by rigid points to surface registration, using the Iterative Closest Point (ICP) algorithm [BM92]. To decrease the search space, bounds to the parameters are applied.

5 Results

5.1 Simulation

Ten right femurs have been used to build the statistical shape model and experiments have been done with the remaining femur, on which 60 points were interactively selected to simulate a realistic intra-operative digitization.

Table 1(a) shows the relative importance of the modes of variation for the knee model. It can be seen from this table that the first four modes already represent more than 90% of the shape variation in the model. Mode 1, which accounts for almost 70% of the total variance within the model, can be seen to be primarily concerned with describing global scaling. Since the iteratively computed mean shape is only an approximation, the 10th eigenvalue is not exactly 0.0 but it is relatively low. Fig.3(b) shows the effect of applying ±3 standard deviations of the first two modes of the obtained model to the mean shape.

After rigid alignment and optimization of the fitting function, the resulting root mean square error (RMS) between the test data and the registered model as well as the RMS between the complete test shape and the registered model are computed. As expected the final RMS between the test data and the registered model decreases using more deformation modes ($\sim 0.7mm$ using one mode to $\sim 0.4mm$ using 5 modes) while this is not always the case for the RMS between the test shape and the registered model. Similar results are obtained by permuting the model in the set of specimen. Fig.4(a) (top) shows the model (triangle mesh) and the test femur after the initial rigid registration with the ICP algorithm. Fig.4(a) (bottom) shows the model and the reference femur after the non rigid registration. The black spots represent the data points.

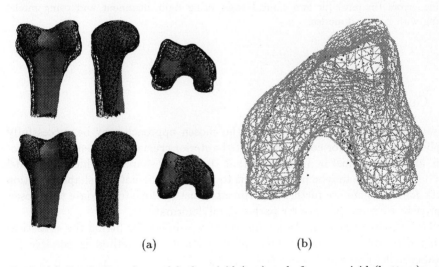

(a)   (b)

Fig. 4. (a) Simulation: the model after rigid (top) and after non rigid (bottom) registration (b) Clinical case: the model after non-rigid fitting using 6 modes in comparison with the sparse set of points.

5.2 Experiments with real intra-operative data

For two clinical cases, the surgeon acquired about 100 points randomly distributed on the femoral notch surface (not limiting the acquisition to a small patch and the anterior border of the notch). Results of fitting the model with those data are provided in Table 1(b). Fig.4(b) shows the deformed statistical model that fits the points collected during surgery. Although additional local deformation of the model would be necessary for perfect fitting, the result is satisfactory.

Nr.	Eigenvalue	Percentage	Sum
1	5500.59	69.40	69.40
2	880.37	11.11	80.50
3	548.97	6.93	87.43
4	227.88	2.87	90.30
5	191.34	2.41	92.72
6	155.18	1.96	94.67
7	128.95	1.63	96.30
8	107.22	1.35	97.65
9	104.08	1.31	98.97
10	81.91	1.03	100.00

(a)

RMS error	Case 1	Case 2
Rigid alignment	2.23	2.82
Model fitting with 2 modes	2.07	2.17
Model fitting with 4 modes	1.75	1.90
Model fitting with 6 modes	1.61	1.83

(b)

Table 1. (a) Relative importance of the modes of variation for the model (b) Residual fitting errors (in mm) for two clinical cases using rigid alignment and using model fitting with 2, 4 or 6 modes.

6 Conclusion

First experimental results show that the chosen approach may be successfully applied to a system for computer-assisted anterior cruciate ligament reconstruction, although it must be mentioned that 10 training shapes of which the model has been built are maybe not sufficient to represent the natural shape variation of the femur. Therefore further experiments must be done to validate the chosen approach, with special care for pathological deformations.

The current implementation requires a few minutes for fitting the statistical model with 100 data points, but optimisation of the method is possible for instance using gradient descent techniques.

The proposed method is a general technique for building specific models that can be applied to any case where the shape is stable and for which only a partial area can be digitized.

One of the key features of this approach is to use a volumetric elastic registration method (using octree-splines) to establish point correspondences between training sets which differ by their density and local distribution of points.

References

[BM92]   P.J. Besl and N.D. McKay. A method for registration of 3-D shapes. *IEEE Transactions on Pattern Analysis and Machine Intelligence*, 14(2):239–256, 1992.

[BV91] R.M. Bolle and B.C. Vemuri. On three-dimensional surface reconstruction methods. *IEEE Trans PAMI*, 13(1):1–13, 1991.

[CCMS97] A. Ciampalini, P. Cignoni, C. Montani, and R. Scopigno. Multiresolution decimation based on global error. *The Visual Computer*, 13(5), 1997.

[CTCG95] T.F. Cootes, C.J. Taylor, D.H. Cooper, and J. Graham. Active shape models - Their training and application. *Computer Vision and Image Understanding*, 61(1):38–59, 1995.

[DLJ+95] V. Dessenne, S. Lavallee, R. Julliard, P. Cinquin, and R. Orti. Computer assisted knee anterior cruciate ligament reconstruction : first clinical tests. In *Conference of Computer Vision, Virtual Reality, Robotics in Medicine (CVRMed'95), LNCS Series 905*, pages 476–480. Springer, 1995.

[DLO+95] V. Dessenne, S. Lavallee, R. Orti, R. Julliard, S. Martelli, and P. Cinquin. Computer assisted knee anterior cruciate ligament reconstruction : first clinical tests. *J. of Image Guided Surgery*, 1(1):59–64, 1995.

[FBF77] J. H. Friedman, J.L. Bentley, and R. A. Finkel. An algorithm for finding best matches in logarithmic expected time. *ACM Trans. Math. Software*, 3(3):209–226, Sept. 1977.

[HDDW92] H. Hoppe, T. DeRose, T.and McDonald J. Duchamp, and Stuetzle W. Surface reconstruction from unorganized points. In Catmull E. E., editor, *Computer Graphics (SIGGRAPH '92 Proceedings)*, pages 71–78, July 1992.

[JLD98] R. Julliard, S. Lavallee, and V. Dessenne. Computer Assisted Anterior Cruciate Ligament Reconstruction. *Clinical Orthopaedics and Related Research*, 1998.

[LSB91] S. Lavallee, R. Szeliski, and L. Brunie. Matching 3-D smooth surfaces with their 2-D projections using 3-D distance maps. In *SPIE Vol. 1570 Geometric Methods in Computer Vision*, pages 322–336, San Diego, CA, July 1991.

[MT96] T. McInerney and D. Terzopoulos. Deformable models in medical image analysis: a survey. *Medical Image Analysis*, 1(2):91–108, 1996.

[PFTV92] W. H. Press, B. P. Flannery, S. A. Teukolsky, and W. T. Vetterling. *Numerical Recipes in C : The Art of Scientific Computing*. Cambridge University Press, Cambridge, England, second edition, 1992.

[PS91] A. Pentland and S. Sclaroff. Closed-Form Solutions for Physically Based Shape Modeling and Recognition. *IEEE Transactions on Pattern Analysis and Machine Intelligence*, 13(7):715–729, July 1991.

[SkBG96] R. Szekely, A. kelemen, C. Brechbuler, and G. Gerig. Segmentation of 2D and 3D objects from MRI volume data using constrained elastic deformations of flexible Fourier surface models. *Medical Image Analysis*, 1(1):19–34, 1996.

[SL96] R. Szeliski and S. Lavallee. Matching 3-D anatomical surfaces with non-rigid deformations using octree-splines. *Int. J. of Computer Vision (IJCV)*, (18)(2):171–186, 1996.

[STA96] G. Subsol, J.P. Thirion, and N. Ayache. Application of an automatically built 3D morphometric brain atlas: study of cerebral ventricle shape. In K.H. Hohne and R. Kikinis, editors, *Visualization in Biomedical Computing (VBC'96) Proc. LNCS 1131*, pages 373–382, Berlin, 1996. Springer-Verlag.

---

[0] Authors wish to thank Dr Rémi Julliard for his active collaboration to this project and the Anatomy Department of Grenoble University (Pr. JP Chirossel) for providing the specimen of femurs.

Constrained Elastic Surface Nets: Generating Smooth Surfaces from Binary Segmented Data

Sarah F. F. Gibson

MERL - A Mitsubishi Electric Research Lab
201 Broadway, Cambridge, MA 02139
Email: gibson@merl.com

Abstract. This paper describes a method for creating object surfaces from binary-segmented data that are free from aliasing and terracing artifacts. In this method, a net of linked surface nodes is created over the surface of the binary object. The positions of the nodes are adjusted iteratively to reduce energy in the surface net while satisfying the constraint that each element in the surface net must remain within its original surface cube. This constraint ensures that fine detail such as cracks and thin protrusions that are present in the binary data are maintained.

1 Background

Image data from 3D Magnetic Resonance Imaging (MRI) or Computed Tomography (CT) scanners can be used to create computer models of human anatomy for visualization and surgical simulation. Volumetric models, which are composed of 3D arrays of sampled values, are more suitable for visualization and physically-based modeling of complex objects than surface-based models because they incorporate internal structure[10]. In particular, volumetric models are necessary for modeling object deformation using mass-spring (e.g. [21, 15, 14]), finite element (e.g. [11, 3, 2]), or other methods (e.g. [4, 6]) and they have significant advantages over surface-based models for modeling the cutting, tearing and joining of objects and soft tissues [8].

Until recently, one of the disadvantages of volumetric models was that they could not represent surfaces well. High quality rendering with lighting and shading effects is important for anatomical structures because it provides shape cues and a sense of realism in visualization and simulation. However, in medical data, image intensities tend to change abruptly at object surfaces, indicating the presence of high spatial frequencies. These high spatial frequencies cause aliasing artifacts in volume rendered images, which are manifested as jagged or irregular surfaces. Such artifacts are particularly noticeable when a highly reflective surface is rendered with a lighting model, such as the Phong lighting model [5].

In [9], a new method for encoding surfaces into volume-sampled data is proposed. In this method, two values are stored for each volume element: an intensity value which is used to calculate color and opacity at each sample point; and a signed distance to the closest surface point, which is used to estimate positions and normal vectors of the object surface. Because the distance function varies slowly across object surfaces, it can be sampled at relatively low rates and still provide alias-free estimates of object surfaces for high quality rendering.

In order to generate the sampled distance map for this representation, a model of the underlying surface is required. In [9] it was shown that when the object originates as an analytic or polygonal model, high quality shading can be accomplished. However, when objects originate in binary-segemented volumes, as often occurs for medical data, the underlying surface and its distance map must be estimated from the binary data. Several methods for estimating distance maps from binary data were analyzed in [7]. However, all of these methods are prone to artifacts. In particular, when the volume is sampled less frequently in one dimension (e.g. in MRI, the distance between image planes is often greater than the in-plane pixel spacing), existing methods for calculating distance maps are subject to terracing artifacts, where sloped surfaces appear as flat terraces separated by sharp elevation changes.

This paper presents a method for generating a smooth surface model from binary segmented data that is constrained to follow the original object segmentation but that reduces aliasing and terracing artifacts. The resultant surface model can be used to generate distance maps for distance-based shading in volume rendering. In addition, it provides an alternative to methods such as Marching Cubes [16] for creating triangulated surface models from binary data.

2 Previous Work

2.1 Binary Segmented Data

Image segmentation, where elements of the volume are labeled according to what structure they belong to, is the first step in creating a computer model from 3D data. Once elements in the volume have been labeled, elements with the same tissue classification are grouped into objects that represent anatomical structures. With CT data, segmentation can be performed relatively automatically using intensity thresholding or other low-level image processing. However, with MRI, image segmentation is challenging and generally requires more sophisticated algorithms and significant human input. The knee data used to illustrate examples in this paper were segmented manually from an MRI data volume of size 512x512x87 acquired at a resolution of 0.25x0.25 mm in-plane and 1.4 mm between planes.

Although surface normals can be estimated from the original grey-scale data [12], in volume rendering, grey-scale shading can fail for the same reasons that automatic segmentation fails. This is illustrated in the MRI image in Figure 1b) where the grey-scale image gradient has been calculated along the manually-segmented surface of the femur, a bone in the knee. Because the real bone surface is smooth and of uniform texture, surface normals along the edge of the femur should have similar magnitudes and slowly varying directions. However, the grey-scale image gradient depends on tissues adjacent to the bone surface, whose

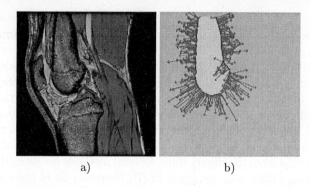

Fig. 1. a) MRI cross section through a human knee. b) Image gradient vectors calculated along the surface of the segmented femur using central differences on the grey-scale data. Image gradients vary much more than bone surface normals would be expected to vary, in some cases pointing inward when an outward facing normal is expected. Hence, applying a gradient operator to the grey-scale data does not provide a good estimate of surface normals. (Data and segmentation courtesy of Surgical Planning Lab, Brigham and Women's Hospital, Boston MA.)

intensities and thicknesses can vary significantly. Hence, both the direction and magnitude of the calculated gradient can vary dramatically around the edge of the femur. For this reason, it can be more accurate to estimate surface normals from a binary segmentation of the data than from the grey-scale image.

Unfortunately, in Volume Rendering, estimating surface normals from binary data poses significant challenges. Because of the high spatial frequencies in binary data, rendered images tend to have significant aliasing artifacts that are particularly apparent in shaded images. In addition, when surfaces lie at a shallow angle to the sampling grid, the rendered image exhibits terracing, in which sloped surfaces appear as a sequence of flat planes separated by sudden elevation changes. These elevation changes can be dramatic when the spacing between image planes is significantly larger than the in-plane spacing, as often occurs in clinical imaging.

2.2 Existing Methods for Rendering Surfaces from Binary Data

There are a number of existing methods for achieving smooth surfaces from binary segmented data. In volume rendering, several approaches have been used to approximate surfaces during rendering (see reviews in [13, 25]) including various methods using look-up tables [17], smoothing filters, and surface estimation filters [22] which approximate surface normals from the state of local neighbors. Alternatively, instead of filtering during rendering the data can be pre-processed by appling a low-pass filter to the binary data [23, 24, 1, 19]. Surface normals are then estimated from gradients of the resulting band-limited grey-scale image. All of these methods reduce aliasing artifacts but, because they are applied to local neighborhoods, they do not eliminate terracing artifacts. As illustrated in Figure

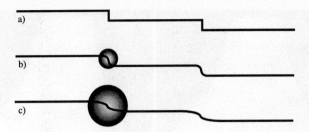

Fig. 2. The effect of filtering on terraces in binary segmented data. a) Original binary terraces. b) and c) Gaussian low-pass filters reduce the slope of the terraces but do not eliminate terraces. In order to eliminate terraces, the filter extent must be comparable to the width of the terraces.

2, local filtering reduces the slopes of terraces. However, unless the filter extent is significantly wider than the terraces, terracing artifacts are not removed. When terraces are wide (i.e. when the slope of the object is small) and deep (i.e. when the distance between planes is significantly larger than the in-plane sampling), a local filter sufficient to eliminate terracing would remove significant detail from the object model. Figure 3 illustrates the effect of a local smoothing filter on the femur data. As filter size is increased, aliasing artifacts are eliminated and the slope of the terrace is reduced. However, even after convolution with a large Gaussian filter of size 19x19x19, unacceptable terracing artifacts remain.

In surface rendering, two basic methods have been used to fit surfaces to binary data. In the first, the binary data is low-pass filtered, and an algorithm such as Marching Cubes is applied, where the surface is built through each surface cube at an iso-surface of the grey-scale data. Unfortunately, the resultant surface is subject to the same terracing artifacts and loss of fine detail as low-pass filtered volumetric representations. In order to remove terracing artifacts and reduce the number of triangles in the triangulated surface, surface smoothing and decimation algorithms can be applied. However, because these procedures are applied to the surface without reference to the original segmentation, they can result in further loss of fine detail.

In the second general method for fitting a surface to binary data, the binary object is enclosed by a parametric or spline surface. Control points on the surface are moved towards the binary data in order to minimize an energy function based on surface curvature and distance between the binary surface and the parametric surface. McInerney and Terzopoulos used such a technique to detect and track the surface of the left ventricle in sequences of MRI data [18] and Takanahi et al. used a similar technique to generate a surface model of muscle from segmented data [20]. This approach has two main drawbacks for general applications. First, it is difficult to determine how many control points will be needed to ensure sufficient detail in the final model. Second, this method does not handle complex topologies easily.

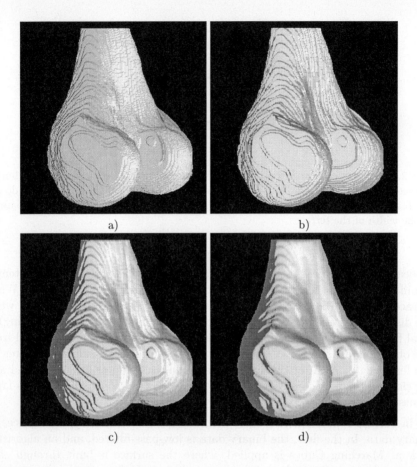

Fig. 3. Shaded, volume rendered images of low-pass filtered binary data of a human femur. a) was rendered from the binary data. In b), c) and d), the data was filtered with a Gaussian filter of size 7^3, 13^3, and 19^3 respectively. Even with a large filter size, significant terracing artifacts are present.

3 Surface Nets

The goal of the surface net approach is to create a globally smooth surface model from binary segmented data that retains fine detail present in the original segmentation. Methods that apply local low-pass filters to the binary data can reduce aliasing but they are not effective at removing terracing artifacts. In addition, low-pass filters can eliminate fine structures that can be especially important in medical applications. In contrast, surface nets produce a smooth surface that is constrained to maintain all of the surface structure present in the original data. Surface nets are constructed by linking nodes on the surface of the binary-segmented volume and relaxing node positions to reduce energy in the surface net while constraining the nodes to lie within a surface cube defined by

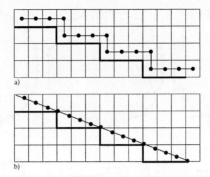

Fig. 4. Terracing artifacts in binary segmented data cause smooth surfaces to appear jagged. a) A linked net of surface nodes is constructed, placing one node at the center of each surface cube. b) Constrained elastic relaxation of the surface net smooths out terraces but keeps each surface node within its original surface cube.

the original segmentation. Figure 4 illustrates how a linked net of surface points can smooth out terracing artifacts.

3.1 Generating Surface Nets

The first step in generating a surface net is to locate cubes that contain surface nodes. A cube is defined by 8 neighboring voxels in the binary segmented data, 4 voxels each from 2 adjacent planes. If all 8 voxels have the same binary value, then the cube is either entirely inside or entirely outside of the object. If at least one of the voxels has a binary value that is different from its neighbors, then the cube is a surface cube. The net is initialized by placing a node at the center of each surface cube and linking nodes that lie in adjacent surface cubes. Each node can have up to 6 links, one each to its right, left, top, bottom, front, and back neighbors.

Once the surface net has been defined, the position of each node is relaxed to reduce an energy measure in the links. In the examples presented here, surface nets were relaxed iteratively by considering each node in sequence and moving that node towards a position equi-distant between its linked neighbors. The energy was computed as the sum of the squared lengths of all of the links in the surface net[1]. Defining the energy and relaxation in this manner without constraints will cause the surface net to shrink into a sphere and eventually onto a single point. Hence, to remain faithful to the original segmentation, a constraint is applied that keeps each node inside its original surface cube. This constraint favors the original segmentation over smoothness and forces the surface to retain thin structures and cracks.

---

[1] Alternative energy measures and relaxation schemes are also feasible. For example, a system that adjusts node positions to reduce local curvature would produce smoother surfaces and with less sharp corners than the method used here.

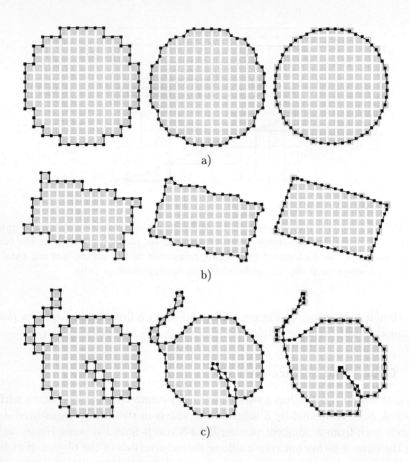

Fig. 5. Examples of surface nets applied to 2D binary objects. Each row contains the surface net superimposed on its 2D binary object for various numbers of relaxations of the surface net. In a) a surface net was fit over a circle and relaxed, from left to right, 0, 1, and 10 times. In b) the surface net was fit over a tilted rectangle and relaxed 0, 1, and 30 times. In c) the surface net was fit over an object with a thin crack and a thin protrusion and relaxed 0, 1, and 20 times. After relaxation, curved surfaces are relatively smooth, corners are sharp, and thin structures are preserved.

Several examples of surface nets applied to binary segmented 2D objects are illustrated in Figure 5. Observe that the surface nets generate relatively smooth surfaces for curves objects, produce sharp corners for rectangular objects, and preserve thin structures and cracks. Figure 5 shows the surface nets after initialization, after 1 relaxation iteration, and after several iterations. The number of iterations is chosen according to the desired result: it can either be chosen interactively or set according to the behavior of the computed energy in the net. In our work, we have observed that the net energy decreases quickly to a minimum and then increases slowly and asymptotically to a slightly higher level. At the

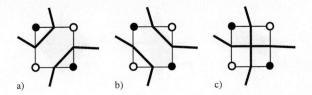

Fig. 6. Possible surface constructions for a 2D surface cube containing matched diagonal elements. a) The two black voxels are separated by the surfaces. b) The surface bridges the space between the two black voxels. In Marching Cubes, one of these two topologies is chosen arbitrarily. c) In surface nets, neither topology is assumed but the surface is pinched together at the ambiguous node.

minimum energy level, the surface appears to be smoothest, but corners become sharper as the energy increases to the final level.

The thin protrusion in Figure 5c) demonstrates that the surface net approach can produce surfaces that are topologically different from surfaces that would be produced by Marching Cubes. When a surface cube contains like elements on opposite corners, there may be more than one topological surface that can be constructed. This is illustrated in 2D in Figures 6a) and b). The separating surfaces in Figure 6a) and the bridging surface in Figure 6b) both keep black voxels inside the constructed surface and white voxels out of the constructed surface but they result in topologically different structures. In Marching Cubes, one of these surfaces would be chosen arbitrarily. In the surface net approach, illustrated in Figure 6c), the surface is pinched in at the net node, but neither a separating nor a bridging surface is created. Because arbitrary topological decisions are not made arbitrarilyly, higher level algorithms could be applied after surface smoothing to separate or bridge the surface at ambiguous surface points.

3.2 Triangulating the Surface and Estimating the Distance Map

Once a smooth surface net has been constructed, the surface net can be triangulated to form a 3D surface model. To create a triangulated surface from the surface net, each node and its links are considered one at a time. As illustrated in Figure 7, there are 12 possible triangles joining each node to pairs of neighbors. By determining which pairs of neighbors are present in the surface, possible surface triangles are identified. In order to avoid creating redundant triangles in the surface model (see Figure 8), only 6 of the 12 possible triangles are considered for each node.

In order to volume render these surfaces, distance maps were generated from the triangulated surfaces by calculating the distances from each point in the distance map to the nearest surface triangle. This was done using a brute force method by considering each triangle one at a time, calculating the distance to each point in the distance map within a local neighborhood of the triangle, and

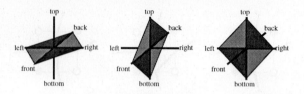

Fig. 7. For each node in the surface net, the center node can be connected to its 6 neighbors with 12 possible triangles. In the triangulation, each of the 12 triangles is created only if the two relevent neighbors are nodes of the surface net.

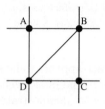

Fig. 8. To avoid redundant triangulation of the surface net, if triangles DAB and BCD are created when considering nodes A and C, then triangles CDA and ABC should not be created when considering nodes D and B.

replacing the current distance value stored at that point with the new distance value if the new magnitude was smaller.

Figure 9 shows images that have been volume rendered with distance maps created from binary data using a simple, front-to-back ray casting algorithm and Phong shading. Surface normals were calculated from the distance map using a 6-neighbor central difference gradient estimator. For purposes of comparison, the images of Figures 3, and 9 were generated using the same rendering algorithm and imaging parameters. Object opacities were set to 1.0 and large diffuse and specular reflection coefficients were used to emphasize surface artifacts.

Figure 9 compares images rendered from distance maps created from a surface net that has been relaxed by 10 and 100 iterations. Compared with Figure 3, there is a significant reduction in terracing artifacts. In addition, the surface net approach is guaranteed to preserve fine structures that can be important in medical applications.

4 Discussion

Applications such as surgical simulation or computer assisted surgery require computer models of patient anatomy. The best models available are often in the form of a binary-segmented MRI or CT image volume[2]. Depending on the

---

[2] A probabilistic classification of the data would help to alleviate some of these artifacts. However generating probabilistic classifiers is still the subject of active research.

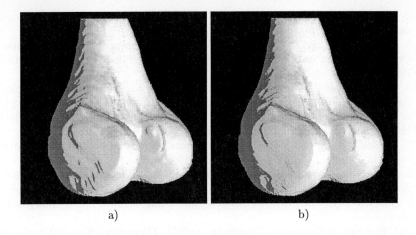

Fig. 9. Femur rendered and shaded using distance maps generated from surface nets after a) 10 relaxations and b) 100 relaxations. Compare with Figure 3, noting a significant reduction of terracing artfacts and that all surface elements have been constrained to lie within 1 voxel of the original binary segmentation.

application, these binary volumes must be converted into volumetric models or triangulated surface models for graphical representation. However, because of the high spatial frequencies in binary data, the surfaces of these models are subject to artifacts known as aliasing and terracing.

In this paper, a method has been presented that produces smooth surfaces with reduced aliasing and terracing artifacts. The resultant surface net can be used to generate either volumetric models or triangulated surface models. The surface net is created by linking surface nodes generated from the binary surface. Node positions are adjusted to reduce energy in the surface net while following constraints set by the original binary surface of the data. This creates a relatively smooth surface that retains fine detail and structures that can be important in medical applications.

References

1. R. Avila and L. Sobierajski. A haptic interaction method for volume visualization. In *Proc. Visualization'96*, pages 197–204. IEEE, 1996.
2. M. Bro-Nielsen and S. Cotin. Real-time volumetric deformable models for surgery simulation using finite elements and condensation. In *Proc. Eurographics*, volume 15, pages 57–66, 1996.
3. D. Chen and D. Zeltzer. Pump it up: computer animation of a biomechanically based model of muscle using the finite element method. In *Proc. SIGGRAPH 92*, pages 89–98., 1992.
4. M. Desbrun and M-P Gascuel. Animating soft substances with implicit surfaces. In *Proc. SIGGRAPH 95*, pages 287–290, 1995.

5. J. Foley, A. vanDam, S. Feiner, and J. Hughes. *Computer Graphics: Principles and Practice*. Addison-Wesley, 1992.
6. S. Gibson. 3D chainmail: a fast algorithm for deforming volumetric objects. In *Proc. Symposium on Interactive 3D Graphics*, pages 149–154. ACM SIGGRAPH, 1997.
7. S. Gibson. Calculating distance maps from binary segemented data. Technical Report WP98-01, MERL – A Mitsubishi Electric Research Laboratory, 1998.
8. S. Gibson. Linked volumetric objects for physics-based modeling. *submitted to IEEE Trans. on Visualization and Computer Graphics*, 1998.
9. S. Gibson. Using distance maps for accurate surface representation in sampled volumes. In *Proc. Visualization'98*. IEEE, 1998.
10. S. Gibson, C. Fyock, E. Grimson, T. Kanade, R. Kikinis, H. Lauer, N. McKenzie, A. Mor, S. Nakajima, H. Ohkami, R. Osborne, J. Samosky, and A. Sawada. Volumetric object modeling for surgical simulation. *Medical Image Analysis*, 2(2), 1998.
11. J.P. Gourret, N. Magnenat-Thalmann, and D. Thalmann. Simulation of object and human skin deformations in a grasping task. In *Proc. SIGGRAPH 89*, pages 21–30, 1989.
12. K. Hohne, M. Bomans, A. Pommert, M. Riemer, C. Schiers, U. Tiede, and G. Wiebecke. 3D visualization of tomographic volume data using the generalized voxel model. *The Visual Computer*, 6(1):28–36, February 1990.
13. A. Kaufman. *Volume Visualization*. IEEE Computer Society Press, Los Alamitos, CA, 1991.
14. R. Koch, M. Gross, F. Carls, D. von Buren, G. Fankhauser, and Y. Parish. Simulating facial surgery using finite element models. In *Proc. SIGGRAPH 96*, pages 421–428, 1996.
15. Y. Lee, D. Terzopoulos, and K. Waters. Realistic modeling for facial animation. In *Proc. SIGGRAPH 95*, pages 55–62., 1995.
16. W. Lorensen and H. Cline. Marching cubes: a high resolution 3D surface construction algorithm. In *Proc. SIGGRAPH 87*, pages 163–169, 1989.
17. S. Lu, D. Cui, R. Yagel, R. Miller, and G. Kinzel. A 3D contextual shading method for visualization of diecasting defects. In *Proc. Visualization'96*, pages 405–407. IEEE, 1996.
18. T. McInerney and D. Terzopoulos. Deformable models in medical image analysis: a survey. *Medical Image Analysis*, 1(2):91–108, 1996.
19. A. Mor, S. Gibson, and J. Samosky. Interacting with 3-dimensional medical data: Haptic feedback for surgical simulation. In *Proc. Phantom User Group Workshop'96*, 1996.
20. I. Takanahi, S. Muraki, A. Doi, and A. Kaufman. 3D active net for volume extraction. In *Proc. SPIE Electronic Imaging'98*, pages 184–193, 1998.
21. D. Terzopoulos and K. Waters. Physically-based facial modeling, analysis, and animation. *Journal of Visualization and Computer Animation*, 1:73–80, 1990.
22. G. Thurmer and C. Wurthrich. Normal computation for discrete surfaces in 3D space. In *Proc. Eurographics'97*, pages C15–C26, 1997.
23. S. Wang and A. Kaufman. Volume sampled voxelization of geometric primitives. In *Proc. Visualization'93*, pages 78–84. IEEE, 1993.
24. S. Wang and A. Kaufman. Volume-sampled 3D modeling. *IEEE Computer Graphics and Applications*, 14:26–32, 1994.
25. R. Yagel, D. Cohen, and A. Kaufman. Discrete ray tracing. *IEEE Computer Graphics and Applications*, 12:19–28, 1992.

Assessing Skill and Learning in Surgeons and Medical Students Using a Force Feedback Surgical Simulator

O'Toole, R.[1,2], Playter, R.[1], Krummel, T.[3], Blank, W.[1], Cornelius, N.[1], Roberts, W.[1], Bell, W.[1], and Raibert, M.[1]

[1] Boston Dynamics Inc., Cambridge, MA, USA.
[2] Harvard Medical School, Harvard-MIT Division of Health Sciences and Technology, Boston, MA, USA.
[3] Department of Surgery, Hershey Medical Center, Penn State University, Hershey, PA, USA.

Abstract. We have developed an interactive virtual reality (VR) surgical simulator for the training and assessment of suturing technique in the context of end-to-end anastomosis. The surgical simulator is comprised of surgical tools with force feedback, a 3D visual display of the simulated surgical field, physics-based computer simulations of the tissues and tools, and software to measure and evaluate the trainee's performance. This study uses the simulator to compare the skills of experienced vascular surgeons to medical students. Eight parameters were measured to evaluate performance during VR suturing tasks. The data indicate significant differences between surgeon and non-surgeon performance, as well as improvement in performance with training. We believe that this study offers support for the use of virtual reality surgical simulators to augment surgical skill assessment and training.

Introduction

Although surgical technique has evolved considerably over time, the process of training surgeons has undergone little change since the inception of the Halstedian technique over a century ago [barnes89]. Surgery is in many ways a traditional hands-on apprenticeship. Surgical residents acquire skill by first observing experienced surgeons in action, and then performing progressively more of the surgical procedures themselves as their training progresses. As their skill levels increase, the residents are given increasing responsibility. The assessment of the trainee's skill is performed subjectively by senior surgeons.

We are exploring the use of interactive virtual reality computer simulations to augment training on patients. Virtual reality (VR) refers to a computer-simulated environment that provides sensory output to the user in an attempt to mimic a real environment. A particularly successful example of virtual reality training is the use of aircraft simulators for the training of commercial and military pilots [Higgens97]. With the exception of one flight in a real aircraft, commercial pilots regularly do all of their training to upgrade from one aircraft to another on simulators. The potential advantages of VR to augment training include:

- ***Quantification*** of performance and progress for training and accreditation.
- ***Standardization*** of training regimens independent of patient population.
- ***Exposure*** to rare but important situations in an era of shrinking training opportunities.
- ***Reduction of risk*** to patients.
- ***Reduction of cost*** through more effective use of operating room time.
- ***Improved*** educational techniques.

The potential benefits of VR training have motivated the development of VR surgical simulators during the past several years [satava96]. These simulators have advanced from fly-through applications [satava93] to more recent work incorporating real surgical tools and force feedback [baumann96, fischer95, singh94, mcdonald95]. Research groups are now beginning to attack the problem of validating surgical simulators [Weghorst98, Taffinder98].

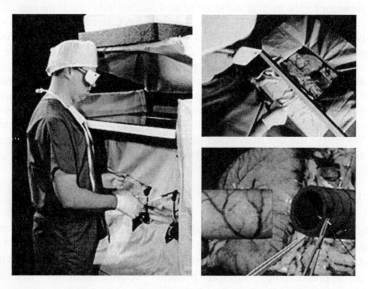

Fig. 1. The BDI surgical simulator lets you see, touch, and feel simulated organs using 3D computer graphics, physics-based simulations, and advanced force feedback. Using a needle holder and forceps attached to force feedback devices, the user can grasp, poke, pluck, and suture flexible tube organs. The user can feel the vessels when touched and the vessels move realistically in response to touch. The surgical station uses a mirror arrangement to place the 3D image of the patient in the correct position relative to the user. This system allows the user to control a virtual needle and thread to perform a simulated end-to-end anastomosis.

We have developed a surgical simulator for the evaluation and training of surgical skills for anastomosis [Playter 1997]. Anastomosis was chosen as a first application as it is a common surgical task that has a high reliance on proper technique. The simulator is an integrated system that allows users to perform a simulated end-to-end anastomosis using a virtual needle and thread [Figure 1]. The simulator is specialized for touch and interactivity. Users feel virtual organs when they touch, probe, grasp, and suture simulated biological tissues. Physics-based simulation is used to make the flexible vessels feel realistic and be responsive to touch. Instrumented surgical tools mounted to force-feedback devices act as two-way connections to the simulated world; they measure the position and configuration of the tools and apply interaction forces to the user's hands. The user's view of the surgical field is created using real-time, 3D computer graphic images of bodily organs, tissues, and surgical tools. The visual image is projected into a natural position relative to the surgeon using a mirror system. The anastomosis simulator is able to measure many aspects of the user's performance including the forces applied to the tissues as well as the actual motions of the tools in space. By recording these values we can quantify the user's performance. A force history plot of the forces exerted by the needle, as well as 3D needle guide vectors to indicate ideal needle orientation, can be displayed during the simulation to guide training. A digital video is automatically created during each training session so that the user may replay performances.

In this paper we describe a preliminary study aimed at investigating two key questions regarding surgical simulation:

1. Can surgical simulation be used to *measure* surgical skill?
2. Can surgical simulation be used to *train* surgical skill?

To address these issues we simulated the essential elements of suturing technique in the context of end-to-end anastomosis and devised metrics for evaluating performances. We then measured and compared the performances of subjects of presumably different surgical skill levels. The skilled and unskilled users of our surgical simulator were experienced vascular surgeons and medical students, respectively. Our hypothesis was that if the trainer could measure surgical skill, then these two groups should have different levels of performance on the simulator. Further, if the trainer can be used to improve surgical skill, then the performances should improve over time, particularly amongst the medical students.

Methods

In an assessment of our surgical simulator we designed and implemented a human performance study to test if the surgical simulator can measure or train surgical skill. We chose suturing on a large flexible vessel as the surgical task. We used a simplified version of the surgical simulator that included only a needle driver, a curved needle and one flexible vessel with four small targets near the edge. The goal of the surgical task was to 'suture' the vessel in sequence at the targeted locations. A 'suture' consisted of passing the needle completely through the vessel. The completion of four sutures is defined as one trial [Figure 2].

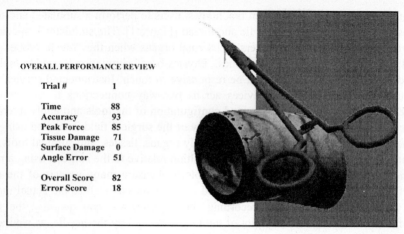

Fig. 2. A performance evaluation is displayed to the user at the completion of each trial. The Overall Score equals 100 minus the Error Score. The four goal target locations for the surgical task are shown on the edge of the vessel. Passing the needle completely through the tissue four times is considered one trial. Note the four goal targets the scratch marks on the surface of the vessel near the target locations.

Seven parameters were used to evaluate performance during the simulated suturing task: total tissue damage, peak force to the tissue, accuracy of stitches, time to complete the task, damage to the surface of the tissue, angular error in needle technique, and an overall error score. The scoring in each category, as well as an overall error score, is displayed to the user at the completion of each trial [Figure 2]. An eighth parameter, the total distance traveled by the tip of the tool, was also measured, but the value was neither displayed to the users at the completion of the task, nor included in the overall error score.

The participants were eight currently practicing vascular surgeons from four Boston hospitals and twelve medical students from Harvard Medical School. The eight surgeons ranged in experience from 7 to 25 years in practice (mean 14.5 years), and had performed between 1100 and 7000 vascular surgeries (mean 3250 surgeries). The surgeons were all right handed, were all male, and had an average age of 43.5 years (range from 31 to 56). The medical students were first, second and third year medical students from Harvard Medical School (three first years, six second years, and three third years). Eleven of the twelve were right handed, and eight of the twelve were male. Two of the third years had already completed their core surgery rotation, but otherwise none of the students had any surgical experience. The medical students' average age was 24.6 years (range of 20 to 30). None of the surgeons or students were involved in the design of the system or associated with our research group, and none had previously used the system. Each participant in the study performed an identical protocol, and was tested in isolation from other test subjects. After collecting demographic data on each subject and a brief initial training period with a non-surgical VR application, the experimental protocol was performed. All experiments were performed between February and March of 1997. The protocol consisted of each user performing the previously described VR task (4 'sutures' into a single large vessel) 15 consecutive times, under varying test conditions. These conditions included using the dominant hand (test condition 1), using the non-dominant hand (test condition 2), and using the dominant hand with some additional visual guidance (test condition 3). For all analyses, statistical significance was defined as a p value <= 0.05 using two-sided Student's t test.

Results

Comparison of Surgeon and Medical Student Performances

For experimental condition 1(dominant hand), the surgeons outperformed the students in all 8 parameters, and 6 of these differences were significant [Figure 3]. There were statistically significant differences, with the average medical student performance being worse than the average surgeon performance, for time, tissue damage, angle error, tip distance, accuracy error, and overall error. Similar results were obtained for the other test conditions, but these data are not included in this text.

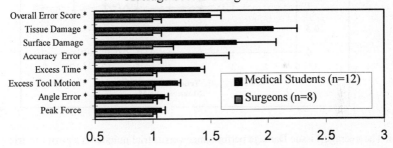

Performance Error Scores
Mean +SEM, Values Normalized to Surgeons' Mean Score
* P<0.05, Medical Students vs. Surgeons

Fig. 3. The bar graph compares the average surgeon and medical student performances for the 8 measured parameters. The average values have been normalized to the surgeons' average score. Larger values indicate worse performance. The surgeons average was better than the medical students average for all 8 parameters. Six of these differences were statistically significant at the p < 0.05 level. This data is for Test Condition 1 where the participants used their dominant hand for the task.

Changes in VR Performance with Training

Both the surgeons and medical students tended to improve during the training session as demonstrated by data for the metric tissue damage [Figure 4]. To determine the magnitude of the users' performance change with training, the scores from trials 1 and

2[1] were compared with trials 13 and 14. All four of these trials were performed under the same test condition (condition 1 - dominant hand). The only difference between these two sets of trials is that the user performed 10 training trials between the two sets. The data demonstrate that for seven of the eight parameters, both the surgeons and the medical student performances improved [Figure 8].

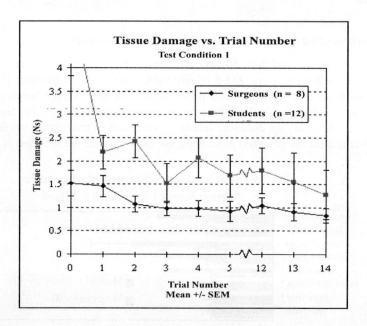

Fig. 4. The average Tissue Damage performance versus trial number is shown for trials 0 to 6, and 12 to 14, the trials under test condition 1. Larger values represent worse performance. Note that the students initially have a very poor performance and improve with time. The surgeons also improve with time, but to a lesser extent as quantified in Figure 5.

The magnitude of performance improvement was larger for the students than the surgeons in six of the eight measured parameters [Figure 5]. In five of these cases these differences were statistically significant. Depending on the parameter, the improvements were of differing magnitudes. For example there was a large improvement by the medical students for the Surface Damage parameter and a very small improvement in the Tip Distance parameter. Only for the case of the surgeons' Angle Error does the average score actually become worse during the training session.

---

[1] Trial 0 was not included in the Before Training data because trial 0 is slightly different than the other trials as the users are not yet familiar with the system. Including trial 0 would only strengthen our conclusions, as the medical students performed poorly in trial 0. Excluding trial 0 is therefore the conservative approach.

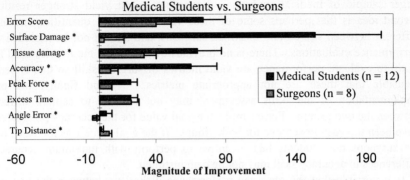

Fig. 5. The bar graph compares the average magnitude of improvement for the surgeons and medical students. Larger values indicate larger amounts of improvement. The values are the raw magnitude of improvement divided by the surgeons' average value before training. The medical students had statistically significant larger improvements for 5 of the cases, indicating that their scores improved more than the surgeons' scores during the training session. The surgeons had a larger improvement for Tip Distance, the only parameter for which the participants were not given feedback concerning their performance during the training sessions.

Discussion

This study aims to test if the surgical simulator can measure or train some component of surgical skill. Assuming that the surgeons and medical students have different levels of skill, one would expect their performances to differ if the simulator measured some component of surgical skill. If the surgical simulator was able to train some component of surgical skill, one would expect that the performance would improve with time and that the medical students would improve more than the surgeons.

There were statistically significant differences between the surgeons' and medical students' average performances on 6 of the 8 test cases. This data demonstrates difference between the two groups, with the surgeons generally outperforming the students. The magnitude of the difference between the two groups varied depending upon the parameter. For example, there were large differences in the two groups in the tissue damage scores, whereas the peak force scores tended to be much more similar. Parameters with large differences between the medical students and surgeons may represent more useful indicators of surgical skill. Tissue damage, excess time, excess tool tip motion, and overall error score all seem to be useful metrics, since there were statistically significant differences between the two groups for all three test conditions.

There are several possible explanations for the cases where there were no significant differences between the two groups. The most obvious explanation is that the present study lacks statistical power to observe these differences. A study with a larger sample of medical students and surgeons might yield stronger results. A second idea is that perhaps some of these values represent quantities that are not different between skilled and unskilled surgeons, and should not be included in the performance evaluations. There is no previous evidence that the metrics used in this study to evaluate performance are valid metrics of surgical skill so this is certainly plausible that these are not appropriate metrics. And finally, the precise implementation of the skills assessment may not be able to capture differences between the two groups. For example, the goal value for the accuracy parameter may have been too easy to achieve for both groups. If the goal value was too easy, neither the surgeons nor students had incentive to perform with maximum accuracy, so differences in accuracy skill may not be demonstrated.

Is it possible that the observed performance dichotomy between the two groups was the basis of some difference between the two groups besides surgical skill? There are several factors that differed between the surgeons and the medical students: age (the medical students were younger), gender (33% of the medical students were women, none of the surgeons were), and having chosen surgery as a career (all of the surgeons chose surgery as a career, only about a fifth of the students would be expected to choose surgery).

Each of these three factors will be considered individually. First, there was a rather large difference in age between the two groups; however, one would not expect the older group to perform better in a manual dexterity task. In fact, there is evidence that manual dexterity skills tend to deteriorate with age [Scheuneman89]. Therefore one would expect the younger medical students to do better, not worse, than the surgeons if the performance differences were based upon age. Second, there were more women in the medical student group. As with age, there is no clear evidence that women would tend to do worse on a manual dexterity task. Again, there is evidence that women tend to do better [Harris94, Scheuneman89], on some components of manual dexterity tasks, so one might expect the gender difference to improve medical student performance, not hinder it.

Finally one might theorize that medical students who choose surgery are self-selected for greater manual dexterity or visuospatial ability than their colleagues who do not choose surgery. Presumably the medical student group in this study contains a large percentage of students who will not become surgeons. However there is evidence debunking the idea that medical students who choose surgery have better manual dexterity or visuospatial skills [Harris94,Squire89]. No study has yet shown differences in general manual dexterity between medical students who chose surgery and those who do not. A task must be very similar to a specific surgical skill for the surgeons to outperform the non-surgeons. It is therefore not likely that either age, gender, or choice of medical career path explain our results.

In addition to the observed differences in performance between the two groups, the data also demonstrate changes in performance with repeated training. During the course of the training session, the medical student average performance improved in all 8 measured categories. Four of the parameters showed statistically significant improvements (time, peak force, tissue damage, and error score), and two more were very close to statistical significance (surface damage (p = 0.06) and accuracy (p=0.07)). The other two values, tip distance and angle error were not significantly improved and had the smallest magnitude of improvement. The fact that tip distance did not improve is not surprising since this is the only parameter about which the participants were given no feedback during the experiment. Without information regarding this parameter they had no incentive to improve the score in this area.

In all of the categories except time and tip distance, the medical students average improved by a larger magnitude than the surgeons. The surgeon average did improve by a statistically significant margin for 4 of the 8 parameters (time, tip distance, tissue damage, and error score). Some improvement in performance is expected as the trainees become accustomed to the test apparatus and the surgical task, so it is not surprising that both the surgeons and medical students showed improvement. However, the larger, statistically significant improvement demonstrated by the students in 5 of the 7 parameters in the surgical score (recall that tip distance was not a component of the overall error score) indicates that the medical student scores improved more during the training session. This result is consistent with the idea that if the surgical trainer can train surgical skill, the medical students would benefit more from a training session than the surgeons.

One explanation for the larger improvements during the trials by the students is that the students were acquiring surgical skills that the surgeons already had. An alternate explanation is that the students were simply faster learners than the surgeons. Whatever the reason, one should be cautious about extrapolating these results to imply that the medical students were learning surgical skill. Since there was no long term follow-up on this single training session, there is no evidence that any of the improvements in performance were permanent. And further, there is not yet evidence that the observed improvements correlate with improvements in surgical skill. Be that as it may, the data are a first step in validating the use of surgical simulators for training of surgical skill.

Conclusions

To our knowledge we have created the first 3D VR surgical simulator to measure suturing skills and have used it to demonstrate significant performance differences between medical students and surgeons. Our VR surgical trainer is unique because it provides quantification and evaluation of a user's performance, and focuses on the realistic sense of touch by allowing users to reach into the virtual environment with tools to touch and manipulate simulated tissues.

Our current research is aimed at answering two broad questions: 1) Can we *measure* surgical skill using VR technology? and 2) Can we *train* surgical skill using VR technology?

Strictly speaking, we have not yet addressed either of these questions directly. To directly answer the first question we must assess surgical skill using some other traditional method of evaluating skill and determine if VR surgical skill is correlated to real surgical skill. To fully answer the second question, we must compare actual surgical skill with and without VR surgical training over time. In this initial study we have avoided the issue of evaluating real surgical skill. Instead we have focused on evaluating skill level and learning using only VR technology.

Our initial study compares the performance of two groups of subjects that are assumed to have different levels of real surgical skill: practicing vascular surgeons and medical students. The performances of these two groups were distinguishable from one another, suggesting that the simulator could be measuring components of surgical skill. Similarly, improvements in performance with practice suggests that the simulator may be capable of teaching components of surgical skill. Future clinical validation studies will be needed to verify that the trainer can be used to measure and train actual surgical skill. However, the current study does provide data indicating that VR technology may play an important role in training tomorrow's surgeons

Acknowledgments

The surgical simulator has been developed as part of DARPA's Advanced Biomedical Technologies Program. We are indebted to Dr. William Quist from the Beth Israel-Deaconess Medical Center who provided significant clinical input and assistance to the project. Many thanks are also due to the Harvard Medical School students and Boston area vascular surgeons who generously gave their time to participate in the study.

References

Barnes, R. W., Lange, N.P., Whiteside, M.F.:],Halstedian Technique Revisited, Annals of Surgery, 210, 1989: 118-121.

Barnes, R. W.,Surgical Handicraft: Teaching and Learning Surgical Skills, The American Journal of Surgery 153, 1987: 422-427.

Playter, R., Raibert, M.,A Virtual Surgery Simulator Using Advanced Haptic Feedback, Journal of Minimally Invasive Therapy, To Appear, 1997.

Satava, R. M., Medical Virtual Reality, The Current Status of the Future. S. Weghorst, H. Siegurg and K. Morgan Eds., Health Care in the Information Age. IOS Press, Amsterdam, 1996: 542-45.

Satava, R. M., Virtual Reality Surgical Simulator: The First Steps, Surg Endosc 7, 1993: 203-05.

Reinig K., C. Rush, H. Pelster, V. Spitzer, and J. Heath, Real-Time Visually and Haptically Accurate Surgical Simulation. S. Weghorst, H. Siegurg and K. Morgan Eds., Health Care in the Information Age. IOS Press, Amsterdam, 1996: 542-45.

Baumann, R., D. Glauser, D. Tappy, C. Bauer, and R. Clavel, Force Feedback for Virtual Reality Based Minimally Invasive Surgery Simulator. S. Weghorst, H. Siegurg and K. Morgan Eds., Health Care in the Information Age. IOS Press, Amsterdam, 1996: 564-579.

Fischer, H., B. Neisius and R. Trapp, Tactile Feedback for Endoscopic Surgery. K. Morgan, R. Satava, H. Sieburg, R. Mattheus, and J. Christensen Eds., Interactive Technology and the New Paradigm for Healthcare, IOS Press, Amsterdam, 1995: 114-117.

Singh, S., M. Bostrom, D. Popa, and C. Wiley, Design of an Interactive Lubar Puncture Simulator with Tactile Feedback. Proceedings of IEEE International Conference on Robotics and Automoation, IEEE, New York, 1994: 1734-1752.

McDonald, J., L. Rosenberg and D. Stredney, Virtual Reality Technology Applied to Anesthesiology. K. Morgan, R. Satava, H. Sieburg, R. Mattheus, and J. Christensen Eds., Interactive Technology and the New Paradigm for Healthcare, IOS Press, Amsterdam, 1995: 237-243.

Steele, R. J. C., Walder, C, and Herbert, M., Psychomoter testing and the ability to perform an anstomosis in junior surgical trainees, Br. J. Surg, 1992, **79**:1065-1066.

Harris, C.J., Herbert, M., and Steele, R.J.C., Psychomotor skills of surgical trainees compared with those of different medical specialists, Br. J. Surg, 1994, **81**: 382-283.

Squire, D., Giachino, A.A., Profit, A.W., Heaney, C., Objective comparison of manual dexterity in physicians and surgeons Can J Surg 1989; **32**:467-76.

Scheueneman, A., Pickleman, J., Freeark, R. Age, gender, lateral dominance, and prediction of operative skill among surgical residents. Surgery 1983; 98: 506-13.

Higgens, G. A., Merrill, G.L., Hettinger, L.J., Kaufman, C.R., Champion, H.R., and Satava, R.M. New Simulation Technologies for Surgical Training and Certification: Current Status and Future Projections, Presence, 6 (2) April 1997, 160-172.

Weghorst, S., Airola, C., Oppenheimer, P., Edmond, C.V., Patience, T., Heskamp, D., and Miller, J., Validation of the Madigan ESS Simulator, In: Westwood, J.D., Hoffman, H.M, Stredney, D. And Weghorst, S.J. Medicine Meets Virtual Reality: Art, Sceince, Technology: Healthcare (R)Evolution, IOS Press, 1998, pg.399-405.

Taffinder, N., Sutton, C, Fishwick, R.J., McManus, I.C., and Darzi, A. Validation of Virtual Reality to Teach and Access Psychomotor Skills in Laparoscopic Surgery: Results from Randomised Controlled Studeies Using the MIST VR Laparoscopic Simulator, In: Westwood, J.D., Hoffman, H.M, Stredney, D. And Weghorst, S.J. Medicine Meets Virtual Reality: Art, Sceince, Technology: Healthcare (R)Evolution, IOS Press, 1998, pg.124-130.

Virtual Reality Vitrectomy Simulator

Paul F. Neumann[1], Lewis L. Sadler[2], and Jon Gieser M.D.[3]

[1] Division of Neuroimage Science, University of Illinois at Chicago,
912 S. Wood St. M/C 799, Chicago IL 60612, USA,
pneumann@uic.edu,
WWW home page: www.neuroimage.uic.edu/people/paul/
[2] sadler@uic.edu
[3] UIC Department of Ophthalmology and Visual Sciences,
jongies@uic.edu

Abstract. In this study, a virtual reality vitrectomy simulator is being developed to assist Ophthalmolgy residents in correcting retinal detachments. To simulate this type of surgery, a three dimensional computer eye model was constructed and coupled with a mass-spring system for elastic deformations. Five surgical instruments are simulated including: a pick, blade, suction cutter, laser, and drainage needle. The simulator will be evaluated by a group of fellows and retinal surgeons with a subjective Cooper-Harper survey commonly used for flight simulators.

1 Background

1.1 Retinal Detachments

Ophthalmology programs generally follow four stages: clinical introduction, researching subspecialities, treating patients, and an optional subspecialty fellowship. Introductory training begins with lectures, surgical texts, prerecorded surgical video tapes, and practice on animal cadavers and sometimes fruits. Participation in surgery is similar to an apprenticeship where residents gradually perform more complex procedures under a surgeon's supervision. Modern vitreous surgery is categorized as a closed divided system in which an operative instrument and a light probe are inserted into the vitreous chamber to repair any abnormalities such as retinal detachments. To correct detachments, a vitrectomy is performed to reattach the retina, stop any bleeding and remove any fibrovascular tissue. Operative instruments range from simple forceps and picks, vitreoretinal scissors and cutting blades, blunt drainage needles, suction cutters; to more complex instruments such as lasers and cryoprobes.

1.2 Virtual Reality Surgical Simulators

Virtual reality surgical simulators generally consist of five components: anatomical models, a physics system, an abnormality simulation, a VR interface, and virtual surgical instruments. Anatomical models are computer representations such as surfaces or volumes which approximate the form of the human body. Models can be constructed from sequential cross-sectional images, physical cadavers slices, or from population statistics. A physics system couples anatomical models with physical properties so they can respond to external and internal forces much like their real world counterparts. Current physics systems range from mass-spring networks to finite element analysis to simulate deformation and fracture. An abnormality simulation is the anomaly or pathology that needs to be corrected through the surgical procedure. The VR interface is the real-world devices of the simulator. Lastly, virtual instruments allow the resident to interact with the anatomical models through the VR interface. Figure 1 shows a possible schematic diagram for a virtual reality surgical simulators.

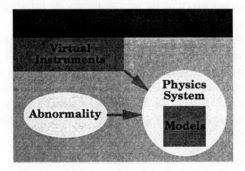

Fig. 1. Surgical simulator schematic diagram

Theoretically, a virtual reality simulator can assist in the surgical training process in a variety of ways such as reinforcing hand-eye coordination, the formation of a 3D mental model, finetuning a resident's performance, providing access to a variety of diseases, and ultimately supporting a uniform accreditation procedure [3]. The expense of a VR simulator could be offset by the surgical time reduction currently needed to train residents and recover from their initial complications. In addition, funding from the federal government to supplement surgical training may be reduced or discontinued in the future to cap health care costs.

1.3 Previous Research

The eye's small size and fine structures make it difficult to reconstruct using standard imaging modalities. An early eye reconstruction with an ocular tumor was created by segmenting and stacking ultra-sound images to visualize a radiation treatment plan [5]. Another model was developed to train surgeons in performing radial keratotomy on a cornea model using finite element analysis [12]. At the Interactive Media Technology Center, an eye simulator was prototyped with a tactile stylus that controlled several virtual instruments [13]. Their software program demonstrated a user cutting the sclera and inserting a phacoemulsifier to remove a cataract.

Of all of surgical instruments functionalities, cutting presents the greatest challenge for simulators. An early related method proposed by [16] propagated fractures by inserting positional discontinuities in regions with the largest elastic displacement. [15] demonstrated a cutting technique using a constrained particle system, but the method appeared to lose surface area when particle bonds were broken. Another method developed by [11] for plastic surgery radially projected a screen based cutting path onto a finite element mesh attached to a laser scanned facial model. Another finite element method by [14] moved a template over a 2D surface to define the cutting incision. In addition, the user's force vector from the input stylus had to overcome the shear strength of the virtual surface for cutting to occur. A more recent method by [6] used a single bilinear reference plane to cut into a voxel array of tetrahedral finite element substructures derived from CT and MRI images. Unfortunately, the algorithm was not within interactive frame rates needed by simulators. Another approach was taken by [2] who used boolean operations on 3D surface geometry, but did not included any underlying physics system. Other researchers have demonstrated cutting techniques but have not published their algorithms [12, 13]. One novel proposal incorporates fuzzy logic to quantitatively evaluate a user's cutting performance within a simulator [8].

1.4 Training Issues

Much of the purported potential attributed to medical simulators is based upon the training success achieved by flight simulators [4]. Correspondingly, a number of performance and training assessment techniques developed for flight simulators can be applied to medical simulators. A trainee's performance is a ranking of their decision-making process and motor skills compared to another session. Training assessment is the amount of skills that trainee has achieved from the simulator that can be applied to real-world tasks. One transference rate measurement is the Transfer Effectiveness Ratio which is the difference between the transfer performance of a control group to a simulator-based group [1]. Imperfections in a simulator may lead to negative transfer or counterproductive behavior that is reinforced by the simulator. Since simulators can only approximate their real-world tasks, they must be judged on their training effectiveness. One subjective method, the Cooper-Harper characteristic scale, allows pilots to determine if a flight simulator is unsatisfactory, needs improvements, or is sufficient for training. Another important aspect of a simulator is its workload which is the amount of mental ability required by the trainee to perform a task. As workload increases, the trainee can initially compensate but with further increases, performance drops rapidly until the trainee is overloaded [7]. Workload assessment can be done subjectively, based on performance measurements or by physiological measures.

2 System

2.1 Overview

The current implementation of our opthalmic surgical simulator was developed to test the system's response time and prototype the functionality of several surgical instruments. Since virtual reality applications require a real-time frame rate, a mass-spring network was initially chosen to perform the necessary physical behaviors of the models. The mass-spring algorithm is also parallelizable. Models were based on cross-sections derived from published statistical averages on anatomical curvature and thickness [10]. Alias Studio software was used to construct and export all surface models. Physically based models were composed of triangle sets for flexibility while static models consisted of triangle meshes for speed. Available surgical instruments are: a pick, blade, suction cutter, drainage needle, and laser. None of the instruments had any moving parts. The current VR interface consists of a 3D mouse and stereo glasses, but a more nonintrusive interface is under development which will consists of two tracked vitrectomy instruments, a microscope-like housing for the stereo glasses, and a wrist support structure. Although tactile feedback is not supported, most vitrectomy maneuvers do not generate strong contact forces. The intersection of an instrument and a model involved testing a general line/sphere intersection routine with each surface vertex. Simple disease simulation consists of a planar fibrovascular tissue with perpendicular traction and a force function to simulate rhegmatogenous detachment. The software is comprised of C++ classes with the OpenGL graphics library and the Electronic Visualization Laboratory's CAVE library [9] running on a duel Silicon Graphics MXE Octane workstation. Figure 3 shows the exterior and interior views of the model.

2.2 Physics System

Flexible structures such as the retina and fibrovascular tissue were modeled as above but the conversion program fitted a vector spring through each edge. Vector springs were developed as a more stable spring algorithm by Alan Millman at the Electronic Visualization Laboratory. Spring stiffness constants and models' mass distribution were based upon local surface area [17]. Vertices can be marked as instances to propagate forces between different models, or they can be marked as fixed to prevent them from being integrated. Global force functions include gravity, intraocular pressure and viscosity. Incorporating measured elasticity material properties for all physical structures is currently under investigation.

2.3 Disease Simulation

A circular fibrovascular tissue model was constructed and attached onto the posterior section of the retina model via common instance vertices. An inward perpendicular contraction force was generated by reducing the natural rest length of the tissue model's springs. This caused the model to shrink inwards pulling the retina with it. To approximate a rhegmatogenous detachment, a simple local force function was implemented which added a radial force towards the center of the vitreous chamber to selected retinal vertices.

2.4 Instrumentation

Pick A pick is primarily used to elevate tissue. When the simulated pick intersects a surface, all of the intersecting vertices are linked its current position. Nearby vertices react by the force propagation of their shared springs. Current work will couple the pick with the light probe so that tissue models can be elevated before being cut. In addition, a fracture algorithm has been planned to subdivide surface springs and triangles when a spring's length exceeds a set limit. Figure 4 shows a screen snapshot of the pick instrument as well as the other instruments available in the simulator.

Blade A new interactive cutting algorithm is currently being implemented to subdivide surface springs and triangles along the path of the blade instrument. The blade's path will be approximated with a set of parallelograms which can be quickly intersected with a model's spring list. Springs will be subdivided about their intersection points and induce adjacent triangles to subdivide. A partial intersection algorithm has also been outlined when a surface slopes away from the cutting path, or when cutting begins or ends within a triangle. Newly created springs' stiffness constants and vertices' mass values will be computed based upon the local surface area of the new triangle configuration. Figure 2 illustrates the steps in the subdivision process.

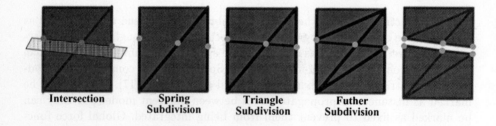

Intersection   Spring Subdivision   Triangle Subdivision   Futher Subdivision

Fig. 2. Cutting subdivision

Suction Cutter The suction cutter attracts nearby vertices to its opening, and then subdivides and removes triangles similar to the blade's cutting algorithm when they are within a certain distance.

Drainage Needle A simple gas-fluid exchange is being implemented with a height ramp function to represent separate gas and fluid regions using different values for intraocular pressure and viscosity. The fluid-gas boundary is initialized at the top of the vitreous chamber and is decremented for each time step while the needle is activated until it reaches the needle's tip position. Individual vertices can quickly determine their region before computing their forces. Drainage of breaks is done by first testing if nearby vertices have the detachment force function and if they are all within the gas region for drainage to occur. If successful, then the deattachment force function's magnitude is decreased until it reaches zero.

Laser After breaks have been successfully drained, the laser instrument is used to adhere the surrounding retina so that fluids cannot reenter. This implementation first performs a ray-cylinder intersection from the laser's position to the retina's spring list to determine if springs are outside, inside or partially intersecting the laser's projection. If a spring is outside or not near its rest position, adhesion cannot occur and the spring is ignored. Internal springs near their rest position will have their vertices marked as fixed and have a small whitish circular map blended at their corresponding texture positions within retinal map to visually indicate adhesion. Partially intersecting springs are subdivided and then processed.

3 Evaluation

As a first step in evaluating the simulator in terms of a training environment for ophthalmology residents, a group of fellows and retinal surgeons will be asked to attend several evaluation sessions in which they will process three simulated surgical cases and rank the simulator's training potential through a modified Cooper-Harper survey. To allow for adjustment to the virtual reality interface, several short practice exercises with each instrument will precede the cases. Once the simulator's ranking is known, subjects will be asked to comment on the image quality, modeling detail, tracking accuracy, physical interface, and instrumentation.

References

1. Arthur S. Blaiwes, Joseph A. Plug, and James J. Reagan. Transfer of training and the measurement of training effectiveness. *Human Factors*, 15(6):523–533, 1973.
2. Scott L. Delp, Peter Loan, Cagatay Basdogan, and Joseph M. Rosen. Surgical simulation: An emerging technology for training in emergency medicine. *Presence*, 6(2):147–159, April 1997.
3. Nathaniel I. Durlach and Anne S. Mavor, editors. *Virtual Reality Scientific and Technological Challanges*. National Academy Press, Washington D.C., 1995.

4. Gerald A. Higgins, Gregory L. Merrill, Lawrence J. Hettinger, Christoph R. Kaufmann, Howard R. Champion, and Richard M. Satava. New simulation technologies for surgical training and certification: Current status and future projections. *Presence*, 6(2):160–172, April 1997.
5. Wayne Lytle. Simulated treatment of an ocular tumor. ACM SIGGRAPH Video Review, July 1989.
6. Andreas Mazura and S. Seifert. Virtual cutting in medical data. In K.S. Morgan, editor, *Transformation of Medicine Through Communication*, volume 39, pages 420–429. Medicine Meets Virtual Reality Conference, IOS Press, January 1997.
7. Robert D. O'Donnell and F. Thomas Eggmeier. Workload assessment methodology. In K. R. Boff, L. Kaufman, and J. Thomas, editors, *Handbook of Perception and Human Performance: Sensation and Perception*, chapter 42. John Wiley & Sons, 1986.
8. David Ota, Bowen Loftin, Tim Saito, Robert Lea, and James Keller. Virtual reality in surgical education. *Computers in Biology and Medicine*, 25(2):127–137, 1995.
9. Dave Pape. A hardware-independent virtual reality development system. *IEEE Computer Graphics and Applications*, 16(4):44–47, July 1996.
10. Robert F. Parshall. Computer-aided geometric modeling of the human eye and orbit. *Journal of Biomedical Communication*, 18(2):32–39, 1991.
11. Steven Pieper, Joseph Rosen, and David Zeltzer. Interactive graphics for plastic surgery: A task-level analysis and implementation. In *ACM Proceedings Interactive 3D Graphics*, volume 3, pages 127–134, 1992.
12. Mark A. Sagar, David Bullivant, Gordon D. Mallinson, Peter J. Hunter, and Ian W. Hunter. A virtual environment and model of the eye for surgical simulation. In *Computer Graphics Proceedings*, pages 205–212. SIGGRAPH, 1994.
13. Micheal J. Sinclair, John Peifer, and Ray Haleblian. Computer-simulated eye surgery. *The Journal of the American Academy of Ophthalmolgy*, 102(3):517–521, March 1995.
14. Gyeong-Jae Song and Narender P. Reddy. Tissue cutting in virtual environments. In Richard M. Satava, Karen Morgan, Hans B. Sieburg, Rudy Mattheus, and Jens P. Christensen, editors, *Interactive Technology and the new Paradigm for Healthcare*, volume 18, pages 359–364. Medicine Meets Virtual Reality, IOS Press, January 1995.
15. Richard Szeliski and David Tonnesen. Surface modeling with oriented particle systems. In *Computer Graphics Proceedings*, pages 185–194. SIGGRAPH, 1992.
16. Demetri Terzopoulos and Kurt Fleischer. Modeling inelastic deformation: Viscoelasticity, plasticity, fracture. In *Computer Graphics Proceedings*, pages 269–278. SIGGRAPH, 1988.
17. Jane Wilhelms and Allen Van Gelder. Anatomically based modeling. In *Computer Graphics Proceedings*, pages 173–180. SIGGRAPH, 1997.

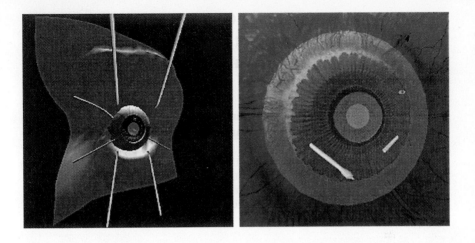

Fig. 3. Exterior and interior views of the VR model

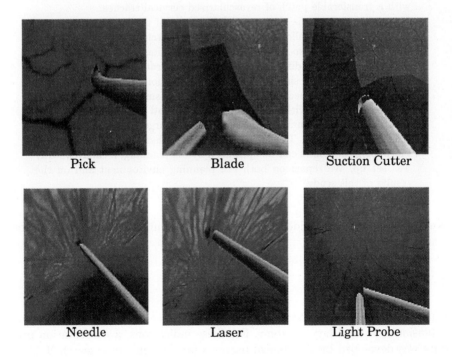

Fig. 4. Instrument screen snapshots

An Experimental Image Guided Surgery Simulator for Hemicricolaryngectomy and Reconstruction by Tracheal Autotransplantation

Filip Schutyser[1], Johan Van Cleynenbreugel[1], Vincent Vander Poorten[2],
Pierre Delaere[2], Guy Marchal[1], and Paul Suetens[1]

[1] Laboratory for Medical Image Computing (ESAT and Radiology) K.U.Leuven,
[2] Departement of Oto-Rhino-Laryngology Head and Neck Surgery
University Hospitals of Leuven, Herestraat 49, B-3000 Leuven, Belgium
Filip.Schutyser@uz.kuleuven.ac.be

Abstract. In this paper we describe the current state of our surgical planning environment for a conservation method for unilateral glottic cancer with significant subglottic extension. The latter consists of a hemicricolaryngectomy and subsequent reconstruction of the laryngeal defect with a transferable patch of revascularized cervical trachea.

In order to restore the three crucial functions of the larynx: airway patency, speech and swallowing, such a tracheal patch has to meet a typical surgical constraint (so-called paramedian position at glottic level). As such constraints are difficult to realise intraoperatively, we designed an image-based surgery simulator for the application. The planning environment visualizes medical image volumes (3D surfaces of the anatomy of interest together with multiplanar reslices) and takes specific surgical constraints into account. The guidance of the surgeon through the planning is menu-driven. To partly test our hypothesis that postoperative morphological results can be optimized by 3D planning, a cadaver study was set up. We report on both the planning environment and on the results of this study.

Keywords Image guided therapy, surgery simulation, hemilaryngectomy, tracheal autograft

1 Introduction

Current surgical treatment for unilateral glottic cancer with significant subglottic extension is a total laryngectomy. For these indications, a conservation procedure was developed by the clinical partners involved in this research [1, 2]. The technique consists of a hemicricolaryngectomy and subsequent reconstruction of the laryngeal defect with a transferable patch of revascularized cervical trachea. The advantage of this technique over the formerly performed total laryngectomy is the absence of a permanent tracheostoma and the preservation of the voice, obviating the need for a voice prosthesis and its accompanying inconveniences.

In this conservation procedure, the position of the patch at the glottic level is pivotal in determining the functional result of the technique with regard to airway patency, speech and swallowing.

We hypothesize that the postoperative morphological results of this technique can be optimized if the procedure is planned in 3D, starting from the CT-images that are routinely made in the diagnostic workup of such patients. A crucial step towards this hypothesis is the ability to respect the constraints on the patch at the glottic level. For this purpose we have developed an image guided surgery simulator. In it, the dimensions and location of the laryngeal resection and of the tracheal patch are planned, taking into account a number of surgical constraints, the one at the glottic level being the most important. From this simulation, actual measurements are obtained of the specimen to be resected and of the patch to be used for the reconstruction. To test that crucial step towards our hypothesis, a cadaver study was set up.

In section 2 some background information is given on the surgical technique. Section 3 outlines our approach towards surgery simulation. The cadaver experiments and their results are described in section 4. Concluding remarks finish the paper in 5.

2 Background

The surgeons involved in this research [1,2] have postulated the paramedian position to be the ideal patch position to provide for the three crucial larynx functions. If the patch is positioned in this way, the reconstructed "larynx" would resemble a situation of one paralyzed and one intact vocal fold at the glottic level, a situation known to give acceptable functional results. This position is however difficult to achieve intraoperatively because variable tumor dimensions in patients with variable laryngeal dimensions demand an individualized resection and an individually tailored tracheal patch for reconstruction.

So far (July 1998) fourteen patients have undergone this operation, the resection and the reconstruction being based on the clinical intuition of the surgeons. All patients did well postoperatively, but varying results with respect to airway patency, speech and swallowing have been observed, the results being better with the definitive patch position being closer to the paramedian position. In order to optimize the postoperative functional results of this new surgical technique, image guided surgical planning was envisaged.

3 Simulation environment

At the core of this simulation environment is the notion of representing the 3D space covered by the medical imaging data volume(s) as a 3D scene. In that scene multiplanar reslices are co-presented with image derived 3D surface triangle mesh representations of the anatomical structures of interest. The concepts of our environment are described in [3] and are currently implemented on top of OpenInventor [4]. As a working hypothesis, we assume that the surfaces

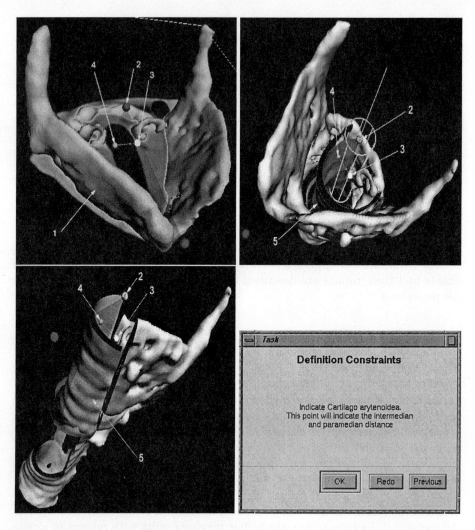

Fig. 1. This figure illustrates our laryngectomy simulation applied to a cadaver larynx. In the upper left part, an axial CT slice at subglottic level and a surface model of the larynx (label 1) are partially shown. Label 2 refers to one of the 3D points defining the symmetry plane of the larynx. Label 3 refers to a 3D point added by the surgeon on an anatomical landmark on the CT slice at glottic level. From this point and from the position of the symmetry plane, the simulator calculates the point labeled by 4. This is the point at paramedian position. In the upper right part, the same structures are labeled and the tracheal patch (label 5) has already been cut and translated to an axis in the symmetry plane through point 2. A manipulator is attached to the patch in order to let the surgeon rotate it towards the paramedian position (4). This result is shown in the lower left part, where the patch (5) is rotated in such a way that it makes contact with point 4. At that moment the patch and the larynx are resected as shown. The lower right part shows a typical example of a menu. This menu asks the surgeon to indicate the cartilago arytenoidea (3).

of anatomical structures are rigid. To simulate resecting actions, cutting algorithms (cutting with a plane, cutting along a free-hand drawn line) on surface representations are developed [5,6]. The basis of these cutting algorithms are classification of triangles and retriangulation along the intersection line.

From the routinely made spiral CT images, 3D surfaces of the larynx and trachea are derived. For real patients, the vicinity of other structures and the large differences in degree of calcification of the larynx, necessitates manual segmentation. Structures like the arythenoids which are hard to see on CT, need extra attention. However, for cadaver larynges, all segmentation can be done by thresholding. All the cadaver larynges used for the study discussed in section 4, are segmented by thresholding.

Constraints typical for success in this new surgical treatment are incorporated in the surgical simulator. The paramedian position is the constraint defining the desirable morphological result. Other constraints define the cutting planes: the position of the radial forearm fascial flap revascularizing the cervical trachea segment, the middle of the cartilago thyroidea, ... These constraints determine different important surgical parameters (e.g. the distance between the upper border of the arythenoid and the lower border of the cricoid determines the cranio-caudal length of the tracheal patch). Based on these constraints, the repositioning of the tracheal patch is determined. These constraints are visualised as geometric entities such as points, planes, axes, allowable transformations, and can be attached as annotations to particular locations of the 3D scene.

To complete the simulation, raw basic tools (cutting objects, annotation tools, ...) alone do not suffice. To supply extra guidance to the surgeon, a menu-based approach pilots the surgeon through a number of subtasks to complete the virtual operation. These subtasks ask the surgeon to instantiate the constraints on the individual anatomy of the patient. Based on his expertise, he indicates a possible configuration for the constraints on the CT-images or the 3D surface representation. When following these subtasks, cutting actions are performed. Once he finishes a first simulation, he can redo some subtasks to optimize some of the previous choices. In figure 1, details of this simulation are pointed out.

Once an optimal configuration is selected, a set of measurements easily reproducible during the actual operation is derived. Measurement tools resembling tools common to the surgeon in the operating theatre are available, e.g. (flexi)rulers.

4 Experiments

To test the crucial step towards our hypothesis mentioned in the introduction, a cadaver study was set up. We tested (on seven cadaver larynges) whether the simulated operation – i.e. the optimal one according to the postulate of the surgeons and thus taking into account the defined constraints and the anatomy of the larynx – could be advantageously employed during actual operation. Therefore post-operative imaging was used to measure how the constraints were met.

To enable post-to-pre registration fiducial markers were attached to the cadaver larynges.

For each cadaver larynx, pre-operative CT imaging was used to plan the operation. The surgeon repeated and adapted the planning until an optimal configuration was reached. Based on this configuration, enough reproducible distances (different measurements on the larynx: length of the tracheal patch, internal "circular" distances on the tracheal patch, see figure 2) were measured to reconstruct the virtual operation during the actual surgery.

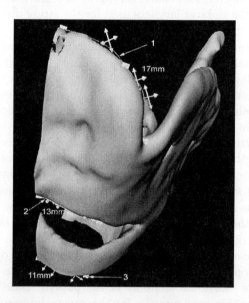

Fig. 2. This figure shows the measurements on the part of the larynx that will be resected. All measurements start from the middle of the larynx, a landmark which can be easily determined intra-operatively. Label 1 and 2 point to distances on the cartilago thyroidea, label 3 points to a distance on the arcus cartilago cricoidea. The measurement tool is a flexiruler (i.e. a planar, but curved distance).

After the actual surgery, post-operative CT imaging of the resected larynges makes it possible to compare the planned and actual results. The post-to-pre registration was done by least squares point based matching on the fiducial markers. After registration, the post-operative images are resampled on the grid of the pre-operative image volume to generate comparable measurements. To apply adequate measurements, magnitudes (see figure 3) presumed to be related to the functional results of the operation were chosen [1].

Based on the seven test cases, a few trends become clear. First of all, the major purpose of the planning, i.e. assuring that the patch meets the paramedian position, is reached. All the tracheal patches were positioned conforming to the paramedian position. However, concerning the anterior-posterior glottic diameter

Larynx Nr	AP simul mm	AP post mm	GL simul mm^2	GL post mm^2	SG simul mm^2	SG post mm^2	Δ PM mm
1	15	17	104	90	125	110	-1
2	20	17	126	111	170	129	0
3	13	16	52	53	178	213	0
4	21	21	95	55	191	121	-2
5	17	20	77	116	89	143	1
6	20	22	80	109	149	157	0
7	19	14	64	45	105	115	0

Table 1. Measurements on seven test larynges.
AP   = anterior-posterior diameter at glottic level
GL   = area of airway lumen at glottic level
SG   = area of airway lumen at subglottic level
Δ PM = difference between simulated paramedian distance and postoperative patch position (negative distance means that the patch is more proximal).

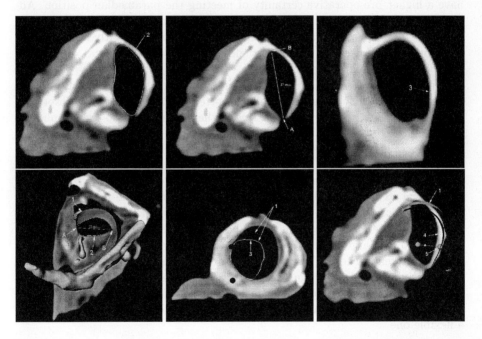

Fig. 3. This figure illustrates, for the particular case of larynx 1, the quantitative measures used in table 1. The upper row shows three slices through the post-operative CT volume. The lower row shows two (left, middle) slices through the pre-operative and one (right) through the post-operative CT volume, in combination with simulation data. Label 1 indicates the planned tracheal patch. Line AB, label 2 and label 3 refer to the anterior-posterior glottic diameter, the area of the airway lumen at glottic level and the area of the airway lumen at subglottic level respectively. Label 4 points to the actual tracheal patch. Label 5 points to the paramedian position. This position is shared by both the planned and the actual patch.

and the airway lumen areas (at glottic level and subglottic level), there are fairly small differences (see Table 1). The fact there is a slight variation in the stitches used to fix the patch to the cricoidal remnant posteriorly and to the vocal cord remnant anteriorly, can explain the differences from the planned configuration. Moreover, in some cases the tracheal patch is stretched in sagittal direction, a situation we will try to foresee in the future.

A more rigorous validation in the near future will investigate the importance of deformable patches in the planning system and the methods of attaching the tracheal patch and the vocal cord. We also consider more advanced methods (video matching) for intra-operative support than a list of measurements.

5 Discussion

When following our approach from planning to surgery, even when resecting cadaver larynges, surgeons report to feel more comfortable, mainly because they have a higher pre-operative certainty of meeting the paramedian position. Additionally they report to obtain a better insight in the particular anatomy and even in sometimes competing constraints, they are only implicitly aware of (e.g. reaching the paramedian position at glottic level versus minimal decrease of airway lumen area at subglottic level).

During the course of the design of the planning system and its use in the cadaver experiments, the surgeons also reported to gain insight with respect to refinement of their technique. Furthermore, the system has also been applied to three patients at this moment (see figure 4). From the experiences gained by this actual use of the laryngectomy simulator, we were forced to reconsider our basic assumptions.

Earlier, we assumed that our simulation environment only had to handle rigid anatomical structures. Rigidity certainly is a property of the larynx. However, for the tracheal patch, this assumption is not always valid. Although the surgery itself can be performed by using an undeformed patch, this way of working can lead to too large a resection. Only in the case where a maximally possible resection is really needed – e.g. for a tumor including the anterior coomissura and crossing the larynx symmetry plane –, a rigid patch would be appropriate. As this is not always needed in clinical practice, future work will investigate the application of deformation techniques turning the rigid tracheal patch into a flexible one.

Acknowledgments

This work is performed, partly under the Flemish government-funded IWT ITA-GBO202, *TeleVisie* project, and partly under the EU-funded Brite Euram III *PISA* project (nr. BRPR CT97 0378). Partners in the latter are Materialise NV, Belgium; Philips Medical Systems BV, the Netherlands: ICS-AD; DePuy International Ltd, UK; Ceka NV, Belgium; K.U. Leuven, Belgium: ESAT/Radiology & Div. Biomechanics; University of Leeds, UK: Research School of Medicine.

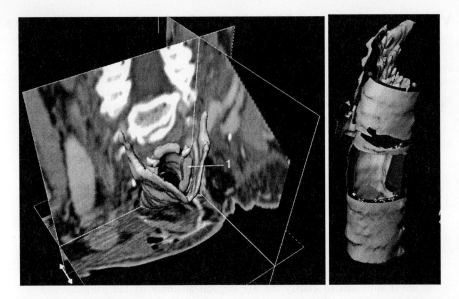

Fig. 4. This figure illustrates the simulator applied to a real patient. On the left, a 3D scene representation of a larynx containing a T3 glottic cancer with vocal fold fixation (label 1) is shown. On the right, the result of laryngeal resection and tracheal patch relocation is depicted.

References

1. P.R. Delaere, V. Vander Poorten, A. Goeleven, M. Feron, R. Hermans: Tracheal Autotransplantation: a Reliable Reconstructive Technique for Extended Hemilaryngectomy Defects. Laryngoscope 108: June 1998, p 929 – 934
2. P.R. Delaere, V. Vander Poorten, R. Hermans: Autotransplantation of the trachea: experimental evaluation of a reconstructive technique for extended hemilaryngectomy defects. *accepted for publication in* Annals of Otology, Rhinology and Laryngology, 1998
3. J. Van Cleynenbreugel, K. Verstreken, G. Marchal, P. Suetens: A flexible environment for image guided virtual surgery planning. Proc. VBC96, Lect. Notes in Computer Science, 1131, 1996, p 501–510
4. J. Werneke: The Inventor Mentor, Programming Object-Oriented 3D Graphics with OpenInventor Addison-Wesley, release 2, 1994
5. F. Schutyser, J. Van Cleynenbreugel, G. Marchal, P. Suetens: An interactive environment for constraint-based pre-operative simulation of rigid tomia procedures. Technical Report KUL/ESAT/PSI/9801, February 1998
6. F. Schutyser, J. Van Cleynenbreugel, G. Marchal, P. Suetens: Implementation of Tomia algorithms on Triangle Strip Sets. Technical Report KUL/ESAT/PSI/9802, February 1998

Virtual Endoscopy of Mucin-Producing Pancreas Tumors

Toshio Nakagohri, Ferenc A. Jolesz, Shigeo Okuda, *Takehide Asano,
*Takashi Kenmochi , *Osamu Kainuma, *Yoshiharu Tokoro *Hiromichi Aoyama,
**William E.Lorensen, Ron Kikinis

Department of Radiology Brigham and Women's Hospital, Harvard
Medical School
*Department of Surgery Chiba University School of Medicine
**General Electric Corporate Research and Development Center
e-mail:nakagori@med.m.chiba-u.ac.jp

Abstract. We have used computer based virtual endoscopy techniques as a novel approach to clarify the 3D surgical anatomy of the pancreas and improve preoperative surgical planning. 13 cases (18 lesions) with mucin-producing pancreas tumors were investigated by "virtual pancreatoscopy". All cystic tumors and the pancreatic ducts were displayed by virtual endoscopy. The surfaces of intraductal papillary adenocarcinomas were illustrated more irregularly than benign cystic lesions. Virtual pancreatoscopy was useful for surgical planning of minimally invasive resection of the pancreas.

Introduction

Virtual Endoscopy is a new technology which can make computer simulated endoscopic images by processing high resolusion MRI/CT data. Preliminaly study about virtual endoscopy revealed that this technique had many promising advantages. For example, virtual endoscopy can generate views that are not possible in an actual endoscopic examination. Clinical applications of virtual endoscopy for pancreas have not been reported. In this study, usefulness of virtual endoscopy of mucin-producing tumor of the pancreas was studied.

Patients and Methods

13 cases with mucin-producing pancreas tumor(MPPT) were studied . Two patients have 3 cystic lesions and one patient have 2 lesions, so we investigated 18 lesions with using virtual endoscopy. All patients underwent resection of the pancreas in Chiba University Hospital from 1996 to 1997. Each patient's profile is in Table 1

Table 1 Patient's profile

no.	age/sex	pathological diagnosis	location	virtual endoscopy	operation
1	37/M	intraductal papillary adenoma	head	smooth	inferior head resection
2	69/M	intraductal papillary adenoma	head	intermediate	DpPHR
3	72/F	intraductal papillary adenocarcinoma	head	irregular	PpPD
4	57/M	intraductal papillary adenocarcinoma	head	irregular	DpPHR
5	59/M	intraductal papillary adenoma	head	intermediate	inferior head resection
6	69/F	1.intraductal papillary adenoma 2.simple cyst	1.head 2.head	1.smooth 2.smooth	inferior head resection
7	65/M	1.intraductal papillary adenoma 2.intraductal papillary adenoma 3.intraductal papillary adenoma	1.head 2.head 3.head	1.irregular 2.smooth 3.smooth	PpPD
8	65/M	1.intraductal papillary adenoma 2.intraductal papillary adenoma 3.intraductal papillary adenoma	1.head 2.head 3.tail	1.intermediate 2.smooth 3.smooth	DpPHR+DP
9	61/M	intraductal papillary adenoma	head	intermediate	inferior head resection
10	72/F	intraductal papillary adenocarcinoma	head	irregular	DpPHR
11	50/M	intraductal papillary adenoma	body	smooth	segmental resection
12	53/M	intraductal papillary adenocarcinoma	body	irregular	DP
13	68/F	intraductal papillary adenoma	body	intermediate	DP

Abbreviation :
DpPHR: duodenum-preserving pancreas head resection
PpPD: pylorus-preserving pancreatoduodenectomy
DP: distal pancreatectomy

The MRI data were acquired by 1.5T Signa MR system(GE) .The diagnosis of MPPT was established by findings during endoscopic retrograde cholangio-pancreatography (ERCP) and pathological findings. Virtual endoscopy images were generated with Virtual Endoscopy Software Aplication (VESA) on UNIX workstations in surgical planning laboratory,Department of Radiology and MRI Unit, Brigham and Women's Hospital/Harvard Medical School.
Each image was visualized by processing cross-sectional MRI date according to the threshold of the signal intensity. We used an automated path planning technique to generate path1,2,3).

Patients and Methods

It was possible to visualize all the pancreatic ducts and cystic lesions of mucin-producing pancreas tumor (MPPT) by virtual endoscopy.The pancreatic ducts and 18 cystic lesions were detected correctly . Virtual endoscopy allowed us to observe the pancreatic duct and the inner surface of the cystic lesions (Fig1,2) .

Fig. 1: Virtual endoscopy image of the pancreatic duct. A normal pancratic duct was visualized.

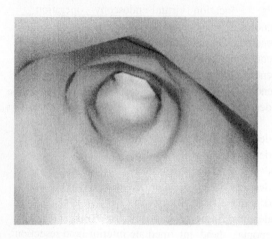

Fig. 2: Virtual endoscopy image of the mucin-producing pancreas tumor. Virtual endoscopy demonstrated the pancreatic duct(right side) and the cystic lesion(left side) simultaneously.

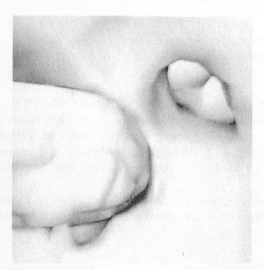

Virtual endoscopy was useful to clarify the anatomical relationship between the cystic tumor ,the pancreatic duct and the bile duct. Eighteen cystic lesions were divided into 3 groups according to the degrees of the irregularity of the surface images rendered by virtual endoscopy: irregular type(n=5)(Fig. 3), intermediate type(n=5)(Fig. 4), and smooth type(n=8)(Fig. 5).

Fig. 3 : Virtual endoscopy image of irregular type(case 4)

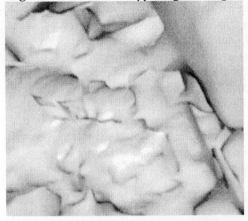

Fig. 4 : Virtual endoscopy image of intermediate type(case 9)

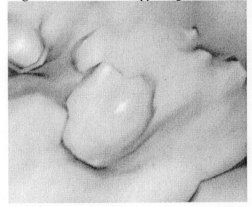

Fig. 5 : Virtual endoscopy image of smooth type(case 11)

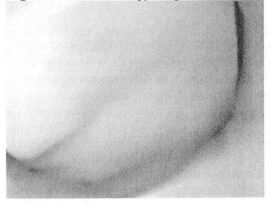

Four lesions of irregular type (n=5) were intraductal papillary adenocarcinomas, and the other irregular lesion was a intraductal papillary adenoma. All five lesions of intermediate type were intraductal papillary adenomas. Six lesions of smooth types were intraductal papillary adenomas, and one lesion of smooth type was a simple cyst. This result revealed that surfaces of adenocarcinomas were illustrated more irregularly than benign cystic lesions by virtual endoscopy. Cystc lesions next to the pancreatic duct were visualized together with the pancreatic duct(Fig.6), because thin septa between cystic lesions and the pancreatic ducts could not be illustrated.

Fig. 6 : A cystic lesion next to the pancreatic duct was generated together with the pancreatic duct. Septum between the panceatic duct and cystic lesion was illustrated like pillars in some cases.

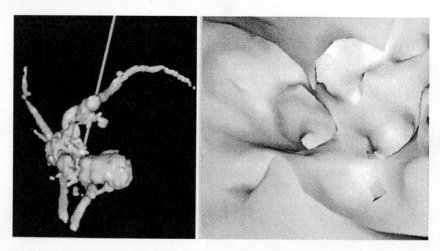

Discussion

There are two technical approaches for virtual endoscopy: Perspective volume rendering and surface rendering. To improve interpretation and exploration, we have made surface-rendered images derived from computer reconstruction of the cross-sectional MRI image data1,2,3). Walls of fluid-containing organs, such as the pancreatic duct and the bile duct are well demarcated in MRI and CT. Virtual endoscopy depicts the surfaces of the pancreatic duct, the bile duct and the cystic lesions in the pancreas. We can explore the inner space of the pancreatic ducts and cystic lesions interactively. Our virtual endoscopy technique can demonstrate not only a surface rendered image but also a three dimensional (3D) reconstructed image of the pancreas. Therefore, the relationship to anatomic structures located outside the surfaces is continuously maintained and displayed at the same time. Changing the transparency of the images assist the operator to view the bile duct and cystic tumors from the inner space of the pancreatic duct. The viewer may penetrate the walls and see the extent of lesions within and beyond the walls as well as the adjacent organs, such as the bile duct and the duodenum. We can also overview the pancreatic duct from the outside at the same time using split screen display (Fig.7).This technique can generate 3D reconstructed images of the pancreatic duct and the bile duct. The operator of virtual endoscopy can perceive his own position. Precise and interactive 3D images also provide information useful for the surgical procedure4,5). Multiwindow display helps surgeons to recognize the anatomical relationship among the cystic lesion, the pancreatic duct and the bile duct. Conventional MRI produce flat, two-dimensional images that give a poor picture of the location and the extent of the tumor in the pancreas.

Fig. 7 : Our virtual endoscopy technique can make 3D reconstructed images of the pancreatic duct and the bile duct. Split screen display helps surgeon to recognize the anatomical relationship among the cystic lesion,the pancreatic duct, and the bile duct. 3-D images and virtual endoscopy images aid diagnosis and surgical planning of mucin-producing pancreas tumors.

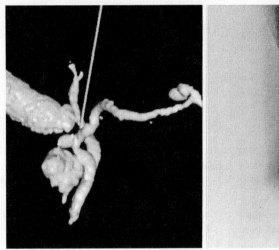
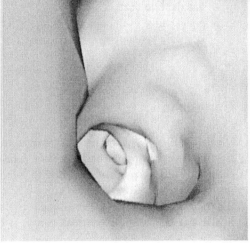

When treating low grade malignant tumors of the pancreas such as mucin-producing intraductal papillary tuomrs, minimally invasive surgical procedures have been advocated these days because of patient's quality of life6). For surgical planning of pancreatectomy, it is necessary to clarify the anatomical relationship among the tumor, the panceatic duct and the bile duct. Whether the bile duct can be preserved or not is one of the most important factor for choosing operative procedures. Preservation of the bile duct depends on the degree of the involvement by the tumors. When the bile duct is not involved by the tumor, we perform resection of the inferior head of the pancreas or duodenum-preserving pancreas head resection (DpPHR) according to the tumor extension to the Santorini"s pancreas. Anatomical identification of the lesion in the head of the pancreas is useful for surgical planning.

Virtual endoscopy proved to have a diagnostic potential for pancreatic disease. The surfaces of the cystic lesions could be visualized in all cases of our serires. Real pancreatoscopy do not always demonstrate the view of inner space of the cystic lesions in the pancreas. All intraductal papillary adenocarcinoma(n=4) had irregular surfaces illustrated by virtual endoscopy. 13 lesions of 14 benign lesions had smooth or slightly irregular surface. Preoperative diagnosis of MPPT is difficult, especially concerning the oncological feature of these kind of tumors. So virtual endoscopy would be useful to evaluate the oncological characters before the operation. The advantages of virtual endoscopy are summarized in Table 2.

Table2: Advantages of virtual endoscopy

1. visualization of inner surface of cystic lesions and the pancreatic duct
2. display of anatomical relationship among the lesion, the pancreatic duct and the bile duct
3. preoperative evaluation of oncological feature by observing the surface of cystic lesions

Conclusion

Virtual endoscopy of the pancreas proved to be a valuable method for clarifying the anatomical relationship between the pancreatic ducts and cystic lesions. Virtual endoscopy had a diagnostic potential to evaluate oncological features by observing the inner surface of the cystic lesions.
It is concluded that virtual endoscopy is useful for surgical planning of minimally invasive resection of the pancreas.

Acknowledgement: This study was supported by Japan association for the advancement of medical equipments.

References

1)Jolesz FA, Lorensen WE, Kikinis R et al. Interactive Virtual Endoscopy. AJR Vol 169: 1229-1235, 1997

2)Jolesz FA, Lorensen WE, Kikinis R, et al. Virtual endoscopy: three-dimensional rendering of cross-sectional images for endoluminal visualization (abst). Radiology 469, 193,1994

3)Lorensen WE, Jolesz FA, Kikinis R. The exploration of cross-sectional data with a virtual endoscope. In: Satava RM, Morgan K, Sieburg HB et al. Interactive technology and the new pardigm for health-care: medicine meets virtual reality III proceedings. Amsterdam, Holland: IOS Press; 221-230. 1995

4)Ron Kikinis ,P. Langham Gleason ,Thomas M. Moriarty et al. Computer Assisted Interactive Three-Dimensional Planning for Neurosurgical Procedures. Neurosurgery, Vol 38: 640-651,1996

5)Shin Nakajima, Hideki Atsumi, Abhir H. Bhalerao, et al. Computer-assisted Surgical Planning for Cerebrovascular Neurosurgery.Neurosurgery.Vol41,403-409,1997

6)Nakagohri T, Asano T, Takayama W et al. Resecton of the Inferior Head of the Pancreas:Report of a case. Surgery Today. Vol 26,640-644,1996

Augmented Reality Visualization for Laparoscopic Surgery

Henry Fuchs[1], Mark A. Livingston[1], Ramesh Raskar[1], D'nardo Colucci[1], Kurtis Keller[1], Andrei State[1], Jessica R. Crawford[1], Paul Rademacher[1], Samuel H. Drake[3], and Anthony A. Meyer, MD[2]

[1] Department of Computer Science, University of North Carolina at Chapel Hill
[2] Department of Surgery, University of North Carolina at Chapel Hill
[3] Department of Computer Science, University of Utah

Abstract. We present the design and a prototype implementation of a three-dimensional visualization system to assist with laparoscopic surgical procedures. The system uses 3D visualization, depth extraction from laparoscopic images, and six degree-of-freedom head and laparoscope tracking to display a merged real and synthetic image in the surgeon's video-see-through head-mounted display. We also introduce a custom design for this display. A digital light projector, a camera, and a conventional laparoscope create a prototype 3D laparoscope that can extract depth and video imagery.

Such a system can restore the physician's natural point of view and head motion parallax that are used to understand the 3D structure during open surgery. These cues are not available in conventional laparoscopic surgery due to the displacement of the laparoscopic camera from the physician's viewpoint. The system can also display multiple laparoscopic range imaging data sets to widen the effective field of view of the device. These data sets can be displayed in true 3D and registered to the exterior anatomy of the patient. Much work remains to realize a clinically useful system, notably in the acquisition speed, reconstruction, and registration of the 3D imagery.

1 Introduction

1.1 Challenges in Laparoscopic Surgery

The success of laparoscopy as a surgical technique stems from its ability to give the surgeon a view into the patient's internal spaces with only small incisions in the skin and body wall. Surgery done through such minimally invasive techniques leads to reduced trauma, shorter hospitalization, and more rapid return to normal activity. Although laparoscopy is a powerful visualization and intervention tool, it suffers from some visual limitations which we believe our proposed system will ameliorate.

- **The imagery is 2D and not 3D.** The surgeon can only estimate the depth of structures by moving the camera (to achieve motion parallax) or

by physically probing the structures. While stereo laparoscopes and stereo displays ameliorate this problem, they still separate the camera from the physician's point of view and fail to provide head-motion parallax.
- **The laparoscope has a small field of view**. The surgeon must frequently adjust the camera position and orientation, which requires skilled coordination with the assistant. A surgeon may opt to operate the camera himself to reduce the discoordination of the actual view with the desired view, but that limits him to only one hand with which to operate. Fixed camera holders can be used, but then the viewpoint and view direction are limited; this introduces risk due to the possible presence of important, vulnerable structures outside the viewing field.
- **The procedure requires significant hand-eye coordination**. The laparoscopic camera does not generally face the direction in which the surgeon is facing. This means that the instruments' on-screen movements will not match the surgeon's hand movements. It requires experience and hand-eye coordination for a surgeon to adjust to this disparity.

1.2 Benefits of Augmented Reality

Augmented reality (AR) refers to systems that attempt to merge computer graphics and real imagery into a single, coherent perception of an enhanced world around the user. Emerging AR technologies have the potential to reduce the problems caused by the visual limitations of laparoscopy. The AR system can display the resulting 3D imagery in the proper place with respect to the exterior anatomy of the patient. By acquiring depth information and rendering true 3D images of the structures visible in the laparoscopic camera, the AR system gives the physician most of the depth cues of natural vision. (Exceptions include focus and visual acuity.) The display of the laparoscopic data is not limited to the current viewpoint of the camera, but can include data acquired from a previous camera location (perhaps subject to a limit on the length of time the data is considered "current"). Thus objects not currently within view of the camera can still be displayed by the AR system.

We want to emphasize that this technology is fundamentally different than coupling a stereo laparoscope with a stereo display system. AR systems allow the surgeon to view the medical imagery from the natural viewpoint, use head-induced motion parallax (instead of hand-eye coordination and camera-induced motion parallax), allow the medical imagery to be visually aligned to the exterior anatomy of the patient, and incorporate proprioceptive (body-relative) cues.

The lack of depth perception in laparoscopic surgery might limit delicate dissection or suturing [Durrani95]. An AR display presents objects in correct perspective depth, assuming that the geometry has been accurately acquired. With an AR guidance system, a laparoscopic surgeon might be able to view the peritoneal cavity from any angle merely by moving his head, without moving the endoscopic camera. AR may be able to free the surgeon from the technical limitations of the imaging and visualization methods, recapturing much of the physical simplicity and direct visualization characteristic of open surgery.

2 Previous Work

2.1 Medical Augmented Reality Systems

The first medical application of AR was to neurosurgery [Kelly86]. Similar systems [Lorensen93,Grimson95] have been developed independently. AR has also been applied to otolaryngology [Edwards95]. These applications demand less of the AR system than laparoscopy for four reasons. The surgical field is small, the patient doesn't move, the view into the patient is from a single viewpoint and view direction, and this viewpoint is external to the patient (e.g. already suitable for a hand-eye coordination). This simplifies the difficult task of building an enhanced visualization system.

Our research on medical applications of AR has until recently concentrated on ultrasound-guided procedures such as fetal examination [Bajura92,State94] and breast biopsy [Fuchs96,State96]. In the latter system, the ultrasound data is captured as a video stream and registered to the patient in real time. The physician's head must be tracked in order to view the dynamic data from any direction. We calibrate the location of the ultrasound data with respect to the probe geometry and track the probe location. These two tasks enable registration of multiple discrete slices to each other and registration of the ultrasound data set to the patient. A virtual pit [Bajura92] within the patient's body provides proper occlusion cues for the registered ultrasound data. We base our proposed system to aid laparoscopic surgery on this system.

2.2 Depth Extraction

The major new technology needed for laparoscopic visualization is acquisition of the depth map associated with the image from the laparoscopic camera. Determination of 3D scene structure from a sequence of 2D images is one of the classic problems in computer vision [Faugeras93]. There are numerous techniques for computing 3D structure, including cues from motion, stereo, shading, focus, defocus, contours, and structured light. We chose structured light for several reasons. It is an efficient and direct computation. It is as robust to shading variations and repeating patterns as other methods (although no method is immune to some features, such as specular highlights) and can be dynamically tuned to increase robustness. It offers a large depth range and allows us to trade speed for spatial resolution in the acquisition.

Structured light has long been used in computer vision to acquire depth information [Besl89,Daley95]. A variety of patterns have been tried: points, lines, multiple points, multiple lines, grids, circles, cross-hairs, thick stripes, binary-coded patterns, color-coded stripes, and random textures. Pseudo-random binary arrays [Lavoie96] are grids with recognizable points based on a pattern of "large" and "small" intersection points. We initially chose binary-coded patterns, but switched to lines since our prototype system cannot acquire images of the pattern fast enough to support depth extraction from dynamic scenes. (See Section 7 for our future plans regarding this issue.)

3 Hardware Configuration

There are four primary hardware components to our system. Three are the standard tools of AR systems: an image generation platform, a set of tracking systems, and a see-through head-mounted display (HMD) that allows the user to see the real environment. The fourth component required for this application is a 3D laparoscope that can acquire both color and range data. As noted above, we have previously applied AR to in-place visualization of ultrasound imagery. The current system is similar to that system [State96,Fuchs96].

3.1 See-Through Head-Mounted Display

We believe that the depth cue of occlusion is vital to the physician in determining the 3D structure of the medical imagery. Video-see-through (VST) displays offer the possibility of complete occlusion of the real world by the computer-generated imagery, which in this case is the medical image data. (The other option, optical-see-through displays, cannot achieve complete occlusion of the real world.) Being unaware of any commercially available VST HMDs, we initially built a simple prototype VST HMD from commercial components [State96]. This device had numerous limitations [Fuchs96]. In response to our experience with that device, we designed and implemented a new VST HMD, which is described in Section 4.

3.2 Image Generation

Having chosen to build a VST system, we needed an image generation platform capable of acquiring multiple, real-time video streams. We use an Onyx Infinite Reality system from Silicon Graphics, Inc. equipped with a Sirius Video Capture™ unit. This loads video imagery from the cameras on the VST HMD directly into the frame buffer. We augment this background image with a registered model of the patient's skin acquired during system calibration [State96]. We then render the synthetic imagery in the usual manner for 3D computer graphics. At pixels for which there is depth associated with the video imagery (e.g. the patient's skin), the depth of the synthetic imagery is compared. The synthetic imagery is painted only if it is closer. This properly resolves occlusion between the synthetic imagery and the patient's skin.

The video output capabilities of the Infinite Reality architecture allow us to output two VGA signals to the displays in the HMD and a high resolution video signal, which contains a user interface and is displayed on a conventional monitor. The system architecture is depicted graphically in Figure 1.

3.3 Tracking Systems

We use UNC's optoelectronic ceiling tracker [Welch96] for tracking the physician's head. It offers a high update rate, a high degree of accuracy, and a large range of head positions and orientations. The large range allows the physician to move freely around the patient and to examine the patient from many viewpoints. We track the laparoscope with the FlashPoint™ 5000 [IGT97] optical tracker from Image-Guided Technologies, Inc. It also offers high accuracy, but over a small range. Since the laparoscope does not move much, this is suitable for our system. Its accuracy enables the registration between multiple laparoscope data images and between the laparoscopic data set and the patient.

3.4 3D Laparoscope

To properly display the 3D structure, the laparoscope must acquire depth information. To properly display the visual texture (e.g. color, shading), the laparoscope must acquire the usual 2D color video image. We can then texture the resulting 3D mesh with the color data. We designed a custom device, described in Section 5. The device requires input of structured light images and outputs images suitable for depth and color processing. We off-load the processing of these image streams to a Silicon Graphics O2, which outputs the structured light and acquires the camera video. After simple image processing, the O2 sends to the Onyx a list of lit pixels, from which the depth is computed.

4 Video-See-Through Head-Mounted Display

We use a miniature HMD custom-designed at the computer science laboratories at the University of North Carolina and University of Utah. This VST HMD has a miniature video camera mounted in each display optic in front of each eye (Figure 4). A pair of mirrors place the apparent centroid of the camera in the same location as the center of the eye when the HMD is properly fitted to the user. A 640 × 480 LCD mounted in the eyepiece is viewed through a prism assembly which folds the optical path within a small cube. This design reduces the problem of unequal depths for the user's visual and tactile senses. The HMD has two eyepieces mounted on a horizontal bar which provides one degree of translational freedom and one degree of rotational freedom. This allows the user to adjust the inter-camera distance and the convergence angle. The entire front bar can be moved out of the way (Figure 3). The complete HMD weighs only twelve ounces, compared to six pounds for our initial prototype.

5 3D Laparoscope

To extract 3D shape, we added a structured light to a conventional laparoscope. Our "structure" is a vertical line in the image plane of the projector. We calibrate the device by building a table of depth values, then use a simple extraction algorithm which interpolates through the table. This technique has performed well on simple geometry such as scenes with little or none of the surface occluded from the projector's view. It has not yet performed well on topologically complex models that have great discontinuities in depth, highly specular reflections, low reflectance, or large patches of surfaces hidden from the projector's viewpoint.

5.1 3D Laparoscope Design

The structured light 3D laparoscope design (Figure 7) uses a conventional laparoscope in a rather unique way. Instead of being the both the illumination source and imaging device, it is only a projector—but of structured light patterns. A digital micromirror device [Hornbeck95] projector displays its image through a custom optic and through a standard laparoscope, projecting its image inside the patient. The image is the dynamic, calibrated structured light image. Alongside the projecting laparoscope is a miniature video camera mounted in a metal tube similar to a second laparoscope. This camera observes the structured light pattern on the scene and sends the image to the host. The two laparoscopes are mounted a fixed distance from each other for accurate and repeatable depth extraction.

5.2 Depth Calibration and Extraction

We measure the reflected light pattern for a set of known depths and store the results in a table. By imaging each potential light stripe from the projector onto a flat grid at a known depth, we can determine the 3D location of the point at each pixel in the camera image. With several depths, we can build a table indexed by the column number from the projector and the u and v-coordinates on the camera image plane. At each cell in the table is a 3D point. Simple thresholding determines which pixels in the camera image are illuminated by the light stripe. We find the centroid of the biggest and brightest 1D blob on each camera scanline. The 3D location of this point is interpolated from the table.

6 Experiments and Results

We have implemented two versions of this system. In the first prototype, we acquired depth via manual digitization. This implies a pre-operative acquisition of the 3D structure of the internal anatomy. Guided by real-time color images textured onto the 3D mesh, the surgeon (Meyer) successfully pierced a small foam target inside the abdominal cavity of a life-sized human model (Figures 2 and 7). This experiment showed the potential of our proposed paradigm for laparoscopic surgery. It also emphasized the importance of extracting the internal 3D structure in real time. For example, a manipulator inserted into the abdomen was severely distorted onto the surface mesh instead of appearing to be above the surface because only imagery was acquired in real time, not the 3D structure.

The second experiment was recently conducted with a system that implements interactive depth extraction. The results of this system have been promising (Figure 7). The augmented images shown to a moving HMD user clearly present the 3D structure. The computer-generated imagery of the internal structure is visually aligned with the exterior patient anatomy.

7 Discussion

We are currently focusing on three issues. First, depth extraction is slow due to inconsistent delay between commanding the projector to emit a pattern and receiving the image of the pattern from the camera. (This is more complex than synchronizing the vertical refresh.) Second, gathering multiple views is difficult due to the rigid connection between the (bulky) projector and the laparoscope. Third, multiple depth images are misregistered due to poor depth calibration.

Our current solution to the slow speed is to wait for the delay to expire. We are developing a tighter, coupled control of the camera and projector. When this is in place, we will be able to extract new data at every frame. We can also return to using binary-coded patterns as the structured light. These algorithmic and hardware improvements, along with a higher-speed projector and camera, will enable us to incrementally update an entire range image with each new video image of the pattern, thus extracting depth from a larger area of the surgical field at each time step. We will investigate methods of adaptive depth acquisition to increase accuracy and resolution in regions of particular concern to the surgeon. For gathering multiple views, we are working with fiberoptic cables and miniature cameras and displays to make the 3D laparoscope smaller and easier to maneuver into multiple positions. By improving depth calibration and merging multiple range images [Turk94], we hope to provide a more complete view of the interior scene than visible from a single laparoscope location, approaching the wide-area surgical field in open surgery. In the future, by registering pre-operative images (e.g. MRI or CT), surgical planning data, and intra-operative (e.g. ultrasound), we hope to provide a more comprehensive visualization of the surgical field than even open surgery.

We postulate that viewing laparoscopic images with our augmented reality paradigm, from outside the body, as if there were an opening into the patient, will be more intuitive than observing laparoscopic imagery on a video monitor or even viewing images from stereo laparoscopes on a stereo video monitor. We expect that the physician will still choose to move the laparoscope frequently (closer to view structures of interest or farther away to view of the entire intervention site), but with our system such movements will not cause confusing changes in the viewpoint requiring mental adaptation. Rather they will change the level of detail and update the visualization of structures that become visible to the laparoscope. We expect the physician's use of the laparoscope to be somewhat akin to exploring a dark room with a flashlight, with the added benefit of visual persistence of the regions of the scene that were previously illuminated.

We hope that our proposed system will eventually offer the following specific benefits. It could reduce the average time for the procedures (benefiting both physician and patient), reduce training time for physicians to learn these procedures, increase accuracy in the procedures due to better understanding of the structures in question and better hand-eye coordination, reduce trauma to the patient through shorter and more accurate procedures, and increase availability of the procedures due to ease of performing them.

References

[Bajura92] Bajura, M., Fuchs, H., and Ohbuchi, R. (1992). Merging virtual objects with the real world: Seeing ultrasound imagery within the patient. In *Computer Graphics (SIGGRAPH '92 Proceedings)*, volume 26, pages 203–210.

[Besl89] Besl, P. J. (1989). Active optical range imaging sensors. In *Advances in Machine Vision*, pages 1–63. Springer-Verlag.

[Daley95] Daley, R. C., Hassebrook, L. G., Stanley C. Tungate, J., Jones, J. M., Reisig, H. T., Reed, T. A., Williams, B. K., Daugherty, J. S., and Bond, M. (1995). Topographical analysis with time modulated structured light. *SPIE Proceedings*, 2488(5):396–407.

[Durrani95] Durrani, A. F. and Preminger, G. M. (1995). Three-dimensional video imaging for endoscopic surgery. *Computers in Biological Medicine*, 25(2):237–247.

[Edwards95] Edwards, P., Hawkes, D., Hill, D., Jewell, D., Spink, R., Strong, A., and Gleeson, M. (1996). Augmentation of reality in the stereo operating microscope for otolaryngology and neurosurgical guidance. *Journal of Image-Guided Surgery*, 1(3).

[Faugeras93] Faugeras, O. (1993). *Three-Dimensional Computer Vision: A Geometric Viewpoint*. MIT Press.

[Fuchs96] Fuchs, H., State, A., Pisano MD, E. D., Garrett, W. F., Hirota, G., Livingston, M. A., Whitton, M. C., and Pizer, S. M. (1996). Towards performing ultrasound-guided needle biopsies from within a head-mounted display. In *Visualization in Biomedical Computing 1996*, pages 591–600.

[Grimson95] Grimson, W., Ettinger, G., White, S., Gleason, P., Lozano-Pérez, T., Wells III, W., and Kikinis, R. (1995). Evaluating and validating an automated registration system for enhanced reality visualization in surgery. In *Proceedings of Computer Vision, Virtual Reality, and Robotics in Medicine '95 (CVRMed '95)*,.

[Hornbeck95] Hornbeck, L. J. (1995). Digital light processing and MEMS: Timely convergence for a bright future. In *Micromachining and Microfabrication '95*.

[IGT97] Image-Guided Technologies, Inc. (1997). *FlashPoint^{TM} Model 5000 3D Localizer User's & Programmer's Manual*. Boulder, CO.

[Kelly86] Kelly MD, P. J., Kall, B., and Goerss, S. (1986). Computer-assisted stereotaxic resection of intra-axial brain neoplasms. *Journal of Neurosurgery*, 64:427–439.

[Lavoie96] Lavoie, P., Ionescu, D., and Petriu, E. M. (1996). 3-D object model recovery from 2-D images using structured light. In *IEEE Instrument Measurement Technology Conference*, pages 377–382.

[Lorensen93] Lorensen, W., Cline, H., Nafis, C., Kikinis, R., Altobelli, D., and Gleason, L. (1993). Enhancing reality in the operating room. In *Proceedings of IEEE Visualization '93*.

[State94] State, A., Chen, D. T., Tector, C., Brandt, A., Chen, H., Ohbuchi, R., Bajura, M., and Fuchs, H. (1994). Case study: Observing a volume-rendered fetus within a pregnant patient. In *Proceedings of IEEE Visualization '94*, pages 364–368.

[State96] State, A., Livingston, M. A., Hirota, G., Garrett, W. F., Whitton, M. C., and Fuchs, H. (1996). Technologies for augmented-reality systems: Realizing ultrasound-guided needle biopsies. In *SIGGRAPH 96 Conference Proceedings*, Annual Conference Series, pages 439–446. ACM SIGGRAPH, Addison Wesley.

[Turk94] Turk, G. and Levoy, M. (1994). Zippered polygon meshes from range images. In *Proceedings of SIGGRAPH '94*, Computer Graphics Proceedings, Annual Conference Series, pages 311–318.

[Welch96] Welch, G. F. (1996). *Single-Constraint-At-A-Time Tracking*. Ph.D. Dissertation, University of North Carolina at Chapel Hill.

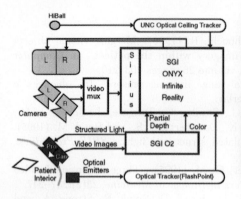
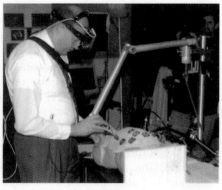

Fig. 1. Diagram of the hardware configuration of the prototype system. The VST HMD consists of two cameras, two displays, and a HiBall tracking sensor.

Fig. 2. The physician (Meyer) uses the system in the preliminary experiment (Dec 96). The mechanical arm he holds is unnecessary in the current implementation. The colored circular landmarks on the "body" surface assist the head tracking subsystem.

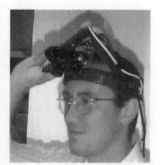
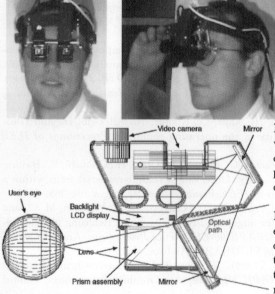

Fig. 3. (*Above*) Custom-designed video-see-through head-mounted display for augmented reality applications. The lightweight unit can be flipped up and down.

Fig. 4. (*Left*) The design of one eyepiece of the VST HMD. The optical paths from the camera to the world and from the user's eye to the LCD are folded in order to match the lengths.

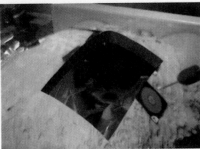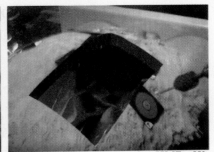

Fig. 5. Wall-eyed stereo pair of images the physician sees in the HMD. We manually digitized the interior structure prior to this experiment (Dec 96).

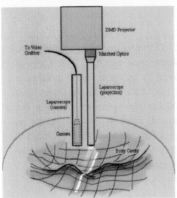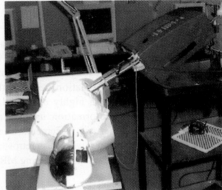

Fig. 6. Our prototype 3D laparoscope combines a conventional laparoscope, a projector emitting structured light in the form of vertical stripes, and a camera to create a laparoscope that acquires depth and color data.

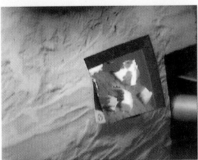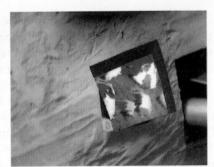

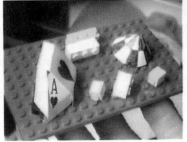

Fig. 7. Stereo augmented view from the second experiment (Feb 98). The test target is visible through the synthetic opening in the phantom. At left is an image of the target outside the phantom. As our real-time depth extraction improves, we hope to approach the quality of the digitized depth in Figure 7.

Evaluation of Control Point Selection in Automatic, Mutual Information Driven, 3D Warping

Chuck Meyer, Jennifer Boes, Boklye Kim, and Peyton Bland

Department of Radiology, University of Michigan, Ann Arbor, MI 48109-0553
cmeyer@umich.edu
http://www.med.umich.edu/dipl

This work was supported in part by DHHS PHS NIH 1R01 CA59412

Abstract. We have implemented automatic 3D thin-plate spline warping as a geometric interpolant to map one dataset volume onto another. Homologous control points in one space are iteratively moved by an optimizer to maximize the global mutual information between the two data volumes. Given two different poses between highly deformed objects we desire to compute the relative geometric deformation using a minimal set of control points as determined by number and placement. The general solution to this problem is not known. In this paper we assess retrospective control point selection for the case of significant patient motion during MRI breast imaging.

1 Introduction

Optimization of mutual information (MI) to drive the automatic affine registration of multimodality data volume sets has been actively pursued for the last 3-4 years [1-6]. Over the last 2 year period we have demonstrated that MI can be used to drive automatic thin-plate spline (TPS) warping as well [7-10]. The process is implemented by allowing an optimizer, the Nelder-Mead simplex algorithm in this case, to drive the positions of homologous control points in the homologous data set, i.e. the data volume to be mapped onto the reference volume, subject to maximizing the resultant MI between the reference volume and the transformed homologous volume.

For cases where the bending energy of the TPS warping is small [11], nearly any evenly distributed, volumetric placement of a few control points, e.g. more than four and fewer than 10, in the reference volume is sufficient to compute a good registration. In our typical implementation only the first 3 homologous control point pairs must be initially placed in the homologous volume. Then the 6 degree of freedom (DOF) rigid body registration is computed by the optimizer's movement of the 3 control points in homologous space to maximize MI. Next, using the optimized rigid body model, the first 4 control points in the reference space are mapped into the homologous space, and then the 12 DOF, full affine registration is subsequently computed, again by optimizing MI through iterative movement of the 4 control points in homologous space. Finally the optimized warping solution is initiated by using the previously optimized full affine solution to map all of the reference control points into the homologous volume.

However, in cases involving significant deformation between initial poses of the data sets, our typical implementation described above may fail. For these problematic circumstances we desire to know the minimal number of homologous control point pairs and the range of their initial placement to subsequently converge to a good geometric model of the warping between the two poses. The remainder of this paper examines criteria for the retrospective evaluation of control point pairs in the situation where the DOF of the warping is initially overdetermined, i.e. more than the necessary number of homologous control point pairs are initially chosen to determine the warp. The physical data set and registered results appear in the latter part of this paper.

2 Methods

Although the algorithm, mutual information for multimodality image fusion (MIAMI Fuse), was developed for multimodality registration, in this case it has been applied to two MRI breast volumes acquired before and after significant patient movement. A case for the use of a multimodality registration algorithm can be made by noting that tissue intensities can vary dramatically depending on changes in tissue positioning with respect to breast coil location, i.e. B1-field inhomogeneitities. Repositioning of the breast occurs with patient movements during a single exam, or more obviously when exams are repeated at 6-12 week intervals. Volume imaging data were acquired in coronal planes over both breasts of the patient lying prone over breast coil wells inside the 1.5T magnet. Voxel dimensions were 1.18 x 1.18 x 5.5 mm^3. Since only the patient's left breast was significantly deformed, 18 nearly homologous control points in the left breast were identified manually in both the pre and post movement data volume. Using these points as the initial starting vector for automatic registration via TPS warping resulted in an initial MI of 1.01 bits, where the entropy in the reference data set was 4.576 bits. The optimization algorithm was repeatedly run from start to finish 8 times using random control point placements up to 3 mm city block metric from the manually chosen starting vector. Each optimization "run" consists of many repeated optimization cycles. Each cycle consists of a single decent to the cost function, i.e. -MI, minimum, where the minimum was detected when the optimizer called for all control points to move less than 0.5 mm in any coordinate axis direction from the previous iteration. The process of repeating optimization cycles stopped (which defined a "run") when the optimized cycle value of MI changed less than 0.0001 bit over 3 previous optimization cycles. This process of repeating optimizations from starting vectors randomly distributed around the previous cycle's solution is used to prevent entrapment by a local minimum.

3 Results

As averaged over the 8 runs, the number of times the objective function was evaluated for each run was 12271 (sem = 1331). Each full run required an average of 2 hours on a 433 MHz DEC Alpha personal workstation running Digital UNIX V4.0C. Figure 1 describes the typical behavior of the cost function vs. number of iterations.

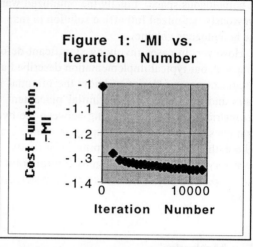

Figure 1: -MI vs. Iteration Number

The variance of each control point's stopping position in each of the coordinate directions was computed and compared to the second partial derivative of the cost function in the same direction at one of the computed solutions for the same control point. Figure 2 illustrates the excellent inverse correlation between the components of the second partials and variance in the final control point positions.

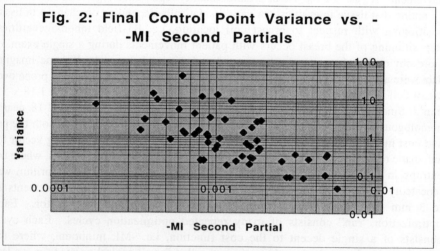

Fig. 2: Final Control Point Variance vs. -MI Second Partials

After removing the control point with the most variance, i.e. rms error for all three vector components, 8 more optimized registrations were completed. The same process was repeated using 16 and 10 control points where the points removed ranked highest in variance. In the original set of 18 control points, the standard error around the average solution for one (outlier) control point was more than 3 times that of the average, while two points were more than 2 times the average. In the distribution of final control point positions for the set of 17, all points had standard errors less than 2 times the average. Figure 3 summarizes the generalized dependence of the final cost function, -MI, vs. number of control points or DOF. Although only the results for ≤16 control points are significantly different from the result using 18 points, there appears to be a smooth trend towards lesser MI values as the number of control points decrease, only.

Finally in an effort to <u>prospectively</u> evaluate which of the set of proposed control points might be the most valuable toward computing a good solution, we examined the initial gradient magnitude of MI for each control point at the manually selected starting vector.

Fig. 4 illustrates the results of this experiment. Note that choosing control points according to rank by MI gradient magnitude at the start vector removes valuable points that had some of the smaller variances around the final solution. The same lack of correlation is

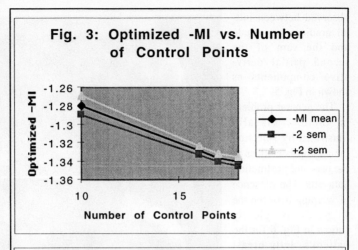

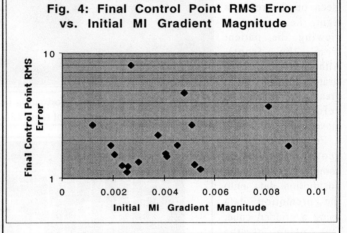

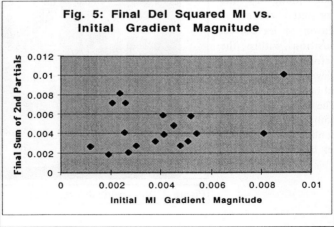

observed between initial gradient magnitude and the sum of the second partial derivative components as shown in Fig. 5.

The general problem is better visually illustrated by selecting the appropriate slices in the pre- and postmotion data sets. The presence of warping between the 2 poses is clearly shown in Fig. 6 for the patient's left breast (seen on the reader's right, i.e. reader is viewing the patient from the front). Although not demonstrated here, the right breast was much less deformed by the movement.

Fig. 7 displays the geometric warping computed to warp the postmotion data onto the premotion data using a gridded cube. One plane of the registered volume is shown in its correct position within the deformation grid (the viewer is now positioned behind the patient). The deformation was computed using 18 control points for the left breast.

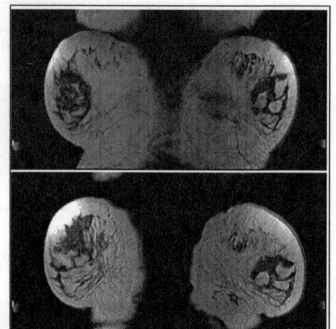

Figure 6. Note significant deformation in left breast (↑) before (upper) and after (lower) patient repositioning.

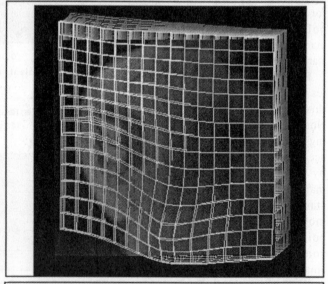

Figure 7. Volumetric deformation required to remove motion.

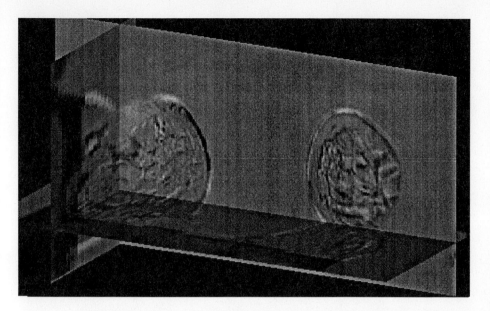

Figure 8. Difference volume obtained after mapping postmotion onto premotion data volume, where mapping was computed using 24 total control points.

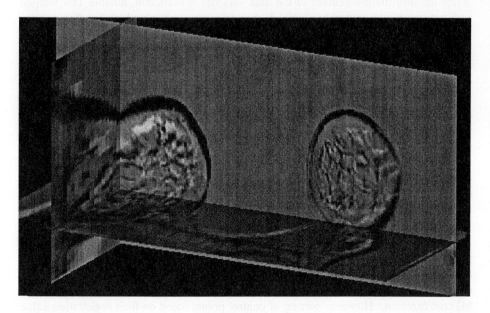

Figure 9. Difference volume obtained after mapping postmotion onto premotion data volume, where mapping was computed using 8 total control points.

Figs 8 and 9 demonstrate the improved spatial registration associated with the increase in number of effective control points or DOF. In Figs. 8 & 9 black-to-white represents a difference range from −128 to +128, respectively; perfect registration would be indicated by midscale gray corresponding to a difference of nearly zero. Essentially the same information is conveyed by Fig. 3 in terms of increasing MI (decreasing −MI) as a function of number of control points, although the consequences are a little less visual. The use of a 6 control point, TPS warping was sufficient to register the right breast (seen in Fig. 9 on the reader's right as viewed from behind the patient). The combined registration was obtained using the separately computed, optimized positions for the 6 control points of the right breast and 18 control points of the left. A single 24 homologous point, TPS warping was computed to register the pre and post motion data sets. Data missing from the warped data set can be seen on the axial and sagittal planes in Fig. 8, where the mapping called for data that was outside the field of view of the postmotion data volume, and was thus rendered as zeros. In such cases of limited fields of view it is important not to penalize the resultant MI for the missing data that maps outside of the reference volume.

4 Conclusions

When the information content of the data volumes is sufficient, reliable TPS warped registrations can be routinely obtained, even in poses containing high bending energy. The minimal subset, i.e. number and placement, of control points in the reference and homologous data volumes is generally unknown to generate an acceptable solution as defined by a minimal mutual information criterion. In a retrospective evaluation of an overdetermined set of manually selected control points we found good inverse agreement between the curvature of the cost function, i.e. -MI, and the variance in the final positions of the control points. The greater the curvature of the cost function at its minimum with respect to movement of a control point in any one direction, the smaller the variance in the final resting position along that direction over repeated random trials. However, prospective evaluation of the local gradient magnitude of the cost function at potential, initial starting positions of the control functions was seemingly uncorrelated with the warping value of the control point as judged by either its variance or curvature at the locus of the final solution position.

Clearly it is desirable to eliminate candidate control points from an automatic instantiation of an overdetermined grid of possible starting points. Just as clearly it is possible to eliminate some control points where one of the pairs lies centrally in a relatively large region of no texture where the optimizer can radically reposition the control point while generating large bending energies with little or no change in the MI cost function. However sorting of control points based on their registration value in computing the desired warping will likely require more than estimates of local MI gradients.

References

[1] A. Collignon, F. Maes, D. Delaere, D. Vandermeulen, P. Suetens, and G. Marchal, "Automated multimodality image registration using information theory," presented at Computational Imaging and Vision, Ile de Berder, FR, 1995.

[2] D. L. G. Hill, C. Studholme, and D. J. Hawkes, "Voxel similarity measures for automated image registration," presented at Visualization in Biomedical Computing, Rochester, MN, 1994.

[3] C. Studholme, D. Hill, and D. Hawkes, "Multiresolution voxel similarity measures for MR-PET registration," presented at Computational Imaging and Vision, Ile de Berder, FR, 1995.

[4] F. Maes, A. Collignon, D. Vandermeulen, G. Marchal, and P. Suetens, "Multimodality image registration by maximization of mutual information," *IEEE Transactions on Medical Imaging*, vol. 16, pp. 187-198, 1997.

[5] P. Viola and W. M. Wells, "Alignment by maximization of mutual information," presented at 5th Int'l. Conf. on Computer Vision, MIT, 1995.

[6] W. Wells, P. Viola, and R. Kikinis, "Multimodal volume registration by maximization of mutual information," presented at Medical Robotics and Computer Assisted Surgery II, Philadelphia, 1995.

[7] B. Kim, J. L. Boes, K. A. Frey, and C. R. Meyer, "Mutual information for automated multimodal image warping," presented at Visualization in Biomedical Computing, Hamburg, Germany, 1996.

[8] B. Kim, J. L. Boes, K. A. Frey, and C. R. Meyer, "Mutual information for automated unwarping of rat brain autoradiographs," *NeuroImage*, vol. 5, pp. 31-40, 1997.

[9] C. R. Meyer, J. L. Boes, B. Kim, P. H. Bland, and K. A. Frey, "Warping normal patients onto the ICBM atlas by maximizing MI," presented at 4th Int'l Conference of Functional Mapping of the Human Brain, Montreal, Quebec, CA, 1998.

[10] C. R. Meyer, J. L. Boes, B. Kim, P. Bland, K. R. Zasadny, P. V. Kison, K. Koral, K. A. Frey, and R. L. Wahl, "Demonstration of accuracy and clinical versatility of mutual information for automatic multimodality image fusion using affine and thin plate spline warped geometric deformations," *Medical Image Analysis*, vol. 3, pp. 195-206, 1997.

[11] F. L. Bookstein, *Morphometric tools for landmark data: geometry and biology*. Cambridge: Cambridge University Press, 1991.

3D/2D Registration Via Skeletal Near Projective Invariance in Tubular Objects

Alan Liu[1], Elizabeth Bullitt[2], Stephen M. Pizer[2]

1. Presently at the Center for Information-Enhanced Medicine
National University of Singapore
liu@ciemed.nus.edu.sg

2. Medical Image Display & Analysis Group
The University of North Carolina at Chapel Hill

Abstract. We present a method of 3D/2D image registration. The algorithm is based on the property of near projective invariance in tubular objects. The skeletons of tubular anatomical structures (e.g., intracerebral blood vessels) are used as registration primitives. Experiments with Magnetic Resonance Angiogram (MRA) patient studies and both simulated and actual X-ray angiograms suggest that the algorithm is very accurate and robust. The algorithm requires only a small number of primitives. In addition, the algorithm is relatively insensitive to the choice of tubular structures used. Experimental results justifying these claims are included.

1 Introduction

The objective of 3D/2D image registration can be described thus: Given a 2D image and a 3D model, determine the position and orientation (i.e., *pose*) of the imaging device when the 2D image was taken. In this paper, we describe an algorithm for registering 3D Magnetic Resonance Angiogram (MRA) images with X-ray angiograms. The imaging device for our application is a digital fluoroscope. Many 3D/2D registration algorithms have the following paradigm. First, image structures common to both 3D and 2D imaging modalities are chosen as *registration primitives*. Examples include the images of external fiducial markers. The images are assumed registered when the projected 3D registration primitives are within a small distance of coinciding with their 2D counterparts. Second, for a given choice of primitives, an objective function is formulated. The objective function has a minimum value when the primitives coincide. Finally, an optimization algorithm to minimize the objective function is chosen.

Registration primitives include points, curves, and surfaces. The projection involved in registering 3D with 2D images complicates the choice of registration primitives. Not all types of primitives can be unambiguously projected. For example, 3D surfaces may overlap and project onto the same part of the 2D plane. In this paper, we show that the property of near projective invariance permits us to use the skeleton curves of tubular objects as registration primitives. With local exceptions, 3D curves can be projected unambiguously as 2D curves. Section 2 describes this property in greater detail.

2 Method

A 3D tubular structure such as a blood vessel generally appears as a 2D tube under projection. This section describes the property of projective invariance and its application in 3D/2D registration. Section 2.1 presents the concept of projective invariance and applicable conditions. Section 2.2 describes conditions where projective invariance is inapplicable.

2.1 Near Projective Invariance

A 3D tube contains a central axis or *skeleton* such that cross sections of the object made perpendicular to the skeleton are circular. A 2D tube contains a skeleton which is equidistant from the tube's boundaries. Tubes are not required to have constant width. Generally, the projection of a 3D tube is a 2D tubular shadow. For a given projection, if the 3D skeleton projects onto the 2D skeleton of the projection's shadow, *projective invariance* is preserved. That is, a 3D tube is said to preserve projective invariance if the projection of the 3D skeleton and the 2D skeleton of the tube's projection are the same.

Strict projective invariance is preserved where the tubular object is not overlapped under projection. Liu [1] enumerates such conditions in detail. In practical situations, intensifier induced image distortions, the resolution of the imaging device, and the characteristics of X-ray image formation affect invariance. While strict invariance is not preserved, it is minimally affected. Tubular objects exhibit the property of *near projective invariance* in this situation. That is, the projected 3D skeleton only differs slightly from the projection's 2D skeleton. Tests using both simulated and actual X-ray angiograms suggest that this difference does not significantly affect registration results, as shown in section 4.

Near projective invariance simplifies the use of tubular objects for 3D/2D registration. The problem is reduced to that of registering sets of curves. Curves are computationally simple structures from which a fast, highly accurate registration algorithm can be developed. This algorithm is described in section 3.

2.2 Exceptions to Near Projective Invariance

A tube may not display near projective invariance throughout its length. The invariance property is not preserved when tubes overlap under projection. Such segments should not be used for registration. Two kinds of overlap are possible: local and non-local overlaps.

A local overlap or self-occlusion occurs when a contiguous portion of the same tube overlaps under projection. Fig. 1 illustrates this case. The object is a tubular helix. The helix's axis is perpendicular to the view direction. The left image shows the tube and its 3D skeleton. The right image is a projection of the tube with the projection's 2D skeleton. The tube's 3D skeleton forms a cusp after projection whereas the 2D skeleton is smooth and does not extend as far out the bend as its 3D complement.

A non-local overlap occurs when portions of two distinct tubes or when two non-contiguous portions of the same tube overlap under projection. Fig. 2 illustrates. The

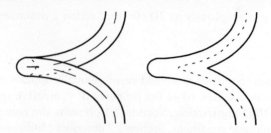

Fig. 1: The effect of self occlusion on projective invariance. Left: projection of the 3D skeleton. Right: The projected tube's 2D skeleton

middle image is an angiogram. The side images are magnified regions where ambiguity arises due to non-local overlaps. From these images, it is not clear whether the projected vessels cross or are just touching.

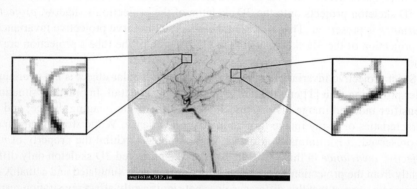

Fig. 2: A lateral X-ray angiogram of the head. Highlighted areas contain overlapping projections of distinct vessels

3 The Registration Algorithm

Our goal is to register 3D MRA studies with X-ray angiograms. By the property of projective invariance, registering blood vessels with their corresponding projections is equivalent to registering the projected 3D skeletons with their 2D analogues. A 3D/2D registration algorithm was developed that uses the skeletons directly. The algorithm accepts as input the set of 3D skeletons extracted from volume data, the set of 2D skeletons extracted from X-ray images, and the correspondence between the 3D and 2D skeletons. The algorithm returns the pose required to register the primitives. The set of 3D skeletons is assumed to be rigid. Liu [1] develops the registration algorithm at length. In this paper, we summarize its key aspects. Section 3.1 describes our method of extracting tubular skeletons. Section 3.2 describes the objective function. Section 3.3 briefly outlines the optimization method.

3.1 Extracting Tubular Skeletons

Tubular skeletons are extracted directly from digital images. Extraction is performed via cores [2], a method of multi-scale object description. For tubular structures, cores encode the object as a curve in $\Re^n \times \Re^+$ space, where n is the dimensionality of the tube. The *core-middle*, or spatial component of the core, corresponds to the tube's skeleton. Fritsch's algorithm [3] is used to extract cores from X-ray angiograms. The 3D extraction of core-middles from MRAs is performed using Aylward's algorithm [4].

3.2 Computing the Disparity Value

From the property of projective invariance, tubular structures are accurately registered with their projections when the projected 3D skeletons overlap their corresponding 2D equivalents. This section describes a method for measuring registration accuracy based on the degree of overlap or *disparity* between skeletons.

Let C be the skeleton of a 3D tubular blood vessel, and c be the skeleton extracted from the vessel's projection. Let P be the perspective projection function. Under perfect registration, projective invariance implies that $P(C)$ perfectly overlaps c. When they are misregistered, c and $P(C)$ will be misaligned. Given a projected 3D and 2D curve pair $(P(C), c)$, take a set of evenly spaced points $p_0, p_1, ..., p_n$ along $P(C)$. For each point p_i, the corresponding point q_i on c is located by computing the intersection of c with the line perpendicular to the tangent of $P(C)$ at p_i. If more than one intersection exists, the closest is selected. If there are no intersections, then p_i does not have an analogue on c. Fig. 3 illustrates a few cases. Note that either c or $P(C)$

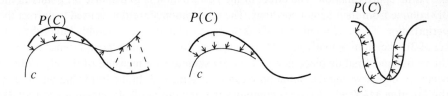

Fig. 3: Computing the disparity between 2D and projected 3D skeletons

may be incomplete. Fig. 3 (middle) illustrates point pairing when c is incomplete.

The disparity value is taken to be the mean-square value of all point pairs (p_i, q_i) for all curve pairs $(P(C), c)$. In our registration algorithm, the association of 3D skeletons with their 2D counterparts is performed by the user. Under perfect registration, the disparity is at most small positive value. When misregistered, a significantly larger non-zero value is obtained. The disparity value changes according to the projection P. We write $Cost(P)$ to denote the objective function.

3.3 Optimizing $Cost(P)$

Various methods for optimizing $Cost(P)$ exist [5]. Liu [1] describes an efficient method based on computing the partial derivatives of P with respect to the pose (registration) parameters. The method is similar to that described in [6]. This section summarizes the discussion in [1].

Since rigid registration is assumed, P can be expressed as a six-parameter function (3 rotations and 3 translations). Let X be the vector of parameters. Let P_X be the projection computed using the parameters in X. Given an approximation X_0 to the final solution, the algorithm uses Newton's method to compute the actual solution X_{sol}. From section 3.2, a set of point pairs (p_i, q_i) for each curve pair $(P(C), c)$ can be computed. The disparity function $Cost(P)$ is minimal when $p_i = q_i$ for all point pairs. A refinement X_1 to X_0 is obtained by computing a least squares solution for ΔX in $q_i = p_i + Jacobian(P)|_{\vec{0}} \bullet \Delta X$ for all points (p_i, q_i). $Jacobian(P)|_{\vec{0}}$ is the partial derivative of P w.r.t. X evaluated at $X = \vec{0}$ and ΔX is a 6-dimensional correction vector. Given ΔX, X_1 can be computed. The process is repeated for $X_2, X_3, ..., X_n$ or until $Cost(P_{X_n})$ falls below an arbitrary threshold.

4 Experiments

This section describes experiments to evaluate the algorithm's accuracy and performance under various conditions. Both simulated and actual X-ray angiograms are used. Using simulated X-ray angiograms with known poses permit registration accuracy to be quantified. The actual pose is perturbed by arbitrary amounts to derive the initial approximation. The effect of the perturbation is to displace all points in the 3D volume from their actual positions. The registration algorithm is used to correct the perturbation. The total number of 3D skeletons available is considerably larger than the set of 3D skeletons actually used for registration. By computing the difference between the initial and final displacements of *all* 3D skeletons, a measure of the algorithm's accuracy in recovering the initial pose can be determined. In the following discussion, the function *MAX(pose1,pose2)* computes the maximum displacement among all 3D skeletons between two states. For example, *pose1* may be the actual pose and *pose2* may be the computed pose returned by the algorithm. The function *MIN(pose1,pose2)* can be similarly defined.

Experiments in sections 4.1 through 4.3 used two 3D MRA studies of the head as input. Study A is a $256 \times 256 \times 61$ scan with voxel size $0.78mm \times 0.78mm \times 1.3mm$. Study B is a $256 \times 256 \times 48$ scan from a different patient. The voxel size for this study was $0.62mm \times 0.62mm \times 1mm$. In both studies, the imaging parameters were chosen to highlight intracerebral vessels. For each study, a set of 3D curves representing the central axis of intracerebral vessels was extracted using Aylward's algorithm (section 3.1). 204 curves were extracted from Study A while 223 vessels were extracted from

Study B. Simulated X-ray angiograms were generated by applying a perspective projection on these segmented vessels.

In contrast, the experiment in section 4.4 used actual patient angiograms. A digitally subtracted angiogram was acquired ($XRAY_1$). A simple algorithm was used to correct for image distortion. In addition, an MRA dataset (Study C) of size $256 \times 256 \times 72$ was acquired from the same patient. The voxel size was $0.86mm \times 0.86mm \times 1.1mm$.

In the following sections, details of each experiment are presented together with the results. Section 4.1 is a test of the algorithm's interactive performance. Section 4.2 evaluates the algorithm's ability to converge. Section 4.3 describes an experiment to test the algorithm's sensitivity to the choice of registration primitives. Sections 4.1 through 4.3 use synthetic 2D images. Section 4.4 describes an experiment to evaluate the algorithm using actual angiograms.

4.1 Interactive Performance Test

This experiment evaluates the algorithm's interactive performance. Three trials were conducted. Trials 1 and 2 were conducted using Study B whereas trial 3 was conducted using Study A. In each trial, a simulated X-ray angiogram was generated from an arbitrary viewpoint and the pose noted. A perturbation was introduced to the actual pose to produce the initial pose. The amount and nature of perturbation differed for each trial. To ensure fairness, the individual generating the angiograms and perturbations was different from the individual performing the registration. The actual pose was not known to the latter until after the experiment. The individual performing the registration was free to extract a number of 2D skeletons from each simulated angiogram. Between 27 and 37 curves per image were extracted using Fritsch's algorithm (section 3.1). Correspondence between the 2D and 3D skeletons was manually established. The registration algorithm was executed until $Cost(P)$ did not show any further improvement. The current solution at that point was noted. The program required approximately 3-5 minutes of run time on an HP 712/80 workstation with 64Mb of memory.

Table 1 shows the results. In each case, *MAX(actual,initial)* was in the range of a few centimeters. That is, the initial misregistration displaced all 3D skeletons on the order of centimeters. After registration, *MAX(actual,final)* was in the range of tenths of a millimeter. That is, the largest amount of misregistration among all 3D skeletons is in the tenths of a millimeter. We emphasize that we measure the misregistration of *all* 3D skeletons (more than 200), not just the skeletons used for the registration (27 to 37). The results indicate that the registration algorithm performs very well in an interactive environment. The set of 2D primitives was selected with no particular limitations other than ensuring that curves were chosen from all parts of the projected image. The algorithm is sufficiently robust to converge to the true solution in each case. This suggests that the algorithm is relatively insensitive to the choice of initial approximation as well as having a strong tolerance to the choice of registration primitives. The next two sections provide additional proof to these claims.

Exp.	Max. initial misregistration (cm)	Max. final misregistration (cm)
1	4.04×10^0	1.16×10^{-2}
2	2.85×10^0	9.60×10^{-2}
3	5.03×10^0	9.59×10^{-2}

Table 1: Results of registration accuracy test.

4.2 Test of Robustness

This is a test of the algorithm's ability to converge to the true solution given a range of initial poses. A good registration algorithm should be relatively insensitive to the choice of starting pose, quantified by the *capture radius*. The algorithm is said to have a capture radius of at least r if it converges to the correct solution from any choice of initial pose that displaces all 3D skeletons by *at least* r. In practice, there are an infinite number of possible starting positions where the initial misregistration is at least r. Moreover, the capture radius is partially dependent on the 2D and 3D images used. An approximation of the capture radius can be determined by using a large number of trials and datasets representative of typical cases.

Two experiments were conducted. The first used Study A, and the second used Study B. For each experiment a simulated angiogram was generated from an arbitrary pose. Thirteen 2D curves were extracted from each angiogram. These curves form the set of 2D registration primitives. Correspondence between 2D and 3D curves was established manually. For each experiment, 100 trials were performed. In each trial, the actual pose was given random perturbations to produce an initial pose. Up to $\pm 30°$ rotation and $\pm 10\ cm$ translation in all three coordinate axis were used for experiments on Study A. Up to $\pm 25°$ rotation and $\pm 5\ cm$ translation in all three coordinate axis were used for experiments on Study B. For each perturbation, $MIN(actual, initial)$ was determined. That is, the set of more than 200 3D skeletons was initially *at least* that distance away from their actual position. The registration algorithm was executed until $Cost(P)$ fell below $1.75 \times 10^{-5}\ cm^2$ or 100 until iterations have occurred. The computed solution was noted. $MAX(actual, comp)$ was determined. That is, the set of all 3D skeletons was displaced *at most* that distance from their final position after registration.

Fig. 4 are scatterplots of the results. The abscissa gives the initial minimum misregistration. That is, all 3D skeletons were displaced from their true position by *at least* that amount. The ordinate gives the maximum final misregistration. That is, all skeletons were displaced by *at most* that amount after registration. Apart from a single outlier in Study B, the capture radius is at least $15\ cm$ in both studies. For each experiment, the set of trials formed two distinct groups. One group terminated with misregistrations in excess of $10\ cm$ whereas the other has misregistrations less than $0.1\ cm$. This suggests that the algorithm's objective function is remarkably free of local minima over a wide region surrounding the actual solution. Either the algorithm converged to the true solution with little residual error or it did not converge at all.

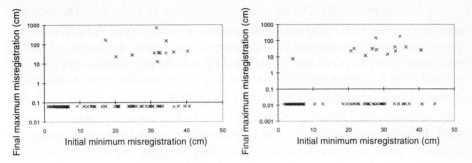

Fig. 4: The results of the capture radius experiment. Scatterplots for Study A (left) and Study B (right)

4.3 Sensitivity to Choice of Primitives

This experiment evaluates the algorithm's performance as a function of the number of curves used and their 3D spatial distribution. Two experiments were performed. The first used Study A whereas the other used Study B. The same angiograms and sets of 2D skeletons described in section 4.2 were used. In each experiment, an initial pose was generated by applying a perturbation to the actual pose. Each experiment has three series of trials. For each series, a random subset of k 2D curves were chosen of the 13 available. In every series, k was chosen to be 4, 8, and 10. Fifty trials were held for each series. Fig. 5 illustrates the organization of this experiment.

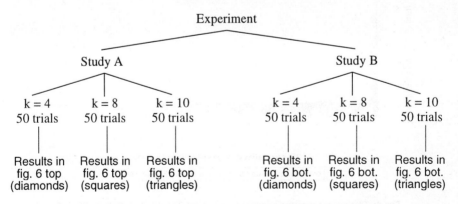

Fig. 5: Organization of experiment to evaluate sensitivity to choice of primitives

In each trial, the 3D spatial distribution of the 3D curve primitives were quantified using $Spread_{3D}$, a moment of inertia measure sensitive to the number of curves used as well as the spatial distribution or "spread" of 3D primitives [1]. The algorithm was executed until $Cost(P)$ fell below 1.75×10^{-5} cm^2 or until 100 iterations have occurred. The computed pose was noted and $MAX(actual, comp)$ determined.

Fig. 6 plots the results. The absicca gives the value of $Spread_{3D}$. The ordinate gives the amount of residual misregistration when the algorithm halts. While four curves converged with submillimeter accuracy in some cases, the number of curves used is too small to be reliable. Using eight curves, the algorithm is very likely to succeed. With ten curves, there is virtual certainty. As the number of curves increased, $Spread_{3D}$ also increased. Having a larger value for $Spread_{3D}$ generally produced more accurate results. Spatial distribution is not just a function of the number of curves used. In both experiments, there is considerable overlap between the range of $Spread_{3D}$ achieved using 8 and 10 curves. This suggests that a well chosen but smaller set of curves can perform just as well as a larger set of poorly chosen curves.

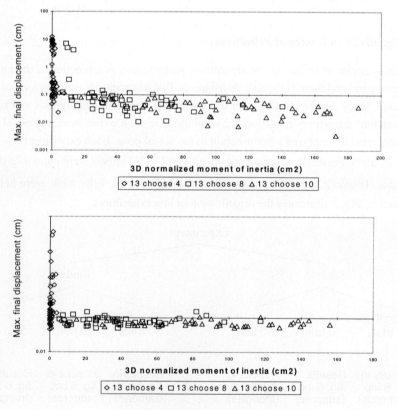

Fig. 6: Choice of registration primitives experiment. Top: Study A. Bottom: Study B

4.4 Clinical Test

Unlike the previous experiments which used synthetic angiograms, this experiment evaluates the algorithm's performance by registering an actual patient angiogram

($XRAY_1$) with its corresponding MRA (Study C). True angiograms have more sources of errors and present a greater challenge to the algorithm. With actual angiograms, the true pose is not known. We evaluated the algorithm's performance by comparing its performance with a manual registration using the same images. A neurosurgeon familiar with the patient registered the projected 3D skeletons against the 2D image. The manual attempt was then compared with the algorithm's solution. Fig. 7 (top) illustrates the results. The attempt used an anterior-posterior (AP) orientation as the starting pose. The effort took approximately one hour. The bottom figure was registered using our algorithm from the same starting pose. The attempt took approximately 10 minutes in total. Approximately 5 minutes of this time was spent by the user determining the correct correspondence between 2D and 3D skeletons.

The registration results appear very similar, indicating that the algorithm performs at least as well as manual registration but requiring only a fraction of the latter's time. In some places (notably vessel "B"), the algorithm performed noticeably better than the neurosurgeon. Since the entire intracerebral circulation was not highlighted, some 3D vessel skeletons did not have a corresponding 2D vessel. For example, vessels "A" and "C".

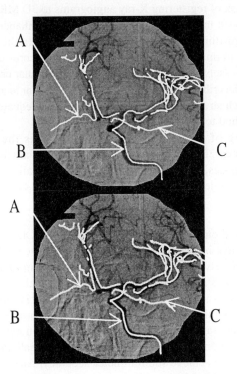

Fig. 7: Results of registration experiment on clinical data. Top: Manual registration by neurosurgeon. Bottom: Registration via our algorithm

5 Discussion

3D/2D registration algorithms have applications in surgical instrument guidance (e.g., [7], [8], and [9]) and in anatomical model synthesis (e.g., [10]). An accurate, robust registration algorithm significantly improves the accuracy of reconstruction and surgical guidance. Sections 4.1 through 4.4 demonstrated our algorithm's accuracy and robustness. The algorithm is capable of submillimeter accuracy over a wide range of starting poses and choice of primitives.

An advantage of our registration method is the use of curves as registration primitives. Point based algorithms (e.g., [11] and [12]) generally rely on a few landmarks for registration. These methods have the advantage of computational simplicity and thus speed. However, errors in locating fiducial points can result in decreased accuracy. Some surface based algorithms register the surface's silhouette with the 2D image. However, determining the silhouette may be computationally expensive or may require auxiliary data structures. In contrast, the projection of a curve is generally still a curve. Curves may be treated as a locus of points. By using curves as registration primitives in our algorithm, we retain the computationally simplicity of point based registration without sacrificing registration accuracy. By the principle of projective invariance, registering the skeletons of tubular structures such as blood vessels is equivalent to directly registering the vessels themselves. Thus, our algorithm is well suited to the task of registering X-ray angiograms to 3D MRA.

The use of cores as a method of extracting primitives enhances the accuracy and robustness of our algorithm. Cores are remarkably robust in the presence of image noise and differences in image resolution [13]. In addition, cores are little affected by variations in normal vessels which do not have perfectly circular cross-sections.

The algorithm as described requires both 2D and 3D tubular anatomical objects. For some applications, such structures may not be available in adequate numbers. We have proposed a novel method to overcome this problem [9].

One shortcoming of our present implementation is the need for manual correspondence between 2D and 3D vessel skeletons. Since angiograms are typically taken from standard poses, it may be possible to automatically associate the vessels based on their relative projected positions on the 2D image [14].

6 Conclusion

This paper described our method of 3D/2D registration. Our algorithm is based on the principle of projective invariance which permits the skeletons of tubular anatomical structures (e.g., blood vessels) to be used as registration primitives. Using curves as registration primitives is computationally straightforward and does not sacrifice accuracy. Experiments under test conditions where truth is known show that our method is capable of submillimeter accuracy. Elaborate preprocessing is unnecessary. Our algorithm is robust, and converges to the true solution even from large initial misregistrations. In addition, our algorithm requires only a small number (typically less than 10) of curve pairs to achieve submillimeter accuracy. An experiment conducted using actual X-ray and 3D MRA studies suggest that the algorithm is at least as accurate as a manual registration performed by an expert, but takes only 20% of the time required by the latter.

7 Acknowledgments

The authors gratefully acknowledge the use of computing facilities at the Center for Information Enhanced Medicine (CieMED), National University of Singapore. We thank Stephen Aylward and Daniel Fritsch for assistance with and the use of programs for core extraction, and UNC hospitals diagnostic radiology department for assistance with acquiring MRI/MRA images. This work is partially supported by R01-CA67812 NCI-NIH, and by PO1 CA47982 NCI-NIH.

References

1. Liu A. "3D/2D registration and reconstruction in image-guided surgery." Ph.D. Dissertation, University of North Carolina at Chapel Hill, 1998.
2. Pizer S.M., Eberly D., Morse B.S., Fritsch D. "Zoom-invariant vision of figural shape: The mathematics of cores" Computer Vision and Image Understanding Vol. 69 No. 1, January, pp. 55-71, 1998, Article No. IV970563. Also available as UNC Technical Report TR96-004.
3. Fritsch D.S., Eberly D.H., Pizer S.M., McAuliffe M.J. "Stimulated cores and their applications in medical imaging" IPMI '95: Information Processing in Medical Imaging, 1995. pp. 365-368.
4. Aylward S., Pizer S., Bullitt E., Eberly D. "Intensity ridge and widths for tubular object segmentation and description." Proc IEEE WWMMBIA (IEEE96TB100056), 1996. Also available as UNC Technical Report TR96-018.
5. Press W.H., et. al. "Numerical recipes in C: The art of scientific computing." Cambridge [Cambridgeshire]: New York: Cambridge University Press, 1992.
6. Lowe D.G. "Three-dimensional object recognition from single two-dimensional images" Artificial Intelligence, Vol. 31, No. 3, 1987. pp. 355-395.
7. Grimson W.E.L., Ettinger G.J., White S.J., Gleason P.L., Lozano-Perez T., Wells W.M., III; Kikinis R. "Evaluating and validating an automated registration system for enhanced reality visualization in surgery." Computer Vision, Virtual Reality and Robotics in Medicine, 1995 pp. 3-12.
8. Lavallee S., Cinquin P., Szeliski R., Peria O., Hamadeh A., Champleboux G., Troccaz J. "Building a hybrid patient's model for augmented reality in surgery: A registration problem." Comput. Biol. Med. Vol 25, No. 2., 1995. pp. 149-164.
9. Liu A., Bullitt E., Pizer S.M. "Surgical instrument guidance using synthesized anatomical structures" CVRMed-MRCAS '97. First Joint Conference, Computer Vision, Virtual Reality and Robotics in Medicine and Medical Robotics and Computer-Assisted Surgery. pp. 99-108.
10. Bullitt E., Liu A., Pizer, S.M. "Three-dimensional reconstruction of curves from pairs of projection views in the presence of error. I. Algorithms." Medical Physics, vol. 24, no. 11, Nov. 1997. pp. 1671-1678.
11. Mellor J.P. "Realtime camera calibration for enhanced reality visualization." Computer Vision, Virtual Reality and Robotics in Medicine. First International Conference, CVRMed '95. Proceedings. pp. 471-475.
12. Uenohara M., Kanade T. "Vision-based object registration for real-time image overlay." Comput. Biol. Med. Vol. 25, No. 2. pp. 249-260.
13. Morse B., Pizer S., Fritsch D. "Robust object representation through object-relevant use of scale", Medical Imaging '94, Image Processing, SPIE 2167. pp. 104-115.
14. Fritsch D., Pizer S.M., Yu L., Johnson, V., Chaney E. "Segmentation of medical image objects using deformable shape loci." IPMI '97, Lecture Notes in Computer Science (Duncan J., Gindi G., eds), 1230, 1997. pp. 127-140.

Measuring Global and Local Spatial Correspondence Using Information Theory

F. Bello and A.C.F. Colchester

Neurosciences Medical Image Analysis Group, Kent Institute of Medicine and Health Sciences, University of Kent at Canterbury, Canterbury Kent CT2 7NT, UK
f.bello@ukc.ac.uk

Abstract. The evaluation of spatial correspondence between binary objects resulting from a segmentation step performed by two different observers or methods is a critical part of the validation of a segmentation criterion or technique. Several global measures of correspondence have been previously proposed, but all of them assume a one-to-one correspondence between objects, thus failing to address local problems such as the splitting of an object by one of the observers. Moreover, such global measures do not distinguish between the reference and the observed objects and most of them lack a solid theoretical foundation. In this paper, we introduce a set of spatial correspondence indices that can evaluate global (many-to-many), local (many-to-one) and individual (one-to-one) spatial correspondence between observed and reference objects and vice versa. The proposed measures, derived from applying information theory concepts to the problem of spatial correspondence, are shown to be well-behaved and suitable to be used in medical imaging applications.

1 Introduction

One of the central problems in the area of medical image computing is the validation of results from a segmentation algorithm. Such validation or comparison always requires at certain levels of abstraction the recognition of similarities or differences between two representations, one representation being considered as the current observation, and the other as some reference model or ground truth. Quantifying these similarities by developing suitable *similarity measures* is often quite difficult.

The concept of pattern similarity is key to many statistical, syntactic and neural pattern recognition techniques [1]. Within the area of medical imaging various measures have been used to assess the similarity or agreement between segmentation algorithms and human observers [2] [3] [4] and between observers [5], but they all have been used as global measures of similarity with some elaborated on an empirical basis without adequate theoretical justification. The spatial correspondence indices introduced here are based on information theory, which has been successfully used to register medical images by maximisation of mutual information [6] [7]. In fact, the main difference between those methods and the concept introduced here is that registration methods assume that the majority of the underlying objects which generated both representations were the same.

The methods then seek the transformation that will maximise spatial correspondence, regardless of the actual values of the objective function. In contrast, we are attempting to directly measure the spatial correspondence and utilise the measures to analyse details of the similarities and differences.

Our immediate motivation is the comparison and validation of lesions segmented by two different observers or segmentation methods on the same, i.e. perfectly registered, magnetic resonance (MR) brain scans of multiple sclerosis (MS) patients. Such comparison must take into account the inherent difference between identifying the presence of a lesion and the accurate placement of a boundary around it. Provision of global and local quantitative measures of agreement can significantly improve the understanding of the lesion identification and delineation process, as well as simplify the analysis and validation of segmentation results in large numbers of scans.

2 Spatial Correspondence

Let X be the set of objects $X_k, k = 1\ldots, K$ in the reference model and Y be the set of objects $Y_j, j = 1, \ldots, J$ in the current observation. Consider X and Y as two different partitions of the same image and assume that there are Q locations equally spaced in G, a lattice extending over the area covered by both partitions. Each point in G can be identified in relation to the objects in X and the objects in Y. Let f_{kj} be the number of lattice points to be found in $X_k \cap Y_j$ with $\sum_{k=1}^{K} \sum_{j=1}^{J} f_{kj} = Q$. Then, $P_{XY}(k,j) = f_{kj}/Q$ is the probability that a point in G falls in objects X_k and Y_j. Similarly, $P_X(k) = f_k/Q$ and $P_Y(j) = f_j/Q$ give the probability that a point in G will fall in object X_k or object Y_j, respectively.

An object Y_j present in the observation is said to correspond to the object X_k in the reference model if and only if the set of all lattice points $\{y_{j1}, \ldots, y_{jL}\} \in Y_j$ is the same as the set of all lattice points $\{x_{k1}, \ldots, x_{kM}\} \in X_K$. As each of the lattice points y_{jl} and x_{km} has a unique spatial location, the correspondence between objects Y_j and X_k implies not only that $P_Y(j) = P_X(k)$, but also that the space occupied by $\{y_{j1}, \ldots, y_{jL}\}$ must be the same as that occupied by $\{x_{k1}, \ldots, x_{kM}\}$. It is only when these two conditions are met that both identification and boundary delineation errors can be avoided.

Of the measures used in the analysis of MS segmentations, the **area error** and the **correlation coefficients** [4] [5] only evaluate the agreement in terms of the total number of elements in each segmentation, thus making a more detailed analysis of the segmentation errors impossible. The **similarity index** [2] and **overlap index** [3] consider the total number of elements and the total overlap to give an overall measure of agreement, but they are still global measures and therefore not capable of discriminating between the different types of segmentation errors.

To address local spatial correspondence we create a joint frequency distribution based on the above definitions by means of a Correspondence matrix O. This matrix is similar in concept to the co-occurrence matrix widely used in texture analysis. Assuming that all the objects in $\boldsymbol{X}$ and $\boldsymbol{Y}$ have been uniquely labelled, the columns of $\boldsymbol{O}$ correspond to the objects $Y_j, j = 1, \ldots, J$ in the observation and the rows to the objects $X_k, k = 1 \ldots, K$ in the reference. Each entry o_{kj} in $\boldsymbol{O}$ indicates the number of lattice points common to objects X_k and Y_j, i.e. $X_k \bigcap Y_j$. The background in each partition, $\overline{\boldsymbol{X}}$ and $\overline{\boldsymbol{Y}}$, is treated as a separate object to allow the computation of a valid joint probability distribution from $\boldsymbol{O}$. The marginal probabilities for each object, $P_X(k)$ and $P_Y(j)$, can then be computed by adding all entries across the rows or columns. Various other global and local measures such as those to be introduced in the next section can be directly computed from $\boldsymbol{O}$. As $P_{XY}(k,j)$, $P_X(k)$ and $P_Y(j)$ are dependent on the density of points in $\boldsymbol{G}$, a relatively dense pattern of points must be used for a reliable estimation.

3 Theoretical Framework

If we interpret $\boldsymbol{X}$ as the input into a noisy discrete channel and $\boldsymbol{Y}$ as the output from the channel, using the information theory concepts introduced by Shannon [8] we know that the information provided about the event X_k occurring at the source by the occurrence of event Y_j at the output is given by their mutual information $I_{X;Y}(k,j) = \log\left(P_{X|Y}(k,j)/P_X(k)\right)$. A special case of $I_{X;Y}$ is when knowledge of the output uniquely determines the input, i.e. $P_{X|Y}(k,j) = 1$. In this case $I_{X;Y}$ is known as the self information of X_k or Y_j (denoted by $I_X(k)$ and $I_Y(j)$). This situation occurs if the discrete channel is noiseless and there is full agreement between $\boldsymbol{Y}$ and $\boldsymbol{X}$. By considering such a situation, it is possible to define C_{jk}, a measure of spatial correspondence between object Y_j and object X_k, as the ratio of the average mutual information between the objects, $I(X_k; Y_j)$, to the average self information or entropy, $H(X_k)$, of the reference object:

$$C_{jk} = \frac{I(X_k; Y_j)}{H(X_k)} = \frac{P_{XY}(k,j)}{P_X(k)} \cdot \frac{I_{X;Y}(k,j)}{I_X(k)} \qquad (1)$$

Similarly, if $\boldsymbol{Y}$ is considered as the reference, C_{kj} measures the correspondence between the objects X_k and Y_j:

$$C_{kj} = \frac{I(X_k; Y_j)}{H(Y_j)} = \frac{P_{XY}(k,j)}{P_Y(j)} \cdot \frac{I_{X;Y}(k,j)}{I_Y(j)} \qquad (2)$$

$C_{jk} = C_{kj}$ if Y_j and X_k have the same number of elements or lattice points, regardless of their spatial location.

Using the average mutual information between Y_j and $X_k, k = 1, \ldots, K$ it is also possible to compute C_j, a measure of the local spatial correspondence between Y_j and all the objects in $\boldsymbol{X}$. Equally, the local spatial correspondence between X_k and all the objects in $\boldsymbol{Y}$ can be estimated by computing C_k:

$$C_j = \frac{I(\boldsymbol{X}; Y_j)}{H(Y_j)} \qquad\qquad C_k = \frac{I(X_k; \boldsymbol{Y})}{H(X_k)} \qquad (3)$$

From the definition of average mutual information we can deduce that C_j and C_k effectively measure the degree of spatial correspondence between the selected object and all those objects in the alternate representation with which it shares at least one element. Furthermore, these measures obey the following relationship:

$$C_j = \sum_{k=1}^{K} C_{kj} \qquad C_k = \sum_{j=1}^{J} C_{jk} \qquad (4)$$

The above measures estimate the spatial correspondence between an individual object and those with which it has common elements. A global measure of spatial correspondence between the observation Y and the reference X can be obtained by dividing the average total mutual information $I(X;Y)$ by the average total self information or entropy of X, $H(X)$.

$$C_Y = \frac{I(X;Y)}{H(X)} = \frac{\sum_{k=1}^{K} \sum_{j=1}^{J} P_{XY}(k,j) \cdot \log \frac{P_{XY}(k,j)}{P_X(k)P_Y(j)}}{\sum_{k=1}^{K} P_X(k) \cdot \log \frac{1}{P_X(k)}} \qquad (5)$$

Similarly, if Y is considered as the reference, C_X estimates the global spatial correspondence between X and Y:

$$C_X = \frac{I(X;Y)}{H(Y)} = \frac{\sum_{k=1}^{K} \sum_{j=1}^{J} P_{XY}(k,j) \cdot \log \frac{P_{XY}(k,j)}{P_X(k)P_Y(j)}}{\sum_{j=1}^{J} P_Y(j) \cdot \log \frac{1}{P_Y(j)}} \qquad (6)$$

4 Experiments

Three types of objects were used to study the new measures: single synthetic 2-D objects, multiple synthetic 2-D objects and 3-D MS lesions segmented by two different observers (Fig. 1). In all the experiments a complement **area error** measure ($ErrA = 1 - 2*|b-c|/(b+c)$), the **overlap index** ($Over = a/(b+c-a)$) and the **similarity index** ($Sim = 2*a/(b+c)$) were also computed. The size of the objects (b,c) and the overlap (a) are expressed in number of lattice points.

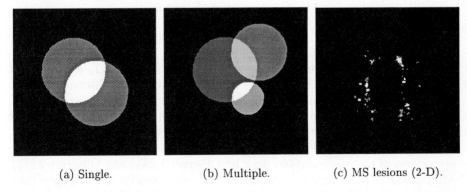

(a) Single. (b) Multiple. (c) MS lesions (2-D).

Fig. 1. Sample synthetic objects and MS lesions. Brighter areas indicate elements common to both images.

4.1 Single Objects

Synthetic objects as those in Fig. 1.a were generated and individually labelled. The size of the objects (b,c), their overlap (a) and the size of the lattice (Q) were varied to observe the response of C_{jk} and C_{kj}. Fig. 2.a shows the behaviour of C_{jk} when both objects have the same size and their degree of overlap is varied from 0.01% to 100%. The different curves correspond to increases in Q. For the bottom curve $Q = b + c$ and for the top curve $Q = b * c$.

4.2 Multiple Objects

The experiments to study the behaviour of C_j and C_k consisted of generating a large single object in the observation image and two small objects in the reference. Their degree of overlap ($a = b \bigcap c$, $e = b \bigcap f$) was simultaneously varied, keeping their size constant and using a lattice size $Q = b + c + f$. Fig. 2.b presents the response of C_j, the spatial correspondence between b and the objects c and f. When segmenting MS lesions in MR scans this situation occurs if an observer subdivides a large lesion identified as a single lesion by the other observer. Because the total area of both segmentations is the same, C_j is an estimate of the boundary placement error.

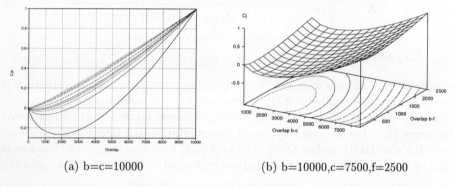

(a) b=c=10000 (b) b=10000,c=7500,f=2500

Fig. 2. Behaviour of C_{jk} and C_j.

4.3 MS Lesions

To evaluate the performance of the new indices in MS, two 3-D T_2-weighted MR brain scans from different MS patients were segmented by two observers. In both cases there was significant disagreement in the total number of lesions (Case 1: $K = 145$, $J = 581$; Case 2: $K = 113$, $J = 278$), but the total lesion volume was significantly different in only one of the cases (Case 1: $Vol_K = 16.49$ml, $Vol_J = 25.69$ml; Case 2: $Vol_K = 13.39$ml, $Vol_J = 14.96$ml). Fig. 3 shows surface projections of the segmentations done by Observer-1 (X_k) and Observer-2 (Y_j). After uniquely labelling all the lesions in each segmentation, a Correspondence matrix was formed and percentage measures of individual (one-to-one), local (many-to-one) and global (all-to-all) spatial correspondences were computed. For simplicity, the 3-D image grid was used as the lattice G.

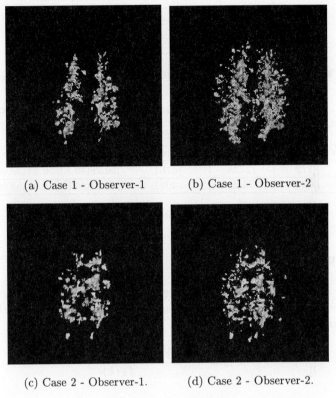

(a) Case 1 - Observer-1 (b) Case 1 - Observer-2

(c) Case 2 - Observer-1. (d) Case 2 - Observer-2.

Fig. 3. Surface rendering of segmented MS lesions.

Table 1 shows the values of the individual spatial correspondence measures between a lesion from Case 1 segmented by Observer-2 (Y_{93}) and all the lesions segmented by Observer-1 with which it overlaps (X_{19}, X_{34}, X_{45}, X_{62}, X_{86}, X_{92}, X_{94}, X_{95} and X_{113}).

Observer-2		Observer-1		$X_k \cap Y_j$	C_{kj}	C_{jk}	$ErrA$	$Over$	Sim
j	Voxels	k	Voxels						
93	1530	19	52	42	2.66	54.58	-86.85	2.72	5.30
		34	28	28	1.83	65.83	-92.81	1.83	3.59
		45	499	349	21.75	58.23	-1.62	20.77	34.40
		62	34	19	1.14	34.58	-91.30	1.22	2.42
		86	20	14	0.87	42.72	-94.83	0.91	1.80
		92	422	270	16.62	51.64	-13.52	16.05	27.66
		94	3	3	0.19	55.28	-99.21	0.19	0.39
		95	4	4	0.26	56.45	-98.95	0.26	0.52
		113	36	33	2.13	60.97	-90.80	2.15	4.21

Table 1. Measures of spatial correspondence between individual lesions.

The local spatial correspondence for the above example of lesion subdivision is presented in Table 2, where a local **overlap index** and a local **similarity index** have been computed by adding all the individual measures.

Lesion	C_j	Over	Sim
Y_{93}	47.45	46.1	80.29

Table 2. Measures of local spatial correspondence for lesion Y_{93}.

Lastly, Table 3 shows the values of the global spatial correspondence measures for the two cases under consideration.

Case	Voxels in X	Voxels in Y	Voxels in $X \cap Y$	C_X	C_Y	ErrA	Over	Sim
1	8172	12735	5761	20.28	39.83	56.34	38.03	55.11
2	6636	7418	4927	57.07	44.37	88.87	53.98	70.11

Table 3. Measures of global spatial correspondence.

5 Results and Discussion

To better understand the characteristics of the new indices and the results of the previous experiments we can express Eq. 1, 3 and 5 in terms of the number of elements in X_k, Y_j and $X_k \cap Y_j$:

$$C_{jk} = \frac{X_k \bigcap Y_j}{X_k} \cdot \frac{I_{X;Y}(k,j)}{I_X(k)} \qquad (7)$$

$$C_j = \sum_{k=1}^{K} \frac{X_k \bigcap Y_j}{Y_j} \cdot \frac{I_{X;Y}(k,j)}{I_Y(j)} \qquad (8)$$

$$C_Y = \frac{\sum_{k=1}^{K} \sum_{j=1}^{J} X_k \bigcap Y_j \cdot I_{X;Y}(k,j)}{\sum_{k=1}^{K} X_k \cdot I_X(k)} \qquad (9)$$

It is then possible to interpret the new indices as a weighted ratio of the number of overlapping elements to the total number of elements in the reference object. The weighting factor is an uncertainty coefficient that indicates the fraction of the information in the observation that is redundant in the reference. The value of this factor depends not only on the degree of overlap between the objects, but also on the size of the sampling lattice G. This dependence of the new indices on the size of the sampling lattice is clearly shown in Fig. 2.a.

Considering G as the space of possible disagreement between the observers, if its size is small relative to the size of the objects, the proposed measures will only be greater than 0 if the overlap between the objects is larger than that expected by mere chance ($P_{XY}(k,j) > P_X(k)P_Y(j)$). If we let Q, the size of the lattice, increase arbitrarily, Equations 7, 8 and 9 are reduced to the following:

$$\lim_{Q \to \infty} C_{jk} = \frac{X_k \cap Y_j}{X_k} \qquad (10)$$

$$\lim_{Q \to \infty} C_j = \sum_{k=1}^{K} \frac{X_k \cap Y_j}{Y_j} \qquad (11)$$

$$\lim_{Q \to \infty} C_\mathbf{Y} = \frac{\sum_{k=1}^{K} \sum_{j=1}^{J} X_k \cap Y_j}{\sum_{k=1}^{K} X_k} \qquad (12)$$

In this situation of maximum uncertainty where $\lim_{Q \to \infty} I_{X;Y}(k,j) = \infty$ and $\lim_{Q \to \infty} I_X(k) = \infty$, the new indices will always be positive as any degree of overlap, however small, will be larger than that expected by mere chance.

Regarding the size of the objects, C_{jk} will be equal to C_{kj} only when both objects are of the same size. This non-symmetric nature manifests the intuitive non-reflexive relationship between a large object and a small object.

The effect of considering the space of possible disagreement and the non-symmetric nature of the new indices becomes evident when comparing them with the more established measures. If the lattice size is small relative to the size of the object, the values of C_{jk} and C_{kj} are well below those of the other measures. This is to be expected as the new indices will penalise large errors when the space of possible disagreement is small. As the lattice size is increased, C_{jk} and C_{kj} tend to bound the values of the **overlap index** and the **similarity index**. If the objects are of the same size ($C_{jk} = C_{kj}$), then $\lim_{Q \to \infty} C_{jk} = Sim$. If the objects have different size and the smaller object (e.g. Y_j) is fully enclosed by the large object (e.g. X_k), then $C_{jk} = Over$.

Table 1 demonstrates the behaviour of the individual correspondence indices for various combinations of lesion size and overlap. The non-reflexive relationship between the larger 'inclusive' object and the smaller 'split' objects is clearly reflected in the different values obtained for C_{jk} and C_{kj}. The relative values of C_{jk} and C_{kj} are a measure of the boundary placement error. The larger the difference in their values, the larger the error. The absolute values of C_{jk} and C_{kj}, on the other hand, quantify the agreement in lesion identification. The larger the values, the more likely it is that the lesions identified by the observers are the same. With this in mind, for the sample lesions in Table 1 it can be said that there is a very large boundary placement error and that, apart from lesions X_{45} and X_{92}, the lesions segmented by Observer-1 should probably be interpreted as completely different lesions with respect to Y_{93}. Comparing the new indices with the other measures in this table, the values of C_{kj} are close to those of the **overlap index** because all of the objects X_k are smaller than the object Y_j and are partly or fully enclosed by it. C_{jk}, on the other hand, shows significantly larger values reflecting the fact that a larger proportion of the elements in each of the small objects X_k is included in the large object Y_j. The values of the **similarity index** are larger than those of C_{kj}, but are still bounded by C_{jk}. Regarding the complement **area error**, its values suggest that it is not well suited to estimate the correspondence when there are large differences in size between the objects. None of these three measures can be used to further study the similarities and differences between the observers as is the case with C_{jk} and C_{kj}.

An example of applying the local spatial correspondence measure C_j to MS is shown in Table 2, where part of the volume segmented by Observer-2 as lesion Y_{93} has been identified as nine separate lesions by Observer-1. From the analysis above, this can be considered as an extreme case of boundary placement disagreement between the observers. C_j is a measure of the local agreement between the observers that is influenced by both the boundary placement error and the lesion identification error. Large values of C_j indicate that there is agreement between the observers as to the location and possible extent of a certain lesion area, even if one of the observers has subdivided the lesion area in various regions. The value of C_j is slightly larger than the local **overlap index** and much smaller than the local **similarity index**, which seems to significantly overestimate the local spatial correspondence.

Lastly, Table 3 presents the global spatial correspondence indices for both examples under consideration. In this case, the relative values of $C_{\boldsymbol{X}}$ and $C_{\boldsymbol{Y}}$ are related to the boundary placement and the lesion identification errors. The larger the difference in their values, the larger the difference in the total number of lesions and the total lesion volume segmented by the observers. The absolute values of $C_{\boldsymbol{X}}$ and $C_{\boldsymbol{Y}}$, on the other hand, are a measure of the overall spatial correspondence between the observers. As expected, $C_{\boldsymbol{X}}$ and $C_{\boldsymbol{Y}}$ are larger for Case 2 (large difference in total number of lesions, but small difference in total volume) than for Case 1 (large difference in total number of lesions and in total volume). This is also true for the other three measures, but closer examination of the new indices also reveals that in Case 1 the area common to both observers has a greater correspondence with the segmentation done by Observer-1 ($C_{\boldsymbol{Y}} > C_{\boldsymbol{X}}$), whereas in Case 2 the area common to both observers has a greater correspondence with the segmentation done by Observer-2 ($C_{\boldsymbol{X}} > C_{\boldsymbol{Y}}$). This reflects an inconsistency between the observers which is not at all apparent from any of the other measures. Moreover, the complement **area error** and the **similarity index** tend to overestimate the spatial correspondence, whereas the values of the **overlap index** are once again bounded by the new indices.

6 Conclusions and Future Work

In this paper we introduced the concept of a Correspondence Matrix that can be used to compute measures of spatial correspondence between binary objects segmented by two different observers and/or segmentation algorithms. Using Information Theory we then derived a set of indices to estimate individual (one-to-one), local (many-to-one) and global (many-to-many) spatial correspondence. The main characteristics of the new indices are the implicit consideration of the space of possible disagreement and their non-symmetric nature.

The behaviour of the new indices was shown to be consistent for both synthetic and real objects regardless of their number and size. Comparing the new individual spatial correspondence indices with the more established measures of similarity illustrated the effect of considering the space of possible disagreement, and their ability to distinguish and quantify the boundary placement and lesion identification errors as a result of their non-symmetric nature. At a local level, the new indices showed the importance of quantifying the correspondence between subdivided objects and the risk of overestimating such correspondence. Globally, the proposed indices proved to be sensitive to the overall spatial correspondence as well as to more subtle inconsistencies between the observers.

In general, the values of the new indices act as bounds to those obtained for the **overlap index**, while the **similarity index** seems to consistently overestimate spatial correspondence and the complement **area error** is either not well suited or overestimates spatial correspondence. This possible overestimation and the proved lack of sensitivity of these three measures to quantify errors and inconsistencies make the proposed new indices highly attractive for medical imaging applications, such as MS lesion segmentation, where validation and comparison of segmentation results obtained by different observers and/or automated algorithms is vital.

Amongst the further work under consideration is the determination of the optimal size of the sampling lattice G, the use of thresholds to establish the number of corresponding and non-corresponding lesions, and the development of a methodology based on the new indices to automatically quantify spatial correspondence and spatial dissimilarity through time or across modalities.

7 Acknowledgements

This work is part of BIOMORPH (Development and Validation of Techniques for Brain Morphometry), project PL95 0845 of the BIOMED programme of the European Commission. Special thanks go to Prof. R. Hughes and Dr. B. Sharrack from the Department of Neurology at UMDS-Guy's Hospital for providing the MR data and the MS lesion segmentations.

References

1. Schalkoff, R. *Pattern Recognition*. J. Wiley & Sons, 1992.
2. Zidjenbos, A P; Dawant, B M; Margolin, R A and Palmer A C. *Morphometric Analysis of White Matter Lesions in MR Images: Method and Validation*. IEEE T.M.I. **13**:716-724, 1994.
3. Brummer, M E; Mersereau, E M; Eisner, R L and Lewine, R R J. *Automatic Detection of Brain Contours in MRI Data Sets*. IEEE T.M.I. **12**:153-166, 1993.
4. Grimaud J; Lai M; Thorpe J; Adeleine P; Wang G and Barker G J. *Quantification of MRI Lesion Load in Multiple Sclerosis: a comparison of Three Computer-assisted Techniques*. Magnetic Resonance Imaging **14**:495-505, 1996.
5. Jackson E F; Narayana P A; Wolinsky J S and Doyle T J. *Accuracy and Reproducibility in Volumetric Analysis of Multiple Sclerosis Lesions*. Journal of Computer Assisted Tomography **17**:200-205, 1993.
6. Wells, W M; Viola, P; Atsumi, H; Nakajima, S and Kikinis, R. *Multi-modal Volume Registration by Maximization of Mutual Information*. Medical Image Analysis **1**:35-51, 1996.
7. Maes, F; Collignon, A; Vandermeulen, D; Marchal, G and Suetens, P. *Multimodality Image Registration by Maximization of Mutual Information*.. IEEE T.M.I. **16**:187-198, 1997.
8. Weaver, W and Shannon, C E. *The Mathematical Theory of Communication*. Univ. of Illinois Press, 1949.

Non-linear Cerebral Registration with Sulcal Constraints

D. Louis Collins, Georges Le Goualher, and Alan C. Evans

McConnell Brain Imaging Centre, Montréal Neurological Institute,
McGill University, Montréal, Canada
{louis,georges,alan}@bic.mni.mcgill.ca
http://www.bic.mni.mcgill.ca

Abstract. In earlier work [1], we demonstrated that cortical registration could be improved on simulated data by using blurred, geometric, image-based features (L_{vv}) or explicitly extracted and blurred sulcal traces on simulated data. Here, the technique is modified to incorporate sulcal ribbons in conjunction with a chamfer distance objective function to improve registration in real MRI data as well. Experiments with 10 simulated data sets demonstrate a 56% reduction in residual sulcal registration error (from 3.4 to 1.5mm, on average) when compared to automatic linear registration and an 28% improvement over our previously published non-linear technique (from 2.1 to 1.5mm). The simulation results are confirmed by experiments with real MRI data from young normal subjects, where sulcal misregistration is reduced by 20% (from 5.0mm to 4.0mm) and 11% (from 4.5 to 4.0mm) over the standard linear and nonlinear registration methods, respectively.

1 Introduction

In medical imaging processing research, correct automatic labelling of each voxel in a 3-D brain image remains an unsolved problem. Towards this goal, we have developed a program called ANIMAL (Automatic Nonlinear Image Matching and Anatomical Labelling) [2] which, like many other non-linear registration procedures, is based on the assumption that different brains are topologically equivalent and that non-linear deformations can be estimated and applied to one data set in order to bring it into correspondence with another. These non-linear deformations are then used (i) to estimate non-linear morphometric variability in a given population [3], (ii) to automatically segment MRI data [2], or (iii) to remove residual alignment errors when spatially averaging results among individuals.

Our previous validation of ANIMAL showed that it worked well for deep structures [2], but sometimes had difficulty aligning sulci and gyri. In a follow-up paper presented at VBC96 [1], we described an extension of the basic non-linear registration method that used additional image-based features to help align the cortex. Simulations showed that L_{vv}-based features and blurred sulcal traces significantly improved cortical registration, however these results were not confirmed with real MRI data. In this paper, we demonstrate the use of automatically extracted and labelled sulci as extra features in conjunction with a chamfer distance objective function [4, 5]. Experimental results presented here (for both simulated and real data) show significant improvement over our previous work.

In contrast to existing methods for cortical structure alignment that depend on manual intervention to identify corresponding points [6, 7] or curves [8–11], the procedure presented here is completely automatic. While other 3D voxel-based non-linear registration procedures exist (e.g., [12–20]), none of these have looked specifically at the question of cortical features for cortical registration. The method presented here explicitly uses sulcal information in a manner similar to surface-matching algorithms described in [10, 21, 22] to improve cortical registration. However, our method is entirely voxel-based, *completely automatic*, and does not require any manual intervention for sulcal identification or labelling.

The paper is organized as follows: Section 2 describes the brain-phantom used to create simulated data, the acquisition parameters for real MRI data, the non-linear registration method, and the features used in the matching process; Section 3 presents experiments on simulated MRI data with known deformations in order to compare our standard linear and non-linear registration procedures with the new technique and to determine a lower-bound for the registration error. Section 3 with experiments on 11 real MRI data sets, comparing the old and new registration methods. The paper concludes with a discussion and presents directions for further research.

2 Methods.

2.1 Input Data

Two sets of experiments are presented below where the first involves simulations to validate the algorithm and the second, real MRI data from normal subjects.

Simulated data: Simulations are required validate any image processing procedure since it is difficult, if not impossible to establish ground truth with in-vivo data. Here, we simulate MRI volumes [23] from different anatomies by warping a high resolution brain phantom [24] with a random (but known) deformation. Since both the deformation and structural information are known a priori, we can directly compute an objective measure of algorithm performance.

Simulated MRIs: Magnetic resonance images are simulated by MRISIM [23], a program that predicts image contrast by computing NMR signal intensities from a discrete-event simulation based on the Bloch equations of a given pulse sequence. A realistic high-resolution brain phantom was used to map tissue intensities into MR images. The simulator accounts for the effects of various image acquisition parameters by incorporating partial volume averaging, measurement noise and intensity non-uniformity. The images in Fig. 1 were simulated using the same MR parameters as those described below (c.f., 2.1) for the real MRI acquisitions.

Simulated deformations: Most non-linear registration algorithms compute a continuous spatial mapping from the coordinate system of a given subject's MRI to that of a target MRI volume. It is assumed that this mapping incorporates all morphological differences between subject and target anatomies. We turn this paradigm around to simulate different anatomies, based on a single target volume. Random spatial deformations were generated and applied to the brain phantom to build a family of homologous, but morphologically different brain phantoms. An MRI volume was simulated for each member of the family.

Random spatial deformations were generated by defining a set of twenty landmarks within the target brain volume. A second deformed set of landmarks was produced by adding a random displacement to each of the landmark coordinates. Since previous work in our laboratory has shown anatomical variability to be on the order of 4-7mm [25], a Gaussian random number generator with a standard deviation of 5mm was used to produce each component of the displacement vector. The two resulting point sets (original and deformed) were then used to define a continuous 3-D thin-plate spline transformation function. Ten such deformations were generated and used to resample the original target data and produce 10 spatially warped source data sets for testing. The average deformation magnitude was 7.7mm with a maximum of 19.7mm. Figure 1 shows transverse slices (after linear stereotaxic registration) through the original and three of the ten warped volumes used in the experiments below. While these images demonstrate extreme deformations, they form a good test for ANIMAL.

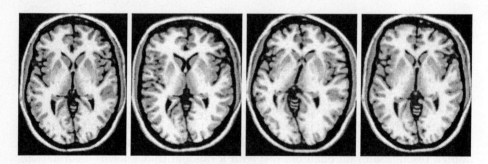

Fig. 1. Simulated data

This figure shows transverse slices at the level of the ventricles for four of the ten simulated test volumes, after resampling with the linear transformation recovered by ANIMAL. While these volumes are perhaps deformed more than one would find on average in the normal population, subjects representing an extreme of normal anatomical variability could be shaped like these examples. Note that while only 2-D images are shown in the figures, all calculations are computed in 3-D on volumetric data.

MRI Acquisition: In order to validate the ANIMAL algorithm with real data, eleven subjects were scanned on a Philips Gyroscan ACS 1.5 Tesla superconducting magnet system at the Montreal Neurological Institute using a T1-weighted 3-D spoiled gradient-echo acquisition with sagittal volume excitation (TR=18, TE=10, flip angle=$30°$, 1mm isotropic voxels, 140-180 sagittal slices). Without loss of generality, one of the 11 MRI volumes was chosen to serve as the target and the other 10 were registered to it.

2.2 Processing Pipeline

A number of processing steps are required to register two data sets together. We have combined preprocessing steps (image intensity non-uniformity correction [26], tube masking), linear registration (ANIMAL in linear mode [27]) and re-sampling into stereotaxic space, cortical surface extraction (MSD [28, 29]), tissue classification (INSECT [30]), automatic sulcal extraction (SEAL [31]) and non-linear registration (ANIMAL in nonlinear mode [2]) into a processing pipeline. After running this basic pipeline, a subject's MRI volume can be visualized in stereotaxic space with its corresponding tissue labels, anatomical structure labels, cortical surface and sulcal ribbons — all in 3D. The following sections describe the registration and sulcal extraction procedures in more detail.

Registration Algorithm: Registration is completed automatically in a two step process. The first [27] accounts for the linear part of the transformation by using correlation between Gaussian-blurred features (described below) extracted from both volumes. After automatic linear registration, there remains a residual non-linear component of spatial mis-registration among brains that is due (mostly) to normal anatomical morphometric variability. In the second step, the ANIMAL program estimates the 3D deformation field [2, 3] required to account for this variability. The deformation field is built by sequentially stepping through the target volume in a 3D grid pattern. At each grid-node i, the deformation vector required to achieve local registration between the two volumes is found by optimization of 3 translational parameters (tx_i, ty_i, tz_i) that maximize the objective function evaluated only in the neighbourhood region surrounding the node. The algorithm is applied iteratively in a multi-scale hierarchy, so that image blurring and grid size are reduced after each iteration, thus refining the fit. (The algorithm is described in detail in [2, 32]).

Features: The objective function maximized in the optimization procedure measures the similarity between features extracted from the source and target volumes. We use blurred image intensity and blurred image gradient magnitude, calculated by convolution of the original data with zeroth and first order 3D isotropic Gaussian derivatives in order to maintain linearity, shift-invariance and rotational-invariance in the detection of features. Since both linear and non-linear registration procedures are computed in a multi-scale fashion, the original

MR data was blurred at two different scales: FWHM=8, and $4mm$, with the FWHM= (2.35σ) of the Gaussian kernel acting as a measure of spatial scale.

The enhanced version of ANIMAL uses geometrical landmarks such as sulci to improve cortical alignment. We have previously detailed a method called SEAL (Sulcal Extraction and Automatic Labeling) to automatically extract cortical sulci (defined by the 2D surface extending from the sulcal trace at the cortical surface to the depth of the sulcal fundus) from 3D MRI [33, 31]. Each sulcus is extracted in a two step process using an active model similar to a 2D Snake that we call an *active ribbon*. First, the superficial cortical trace of the sulcus is modeled by a 1D snake-spline [34], that is initialized to loci of negative curvature of the cortical surface. Second, this snake is then submitted to a set of forces derived from (1) tissue classification results, (2) differential characteristics of the image intensities near the cortex and (3) a distance-from-cortex term to force the snake to converge to the sulcal fundus. The set of successive iterative positions of the 1D snake define the sulcal axis. These loci are then used to drive a 2D active ribbon which forms the final representation of the sulcus.

When applied to an MRI brain volume, the output of this automatic process consists of a set of *Elementary Sulcal Surfaces* (ESS) that represent all cortical sulcal folds. A number of these ESSs may be needed to represent a sulcus as defined by an anatomist. Simply blurring the voxel masks that represent the sulci at scales of FWHM=16 and $8mm$ so that they could be directly incorporated into the standard ANIMAL procedure for correlative matching was found not to improve cortical registration for real MRI data [1]. Here, in order to incorporate the geometric sulcal information represented by the ESS, the sulcal ribbons are voxelated. Like Sandor et. al.[10], we use a chamfer distance function to drive sulci together. This methods brings sulci that are initially far apart into registration.

2.3 Error measures

In order to quantitatively evaluate the methods and compare them with previously published results [1], a 3D root-mean-squared (rms) minimum distance measure, D_{surf}, was computed for the ESS of selected sulci[1] that were identified manually by a medically-trained expert on the phantom volumes and on the real MRI volumes. The 3D rms minimum distance measure is defined on a point-wise basis, computing the root mean square (over all nodes in the ESS defining the

---

[1] The following 16 sulci were traced bilaterally using a visualization tool that shows a 3D surface rendering of the cortex and orthogonal slices through the brain volume: (a) central sulcus and (b) the Sylvian fissure; (c) the superior, (d) the middle, and (e) the inferior frontal sulci; (f) the vertical (a.k.a. ascending) and (g) the horizontal rami of the Sylvian fissure, as well as (h) the incisura (located between these other two rami); (i) the olfactory sulcus as well as (j) the sulcus lateralis, (k) the sulcus medialis, (l) the sulcus intermedius, and (m) the sulcus transversus (all found along the orbitofrontal surface of the brain); (n) the precentral and (o) the postcentral sulci; and finally (p) the intraparietal sulcus.

sulcus) of the minimum distance between each node in the transformed source sulcus and closest point on the target sulcus surface.

3 Experiments and Results

Two series of three experiments were completed varying only the features used by ANIMAL where the first series was completed for simulated data, and the second series, for real MRI data. In each experiment, 10 MRI volumes were registered to the chosen target volume. The 3 different experiments were defined as follows: (1) ANIMAL in standard non-linear mode, (2) ANIMAL+selected sulci, (3) ANIMAL+all sulci after using selected sulci.

In method 2, the problem of establishing correspondence is addressed by using ten extracted sulci (superior and middle frontal, Sylvian, olfactory and central, on both hemispheres) as features in addition to the blurred MRI intensity volume already used by ANIMAL, The third method is an attempt to improve the second, by adding all sulci automatically extracted by SEAL into the registration process after completing the ANIMAL+selected sulci registration. A linear transformation is also presented for comparisons. Figures 2 and 3 summarize the results qualitatively for simulated and real data, respectively. Tables 1 and 2 present quantitative results for the measure described above.

TABLE 1   TABLE 2

	simulations				real MRI			
	lin	∇	$\nabla+5$	$\nabla+all$	lin	∇	$\nabla+5$	$\nabla+all$
Central	3.2;1.5	1.2;1.4	0.7;0.3	0.7;0.4	4.7;1.3	4.1;1.4	2.5;1.2	2.5;1.2
Postcentral	4.2;2.3	2.2;2.4	1.3;1.5	1.3;1.5	6.4;1.7	6.1;2.0	5.0;1.7	5.0;1.8
Middle Frontal	3.2;1.0	1.4;1.2	0.7;0.6	0.7;0.6	6.2;3.5	5.4;3.2	4.5;3.1	4.7;3.2
Superior Frontal	3.4;1.9	1.8;2.1	1.6;2.1	1.7;2.1	6.2;3.8	5.6;3.6	4.4;3.9	4.4;4.0
Sylvian	4.0;1.3	3.0;1.2	2.4;0.9	2.4;1.0	5.2;1.6	5.0;1.4	3.6;0.9	3.7;1.0
Olfactory	3.2;4.2	1.7;2.8	1.5;2.9	1.6;2.8	2.1;1.7	1.6;1.9	1.3;1.6	1.4;1.8
average (n=16)	3.4;2.3	2.1;2.1	1.6;1.7	1.5;1.7	5.0;3.2	4.5;3.1	4.0;3.1	4.0;3.1

Quantitative results for simulations and real data. Mean and standard deviation of D_{surf} minimum distance results (mean(D_{surf});std(D_{surf})) for linear (lin), ANIMAL (∇), ANIMAL+selected sulci ($\nabla+5$), ANIMAL with all sulci ($\nabla+all$) registration methods. Average is computed for both left and right hemispheres for 16 sulci on 10 subjects. All measures in millimeters.

3.1 Simulations

Standard ANIMAL: In the first experiment (Fig. 2-b) we can see that the global brain shape is properly corrected and that the main lobes are mostly aligned since the central and Sylvian sulci are better aligned than in the linear registration. Even though previous experiments in [2] have shown that basal ganglia structures (e.g., thalamus, caudate, putamen, globus pallidus) and ventricular structures are well registered (with overlaps on the order of 85% to 90%) for both simulated and real data, the simulations presented here indicate that the standard ANIMAL technique cannot always register cortical structures by using only blurred image intensities and gradient magnitude features.

ANIMAL+selected sulci: In Fig. 2-c, 10 extracted sulci (superior and middle frontal, Sylvian, olfactory and central, on both hemispheres) were used as additional features in ANIMAL to address problems in establishing correspondence. Visual inspection of Fig. 2-c shows that the previous misalignments in the motor-sensory area have been corrected, and alignment for neighbouring structures has improved greatly. Indeed, when evaluated on the central sulcus, the D_{surf} measure improves dramatically: $3.2mm$ for linear; $2.0mm$ for standard non-linear; $0.7mm$ for ANIMAL with labelled sulci. The standard deviation of D_{surf} decreases as well, indicating tighter grouping around the target sulci. The 0.54mm average D_{surf} reduction is highly significant ($p < 0.0001$, $T = 157$, $d.o.f. = 320$, paired T-test over all sulci and all subjects).

ANIMAL+selected sulci+all sulci: In this experiment, the ANIMAL+selected sulci transformation is used as input where all sulci extracted by SEAL are used as features in an attempt to further improve cortical alignment in regions that are not close to the previously selected sulci. The improvement is evident qualitatively in Fig. 2-d and quantitatively in Table 1 where the average D_{surf}, evaluated over all sulci and all subjects drops from $1.6mm$ for the standard ANIMAL to $1.5mm$ when using all sulci. While this improvement is small, it is statistically significant ($p < 0.0001$, $T = 88.5$, $d.o.f. = 320$, paired T-test).

3.2 Real MRI data

Standard ANIMAL: When applied to real data, the image in Fig. 3-b shows that that the standard ANIMAL non-linear registration is not enough to align cortical structures. In fact, it does not appear to be much better than the linear registration. This is confirmed by the quantitative results in Table 2, where the average D_{surf} value for the standard ANIMAL registrations is only slightly better than that for linear registrations.

ANIMAL+selected sulci: The use of 5 paired sulci improves cortical registration significantly in the neighbourhood of the chosen sulci as shown in Fig. 3-c. The central sulcus (purple), superior frontal (orange), middle frontal (red), olfactory (black) and Sylvian (red) (arrows) are well defined, and this is confirmed by improved D_{surf} values in Table 2, when compared to the standard ANIMAL registrations. Unfortunately, the effect appears to be relatively local in that alignment of neighbouring sulci are only somewhat improved (e.g., postcentral sulcus). This is probably because there is no explicit representation of the other sulci in the registration, so they do not participate in the fitting process. However, using some labelled sulci yields a 0.50mm average D_{surf} reduction (from 4.5 to 4.0mm) that is highly significant ($p < 0.0001$, $T = 157$, $d.o.f. = 320$, paired T-test).

ANIMAL+selected sulci+all sulci: When the previous result is used as input for a registration using all sulci as features, then some of the other sulci (e.g., postcentral) come into alignment, however others may be attracted to non-homologous sulci, since no explicit labelling of sulci is used in this step.

4 Discussion and Conclusion

The simulation results indicate clearly that the registrations computed by ANIMAL improve substantially when using the extra cortical features. The random deformations used to simulate different anatomies (section 2.1) only model one aspect of anatomical variability, namely the second-order morphological difference between subjects (i.e., a difference in position for a given structure after mapping into a standardized space). The simulations do not account for different topologies of gyral and sulcal patterns. For example, it cannot change the region corresponding to Heschl's gyrus, to contain double gyri when the phantom has only a single. Still, the value of these simulations is not diminished since they can be used to determine a lower-bound on the registration error — corresponding to the optimal case when a 1-to-1 mapping exists between two subjects.

The experiments with real data indicate that the use of automatically extracted and labelled sulci in conjunction with a chamfer distance function can significantly improve cortical registration. One must keep in mind that the D_{surf} measure includes possible sulcal mis-identification and sulcal extraction errors (from SEAL) in addition to ANIMAL's mis-registration error. We are working on quantifying the performance of SEAL in order to improve the error measure. Further improvements to the registration algorithm will require a slight change in fitting strategy to account for different cortical topologies apparent in real MRI data. We envision using a number of different targets simultaneously, where each target will account for a particular type of sulcal pattern [35].

The current version of ANIMAL now allows the use of a chamfer-distance objective function to align sulci, however nothing in the implementation is sulci-specific. Indeed, any geometric structure that can be voxelated can be incorporated into the matching procedure to further refine the fit. We are currently evaluating the incorporation of explicitly extracted cortical surfaces [28, 29] into the registration process.

Acknowledgments: The authors would like to express their appreciation for support from the Human Frontier Science Project Organization, the Canadian Medical Research Council (SP-30), the McDonnell-Pew Cognitive Neuroscience Center Program, the U.S. Human Brain Map Project (HBMP), NIMH and NIDA. This work forms part of a continuing project of the HBMP-funded International Consortium for Brain Mapping (ICBM) to develop a probabilistic atlas of human neuroanatomy. We also wish to acknowledge the manual labelling of sulcal traces completed by Rahgu Venegopal.

References

1. D. Collins, G. LeGoualher, R. Venugopal, Z. Caramanos, A. Evans, and C. Barillot, "Cortical constraints for non-linear cortical registration," in *Visualization in Biomedical Computing* (K. Höene, ed.), (Hamburg), pp. 307–316, Sept 1996.
2. D. Collins, C. Holmes, T. Peters, and A. Evans, "Automatic 3D model-based neuroanatomical segmentation," *Human Brain Mapping*, vol. 3, no. 3, pp. 190–208, 1995.

3. D. L. Collins, T. M. Peters, and A. C. Evans, "An automated 3D non-linear image deformation procedure for determination of gross morphometric variability in human brain," in *Proceedings of Conference on Visualization in Biomedical Computing*, SPIE, 1994.
4. G. Borgefors, "Distance transformations in arbitrary dimensions," *Computer Graphics, Vision and Image Processing*, vol. 27, pp. 321–345, 1984.
5. G. Borgefors, "On digital distance transforms in three dimensions," *Computer Vision Image Understanding*, vol. 64, pp. 368–76, 1996.
6. A. C. Evans, W. Dai, D. L. Collins, P. Neelin, and T. Marrett, "Warping of a computerized 3-D atlas to match brain image volumes for quantitative neuroanatomical and functional analysis," in *Proceedings of the International Society of Optical Engineering: Medical Imaging V*, vol. 1445, (San Jose, California), SPIE, 27 February – 1 March 1991.
7. F. Bookstein, "Thin-plate splines and the atlas problem for biomedical images," in *Information Processing in Medical Imaging* (A. Colchester and D. Hawkes, eds.), vol. 511 of *Lecture Notes in Computer Science*, (Wye, UK), pp. 326–342, IPMI, Springer-Verlag, July 1991.
8. Y. Ge, J. Fitzpatrick, R. Kessler, and R. Margolin, "Intersubject brain image registration using both cortical and subcortical landmarks," in *Proceedings of SPIE Medical Imaging*, vol. 2434, pp. 81–95, SPIE, 1995.
9. S. Luo and A. Evans, "Matching sulci in 3d space using force-based deformation," tech. rep., McConnell Brain Imaging Centre, Montreal Neurological Institute, McGill University, Montreal, Nov 1994.
10. S. Sandor and R. Leahy, "Towards automated labelling of the cerebral cortex using a deformable atlas," in *Information Processing in Medical Imaging* (Y. Bizais, C. Barillot, and R. DiPaola, eds.), (Brest, France), pp. 127–138, IPMI, Kluwer, Aug 1995.
11. D. Dean, P. Buckley, F. Bookstein, J. Kamath, and D. Kwon, "Three dimensional mr-based morphometric comparison of schizophrenic and normal cerebral ventricles," in *Proceedings of Conference on Visualization in Biomedical Computing*, Lecture Notes in Computer Science, p. this volume, Springer-Verlag, Sept. 1996.
12. R. Bajcsy and S. Kovacic, "Multiresolution elastic matching," *Computer Vision, Graphics, and Image Processing*, vol. 46, pp. 1–21, 1989.
13. R. Dann, J. Hoford, S. Kovacic, M. Reivich, and R. Bajcsy, "Three-dimensional computerized brain atlas for elastic matching: Creation and initial evaluation," in *Medical Imaging II*, (Newport Beach, Calif.), pp. 600–608, SPIE, Feb. 1988.
14. M. Miller, Y. A. G.E. Christensen, and U. Grenander, "Mathematical textbook of deformable neuroanatomies," *Proceedings of the National Academy of Sciences*, vol. 90, no. 24, pp. 11944–11948, 1990.
15. J. Zhengping and P. H. Mowforth, "Mapping between MR brain images and a voxel model," *Med Inf (Lond)*, vol. 16, pp. 183–93, Apr-Jun 1991.
16. K. Friston, C. Frith, P. Liddle, and R. Frackowiak, "Plastic transformation of PET images," *Journal of Computer Assisted Tomography*, vol. 15, no. 1, pp. 634–639, 1991.
17. G. Christensen, R. Rabbitt, and M. Miller, "3D brain mapping using a deformable neuroanatomy," *Physics in Med and Biol*, vol. 39, pp. 609–618, 1994.
18. J. Gee, L. LeBriquer, and C. Barillot, "Probabilistic matching of brain images," in *Information Processing in Medical Imaging* (Y. Bizais and C. Barillot, eds.), (Ile Berder, France), IPMI, Kluwer, July 1995.

19. J. Gee, "Probabilistic matching of deformed images," Tech. Rep. Technical report MS-CIS-96, Department of Computer and Information Science, University of Pennsylvania, Philadelphia, 1996.
20. G. Christensen, R. Rabbitt, and M. Miller, "Deformable templates using large deformation kinematics," *IEEE Transactions on Image Processing*, 1996.
21. P. Thompson and A. Toga, "A surface-based technique for warping 3-dimensional images of the brain," *IEEE Transactions on Medical Imaging*, vol. 15, no. 4, pp. 383–392, 1996.
22. C. Davatzikos, "Spatial normalization of 3d brain images using deformable models," *J Comput Assist Tomogr*, vol. 20, pp. 656–65, Jul-Aug 1996.
23. R. Kwan, A. C. Evans, and G. B. Pike, "An extensible MRI simulator for postprocessing evaluation," in *Proceedings of the 4th International Conference on Visualization in Biomedical Computing, VBC '96:*, (Hamburg), pp. 135–140, September 1996.
24. D. Collins, A. Zijdenbos, V. Kollokian, J. Sled, N. Kabani, C. Holmes, and A. Evans, "Design and construction of a realistic digital brain phantom," *IEEE Transactions on Medical Imaging*, 1997. submitted.
25. C. Sorlié, D. L. Collins, K. J. Worsley, and A. C. Evans, "An anatomical variability study based on landmarks," tech. rep., McConnell Brain Imaging Centre, Montreal Neurological Institute, McGill University, Montreal, Sept 1994.
26. J. G. Sled, A. P. Zijdenbos, and A. C. Evans, "A non-parametric method for automatic correction of intensity non-uniformity in MRI data," *IEEE Transactions on Medical Imaging*, vol. 17, Feb. 1998.
27. D. L. Collins, P. Neelin, T. M. Peters, and A. C. Evans, "Automatic 3D intersubject registration of MR volumetric data in standardized talairach space," *Journal of Computer Assisted Tomography*, vol. 18, pp. 192–205, March/April 1994.
28. D. MacDonald, D. Avis, and A. C. Evans, "Multiple surface identification and matching in magnetic resonance images," in *Proceedings of Conference on Visualization in Biomedical Computing*, SPIE, 1994.
29. D. MacDonald, *Identifying geometrically simple surfaces from three dimensional data*. PhD thesis, McGill University, Montreal, Canada, December 1994.
30. A. P. Zijdenbos, A. C. Evans, F. Riahi, J. Sled, J. Chui, and V. Kollokian, "Automatic quantification of multiple sclerosis lesion volume using stereotaxic space," in *Proceedings of the 4th International Conference on Visualization in Biomedical Computing, VBC '96:*, (Hamburg), pp. 439–448, September 1996.
31. G. L. Goualher, C. Barillot, and Y. Bizais, "Three-dimensional segmentation and representation of cortical sulci using active ribbons," in *International Journal of Pattern Recognition and Artificial Intelligence*, 11(8):1295-1315 1997.
32. D. Collins and A. Evans, "Animal: validation and applications of non-linear registration-based segmentation," *International Journal and Pattern Recognition and Artificial Intelligence*, vol. 11, pp. 1271–1294, Dec 1997.
33. G. L. Goualher, C. Barillot, Y. Bizais, and J.-M. Scarabin, "Three-dimensional segmentation of cortical sulci using active models," in *SPIE Medical Imaging*, vol. 2710, (Newport-Beach, Calif.), pp. 254–263, SPIE, 1996.
34. F. Leitner, I. Marque, S. Lavalee, and P. Cinquin, "Dynamic segmentation: finding the edge with snake splines," in *Int. Conf. on Curves and Surfaces*, pp. 279–284, Academic Press, June 1991.
35. M. Ono, S. Kubik, and C. Abernathey, *Atlas of Cerebral Sulci*. Stuttgart: Georg Thieme Verlag, 1990.

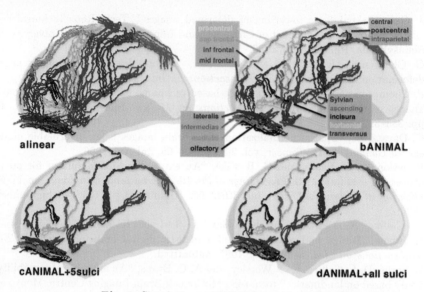

Fig. 2. Simulations: ANIMAL-only vs ANIMAL+sulci

Left-side view of the cortical traces of 16 sulci from 10 simulated volumes overlaid on an average cortical surface after mapping into stereotaxic space with the different transformations indicated. These simulations show that extracted and labelled sulci improve the standard ANIMAL registrations.

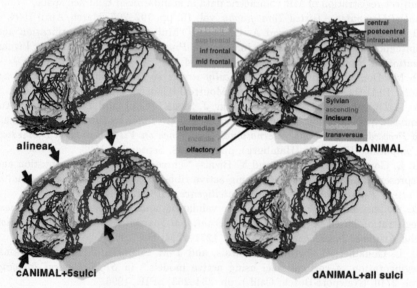

Fig. 3. Real data: ANIMAL-only vs ANIMAL+sulci

Left-side view of the cortical traces of 16 sulci from 10 real subjects overlaid on an average cortical surface after mapping into stereotaxic space. It is easy to see that the standard registration technique does not deal well with cortical structures, however addition sulcal constraints improve cortical registration significantly for real data near sulci participating in the registration process (arrows).

A Double Scanning Procedure for Visualisation of Radiolucent Objects in Soft Tissues: Application to Oral Implant Surgery Planning

Kris Verstreken[1], Johan Van Cleynenbreugel[1], Guy Marchal[1], Daniel van Steenberghe[2], Paul Suetens[1]

[1]Laboratory for Medical Image Computing, ESAT/Radiology, University Hospital Gasthuisberg, Herestraat 49, 3000 Leuven, Belgium
[2]Holder of the P-I Brånemark Chair in Osseointegration, Department of Periodontology, Faculty of Medicine, Katholieke Universiteit Leuven, Capucijnenvoer 7, 3000 Leuven, Belgium
Kris.Verstreken@uz.kuleuven.ac.be

Abstract. A procedure for visualization of radiolucent objects in CT scan images is proposed and applied to endosseous oral implant surgery planning. Many of these patients have a removable prosthesis, and visualisation of this prosthesis proves to be advantageous during planning. Such a prosthesis is usually quite radiolucent and thus not distinguishable on CT. The technique glues small markers on the prosthesis, and then scans it, giving a first image set. A second image set of the patient with the intraoral marked prosthesis is then acquired. From the first set, a surface rendered model of the prosthesis can be constructed. From the second set, a surface model of the bone can be made, and the markers indicate the position of the prosthesis in the mouth of the patient. The prosthesis model is then orthogonally transformed so that it fits the bone model. The views obtained are clinically very relevant since they indicate where the teeth of a later fixed prosthesis will come, and the planner can orient the axes of the implants towards the occlusal plane of the teeth. This double scanning procedure is a low-cost technique that nevertheless has significant clinical benefits.

Introduction

When patients with compromised bone quality are to receive oral implants, a preoperative plan is often made to assure optimal use of the remaining bone. This plan can be based upon computed tomography (CT), orthopantomography, or other scanning techniques (Jacobs and van Steenberghe (1998)). The available bone quality and -quantity are the most important parameter assessed as yet. However, the ability to evaluate the esthetics and biomechanics of a proposed implant configuration provides an added value. Many patients already have a removable prosthesis indicating optimal tooth position, which could be kept in the mouth during scanning to visualise it on the CT scans instead of a custom designed template. This is not evident however: Most prostheses, if they contain no metal, are not well visible when scanned intraorally. They have the same radiodensity as the soft tissues around them, making them undistinguishable from these tissues Even painted with a contrastmedium for CT, they suffer from streak artifacts due to the dental fillings in eventual remaining teeth. In standard jaw acquisitions where bone quality is to be judged these artifacts cause no problems because the scatter lies mainly in the occlusal plane, but for prosthesis design the position of the teeth in the occlusal plane is essential information that should not be lost.

A second acquisition of the prosthesis alone, scanned in the surrounding air, could be used to obtain its structure: The contrast with the surrounding medium is now sufficient, but a new problem is created: The position of the prosthesis relative to the patient's anatomy is lost.

To combine the best of both worlds, we use a *double scan technique*: Small radioopaque markers are attached to the prosthesis. A first scan of the marked prosthesis shows the prosthesis surface clearly enough together with these markers (Fig 1), and allows a good surface rendering of the removable prosthesis (Fig 2). Then a second scan of the patient and the intraoral marked prosthesis is made (Fig 3), showing the location of the markers with respect to the bone, but not the prosthesis itself. A surface model of the bone can be constructed however (Fig 4). The markers are visible in both sets and so allow the transformation between the two sets to be computed. Once this transformation is known, the scan of the prosthesis can be realigned with the scan of the patient, and both can be inspected together. When following this procedure, several things must be kept in mind however. We will now go into more detail.

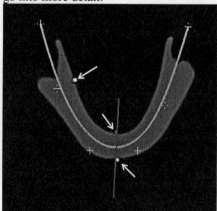 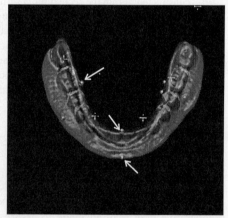

Fig. 1. Prosthesis scanned separately. The arrows point at the attached markers.

Fig. 2. The model made from the previous images, showing the markers from (Fig 1) as small balls on the structure.

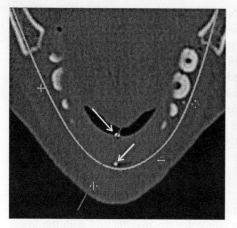 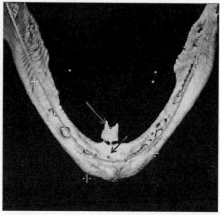

Fig. 3. The markers from (Fig 1) are visible on the patient scan images.

Fig. 4. The markers are manually indicated by small annotation spheres.

Methodology

Equipment

For the acquisition, a Somatom Plus CT (Siemens, Erlangen, Germany) is used, in spiral mode with a table feed of 1 mm/rotation together with an aperture of 1 mm. Reconstruction is at the theoretically optimal interslice distance of 0.5 mm. A maximum height of 40 mm can be scanned with this CT and these settings, but this is sufficient for these structures.

The reconstructed data are transferred to the workstation over the intranet of the hospital. The fiducials are Gutta-Percha balls and are attached to the prosthesis with simple pieces of adhesive tape. They are disposable.

Scanning Procedure

Prosthesis CT

Meticulous execution of the steps in the sequence avoids some pitfalls. The prosthesis should indicate optimal teeth location and -angulation, and it should not contain large metal parts because they will create streak artifacts that obscure the fiducials and even the bone of the jaw. A uniform distribution of the markers over the available height and width is ideal, but if the patient is not edentulous he might have fillings, and in that case it is best to avoid placing markers within the occlusal plane. The available space for the markers is then much less in height and care must be taken to attach enough markers to avoid coplanarity. The prosthesis is fixed to the scanner table with approximately the same angulation as it will have in the mouth of the patient, to avoid distortions comparable to those introduced by gantry tilt. If all requirements are fullfilled, the prosthesis is scanned. Streak artifacts in the images will warn the technician if any invisible larger metal parts were overlooked. If this is the case, the procedure cannot be used and the patient is scanned without the prosthesis, as for the normal dental CT. If there are no such problems however, the patient is scanned with the prosthesis intraorally.

Patient CT

The marked prosthesis is placed into the mouth of the patient as it is usually worn. The head of the patient is aligned with the palate for the maxilla and with the lower mandibular border for the mandible. If there are dental fillings present, this orientation will keep the streak artifacts out of the plane of the jawbones. Once proper alignment is reached, the head is immobilized relative to the scanner table. Patient and prosthesis are scanned together using the normal settings for this type of acquisition.

Data Handling

Both data sets are reconstructed on the CT console and the images are transferred to the workstation by any suitable means. Several preprocessing steps prepare the data (Schroeder and Lorensen (1996)), amongst them the creation of the surface renderings for bone and prosthesis, using the marching cubes algorithm (Lorensen and Cline (1987) or Udupa and Gon÷alves (1996)).

Fiducial Indication

The images are inspected on the workstation. In each of the datasets the coordinates of the visible fiducials are indicated by putting a spherical marker on them. These coordinates could just as well be determined on the scanner console, but care should be taken that a reslice along the z-axis is taken for this selection, since otherwise a rounding on the slice position will occur, resulting in coordinates that are a multiple of the interslice distance.

Two sets result, called X_1 and X_2, for the patient and the prosthesis scans respectively. The center of the marker is indicated manually on the reslices along the z-axis, but the images should be zoomed out sufficiently to increase the accuracy. Visual comparison of both marker sets provides a first check on the correctness of the indications. Sometimes scatter artifacts make marker selection difficult in the patient data set, but the prosthesis data serve as a map that gives a hint as to where the user should look for the markers in the patient set.

Registration Procedure

Statement as a multidimensional Least Squares Problem

Adjusting the position and orientation of the prosthesis relative to the bone of the patient is called registration. This registration problem can be stated as follows:

Given two sets of coordinates X_1 and X_2 for the same points in two different reference frames, that of the patient and that of the prosthesis, a matrix T is sought that transforms one set into the other, where $X_1, X_2 \in \Re^{4 \times m}$ and $T \in \Re^{4 \times 4}$:

$$X_1 = TX_2 \tag{1}$$

Solving (1) for the transformation matrix T is similar to the following mathematical problem:

Given a data matrix $A \in \Re^{m \times n}$ and an observation matrix $B \in \Re^{m \times d}$, find a matrix $X \in \Re^{n \times d}$ such that $AX = B$. If $m > n$ there are more equations than unknowns and the problem is overdetermined. In almost all cases there are errors on the data so that $B \notin R(A)$ and there is no exact solution. The notation then used is $AX \approx B$. Solution methods can be found by considering the problem as a multidimensional Least Squares (LS) problem:

Definition: Multidimensional Least Squares Problem:

$$\text{Find the } X \in \Re^{n \times d} \text{ that minimizes } \|AX - B\|_{Frob} \tag{2}$$

X is then called a LS solution of the set $AX \approx B$. This solution is in a sense ideal since it has been shown in (Gauss (1823)) that the X that can thus be found has the smallest variance that can be produced if there is no systematic error in the result and X depends linearly on B.

Solutions for the LS Problem

For a solution of (2) to exist, B has to be a part of the range of A. If the problem is overdetermined this is not likely to be the case. The equations are first converted to the so-called normal equations:

$$A^T AX = A^T B \text{ with their solution } X = \left(A^T A\right)^{-1} A^T B \tag{3}$$

This is not a solution that is numerically ideal. A better solution is given by the Singular Value Decomposition (SVD), a powerful computational tool for solving LS problems (Golub and Van Loan (1989)). This decomposition is defined as:

Definition: Singular Value Decomposition:
Every matrix $A \in \Re^{m \times n}$ can be factorized as

$$A = U\Sigma V^T \qquad (4)$$

Where $U \in \Re^{m \times m}$ and $V \in \Re^{n \times n}$ are orthonormal matrices and Σ is a real $m \times n$ matrix containing $\Sigma_r = diag(\sigma_i)$. The $\sigma_i \in \Re_0^+$, with $\sigma_1 \geq \sigma_2 \geq ... \geq \sigma_r \geq 0 \;\; \forall i$ are called the singular values of A. The corresponding columns of U and V are called the left and right singular vectors.

Application of this SVD factorization for A yields another solution that is numerically more stable:

$$A = U\Sigma V^T = \begin{bmatrix} U_1 & U_2 \end{bmatrix} \begin{pmatrix} S & 0 \\ 0 & 0 \end{pmatrix} \begin{bmatrix} V_1^T \\ V_2^T \end{bmatrix} = U_1 S V_1^T \qquad (5)$$

with $S \in \Re^{r \times r}$, $r = rank(A)$ and U and V partitioned accordingly. Insertion into the normal equation (3) results in the expression

$$\left(V_1 S^T S V_1^T\right) X = V_1 S U_1^T B \qquad (6)$$

so that a general solution can be written as

$$X = V_1 S^{-1} U_1^T B \qquad (7)$$

Decoupling of the Parts of the Transformation Matrix

The solution methods seen will yield a solution for the transformation matrix but the rotational part of this matrix will not necessarily be orthogonal, meaning that the transformation might induce deformations into the prosthesis model. This is an undesirable effect and can be avoided by separately determining the translation and rotation, and solving for the rotational part by an extension of the LS method. Differences in scaling will normally not occur since the CT scanner will mention the zoom factor used in the images, so that an eventual different zoom factor can be corrected in a preprocessing step.

The first step will be to determine the centers of inertia for both coordinate sets and to translate each set so that its center of inertia coincides with the origin:
For the m markers of each set:

$$\text{If } A = [a_1, ..., a_n]: \;\; \mu_A = \frac{1}{n} \sum_{i=1}^{n} a_i \text{ and } \forall a_i \in A: a_i = a_i - \mu_A \qquad (8)$$

Once both sets are centered around the origin, the orthogonal rotation matrix that rotates one set into the other has to be found. This is called an Orthogonal Procrustes problem (Golub and Van Loan (1989)), and is a special case of the LS problem above, with an additional constraint:

Definition: Orthogonal Procrustes Problem
Given a data matrix $A \in \Re^{m \times n}$ and an observation matrix $B \in \Re^{m \times d}$, find a matrix $X \in \Re^{n \times d}$ that

$$\text{minimizes } \|B - AX\|_F \text{ subject to } X^T X = I_d \qquad (9)$$

The solution to this problem can be derived by noting that if X is orthogonal, then

$$\|B - AX\|_F^2 = trace(B^T B) + trace(A^T A) - 2 trace(X^T A^T B), \qquad (10)$$

so that minimizing (10) is equivalent to maximizing $trace(X^T A^T B)$. The X that maximizes this expression can be found through the SVD factorization of $A^T B$:

$$U^T (A^T B) V = \Sigma = diag(\sigma_1, \ldots, \sigma_p) \qquad (11)$$

Define $Z = V^T X^T U$ so that

$$trace(X^T A^T B) = trace(X^T U \Sigma V^T) = trace(Z\Sigma) = \sum_{i=1}^{d} z_{ci} \sigma_i \leq \sum_{i=1}^{d} \sigma_i \qquad (12)$$

The upper bound of this expression is attained by setting $X = UV^T$, for then $Z = I_d$. So the orthogonal rotation that turns one set into the other will be given by

$$X = UV^T \qquad (13)$$

Error Analysis

Error Sources

The whole procedure involves several steps, ranging from acquisition to registration, and each of these may introduce some errors in the data:
- *Acquisition errors*:
1. Distortions in CT images.
2. Patient movement artifacts.
3. Loosening of the fiducials.
- *Registration errors*
1. Badly conditioned problem, due to coplanarity of markers.
2. Distorting transformation matrix.
3. Numerical errors.
- *Errors in fiducial coordinate determination*
1. Markers are indicated off-center (Not zoomed in during indication).
2. Indication of markers on axial plane with corresponding rounding to a multiple of the interslice distance.

3. Erroneous correspondency between fiducial sets (wrong order).
4. Wrong coordinates for one or more fiducials, often due to streak artifacts obscuring the markers.

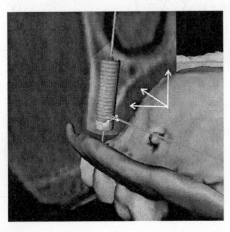
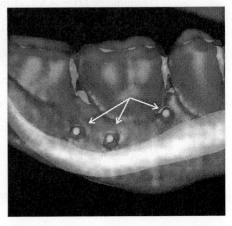

Fig. 5. A small error in the registration would show in the gap between the palate and the prosthesis (arrows).

Fig. 6. After transformation, the prosthesis fiducials nicely surround the points that represent the patient fiducials (arrows).

Checks on the accuracy

It is very important to ensure that no insidious errors are overlooked. Several precautions can be taken to warn about some of the error sources mentioned above:

1. Visual check of surface models: Prosthesis must fit to the bone and to the soft tissue visible on the grey value slices. Prosthesis fiducials must surround points indicated on patient scan.
2. Visual check of point sets on fiducials: Overlay of point sets is more sensitive to errors.
3. Distances between consecutive points within the same set should be the same when compared between both sets.
4. The determinant of the resulting rotation matrix should be 1 and not −1 (equivalent to mirroring the model).
5. The condition number of a matrix can be defined in terms of its SVD and is then given as $\kappa(A) = \sigma_1 / \sigma_n$. A large $\kappa(A)$ means that a small error on the measurements will be amplified in the solution of the LS problem. This is an indicator that more points must be collected to improve the condition.

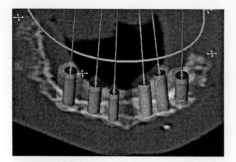 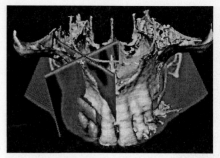

Fig. 7. Combination of 2D grey value slices, CAD models of implants and the curve guiding the reslices.

Fig. 8. 2D and 3D information together, adding soft tissue information to the surface models.

Results and Discussion

The Planning System

In our center we use a generic library suitable for planning many different types of surgery, that is specifically instantiated and extended for implant surgery (Verstreken et al. (1996)). This package allows all standard visualization methods available on the scanner console, and adds multiplanar reslicing, eventually along a curviform path. 3D CAD models of implants can be added to the scenery and manipulated within it (Fig 7). Two-dimensional (2D) grey value information and the implant models are shown together with three-dimensional (3D) surface rendered models (Fig 8).

Benefits of the Prosthesis Model for the Planning

The advantages are manyfold. The superstructure is now included in the planning stage, and the surgeon can adjust his plan to facilitate the work of the prosthodontist, where the bone allows it. A number of problems may otherwise occur, making a prosthesis difficult to design or more expensive to make. Axes may come out of the gums at the labial side of the teeth (Fig 9-10), which may be very difficult to hide. For the same reason, interdental implant axes are to be avoided, especially in the frontal area.

Other construction problems can be caused by axes that are too palatal, since they come in a prosthesis part that is too thin to provide support for the abutment (Fig 11-14). It is nearly impossible to predict such complications from the normal 2D planning, or even from the 3D bone surface model.

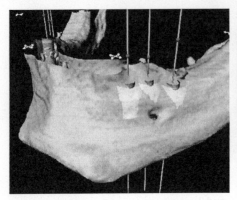

Fig. 9. This seems a good configuration for bone and implants.

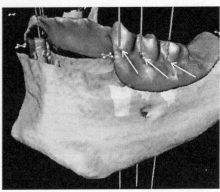

Fig. 10. But her it is seen that the axes are at the outside of the teeth (arrows).

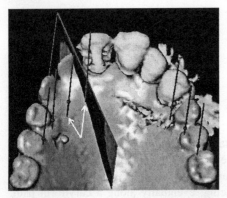

Fig. 11. These axes (arrows) are too palatal. The prosthesis is too thin in this area.

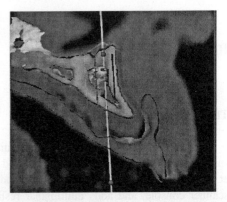

Fig. 12. The 2D slice shows how the prosthesis extends in front of the bone.

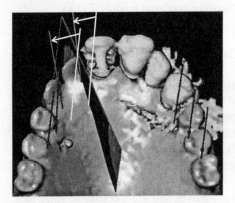

Fig. 13. The axes from (Fig 13) are shown by the lines. Adjustments to the orientation were made on this view.

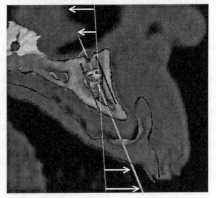

Fig. 14. Further corrections were needed here to keep the implant within the bone.

In many larger centers there is a preoperative consultation where both the prosthodontist and the oral surgeon are present. The images from the bone with the matched prosthesis include elements from both subfields and may be an ideal discussion and demonstration tool. A deliberation considering the relative importance of all design factors: Bone, biomechanics and superstructure is now greatly facilitated.

Conclusion

The double scanning procedure that is proposed is a technique that yields impressive benefits at a very low cost. There is no additional radiation dosage for the patient and no expensive radioopaque temporary prosthesis has to be made. Streak artifacts pose no problems and inaccuracies are immediately visible. The algorithm for the registration is straightforward while the planning advantages are clear. In our opinion this is a technique worth incorporating into routine dental scanning procedures, whereever 3D visualization technology is available.

References

Gauss CF (1823) Theoria Combinationis Observationum Erroribus Minimis Obnoxiae. Comment. Soc. Reg. Sci. Gotten. Recent., 5, 33-90.

Golub GH and Van Loan CF (1989) Matrix Computations. John Hopkins University Press, Baltimore, MD.

Jacobs R and van Steenberghe D (1998) Radiographic Planning and Assessment of Endosseous Oral Implants. Springer-Verlag, Berlin Heidelberg, 31-44.

Lorensen WE and Cline HE (1987) Marching cubes: A high resolution surface construction algorithm. Comput. Graphics **21**(4), 163-169.

Neider J, Davis T and Woo M (1993) OpenGL Programming Guide. The Official Guide to Learning OpenGL. Addison-Wesley, California.

Schroeder W, Martin K and Lorensen B (1996) The Visualisation Toolkit: An Object Oriented Approach to 3D Graphics. Prentice-Hall, New Jersey.

Udupa JK and Gon÷alves RJ (1996) Imaging transforms for volume visualization. In: Computer-Integrated Surgery, Taylor RH, Lavallée S, Burdea GC and M¬sges R (eds), The MIT Press, Cambridge, Massachusetts, 33-57.

Verstreken K, Van Cleynenbreugel J, Marchal G, Naert I, Suetens P, van Steenberghe D (1996) Computer-assisted planning of oral implant surgery: A three-dimensional approach. Int J Oral Maxillofac Implants, **11**, 806-810.

Interactive Pre-operative Selection of Cutting Constraints, and Interactive Force Controlled Knee Surgery by a Surgical Robot

S.J.Harris*, M. Jakopec*, R.D.Hibberd*, J.Cobb†, B.L. Davies*

* Mechatronics in Medicine Laboratory,
Department of Mechanical Engineering
Imperial College of Science, Technology and Medicine,
Exhibition Road, London SW7 2BX, England

† Department of Orthopædic Surgery,
The Middlesex Hospital,
Mortimer Street, London W1N 8AA, England

email: s.j.harris@ic.ac.uk

Abstract. This paper describes a low-cost computer system that takes CT images of the knee, and with three-dimensional models of knee prostheses allows a surgeon to position the prosthesis correctly pre-operatively in an interactive manner. Once in position the computer can process bone and prosthesis geometry to derive a set of constraint boundaries that constitute a safe cutting area for a force controlled robot (i.e. that avoids soft tissue such as ligaments), and provides the correct cutting planes for good prosthesis/bone alignment. This boundary information is used to program the robot, allowing a surgeon to move the robot within predefined regions to machine away bone accurately whilst preventing damage to soft tissue.

Keywords: robotics, orthopædics, force control, imaging

1. Introduction

Total knee replacement is a common surgical procedure used particularly with the elderly to replace worn and painful arthritic joints. To achieve good, pain-free mobility with a reliable joint, a degree of precision is necessary both with regard to the positioning of the prosthesis components relative to the bone axes and to each other, and with regard to the mating surfaces of the bone and prosthesis. The prosthesis components are complex shapes. To achieve the correct cuts in the bone, a series of jigs and fixtures are applied sequentially which ideally should produce a set of accurate cuts. However, the sequential nature of the application can result in small errors becoming compounded, as the reference frames are changed, compromising the requirement for accuracy.

To reduce the cumulative errors, a robotic aid is being developed which measures its position for each cut from a single reference frame. This removes the need for a series of jigs and fixtures as the surfaces of the bone for cutting are held within a computer's memory. Emphasis should be placed on the fact that the robot is an aid to the surgeon rather than a replacement. Automated surgical procedures have been tried by this group [1][2] and others [3], however, it has been found after discussions with surgeons that there has been some resistance to them, due to the lack of continuous control and tactile sensation by the surgeon during the operation. The robotic aid under development can be used by the surgeon to locate a bone-cutting rotary milling-bit in the correct position for each cut and prevent it from being moved into dangerous regions and from removing too much bone. The surgeon has a 'hands-on' approach, enabling him to feel the quality of the bone being cut, and adjust his cutting forces and speed appropriately. Thus, the surgeon uses his skills and senses to the full, while the robot provides the geometrical accuracy required for a good fit and the physical constraints to avoid soft tissue damage.

2. Image Acquisition

Before the bones can be cut to fit the prosthesis, images of the joint and surrounding area are necessary to allow the surgeon to position the prosthesis optimally on the bone. For manual surgery assessing the optimal component sizes is done with templates positioned on x-ray images of the joint while the optimal position is found per-operatively.

For the robotic system it was decided that CT images of the leg would be used. These have a number of advantages over normal x-rays, particularly of use in a robotic system: (1) there is no variable, depth related image magnification, thus accurate measurements can be made; (2) full three dimensional data is available, so x-ray images and bone cuts can be simulated from any angle and three dimensional reconstructions made; (3) the positions of fiducial markers can be found in three dimensions allowing registration of the CT data and physical bone.

Because of the accuracy required for positioning the prosthesis, CT images are needed with a fine slice spacing (1 mm or better). The use of CT images gives the surgeon the ability to perform all prosthesis sizing and positioning pre-operatively, reducing the amount of time required during surgery and allowing him to plan the optimal cutting sequence. The imaging, modelling and planning phases have been implemented on a low-cost PC which is robust enough for clinical use, but nevertheless is adequate for the modelling, planning and implementation procedures.

3. CT pre-processing

Before the images can be used, they must be processed to distinguish between soft tissue, femur, tibia and fiducial markers. To distinguish between bone and soft tissue, a bone threshold level is set. A flood fill procedure is then run on each image, starting from outside of any bone, set to replace any pixels with black up to a border of intensity greater than the threshold. This preserves the medullary canal within the bone. Often this has an intensity level similar to that of soft tissue and would hence be removed by normal thresholding methods. This procedure preserves it because the surrounding high intensity bone image provides a border that prevents the flood-fill from reaching it. Once soft tissue has been removed, the bone is thresholded to black and white. This is processed interactively to distinguish between femur, tibia and other leg bones. Starting from the top of the leg, the bone image is taken and each individual area of bone is coloured separately. The surgeon can then re-colour the areas in one of four colours depending on bone type (figure 1). He also has basic painting and deleting tools to remove artefacts, separate touching bones, and replace bone in the image that was below the threshold level (this can happen if the x-ray beam just skims the surface of bone). Having completed the first slice, the next is presented. However, on this one the computer checks each bone area in the image, comparing it with the image above. Regions in the current slice that contact regions that the surgeon has marked in the previous slice are coloured to match those already marked. Because of the need for small slice spacing, and hence many images, this semi-automatic process speeds up the bone identification procedure, as the surgeon only needs to take action when the bone types change, or when the image requires correction for artefacts.

To give the surgeon more complete landmark information, as each bone image is displayed, the unprocessed CT slice is shown alongside, allowing him to determine whether the computer has mistakenly joined two bones or deleted bone material.

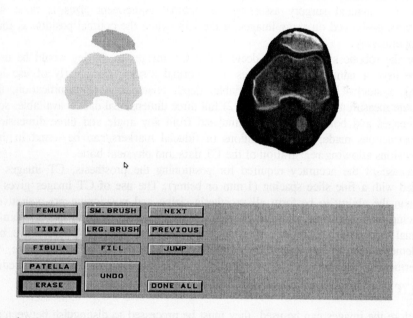

Figure 1 - Annotation of CT images to discriminate between bone. Note the simplified image (left) and the original CT (right) to provide the surgeon with landmark features

4. Detection of fiducial markers

For initial trials, it is intended that metal screws are used as fiducial markers. These indicate reference points that can be used to align the coordinate frames of the robot with the CT images. Trials with different screw types have revealed that stainless steel screws have a much greater intensity than bone, and hence should be easy to find. However, they are too bright, and can cause the following problems with the image: *blooming* - the region around the screw becomes very bright, resulting in an uncertainty in the screw position; *image distortion* - bone intensities in the image near the screw are elevated, so bone/soft tissue discrimination may give errors in such regions; *image interference* - reflections off the screws results in patterns of dark and bright banding across the image that can make image processing difficult. These problems can be seen in figure 2. Note that the CT image has been inverted to show bone in darker intensities as this appears more clearly in printed images.

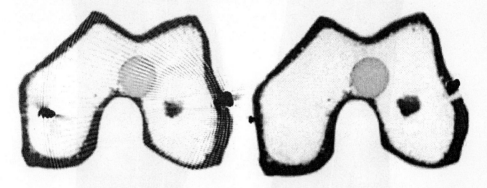

Figure 2 - Comparison of the effects of steel (left) and titanium (right) fiducial pins on the image quality. Note the blooming of steel pins and the pattern superimposed over the image.

As an alternative, titanium screws have been tried. These have an intensity in the CT image not much greater than bone (although still distinguishable by thresholding) and do not cause so much distortion or interference. Because of the small intensity difference, artefacts such as noise in the image can cause false detection of pixels above the screw detection threshold. To discriminate between this noise and real screws, pixels above the threshold are checked with the images above and below in the CT record. If either of these images also contains pixels at the same coordinates which are above the screw threshold, then the pixels under test are assumed to be screws. As the CT scan is processed, a record is made of the coordinate of every remaining pixel found to be above the screw threshold.

Clusters are created by grouping pixels that are close together. Each cluster is then processed in turn to compute its position and major axis. The outermost end point of the cluster along the major axis is chosen as the contact point for mechanical registration of the robot during surgery. Very small clusters are ignored as they are assumed to be noise or artefacts.

5. Initial positioning of the prosthesis

After pre-processing the CT to determine bone types and fiducial marker positions, the surgeon provides an initial estimate of the prosthesis position. For normal posture, there should be approximately 5 to 8° valgus angle between the long axes of the tibia and femur, while for the prostheses used there should be a varus tilt of approximately 0 to 2°, and a posterior slope of 5° [4]. For initial positioning of the prosthesis, the surgeon can mark on X-ray images computed from the CTs where the long bone axes are and specify the appropriate angles using a simple graphical interface. An example of long bone axis selection can be seen in figure 3.

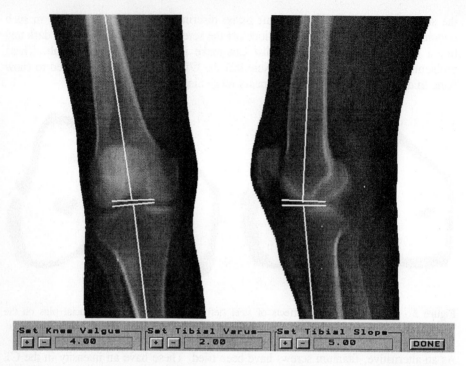

Figure 3 - Interactive alignment of prosthesis with long bone axes. Axes are selected by dragging marker lines on the simulated X-rays. Angles are selected using the control panel

Having obtained an initial estimate of the prosthesis position the surgeon can fine tune it by moving the prosthesis parts on the CT images, and selecting appropriately sized components to find a good match with the bone geometry. During this procedure the bone can be viewed either as X-ray images (as shown in figure 4) or CT slices to give an overall view or fine detail at particular depths, and in any of three orientations (slice by slice, medial-lateral or anterior-posterior). The prosthesis can be viewed as a wire-frame or as a solid model (figure 4). This process mimics quite closely the procedure currently used by surgeons manually to size the prosthesis components, presenting them with a task with which they are already familiar. It does, however, allow them to assess the prosthesis size and position from views that would otherwise be impossible (e.g. the CT slice views allow the tibial component to be matched to the shape and orientation of the tibial plateau). In addition the interference between the prosthesis and the bone in individual CT slices can be shown. This allows the surgeon to detect whether, for example, the top of the femoral component is notching the femur, and creating a weak point in the bone. To visualise the completed procedure, the surgeon can view a three-dimensional rendering of the bone with the appropriate cuts made and the prosthesis in position.

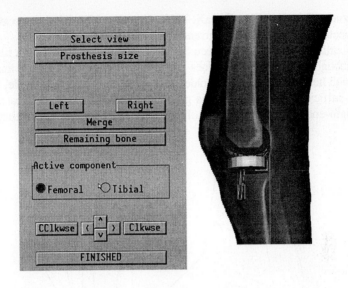

Figure 4 shows a simulated X-ray with a model of the prosthesis components superimposed

6. Computing the cutting boundary

When cutting leg bones to accept a prosthesis, it is usual to cut to the edge of the bone rather than to the edge of the prosthesis. Since prostheses come in a limited number of sizes, this prevents the generation of a brittle bony lip around the prosthesis that could both interfere with prosthesis component mating and be susceptible to breaking and damaging nearby tissue. Once the prosthesis position has been finalised, it is therefore necessary to compute the cutting planes required to generate the five surfaces on the femur and the one surface on the tibia, and to find the outline of bone required to be cut on these surfaces.

The current requirement (neglecting fixation and stabilisation shafts and vanes) for each mating surface is that they are flat planes. Therefore, each surface has a coordinate (its centre point) and a pair of unit vectors associated with it (figure 5 shows a typical component). These unit vectors describe the direction taken in the space of the CT image to move one unit on a cutting plane in the X and Y direction, assuming the plane is being viewed along its perpendicular. The cutting boundary will then be defined by points in this plane and the orientation and position of the plane. Initially the centre point and unit vectors are set up with the prosthesis not rotated and referenced to the CT origin. They are subjected to the same transformations as the prosthesis components as they are moved into position on the CT. To generate the cutting outline a two-dimensional image array is set up and voxels in the CT bone data record mapped onto the plane using the centre point and unit vectors. If the centre point for a plane is (C_x, C_y, C_z) and the two unit vectors are (X_x, X_y, X_z) and (Y_y, Y_y, Y_z), then a point (a,b) on the cutting plane is taken from the CT bone data record at point $(C_x+aX_x+bY_y, C_y+aX_y+bY_y, C_z+aX_z+bY_z)$. Any bone other than the one expected to be cut for the current plane is ignored.

Once the cutting plane image has been created a Roberts edge extraction filter is run over it. Although the Roberts filter does not fare well with low contrast images, the ones dealt with here are already thresholded to a high contrast so this simple, fast edge extractor is sufficient for the task. This gives an outline for the bone area to be cut, which is chain-encoded to follow its outline and produce an ordered cutting region.

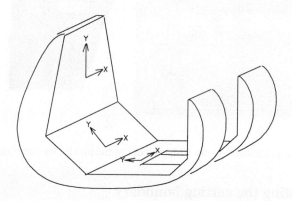

Figure 5- Directions of unit vectors for three of the cutting planes required for a typical femoral component, relative to the component itself. These vectors are rotated to match the rotation of the prosthesis as it is moved into position

An additional task performed is to run through the mapping of CT data onto the cutting plane, but this time to scan outwards along the perpendicular to the cutting plane until the CT data registers that the edge of the bone has been reached. A count of the number of voxels passed through from the cutting plane to the bone edge is recorded for each pixel in the cutting plane. This procedure generates a height map, indicating the shape of the region of bone that will be removed.

These processes are repeated for each of the six cutting planes and the resulting data stored before it is passed onto the robot.

7. The Acrobot active constraint robot

The robot aid is a four axis system (vertical motion, in-out motion, yaw and pitch) as shown in the photograph of figure 6 with a rotating milling bit as the end-effector. The mechanical and electrical arrangement has been described in detail elsewhere [5][6]. Backdriveable gearboxes on the motors enable it to be moved around by hand as well as under computer control, or using servo assist as some mixture of the two. A 6-axis force sensor with joystick type handle allows the robot to sense the surgeon's movement forces and move accordingly. This provides the robot with the surgeon's force requests in all three dimensions, and torque measurements around three axes.

Under normal operation the robot is controlled by the surgeon, who can direct its movements using the joystick handle, but is constrained to resist movements outside of a safe region, as defined by the pre-operative processing described above. This is achieved using a variable force control strategy. It should be emphasised that the low and equal impedance which gives sensitivity of force control, together with good stiffness when required is a compromise which is quite different from the requirements for, say, registering the tip of a conventional industrial robot under force control.

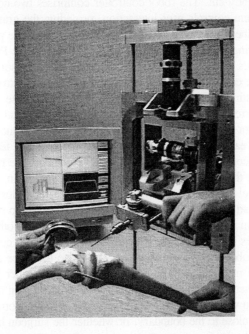

Figure 6 - Photograph of the Acrobot knee surgery robot in bench trials showing the robot (right) and a typical interactive display (left)

For yaw and pitch motions, the gear ratios were chosen to give approximately equal backdriveable force, so the surgeon has no sensation of being 'guided' in a specific direction unless at a boundary. The in-out axis requires a greater backdriving force, but preferential motions in other axes are compensated for by servo assistance on this axis. The vertical motion axis is not driven under surgeon control. The position on this axis is selected by the computer to allow optimum access to each cutting surface.

Movement of the cutting robot is limited to a small operating environment. Thus to position and align it correctly with respect to the knee, a passive positioning system is used. This carries the robot and allows it to be moved under manual control in three linear axes until the surgeon is satisfied that the cutter is correctly placed to obtain the desired cutting planes. A fourth axis allows the robot to be rotated by $\pm 45°$ with respect to the vertical (orientation shown in figure 6). This allows it easy access to all bone surfaces. The milling cutter and control strategy allow the robot to mill away bone with the cutter perpendicular, at an angle, or parallel to the required cutting plane. The latter method is fastest and is used preferentially where the geometry of the cuts and bone access allows.

8. Control of the robot

As with the pre-operative processing functions, the real-time robot control system uses graphics interactively with the surgeon, allowing him to select cutting planes using a simple set of on-screen control buttons and graphics. These provide views of the position of the robot's cutter in relation to the plane currently being cut, and the depth of bone currently cut. The robot controller comprises two computer systems. A PC compatible system controls user interaction, providing the graphical interface and storage for the outline database as generated by the pre-operative process, and overall control and monitoring. A DSP controlled system, hosted by the PC, provides control of the robot's motors and signal processing from the force sensor system.

The robot is force controlled on the yaw, pitch and in-out control motors (as shown in figure 6) by adjusting the torque of the motors depending on the force applied by the surgeon, and the current position of the robot in relation to the cutting boundaries. The vertical motion motor is under position control, and is used to move the cutter to the optimum height for each cutting plane. To allow the surgeon to feel how close to the boundary he is, the control strategy varies the admittance (i.e. the relationship between the force applied by the surgeon and the torque of the motors) in varying regions, by providing a two level control system. At the lower level is a closed-loop PD system whose gains can be adjusted to control stiffness. This control loop includes friction and gravity compensation to remove preferential motion that would otherwise result from gravity or differences in friction in each motor linkage. An outer control loop monitors the position of the robot relative to boundaries, and also the force and direction of the surgeon's requested movements. The controller adjusts the inner loop parameters to allow a strategy of servo assistance or neutral control, increasing stiffness or position control depending on whether the robot is in a safe region far from boundary regions, getting increasingly close to the boundary, or whether the surgeon has forced the robot over the boundary. In the first case, the surgeon is free to move anywhere within this region without constraint, and servo assist is used to balance the admittances on the various movement axes. In the second case, as the surgeon moves towards the boundary, the stiffness is increased, making it difficult to cross into a dangerous region, and providing force feedback to the surgeon that he is nearing the boundary. In the last case if the surgeon has overstepped the boundary (a situation that can't be completely eliminated as this would otherwise require very large, powerful motors) the robot provides position control normal to the constraint boundary to bring the cutter back to a safe region, while giving low resistance force control tangential to the boundary. Thus it is possible to move around the constraint boundary while the computer resists movement outside it.

Because of the nature of the prosthesis used, the control regime is set up to allow each plane to be cut in sequence. This simplifies the control task since each constraint region can be reduced to a two-dimensional boundary of coordinates from the pre-operative planning system and a flat plane. These two cutting constraints can be controlled individually and result in a prismatic (or 'tunnel-like') constraint, terminated in a flat plane. Considering the plane part of the regime, the stiffness is adjusted in the direction of the normal to the plane. This increases as the distance to the plane decreases if the cutter is pushed towards the plane. For the prismatic boundary, the nearest point on the constraint curve is found (i.e. when projected onto the cutting plane, how close would the cutter be to the edge of the safe region). The stiffness of the robot is then adjusted independently in normal and tangential directions to the boundary curve at this nearest point. These stiffnesses, each of which are computed along three orthogonal axes (normal to the appropriate constraint surface and in two directions along the surface), from the two control calculations are then combined before being passed to the inner loop.

9. Positional accuracy of the robot and control algorithm

Preliminary tests have been performed to acquire information about the robot's accuracy and repeatability in terms of positioning, and its ability to cut flat planes.

To test positional accuracy, the milling tip was replaced by a 4mm diameter ball-ended probe. This probe was then placed in 30 holes of 3mm diameter in known positions in a perspex panel. Being ball ended, the probe tip is automatically centred on the hole. This process was repeated 10 times for each hole. From this test it was found that each hole could be found to within 0.13mm of its expected position on average, while the repeatability was measured to be 0.16mm (1 standard deviation).

Tests were made of the robot's accuracy when cutting flat planes in three modes - with the cutter axis perpendicular to the plane, with the cutter axis at 45° to the plane, and with the axis parallel to the plane. During the cutting process, position data from the robot was obtained and the positions of the deepest cuts, along the length of the milling cutter, were logged on a 0.1mm resolution grid covering the cutting plane. It was found that the cutter could be used to cut with little deviation from the cutting plane. For each of the cutting regimes, results were as follows:

Cutting method	Average distance of cut from plane	Max distance of cut from plane	Standard deviation
Perpendicular	-0.19mm	-0.35mm	0.039mm
Parallel	-0.15mm	-0.38mm	0.065mm
45° to plane	-0.15mm	-0.28mm	0.034mm

Negative values indicate depths past the required cutting plane. These results show that cuts are on average less than 0.2mm deeper than required. Although deeper than the required cutting plane, they are still well within the tolerances demanded by surgeons. The small standard deviations indicate that there is very little 'waviness' over the surface of the plane.

10. Conclusions

The pre-operative system provides a user-friendly method of setting up the information required by the robot for its cutting outline. Where ever possible, the procedures performed on screen have been designed to mimic those that the surgeon would normally do manually with x-ray images. The use of CT instead of x-ray images enables the surgeon to do pre-operatively many of the functions that were previously done during surgery (e.g. final decisions as to the prosthesis size).

The accuracy of the robot is well within the required accuracy required by surgeons (who have indicated that a 1mm error is acceptable overall). It should be emphasised however that this is only one link in the chain. For accurate imaging and modelling CT image sets are required with sub-millimetre slice spacings, which generates large amounts of data, and exposes the patient to increased radiation (although this accuracy is only needed in the immediate vicinity of the knee). The control strategies have been found to enable planes to be cut with a good degree of flatness.

Initial tests indicate that the robot can match the shape of the prosthesis allowing a good match between prosthesis component and bone. Further tests are required to determine the accuracy of the complete system, in addition to that of the robot.

The approach of co-operation between surgeon and machine enables both the accuracy of the robot and the senses and intelligence of the surgeon to be used together for maximum effect, and provides a more acceptable solution than that of an autonomous system.

11. Acknowledgements

We would like to acknowledge the financial assistance of the UK Department of Health and the 'LINK' Medical Implants Fund in support of this project.

12. References

1. Harris, S.J. *et al.*: Transurethral Resection of the Prostate: The evolution of a robotic system to meet users' needs, Proceedings of the First International Symposium on Andrology Bioengineering and Sexual Rehabilitation (1995), 73-80

2. Davies, B.L.: Safety of Medical Robots, Safety Critical Systems, Chapman Hall Press, Part 4, chapter 15 (1993) 193-201

3. Taylor, R.H, *et al*: An Image-Directed Robotic System for Precise Orthopaedic Surgery, Computer Integrated Surgery, Chapter 28, The MIT Press (1996) 379-396

4. Howmedica: Kinemax modular total knee system - Instrument Surgical Technique (1995)

5. Harris, S.J., *et al.*: Experiences with Robotic Systems for Knee Surgery, Proceedings of CVRMed-MRCAS'97, Springer-Verlag (1997) 756-766

6. Davies, B.L. *et al.*: Active compliance in robotic surgery - the use of force control as a dynamic constraint, Proceedings of the Institution of Mechanical Engineers, Part H (1997) 285-292

Multimodal Volume-Based Tumor Neurosurgery Planning in the Virtual Workbench

Luis Serra[1], Ralf A. Kockro[1,2], Chua Gim Guan[1], Ng Hern[1]
Eugene C.K. Lee[1], Yen H. Lee[1], Chumpon Chan[2] and Wieslaw L. Nowinski[1]

[1]Kent Ridge Digital Labs (formerly, the Institute of Systems Science, ISS),
21 Heng Mui Keng Terrace, Singapore 119613
{luis, ralf, ggchua, nghern, cklee, yhlee, wieslaw}@krdl.org.sg
[2]Dept. of Neurosurgery, Singapore General Hospital, Singapore

Abstract. We present a multimodal volume-based pre-operative surgical planning system developed around the KRDL Virtual Workbench, a mirror-based Virtual Reality system for precise work with 3D data. The planning system is being developed in collaboration with the Singapore General Hospital (SGH), and is undergoing clinical evaluation at SGH and Tan Tock Seng Hospital where 16 cases have been planned. We give a systems perspective on the user interface, introduce the multimodal aspects of the volume rendering technique, and describe the stages involved in creating the final multimodal image for planning with a clinical case: registration, segmentation of tumors, bone removal, path planning and measurements.

Keywords. Virtual Reality, neurosurgery planning, multimodal volume rendering

1 Goal: Patient-Specific Tumour Neurosurgery Planning

Effective planning of neurosurgery requires interaction with a complete and accurate picture of the patient's 3D pathology and surrounding anatomy. This involves two kinds of technologies: one for presenting the anatomy in many different, combined ways and seeing it from many viewpoints, and another for interacting with it. Multimodal volumetric rendering in real-time is thus our visualization of choice. Volume rendering works directly from the available scan images, and delivers a good degree of fidelity to the original images (unlike surface rendering). This is essential to show the interrelations of the different tissues for a same patient. Real-time rendering is obviously desirable to allow quick exploration of the volume, inviting the surgeon to explore viewpoints.

It is also important in planning to be able to perform operations that are 3D in nature, such as segmenting the tumor, measuring distances, areas and volumes, specifying cross-sections at non-orthogonal angles and planning of the path of approach. This combination of accuracy (in reporting detail from the original) and the need for a way to interact in three dimensions demands a system that can integrate volumetric rendering and 3D interaction.

We have been applying a Virtual Reality (VR) interface to the field of neurosurgery in collaboration with the department of neurosurgery Singapore General Hospital. The interface is called The KRDL Virtual Workbench [7][11], a mirror-based system: the user sits comfortably wearing stereoscopic glasses and enjoys precise hand-eye coordination by 'reaching in' into a 3D virtual image behind the mirror, with both hands. In this paper, we describe VIVIAN (Virtual Intracranial Visualization and Navigation), a tumor (frameless) neurosurgery patient-specific planning system built around the Virtual Workbench. Our approach to planning is more efficient, faster and natural than conventional methods clinically available.

2 Background

Neurosurgery is inherently a 3D activity, where surgical instruments have to be reliably guided to targets with millimetric accuracy. Although computer generated 3D views are common in clinical planning, precise 3D interaction with them is still rare. This is because the manipulative capabilities of common input devices such as the 2D mouse and keyboards do not match the volumetric manipulation. Moreover, the possibilities of 3D interaction go beyond what is practical using the mouse.

Great progress has been made in planning neurosurgery (see for example [6]). There are several commercially available packages that support neurosurgical patient-specific planning (pre- and intra-operative) using 3D views: e.g, Elekta's *SurgiPlan*, Radionics' *Stereoplan*, BrainLAB's *BrainMAP 3D*, Philips' *EasyVision CT/MR* and *VolumeView CT/MR*, Leibinger's *STP* [12]. All these systems display 3D views of the preoperative data co-registered with the patient and stereotactic equipment. However, user interaction with the planning software is achieved with a conventional mouse-screen setup. Three-dimensional interaction with the preoperative data takes place during surgery, where the software guides the neurosurgeon, who holds a 3D pointer (tracked by video cameras, infrared, or other methods) that is displayed registered with the preoperative data. These interaction, although 3D, is usually limited due to the constrains of surgery to pointing at structures of interest (with the pointer or with the focus of the microscope) and little manipulation of the data and models is available to the neurosurgeon.

Interaction in 3D is not only more natural but provides a wider spectrum of operations. Three dimensional interfaces have been proposed for the planning: for example, Goble et al. 1995 [4] describe a 3D interface for image exploration, using hand-held props. The props approach is intuitive but the 3D interactions rely entirely on relative visual parallax and other non-stereoscopic depth cues, which tends to be inefficient due to unnecessary to and fro movement when approaching an object. Systems like Boston Dynamics [1] or SRI International [5], although using a similar setup to ours (with the addition of force feedback), concentrate in training dexterity skills and not patient-specific planning.

In the Brain Bench [8] we used the Virtual Workbench to integrate an electronic atlas of brain structure with a virtual stereotactic frame in a system which allowed faster specification of target points, improved avoidance of sensitive structures and speedier, more effective training. The Brain Bench had limited visualization capabilities (only triplanar support) and concentrated on planning the path of the virtual probe of the stereotactic frame relative to the brain atlas structures.

3 VIVIAN - An Overview

VIVIAN combines a VR user interface with a volume rendering graphics engine to provide an environment for neurosurgical planning (see [3] for a short description). In VIVIAN, one of the user's hands controls the patient's volume data, turning and placing it as one would do with an object held in real space. The tool in the other hand appears as an 'stylus' or virtual tool, and performs detailed manipulation, using 3D widgets (interaction gadgets) to interact with the surgical planning tools (refer to Fig. 1 during this discussion). In all interactions, the approach is 'reach in for the object of interest and press the switch on the stylus to interact with it'. When the tip of the virtual tool enters the volume of influence around an object, the object signals that it is reactive by a colour change or other highlighting. When the tool enters a widget's volume of influence, the tool becomes the manipulator associated with that widget, and knows how to interact with it.

A 'toolrack' menu at the bottom switches between stylus modes. The buttons display their function, which may then be enabled by clicking. A slider scales the whole head ensemble, allowing detailed or overall inspection and manipulation.

Since VIVIAN deals with a variable number of objects of different and overlapping sizes (volumetric as well as polygonal), efficient selection of the working object with the stylus is important. A pop-up menu appears when clicking is done outside all objects, and remains visible while the digital switch is pressed. While the pop-up menu is up, the user can directly select an object. The list of available objects is overlaid on the display at the top-left corner. This provides feedback on the status of the objects: visible or hidden, 'selected' (indicated by a small arrow on the left), object closest to the tip of stylus (indicated by a highlight of the name) and order of alignment for registration. When objects occupy the same space (a common occurrence) highest priority is given to the object which is currently selected, followed by the position in the object list.

3.1. Volume Rendering with 3D Textures

We achieve real-time volume rendering by means of 3D textures [2]. This approach achieves real-time performance by relying on the Silicon Graphics hardware-accelerated 3D texture mapping. Briefly, the algorithm takes a volume and generates sample planes orthogonal to the viewing direction, in back to front order, mapping a texture to each sample plane and blending it with the rest. The texture is obtained from the intersection between the sample plane and the volume, by trilinear interpolation. Our implementation enables free movement of the volume in 3D space and speeds up the display by having a number of sample planes that decreases with the distance to the viewpoint [9].

Multimodal support is necessary to simultaneously display complementary images in the same virtual space. Volume rendering with 3D textures has an inherent problem with this, since the shape of the volume is not accounted for in the depth buffer, which receives only polygons (the sampled planes). When a second set of sampled planes is rendered over another, the depth buffer disables the write over the first volume's planes, which results in an incorrect image (see Fig. 2a: MRI and MRA extents overlap, but since MRA is rendered first, MRI is excluded within the MRA's extent). Even if the depth buffer is disabled, the composition would still be incorrect, since the blending function used to composite the image is order dependent (back to front).

To avoid this depth buffer problem, the traditional solution is to interleave the sample planes of the overlapping volumes, sorting them by depth value. This method composites the volumes producing a correct picture at the expense of texture binding time. Binding, the process of getting the volume texture ready for operation, is time consuming if the texture has to be reloaded, and therefore should be avoided when possible. This reloading is very likely to happen in the interleaving method given that, although a volume by itself might fit into texture memory, the combination of two (or more) is less likely to do so. The main drawback of the interleaving approach is that it requires one bind per sample plane per volume.

Another method is to composite the volumes at the image level (combining slices of the different volumes into a single set of slices). This method is not applicable if the positions of the volumes have to be controlled independently (registered together, for example). Also, it is hard to find the extent of overlap of the texels, specially from volumes that have different orientations.

Our solution capitalizes on the 'multisampling mask' option available in SGI workstations which then enables to render the volumes one at a time. When multisampling is enabled, each pixel is allocated n 'samples', in effect dividing it into n subpixels. Depending on the transparency value of each voxel (ranging from 0.0 to 1.0), the mask is modified so that [*transparency*n*] of the subpixels is written. This method is efficient in terms of texture bindings (one volume is bound at a time), is easy to implement, and most importantly for surgical planning, gives a correct visual position of the volumes. Since this method combines volumes based on a limited number of samples per pixel with a mask, one objection would be how faithful the resulting image is (compared to what would be obtained using traditional volume rendering). Another shortcoming is that the approach is volume-order dependent (different order in the rendering can produce different images). These two problems are not significant for our purposes. Firstly, the images produced are almost identical: compare Fig. 2c and d, which use four samples per pixel, the maximum available to us — better images can be obtained if more samples per pixel are available. Fig. 2c renders MRI first, and (d) MRA first. Second, since our main objective is to determine positional relationships, fidelity to the traditional volume rendering is not the issue, as long as positional accuracy is preserved. Fig. 2b shows an image obtained by combining the same two volumes but having the MRA displayed without the mask enabled: the resulting image shows more detail. But if we reverse the order of rendering, this produces the wrong picture (Fig. 2a is an example of that).

3.1.1 Volume Exploration Tools. Planning involves patient data (volumetric) exploration. A *roaming* tool was added to the standard volume tools (*cut-box* tool to provide mixed orthogonal and volumetric views by removing a wedge of the volume, or a *clip* tool to position and orient of six arbitrary-orientation clipping planes). This tool allows to cut and roam inside several multimodal data sets cropping them simultaneously. Real-time performance is maintained by displaying only a part of the total volume while keeping all objects in view. In this way, a cross section of all objects can be studies to reveal where and how tumors and vessels intersect (see Fig. 3a).

3.2. Registration

VIVIAN provides a set of tools for performing direct transformations on an object, such as translation, scaling and rotation. Additionally, an automatic n-point alignment tool to register more difficult cases is available. This requires at least four corresponding landmarks from source and destination objects, and uses the least-square approximation method. The more landmarks specified, the better the fit.

3.3. Segmentation: Highlighting Pathology

VIVIAN features a user-controlled crop-and-clone facility to segment out volumetric objects from the MRI volume. Each volume has its own Colour Look-Up Table (CLUT), a 3D widget that interactively maps scan values to external appearance. The transparency control of this widget is an effective segmentation tool to make invisible specific regions and isolate regions of interest. (This is possible with tumors that have significant density contrast against the surrounding tissue). Fig. 4 illustrates how to segment a tumor by increasing the transparency (lower white control line) of the surrounding tissue. Fig. 1 shows CT, MRA and a tumor all segmented this way.

3.3.1 Outlining Tumors. When there is no significant density contrast between a tumor and the surrounding tissue, an outlining tool is available to let the surgeon decide the extent of the tumor. The outlining tool lets the surgeons draw outlines over the original scan slices (see Fig. 5). Although the drawing is done on a slice-by-slice basis, the volume of interest remains in context during the outlining, facilitating the appreciation of the shape of the tumor.

Once the outline is completed, the surgeon can verify its extent against the volume, and correct it. Additionally, the outline can be displayed as a surface, and can be coloured and rendered with different degrees of transparency to study its relationship to the rest of the anatomy. The surgeon can then go back to the outlining tool and adjust its contours to achieve a better fit.

3.4. Planning: Interacting with the Data

3.4.1 Voxel Editing. The ability to interactively change the properties of individual voxels or groups of voxels is useful in planning. This allows turning voxels transparent, to see through them (thus simulating a craniotomy or a suction tool), or painting them in a different colour (for marking purposes), or restoring their original values (to correct interaction errors): Fig. 3b.

The surgeon can select the shape of the voxel tool (rectangular, cylindrical and spherical) and its size (pointing upwards and clicking to make it bigger, or downwards to make it smaller). Without pressing the switch, the voxel tool works in 'inspect' mode: the voxels covered by the tool's shape are not shown, revealing the tissue behind. When the switch is pressed, the tool removes the voxels.

3.4.2 Measurement and Trajectory Planning. It is important in surgical planning to measure distances between points in 3D space and to draw lines that guide surgical approaches. VIVIAN uses markers (adjustable line segments that display length) for both purposes. The marker end-points can be moved by reaching into them with the stylus, and are either free-moving, or snapped to the nearest orthogonal axis. This is a simple and yet essential feature that capitalizes on the ease and directness of reach on the Virtual Workbench. Fig. 1 shows several trajectory paths planned on the lower-left side of the head.

4 Case Example

Our planning system has been used by neurosurgeons from the Singapore General Hospital and the Tan Tock Seng Hospital to plan neurosurgical approaches in 16 cases. We illustrate the planning procedure with a clinical case of a 65 year old male with a skull base tumor (meningeoma) in the petroclival region.

Three days before surgery, the patient was scanned with a contrast enhanced MRI (gradient echo) and a MRA (time of flight) both extending over the same field of view (FOV). The patient's head was fixed firmly during the scanning procedure to ensure a good registration. To visualize the bone, the skull base was scanned with a CT of 1mm slice thickness. During both MR and CT procedures the patient had fiducial markers attached to his skin.

Once the data was available in VIVIAN, fusion of MRI and MRA was achieved easily since the orientation and the FOV were the same. The position and extent of coverage in the z-axis differed and were adjusted manually (moving exclusively along z; MRA displayed as volumetric vessels, MRI made semi-transparent, or as triplanar structure). Subsequently MRI/MRA and CT were fused by manually placing landmarks on the fiducials.

The tumor was segmented easily using the CLUT method, since the meningeoma showed uniform contrast-enhancement (Fig. 4).

Two possible approaches to the lesion were outlined and measured. Using the voxel editing tool, a suboccipital and a temporal craniotomy were simulated and parts of the tumor were removed respectively (Fig. 3b). It was concluded that complete removal could probably only be achieved by approaching the lesion along those two trajectories and this assumption was intra-operatively confirmed to be correct.

5 Implementation

VIVIAN is written with the KRDL BrixMed C++/OpenGL software toolkit [10] and runs on a Silicon Graphics Onyx2 (1 R10000 180 Mhz CPU, 1 Raster Manager with 64MB texture memory). The input devices used are the FASTRAK from Polhemus, with two receivers: one stylus, and one normal receiver with a digital hand switch attached. For multimodal volumes of less than 64 MB (the available hardware texture) that occupy a quarter of the total screen space (1024x768 pixels) we obtained an average performance of 10 frames per second, in stereo. When the volumes occupy more than half of the screen space, the speed falls to 5 frames per second, due to overloading of the single Raster Manager.

6 Conclusions and Further Work

Neurosurgeons value the efficient and comprehensive way in which the system allows them to understand the complexity of anatomical and pathological relationships surrounding a lesion. They all agreed that the preoperative experience of planning the approach virtually remains in the neurosurgeon's mind and is supportive during the operative procedure.

It takes less than two hours to prepare the images for the neurosurgeon (such as the ones presented in this paper), from the moment the images are available from the scanners until the neurosurgeon can start the planning. This includes off-line image conversion, registration, CLUT control, and tumor segmentation. We intend to carry the planning into the operating theatre by modifying the interface to suit a microscope.

Neurosurgeons with no prior experience with the Virtual Workbench can reach a sufficient level of familiarity with the system in approximately 20 minutes. The interface is undergoing simplification, but still maintaining the tools necessary to plan a complex procedure.

Acknowledgments. We would like to acknowledge the contribution to the project of Dr. Yeo Tseng Tsai (Dept. Neurosurgery) and Dr. Robert Tien and Dr. Sitoh Yih Yian (Dept. Radiology) of the Tan Tock Seng Hospital, and also of Dr. Tushar M. Goradia, Dept. Neurosurgery, Johns Hopkins Hospital.

References

1. Boston Dynamics, Inc. 614 Massachusetts Avenue, Cambridge, MA 02139, USA
2. Cabral, B., Cam, B., Foran, J.: Accelerated Volume Rendering and Tomographic Reconstruction Using Texture Mapping Hardware, Proc. ACM/IEEE 1994 Symposium Volume Visualization., (1994) 91-98 and 131.
3. Chua, G.G., Serra, L., Kockro, R.A., Ng, H., Nowinski, W.L., Chan, C., Pillay, P.K.: Volume-based tumor neurosurgery planning in the Virtual Workbench, Proc. IEEE VRAIS'98, (1998) 167-173.
4. Goble, J. C. Hinkley, K., Pausch, R., Snell, J. W. and Kassell, N. F.: Two-handed spatial interface tools for neurosurgical planning, IEEE Computer, 28 (7), (1995) 20-26.
5. Hill, J.W., Holst, P.A., Jensen, J.F., Goldman, J., Gorfu, Y., Ploeger, D.W., Telepresence Interface with Applications in Microsurgery and Surgical Simulations, Proc. MMVR:6, (1997) 96-102.
6. Kikinis, R., Gleason, P.L., Moriarty, T.M., Moore, M.R., Alexander, E., Stieg, P.E., Matsumae, M., Lorensen, W.E., Cline, H.E., Black, P., and Jolesz, F.A.: Computer Assisted Interactive Three-Dimensional Planning for Neurosurgical Procedures. Neurosurgery, 38 (4) (1996) 640-651.
7. Poston, T. and Serra, L.: Dextrous Virtual Work, Communications of the ACM, 29 (5), (1996) 37-45.
8. Serra, L., Nowinski, W.L., Poston, T., Chua, B.C., Ng H., Lee, C.M., Chua, G.G., Pillay, P.K.: The Brain Bench: Virtual Tools for Neurosurgery, J. Medical Image Analysis, 1 (4), (1997) 317-329.
9. Serra, L., Ng, H., Chua, B.C. and Poston, T.: Interactive vessel tracing in volume data, Proc. ACM Symposium of Interactive 3D Graphics, (1997) 131-137.
10. Serra, L. and Ng, H.: The BrixMed C++ Applications Programming Interface, ISS Internal Technical Report. (1997)
11. The Virtual Workbench Web Page: http://www.krdl.org.sg/RND/biomed/virtual/index.html
12. The 65th Annual Meeting of the American Association of Neurological Surgeons, Scientific Program, (1997) 71-81.

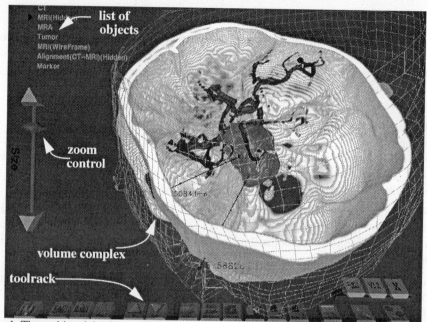

Fig. 1. The multimodal volume: CT, MRA and MRI fused. Markers show the approach

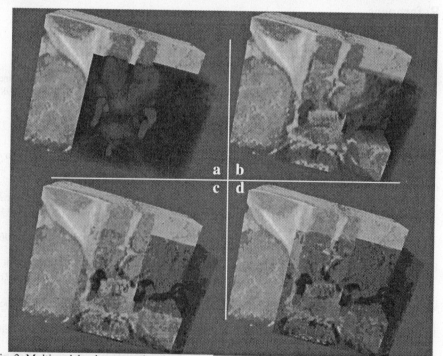

Fig. 2. Multimodal volumes rendered using 3D textures: (a) MRA without mask; (b) MRA with mask; (c, d) using the 'multisampling mask' approach, (c) MRI rendered first, (d) MRA first

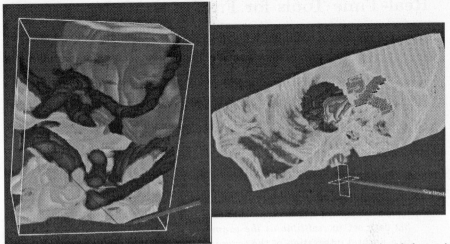

Fig. 3. Volume tools: (a) Roaming around objects; (b) Voxel editor: eraser and paint (dark cross)

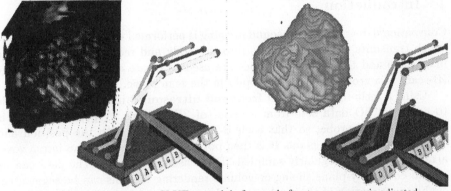

Fig. 4. Tumor highlighting using CLUT control: before and after transparency is adjusted

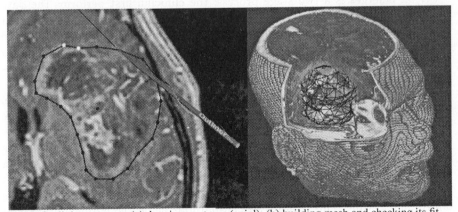

Fig. 5. Outlining a tumor: (a) drawing contours (axial); (b) building mesh and checking its fit

Real-Time Tools for Freehand 3D Ultrasound

Richard Prager[1], Andrew Gee[1], and Laurence Berman[2]

[1] Department of Engineering, University of Cambridge, UK
[2] Department of Radiology, University of Cambridge, UK

Abstract. One of the drawbacks of many 3D ultrasound systems is the two-stage nature of the process. The strict separation of data acquisition and visualisation disturbs the continuity of the ultrasound examination. Furthermore, some systems require the clinician to wait for an unacceptable amount of time while the voxel array is constructed. In this paper, we describe tools which allow arbitrary slices to be viewed through the 3D data set *in real-time as the examination is taking place*. This leads to a natural integration of the scanning and visualisation processes.

1 Introduction

Conventional diagnostic ultrasound imaging is performed with a hand-held probe which transmits ultrasound pulses into the body and receives the echoes. The magnitude and timing of the echoes are used to create a 2D grey scale image (B-scan) of a cross-section of the body in the scan plane.

Using a technique called **3D freehand ultrasound imaging**, it is possible to construct 3D data sets from a series of 2D B-scans. A position sensor is attached to the probe, so that each B-scan is labelled with the position and orientation of the scan plane. It is then possible to slot each B-scan into a voxel array, producing a regularly sampled 3D ultrasound data set. The data can be visualised by any-plane slicing or volume rendering. Organs can be segmented, enabling estimation of their volumes and graphical rendering of their surfaces.

What emerges is a two stage process: the clinician first performs the data acquisition and then, when this is complete, uses a separate set of controls for reslicing and visualisation. This disturbs the interactive nature of the ultrasound examination. In this paper, we describe two tools for real-time display of data from a freehand 3D ultrasound system. These tools enable the clinician to visualise any slice taken at any angle while the scan is actually taking place.

The first tool enables the visualisation of a long structure in a single plane. It involves extracting vertical strips from a series of ultrasound images as the probe is moved over the structure, and aligning them to produce a composite, panoramic picture of the complete length of the structure. Recent interest in this type of imaging has been triggered by the release of the Siemens Sonoline Elegra ultrasound machine, which offers a panoramic imaging facility called "SieScape". The Siemens machine achieves accurate registration by correlating consecutive images in real-time. This requires special-purpose, dedicated hardware that contributes to the high cost of the machine. We achieve a similar result using the 3D position and orientation of the probe provided by the position sensing device.

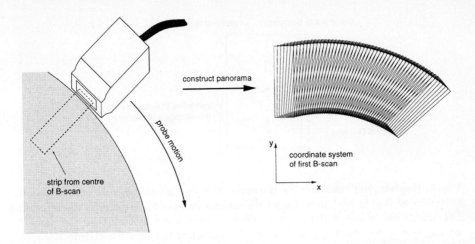

Fig. 1. Panoramic ultrasound. As the probe is moved in the plane of the B-scans, thin strips from the centre of the B-scans are used to construct a panorama in real-time.

The second tool uses the same live information about the current position of the probe to build up a picture showing a slice through the body in any required direction. The clinician defines the position of the slice and then, as the probe is moved along, the slice image is gradually built up on the computer screen.

2 Panoramic ultrasound

Data for a panoramic image is acquired by translating the probe in the plane of the B-scans. The B-scans are then accurately registered and stitched together to produce a seamless composite — see Figure 1. This is performed in real-time, so the clinician sees the panorama as the probe is moved over the region of interest.

2.1 Registration

We use the readings from the position sensor to register sequential B-scans and hence construct a panoramic image. Consider B-scans n and $n+1$. Since we know the 3D position and orientation of both scans, it is straightforward to calculate the rigid body transformation **T** between the local coordinate systems of the two images. We can then map pixels in B-scan $n+1$ into B-scan n's coordinate system, and display both images on the same axes.

There is one complication. Unless the probe is moved perfectly in the plane of the B-scans, **T** will involve not only a within-plane translation and rotation, but also an out-of-plane transformation. We need to "flatten" this transformation to warp the surface traced out by the B-scans onto a flat plane. This can be achieved as follows. We use **T** to transform the centerline of B-scan $n+1$ into B-scan n's coordinate system. The centre and endpoints of the centerline will not

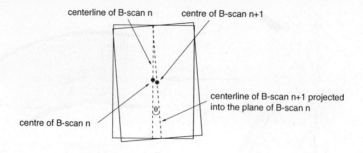

Fig. 2. Registering consecutive B-scans. The position readings are used to map the centerline of B-scan $n+1$ into B-scan n's coordinate system. In general, the centerline lies outside the plane of B-scan n, so its endpoints are projected onto the plane by zeroing their z-coordinates. It is then simple to measure the angle θ and deduce $(\delta x, \delta y)$, such that an in-plane rotation θ followed by a translation $(\delta x, \delta y)$ maps the centre of B-scan $n+1$ on to its projected position in B-scan n's coordinate system.

generally have zero z-coordinates in the new coordinate system. We flatten the transformation by setting these coordinates to zero. We then calculate the angle θ and the displacement $(\delta x, \delta y)$, such that a within-plane rotation θ followed by a translation $(\delta x, \delta y)$ maps the centre of B-scan $n+1$ on to its projected position in B-scan n's coordinate system — see Figure 2. We can easily construct a planar Euclidean transformation matrix $\mathbf{T}'$ from θ and $(\delta x, \delta y)$. The panorama is then created using $\mathbf{T}'$ to map pixels in B-scan $n+1$ into B-scan n's coordinate system.

We do not need to render every B-scan in its entirety to construct the panoramic image. Consecutive B-scans will overlap, and it suffices to use only a narrow strip from the centre of each B-scan. The panorama is constructed in the coordinate system of the *first* B-scan. $\mathbf{T}'$ is calculated for each pair of consecutive B-scans, and the frame-to-frame transformations are concatenated to refer the current B-scan back to the coordinate system of the first B-scan.

2.2 Wedge-based interpolation

Where adjacent strips overlap, we would like to see pixels from the centre of the strips and not the edges. This can be achieved by mapping the intensity data not onto a flat strip, but a wedge, such that the projection of the wedge onto the plane is the same as the original strip — see Figure 3. To an observer viewing the plane from above, a single wedge looks exactly the same as the flat strip. However, intensities associated with the centre of each strip are close to the viewer, while those closer to each edge are further away. If the graphics system renders the wedges with hidden surface removal, then the panorama will reveal only those portions of the strips that are as close as possible to their centerlines.

This technique is free of parameters. It is necessary to specify the width of each strip, but this can be determined automatically, using $\mathbf{T}'$ to calculate the minimum width such that there are no gaps between adjacent strips. Since the

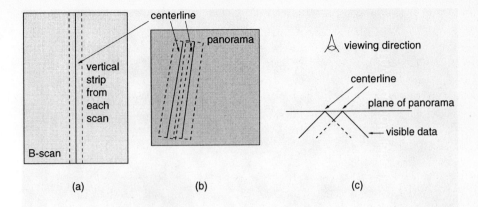

Fig. 3. Correct treatment of overlapping strips. Where strips overlap, the panorama should show data from the centre of the B-scan, not the edges. This can be accomplished by "folding" each strip around its centerline to form a wedge. If the graphics system renders the wedges with hidden surface removal, then the slice will reveal only those portions of the strips that are as close as possible to their centerlines.

wedges determine the parts of each strip that are displayed, using slightly too wide a strip only affects the rendering speed, not the image quality.

2.3 Implementation

Central to the success of this approach is the need to develop a *fast* implementation. To this end, we exploit the standard graphics accelerator hardware found in many of today's desktop computers.

The wedges can be rendered using one of two techniques. The first, 2D texture mapping, defines each wedge as two rectangles and projects the appropriate grey level pattern from the B-scan onto the rectangles. This is the preferred technique with hardware that offers flexible, accelerated texture mapping. Alternatively, we can extract adjacent columns of pixels from the B-scans, and place each pixel at its correct position on the wedge. These points can then be rendered as the vertices of a dense mesh of triangles, using Gouraud shading to fill in the gaps.

Given suitable (but not extravagant) graphics hardware, the panorama can be rendered very rapidly. For instance, using the Gouraud technique, the panorama is easily rendered on a Silicon Graphics Indy workstation at the video frame rate. Typical panoramas constructed using this technique can be found in Figure 4.

3 Real-time any-plane slicing

The normal way to produce an arbitrary slice through a 3D ultrasound data set is to resample the data onto a regular grid [1] and then use fast, integer arithmetic to extract the voxels straddling the desired slice. If we are to compute the slice

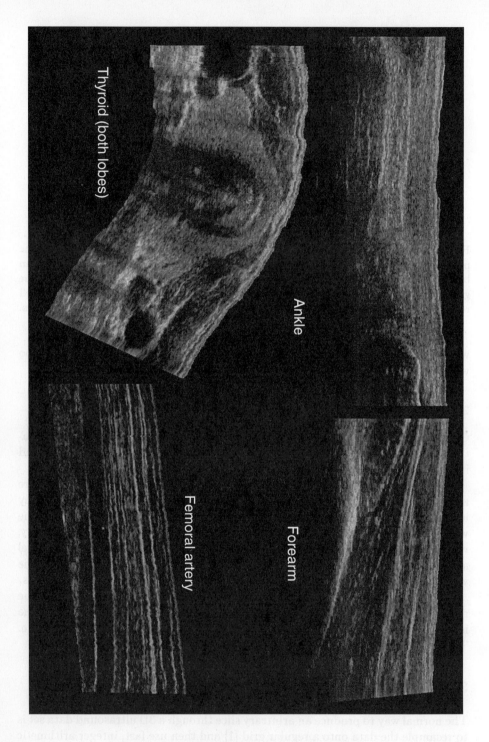

Fig. 4. Typical real-time panoramic images.

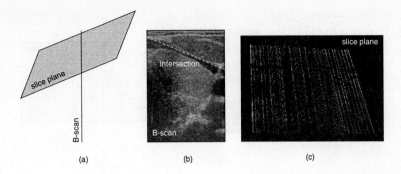

Fig. 5. Reslicing thin B-scans. The slice plane intersects each B-scan along a line, as shown in (a) and (b). Intensities can be extracted from the B-scans along these lines and drawn on the slice plane. However, this produces a fragmented image (c).

as the data is acquired, we cannot perform the initial voxelisation procedure. The system must work only with the raw B-scans and their positions.

We also need to design a suitable tool which allows the clinician to define the desired slice plane without reference to the full 3D data volume (which has not yet been acquired). In our current implementation, the clinician places the probe orthogonal to the required slice and then uses a touch screen to draw a line at a suitable position on the current B-scan: this defines the line of intersection of the slice with the current B-scan. The clinician can then sweep the probe over the volume of interest, while the slice appears in real-time on the computer monitor.

A naive reslicing algorithm might extract intensity values along the lines of intersection of each B-scan with the slice plane, and paint these intensities onto the slice plane — see Figure 5. The problem with this approach is that the slice comprises a set of fragmented line segments, as shown in Figure 5(c).

To improve the quality of the slice we clearly need to interpolate between the line segments. Figure 6 illustrates an interpolation scheme which takes into account the anisotropic resolution of the 3D ultrasound data. Since the ultrasound beam has a finite thickness, perhaps as much as 10 mm [2], we should think not of a single, thin B-scan in space, but a continuum of repeated B-scans smeared across the width of the ultrasound beam[1]. The intersection of the slice plane with the smeared B-scan is now a polygon. Intensity values can be extracted within this polygon and drawn at the appropriate position on the slice plane. Repeating this process for all B-scans tiles the slice plane with a set of overlapping polygons filled with intensity data.

It is only left to decide which intensity to display where two or more polygons overlap on the slice plane. Intuitively, we would like to see data gathered along the centerline of the ultrasound beam, and not the periphery. We therefore use the wedge-based strategy described in Section 2.2 above.

---

[1] For simplicity, we assume that the width of the ultrasound beam is constant, though in reality the width varies with distance from the probe face [2].

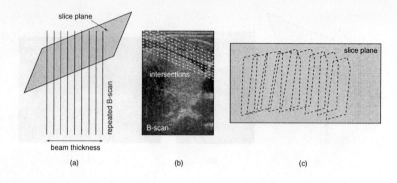

Fig. 6. Reslicing thick B-scans. In practice, the ultrasound beam is not focussed out of the plane of the B-scan. In effect, the B-scan can be imagined repeated in space over the extent of the beam thickness (a). The intersection of each B-scan with the slice place is now a polygon (b). Intensities can be extracted from within the polygons and drawn on the slice plane. This typically produces a set of filled, overlapping polygons (c).

Orthogonal slices, rendered using the Gouraud scheme, are shown in Figures 7(d)–(f)[2]. For comparison, Figures 7(a)–(c) show similar slices through a regular voxel array constructed off-line from the same data. The voxels were cubic, with the same dimension as a pixel in the original B-scans. Gaps in the voxel array were filled by averaging intensities in a $5 \times 5 \times 5$ local neighbourhood (this took several minutes on a powerful workstation). Close inspection of the two sets of slices shows that the grey scale texture is better preserved by the voxel-less scheme, since there is *no* averaging of the raw intensity data.

4 Conclusions

We have described two tools for real-time visualization of data from a 3D ultrasound system. By using an interpolation strategy that requires information from only one B-scan at a time, we are able to produce large panoramic images and interactively compute slices through the body at any angle. As the 3D ultrasound data does not need to be stored, this greatly reduces the amount of computer memory required to reconstruct an image.

References

1. T. R. Nelson and T. T. Elvins. Visualization of 3D ultrasound data. *IEEE Computer Graphics and Applications*, pages 50–57, November 1993.
2. M. L. Skolnick. Estimation of ultrasound beam width in the elevation (section thickness) plane. *Radiology*, 180(1):286–288, 1991.

---

[2] In order to facilitate comparison with the voxel-based slices, these images have been constructed off-line from a single set of recorded B-scans. They are, however, mathematically and visually identical to those we generate in real-time.

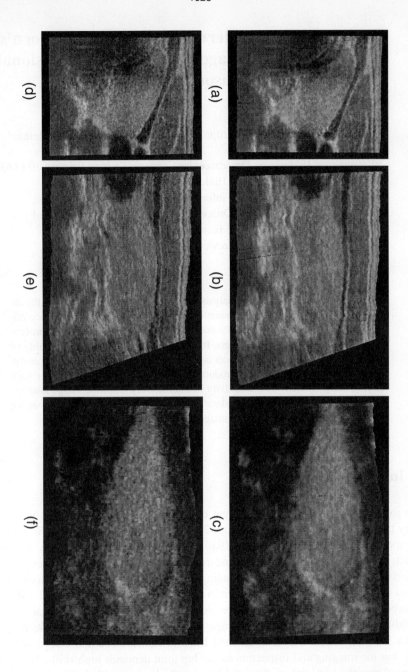

Fig. 7. Any-plane slicing of a human thyroid gland. The figure shows results of a voxel-based (a)–(c) and voxel-less (d)–(f) approach. Slices (a) and (d) are virtually parallel to the B-scans. Slices (b) and (e) are orthogonal to these but the skin is still at the top: similar B-scans could have been obtained by rotating the probe through 90°. Slices (c) and (f) are located a constant depth below the skin, and could not have been obtained using conventional 2D ultrasound.

Computer-Based Determination of the Newborn's Femoral Head Coverage Using Three-Dimensional Ultrasound Scans

Heinrich M. Overhoff[1], Djordje Lazovic[2], Ute von Jan[1], Peter Heinze[1]

[1] University of Hildesheim, Department for Computer Science, Postfach 10 13 63,
D-31113 Hildesheim, Germany
martin@med-informatik.uni-hildesheim.de

[2] Hannover Medical School, Orthopedic Department, Heimchenstraße 1 - 7,
D-30625 Hannover, Germany
lazovic@t-online.de

Abstract. An automatic image analysis method is presented, which finds the diagnostic landmarks for the determination of the femoral head coverage according to Graf's method in a 3-D ultrasound image volume. Some of the process steps depend on tuneable parameters. It is a typical experience that the quality of images differs between investigators and patients respectively. An image analysis algorithm therefore should produce results which are robust against such varying image quality. The sensitivity of intermediary and final image analysis process steps versus expert defined parameters is investigated. This analysis are performed in a pilot study on 3-D image data of 10 newborns.

1 Introduction

Hip joint dysplasia is the most frequent congenital skeletal disease [1], with exemplary prevalences in newborns are about 2 % in the USA and the UK, 4 % in Central Europe, and 10 % in Japan. In the 1980's Graf developed a diagnostic technique, which is meanwhile established as standard method for the investigation and quantification of the newborn's hip joint findings in Central Europe. Graf's technique is based on a 2-D ultrasound image taken in the so-called standard plane [2], [3], [4]. It focuses on the analysis of the relative location of the newborn's femoral head and acetabulum. The femoral head coverage is then quantified by geometric measures taken from the 2-D image. This method leads to standardised and comparable findings, but the imaging and inspection of the hip joint demands high skills. It has to be claimed that the hip joint of the newborn usually is not ossified. Therefore, the hip joint itself is invisible in the ultrasound images: the femoral head of the newborn is cartilaginous, and the same holds for the non-ossified junction of iliac, ischial and pubic bone, the so called hypsiloid cartilage. These structures can only be identified indirectly by bounding landmarks. Another disadvantage is the systematic reduction of a spatial geometry to a single or a few 2-D plane cuts. Thus, findings visible in non-standardised image planes must be interpreted and documented individually, which reduces the comparability of clinical reports.

The use of 3-D ultrasound for several diagnostic investigations has been studied in the past few years including the visualisation of the newborn's hip joint [5], [6]. The reporting of 3-D ultrasound image data sets primarily aims on a more precise inspection. An automatic processing of Graf's diagnostic method or a quantification of the femoral head coverage, e.g. the derivation of geometric measures of the joint based on a spatial representation, to our knowledge has not been reported so far (cf. [7]).

In this study, an automatic image analysis method is presented, which finds the diagnostic landmarks for the determination of the femoral head coverage according to Graf's method in a 3-D ultrasound image volume. To ensure the robustness of the image analysis algorithm, the sensitivity of intermediary and final image analysis process steps versus central process parameters was investigated. This analysis are performed in a pilot study on 3-D image data of 10 newborns. Final results were taken for a robust parametrization.

2 Materials and Methods

For data sets of 10 newborns (2 days - 12 weeks) an image analysis was performed automatically. In this application certain structures with typical shapes are expected in the images. Therefore the automatic image analysis is organised in two steps. First a data-driven image pre-processing is performed, and their results are investigated in a second step using mathematical functions which model the expected forms. From a methodical point of view the sensitivity of model-based image processing vs. the pre-processed raw-data is investigated. Implicitly the assumption is made that data-driven image processing tends to be error sensitive, while model-based approaches are more robust. Therefore only the robustness of the image analysis vs. the pre-processing steps is analysed. Thus the location of resulting landmarks and sphere parameters is investigated vs. pre-processing parameters.

2.1 Image processing

Image acquisition. Images of the newborn's hip are taken during a free-hand sweep around the coronal plane. A typical image data set includes about 30 images of about $200\,pixel \times 200\,pixel$ size. A conventional ultrasound imaging system (Kontron AI 5200) with a 7.5 MHz-Linear Array transducer is used. The pixel's edge measures are about $0.23mm \times 0.23mm$. The image contrast is manually controlled by a depth-dependent signal gain.

For the determination of the transducer motion a specially developed sensing system is used. By the parallel orientation of transducer and image, the spatial image positions can directly be determined from the transducer movement measurements.

The sensing system is optimised for rotation measurements, its accuracy is $\leq 0.1°$. During the image data collection, the scan head is only rotated around two axes.

The data are acquired by an IBM-PC. The images are provided by the video output of the US system and digitised with a video grabbing card. The image processing, the automatic determination of a sphere approximating the femoral head, and the identification of the acetabular landmarks were performed on an IBM-compatible PC (166 MHz, 64 MBytes RAM).

Transducer kinematics. The motion of the transducer is described according to the kinematics of masspoints known from mechanics [8]. As the transducer's object co-ordinate system only rotates in the world co-ordinate system, a spherical co-ordinate system is adequate to express the relative motion parameterized by the two angles ϑ and φ. With these data the spatial location of the image pixels can be calculated.

Image analysis. The interpretation of a hip joint dysplasia using 2-D standard plane images is based on ultrasound reflecting structures, which have a fix relation to the hip joint. These landmarks must be identified to derive coverage measures. According to Graf's diagnostic method, these landmarks are the contour of the iliac bone as reference axis (1), the osseous edge of the acetabulum (2), the most distal osseous edge of the ilium (3), the cartilaginous acetabular labrum (4), and the reflection of the capsule (5); the numbers refer to Fig. 1. The image analysis itself is dissected into three major steps:
1. identification of the iliac bone and a region of interest, where the femoral head is suspected,
2. estimation of a sphere approximating the femoral head and determination of the β-angle, which is a criterion for the cartilaginous head coverage, and
3. calculation of the iliac part of the already ossified acetabulum and determination of the α-angle, which is an indicator for the quality of the head coverage (Fig. 2).

An automatic image analysis for the femoral head approximation [7] was extended by an algorithm identifying the acetabular landmarks (2) and (3). The entire procedure is described in the following. For each process step their detail results and major process parameters are listed. The sensitivity of the image analysis results vs. these parameters is investigated to find optimal values for a robust image processing.

Formally, some notations for images are introduced. An image itself is noted as a $N_{line} \times N_{row}$-matrix $\mathbf{P} = [p(i,j)]$, $1 \leq i \leq N_{line}$, $1 \leq j \leq N_{row}$, having grey-values $g_{min} \leq g \leq g_{MAX}$ (here: $g_{min} = 0$, $g_{MAX} = 255$). A histogram is given by $h(g) = card(p(i,j) = g)$, and $H(g)$ denotes cumulated grey-value frequencies normalised by $N_{line} \cdot N_{row}$.

Determination of the region of interest for the femoral head and acetabulum. To detect the echo of the iliac bone, the image volume is binarized using a threshold $g_{THRES,SKELETON}$. A skeletonization is then performed on each plane of the binarized volume, and all skeletons except the medial-most one on the proximal side of each image are discarded. These skeletons coincide with the iliac bone and are idealised as proximal-distal lines. The distal end points of these lines serve to approximate the position of the most distal osseous edge of the ilium.

The cumulative frequency $H(g_{THRES,SKELETON})$ is the major parameter.

Detection of the femoral head approximating sphere and the β-angle. At the most distal osseous edge of the ilium, a region of interest (ROI) in the form of a mirrored "C" is introduced. The diameter-range of the "C" was chosen to $20 \leq D/pixel \leq 60$, as $D \approx 40\,pixel$ is a typical femoral head radius (cf. [7]). Its centre is taken as provisional centre of the femoral head approximating sphere. A gradient image is constructed in the ROI, where the gradient's directions are determined from the provisorial centre. The cumulated grey-value frequencies $H(g)$ are calculated for the gradient image, which then is binarized using a threshold $g_{THRES,CONTOUR}$. The remaining pixels contour the only implicit visible femoral head circle. Pixels in the ROI which are located most to the provisorial centre and have restricted relative angle positions to this point are taken to construct a four-dimensional Hough-accumulator for sphere surfaces. This accumulator then is normalised by the sphere surfaces, cluster analysed and finally investigated for the most frequent sphere parameter combination. For details cf. [7].

The result of the sphere detection is a parameter vector $[x_{centre}\ y_{centre}\ z_{centre}\ D]$. To ease its interpretation, intersections of this sphere with each original image, i.e. circles, are visualised on the computer screen. Fig. 3 additionally shows the intersection with the expert placed reference sphere.

The cumulative frequency $H(g_{THRES,CONTOUR})$ is considered to be the major parameter.

Acetabulum lines and α-angle. From anatomy the special geometric structure of the acetabular part of the iliac bone is known. The voxels bounding the femoral head in the acetabular region construct a ROI, where the osseous edge of the acetabulum and the most distal osseous edge of the ilium are found. Here only those pixels are used, which are brighter then the grey-value $H(g_{THRES,ACE})$. The result of this processing step are the spatial co-ordinates of the two landmarks necessary for the calculation of Graf's α-angle by the use of the most distal osseous edge of the ilium.

2.2 Verification

The results of the image analysis were tested for correctness and robustness vs. the image processing parameters. This analysis was performed to gain stable reliable results independent of image contrast. An objective determination of the parameters of the coverage parameters was not possible, as none of the children was treated surgically. Therefore, to control the automatically determined landmarks and measures, the placement of the distal iliac crest points was compared to pixels determined by three experienced experts. The same was done for the most distal edge of the ilium and the acetabular edge. To control the automatically determined femoral head approximating sphere, an expert placed virtual spheres in a 3D-scene and parametrised their origin and diameter. For control the original image slices intersected the virtual sphere. The section figure in each image is a circle. These circles were inserted into the images and controlled for their location. The location of the virtual femoral head sphere was corrected until this control yielded a plausible result.

The analysis of the first two process steps, defining the hip joint ROI and determination of a femoral head approximating sphere, were statistically analysed even for additional data sets [9]. Due to the smaller number of cases in this study the results of the acetabular landmarks identification was only described statistically.

3 Results

We could obtain data from 10 hip joints and evaluated them for this study. The mean processing time was about 8 minutes for an entire image data set.

The measurement errors for the co-ordinates of the most distal point of the iliac crest line ranged between -1 and 33 pixels for $0.7 \leq H(g_{THRES,SKELETON}) \leq 0.95$ and -1 and 10 for $0.8 \leq H(g_{THRES,SKELETON}) \leq 0.95$ joints. A statistical analysis (t-test) over 20 hip joints did not reject the null-hypothesis of a mean measurement error of 0 pixels ($\alpha = 5\%$). The parameters of the approximating spheres ranged between -4 and 3 pixels for $0.7 \leq H(g_{THRES,CONTOUR}) \leq 0.95$. Significantly ($\alpha = 5\%$) the sphere centre's y- and z-co-ordinate and the sphere diameter measurement errors were between -2 and 2 pixels. As example for the robustness the displacement of the proximal-distal y-co-ordinate of the distal-most point of the pelvic crest line is presented in Fig. 4 (cf. [9]). The figure underlines the correct choice of the thresholds in [7], as for the ranges $0.8 \leq H(g_{THRES,SKELETON}) \leq 0.95$ and $0.85 \leq H(g_{THRES,CONTOUR}) \leq 0.95$ significantly high correctness can be gained.

The automatically determined and the expert defined co-ordinates for the acetabular edge and the most distal edge of the ilium yielded displacements ranging from -5 to 3 pixels for all co-ordinates independently of reasonably chosen parameters $H(g_{THRES,ACE})$.

The median errors for the co-ordinates ranged between -1 and 1 pixel (-0.23mm resp. 0.23mm) in a detail image of about $20\,pixels \times 20\,pixels$ size, and their 75%-quantiles were 0 to 3 pixels (0.23mm resp. 0.0mm). We found a systematic underestimated y-co-ordinate of the acetabular edge.

4 Discussion

The presented automatic analysis of a 3-D US image volume is an attractive supplement to the conventional 2-D investigation according to Graf's method. It could be shown that the image pre-processing bases on robust methods and yields accurate results for the essential intermediary process parameters. These are the most distal osseous edge of the ilium, which serves to locate a ROI, in which the hip joint is expected, a femoral head approximating sphere, and the boundaries of the iliac bone in the proximal acetabulum. By the statistical analysis it turned out that the process parameter choices for the ROI-definition of the expected joint location and the determination of the approximating sphere's parameters in [7] were reasonable. The determined parameters were accurate, only the centre of the sphere tends be located imprecisely in the transducer main sweep direction.

To rate the measurement errors of the acetabular landmarks it should be mentioned that in the investigation the median of the acetabular index is $\alpha = 63°$. Assuming measurement errors with median deviations of the co-ordinates the angles are misinterpreted by $\Delta\alpha_{median} = 5.3°$, and for 75%-quantile measurement deviations by $\Delta\alpha_{75\%-quantile} = 7.1°$. These error measures exemplary can be related to the correctness of landmark identification an experienced physician can reach in clinical routine diagnostics of about 4 pixels for the most distal osseous edge of the ilium [10]. At the moment an interpretation of the systematic measurement error of the y-co-ordinate of the acetabular edge is not possible. More data sets must be investigated to analyse its origin.

As further work, robust statistical methods will be used to evaluate the femoral head parameters due to the inaccurate centre location orthogonal to the image planes. Furthermore, the geometric results should be controlled in a cadaver study to obtain objective measures.

References

1. Tönnis, D.: Die angeborene Hüftdysplasie und Hüftluxation im Kindes- und Erwachsenenalter, Springer-Verlag, Berlin Heidelberg New York (1984)
2. Exner, G.U., Mieth, G.: Sonographische Hüftdysplasie beim Neugeorenen, Schweiz Med Wochenschr (1987) 1015-1020
3. Graf, R.: The Diagnosis of congenital hip joint dislocation by the ultrasonic compound treatment. Arch Orthop Trauma Surg (1980) 117-133
4. Graf, R.: New possibilities for the diagnosis of congenital hip joint dislocation by ultrasonic compound treatment. J Ped Orthop (1983) 354
5. Graf, R., Lercher, K.: Erfahrungen mit einem 3-D-Sonographiesystem am Säuglingshüftgelenk. Ultraschall Med (1996) 218-226
6. Gerscovich, E.O., Greenspan, A., Cronan, M., Karol, L., McGahan, J.P.: Three-dimensional Sonographic Evaluation of Developmental Dysplasia of the Hip: Preliminary Findings. Radiology (1994) 407-410
7. Overhoff, H.M., Lazovic, D., Franke, J., Jan, U. von: Automatic Determination of the Newborn's Femoral Head from three-dimensional Ultrasound Image Data. In: Lecture Notes in Computer Science, Vol. 1205 Springer-Verlag, Berlin Heidelberg New York (1997) 547-556
8. Wittenburg, J.: Dynamics of Systems of Rigid Bodies, Verlag B.G. Teubner (1977)
9. Overhoff, H.M., Jan, U. von: Robustheitseigenschaften eines Algorithmus zur automatischen Vermessung des Femurkopfes in 3D-Ultraschallbildvolumina der Säuglingshüfte. In: Muche, R. et.al. (eds.), Medizinische Informatik, Biometrie und Epidemiologie: GMDS '97, MMV Medizin Verlag, München (1997) 106-110
10. Graf, R.: Sonographie der Säuglingshüfte und therapeutische Konsequenzen: ein Kompendium. 4th edition, Enke-Verlag Stuttgart (1993)

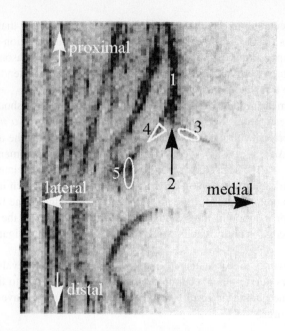

Fig. 1. Ultrasound image of the newborn's hip joint in Graf's standard plane (grey-scale inverted): anatomic orientation and landmarks according to Graf [3], [4]; numbers see text.

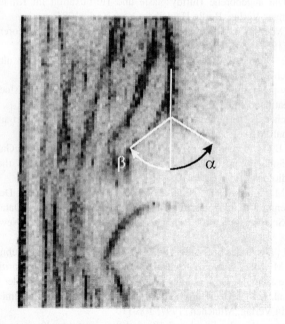

Fig. 2. Ultrasound image with diagnostic angles α and β.

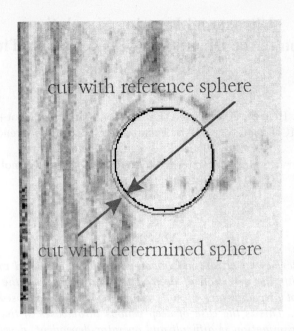

Fig. 3. Automatically determined femoral head approximating (dark grey) and reference sphere (black) intersecting an ultrasound image plane. The difference of the sphere diameters here is about 0.75 *mm*.

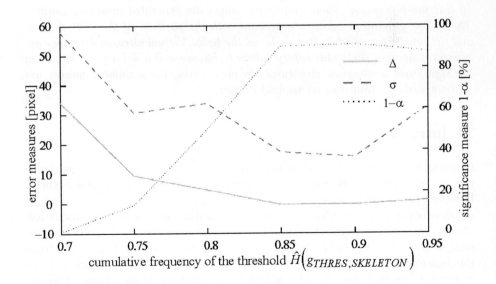

Fig. 4. Displacement of the *y*-co-ordinate of the most distal point of the iliac crest line. Δ: displacement error, σ: standard deviation of Δ, α: significance level

Ultrasound Imaging Simulation: Application to the Diagnosis of Deep Venous Thromboses of Lower Limbs

D. Henry*, J. Troccaz*, J.L. Bosson+ and O. Pichot+
*TIMC Laboratory - IAB, Faculté de Médecine de Grenoble
38706 LA TRONCHE, FRANCE
+Service Médecine interne et Angiologie - CHU Grenoble
38043 GRENOBLE CEDEX, FRANCE
Jocelyne.Troccaz@imag.fr

Abstract

This paper describes an ultrasound imaging simulator dedicated to the training of physicians for the detection of deep venous thromboses of the lower limbs. Currently, a lot of pathologies of soft tissue are readily diagnosed using ultrasound imaging. This is the case of deep venous thromboses of the lower limbs. Because this examination is difficult and operator-dependent, developing a simulator is very useful to give common databases of pathological samples on which physicians can both experiment image acquisition and evaluate their understanding of clinical cases. An ultrasound imaging simulator has been developed. An ultrasound volume is constructed from real images of any typical patient in an off-line pre-processing. Then, simulated images are generated from this volume. The image generation takes into account both the position of the virtual probe and the pressure applied by this probe on the body. Virtual ultrasonic images are generated using a particular interpolation technique and a deformable model of the significant anatomical structures. In most cases, the simulated images are indistinguishable from real ultrasound images.

1 Introduction

Echography has become one of the preferred mean of diagnosis in several pathologies of soft tissues. This comes mainly from its low cost, and non invasiveness. However, compared to conventional radiology, it does not permit later re-reading which raises a major problem for training, evaluation and for differed discussion of cases. Moreover, diagnosis from echographic images may be difficult because images are often of poor quality. Part of the image understanding comes from the dynamic character of the acquisition. This dynamic aspect is important both in terms of probe position and reaction of the anatomical structures. This reaction results from the pressure exerted by the probe over the body. Regarding diagnosis of thromboses, it is generally considered that the number of necessary examinations before having a good technical competence is around 1000. The first 500 examinations made by a student have to be supervised by a senior physician. The possibility of virtual echography, providing intensive training of students. Thus, they could train themselves to acquire images and evaluate their understanding of clinical cases. The virtual echography would allow an increase in the extensive training skills including rare cases, independently of the number of patients of a given medical department. Besides, such a virtual echographic system could speed up new treatment evaluation since it would allow to establish evaluation standards [8].

This paper introduces a computer-based simulator designed to train physicians using ultrasound systems in the diagnosis of deep venous thromboses. In the following sections, we present the medical context of the study (section 2) and an overview of different approaches which can be considered in order to generate virtual ultrasonic images (section 3). In section 4, we present our technical approach and describe the image generation (interpolation and deformation methods). Results are compared to real ultrasound images in section 5. We conclude in section 6.

2 Medical protocol

Our study focuses on the simulation of echographic acquisitions for the diagnosis of deep venous thromboses of the thigh. Ultrasound examination for deep venous thrombosis detection consists in scanning the whole deep venous network perpendicular to vessels (Figure 1). An increasing pressure is applied by the probe on the thigh to observe the vein deformation in the ultrasonic images. From this behaviour, one can decide whether or not a vessel is partly or totally obstructed without necessarily directly seeing a blood clot on a static image.

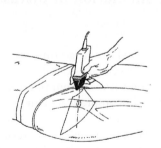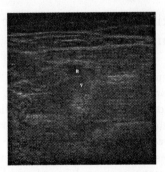

Fig. 1. Examination position (left) and typical ultrasonic image (right)

Deep venous thromboses of lower limbs can be detected by analyzing the vein collapsing when applying increasing pressure on the thigh with the echographic probe. Figure 2 sketches out different echographic images that would be obtained by applying increasing pressure in a non-pathological case. The typical image sequence observed along the arterio-venous axis during the examination is the

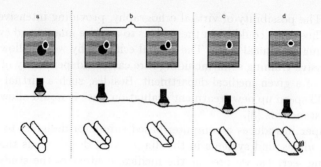

Fig. 2. Echographic aspect of a non pathological vein

following. Vein in relaxation during the initial situation where there is no exerted pressure (cf. fig. 2.a). Figure 1 shows a typical image echographic image of the thigh in state a. Progressive flattening of the vein as the pressure increases (cf. fig. 2.b). Complete venous collapsus when probe pressure is bigger than veinal blood pressure. The vein disappears from the image (cf. fig. 2.c). Arterial hyperpulsatility occurs if probe pressure goes over arterial pressure (cf. fig. 2.d).

Vein incompressibility, detected from the image deformation, is the pathological sign of a thrombosis. In a pathological case, the image would remain in the state described in figure 2.b or somewhere between the states b and c. When arterial hyperpulsatility is reached (state d), the vein may collapse even if obstructed. This state should be avoided as much as possible to avoid both wrong diagnosis and the effect of potential motion of a blood clot in the venous tree.

3 Existing approaches for the simulation of ultrasound imaging

The simulation process can be split into a visual and a gestural part. Existing simulators focus on the visual part of this process. It concerns the real-time generation of realistic images to be displayed on a screen from the position of the probe relatively to the anatomical structures. Two approaches can be considered to generate such images.

Ultrasound imaging is based on ultrasonic wave propagation inside matter. The generative approach is a physical approach consisting in modelling this propagation. Therefore, in order to generate images, we need an accurate model of the probe, a description of organs to be observed and a model of the interaction between the ultrasonic wave and the tissues. This is a very complex problem which has been tackled in several ways depending on the objectives of the simulation (cf. [7], [2], [5], [11]). Generative approaches have the avantage of being applicable to any type of organs provided that a model of them is available. However, the phenomena which have to be modelled are extremely complex and time-consuming. In our context where real-time simulation is needed, a large computational time is totally prohibitive. The compromise which has been proposed by E. Varlet reduces the computing time but does not allow yet to generate textured images.

The second approach is based on the acquisition of a more or less dense volume of ultrasonic data from which new images can be computed (see [1], [3]). The 3D volume of data is acquired in an off-line preprocessing and images are generated during simulation, by computing a slice in the volume. Such images can be generated very rapidly. As they come from real ultrasound images, there is no realism problem.

As stated previously, ultrasonic imaging is a dynamic examination. Images does not only depend on the probe position and orientation but also on the pressure exerted onto the body. The simulation has to take into account deformations induced by this pressure. Very few attention has been paid to this problem in the existing simulators. UltraSim [1] includes elastic registration tools to build a coherent volume from data acquired under different probe positions therefore involving different local deformations. Nevertheless, during simulation no deformation is applied onto the images when the computed pressure of the virtual probe varies. Varlet [11] proposes a local non-linear model of deformation of the computed image allowing to deal with the constraints applied by the tip of the echo-endoscope to the local tissues.

4 Our approach

We have chosen an approach based on the computation of virtual images from a 3D ultrasound data volume. This approach seems to be well-suited to our requirements: realism and real-time. Also for real-time reasons, a deformation model operating on 2D images without pressure consideration has been selected. The system works has follows. Let consider a pathological case of interest. A volume of 3D ultrasonic data is acquired with no significant pressure for database construction. The ultrasound probe is instrumented with infrared diodes which position is tracked using an optical localizer. Using this system, the position and orientation of the echographic plane can be recorded simultaneously to the image. No specific constraints on the position and orientation of the images apply during data acquisition. Regions with thromboses are localized using the protocol described previously and the corresponding images with pressure are also recorded with their position. These sets of images are segmented to compute 3D surfaces of the relevant anatomical structures (cf. [4]) with and without pressure. During simulation, after initialization, the position of the virtual probe is tracked by a localizing device. From the detected position of the virtual echographic plane, a first image is computed using an interpolation method with no consideration of pressure. This image is deformed in a second step to take pressure into account. This second image is displayed to the user.

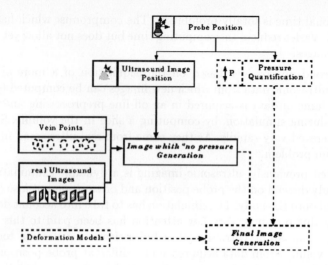

Fig. 3. Image generation

4.1 Interpolation

As already mentioned, firstly, an ultrasound image with no pressure consideration has to be generated. This requires the implementation of an interpolation method which is able to reconstruct an image in a given position from a 3D ultrasound data set. Images from this set have any orientations. Therefore, it is difficult to find an interpolation direction. Due to the image poor quality, it is also very difficult to use interpolation methods such as the shape-based interpolation [9]. Discontinuities due to speckle and to our volume low-density do not allow to use classical interpolation methods for instance using a spline function of the grey level over the volume of data. In order to deal with these problems we have chosen to develop a new interpolation method; we have tested different methods which common point is to focus on the vein principal direction. Because deep venous thrombosis examination is mainly based on vein image observation, its looks reasonable to take the vein as our interpolation direction.

The developed method has been inspired by J. Lengyel's work on 3D reconstruction of intravascular ultrasound slices [6]. Let consider the spline curve C interpolating the centers of the vein in the acquired images. The interpolation method consists in firstly transforming the initial reference system related to the vein (represented by the C curve) into an orthogonal reference system where the vein is represented as a line D (cf. figure 4). In this new space, images can be generated using a linear interpolation method on pixel grey levels: each pixel of the transformed images is linked to its two closest neighbours along D in a suitable database. For each pixel of the synthesized image, the grey intensity is obtained very rapidly by linear interpolation of the closest pixels found in the database.

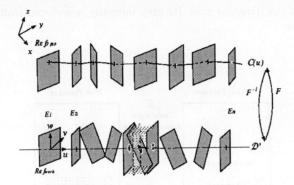

Fig. 4. From a curval reference system to an orthogonal reference system

4.2 Deformation

To represent the deformation due to the probe pressure, we need to find a model which input is this 2D image with no pressure consideration and which output is another 2D image taking into account tissue deformation due to the probe pressure. The main difficulty of this modelling lies in the fact that each structure has its own way to react under pressure. Arteries have almost no deformation. Non pathological veins flatten. Superficial soft tissues have a linear deformation. Deep tissues have almost no deformations. Due to these differences we can not apply the same deformation to the whole image. We have tested a first method which involved different functions of deformations depending on the position of the pixel into these four types of structures. The major problem we had to face lied in the discontinuities obtained in the synthetic image at the boundaries of the structures. Therefore, we propose a more general deformation model based on the elastic registration of images acquired at different levels of pressure. The idea is to deform the 2D image using an elastic transformation computed from relevant anatomical contours. The process is the following (cf. figure 5) :

- Selection of the sets of points to be matched : in our case, the vein, the artery and the skin surface. This provides two sets of 2D points. They are computed from two pre-processed 3D models of the structures of interest (with and without pressure) (cf. [4]).
- Computation of the non-rigid transformation between these sets of points : we propose to represent this transformation using octree-splines (here a quadtree-spline) as described in [10].
- Image generation : A regular grid is associated to the "pressure image" that has to be computed. It is transformed by the elastic transform found in the previous stage into another irregular grid super-imposed to the "non-pressure image" computed using the interpolation methods described previously. Each pixel from the regular grid may be mapped into a pixel or a neighbourhood

of pixels of the irregular grid. Its grey intensity is deduced from them as the mean value.

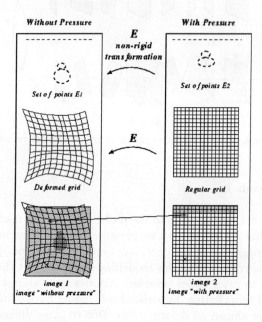

Fig. 5. Image generation including deformations induced by pressure exerted by the probe over the body

5 Results

Interpolation and deformation methods have been implemented and tested in real conditions. The different interpolation methods have been tested using both synthetic and real 3D ultrasound data sets. Given those results, we have chosen the presented interpolation method. To compare real images to virtual ones, we have decided to test our methods at a real acquisition position. The real ultrasound image is removed from the 3D ultrasound data set. Then for this position, an ultrasound image is generated using our interpolation method. The result can be seen on the figure 6. Another image has been generated at an arbitrary position in the ultrasound volume as illustrated on figure 7).

To test the selected deformation method, we have generated an ultrasound image corresponding to a really acquired image. The pressure which has been selected corresponds to a medium pressure for which the vein is still visible in the image. Results can be seen Figure 8.

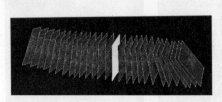 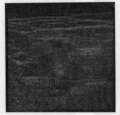 

Fig. 6. (left) Ultrasound images from a thigh ultrasound examination (the image to be generated is represented in white) - (middle) Real image - (right) Interpolated image

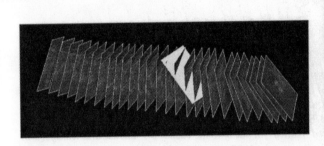 

Fig. 7. (left) Ultrasound images from a thigh ultrasound examination. The image to be generated is represented in white. (Right) Virtual image generated by our interpolation method

Concerning realism, virtual images are similar to real ones. Concerning real-time constraint, images (512x512 pixels) have been computed on a DEC Alpha workstation with a 500 Mhz processor. Generating an image with the interpolation method takes about 0.3 s and deforming it takes less than 0.1 s, if the non-rigid registration is computed in an off-line process.

6 Conclusion

This paper has presented different tools necessary to implement a simulator of ultrasound imaging based on a simple and effective concept where a data volume is constructed from real ultrasound images in an off-line process. Then, during the simulation stage, arbitrary slices of the volume are interpolated and postprocessed to simulate ultrasound images rendering deformation phenomena. Interpolated images have been computed and compared to actual images and the results are very promising. Nevertheless, further steps will be necessary to address other pathologies elsewhere in the body and to be able to render force and tactile feeling to the operator.

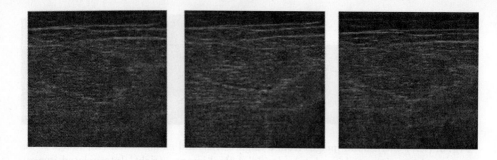

Fig. 8. Generating images with pressure : (left) real image without pressure - (middle) real image with pressure - (right) virtual image synthesized using the deformation model

References

1. D. AIGER AND D. COHEN, *Real-time ultrasound imaging simulation*, RTI, (1997). trouver sur le web http://www.math.tau.ac.il/ daniel/Default.html.
2. J. BAMBER AND R. DICKINSON, *Ultrasonic B-scanning : a computer simulation*, Physics in Medicine and Biology, 25 (1986), pp. 41–60.
3. T. BERLAGE, *Augmented reality for diagnosis based on ultrasound images*, in CVRMed-MRCAS'97, Springer, ed., 1997, pp. 253–262.
4. G. CHAMPLEBOUX AND D. HENRY, *Parametric two-dimensional B-Spline representation of vein and artery from 2.5D echography used to aid virtual echography.*, in CVRMed-MRCAS'97, R. M. J. Troccaz, E.Grimson, ed., LNCS 1205, Springer, 1997, pp. 263–272.
5. J. JENSEN, *Field : A program for simulating ultrasound systems*, in 10th north-baltic conference on biomedical imaging, 1996, pp. 351–353. trouver sur le web.
6. J. LENGYEL, D. GREENBERG, A. YEUG, AND E. ALDERMAN, *Three-dimensional reconstruction and volume rendering of intravascular ultrasound slices imaged on a curved arterial path*, in Computer vision, Virtual Reality, and Robotics in Medicine, CVRMed, 1995, pp. 399 – 405.
7. J. MEUNIER, *Analyse des textures d'échocardiographie bidimensionnelles du myocarde*, PhD thesis, Université de Montreal, avril 1989. in french.
8. O. PICHOT AND AL., *An echographical score for the quantification of deep vein thrombosis. Interest in the follow-up examination.*, Advances in vascular pathology, 3 (1990), p. 471.
9. S. RAYA AND J. UDUPA, *Shape based interpolation of Multidimensional objects*, IEEE transactions on medical imaging, 9 (1990), pp. 32–42.
10. R. SZELISKI AND S. LAVALLEE, *Matching 3-D anatomical surfaces with non-rigid deformations using octree-splines*, Int. J. of Computer Vision (IJCV), (18) (1996), pp. 171–186.
11. E. VARLET, *Etude d'un simulateur pédagogique d'écho-endoscopie digestive, modélisation et réalisation*, PhD thesis, Université Sciences et Techniques de Lille, octobre 1997.

Isolating Moving Anatomy in Ultrasound Without Anatomical Knowledge: Application to Computer-Assisted Pericardial Punctures

A. Bzostek[1], G. Ionescu[2], L. Carrat[2], C. Barbe[2], O. Chavanon[2,3], J. Troccaz[2]

[1] CIS Laboratory, Department of Computer Science, The Johns Hopkins University
[2] TIMC Laboratory, Faculté de Médecine de Grenoble
[3] Cardiac Surgery Department, Grenoble University Hospital

Abstract. This paper presents an approach to semiautomatic segmentation over a time series without the use of *a priori* geometric anatomical knowledge, and demonstrates its applicability to pericardial effusion segmentation from ultrasound. The described technique solves the problem in two stages, first automatically calculating a set of exclusion zones, then leveraging the surgeon's anatomical knowledge, simply and interactively, to create a region which corresponds to the stable region within the target effusion. In preliminary testing, the system performs well versus manual segmentation, outperforming it both in terms of perceived quality, as measured in a blinded comparison by an expert, and in terms of time required for generation.

1 Introduction

Significant work has been devoted to the extraction of anatomical contours in medical imagery from various modalities. Ultrasound imaging poses particular challenges because of its inherently low signal-to-noise ratio, and the dependence of its images on the angle and texture of the target anatomy. Its safety and non-invasiveness, however, maintain this technique's popularity among practitioners. In order to overcome ultrasound's difficulties, most previous attempts at automated segmentation have either relied upon the coding of anatomical knowledge into the recognition procedure, or involved a user heavily in the segmentation process, especially in its initialization. In this paper we present a technique for segmenting moving anatomy which does not rely on any coded knowledge about the target anatomy save that that it is moving cyclically. Instead of in-depth knowledge of the anatomy, the presented algorithm uses knowledge about the ultrasound image formation, and two simple pieces of user input to generate a "safe" segmentation of a pericardial effusion. Because this input is used as the last step of the segmentation process, as opposed to its initialization, the inputs' affects can be viewed and adjusted interactively. By combining simple information over time with this small amount of interactive input, the system is able to achieve a general segmentation of anatomy, even when segmentation of that anatomy within the individual images is quite difficult. Not only is the presented technique nearly automatic, but it produces segmentations which appear to be at least as good as those produced by expert humans, in less time as well. This paper will first present a short overview of previous, related work and an outline of the target procedure. After presenting the technique, we will then present the results from preliminary validation experiments, and will conclude with possible directions for further work.

2 Background

Pericardial effusions are created when, due to disease or injury, fluid collects between the heart and the pericardium, an outer, sack-like sheath that surrounds it. It is particularly common after cardiac surgery [1]. In order to avoid complications, including cardiac tamponade and constrictive pericarditis, the fluid must be drained. This can be achieved through access established percutaneously, using a needle under ultrasound guidance. The minimally invasive puncture poses many difficulties to the surgeon relating both to the difficulty of the task and the extreme sensitivity to errors, particularly in overinsertions, where the epicardium can be punctured. Consequently, surgeons are often reticent to approach small (< ~15mm) or badly placed effusions percutaneously and thus open surgery is preferred in these cases.

2.1 Computer-Assisted Pericardial Puncture

In order to assist surgeons in this task, a system, CASPER, was developed by Barbe, et al [2,3] which provides computer-based guidance during the puncture. They have shown that there exists, for these effusions, a stable target area which remains within the effusion throughout the cardiac cycle. Using CASPER, a surgeon defines this "safe" target area for the needle insertion based on ultrasound imagery registered using an Optotrak IR tracking system. This is accomplished by first, allowing the user to segment the effusion in each of a set of nearly parallel images, then, combining these segmentations to generate the minimal common target area. Again using the IR tracker, the system follows the puncture needle and provides feedback to the surgeon. The feedback combines this positional information with the "safe" target and an insertion trajectory defined intraoperatively. This process was satisfactory for validation, but is labor intensive and needs to be more automated to allow the use of the system clinically. The work presented in this paper attempts to automate this segmentation process.

2.2 Related Work

Automation of image-based medical tasks has been a target of research for some time. Consequently, there is a large body of work dedicated to this sometimes difficult task. Potentially applicable groundwork has been done in texture analysis [4-12] and optical flow [13-19].

Quite a bit of work has been particularly focused on the segmentation of the beating heart from time-sequences of ultrasound images. Though the modality and target anatomy of these systems are the same, their objective and restrictions are different from ours. Previous work has focused primarily on the segmentation of the left ventricle (LV) for geometric and functional analysis [20-28]. Many of these techniques [21-23,25,27] rely on user input for initialization information, and all of them rely on the fact that the image of the target (LV) has some known geometric properties. Additionally, none of these technique are intraoperative, and thus do not have tight time constraints. While our required segmentation is simpler than those used for LV analysis, the lack of known view orientation and target geometry, as well as the time requirements imposed intraoperatively make the problem an interesting one.

3 Methods

The method we have developed is divided into two stages. First, a set of "safe" regions are generated automatically. Using only our knowledge that the target anatomy (heart and pericardium) will either be moving cyclically, or stable and give high response, these regions are created as to not contain any such anatomy in any of the used images. Second, using three pieces of user input, a target zone is calculated which stays within the "safe" regions. Because the first component is computed completely automatically, interactive manipulation of the input and viewing of the resulting target area is possible.

3.1 Image Collection

Images are from a PAL video stream generated by the ultrasound imager. When using a curved probe, imager calibration techniques described in [3] are used to calbrate the imager and covert the image into its inherant polar coordinates.

3.2 Safe Region Generation

The generation of anatomy-free regions is accomplished in three steps:

- *Segmentation:* A rough segmentation, which includes the target anatomy, is generated for each image.
- *Selection:* A set of pixels, or *seeds*, which touch regions of target anatomy are selected for the set of images.
- *Summation:* Portions of the segmentations which are touched by seeds are summed to generate "unsafe" areas which contain target anatomy.

Segmentation. Each rough segmentation is generated using a non-isotropic Laplacian of Deriche (LoD) filter [28], applying a high-pass horizontal run-length filter, and then removing very small groups.

Ultrasound image response falls off dramatically as the angle between the measurement wave and the imaged surface decreases below 45°. Thus, only anatomy whose surface is near perpendicular to the probe direction will be well imaged. Systematic image components (connected groups of high response), which run vertically can thus be considered noise. By applying a non-isotropic LoD, with a small α (large standard deviation, β of the corresponding Gaussian Curve) in the horizontal direction, and large α vertically, the width of near vertical image components is highly reduced. Then, using a horizontal run-length filter, narrow, vertical segmented regions are removed.

Finally, the remaining groups with less than a low threshold size are removed. The resulting segmentation removes much of the systematic noise inherent in the ultrasound images (see **example 1**). This segmentation captures the target anatomy to a very high degree. Unfortunately, it also segments other components in the image.

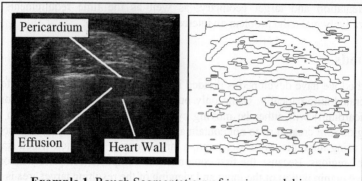

Example 1. Rough Segmentatioin of *in vivo* model image

Selection In order to find important areas in the image, sets of seed pixels are selected, based on sets of attributes calculated per pixel. Two sets of seeds are generated, one corresponding to static, one to moving anatomy. Together, these seed pixels touch both the parts of the image which are strong and stable (pericardium), and those whose strength varies cyclically (heart).

The static seeds are generated simply by calculating the energy (sum squared of activation) at each pixel over all images, and thresholding these values so that a target percentage of the image is covered.

The dynamic seeds are calculated using a similar procedure, except instead of measuring a single attribute, each pixel's value is calculated as the product for four separate, but related measures:

- S/N Ratio of maximum Harmonic
- Power of maximum Harmonic
- Log of the size of the pixel's uniform max harmonic frequency group
- Edge "Pass Over" Count

These attributes measure, respectively, how strongly a pixel's response over time corresponds to a cycle, how strong that cycle is, how large of a connected group is moving in the same cycle, and how much segmented edge motion passes over the pixel. Pixels with high values in all of these attributes are highly likely to lie in regions of the image which contain cyclically moving anatomy, though these pixels will not cover all such regions (see **example 2**).

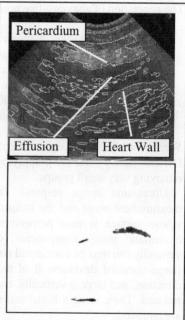

Example 2. Human Images: *TOP*: Image w/ rough segmentation, *BOTTOM*: Dynamic Seeds from the same image set (corrected for curvature)

Summation Once the seeds are determined, we use these, in conjunction with the segmented regions, to generate areas which could contain target anatomy. For each image, a set of pixels is marked which, moving only through regions marked as "inside" by the segmentation, are within a threshold distance of a seed pixel, and which belong to connected marked groups larger than a small threshold size. Any pixel that is marked for any image is considered "unsafe". Thus, those pixels not marked in any image comprise the "safe" zones (see **example 3**).

3.3 Target Area Selection

The automatically generated "safe" zones now constrain the choice of a target area, but in order to actually select a target from the image, anatomical knowledge is necessary. By allowing the user to select a target area in a simple way, we leverage the surgeon's anatomical knowledge in a non-obtrusive manner.

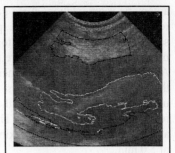

Example 3. Human Image w/ contours of "Unsafe" regions *Black contours-* generated from static seeds, *white regions-* generated from dynamic ones

User Input

User input consists of three things: a center point, a maximum radius, and a smoothing value for the target area. Because the creation of the "safe" zones from the *summation process* need not be repeated, the values specifying the target area can be inputted and modified interactively until the user is satisfied.

Area Generation

Given the user input, a target zone is generated by marking all pixels within the safe zone within the inputted radius from the center, as calculated by traversing only pixels in this zone (similar to the procedure for the seeding of the segmentations in the previous section). An opening of the specified size is then applied and the unconstrained, rounded ends are removed. (see **Example 4**).

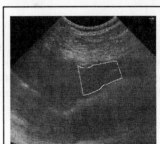

Example 4. Human Image w/ generated target area

4 Results

In order to validate this technique and compare it to manual segmentation, three approaches have been used to date. First, manual segmentations of recorded image sets have been compared directly to segmentations generated automatically (using the center point and radius from the manually generated regions instead of user input). Second, using these same segmentations, a human expert has been asked to rate and compare the segmentations without knowing how they were generated. Third, in order to compare times, automated segmentations were generated on the intra-operative system, using prerecorded data.

4.1 Difference Comparison

Using the center point and maximum radius from manually generated segmentations, automatic segmentations were generated for 10 recorded data sets. The parts of the segmentations corresponding to the inner and outer walls of the effusion were then compared. A difference measure was generated by filling the area between the contours (inner-to-inner, outer-to-outer), then dividing the area of these regions by their length. The differences averaged 3.5 mm, with a maximum difference of 5.0 mm.

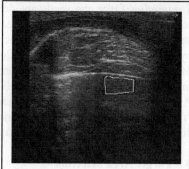

Example 5. Model Image: Manual (*black*) and Generated (*white*) target areas.

4.2 Blinded Survey

The differences found in the last test cannot necessarily be taken as errors on the part of the automatic procedure. It is possible that they fall within the range of acceptable segmentations. To test the quality of the generated segmentations, an expert human (a cardiac surgeon), was asked to compare the segmentations (both automatic and manual) without knowledge as to how the segmentations were generated. As rated by this surgeon, the automatic segmentations were favored overall, and individually in 8 of 10 cases. In the two cases in which the manual segmentation was rated as better, the surgeon rated the automated segmentation as "too conservative".

4.3 Comparison in Intra-Operative System

Running on the same system, the time required for the semi-automatic segmentation was compared against that for the manual segmentation. The semi-automated system requiried approximately 5 minutes (4 minutes of automatic processing, 1 minute of manual selection), while the purely solution required 10.

5 Future Work

More work needs to be done in order to validate the proposed system. Investigations need to be conducted in an *in-vivo* environment and more extensive work needs to be conducted on human effusion images. We are very encouraged by the current results and do not foresee any significant obstacles.

Additionally, there are many ways to extend this work, some of which are being actively investigated. The choice of selection measures is heuristic and thus open to significant extension. Work is currently being done to assess time-texture measures, particularly simple measures such as entropy, as components for this measure.

The automated component of the system could be applied as an initial processing step for a more complete segmentation, allowing a region of interest and geometry approximation to be constructed before a detailed image-by-image segmentation is conducted. The complete system could also be applicable to other procedures where segmentation of each of a series of images is difficult, but where a composite segmentation is the objective.

6 Conclusions

We have presented an approach to semi-automatic segmentation which seeks not to capture the anatomical knowledge of a surgeon, but to utilize it efficiently. As applied to pericardial effusion segmentation, it seeks to generate a composite segmentation from a series of images none of which can be well segmented individually. Rather than an initialization, user interaction is utilized as a final step allowing the interactive manipulation of the inputs and the watching of their affects on the final result. In the preliminary testing so far conducted, the system has performed well and takes less time than manual segmentation. And, while its segmentations sometimes differ from those generated manually by small amounts, it appears that those it generates are not only adequate, but usually better than those created by hand, and, in those cases where they are worse, the segmentations are more conservative. Combining this with the CASPER system's already demonstrated guidance capability could give surgeons the confidence to approach a variety of effusions percutaneously.

Acknowledgements

Supported by NSF Whitaker Foundation Program on Cost-Reducing Health Care Technologies (grant # BES9520501) and INSERM PSTRC grant (GMCAO project # PARMPSTRC9607).

References

1. J. Sahni, T. Ivert, I Harzfeld and L. Bodin. "Late cardiac Tamponade after Open-Heart Surgery," *Scan J. Thorac Cardiovasc Surg* 25, pp. 63-68, 1991.
2. Barbe, C., Carrat L., Chavanon O., and Troccaz, J., "Computer Assisted Pericardic Surgery," *Computer Assisted Radiology*, pp. 781-786, 1996.
3. Chavanon, O., Barbe, C., Troccaz, J., Carrat, L., Ribout C., Blin, D.," Computer Assisted PERicarial punctures: animal freasability study," *Proc. CVRMed-MRCAS '97*, pp. 285-294, 1997.
4. Mir, A.H.; Hanmandlu, M.; and Tandon, S.N.; "Texture analysis of CT images"; *IEEE Engineering in Medicine and Biology*; 781-786; December 1985
5. Bleck, J.S.; Ranft, U.; Hecker, H.; Bleck, M.W.; Thiesemann, C.; Wagner, S.; and Manns, M.;, "Random field models in textural analysis on ultrasonic images of the liver" *IEEE Trans. Medical Imaging*, vol. 15, no. 6, pp. 796-801, Dec. 1996.
6. Conners, R.W.; and Harlow, C.A.; "A theoretical comparison of texture algorithms"; *IEEE Trans. Pattern Analysis and Machine Intelligence*; Vol. PAMI-2; No. 3; pp. 204-222; May 1980.
7. Hall, E.L.; Crawford, W.O.; and Roberts, F.E.; "Computer classification of pneumoconiosis from radiographs of coal workers"; *IEEE Trans. Biomedical Engineering*; vol. BME-2; No. 1; pp. 518-52; Nov 1985.
8. Lizzi, F.L.;, "Relationship of ultrtasonic spectral parameters to features of tissue microstructure" *IEEE Trans. Sonics and Ultrasonics*, vol. UFFC-33, no. 3, pp. 319-329, May 1986.
9. Sutton, R.; and Hall, E.L.; "Texture measures for automatic classification of pulmonary diseases; *IEEE Trans. on Computers*; Vol. C-2; No7; pp667-676; July 1972.
10. Tsatsanis, M.K.; and Giannakis, G.B.;, "Object and texture classification using higher order statistics" *IEEE Trans. Pattern Analysis and Machine Intelligence*, vol. 14, no. 7, pp. 733-749, July 1992.

11. Wu, C.M.; Chen, Y.c.; and Hsieh, K.S., "Texture features for classification of ultrasonic liver images", *IEEE Trans. Medical Imaging*; vol 11; no. 2; pp. 141-152; June 1992.
12. Kruger, R.P.; Thompson, W.B.; and Turner, A.F.; "Computer diagnosis of Pneumoconiosis"; *IEEE Trans. Systems, Man and Cybernetics*; vol. SMC-4; no 1 ;pp 40-49; Jan .1974.
13. Meunier, J.; Sehboub, Z.; Bertrand, M.; and Lesperence, J.; "Estimation of the left ventricle 3-D motion from single plane cineangiograms"; *Not. Av.* 1993
14. Mailloux, G.E.; Bleau, A.; Bertrand, M.; and Petitclerc, R.; "Computer analysys of heart motion from two-dimensional echocardiograms"; *IEEE Trans. Medical Imaging*; vol BME34; no4; pp356-364; May 1987.
15. Mailloux, G.E.; Langlois, F.; Simard, P.Y.; and Bertrand, M.; "Restauration of the velocity field of the heart from two-dimensional echocardiograms"; *IEEE Trans. Medical Imaging*; vol8 no 2, pp. 143-153; June 1989.
16. Thomson, W.B.; Mutch, K.M.; and Berzins, V.A.; "Dynamic occlusion analysis on optical flow fields"; *IEEE Trans. Pattern Analysis and Machine Intelligence*; PAMI-7; no 4. pp 373-383, July1985.
17. Meunier, J,; and Bertrand, M.;, "Caracterisation des tissus par analyse de mouvement de la granularite echographique" Innov. Tech. Biol. Med., vol. 15, no. 3, pp. 268-280, 1994.
18. Meunier, J.; and Bertrand, M.;, "Ultrasonic texture motion analysis : theory and simulation" IEEE Trans. Medical Imaging, vol. 14, no. 2, pp. 293-300, June 1995.
19. Schunk, B.G.;, "Image flow segmentation and estimation by constraint line clustering" IEEE Trans. Pattern Analysis and Machine Intelligence, vol. 11, no. 10, pp. 1010-1027, Oct. 1989.
20. Han, C.Y., Kwun, N.L., Wee, W.G., Mintz, R.M., Porembka, D.T., "Knowledge-Based Image Analysis for Automated Boundary Extraction of Transesophogeal Echocardiographic Left-Ventricular Images," *IEEE Transactions on Medical Imaging*, vol. 10, No. 4, pp. 602-610, December 1991.
21. Kingler, J. W., Vaughn, C. L., Fraker, T. D. Andrews, L. T., "Segmentation of Echocardiographic Images Using Methematical Morphology," *IEEE Transactions on Biomedical Engineering*, vol. 35, no. 11, pp. 925 – 934, November, 1988.
22. Chu, C. H., Delp, E. J., Buda, A. J., "Detecting Left Ventricular Endocardial and Epicardial Boundaries by Digital Two-Dimensional Echocardiography", *IEEE Trans. On Medical Imaging*, vol. 7, no. 2, June 1988.
23. Teles de Figueiredo, M., Leitão, J. M. N., "Baysian Estimation of Ventricular Contours in Angiographic Images", *IEEE Transactions on Medical Imaging*, vol. 11, no. 3, September 1992.
24. Dias, J. M. B., Leitão, J. M. N., "Wall Position and Thickness Estimation from Sequences of Echocardiographic Images," *IEEE Trans. On Medical Imaging*, vol. 15, no. 1, February 1996.
25. Lilly, P, Jenkins, J., Bourdillon, P., "Automatic Contour Definition on Left Ventriculograms by Image Evidence and a Multiple Template-Based Model," *IEEE Trans. On Medical Imaging.* Vol. 8, no. 2, June 1989.
26. Friedland, N, Adam, D., "Automatic Ventricular Cavity Boundary Detection from Sequention Ultrasound Images Using Simulated Annealing," *IEEE Trans. On Medical Imaging*, vol. 8, no. 4, December 1989.
27. Detmer, Paul R., Bashein, G., Martin, R. W., "Matched Filter Identification of Left-Ventricular Endocardial Borders in Transesophageal Echocardiograms," *IEEE Trans. On Medical Imaging*, vol. 9, no. 4, December 1990.
28. Deriche, R, "Fast Algorithms for Low-Level Vision", *IEEE Transactions of Pattern Analysis and Machine Intelligence*, vol. 12, no. 1, January 1990.
29. Press, W. H., Teukolsky, S. A., Vetterling, W. T., *Numerical Recipes in C: The Art of Scientific Computing*, 2nd Edition, Cambridge Univ. Pr., January 1993.

A New Branching Model: Application to Carotid Ultrasonic Data

Alexandre Moreau-Gaudry[1], Philippe Cinquin[1] and Jean-Philippe Baguet[2]

[1] TIMC-IMAG, Institut Albert Bonniot, 38706 La Tronche cedex, FRANCE
{Alexandre.Moreau-Gaudry, Philippe.Cinquin}@imag.fr
[2] Department of Internal Medicine and Cardiology, Hôpital Michallon, CHU Grenoble, FRANCE

Abstract. Ultrasonic acquisition, by its simplicity, low cost and non invasiveness, emerged as an essential supplementary examination for cardiovascular diseases. The aim of this study is to demonstrate the feasibility of a global branching artery modelling. A geometrical approach is used for that purpose. A surface, based on a deformable skeleton and envelope, is defined. Including the shape as an a priori knowledge, this surface is fitted with 3D ultrasonic data by an iterative downhill gradient descent. Quality of the fit is illustrated by figures and numerical results. This tool could be used for objective spatial quantification and can be a useful instrument for blood flow modelling.

1 INTRODUCTION

In industrialized countries, cardiovascular diseases are the most significant mortality causes. In terms of frequency, morbidity and mortality, coronary diseases represent the most important part. Infraclinic atherosclerosis is an abnormality in-between cardiovascular risk factors and athero-thrombotic complications. Its ultrasonic diagnosis on peripherical arteries, particularly carotid, is going to benefit from the introduction of 2.5D ultrasound (2D ultrasonic data located in 3D space [4]). Our objective is to initialize a 3D automatic analysis of the whole artery by fitting a global branching model to the branching of the carotid. This defines an absolute reference system, that can improve the reproductibility of the ultrasonic exploration: tissular modifications can be followed in this reference system. Such a system would be a potentially useful and objective tool to follow disease outcome or to describe therapeutic treatment efficiency.

2 A NEW BRANCHING MODEL

In the first approximation, an arterial branching is a volumetric **"Y"**. From this ensues one of the principal modelling difficulties: the shape is not homotopic to a cylinder, a sphere, or a torus. So, we can not use deformable models like [5, 9] only defined for one of these different topologies. Furthermore, generalization of these approaches to a branching topology appears as a difficult problem.

A branching rebuilding was considered in [6] but it doesn't deal with it globally: each branch of the branching artery is rebuilt independently from the two others. The branching heart is then obtained by an interpolation between the three branches. In this context, the a priori knowledge intrinsically contained in the branching is not used for data fitting.

Another approach for rough branching reconstruction was presented in [1] by the use of implicit iso-surfaces generated by skeletons. In this rebuilding, we find again the previously described pitfall, but it could be interesting to establish relations between different parts of skeletons to integrate the a priori knowledge.

Topologically adaptative deformable models are quoted in [8]. These have been shown to be promising in segmenting vascular structures in 2D and 3D images and in dealing effectively with branching. But contrary to these last two approaches, we focus on an explicit modeling of branches.

The model that we developed includes the shape as an a priori knowledge. Its presentation is divided in two parts: the first one describes shape building, and the second one presents the classical rigid transformations applied to our model.

2.1 THE SHAPE

A shape description is presented figure 1. A surface $M(t,v)$ is a function of two parameters t and v. Because a branching appears to be characterized by its upper convexity, we model it by a plane curve, named **external skeleton S_e** and parameterized by t. To create the surface delimiting the branching, plane closed curves, parameterized by v, are built continuously on S_e: their mathematical envelope then defines the branching. Each plane containing the plane curve is characterized by only one t; coefficients defining the curve are a function of t because of the continuous building.

As regards the look of our plane curve, because we want to be synthetic and realistic, a plane superquadric seems to be a good candidate. Three elements are essential for its definition: the center and the two axis. One axis is defined in direction and norm by the center C of the superquadric and the point M_e of S_e on which the superquadric is built. Now, if we consider the set of all centers when t is varying, we are naturally driven to the notion of the **internal skeleton S_i**.

So, the shape is made up of a skeleton and an envelope. This envelope is supported by the skeleton. The skeleton is split in two components, internal and external.

The external skeleton S_e. To keep the complexity down, S_e must have a minimal number of degrees of freedom. We choose a "polynomial" parametric plane curve coming from the cissoïd family [7] according to our modelling concept of the branching convexity and its simple definition by three shape parameters. The coordinates of the current point $Me(t)$ $t \in [-1..1]$ are shown in the equation (1).

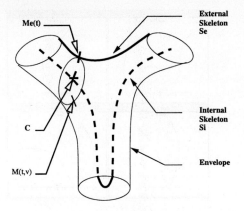 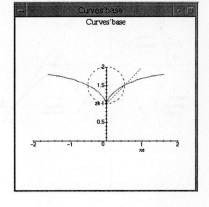

Fig. 1. Description of the shape   **Fig. 2.** Plane curves' base

$$Me(t) = \begin{pmatrix} \frac{a_1*t+a_2*t^2+a_3*t^3}{1+t^2} \\ 0 \\ 1 + \frac{t^2}{1+t^2} \end{pmatrix} = C + a1 * M1(t) + a2 * M2(t) + a3 * M3(t) \ . \quad (1)$$

$M3(t)$ covers a cissoïd and gives the branching idea. $M2(t)$, describing a line, creates asymmetry. $M1(t)$ is on a circle, making round S_e (see figure 2). This decomposition shows advantages of this external skeleton parameterization: we are "polynomial" with natural basic deformations. For the same degrees of freedom, to build a model from a parabolic curve, for example, is not so obvious. Figure 4 shows different forms of S_e (thin upper curves).

The internal skeleton S_i. The middle part of S_i is defined by a plane curve coming from the cissoïd family (parameterized by u). Two splines with four control points are added on each side to take information along upper branches into account. $C1$ continuity is assured. At this development state of the model, it is characterized by 14 parameters: three for S_e, three for the central part of S_i, and four parameters for each lateral splines. Figure 3 presents the building. Figure 4 shows different forms of S_i (thick lower curves).

Consistency of the skeleton. To guarantee the model definition, we must avoid geometric intersections between S_e and S_i. For this reason, constraints on different shape parameters are imposed: S_i is then characterized by five parameters. Figure 3 shows examples of constraints on control points: points at the ends of S_i P_{4r} and P_{4l} are forced to travel on the half line orthogonal to the speed vector in $Me(1)$ and $Me(-1)$. Points P_{3r} and P_{3l} cover segments of horizontal line. $P_{1r}, P_{1l}, P_{2r}, P_{2l}$ are fixed by $C1$ continuity. Figure 4 shows different forms of skeleton.

Furthermore, to build a surface parameterized by t, we have to establish a one-to-one mapping between S_i and S_e. Let $M_i(u)$ be the unique point of S_i

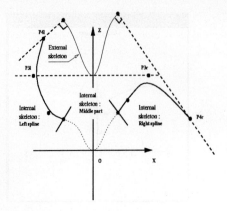
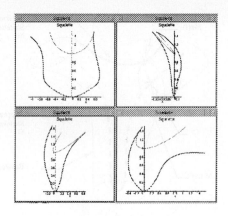

Fig. 3. Internal skeleton building with constraints on control points

Fig. 4. Example of skeleton for different shape parameters

corresponding to $M_e(t)$, one point of S_e. We propose to define $M_i(u)$ by the equation (2) :

$$\overrightarrow{M_i(u)M_e(t)} \cdot \frac{\overrightarrow{dM_e(t)}}{dt} = 0 \ . \qquad (2)$$

This last equation is cubic in u. Thanks to the constraints on parameters, we obtain an explicit solution u of t by the use of CARDAN's formula. Each point of S_i is then located by a unique t (see figure 5). An explicit relation between these two curves is a main point for the model efficiency, because no numerical estimations are needed for describing exactly the surface.

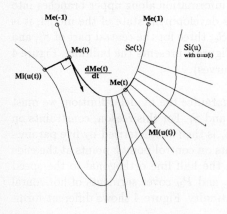
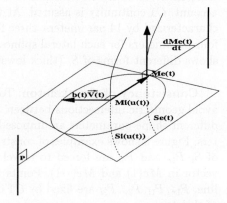

Fig. 5. Illustration of the one-to-one mapping between S_e and S_i

Fig. 6. Representation of the minor axis

The envelope. The final surface is obtained by a continuous juxtaposition of 2D superquadrics [3]. Each superquadric i is bound to the external skeleton at point $M_e(t_i)$. Its center is the image $M_i(u(t_i))$ by the bijection defined in (2). Thus, the branching surface is defined by the following 3D vector:

$$M(t,v) = \vec{A}(t,v) + \vec{B}(t,v) .$$
$$\vec{A}(t,v) = \overrightarrow{M_i(u(t))M_e(t)} * cos(v)^{\epsilon(t)} . \quad (3)$$
$$\vec{B}(t,v) = b(t) * \overrightarrow{V(t)} * sin(v)^{\epsilon(t)} .$$

$\overrightarrow{V(t)}$ is the unit vector normal to the plane $\mathcal{P}$ in $M_i(u(t))$. $\mathcal{P}$ is defined by the equation (4). An illustration is shown in the figure 6.

$$\mathcal{P} : (M_i(u(t)), \overrightarrow{M_i(u(t))M_e(t)}, \frac{d\overrightarrow{M_e(t)}}{dt}) . \quad (4)$$

$b(t)$ represents the "minor" axis norm of the 2D superquadric: it is defined for $t \in [-1,1]$ by two splines with four control points, with a $C1$ continuity in $t = 0$. Six constraint parameters are necessary to characterize it.

$\epsilon(t)$ is a function defined for $t \in [-1,1]$ with values in $]0,1]$. This function allows deformations of 2D superquadrics from an ellipse to a rectangle: a better fit can then be reached in the central region of the artery. Its definition using three parameters α, β, γ is the following:

$$\epsilon(t) = \alpha + (1-\alpha) * \frac{\frac{\delta^2(t)}{1+\delta^2(t)}}{\frac{\beta^2}{1+\beta^2}} . \quad (5)$$
$$\delta(t) = \beta * (t+\gamma) .$$

Finally, we build a branching shape with 17 parameters (shape parameters). Each parameter value has been specifically restricted according to geometric model properties to maintain a meaning shape. Examples of surfaces are presented in the figure 7.

2.2 RIGID TRANSFORMATIONS

The rigid transformations applied to our model are classically defined by 7 parameters (spatial parameters): three Euler angles ψ, θ, φ, three translation parameters T_x, T_y, T_z and one size factor S.

3 MINIMIZATION METHOD

Let N_d data points M_i $_{i=1..N_d}$ extracted from ultrasonic data (see section 4). An energy $\mathcal{E}$ is defined in (6) as the euclidean distance of data points to the surface.

$$\mathcal{E} = \sum_{i=1}^{N_d} ||\overrightarrow{M_i \mathcal{P}_{M_i}(t_i, v_i, X)}||^2 \ . \tag{6}$$

It is a function of 24 parameters X_j $_{j=1..24}$: 17 shape parameters and 7 spatial parameters. $\mathcal{P}_{M_i}(t_i, v_i, X)$ represents the projection of M_i on the surface, t_i, v_i its parameters. An explicit derivative of the cost function according to each parameter X_j is computed by Maple software (Maple V Release 4). We use a Fletcher-Reeves-Polak-Ribiere minimization [10]. During this iterative descent method, we respect the constraints on each parameter by a simple projection according to the descent direction. To decrease time consuming, we do not estimate the energy function during a descent step. All spatial and shape parameters are adjusted simultaneously, so most of the given data points lie close to the model's surface. Initial spatial position is defined manually by selection of the three branching ends. Initial shape parameters are fixed to neutral position according to the definition field. Because of the non convexity of the cost function, and the non convexity of the constraints domain, this minimization drives us to the nearest local minima.

4 DATA COLLECTION

Data are obtained with collaboration of the Department of Internal Medicine and Cardiology at the Grenoble University Hospital. Echographic images are acquired by a HP SONOS (Hewlett-Packard, Santa Clara, California, USA) ultrasonic system. They are stored on an optical disk and computed on a workstation (HP 715/100). A set of 4366 2D points are generated by a semiautomatic segmentation step.

During the medical exploration, the ultrasonic system is connected to an optical localizer (Optotrak Northern Digital Inc.). To collect 2.5D data [4], a six degrees-of-freedom optical tracking device attached to the ultrasound probe is used. The optical tracking system works with infrared diodes put on the probe which are then located by three fixed CCD cameras (Optotrak Northern Digital Inc.). Position and orientation of the echographic planes are thus obtained during all the exploration. Thanks to a temporal synchronization between echographic and spatial data, 3D spatial coordinates for each previous 2D points are computed.

5 RESULTS

Thanks to the a priori knowledge contained in the model, the initialization of the minimization process is easy. Figure 7c shows distance from data to surface resulting from the minimization process. Compared to the figure 7a, one can clearly notice a visual improvment with regard to the data fitting. Numerically, with the previously described data collection, the rms for the cost function decreases from 1.17 to 0.56. Because of the great number of data, the time limiting element of the minimization process is the downhill direction evaluation.

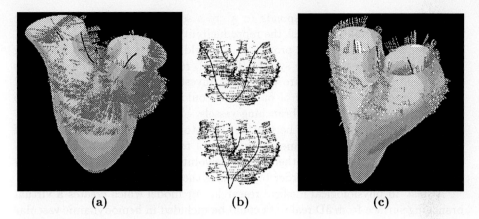

Fig. 7. (a) shows initial surface, distance (gray lines) from data (white points) to the initial surface and parts of the skeleton (black lines). (b) represents data (black points) and deformations of the skeleton (black lines): the top part of the figure shows the initial skeleton; the bottom part, the final skeleton resulting from the minimization process. (c) illustrates final surface, distance (gray lines) from data (white points) to the final surface, and parts of the skeleton (black lines).

6 DISCUSSION AND CONCLUSION

6.1 ADVANTAGES AND PITFALLS

In medical ultrasonic investigation, image analysis is in progress, but only few methods are able to describe automatically the division of one artery in two branches [6, 2]: the first one uses an interpolation of explicit generalized cylinders; the second one uses an implicit approach. To our knowledge, no explicit deformable branching model incorporating the shape as an a priori information had been developed. The aim of this geometric model is to demonstrate the feasibility of modelling the branching artery globally. This region of interest is fitted in one step by 24 parameters. Our tool takes into account the angle between the two derived arterial branches. A potential asymmetry between the branches is included by our model, which confirms its deformation capacity.

One of the pitfalls of our model is the relatively high number of parameters. Pertinence of model's parameters must be tested in the future. In the same time, parameters constraints may be reviewed to impose identifiability of the model.

6.2 PERSPECTIVES

The top part of the figure 7b shows data and initial skeleton; the bottom, the same data, the skeleton resulting from the minimization process and an unappropriatness between the size of each branch and the deepest point of the branching convexity. This remark could explain the relatively bad value of the residual error. The minimization result seems overevaluated. It could be easily improved by adding another longitudinal scale parameter for the external skeleton.

Our data collection corresponds to a cross sectional study. We need some longitudinal information to test the reproducibility and the parameters sensibility of our model. This tool is promising. It could be used for all the branching vessels acquired by ultrasonic system (femoral, renal, popliteal divisions). It is known that ultrasonic slices are very noisy. Investigations by CT scan or MRN could be interesting. The use of our model could be extended, particularly to cerebral, coronary or hepatic branching vessels.

Our geometric model will be the first step to an accurate quantification of this artery part. It will be a measurement tool to evaluate new medical therapeutics tested to slow down atherosclerosis evolution. It could be an element in medical decision making, in order to optimize the cost/benefit equation.

At last, in physiological medical research, our model which creates a virtual branching surface from 3D real data could be included in hemodynamic vascular model to test the local repercussion of turbulence on the atherosclerosis outcome.

Acknowledgments: This work was supported by Hewlett-Packard and Medasys Digital Systems.

References

1. E. Bittar, N. Tsingos, and M-P. Gascuel. Automatic Reconstruction of Unstructured 3D Data: Combining a Medial Axis and Implicit Surfaces. *Computer Graphics forum (Eurographics'95)*, 14(3):457–468, August 1995.
2. D.Attali E.Ferley, M.P.Cani-Gascuel. Skeletal Reconstruction of Branching Shapes. *The Eurographics Association*, 1997.
3. F.Solina and R.Bajcsy. Recovery of parametric models from range images : The case for superquadrics with global deformations. *IEEE Transactions on Pattern Analysis and Machine Intelligence*, 12(2):131–147, February 1990.
4. G.Champleboux and D.Henry. Parametric two-dimensional b-spline, representation of vein and artery from 2.5d echography used to aid virtual echography. *CVRMed-MRCAS'97-LNCS*, pages 285–294, 1997.
5. Lawrence H.Staib and James S.Duncan. Model-based deformable surface finding for medical images. *IEEE Transactions on Medical Imaging*, 15:720–731, October 1996.
6. V.Juhan B.Nazarian K.Malkani R.Bulot J.M.Bartoli and J.Sequeira. Geometrical modelling of abdominal aortic aneurysms. *CVRED-MRCAS*, pages 243–252, 1996.
7. VEB Bibliographisches Intitut Leipzig, editor. *Mathematics at a glance*. 1975.
8. T. McInerney and D. Terzopoulos. Deformable models in medical image analysis: a survey. *Medical Image Analysis*, 1(2):91–108, 1996.
9. S. Benayoun C.Nastar N.Ayache. Dense non-rigid motion estimation in sequence of 3d images using differential constraints. *CVRMed*, 1995.
10. W.H.Press W.T.Vetterling S.A.Teukolsky and B.P.Flannery. Numerical recipies in c : Second edition.

Multi-modal Volume Registration Using Joint Intensity Distributions

Michael E. Leventon and W. Eric L. Grimson

Artificial Intelligence Laboratory,
Massachusetts Institute of Technology, Cambridge, MA
leventon@ai.mit.edu
http://www.ai.mit.edu/projects/vision-surgery

Abstract. The registration of multimodal medical images is an important tool in surgical applications, since different scan modalities highlight complementary anatomical structures. We present a method of computing the best rigid registration of pairs of medical images of the same patient. The method uses prior information on the expected joint intensity distribution of the images when correctly aligned, given *a priori* registered training images. We discuss two methods of modeling the joint intensity distribution of the training data, mixture of Gaussians and Parzen windowing. The fitted Gaussians roughly correspond to various anatomical structures apparent in the images and provide a coarse anatomical segmentation of a registered image pair. Given a novel set of unregistered images, the algorithm computes the best registration by maximizing the log likelihood of the two images, given the transformation and the prior joint intensity model. Results aligning SPGR and dual-echo MR scans demonstrate that this algorithm is a fast registration method with a large region of convergence and sub-voxel registration accuracy.

1 Introduction

Medical scans such as Magnetic Resonance (MR) and computed tomography (CT) are currently common diagnostic tools in surgical applications. The intensity value at a given voxel of a medical scan is primarily a function of the tissue properties at the corresponding point in space. Typically, various anatomical structures appear more clearly in different types of internal scans. Soft tissue, for example, is imaged well in MR scans, while bone is more easily discernible in CT scans. Blood vessels are often highlighted better in an MR angiogram than in a standard MR scan. Figure 1 shows three different acquisitions of MR scans. Notice that some anatomical structures appear with more contrast in one image than in the others. Anatomical structures in these various modalities can be segmented and displayed separately. However, it is most convenient for the surgeon to have information about all the structures fused into one coherent dataset. To perform the multi-modality fusion, the different volumetric images are automatically registered to a single coordinate frame.

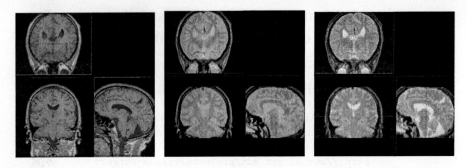

Fig. 1. SPGR, Proton Density, and T2 Weighted Magnetic Resonance images of a brain. Notice that some anatomical structures appear with more contrast in one image than the others.

1.1 Alignment of Features or Fiducials

One method of aligning two medical images is to extract features from the images, then compute the best alignment of the features [7]. This approach depends greatly on the ability to automatically and accurately extract reliable image features. In general, methods of feature extraction such as intensity thresholding or edge detection do not work well on medical scans, due to non linear intensity biases and highly textured structures. Without the ability to accurately localize corresponding features in the images, alignment in this manner is difficult.

A second registration method uses fiducial markers attached to a patient throughout the various acquisitions. If the markers can easily be located in the images, the volumes can be registered by computing the best alignment of the corresponding fiducials [8, 12]. The main drawback of this method is that the markers must remain attached to the patient throughout all image acquisitions.

1.2 Maximization of Mutual Information

Maximization of mutual information is a general approach applicable to a wide range of multi-modality registration applications [1, 2, 6, 11]. One of the strengths of using mutual information (and perhaps in some special cases, one of the weaknesses) is that MI does not use any prior information about the relationship between joint intensity distributions.

Given two random variables X and Y, mutual information is defined as [1]:

$$MI(X, Y) = H(X) + H(Y) - H(X, Y) \tag{1}$$

The first two terms on the right are the entropies of the two random variables, and encourage transformations that project X into complex parts of Y. The third term, the (negative) joint entropy of X and Y, takes on large values if X and Y are functionally related, and encourages transformations where X explains Y well. Mutual information does not use an *a priori* model of the relationships between the intensities of the different images. Our method not

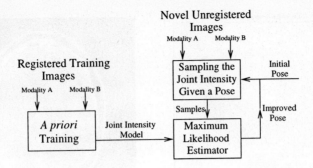

Fig. 2. Flowchart of the *a priori* training and the online registration.

only expects the relationship between the intensity values of registered images to be maximal in mutual information, but also to be similar to that of the pre-registered training data of the same modalities. The prior joint intensity model provides the registration algorithm with additional guidance which results in convergence on the correct alignment more quickly, more reliably and from further initial starting points.

1.3 Incorporating a Prior Model

The framework for our registration process is illustrated in Figure 2. The method requires a pair of registered training images of the same modalities as those we wish to register in order to build the joint intensity model. To align a novel pair of images, we compute the likelihood of the two images given a certain pose based on our model by sampling the intensities at corresponding points. We improve the current hypothesized pose by ascending the log likelihood function.

2 Learning the Joint Intensity Model

We consider two models of joint intensity: mixture of Gaussians and Parzen Window Density. In both methods, we seek to estimate the probability of observing a given intensity pair at the corresponding point in the two images.

2.1 Mixture of Gaussians Model

Given a pair of registered images from two different medical image acquisitions, we can assume that each voxel with coordinate $x = [x_1, x_2, x_3]^T$ in one image, I_1, corresponds to the same position in the patient's anatomy as the voxel with coordinate x in the other image, I_2. Further, consider that the anatomical structure S_k at some position in the patient will appear with some intensity value i_1 in the first image and i_2 in the second image with joint probability $P(i_1, i_2 \mid S_k)$. We also define $P(S_k) = \pi_k$ to be the prior probability that a random point in the medical scan corresponds to structure S_k.

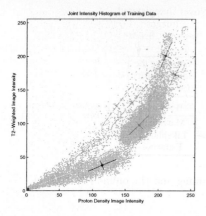 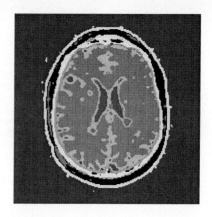

Fig. 3. LEFT: Joint intensity histogram of the registered MR PD/T2 training images used to fit a mixture of Gaussians. RIGHT: Rough segmentation of a registered image pair. Each voxel is classified based on which Gaussian it most likely belongs to, based on the mixture of Gaussian model.

By making the assumption that voxels are independent samples from this distribution (and ignoring relative positions of voxels), we have

$$P(I_1, I_2) = \prod_{x \in I} P(I_1(x), I_2(x)) \qquad (2)$$

$$= \prod_{x \in I} \sum_k \pi_k P(I_1(x), I_2(x) \mid S_k) \qquad (3)$$

We model the joint intensity of a particular internal structure S_k to be a two dimensional (dependent) Gaussian with mean μ_k and full covariance matrix Σ_k. Letting i be intensity pair $[i_1, i_2]^T$,

$$P(i \mid S_k) = \left(\frac{1}{2\pi |\Sigma_k|^{\frac{1}{2}}} e^{-\frac{1}{2}(i-\mu_k)^T \Sigma_k^{-1}(i-\mu_k)} \right) \qquad (4)$$

This model of the intensities corresponds to a mixture of Gaussians distribution, where each 2D Gaussian G_k corresponds to the joint intensity distribution of an internal anatomical structure S_k. Thus, the probability of a certain intensity pair (independent of the anatomical structure) given the model, M is

$$P(i \mid M) = \sum_k \left(\frac{\pi_k}{2\pi |\Sigma_k|^{\frac{1}{2}}} e^{-\frac{1}{2}(i-\mu_k)^T \Sigma_k^{-1}(i-\mu_k)} \right). \qquad (5)$$

To learn the joint intensity distribution under this model, we estimate the parameters π_k, μ_k, and Σ_k using the Expectation-Maximization (EM) method [3].

The mixture of Gaussians model was chosen to represent the joint intensity distribution because we are imaging a volume with various anatomical structures that respond with different ranges of intensity values in the two acquisitions. We

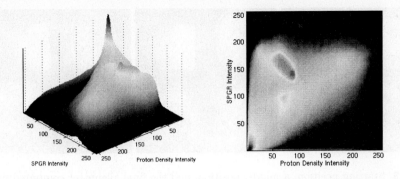

Fig. 4. Two views of the joint intensity distribution function computed using Parzen estimation with a Gaussian windowing function.

assume that those ranges of responses are approximately Gaussian in nature. Therefore, one might expect that each Gaussian in the mixture may correspond roughly to one type of anatomical structure. In other words, the model produces an approximate segmentation of the structures in the images. Figure 3b shows the segmentation of a registered pair of MR images using the Gaussian mixture model prior. Gerig, et al. [5] used similar methods of statistical classification to produce accurate unsupervised segmentation of 3D dual-echo MR data.

Segmentation of medical images based solely on intensity classification (without using position or shape information) is, in general, very difficult. Often different tissue types may produce a similar or overlapping range of intensity responses in a given medical scan, making classification by intensity alone quite challenging. MR images include nonlinear gain artifacts due to inhomogeneities in the receiver or transmit coils [4]. Furthermore, the signal can also be degraded by motion artifacts from movement of the patient during the scan.

The segmentation produced by this method shown in Figure 3b suffers from the difficulties described above. For example white matter and gray matter have overlapping ranges of intensities in both image acquisitions. Furthermore, note that the distinction between gray and white matter on the right hand side is not segmented clearly. This is most likely due to the bias field present in the image.

Despite these difficulties, the segmentation does a reasonable job of picking out the major structures, although it is inaccurate at region boundaries. Therefore, we do not intend to use this method alone to compute an accurate segmentation of the underlying structures. Instead, we could use the mixture model in combination with a more sophisticated algorithm to solve for segmentation, or for registration purposes, as described in section 3.

2.2 Parzen Window Density Estimation

The prior joint intensity distribution can also be modeled using Parzen window density estimation. A mixture of Gaussians model follows from the idea that the different classes should roughly correspond to different anatomical structures

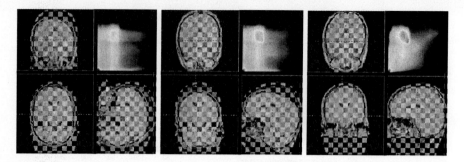

Fig. 5. Starting position, a middle position, and the final alignment computed by the registration gradient ascent algorithm. Each image shows the SPGR and PD overlayed in block format in the three orthogonal slices. The images in the upper right depict the histogram of the intensity pairs at that alignment. When the images are aligned, the histogram should resemble the distribution in Figure 4.

and thus provides an approximate segmentation into tissue classes. However, the EM algorithm for estimating the parameters of a mixture of Gaussians is sensitive to the initialization of the parameters and in some cases can result in an inaccurate prior model of the joint intensities.

We therefore also consider modeling the joint intensity distribution based on the Parzen window density estimation using Gaussians as the windowing function. In practice, this model defined by directly sampling the training data provides a better explanation of the intensity relationship than the Gaussian mixtures that require the estimation of various parameters.

Consider our registered training image pair $\langle I_1, I_2 \rangle$. We estimate the joint intensity distribution of an intensity pair $i = [i_1, i_2]^T$ given the prior model, M:

$$P(i \mid M) = \frac{1}{N} \sum_{\mu \in \langle I_1, I_2 \rangle} \left(\frac{1}{2\pi\sigma^2} e^{-\frac{1}{2\sigma^2}(i-\mu)^T(i-\mu)} \right), \qquad (6)$$

where the μ's are N samples of corresponding intensity pairs from the training images. Figure 4 illustrates this estimated joint intensity distribution.

3 Maximum Likelihood Registration

Given a novel pair of unregistered images of the same modalities as our training images, we assume that when registered, the joint intensity distribution of the novel images should be similar to that of the training data. When mis-registered, one structure in the first image will overlap a different structure in the second image, and the joint intensity distribution will most likely look quite different from the learned model. Given a hypothesis of registration transformation, T, and the Gaussian mixture model, M, we can compute the likelihood of the two images using Equation 2:

$$P(I_1, I_2 \mid T, M) = \prod_x P(I_1(x), I_2(T(x)) \mid T, M). \qquad (7)$$

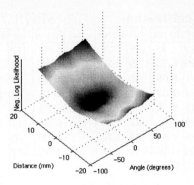

Fig. 6. Samples from the negative log likelihood function over various angles and x-shifts. Note that over this range, the function is very smooth and has one distinct minimum, which in this case occurs 0.86 mm away from the correct alignment.

We register the images by maximizing the log likelihood of the images, given the transformation and the model, and define the maximum likelihood transformation, T_{ML}, as follows:

$$\hat{T}_{ML} = \underset{T}{\operatorname{argmax}} \sum_x \log(P(I_1(x), I_2(T(x)) \mid T, M)) \tag{8}$$

The likelihood term in this equation can be substituted with either Equation 5 or 6, depending on which joint intensity model is chosen. For the results presented here, the Parzen model is used, as it better explains the intensity relationship between the two modalities. However, the mixture of Gaussians model encodes coarse tissue type classes and thus provides a framework for later incorporating into the registration process prior knowledge of the relative positions and shapes of the various internal structures.

To find the maximum likelihood transformation, T_{ML}, we use Powell maximization [9] to ascend the log likelihood function defined in Equation 8, finding the best rigid transformation. In both the mixture of Gaussian and Parzen window models of the distribution, the log likelihood objective function is quite smooth. Figure 6 illustrates samples from the negated objective function for various rotation angles (along one dimension) and x position shifts of the transformation. Over this sampled range of ±60 degrees and ±20 mm, the function is always concave and has one minimum which occurs within a millimeter of the correct transformation. Computing the registration by maximizing the likelihood of the image pair given the transformation and the model seems to be an efficient, accurate method of registration.

PD / T2 Registration									SPGR / PD Registration							
#	Error	#	Error	#	Error	#	Error	#	Error	#	Error	#	Error	#	Error
1	0.74	10	0.79	19	1.42	28	1.26	1	4.87*	10	1.47	19	2.57	28	1.54
2	0.89	11	0.73	20	0.75	29	0.76	2	2.69	11	3.17	20	2.67	29	2.15
3	0.86	12	0.68	21	0.69	30	2.24	3	0.16	12	1.32	21	2.77	30	1.50
4	0.79	13	1.52	22	1.33	31	0.90	4	0.78	13	1.18	22	3.47	31	1.43
5	0.90	14	0.63	23	0.66	32	0.78	5	1.69	14	1.59	23	3.87	32	1.83
6	0.80	15	0.80	24	1.01	33	1.28	6	5.59*	15	1.25	24	6.03*	33	1.64
7	0.81	16	0.89	25	1.07	34	0.74	7	3.02*	16	1.26	25	9.72*	34	3.18
8	0.80	17	0.82	26	0.70	35	1.08	8	1.36	17	1.19	26	2.03	35	2.01
9	0.82	18	1.36	27	0.81	36	0.89	9	0.73	18	1.85	27	5.03*	36	2.46

Table 1. The results of registering 36 test images. The registration error (in mm) was computed by taking the average error of the eight vertices of the imaging volume.
*The patient moved between scans and thus the ground truth is wrong. By inspection, our alignment looks better aligned than the "ground-truth" registration.

4 Results of Registration

The training and registration algorithms described above were tested using MR datasets from 37 patients[1]. Each patient was scanned using two protocols, a coronal SPGR scan of 256 × 256 × 124 voxels with a voxel size of 0.9375 × 0.9375 × 1.5 mm and a dual echo (proton density and T2-weighted) axial scan of 256 × 256 × 52 voxels with a voxel size of 0.9753 × 0.9375 × 3.0 mm. One of the patients' datasets was used for training purposes and the remaining 36 were used for testing. The two types of registration performed in these experiments were PD with T2 and SPGR with PD. The joint intensity distribution for each modality pair was modeled using a Parzen estimation. The initial pose in all cases was about 90° and a few centimeters away. Each registration converged in 1–2 minutes on a Pentium Pro 200. Table 1 shows the results of the registrations.

4.1 Proton Density and T2-Weighted Volume Registration

We first consider the problem of registering PD images to transformed T2 as a means of testing the registration algorithm. Each T2-weighted scan was rotated by 90° and translated 5 cm and then registered with the corresponding PD scan. Since these T2 and PD images were acquired at the same time and are originally in the same coordinate system, by perturbing one scan by a known amount, we have accurate ground-truth upon which to validate the registration process. All 36 test cases registered with sub-voxel, and in most cases with sub-millimeter accuracy. Note that the method has a large region of convergence and thus does not require the starting pose to be very near the correct solution.

---

[1] The MR datasets were provided by M. Shenton and others, see acknowledgments.

4.2 SPGR and Proton Density Volume Registration

A more interesting and more challenging alignment problem consists of registering each patient's coronal SPGR scan with the same patient's PD image. This registration problem is more challenging given that the two modalities were not acquired simultaneously and also do not contain the same region of the head: the PD/T2 images are cropped at the chin (see Figure 1).

Since each patient had the scans performed during the same sitting in the scanner, the headers of the scans provide the ground-truth alignment between the various acquisitions, assuming the patient did not move between acquisitions. However, since the patients' heads were not fixed in the scanner, patients could move between acquisitions. Despite this issue, we use the scanner poses as ground truth, since in most cases it seems that the patient did not move significantly. By visually inspecting the SPGR registered with the PD images using the ground truth, one notices a discrepancy of as much as a centimeter in six of the patients' scans (marked with an ∗ in Table 1). In these cases, the error values reported are not valid, and our registration qualitatively appears better aligned than the "ground-truth" registration. Of the 36 cases we have used in our initial tests of this method, almost all of the cases automatically registered to within one voxel, from a starting position of about 90° and a few centimeters away.

5 Future Work

The promising initial registration results described herein provide various directions of future work. To date, we have tested this registration algorithm only on MR images, primarily due the availability of this particular set of data. There is interest in acquiring more datasets of different modalities, including MR Angiogram, CT, and PET to further examine this registration technique by means of the Retrospective Registration Evaluation Project [12].

Another area of further investigation is to include additional statistical models to the current framework. Non-linear bias fields present in the MR data can cause mismatches in intensity histograms between the training and test images. Registration using a prior on joint intensity information can be sensitive to these differences. Thus, there is interest in integrating the statistical intensity correction work of Wells, *et al.* [10] into this registration technique to both provide a more reliable intensity correspondence between training and test data, and perhaps assist in the process of segmenting the anatomical structures in the images.

Additional information such as prior knowledge of the shapes or relative positions of internal structures may help in the registration process. Such information certainly aids in segmentation, by offering guidelines such as what structures are most likely to appear next to other structures. Given that segmentation and registration are related in that the knowledge of one greatly assists in the computation of the other, this would imply that the addition of these types of priors may also assist in registration.

6 Acknowledgments

This article describes research supported in part by DARPA under ONR contract N00014-94-01-0994 and a National Science Foundation Fellowship. This work was developed using MRI data provided by Martha Shenton, Jane Anderson, and Robert W. McCarley, Department of Psychiatry and Surgical Planning Lab of Brigham & Women's Hospital, and Brockton VA Medical Center. The authors would like to acknowledge Dr. Shenton's NIMH grants, K02 M-01110 and R29 MH-50747, and Dr. McCarley's grant, R01-40799, and the Brockton Schizophrenia Center for the Department of Veterans Affairs.

References

1. A.J. Bell and T.J. Sejnowski. "An information-maximisation approach to blind separation." In *Advances in Neural Information Processing* **7**, Denver, 1994.
2. A. Collignon, D. Verndermeulen, P. Suetens, and G. Marchal. "3D multi-modality medical image registration using feature space clustering". In *First Conf. on Computer Vision, Virtual Reality and Robotics in Medicine*. Springer, 1995.
3. R. Duda and P. Hart. *Pattern Classification and Scene Analysis*. John Wiley & Sons.
4. T. Kapur, W.E.L. Grimson, R. Kikinis, "Segmentation of Brain Tissue from MR Images", in *First Conf. on Computer Vision, Virtual Reality and Robotics in Medicine*, Nice France, April 1995, pp. 429–433.
5. G. Gerig, J. Martin, R. Kikinis, O Kubler, M. Shenton, F. Jolesz. "Unsupervised tissue type segmentation of 3D dual-echo MR head data." Image and Vision Computing, IPMI 1991 special issue, **10**(6):349-360, 1992.
6. F. Maes, A. Collignon, D. Vandermeulen, G. Marchal, and P. Suetens. "Multi-modality image registration by maximization of mutual information", in *Mathematical Methods in Biomedical Image Analysis*. IEEE Computer Society Press, 1996.
7. J.B. Antoine Maintz, P.A. van den Elsen, and M.A. Viergever. "Comparison of Feature-Based Matching of CT and MR Brain Images." *Computer Vision, Virtual Reality and Robotics in Medicine*, Nice France, April 1995, pp. 219–228.
8. V.R. Mandava, J.M. Fitzpatrick, C.R. Maurer, Jr., R.J. Maciunas, and G.S. Allen. "Registration of multimodal volume head images via attached markers." *Medical Imaging VI: Image Processing*, Proc. SPIE 1652:271-282, 1992.
9. W.H. Press, S.A. Teukolsky, S.T. Vetterling, B.P. Flannery, *Numerical Recipes in C, 2nd Edition*, Cambridge University Press, 1992.
10. W. Wells, R. Kikinis, W. Grimson, F. Jolesz. "Statistical Intensity Correction and Segmentation of Magnetic Resonance Image Data." *Third Conf. Visualization in Biomedical Computing*, Rochester MINN:SPIE 1994.
11. W.M. Wells III, P. Viola, H. Atsumi, S. Nakajima, R. Kikinis. "Multi-Modal Volume Registration by Maximization of Mutual Information". *Medical Image Analysis*, **1**(1):35–51, 1996.
12. J. West, J. Fitzpatrick, *et al.* "Comparison and evaluation of retrospective intermodality image registration techniques." In *Medical Imaging: Image Processing*, volume 2710 of *Proc. SPIE*, Newport Beach, California, February 1996.

Multimodality Deformable Registration of Pre- and Intraoperative Images for MRI-Guided Brain Surgery

Nobuhiko Hata[1,2], Takeyoshi Dohi[2], Simon Warfield[1], William Wells III[1,3]
Ron Kikinis[1], Ferenc A. Jolesz[1]

[1]Image-guided Therapy Program, Department of Radiology
Brigham and Women's Hospital and Harvard Medical School
75 Francis St., Boston, MA 02115, USA
{noby, simonw, sw, kikinis, jolesz}@bwh.harvard.edu
[2]Department of Precision Machinery Engineering, Faculty of Engineering
dohi@miki.pe.u-tokyo.ac.jp
[3]Artificial Intelligence Laboratory, Massachusetts Institute of Technology

Abstract. A method by which to register multimodality medical images accommodating soft tissue deformation is presented in the context of interventional therapy with a MR scanner. Accuracy testing with arbitrarily deformed MR images and application studies of a pig's brain were undertaken to evaluate the feasibility of the method. When Mutual Information is employed as the voxel similarity measure in the matching energy function, the algorithm can accommodate multimodality images. Coupled with rigid registration, the deformable registration of pre- and intra-operative multi-modality images enables surgeons to precisely define critical anatomical structures, such as vessels and functional areas, and to localize and optimize trajectories. The method directly and automatically works on volumetric multimodality images. Thus the algorithm is suitable for intra-operative registration, where stability and simplicity are desirable.

1. Motivation

The advantages of intraoperative MRI [1] as a guidance tool have been well acknowledged in neurosurgical procedures [2], including biopsy [3], drainage, and tumor resection in which the aim is to perform the least invasive surgery possible with MRI-specific imaging capabilities (multiplane imaging, soft tissue discrimination and temperature mapping). Despite its obvious advantages in terms of accessibility, the surgical requirements for interventional MRI limit its imaging capability in comparison to that of conventional diagnostic MRI.

Our proposal to overcome this problem as detailed elsewhere [4] is the rigid registration of preoperative images to intraoperative MR images. Images obtained by preoperative computed tomography (CT), T1- and T2-weighted MRI, magnetic resonance angiography (MRA), and single photon emission computed tomography (SPECT) are registered to the intraoperative MR images, in order to show the preoperative anatomical and pathological tissue discrimination in the interventional field. This approach also permits simultaneous access to various preoperative scans and intraoperative images. The incorporation is achieved by the rigid multimodality registration algorithm "Maximization of Mutual Information" [5, 6].

Provided that the patient's position with respect to the scanner is stable, the geometric relation between the (preoperatively defined) master space and the intraoperative scanner coordinate system remains fixed. This assumption is valid early in part brain surgery, since patients are fixed to the MRI table with a Mayfield clamp.

However, as Kato et al. have reported [7], the brain deforms during surgery, primarily because of cerebrospinal fluid leakage and tissue resection. In our experience intraoperative MRI has revealed that the brain shifts at most approximately 17 mm after craniotomy, biopsy, and tumor resection.

This problem motivated us to work on a deformable registration to accommodate any deformations that occur in soft tissues. The deformable registration method developed should be fully automated and accurate in multimodality image settings.

2. Deformable registration with "Maximization of Mutual Information"

2.1 Definition of the problem

Deformable registration using a correlation-based approach divides a volume into subvolumes, searching for optimal translation for each subvolume $p = (x, y, z)^T \in \Re^3$. Several groups of investigators [8-12] have reported that the energy function measuring goodness-of-matching can be formulated as the sum of a voxel similarity and an elastic regularization energy, i.e.

$$F(d) = \sum_{n=1}^{N} \int_{\Omega} -I(r(p), s(p+d)) dx + \omega U(d) , \qquad (1)$$

where d denotes displacement of a subvolume p, or with a transformation function: $T(p) = p(x, y, z)^T + d(u, v, w)^T$.

In equation (1), $I()$ counts a similarity measure of a subvolume p in the reference data r and the sample data s. The second term $U()$ denotes a regularization energy, which imposes a local elasticity constraint on displacement of subvolumes. ω is a weighing coefficient that controls the level of the regularization, or elasticity, effect.

The general problem of deformable registration is to find a set of d that minimizes the matching energy function $F()$.

2.2 Optimization of matching energy function

We employ a stochastic gradient search approach for the optimization of matching energy (1). The local maximum of F is computed with a gradient descent optimization scheme incorporating many steps:

$$T_n \leftarrow T_{n-1} + \lambda \frac{dF}{dT} = T_{n-1} + \lambda \frac{d}{dT}(-I + \omega U) = -\frac{dI}{dT} + \omega \frac{dU}{dT} \quad (2)$$

where λ is a step size parameter. At each step new samples r and s are drawn based on T_n, and the steps are taken until convergence is obtained.

2.3 Mutual information as a voxel similarity measure

We employed Mutual information [13] as the voxel similarity measure in the right term of (1). Mutual information was introduced by Viola and Wells for multimodality medical image registration [5, 6]. This method works automatically and directly on medical images, in contrast to other methods that require the setting of fiducial markers or some other types of manual interaction for registration. Thus, the algorithm is suitable for intraoperative registration, where stability and simplicity are desirable.

Mutual information is formulated as

$$I(r(x), s(T(x))) \equiv H(r(x)) + H(s(T(x))) - H(r(x), s(T(x))), \quad (3)$$

where $r(x)$ and $s(x)$ denote observations of the reference data and the sample data, respectively, and x represents the coordinates of the voxel treated as a random variable over coordinate locations in the reference data. $H(\cdot)$, the entropy of a random variable, is formulated as

$$H(A) = -\int_{-\infty}^{\infty} P(z) \ln P(z) dz \approx -\frac{1}{N_A} \sum_{z_i \in \Omega_A} \log P(z_i), \quad (4)$$

which represents an expectation of the negative logarithm of the probability density $P(z)$ of the observation A. The probability $P(z)$ is computed from a histogram of an image r or s, or from a joint histogram of r and s in which each voxel contains two pixel values from r and s. Thus the dimension of the joint histogram is two, while that of a single histogram is one.

We will construct the derivative of the Mutual Information in (2) with respect to the transformation variable T in order to use it in stochastic optimization:

$$\frac{dI}{dT} = \sum_{i \in \Omega_A} \left(\frac{\partial I}{\partial s_i} \frac{ds_i}{dT} + \frac{\partial I}{\partial r_i} \frac{dr_i}{dT} \right) = \sum_{i \in \Omega_A} \left(\frac{\partial I}{\partial s_i} \frac{ds_i}{dT} \right), \quad (5)$$

where the term $\frac{ds_i}{dT}$ is the gradient of the image intensity of a voxel in the sample data, with respect to transformation T. In the simple case where T is a linear operator [14], (5) is then formulated as follows:

$$\frac{dI}{dT} = -\frac{1}{N} \sum_{i \in \Omega_A} \left(\frac{1}{P(s_i)} \frac{\partial P(s_i)}{\partial s} - \frac{1}{P(r_i, s_i)} \frac{\partial P(r_i, s_i)}{\partial s} \right) \nabla s(T(x_i)) x_i^T. \quad (6)$$

2.4 Elastic energy as regularization energy measure

With the application of external force, an object deforms until equilibrium is reached at which point external force and internal stress are balanced. At the same, time the stress causes strain or displacement, which eventually causes the object to deform. If we hypothesize that the object deforms only elastically (and not plastically), we can assume a potential energy that measures the work by the external force. In an ideal situation in which the object deforms elastically, this potential energy should be minimized according to the principle of minimum potential energy [15].

Elastic deformation principles [15] introduce other terms: Young's modulus E, shear modulus of elasticity G, shear strain γ. If we assume $\gamma = 0$, the derivative of elastic energy U with respect to transformation T of a subvolume $p(x,y,z)$ is formulated as

$$\frac{dU}{dT} = \nabla_T U$$
$$= \left(\frac{E}{2} + 2G\right)\left(2\frac{\partial u}{\partial x}\frac{\partial^2 u}{\partial x^2} + 2\frac{\partial v}{\partial y}\frac{\partial^2 v}{\partial y^2} + 2\frac{\partial w}{\partial z}\frac{\partial^2 w}{\partial z^2}\right)$$
$$+ (E+G)\left(\frac{\partial^2 u}{\partial x^2}\left(\frac{\partial v}{\partial y} + \frac{\partial w}{\partial z}\right) + \frac{\partial^2 v}{\partial y^2}\left(\frac{\partial u}{\partial x} + \frac{\partial w}{\partial z}\right) + \frac{\partial^2 w}{\partial z^2}\left(\frac{\partial u}{\partial x} + \frac{\partial v}{\partial y}\right)\right) \quad (7)$$

3. Results

3.1 Experimental overview

In the first experiment, the evaluated the accuracy of the algorithm by synthesizing sample images from the reference (target) images. Matching error was estimated on the basis of the hypothesis that perfect registration would deform the synthesized image back to its original shape (reference image).

In the second experiment, we evaluated the feasibility of the algorithm, registering MRI scans of a pig's brain before and after a clay weight was placed on the brain.

3.2 Accuracy test: preoperative MRI vs. synthesized intraoperative MRI

The first study registered synthesized deformed images with the original image and numerically compared the result with the known data. The original data were obtained by T1-weighted MRI (3D SPGR, TR/TE = 35/5, Sagital, 256^2 pixels x124 slices, 0.78125^2 x1.5 mm) with contrast agent (Gadolinium-DTP Areg).

Voxels were displaced in a normal distribution. Given the center of force in the image at (x_0, y_0, z_0), a displacement (u,v,w) at (x_0+dx, y_0+dy, z_0+dz) was

$$(u,v,w) = (k\frac{1}{\sqrt{2\pi}}e^{-dx^2/2}, k\frac{1}{\sqrt{2\pi}}e^{-dy^2/2}, k\frac{1}{\sqrt{2\pi}}e^{-dz^2/2}) \quad (8)$$

where k is a constant coefficient to magnify the displacement.

Comparing the result with known data, root-mean-square and standard deviation of the error along the sagital (RL-), colonal (AP-) and axial (SI-) axis's are summarized in Table 1.

The initial displacement of the pixels, 3.39±2.72 mm (in-plane direction), corrected by the deformable registration with an error of 1.58 ± 0.91 mm, or double the voxel size of 0.78125^2 mm. A similar result was obtained in the outplane direction.

A coarse-to-fine multiresolution scheme was employed in direct descending optimization to avoid a matching energy value in the local minimal. The resolution was changed from 1/8, 1/4, 1/2 to the original size (256^2 pixel x124 slices). Ten iterations were performed in each resolution. The parameters given were $\omega = 2.0$ and $\lambda = 100000$, and the computation time was approximately 21 minutes by UltraSPARC 2 (dual 200MHz, 256MB, SUN Microsystems, Mountain View, CA).

Table 1: Result of accuracy testing with synthesized deformed T1-weighted MRI.

	Displacement [mm]	Registration error [mm]
In-plane direction (AP, IS-axis)	3.39±2.72	1.58 ± 0.91
Out-plane direction (LR-axis)	4.75±3.13	2.44 ± 1.21

3.3 Animal study: deformed vs. original pig brain MRI

In the second experiment, we undertook the deformable registration of MRI scans of a pig's brain.

After anesthesia (isoflurane 2% and oxygen 5 L) and KCL 20ml injection, the pig was decapitated. Craniotomy was performed to open a bur hole (approximately 100 mm in diameter) at the top of the head and the brain surface was exposed after the dura had been partially removed. The head was rigidly fixed in a coil for brain scan and placed in the gantry of a MR scanner (0.5T, MRH-500, Hitachi Medico, Japan). After the fixation of the brain in a coil, the initial T1-GFE scan (TR/TE 60/16, FOV 128mm, 128x128x64 pixels, 1.0 x 1.0 x 1.5 mm/voxel, data acquisition 4 times) was performed.

Next, the pressure was applied to upper left section of the brain with a specially developed acrylic bar with clay at the top. MRI scans were performed with a weight of 20.3 g and then 30.1 g (Figure 1).

The deformable registration was applied to fuse (1) the initial scan without the weight vs. The second scan made after placing of the first weight (total, 20.3 g), and (2) the initial scan vs. The third scan after placing the additional weight (total, 30.1 g). The latter result is presented in Figure 2.

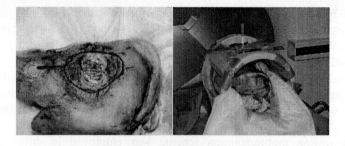

Figure 1: [Left] Bur hole approximately 100 mm in diameter was made to expose the brain of a pig (male, 48.5 kg, 100 days old). [Right] A specially developed acrylic frame with a clay weight was fixed to the MRI head coil, which also rigidly holds the pig's head.

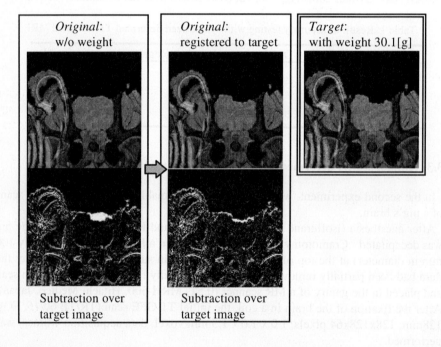

Figure 2: Registered MR images of a pig's brain. The target images are scanned while pushing the top of the brain with a weight (20.3 g). The original MRI is registered to the target image allowing elastic deformation.

As in the first experiment, a coarse-to-fine multiresolution scheme was employed in optimization to avoid a matching energy value in local minimal; the resolution was changed from 1/8, 1/4, 1/2 the original size of 128^2 pixels x 64 slices; and 10 iterations were performed in each resolution. The parameters given were $\omega = 2.0$

and $\lambda = 100000$ and the computation time was approximately 11 minutes by UltraSPARC 2 (dual 200MHz, 256MB, SUN Microsystems, Mountain View, CA).

4. Discussion

In application of MRI-guided therapy, deformable registration must deal with a variety of imaging modalities and protocols. For instance, the direct deformable registration of SPECT and MRI will superimpose the tumor tissue characterization onto the intraoperative images. Therefore, the voxel similarity measure $I()$ in (1) should be carefully selected, as in rigid registration.

Most previously reported methods of deformable registration have used a regularized pixel value, or root mean square, as the voxel similarity measure [8, 10, 11, 16]. This approach works fine if we can restrict the image modalities (e.g., anatomical template, MRI, and CT) and can approximate the intensity value of tissues.

In the next stage of our investigations, we will examine the application of the method to a multimodality setting, accuracy testing with a single-modality image (T1-weighted MRI).

As reported elsewhere [4], we have set up a surgical navigation system for MRI-guided therapy that rigidly registers preoperative images to intraoperative images by the "Maximization of Mutual Information" method [5, 6]. Guided by multiple modalities (T1- and T2-weighted MRI and intraoperative MRI), surgeons and interventional radiologists can localize and optimize trajectories. The approaching path is evaluated by interactively choosing the scan plane with an optical locator device and re-slicing the registered multimodality preoperative images, with a refresh rate of 29 Hz. The registration of preoperative T1-weighted MRI to intraoperative T1-weighted images takes approximately 9 minutes.

In the future, the deformable registration technique presented in this paper will be implemented in this system to accommodate the soft tissue deformation, which cannot be tracked by rigid registration alone.

Acknowledgment

Nobuhiko Hata was supported in part by Japan Society for the Promotion of Science, William Wells III by the The Whitaker Foundation, Ron Kikinis and Ferenc A. Jolesz by NIH grant P01-CA67165.

References

[1] Schenck, J. F., Jolesz, F. A., Roemer, P. B., Cline, H. E., Lorensen, W. E., Kikinis, R., Silverman, S. G., Hardy, C. J., Barber, W. D., Laskaris, E. T., and et al.: Superconducting open-configuration MR imaging system for image-guided therapy. Radiology 195 (1995) 805-814

[2] Black, P. M., Moriarty, T., Alexander, E., 3rd, Stieg, P., Woodard, E. J., Gleason, P. L., Martin, C. H., Kikinis, R., Schwartz, R. B., and Jolesz, F. A.: Development and

implementation of intraoperative magnetic resonance imaging and its neurosurgical applications. Neurosurgery 41 (1997) 831-845

[3] Moriarty, T. M., Kikinis, R., Jolesz, F. A., Black, P. M., and Alexander III, E.: Magnetic resonance imaging therapy. Intraoperative MR imaging. Neurosurg Clin N Am 7 (1996) 323-331

[4] Hata, N., Dohi, T., Kikinis, R., Jolesz, F., and Wells III, W. M.: Computer assisted intra-operative MR-guided therapy: pre- and intra-operative image registration, enhanced three-dimensional display, deformable registration. 7th Annual meeting of Japan Society of Computer Aided Surgery, Sapporo, Japan, (1997) 119-120

[5] Viola, P. A.: Alignhment by Maximization of Mutual Information. *Artificial Intelligence Laboratory*. Cambridge, MA: Massachusetts Institute of Technology (1995) 155.

[6] Wells III, W. M., Viola, P., Atsumi, H., Nakajima, S., and Kikinis, R.: Multi-Modal Volume Registration by Maximization of Mutual Information. Medical Image Analysis 1 (1996) 35-51

[7] Kato, A., Yoshimine, T., Hayakawa, T., Tomita, Y., Ikeda, T., Mitomo, M., Harada, K., and Mogami, H.: A frameless, armless navigation system for computer-assisted neurosurgery. J Neurosurg 74 (1991) 845-849

[8] Bajcsy, R. and Kovacic, S.: Multiresolution elastic matching. Comp Vis Graph Image Proc 46 (1989) 1-21

[9] Gee, J. C., Reivich, M., and Bajcsy, R.: Elastically deforming 3D atlas to match anatomical brain images. J of Compt Assist Tomogr 17 (1993) 225-236

[10] Collins, D. L., Peters, T. M., Dai, W., and Evans, A. C.: Model based segmentation of individual brain structures from MRI data. Visualization in Biomedical Computing, Chapell Hill, NC, (1992) 10-23

[11] Christensen, G. E., Rabbitt, R. D., and Miller, M. I.: 3D brain mapping using a deformable neuroanatomy. Physics in Medicine and Biology 39 (1994) 609-618

[12] Miller, M. I., Christensen, G. E., Amit, Y., and Grenander, U.: Mathematical textbook of deformable neuroanatomies. National Academy of Sciences, (1993) 11944-11948

[13] Papoulis, A.: Probability, Random Variables, and Stochastic Processes, Third Edition. McGraw-Hill,New York, NY (1991)

[14] Wells III, W. M., Halle, M., Kikinis, R., and Viola, P.: Alignment and tracking using graphics hardware: demonstration with software. RSNA annual meeting, Chicago, IL, (1996)

[15] Washizu, K.: Variational methods in elasticity and plasticity. Pergamon Press,Headington Hill Hall, Oxford (1968)

[16] Christensen, G. E., Miller, M. I., and Vannier, M.: A 3D deformable magnetic resonance textbook based on elasticity. Applications of computer vision in medical image processing, Stanford Univ., (1994) 153-156

[17] West, J., Fitzpatrick, J. M., Wang, M. Y., Dawant, B. M., Maurer, C. R. J., Kessler, R. M., Maciunas, R. J., Barillot, C., Lemoine, D., Collignon, A., Maes, F., Suetens, P., Vandermeulen, D., van den Elsen, P. A., Napel, S., Sumanaweera, T. S., Harkness, B., Hemler, P. F., Hill, D. L., Hawkes, D. J., Studholme, C., Maintz, J. B., Viergever, M. A., Malandain, G., Woods, R. P., and al., e.: Comparison and evaluation of retrospective intermodality brain image regsistraion techniques. J Comput Assist Tomogr 21 (1997) 554-566

A Novel Approach for the Registration of 2D Portal and 3D CT Images for Treatment Setup Verification in Radiotherapy

Ravi Bansal[1], Lawrence H. Staib[1], Zhe Chen[2], Anand Rangarajan[1], Jonathan Knisely[2], Ravinder Nath[2], and James S. Duncan[1]

[1] Departments of Electrical Engineering and Diagnostic Radiology,
[2] Department of Therapeutic Radiology, Yale University, New Haven, CT 06520-8042

Abstract. In this paper we present a framework to simultaneously segment portal images and register them to 3D treatment planning CT data sets for the purpose of radiotherapy setup verification. Due to the low resolution and low contrast of the *portal image*, taken with a high energy treatment photon beam, registration to the 3D CT data is a difficult problem. However, if some structure can be segmented in the portal image, it can be used to help registration, and if there is an estimate of the registration parameters, it can help improve the segmention of the portal image. The minimax entropy algorithm proposed in this paper evaluates appropriate entropies in order to segment the portal image and to find the registration parameters iteratively. The proposed algorithm can be used, in general, for registering a high resolution image to a low resolution image. Finally, we show the proposed algorithm's relation to the mutual information [19] metric proposed in the literature for multi–modality image registration.

1 Introduction

Registration is the process that maps pixels from one image, called the *reference image*, to the pixels in another image, called the *test image*. For clinical diagnosis, treatment planning and delivery of a therapy, images from different modalities are often acquired as they provide complementary information about a disease and also can give graphical verification of a delivered therapy. [1]

In radiotherapy for cancer patients, registration of images from different modalities, such as computed tomography (CT) and magnetic resonance imaging (MRI), is often used in treatment planning to delineate the correct spatial extent of the tumor and the surrounding normal structures. Furthermore, registration of images from the same modality is also used for routine radiographical verification of the radiation treatment. In this case, X–ray images are taken at

---

[1] Good reviews of medical image registration, with classification, for multi-modal images can be found in [18], whereas [12] is an excellent review of registration methods in computer integrated surgery.

different energies, one at diagnostic energy (40 – 100 KV) (called the simulation image) when the treatment setup is initially simulated and others using a high energy (4 – 20 MV) treatment beam (called portal images) throughout the treatment course. Due to the high photon energy, portal images are intrinsically of low contrast and poor sharpness. It has remained a difficult task to automate the registration of the simulation and portal images. In fact, such registration is still performed by visual comparison in most radiotherapy centers. Many treatment centers are moving toward offering full 3D conformal treatments that are initially planned from 3D treatment planning CT data sets. Registration of the 3D image set to 2D portal images is therefore necessary to fully quantify the three–dimensional patient setup before treatment [7, 13, 3, 6].

Related Work. To register the portal image to a 3D pre–treatment image, the methods proposed in the literature are either semi–automated or require feature extraction from the portal image. The poor quality of the portal image makes this a difficult problem. However, many registration algorithms require feature extraction as a preprocessing step. Thus, the accuracy of these registration methods is limited by the accuracy of the method to segment features from the portal image. These methods are also called *sparse field* methods.

Instead of using features, some registration methods work directly with the gray scale pixel values of the images [21, 19, 20]. The authors use cross–correlation of pixel intensities has been used as the match metric for aligning portal and simulation images [14]. Woods et al. [21], measure the mis-registration between two images as the dispersion, or variance, of intensities in the 2D histogram. However, this metric is largely heuristic. An information theoretic match metric has been proposed [19] which can be used for multi–modality image registration. These methods which directly manipulate image intensities are called *dense field* methods. The dense field methods, as compared to the sparse field methods, are more robust to noise as these methods do not require extraction of features to be registered.

Our Approach. If the 2D portal and 3D CT images are properly aligned, then the information from the high resolution 3D CT can be used to segment the portal image. On the other hand, if we have an accurate segmentation of the portal image, an accurate registration can be obtained. Thus, this becomes a problem of deciding whether to try to locate structure in the portal film for registration purposes or to perform a crude registration first that might help to look for structure which could be used for better registration. In this paper we propose that there is no clear answer, and the registration and segmentation should be carried out simultaneously, each helping the other.

Thus, we propose an iterative framework in which the segmentation and the registration of two images are estimated in a two stage algorithm using two different entropies, termed *minimax entropy*. In the entropy maximization step, the segmentation of the portal image is estimated, using the current estimates of the registration parameters. In the entropy minimization step, the registration parameters are estimated, based on the current estimates of the segmentation.

The algorithm can start at any step, with some appropriate initialization on the other. We derive this strategy starting from the EM algorithm and show the relationship to the mutual information metric.

2 Problem Definition and Motivation

Patient setup verification, before performing radiotherapy, using a portal and a 3D CT image, is a classical pose estimation problem in computer vision. In the pose estimation problem, the pose of a 3D model is to be determined from a set of 2D images such that the model is aligned with the images. We assume that a rigid transformation of the 3D CT data set will bring it in to alignment with the portal image and hence there are only six transformation parameters to be considered. Since our algorithm works directly on the pixel intensity values, we classify our algorithm as an automated, intrinsic, global, dense–field based algorithm based on the classification in [18].

In the next subsection, we formulate the pose estimation as a maximum likelihood estimation (MLE) problem. This formulation requires the knowledge of the joint density function between the portal and the DRR pixel intensities, denoted as $p(x_i, y_i(T))$ below. As noted earlier in the paper, we want to estimate a segmentation of the portal image in order to help in the registration process. The problem of segmenting the portal image is formulated as a labeling problem in which each pixel is labeled either as bone or background. To incorporate the segmentation information, the joint density function is written in a *mixture density* form where the labels on the portal image pixels are not known. Hence, the segmentation labels are treated as the missing information, and the parameters to be determined are the pose parameters. We formulate our problem as a maximum–likelihood estimation (MLE) problem in section 2.1. An algorithm for computing the MLE from incomplete data is presented in [5] and is called the expectation–maximization (EM) algorithm. Our first thoughts were to select EM algorithm to compute the estimates, are due to its proven monotonic convergence properties, ease of programming and unlike other optimization techniques, it is not necessary to compute Hessians nor it is necessary to worry about setting the step–size. Thus, the EM algorithm may be used to estimate both the pose parameters and the segmentation labels. However, there are several problems with the EM approach that restrict its use in this problem. These are explained in subsection 2.2 and a minimax entropy strategy that addresses these restrictions is described in section 3.

2.1 Problem Definition

Let, $X = \{x(i)\}$, for $i = 1, \ldots, N^2$ be the $N \times N$ portal image. Similarly, let $Y(T) = \{y(i, T)\}$ for $i = 1, \ldots, N^2$ be the $N \times N$ projected 3D CT image, at the given transformation parameters T. Let, $G = \{g(i)\}$, for $i = 1, \ldots, N^3$ be the 3D CT image. Note here we index pixels in the images using a single index, even though the images are 2D (or 3D) images. For simplicity in the formulations below, we have assumed that the portal and the projected 3D CT are of the same dimensions. However, this need not be true. The projected 3D CT image is also called the *digitally reconstructed radiograph* (DRR). Each pixel in the portal image is classified to belonging to one of two classes, bone or background. Thus, we formulate the pose estimation problem as a maximum likelihood estimation problem:

$$\begin{aligned}
\hat{T} &= \arg\max_T \ \log p(X, G|T) \\
&= \arg\max_T \log \left(\frac{p(X, G, T)\, p(G|T)}{p(G, T)} \right) \\
&= \arg\max_T \ [\log p(X, Y(T)) - \log p(Y(T))] \\
&= \arg\max_T \sum_i [\log p(x_i, y_i(T)) - \log p(y_i(T))]
\end{aligned} \quad (1)$$

where we ignore the term $p(G|T)$, since the 3D CT data set, G, is independent of the transformation parameters, T. In equation (1) we assume that the image pixels are independent. The logarithm of the likelihood function is taken to simplify the mathematical formulation. Note that for notational simplicity, we shall now write $x(i) = x_i$ and $y(i, T) = y_i(T) = y_i$, where the current transformation parameters for which the DRR is obtained should be clear from the context, otherwise it will be made explicit.

Mixture Model and the EM. Letting $A = \{1, 2\}$, be the set of classes (i.e. bone, background), where non–bone pixels are defined to be background and using a mixture density model, we can now write the joint mixture density model, from equation (1), for the portal image and DRR as, at pixel i, $p(x_i, y_i) = \sum_{a \in A} p(m_i = a) \ p_a(x_i, y_i) = \sum_{a \in A} p_i(a) \ p_a(x_i, y_i)$, where m_i is a random variable for the ith pixel taking values in A and $p_a(x_i, y_i)$ is the joint density function of the pixel intensities, given that the portal image pixel is labeled a. Classifying the pixels in the portal image is equivalent to the determination of the probability mass function of m_i. Let Z be the $N^2 \times 2$ *classification matrix* with z_{ai} its ith row and ath column entry satisfying the constraints $\sum_{a=1}^{2} z_{ai} = 1$, for $i = 1, \ldots, N^2$. Note that $z_{ai} = 1$ if the ith pixel of the portal image belongs to the class a, i.e., $z_{ai} \in \{0, 1\}$. Thus, z_{ai} are the indicator variables. For each indicator variables, we shall define the expected value as $< z_{ai} > \equiv p_i(a)$.

Using this notation, the EM algorithm [5] for the mixture model can be written as, at the kth iteration,
E–Step:

$$Q(T, T^{(k-1)}) = \sum_i \sum_{a \in A} < z_{ai} >^k \ \log p_a(x_i, y_i) - \sum_i \log p(y_i) \quad (2)$$

M–Step:
$$T^k = \arg\max_T \ Q(T, T^{(k-1)}) \quad (3)$$

where,
$$<z_{ai}>^k = \left(\frac{<z_{ai}>^{k-1} p_a(x_i, y'_i)}{\sum_{b \in A} <z_{bi}>^{k-1} p_b(x_i, y'_i)}\right) \quad (4)$$
where, $y'_i = y(i, T^{(k-1)})$.

2.2 Limitations of EM Approach and Alternative Strategies

For our purposes, the EM algorithm has two key restrictions. First, in the EM algorithm for the mixture model as formulated in equation (2), the function $Q(T, T^{(k-1)})$ is defined only if the component density functions $p_a(x_i, y_i)$, $\forall a$ are specified. The component density functions need to be determined for the specific problem. Thus, for the images used in prostate cancer radiotherapy, the joint density functions need to be determined from the projection model, taking into account the physics of interaction of high energy X-rays with matter. If the joint density functions are not known, then usually a simplified model has to be assumed. In this paper, we propose to estimate the unknown density functions from the given data instead of using simplified models. The second observation comes from Neal and Hinton [15] who provide a view of the general EM algorithm as a coordinate descent algorithm where the coordinates axes are the joint density functions on the missing information and the parameters to be estimated. (A similar view of the EM algorithm for parameter estimation of mixture density models has been given [8] as well). In the E–Step of the EM algorithm, the expected value is calculated, as the missing information is not known. However, this implies that the expected value in equation (2) should be taken with respect to the density function $p(Y)$, instead of $p(Y|X; T^{(k-1)})$. However, Neal and Hinton [15] show that at each iteration of the EM algorithm, the density function $p(Y)$ is estimated to be $p(Y|X; T^{(k-1)})$ and the question still remains as to the relationship between the two density functions. In our approach described in section 3, the *max* step in the *minimax algorithm* formalizes this relation. The *max* step can be viewed as a step for determining the density function on the missing information. The *principle of maximum entropy* [10] (or the *principle of maximal non–committance*) states that in making inferences on the basis of partial information we must use that probability distribution which has maximum entropy subject to whatever is known. This is the only unbiased assignment we can make; to use any other would amount to an arbitrary assumption of information which by hypothesis we do not have.

We overcome the restrictions of the EM algorithm by borrowing the idea of averaging over the estimated density function from *mutual information*. Mutual information as a match metric has been first proposed and successfully applied for multi–modality image registration by [19, 4]. However, the mutual information match metric formulation in the literature assumes that all the pixels in the image are i.i.d., an assumption not true in general. The proposed minimax entropy algorithm described below thus aims at combining the strengths of both the EM algorithm and the mutual information based registration approach to simultaneously segment and register images.

3 Minimax Entropy Approach

The proposed minimax algorithm for solving the basic problem posed by equation (1), in a computational form similar to the EM strategy described by the equations (2), (3) and (4) has two steps, the max step and the min step, which are evaluated iteratively to determine the registration parameters and the probability density function (pdf) of the portal image segmentation. The details of the development of the proposed algorithm are discussed elsewhere [1]. Again, using the notation from section 2, we see the steps mathematically as follows:

Max Step:

$$p^k(m) = \arg\max_{p(m)} \left[-\int p(m) \log p(m) \, dm \right.$$
$$\left. + \int p(m) \, \log p(m|X, Y; T^{(k-1)}) \, dm \right] \quad (5)$$

under the constraint $\int p(m) \, dm = 1$, where m is the random variable whose domain is the set of possible segmentations of the portal image, where each pixel can be labeled from the set of labels A. We assume that pixel labels are statistically independent, i.e., $p(m) = \prod_i p(m_i = a) = \prod_i p_i(a)$.

As formulated above, the max–step simply states that the maximum entropy estimate of the density $p(m)$ is simply $\log p(m|X, Y; T^{(k-1)})$ [2]. This simple formulation of the estimated segmentation density function allows us to systematically put constraints on the density function, as we show below.

Min Step:

$$T^k = \arg\min_T H(m, X|Y)$$
$$= \arg\min_T \left(\sum_{a \in A} <\overline{z_a}>^k H_a(x, y) - H(y) \right) \quad (6)$$

where $<\overline{z_a}>^k = (\frac{1}{N^2}) \sum_{i=1}^{N^2} <z_{ai}>^k$. See [1] for the development of the min–step. The component density function for class a, $p_a(x, y)$, is estimated as the weighted sum of Gaussian kernels using the Parzen window method:

$$p_a(w) = \frac{1}{\sum_{w_i \in D} p_i(a)} \sum_{w_i \in D} p_i(a) \, G_\Psi(w - w_i)$$

where, $w = \begin{pmatrix} x \\ y \end{pmatrix}$ and $p_i(a) = p(m_i = a)$ is the probability that the ith pixel in the portal image belongs to class a, estimated in the *max* step, equation (5), Ψ is 2-by-2 covariance matrix, which is assumed to be diagonal and D is the set of pixels sampled from portal image and the DRR to estimate the conditional density functions. Thus, $H_a(x, y) = -\int\int p_a(x, y) \log p_a(x, y) \, dx \, dy$. In the *min* step, we have chosen the mutual information (MI) metric currently popular in the medical image analysis community. We have found it to be more robust than other interesting metrics (e.g. correlation. See [1] where we present the relation between the two metric and show that the MI is more sensitive to mis–registration then correlation). Because MI assumes that pixels are i.i.d., in general this is a problem, which we get around by using a mixture densities. We note that in [17], the authors register images with mutual information as a match metric while incorporating segmentation information on one of the images. However, the image was pre–hand segmented and thus remains fixed throughout the registration. In our proposed algorithm, the portal image segmentation is estimated simultaneously with the transformation parameters.

An annealing schedule [11] is imposed on the estimated portal image pixel segmentation distribution. The modified *max step*, equation (5), can thus be written as:

Max Step:

$$p^k(m) = \arg \max_{p(m)} \left[-\frac{1}{\beta} \int p(m) \log p(m) \, dm \right.$$
$$\left. + \int p(m) \, \log p(m|X, Y; T^{(k-1)}) \, dm \right] \quad (7)$$

under the constraint $\int p(m) \, dm = 1$, where $\beta = \frac{1}{t}$, and t is the *temperature*, which determines the annealing schedule.

4 Results

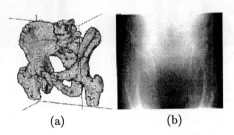

(a) (b)

Fig. 1. (a) Volume rendered 3D CT phantom for which the simulated portal images were calculated. (b) Real portal image of the phantom obtained by taking the high energy X–ray of the phantom in the treatment room.

The experiments were carried out on simulated and real portal images. To obtain simulated portal images, the 3D CT data set was first rotated or translated in the 3D space, by a known amount, and then a perspective projection was computed. These simulated portal images, rendered under known parameters, are used to study the accuracy of the algorithm. Note that we assume that the perspective parameters are known.

The 3D CT data set, shown in figure 1 (a), is a high resolution diagnostic energy data set obtained by scanning a pelvic phantom. The phantom is made of real human pelvic bone enclosed in plexi-glass with density close to soft tissue. After the CT data set was obtained at diagnostic energy X-rays (40 KeV), its voxel values were mapped to high energy X-rays (6MeV), using attenuation coefficient tables [9], to generate projection images close to the quality of the portal image. Since the diagnostic energy is known, the attenuation coefficient tables are used to estimate the tissue type in each voxel. Once the tissue type is known, the attenuation coefficient for that tissue at high energy can be estimated from the tables. These attenuation coefficients are used to map the phantom voxel values to their high energy values. In figure 1 (a), the 3D CT data set was rendered with the opacity value for soft tissue set close to zero.

Figure 1 (b) shows the portal image obtained by imaging the phantom with X-rays at treatment energy level (6 MeV). The portal image was contrast enhanced by histogram equalization. Experimentally, we found that histogram equalized portal images lead to more accurate results. The images shown in figure 4 are simulated portal images obtained at known transformation parameters to validate the proposed algorithm. Scattering of high energy X-ray photons leads to noise and poor contrast in the portal image. To simulate photon scattering, varying amounts of independent and identically distributed (i.i.d.) Gaussian noise were added to the pixels in the simulated portal image.

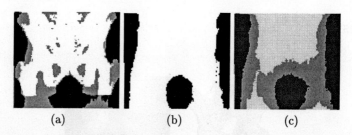

Fig. 2. Estimated segmentation results of the true portal image. (a) Results of using proposed minimax entropy algorithm. (b) Simple threshold. (c) Clustering algorithm in MEDx [16].

Figure 2 shows the segmentation of the real portal image, figure 1 (b), estimated by different segmentation algorithms. Figure 2 (a) shows the segmentation as estimated by the proposed algorithm. The pixel labels are estimated based on the joint density distribution. The bright pixels are labeled bone. The dark pixels are labeled background. Gray pixels are the pixels whose labels cannot be decided based on the joint probability density functions. Figure 2 (b) is the segmentation of portal image under simple, manually selected, threshold. Figure 2 (c) is segmentation using a clustering algorithm, from MEDx. In this clustering algorithm, the image is segmented into three classes based on the nearness of the gray values to the user specified values.

Figure 3 shows the result of registering the real portal image, figure 1 (b), to the 3D CT data set, figure 1 (a). The image in figure 3 (b) is the DRR rendered at the registration parameters estimated by the minimax entropy algorithm. To see the goodness of the estimated parameters, contours were hand drawn on the portal image by an expert, matching closely to key features. These contours were then mapped onto the DRR, using the estimated parameters determined by the proposed algorithm. The contours match closely to the feature points in the DRR, at least showing the accuracy of the estimated transformation parameters in mapping this expert-traced estimate of bone boundaries.

Estimated Parameters					
t_x (vox)	t_y (vox)	t_z (vox)	α (deg)	β (deg)	γ (deg)
2.56	-6.69	2.34	2.51	-1.24	0.73

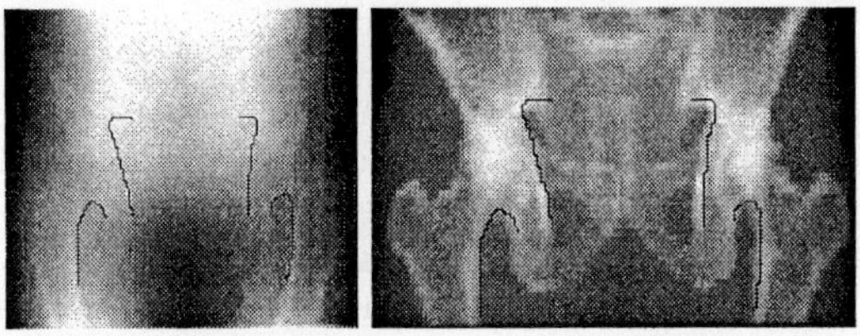

Fig. 3. (a) Portal image with contours. The reference contours shown are drawn, on the portal image, by an expert, matching anatomical features of interest, to study the registration result. (b) The contours are then mapped on to the DRR rendered using the parameters estimated by the proposed minimax entropy algorithm.

Figure 4 (c) shows the initial results obtained for registration of simulated portal images. Each graph corresponds to the variation of one transformation parameter in the rendering of the simulated portal image. For the graph labeled X-Trans, for example, the 3D CT data set was translated along the X-axis by 5 voxels and then a projection was rendered with varying noise. To register the simulated portal image to the 3D CT data set, the transformation parameters were reset to zeros. The results can be summarized as follows. The minimax entropy algorithm is quite robust against noise for in-plane translations along the x-axis and y-axis. The performance of the method deteriorated gracefully for rotations, both in-plane and out-of-plane, as the noise was increased. In the initial steps of the proposed algorithm, when most of the labels have equal probability of belonging to either class, the algorithm is increasing the mutual information between the entire images. Later in the iterations, as the portal image pixels get classified as belonging to one of the two classes, the algorithm is increasing the mutual information of each of the two classes separately.

Overall, for the simulated portal images, where the true registration parameters were known, the estimated parameters converged to the true parameters after only a few iterations. The later iterations of the algorithm led to better segmentation of the (simulated) portal image, which in turn helped registration to lock into a minimum. The proposed algorithm, as implemented, took about 5 to 10 minutes on SGI Indigo 2 R10K machine.

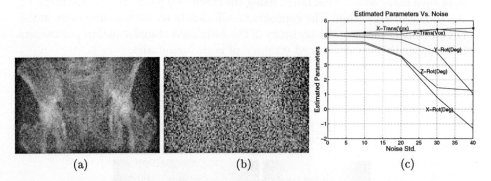

Fig. 4. Digitally rendered simulated portal images from the 3D CT data set in figure 1. The 3D CT data set was rotated by $5°$ about the z–axis before taking the perspective projection. Varying amounts of i.i.d. Gaussian noise were added. The maximum pixel value of the simulated portal image is 296. (a) 2D rendered portal image, noise, std $(\sigma) = 10$. (b) Std $(\sigma) = 30$. (c) This figure shows the graph of estimated parameters against increasing noise added to the simulated portal image.

5 Discussion and the Future work

In this paper we presented an information theoretic framework in which segmentation and registration are carried out together iteratively, with segmentation results helping in the registration and vice–versa. Most registration methods proposed in the literature carry out portal image segmentation as a pre–processing step in the registration process, if at all. Our approach of simultaneously segmenting and registering the images, using a unified framework, leads to a novel and robust algorithm. We need to demonstrate the accuracy of the algorithm in comparison to mutual information based algorithm using raw intensity information only.

The mutual information match metric overcomes the assumption of a linear relationship between the pixel intensities of the images to be registered, an underlying assumption in the correlation match metric. In mutual information based registration, the relationship between the pixel intensities is estimated from the given data itself and thus can register images from different modalities. At an estimated set of transformation parameters, a joint density between the images to be registered can be estimated, from the given data. The mutual information metric assigns a number to each such estimated density, estimated for different transformation parameters The transformation parameters corresponding to the density having the largest mutual information are chosen as the estimated parameters by the algorithm. The EM algorithm provides an iterative framework to estimate the parameters of a distribution, in the presence of missing data. However, the EM algorithm requires that the parametric form of the distribution to be known.

The proposed minimax entropy algorithm overcomes this restriction of the EM algorithm, by borrowing the idea from the mutual information method of estimating the joint distribution from the given data, and emphasizes the fact that the distribution on the segmentation labels is the maximum entropy distribution, satisfying the given constraints. This fact allows us to invoke other constraints on the distribution systematically, which we used to impose an annealing schedule. In the proposed algorithm, if the joint densities are not known, then instead of assuming some simplified parametric form, we estimate the densities from the data given. Then we use the information theoretic framework to estimate the transformation parameters.

Also, we note the relationship of our algorithm to the mutual information match metric which recently has been shown to be applied successfully to multi-modality image registration.

Our future research includes algorithm speed-up, validation of the accuracy and robustness of the algorithm, especially in comparison to the mutual information based registration and the ridge based algorithm proposed in [6]. Our experiments demonstrated that the estimated registration was not as accurate for out of plane rotations and translations, especially as the noise was increased. Thus, we propose using two orthogonal views, anterior–posterior and lateral views, commonly taken in the treatment room, for more accurate registration results. We will then extend the algorithm to make use of portal images acquired from more that two views which need not be orthogonal.

References

1. R. Bansal, L. Staib, et al. A novel approach for the registration of 2D portal and 3D CT images for treatment setup verification in radiotherapy. Technical Report 1998-1, Dept. of Electrical Engineering and Diagnostic Radiology, Yale University, Jan 1998. (http://noodle.med.yale.edu/~bansal/techreps/regis.ps.gz).
2. R. M. Bevensee. *Maximum Entropy Solutions to Scientific Problems.* P T R Prentice Hall, 1993.
3. J. Bijhold. Three-dimensional verification of patient placement during radiotherapy using portal images. *Med. Phys.*, 20(4):347–, March/April 1993.
4. A. Collignon, F. Maes, et al. Automated multimodality image registration using information theory. *Info. Proc. in Med. Imaging (IPMI)*, pages 263–274, 1995.
5. A. P. Dempster, N. M. Laird, and D. B. Rubin. Maximum likelihood from incomplete data via EM algorithm. *J. Royal Statistical Soc., Ser. B*, 39:1–38, 1977.
6. K. Gilhuijs. *Automated verification of radiation treatment geometry.* PhD thesis, Univ. of Amsterdam, Radiotherapy dept., the Netherlands, 1995.

7. K. G. A. Gilhuijs et al. Interactive three dimensional inspection of patient setup in radiation therapy using digital portal images and computed tomography data. *Int. J. Radiation Oncol. Biol. Phys.*, 34(4):873–885, 1996.
8. R. J. Hathaway. Another interpretation of the EM algorithm for mixture distributions. *Statistics & Probability Letters, North Holland*, 4:53–56, 1986.
9. J. H. Hubble. *Photon Cross Sections, Attenuation Coefficients, and Energy Absorption Coefficients From 10KeV to 100 GeV*. Nat. Stand. Ref. Data. Ser., Nat. Bur. Stand. (U.S.), August 1969.
10. E. T. Jaynes. Information theory and statistical mechanics I. In R. D. Rosenkrantz, editor, *E. T. Jaynes: Papers on probability, statistics and statistical physics*, volume 158, pages 4–16. D. Reidel Publishing Company, Boston. USA, 1983.
11. S. Kirkpatrick, C. Gelatt, and M. Vecchi. Optimization by simulated annealing. *Science*, 220:671–680, 1983.
12. S. Lavallee. Registration for computer–integrated surgery: Methodology, state of the art. In Russell H. Taylor et al., editors, *Computer–Integrated Surgery: Technology and Clinical Applications*, pages 77–97. The MIT Press, Cambridge, 1996.
13. S. Lavallee, R. Szeliski, and L. Brunie. Anatomy–based registration of three–dimensional medical images, range images, X–ray projections, and three–dimensional models using octree–splines. In Russell H. Taylor et al., editors, *Computer–Integrated Surgery: Technology and Clinical Applications*, pages 115–143. The MIT Press, Cambridge, Massachusetts, 1996.
14. J. Moseley and P. Munro. A semiautomatic method for registration of portal images. *Med. Phys.*, 21(4), April 1994.
15. R. M. Neal and G. E. Hinton. A view of the EM algorithm that justifies incremental, sparse, and other variants. In M. I. Jordan, editor, *Learning in Graphical Models*. Kluwer Academic Press. To Appear. Web address: http://www.cs.toronto.edu/~radford/papers-online.html.
16. Sensor Systems, Inc. $MEDx^{TM}$: *Multimodality Radiological Image Processing For Unix Workstations*, 1998. Version 2.1.
17. C. Studholme et al. Incorporating connected region labelling into automated image registration using mutual information. In *Proc. of MMBIA '96*, pages 23–31, 1996.
18. P. A. van den Elsen, E. D. Pol, and M. A. Viergever. Medical image matching– a review with classification. *IEEE Eng. in Med. and Biol.*, 12(1):26–39, 1993.
19. P. Viola and W. M. Wells. Alignment by maximization of mutual information. *Fifth Int. Conf. on Computer Vision*, pages 16–23, 1995.
20. J. Weese et al. 2D/3D registration of pre–operative ct images and intra–operative x–ray projections for image guided surgery. In H.U.Lemke et al., editors, *Comp. Assist. Rad. and Surgery*, pages 833–838. 1997.
21. R. Woods, S. Cherry, and J. Mazziotta. Rapid automated algorithm for aligning and reslicing PET images. *J. Comp. Assist. Tomography*, 16(4):620–633, 1992.

Multimodality Imaging for Epilepsy Diagnosis and Surgical Focus Localization: Three-Dimensional Image Correlation and Dual Isotope SPECT

Benjamin H. Brinkmann, Richard A. Robb, Terence J. O'Brien,
Michael K. O'Connor, Brian P. Mullan

*Biomedical Imaging Resource, Dept. of Neurology, and Dept. of Nuclear Medicine,
Mayo Foundation, Rochester, MN 55905*

Abstract

Peri-ictal SPECT is a potentially powerful tool to study changes in regional cerebral blood flow during a partial seizure and to localize the seizure focus for pre-surgical evaluation. Recently we have developed and validated a method for co-registering and normalizing 3D interictal SPECT images to 3D ictal SPECT images and deriving a difference image co-registered to the patient's 3D MRI. This method has been shown to significantly improve clinical outcomes in surgery patients. In order to improve the method's sensitivity and specificity a number of enhancements have been added to the basic technique, including using voxel-based registration to better align ictal and interictal images, dual isotope (Tc-99m and I-123) SPECT for effective tissue discrimination, and a custom software interface written to facilitate the entire process. We report results that show significant improvement over the original method, and we discuss future work which should continue to improve the method as a clinical tool.

Introduction

Localizing the epileptogenic zone, or seizure focus, in partial epilepsy is a challenging clinical problem. Currently 20-50% of intractable partial epilepsy cases are unlocalized by conventional methods, which include scalp-recorded electroencephalography (EEG), magnetic resonance imaging (MRI), and side-by-side visual analysis of peri-ictal (during or immediately after the seizure) and interictal (baseline, non-seizure) single photon emission computed tomography (SPECT) images. EEG gives functional information with high temporal resolution, but provides only vague anatomical seizure localization. MRI gives excellent soft tissue contrast but fails to identify the epileptogenic zone in the absence of an obvious structural lesion. Intracranial EEG is generally reserved for only the most difficult cases because of its invasiveness and potential for morbidity. Positron emission tomography (PET) may also be used, but is not available to most epilepsy centers due to its high cost and the difficulty of obtaining positron emitting isotopes.

Subtraction ictal SPECT coregistered to MRI (SISCOM) [1] is a recent advance in the field of peri-ictal functional imaging and has been shown to significantly improve surgical outcomes in epilepsy patients [2]. Several groups have simultaneously developed comparable methodologies for studying regional cerebral blood flow (rCBF) during and after epileptic seizures [3-5]. The SISCOM technique involves the intravenous injection during a partial seizure (ictal SPECT) or immediately following one (post-ictal SPECT) of a radiotracer exhibiting a high first pass cerebral extraction rate and a low back diffusion. Radiotracers with these properties include Tc-99m hexamethylpropylene amine oxime (HMPAO), Tc-99m ethyl cysteinate diethylester (ECD) and I-123 iodoamphetamine (IMP). The SPECT images can be acquired up to several hours following the event, providing a semi-quantitative image of the rCBF present between 30 and 120 seconds after the injection [6, 7]. A second SPECT image is acquired at a later time under resting conditions (interictal SPECT) to serve as a baseline image. The peri-ictal and interictal images are co-registered, normalized, subtracted, and thresholded to produce an image representing focal activation sites during the seizure. This image is then registered to the patient's MRI and displayed to provide an anatomical context for the func-

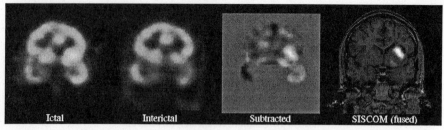

Figure 1A: SISCOM and its component images: ictal SPECT, registered interictal SPECT, subtraction (ictal-interictal) SPECT, and the thresholded subtraction image fused with the patient's MRI. The SISCOM image shows a clear right insular focal activation site. Ictal-interictal registration was performed with AIR, while surface matching was used for SPECT-MRI registration.

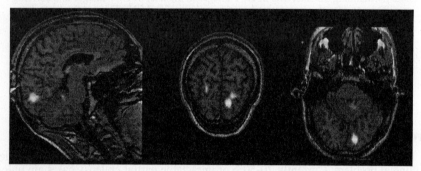

Figure 1B: SISCOM images allow three-dimensional perspectives on the anatomic context of the functional activation site and can be viewed in sagittal (left), coronal (middle), transverse (right), or oblique orientations.

tional activation sites. Figure 1 illustrates the SISCOM image and its component images, as well as its capacity for providing three-dimensional functional and anatomical information.

While conventional SISCOM is a powerful tool for studying neuroactivation in partial epilepsy, it has a number of limitations which advanced image processing and analysis techniques can improve. One important limitation is that while seizures are dynamic phenomena, SPECT is only able to give a single snapshot of the blood flow pattern during a limited time window of the seizure. It is therefore very difficult with current SPECT methods to study the evolution of blood flow changes occurring during and after an epileptic seizure. Another limitation arises from small inaccuracies in the interictal to peri-ictal registration, which can significantly degrade focal spot intensity, accuracy, and detectability [8]. A further limitation of the method is the processing time required for producing the SISCOM images, which can easily approach an hour for an experienced physician. To date at our institution we have evaluated over three hundred forty epilepsy patients using the SISCOM method, which has created a significant time burden on clinicians and residents.

To address these limitations, we have undertaken a number of studies directed at improving the accuracy, reliability, and speed of the SISCOM technique. This paper reports the development and validation of several enhancements to the basic SISCOM method. These developments include voxel-based registration to align the peri-ictal and interictal SPECT images, dual-isotope I-123 and Tc-99m SPECT to provide multiple rCBF maps during a single seizure, and customized software to reduce operator time requirements. We also present several additional improvements we plan to implement in the near future.

Voxel-based SPECT Registration

One of the major factors in the quality and diagnostic utility of the SPECT subtraction image is the accuracy of interictal and peri-ictal SPECT image co-registration. It has been shown that even small misregistrations may reduce the focal spot intensity significantly in paired functional activation images [8]. The original SISCOM method uses surface matching co-registration [10] and consistently matches images with better than 1 voxel dimension of accuracy [1], but it is desirable to extend this accuracy as much as possible to improve the sensitivity and specificity of epileptogenic localization. Voxel-based registration methods have been shown to be more accurate than surface matching methods at a variety of coregistration tasks [11]. However, few have been quantitatively compared for functional SPECT rCBF images, and the performance of different algorithms depends greatly on the registration task to be performed. It has been unclear whether the large changes in image contrast that accompany ictal activation could confound voxel-based registration.

An approach to image matching by maximization of mutual information was described by Wells [12] in 1996. The implementation we used is available in the AnalyzeAVW software package [9] and uses the simplex method to maximize the mutual information of the two images. In contrast, the well-known AIR (or Woods') algorithm [14,15] aligns two images by first thresholding to remove background noise and then using a Newton-Raphson method to minimize the standard deviation of the ratio of corresponding image gray values. We conducted experiments to examine and compare surface matching, mutual information, and AIR registration algorithms and provide a quantitative estimate of their accuracy for aligning peri-ictal and interictal patient SPECT images.

Methods

For surface matching, binary images were created by thresholding. Ventricle and other interior holes were filled using two-dimensional math morphology [9]. Matches were performed with one thousand sample points on the match volume surface. For the mutual information algorithm, default parameters were used (parameter tolerance 1x10-8, function tolerance 0.001, 1000 iterations per step) with the exception of the subsampling parameters, which were found to give superior results with 1:1 sampling for all steps. For Woods' algorithm we used AIR 3.0, obtained from the author. The default convergence change threshold (0.00001) was used, as was the default sampling (81:1 with a factor of 3 decrement at each step) as this sampling approach was found to give better results than the 1:1 sampling used with mutual information. The same intensity thresholds were used for the AIR algorithm as were used in the surface matching algorithm. No smoothing kernel was used. Computation time was not formally considered in this study.

Image	X Rot	Y Rot	Z Rot	Z Trans
1	0.0	0.0	0.0	0.0
2	-14.9	-14.9	1.5	-2.5
3	-10.0	-10.0	3.0	-2.0
4	-5.0	-5.0	5.0	-1.5
5	-3.0	-3.0	10.0	-1.0
6	-1.5	-1.5	14.9	-0.5

Table 1: Misregistrations applied to the brain phantom and patient simulation images. Rotations are given in degrees, while translations are given in voxel units.

Six sequential scans of a realistic 3D volumetric brain phantom (Hoffman 3D brain phantom, Data Spectrum Corp., Hillsborough, NC) containing 15 mCi of Tc-99m were taken, with rotations applied about the central axis of the scanner to the phantom in a headrest. A digital spirit level (Pro Smart Level, Wedge Innovations, San Jose, CA) was used to measure rotation angles, and images were acquired at 0.0, 1.5, 3.0, 5.0, 10.0, and 14.9 degrees. The images were reconstructed on a 64x64 grid with cubic voxel dimensions of 4.4 mm per side using a third-order Metz filter (6mm FWHM). To provide a more challenging registration task using four degrees of freedom, the reconstructed images were then misaligned by known X and Y rotations and Z translations (Table 1) using the AnalyzeAVW software system [9]. Each scan was then registered to the other five, creating fifteen registration tasks to be evaluated for each of the three algorithms. Reference 4x4 transformation matrices were constructed using the known rotation and translation parameters, and these matrices were inverted and multiplied by the matrices given by the registration algorithms, producing residual error matrices. These matrices were evaluated to find the distance in millimeters by which a point on the cortical surface would be misaligned relative to its true position, at the maximum measured radius on the phantom's surface of 79.3 mm.

The phantom images approximate patient SPECT scans with very little functional rCBF change. To approximate a patient SPECT with severe ("worst case") rCBF changes, we obtained a true ictal patient image (patient #2 below) and manually replaced apparent focal activation sites with the mean cerebral pixel intensity. We then systematically modified the contrast in various parts of the image by adding areas of increased and decreased rCBF (bright and dark pixels, respectively). The image was blurred in the transverse plane with a 3x3 mean filter, and zero-mean Gaussian noise (18% of mean cerebral pixel count) was added. The resulting image had very different contrast (and hence rCBF patterns) and reduced resolution compared to the patient's ictal image, but had identical shape and was in perfect coregistration to it. The registration experiment used with the phantom was repeated using the ictal and simulated patient images. The rotations and translations listed in Table 1 were applied to both the ictal and simulated images and the fifteen matching tasks were performed using the ictal image as the base volume and the simulated image as the match volume in each experiment.

Interictal and peri-ictal Tc-99m SPECT images were obtained from fifteen sequentially enrolled epilepsy patients. Informed consent was obtained. Each patient's interictal scan was matched to the corresponding ictal or post-ictal image using each of the three registration algorithms. A SISCOM subtraction image was created for each image pair, and the standard deviation of non-zero pixels in this image was recorded for each of the registration algorithms. This value is comparable to the root mean squared difference between the two images, and would be expected to be small when the images are well registered [16].

Results and Discussion: Registration

Registration results for the six brain phantom SPECT images and for the simulation image are shown in Table 2. For the phantom data the voxel-based methods showed a statistically significant improvement over the surface-based method with $p<0.0005$ (analysis of variance (ANOVA) for repeated measures), while there were no significant differences between mutual information and the AIR algorithm (ANOVA for planned comparisons). For the simulation experiment, the voxel-based methods were significantly better than surface matching with $p<0.0001$ (ANOVA for repeated measures) and AIR showed a statistically significant improvement over mutual information with $p<0.05$ (ANOVA for planned comparisons).

The fifteen patient peri-ictal and interictal SPECT subtraction images had standard deviations of 12.18±1.16, 11.38±1.33, and 10.98±1.24 (mean ± st.dev.) for surface matching, mutual information, and the AIR algorithm, respectively. The improvement in patient standard deviation data for voxel matching over surface matching is statistically significant with $p<0.0001$ (ANOVA for repeated measures), and AIR's results show sta-

	Phantom		Simulation	
	Mean±St.Dev	Range	Mean±St.Dev	Range
Surface Matching	3.08±1.16	1.09-4.47	2.49±1.22	0.30-4.54
Mutual Information	1.84±0.68	0.70-3.20	0.88±0.81	0.03-2.57
AIR 3.0	1.98±1.01	0.77-4.95	0.54±0.40	0.22-1.77

Table 2: Mean, standard deviation, and range results from the phantom and patient simulation registration experiments. All values are given as total error in millimeters.

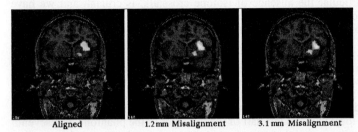

Figure 2: The effects of misregistration on SISCOM images. As the ictal and interictal SPECT images are misaligned, the intensity of the focal spot decreases and its shape changes.

Aligned   1.2 mm Misalignment   3.1 mm Misalignment

tistically significant improvement over mutual information with $p<0.05$ (ANOVA for planned comparisons).

Figure 2 illustrates the importance of accuracy in the ictal-interictal SPECT coregistration. With even small misregistrations the apparent intensity and position of the focal activation spot may change. The superiority of voxel-based methods over surface matching corresponds with findings in the current literature [11] and suggests that in spite of the rCBF differences between ictal and interictal SPECT images, voxel intensity based measures are still more reliable than the cortical surface shape for registration, particularly in low-resolution SPECT images. This data also highlights the differences between mutual information and AIR. The phantom results (no rCBF changes) show a statistically insignificant trend in favor of mutual information, suggesting that further study might show it to be more accurate than AIR for static contrast images. However, AIR is more robust to the ictal-interictal rCBF changes than mutual information, although further study is necessary to determine whether this statistically significant result is clinically significant. The mutual information cost function tends to align images such that voxel intensity values in one image are maximally predictive of intensity values in the other, which does not necessarily hold with large rCBF changes. AIR tends to reduce variation in the ratio image, which is dominated by contributions from misregistration around sharp intensity transitions, such as the ventricles and image edges.

Dual-Isotope SPECT

A dual-isotope, double-injection technique using sequential injections of two radiopharmaceuticals with different energy photopeaks would provide a number of advantages to the SISCOM method by producing two different simultaneously-acquired rCBF images. First, such a method could be used to document the changes occurring over time during a single seizure. As both Tc-99m-ECD and I-123-IMP show similar brain uptake kinetics that closely reflect the pattern of cerebral blood flow shortly after their injection [17-22], the differences between the images should reflect changes in rCBF between the injections. Second, the dual isotope method would allow the subtraction of a post-ictal image from a simultaneously-acquired and perfectly coregistered ictal image. This completely eliminates misregistration noise from the SISCOM subtraction image and furthermore avoids the inconvenience and expense to the patient of returning to the institution for a separate interictal SPECT. In addition, the magnitude of the focal hypoperfusion in the post-ictal seizure focus is believed to be greater and more reliable than interictal epileptogenic hypoperfusion [23-26]. As a result, the magnitude of the focal difference in the subtraction images in the region of the epileptogenic zone should be greater by subtracting from the ictal SPECT a post-ictal SPECT rather than an interictal SPECT.

The purpose of these experiments is to develop and validate an accurate method for performing dual isotope Tc-99m ECD and I-123 IMP SPECT imaging in epilepsy patients. Previous authors have attempted dual isotope SPECT for studying cerebral ischemia [27,28], cerebrovascular interventions [29], and ratio images for cognitive activation studies [30,31]. In quantitative SPECT studies of epilepsy patients the accuracy of rCBF maps, in particular the absence of isotope crosstalk, is crucial, and we have found previous methods [27-32], which have used asymmetric I-123 energy windows offset by varying amounts, inadequate for these purposes.

Methods

A Hoffman brain slice phantom (Data Spectrum Corp., Chapel Hill, NC) was used, which consisted of two flat layers with seven independent fluid compartments simulating realistic cortex and white matter areas in a two-dimensional transaxial slice through the lentiform nucleus and corpus collosum (Figure 3). Six of the compartments were relatively small and were located in the left half of the top layer of the phantom. The seventh compartment was large, spanning the entire bottom layer of the phantom and protruding through to the top layer in the right hemisphere of the phantom (Figure 3A). Compartments 1-4 (total volume 18.6 ml) in the anterior left of the phantom were designated I-123 only compartments, whereas compartments 5 and 6 (total volume 12.3 ml) in the posterior left of the phantom were designated Tc-99m only compartments. The large compartment, No. 7 (96.3 ml), was designated for mixed isotopes. The phantom's perimeter was surrounded by a layer of simulated bone to replicate bone scatter in tomographic acquisitions.

Planar images of the brain phantom were taken with one head of a dual-headed gamma camera system (Helix, Elscint Inc., Haifa, Israel) and were used to develop the dual isotope acquisition technique. Acquisitions were performed using a high resolution parallel hole collimator, obtaining 32 energy band images 2 keV in width, from 120 keV to 184 keV. Intensity parameters were measured using regions of interest in AnalyzeAVW [9] on each of the 2 keV band images. The ROI areas measured are shown in Figure 3: Tc-99m only (T), I-123 only (I), both isotope (B), white matter or cerebral background (BG), and extracerebral background areas (A). These parameters were then plotted across the 32 energy bands and were used to determine the best combination of energy window settings for the Tc-99m and I-123 images. Figure 3A illustrates that it is

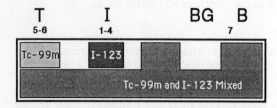

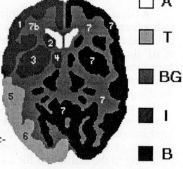

Figure 3: A) A simulated cross section through the Hoffman brain slice phantom. Labels and chamber numbers correspond to those shown in Figure 3B. **B)** A planar diagram of the Hoffman brain slice phantom. Areas are mixed isotopes (B), I-123 (I), bottom layer mixed isotopes (BG), Tc-99m (T), and air or isotope-free areas (A).

necessary to subtract the BG signal from the T and I signals to isolate the Tc-99m and I-123 signals from the large, underlying mixed-isotope compartment. Hence, signal above baseline (SAB)

$$SAB_I = I - BG \qquad SAB_{Tc} = T - BG$$

represents the signal in the single isotope compartments, while percent crosstalk (PC)

$$PC_I = \frac{SAB_{Tc}}{SAB_I} \qquad PC_{Tc} = \frac{SAB_I}{SAB_{Tc}}$$

represents crosstalk from the opposing isotope as a percentage of each isotope's signal.

Energy bands were added together using AnalyzeAVW and specialized software written in Tcl/Tk with the AVW image processing libraries. The energy band images were summed to create images with different energy window settings, allowing us to replicate and compare results from the literature [27-32] to within 1 keV. Optimal settings were chosen based upon SAB and PC, as well as signal to noise ratio (SNR), defined as the isotope SAB divided by the extracerebral background signal. The dual-isotope images were compared to reference Tc-99m only (130-146 keV, phantom containing no I-123) and I-123 only (152-168 keV, phantom containing no Tc-99m) images for validation.

Crosstalk from Tc-99m represents a significant problem in the relatively count-poor I-123 image. To compensate for this, a 4% asymmetric window (134-140 keV) was used to isolate the Tc-99m signal from I-123 contamination and septal penetration, and this then provided a spatial map for subtracting the Tc-99m crosstalk from the I-123 window. The contamination correction fraction was calculated by filling the phantom with Tc-99m only, measuring the counts in the Tc-99m compartment of the phantom across the energy spectrum, and dividing the counts in each energy band by the number of counts in the same ROI in the 4% photopeak image (Table 3). Correction values less than 0.0005 were observed to consist primarily of background noise and were therefore set to zero. The total correction factor for a given energy window is obtained by summing the energy band correction factors over the energy range used.

Tomographic images of the phantom containing I-123 only, Tc-99m only, and a 3:1 Tc:I mixture were acquired using a high-resolution fan beam collimator with the energy windows set according to the arrangement determined with the planar data. Image data was reconstructed using a standard filtered-back-projection algorithm in word mode

Energy Band	Correction Factor
144-146	0.2417
146-148	0.1518
148-150	0.09572
150-152	0.04291
152-154	0.02575
154-156	0.008773
156-158	0.003661
158-160	0.001707
160-162	0.0008535

Table 3: Correction factors for Tc-99m crosstalk in the energy windows used to construct the I-123. Correction factors above 162 keV were negligible.

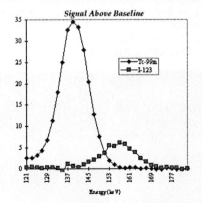

Figure 4: Signal above baseline plotted against gamma ray energy.

| | Brinkmann | | Asymm. I-123 [29-31] | | Shifted I-123 [27,28,32] | |
	Tc-99m	I-123	Tc-99m	I-123	Tc-99m	I-123
Window (keV)	130-146	152-168*	133-147	153-169	133-147	159-175
PC	2.79%	1.33%	3.60%	19.68%	3.60%	3.65%
SNR	180.10	14.73	185.67	15.25	185.67	7.98

*Subtractive crosstalk correction was applied

Table 4: Comparison of the reported dual isotope acquisition method with previously-reported methods in percent crosstalk (PC) and signal to noise ratio (SNR).

with a third-order Metz smoothing filter (6mm FWHM). No attenuation correction has been used to this point, but we expect that some attenuation correction may be useful for the Tc-99m image. The Tc-99m-only and I-123-only images were created with simple energy windows (130-146 keV and 152-168 keV, respectively) as references. The dual isotope images were compared to the reference I-123 and Tc-99m images using ROI intensity ratios. To estimate isotope crosstalk, the ratio of the opposite isotope compartment to the mixed isotope compartment (T/B for the I-123 image, and I/B for the Tc-99m image) was calculated for each dual isotope image, and these ratios were compared to the corresponding ratios for the reference single-isotope images.

Results and Discussion: Dual Isotope

Figure 4 plots the signal above baseline for Tc-99m and I-123 across the acquired energy spectrum. It illustrates that the Tc-99m and I-123 signals show significant overlap and crosstalk between 145 and 155 keV. For the Tc-99m image we used a 12% (130-146 keV) asymmetric window which maximized the Tc-99m counts in the image while minimizing I-123 crosstalk. The optimum I-123 image was obtained using an energy window of 152-168 keV (10%) with crosstalk correction by subtracting 0.041 of the Tc-99m correction image (134-140 keV) from the I-123 image. Figure 5 illustrates planar images formed from a portion of the overlap region (145-155keV), as well as the I-123 (center) and Tc-99m (right) dual isotope images formed using these methods.

Table 4 compares our planar dual isotope images to images created by replicating previously-reported methods [27-32] to within 1 keV in terms of PC and SNR. The Tc-99m images are all fairly comparable, with our strategy reducing counts slightly in favor of minimizing crosstalk. The I-123 image is the challenging part of the dual isotope strategy. Our reported acquisition shows a great deal less crosstalk than other methods and, in fact, offers nearly a tenfold reduction over most other methods [27-31]. Some methods [27,28,32] have reduced crosstalk by excluding nearly half the I-123 photopeak, reducing the SNR commensurately.

Crosstalk correction for the I-123 image was applied before and after image recon-

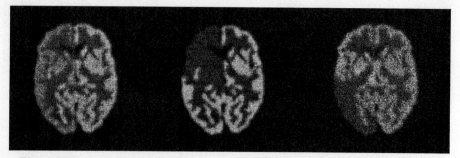

Figure 5: Planar images showing equal amounts of Tc-99m and I-123 signal (left) and the Tc-99m (center) and I-123 (right) dual isotope images using the reported acquisition strategy.

struction with essentially identical results. Post-reconstruction crosstalk correction is preferred for its practical ease and lower computation time. The tomographic dual isotope Tc-99m and I-123 images are shown in Figure 6. The reference I-123 image had a ratio of 0.3155, while the crosstalk-corrected dual isotope image had a ratio of 0.3202, i.e. a difference of 1.51%. A dual isotope I-123 image acquired using a simple energy window (152-168 keV) and no crosstalk correction had a ratio of 0.3547, a difference of 12.44% from the reference I-123 image. The dual isotope Tc-99m image had a ratio of 0.2657 compared to the reference Tc-99m image ratio of 0.2759, a difference of 3.70%. The dual isotope tomographic images differ only slightly from their single-isotope reference counterparts (and are visually indistinguishable), which suggests that accurate quantitative rCBF studies of epileptic seizures may be performed with this technique.

Customized Software

To alleviate the time requirements associated with performing SISCOM using a comprehensive general image analysis software package, a specialized software tool was created. This tool performs the SPECT processing, co-registration, subtraction, and analysis portion of SISCOM. The program has a graphical user interface that is simple and easy to use, and it places

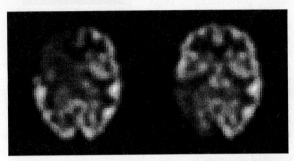

Figure 6: The tomographic dual isotope Tc-99m (left) and I-123 (right) images acquired using the reported method.

tools for the interactive portions of the SPECT image processing within easy reach while automating a large portion of the processing. The software was written in Tcl/Tk with the AVW image processing function libraries [13]. Tcl/Tk allows fast and simple graphical user interface design with a great deal of configurability, while the AVW library contains optimized imaging functions compiled in C. These imaging functions are called by the Tcl/Tk interpreter, providing fast execution. A synopsis of the program flow is as follows:
1. Interactively load ictal and interictal SPECT images
2. Interactively threshold images leaving only the cortical mantle
3. Use chosen thresholds and 2D (transaxial) morphology to create binary images with interior spaces filled
4. Register interictal SPECT to ictal SPECT using surface matching, mutual information, or Woods' AIR algorithm
5. Display registered images with linked cursors to allow the user to visually assess the success of the registration (see Figure 7)
6. Mask the ictal and registered interictal SPECT volumes using their respective binary images
7. Normalize ictal and registered interictal SPECT images to mean cerebral pixel intensity of 100 (for 8-bit images)
8. Subtract interictal SPECT from ictal SPECT
9. Calculate the standard deviation of the nonzero pixels in the subtraction image
10. Threshold the subtraction image at two standard deviations to identify significant activation sites
11. Display final and intermediate images for review

This can take under two minutes for an experienced user on a Silicon Graphics Indy workstation, compared with around 40 minutes for the same tasks using generalized software. Most of this time is spent switching between programs, saving intermediate image volumes to disk, and performing tasks which are easily automated. It is not possible at this time to train technicians to perform these functions, as the physician must screen the procedure for errors, including misregistration, left-right image transposition, and image artifacts or inaccurate header (voxel size, image orientation, etc.) information. The MRI coregistration portion of SISCOM is in the process of being added to the customized software.

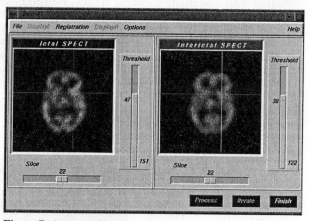

Figure 7: A screen shot from the customized SISCOM software program. Registration accuracy is visually assessed using the linked cursor tool shown.

Future Work

In a previous study [33] we described and validated a method for coregistering scalp EEG electrode positions to a patient's volumetric MRI. Subsequently we have begun using this procedure on epilepsy patients and have improved our methods for EEG topographic mapping. The next step in extending the diagnostic power of SISCOM is to add scalp-recorded EEG topographic maps and neural source dipole estimates to SISCOM, creating a more comprehensive picture of neurological activity during an epileptic seizure.

Conclusions

We have developed and evaluated imaging methods which have improved diagnostic accuracy and speed for a clinically-useful [2] method which is currently being used to evaluate epilepsy patients at our institution. First, voxel-based registration algorithms have been shown to significantly improve the accuracy of registering patient peri-ictal and interictal SPECT scans, which should increase the diagnostic capability of SISCOM. Second, the dual-isotope double-injection method allows dynamic studies of seizure propagation patterns and demonstrates promise for enhancing SISCOM's sensitivity by taking advantage of post-ictal epileptogenic hypoperfusion and by eliminating misregistration noise. Third, the development of customized software has allowed more epilepsy patients to benefit from the SISCOM methodology and has reduced the time requirements on physicians for image processing and analysis. The synergistic effect of these advances is to provide a more comprehensive picture of epileptic neurophysiology and to improve the capacity of physicians to effectively diagnose and treat focal epilepsy.

References

1. O'Brien TJ, O'Connor MK, Mullan BP, Brinkmann BH, Hanson DP, Jack CR, So EL. Seduction ictal SPECT co-registered to MRI in partial epilepsy: Description and technical validation of the method with phantom and patient studies. *Nuc Med Comm* 1998;19:31-45.
2. O'Brien TJ, So EL, Mullan BP, et al. Subtraction Ictal SPECT Co-Registered To MRI Improves Clinical Usefulness Of SPECT In Localizing The Surgical Seizure Focus. *Neurology* 1998;50:445-454.

3. Zubal IG, Spencer SS, Imam K, Smith EO, Wisniewski G, Hoffer PB. Difference images calculated from ictal and interictal technetium-99m-HMPAO SPECT scans of epilepsy. *J Nuc Med* 1995;36:684-689.
4. Weder B, Oettli R, Maguire RP, Vonesch T. Partial epileptic seizure with versive movements examined by [99mTc]HM-PAO brain single photon emission computed tomography: An early postictal case study analyzed by computerized brain atlas methods. *Epilepsia* 1996;37:68-75.
5. Chiron C, Jaminska A, Cieuta C, Vera P, Plouin P, Dulac O. Ictal and interictal subtraction ECD-SPECT in refectory childhood epilepsy. *Epilepsia* 1997;38 (Suppl. 3):9.
6. Berkovic SF, Newton M, Chiron C, Dulac O. Single photon emission tomography. In: Engel J Jr, ed. *Surgical treatment of the epilepsies*. New York: Raven Press, 1993:233-243.
7. Mullan BP, O'Connor M, Hung J. Single photon emission computed tomography. *Neuroimaging Clinics of North America* 1995;5:647-673.
8. Sychra JJ, Pavel DG, Chen Y, and Jani A. The accuracy of SPECT brain activation images: Propagation of registration errors. *Medical Physics* 1994. 21(12):1927-32.
9. Hanson DP, Robb RA, Aharon S, Augustine KE, Cameron BM, Camp JJ, Karwoski RA, Larson AG, Stacy MC, Workman EL. New software toolkits for comprehensive visualization and analysis of three-dimensional multimodal biomedical images. *J Digital Imaging* 1997. 10(2)(Suppl. 1-August):31-35.
10. Jiang, H., Robb, R. A., and Holton K. S. "A new approach to 3-D registration of multimodality medical images by surface matching." *Proc VBC '92*, 1992. Vol. 1808, pp. 196-213.
11. West, J., Fitzpatrick, J.M., Wang, M.Y., et. al. Comparison and evaluation of retrospective intermodality brain image registration techniques. *Journal of Computer Assisted Tomography*, 1997, 21(4):554-566.
12. Wells, W. M. III, Viola, P., Atsumi, H., Nakajima, S., and Kikinis, R. Mulit-modal volume registration by maximization of mutual information. *Medical Image Analysis*, 1996. 1(1):35-51.
13. Robb RA, Aharon S, Augustine KE, Cameron BM, Camp JJ, Hanson, DP, Karwoski RA, Larson AG, Stacy MC, Workman EL. *AVW Reference Manual* Technical Report, 1997.
14. Woods, R.P., Cherry, S.R., and Mazziotta, J.C. Rapid automated algorithm for aligning and reslicing PET images. *J Comp Asst Tomo*, 1992. 14(4):620-633.
15. Woods RP, Mazziotta JC, Cherry SR. MRI-PET registration with automated algorithm. *J Comp Asst Tomo* 1993. 17:536-46.
16. Lange N. Some computational and statistical tools for paired comparisons of digital images. *Stat Meth Med Res* 1994. 3:23-40.
17. Greenberg JH, Araki N, Karp A, et al. Quantitative measurement of regional cerebral blood flow in focal cerebral ischemia using Tc-99m-ECD. (Abstract). *J Nucl Med* 1991;32:1070.
18. Devous MD, Payne JK, Lowe JL, Leroy RF. Comparisons of 99mTc-EDC to 133Xe SPECT in normal controls and in patients with mild-moderate regional cerebral blood flow abnormalities. *J Nucl Med* 1993;34:754-761.
19. Kuhl D, Barrco J, Huang S, et al. Quantifying local cerebral blood flow with N-isopropyl-p-I-123 iodoamphetamine (IMP) tomography. *J Nucl Med* 1982;23:196-203.
20. Takeshita G, Maeda H, Nakane K, et al. Quantitaive measurement of regional perfusion using N-isopropyl-(iodine-123)p-iodoamphetamine and single photon emission computed tomography. *J Nucl Med* 1992;33:1741-1749.
21. Greenberg JH, Kushner M, Rangi M, et al. Validation studies of iodine-123 iodoamphetamine as a cerebral blood flow tracer using emission tomography. *J Nucl Med* 1990;31:1364-1369.
22. Matsuda H SH, Sumiya H, et al. Quantifying local cerebral blood flow by N-isopropyl-(iodine-123)p-iodoamphetamine and single photon emission computed tomography with rotating gamma camera. *Am J Physiol Imaging* 1986;1:186-194.6.
23. Newton MR, Berkovic SF, Austin MC, Rowe CC, McKay WJ, Bladin PF. Postictal switch in blood flow distribution and temporal lobe seizures. *J Neurol Neurosurg Psychiatry* 1992;55:891-894.
24. Newton MR, Berkovic S, Austin M, Rowe C, McKay W, Bladin P. Ictal postictal and interictal single-photon emission tomography in the lateralization of temporal lobe epilepsy. *Eur J Nuc Med* 1994;21:1067-1071.
25. Rowe CC, Berkovic SF, Austin MC, McKay WJ, Bladin PF. Patterns of postictal cerebral blood flow in temporal lobe epilepsy: Quanlitative and quantitative analysis. *Neurology* 1991;41:1096-1103.
26. Rowe CC, Berkovic SF, Sia STB, Austin M, McKay WJ, Kalnins RM, Bladdin PF. Localization of epileptic foci with postictal single photon emission computed tomography. *Ann Neurol* 1989;26:660-668.

27. Devous MD Sr., Lowe JL, Payne JK. Dual-isotope brain SPECT imaging with Technetium-99m and Iodine-123: Clinical validation using Xenon-133 SPECT. *J Nucl Med* 1992. 33(11): 1919-24.
28. Devous MD Sr., Lowe JL, Payne JK. Dual-isotope brain SPECT imaging with Technetium-99m and Iodine-123: Validation by phantom studies. *J Nucl Med 1992*. 33(11): 2030-35.
29. Mathews D, Walker BS, Allen BC, Batjer H, Purdy PD. Diagnostic applications of simultaneously acquired dual-isotope single-photon emission CT scans. *AJNR* 1994. 15:63-71.
30. Madsen MT, O'Leary DS, Andreasen NC, Kirchner PT. Dual isotope brain SPECT imaging for monitoring cognitive activation: Physical considerations. *Nuc Med Comm* 1993. 14:391-6.
31. O'Leary DS, Madsen MT, Hurtig R, Kirchner PT, Rezai K, Rogers M, Andreasen NC,. Dual isotope brain SPECT imaging for monitoring cognitive activation: Initial studies in humans. *Nuc Med Comm* 1993. 14:391-6.
32. Ivanovic M, Weber DA, Loncaric S, Franceschi D. Feasibility of dual radionuclide brain imaging with I-123 and Tc-99m. *Medical Physics* 1994. 21(5):667-74.
33. Brinkmann BH, O'Brien TJ, Dresner MA, Lagerlund TD, Sharbrough FW, Robb RA. Scalp-recorded EEG Localization in MRI Volume Data. *Brain Topography* 10(4):245-253.

Non-rigid Multimodal Image Registration Using Mutual Information

Tom Gaens, Frederik Maes, Dirk Vandermeulen, Paul Suetens

Laboratory for Medical Imaging Computing, ESAT/Radiology, Univ. Hosp. Gasthuisberg, Katholieke Universiteit Leuven, Herestraat 49, B3000 Leuven, Belgium
e-mail: Tom.Gaens@uz.kuleuven.ac.be

Abstract. A fully automated voxel-based algorithm for multimodal non-rigid image registration using a mutual information based similarity criterion is presented. The image deformation vector field is found by dividing images into overlapping neighborhood regions and translating these regions to locally increase the similarity criterion. The calculated displacement in each region is assigned to the centered pixel of each neighborhood region and propagated to its neighbors with a Gaussian window function assuring continuity and smoothness of the deformation field. Initial experiments on 2D test data qualitatively demonstrate the feasibility of this approach.

1 Introduction

Images from different medical imaging modalities often provide complementary information to the clinician, and therefore image alignment or registration has found several applications in diagnosis, treatment planning, and therapy follow-up. Registration algorithms (see [18] [20] for an overview) can be classified as being either *stereotactic frame based*, *landmark based*, *surface based*, or *voxel based*. Voxel-based methods optimize a metric measuring the similarity of all geometrically corresponding voxel pairs for some feature. Until recently, research was mainly focused on the search for an adequate voxel-based similarity measure as an optimization functional. Proposals for new and better alignment measures culminated in the use of information-theoretic matching criterions. An example of this approach is the concept of *mutual information*, which was introduced independently by Collignon et al. [8] and Viola and Wells [21].

Traditional registration methods apply global and *rigid* transformations, which is useful in cases where rigid body assumptions are likely to hold. However, they cannot account for non-rigid morphological variability between and within subjects. For applications where this variability matters, e.g. segmentation of brain structures by matching an individual brain to a labeled brain template, *non-rigid* matching must be used. Other applications include registration of intra-operative imaging data with pre-operative images that delivers intra-operative guidance.

In non-rigid matching, a deformation vector is determined for each image voxel in such a way that, applying the total *deformation vector field*, causes the similarity criterion to reach an optimal value and both images to get geometrically aligned. The vast amount of degrees of freedom introduced in non-rigid matching can be reduced by imposing constraints on the deformation field.

Static constraints are imposed via landmark or control points. The deformation in a certain point is then obtained by interpolation of the known deformations in the landmark points (e.g. by calculating a spline through the landmarks [2]). Succesful work on using mutual information as a similarity measure and thin-plate spline algorithms as static constraints on the deformation field are found in [15] for intra-operative guidance, and more generally in [16]. However, the corresponding control points need to be found manually or semi-automatically, and their limited number is too restrictive.

This problem can be alleviated by formulating registration as a *dynamics* problem, where dynamic constraints are imposed on the deformation field by modeling the imaged objects to be aligned as deformable solid bodies. External forces trying to deform objects are gradients of a similarity criterion, causing the similarity to increase. The deformation is constrained by internal forces generated because of the physical properties of the object. Early work using Navier-Lamé equations found in elasticity theory was reported by Bajcsy et al. [1], based on work by Burr [6] and Broit [3]. Plastic registration [10], has even more degrees of freedom than elastic registration. Very little constraints are imposed on the possible deformations, except that topology must be preserved and that the transformation must be continuous and smooth. Plastic registration can be thought of as deforming a viscous fluid. The more viscous the fluid is, the more it will resist deformation and consequently the more smooth the transformation will be. Because of this kind of interpretation, plastic registration algorithms have also been called *Fluid Transforms* in the literature. Christensen [7] therefore uses Navier-Stokes equations found in hydrodyamics theory to regularize the computed deformation field. In developing a speeded-up implementation of the fluid approach of [7] Bro-Nielsen [4] noticed the correspondence between these Tikhonov-type of regularization methods and the Gaussian scale space. Note that Thirion's [19] so-called Maxwellian 'demon'-based method in [19] makes effectively use of this correspondence. In a practical and approximative implementation, the problem of regularization boils down to the choice between Gaussian smoothing of either the total calculated deformation field (i.e. elastic registration) or the incremental deformation field (i.e. fluid registration), since the Gaussian function is the Green's function of the heat or diffusion equation. In this case, the regularizer is the diffusion equation, that propagates deformations to neighboring points [12]. Hence, one can say that the demons method is a trade-off between speed of calculations and accuracy of the results.

Most of the above mentioned non-rigid matching methods use a least squared-error distance measure as a similarity metric (the so-called Gaussian sensor model). As a lot of clinical applications ask for inter-individual and multi-modal matching, several more effective matching criteria were proposed (e.g. correlation measures [10], or feature-based potentials [7]). Recently, mutual information has been used as a similarity criterion in a dynamics based method, presented by

Maintz et al. [17]. The main drawback of their method is the implicit assumption that probabilities computed after rigid registration are good approximations of the same probabilities after fluid matching.

In this paper, we propose a dynamics based registration algorithm [12] using mutual information, and without these limitations. It's a variant of the uni-modal image registration method explored by D. Collins [10], where image transformations are found by dividing images into regions and translating these regions to increase the local similarity criterium. The theoretical aspects of our algorithm and implementation issues are described in section 2. In section 3, some results on artificial and real images are presented, followed by a discussion in section 4.

2 Algorithm

2.1 Similarity metric

The information-theoretic measure of mutual information [11] measures the amount of information one random variable contains about another random variable. The mutual information of two images is maximal when they are geometrically aligned (see [9] for a rigorous discussion). The advantage of this criterion is its generality, since it does not assume a certain relationship between the grey-values in the images to be registered [14].

Let A and B be two images with marginal entropies $H(A)$ and $H(B)$, and joint entropy $H(A, B)$ then the expression of *mutual information* can be written as: $I(A, B) = H(A) + H(B) - H(A, B)$. Marginal entropies $H(A)$ and joint entropy $H(A, B)$ are defined using joint and marginal probability distributions, which are in turn estimated using image histograms (see [14] for definitions).

2.2 Outline

The goal of our method is to calculate a deformation field that maximizes the mutual information functional. Calculating a displacement separately for each image voxel, makes the problem ill-posed. Because of the statistical nature of mutual information, centered neighboorhood regions are defined in each point of a discrete lattice $\{x_i | i = 1, ..., N\}$, of the image to be registered (N is the number of dimensions). This image is then locally transformed by translating every neighborhood region so that the total mutual information increases. Therefore the incremental changes to the joint histogram and marginal histograms are computed.

The calculated displacement in x_i is then propagated to each point in the neighborhood region by a propagation function, which in practice can be a Gaussian kernel. This deformation propagation can be interpreted in 3 ways. The most direct interpretation is to consider the image as a viscous fluid and the deformation propagation as the viscosity of this fluid. Alternatively one can interpret the Gaussian as a low pass filter and deformation propagation as convolving the deformation field with this low pass filter. Finally one can interpret the Gaussian as a radial basis function and the deformation propagation as a radial basis function spline expansion of the deformation field. Note that the deformation propagation ensures continuity and smoothness of the deformation field.

Because the deformations of neighbouring nodes are not independent, the deformation in every node cannot be estimated in one pass, so this process is repeated iteratively. The iterative process is stopped when the incremental change to mutual information falls below a threshold.

As topology must be preserved, $D(x_i)$ may not 'jump' over any of its transformed neighboring nodes: this is accomplished by appropiately rescaling the incremental updates of the deformation field (for a more rigorous treatment of topology violation, see [13]).

2.3 Implementation issues

In order to speed up the algorithm, some approximations were made to the above outlined method. Sub-voxel translations were not considered in moving the neighborhood region, to avoid additional interpolations. Another change was to consider translations only in the direction of the image gradient of the floating image, hereby assuming that iso-intensity curves deform only in the direction of the normal onto these curves. Note the equivalence with the optical flow based demons method described in [19], and the fact that the number of evaluations of the criterion is hereby reduced.

By translating the neighorhood region around each image voxel, *local* transformations are found, that are propagated into a continuous and smooth transformation. Because macroscopic features are generally more stable than microscopic ones (for human anatomy), it would be useful to recover first more global deformations and in a later stage fine and detailed deformations. This can be controlled in three ways: by using multi-resolution pyramids, by varying the neighborhood region size, and by varying the number of bins in calculating histograms.

Using multi-resolution image pyramids, calculation proceeds from coarse to fine, i.e. from the images with the lowest resolution to the highest resolution. Because of the fact that, by filtering the image the cost function is also smoothed (i.e local minima are filtered away) faster convergence to a *global* optimal value will be made easier. In practice only few levels suffice. The size of the neighborhood region can also be varied on a large-to-small basis. In doing so, large deformations are propagated at low resolution levels, and fine and detailed deformations are recoverd at high resolution levels. As *binning* corresponds to a raw labeling of the imaged objects, the number of bins to build up the histograms can be chosen on a small-to-large basis. In this way, one considers large 'objects' at the coarsest resolution levels and small detailed 'objects' at the finest resolution levels.

3 Results

3.1 Test on Artificial Multi-Modal Images

To evaluate the registration algorithm the image grid of an MR slice (size 256 x 256 pixels) was deformed using an analytically known transformation. In order to simulate multi-modality, the intensities of this deformed image were changed with a sine function: $sin(\pi * intensity)$. In this way, the reference image was created artificially, depicting a similar object imaged with a different modality, with a non-linear and one-to-many relationship between the image intensities of floating and reference images.

To be able to compare the images quantitatively, the theoretical deformation field was applied to the original MR slice, hereby creating a uni-modal equivalent to the reference image. Test setup and results are depicted in figure 1.

3.2 Test on Real Multi-Modal Images

Tests were also carried out on real multi-modal images. Therefore a pair of proton-density and T2 images was used, because they are already optimally registered at acquisition. The T2 image was taken as floating image, while the proton-density image was deformed using a similar exponential deformation field as used for the artificial images.

The comparison of the result with the theoretical solution was possible because of the fact that the original PD and T2 images were aligned from the start, and was made in the same way as with the artificial images: the theoretical deformation field was applied to the original T2 slice, hereby creating a uni-modal equivalent to the reference PD image. Test setup and results are depicted in figure 2.

3.3 Application: Atlas-driven Segmentation

One could use non-rigid registration to match images to a digital anatomical atlas for the segmentation of brain (sub)structures. In the ideal case, this could be accomplished automatically by an adequate registration algorithm, that brings images into correspondence within the same reference frame of the atlas.

As a test case for our algorithm, we made a segmentation map of a set of T2 and proton-density images of one patient A. The image created in this way was considered the 'atlas'. This map was then registered non-rigidly to a T2 image of another patient B (together with a corresponding proton-density image, considered 'study' images). Evaluation of the result is then possible by comparing the deformed 'atlas' to the segmentation of the 'study' images of patient B. Qualitative results are shown in figure 3. Notice that the result could still improve by registering the segmentation map to both study images (this requires building a 3D joint histogram from the atlas and both T2 and PD study images).

4 Discussion and Conclusion

In this work, a non-rigid registration algorithm using an information-theoretic criterion has been presented. The image transformation was found by dividing the image into small regions and translating these regions to increase the local

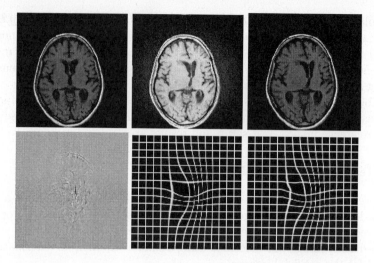

Fig. 1. Test setup and results for artificial images; from top left to bottom right: floating image, reference image, deformed floating image, difference between calculated deformed floating image and theoretically deformed floating image (intensities rescaled to [0,1]), theoretical grid deformation (subsampled detail), calculated grid deformation (subsampled detail)

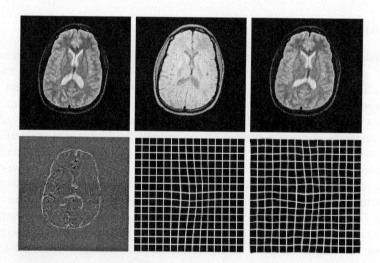

Fig. 2. Test setup and results for real images; from top left to bottom right: T2 floating image, PD reference image, deformed floating image, difference image between calculated T2 image and theoretically deformed T2 image (intensities rescaled to [0,1]), theoretical grid deformation field (subsampled detail), calculated grid deformation (subsampled detail)

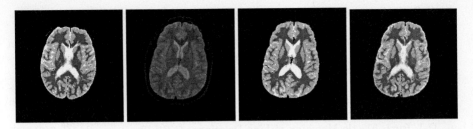

Fig. 3. Preliminary result for atlas segmentation; from left to right: segmentation map of patient A, i.e. the 'atlas' (floating image), T2 reference image of patient B, segmentation map calculated from T2 reference image and corresponding PD image of patient B, deformed floating image

similarity criterium. The floating image was considered a viscous fluid and the deformation propagation the viscosity of this fluid.

Because the resulting deformation field is smooth and continuous, the algorithm cannot account for topological differences (as can be seen in the results of figure 3.

One has to bear in mind that the 'physical' descriptions of elastic and fluid registration model the whole image grid as one physical object, and *not* the separate objects seen in the image. Modelling the different imaged objects as separate tissues would require an a priori segmentation, and a physically correct model for each of the segmented objects depending on the application (for intra- and inter-individual morphometric studies, e.g. based on physical growth models [5] or morphogenesis). It also implies the modeling and calculation of discontinuous and non-smooth deformation fields for applications in intra-operative guidance.

Acknowledgements

This research was performed within the context of the EASI project "European Applications for Surgical Interventions", supported by the European Commission under contract HC1012 in their "4th Framework Telematics Applications for Health" RTD programme, and using research grant KV/E/197 (Elastische Beeldregistratie voor Medische Toepassingen) of the FWO-Vlaanderen to Dirk Vandermeulen, research grant COF 96/12 - AO655 (Actie van de Vlaamse Minister van Wetenschapsbeleid ter stimulering van de Vlaamse Deelname aan EU-programma's), and research grant G-0340-98 of the FWO-Vlaanderen.

References

1. R. Bajcsy and S. Kovacic, Multiresolution elastic matching, *Computer Vision, Graphics, and Image Processing*, 46:1-21, Academic Press, 1989.
2. F.L. Bookstein, Morphometric tools for landmark data. Geometry and biology, Cambridge University Press, 1991.

3. C. Broit, Optimal registration of deformed images, *PhD thesis*, University of Pennsylvania, August 1981
4. M. Bro-Nielsen and C. Gramkow, Fast fluid registration of medical images, in *Proc. Visualization in Biomedical Computing (VBC'96)*, Springer Lecture Notes in Computer Science, 1131:267-276, September 1996.
5. M. Bro-Nielsen, C. Gramkow, and S. Kreiborg, Non-rigid image registration using bone growth model, in *Proc. CVRMed/MRCAS'97*, Springer Lecture Notes in Computer Science, 1205:3-12, 1997.
6. D.J. Burr, Elastic Matching of Line Drawings, *IEEE Trans. on PAMI*, 3(6):708-713, November 1981
7. G.E. Christensen, Deformable shape models for anatomy, *PhD thesis*, Washington University, Sever Institute of Technology, 1994.
8. A. Collignon, F. Maes, D. Delaere, D. Vandermeulen, P. Suetens, and G. Marchal, Automated multimodality medical image registration using information theory, in Y. Bizais, C. Barillot, and R. Di Paola (Eds.), *Proc. XIV'th Int. Conf. Information Processing in Medical Imaging*, Computational Imaging and Vision 3, pp. 263-274, Kluwer Academic Publishers, June 1995.
9. A. Collignon, Multi-modality medical image registration by maximization of mutual information, *PhD thesis*, K.U. Leuven, 1998
10. D.L. Collins, 3D Model-based segmentation of individual brain structures from magnetic resonance imaging data, *PhD thesis*, McGill University, 1994.
11. T.M. Cover and J.A. Thomas, Elements of Information Theory, John Wiley & Sons, 1991.
12. T. Gaens, S. Sagaert, D. Vandermeulen, Non-rigid registration using mutual information, *ESAT/PSI Technical Report* nr. 97/10, 1997.
13. H. Lester, S. Arridge, Summarising fluid registration by thin-plate spline warps with many landmarks, in *Proceedings of Medical Image Understanding and Analysis 1997*, Oxford, July 1997.
14. F. Maes, A. Collignon, D. Vandermeulen, G. Marchal, and P. Suetens, Multi-Modality Image Registration by Maximization of Mutual Information, *IEEE Trans. on Medical Imaging*, 16(2):187-198, April 1997.
15. D. McGarry, T. Jackson, M. Plantec, N. Kassell, J.H. Downs, Registration of functional magnetic resonance imagery using mutual information, *Proc. SPIE Medical Imaging 1997*, pp. 621-630.
16. C. Meyer, J. Boes, B. Kim, P. Bland, K. Zasadny, P. Kison, K. Koral, K. Frey, R. Wahl, Demonstration of accuracy and clinical versatility of mutual information for automatic multimodality image fusion using affine and thin-plate spline warped geometric deformations, *Medical Image Analysis*, 1(3):195-206, April 1997.
17. J.B. Maintz, E. Meijering, M. Viergever, General multimodal elastic registration based on mutual information, to appear in *Proc. SPIE Med. Imaging*, 1998.
18. C. Maurer, and J. Fitzpatrick, A review of medical image registration, in R. Maciunas (Ed.), *Interactive Image-guided Neurosurgery*, pp. 17-44, American Association of Neurological Surgeons, 1993.
19. J.-P. Thirion, Fast non-rigid matching of 3D medical images, *INRIA Technical Report*, nr. 2547, May 1995.
20. P. van den Elsen, E.-J. Pol, and M. Viergever, Medical image matching - a review with classification, *IEEE Eng. in Medicine and Biology*, pp. 26-38, March 1993.
21. P. Viola and W.M. et al. Wells III, Multi-modal volume registration by maximization of mutual information, *Medical Image Analysis*, 1(1):35-51, March 1996.

Feature-Based Registration of Medical Images: Estimation and Validation of the Pose Accuracy

Xavier Pennec[1,2], Charles R.G. Guttmann[3], and Jean-Philippe Thirion[4,1]

[1] INRIA Sophia Antipolis, EPIDAURE project, France
Xavier.Pennec@sophia.inria.fr,
http://www.inria.fr/epidaure/personnel/pennec/pennec.html
[2] MIT, A.I.Lab, Cambridge, USA
[3] Brigham and Women's Hospital, Harvard Medical School, Boston, USA
[4] Focus Imaging SA, France

Abstract. We provide in this article a generic framework for pose estimation from geometric features. We propose more particularly two algorithms: a gradient descent on the Riemannian least squares distance and on the Mahalanobis distance. For each method, we provide a way to compute the uncertainty of the resulting transformation. The analysis and comparison of the algorithms show their advantages and drawbacks and point out the very good prediction on the transformation accuracy. An application in medical image analysis validates the uncertainty estimation on real data and demonstrates that, using adapted and rigorous tools, we can detect very small modifications in medical images. We believe that these algorithms could be easily embedded in many applications and provide a thorough basis for computing many image statistics.

1 Introduction

Registration is a fundamental task in medical imaging to compare images taken at different times for diagnosis or therapy. In the case of images of the same patient, one often assume that the motion between the images is rigid, and registration consists in estimating the six parameters of the 3D rotation and translation. When registration is based on features extracted from the images, the problem can be separated into two steps: (1) finding the correspondences between features (matches) and (2) computing the geometric transformation that maps one set of features to the other. In this article, we do not discuss matching methods per se, but rather the estimation of the geometric transformation from matched features. The quantification of the registration quality is also an important problem as most measurements are done after registration. For instance, registration errors can have a strong influence on the quantification of the lesion evolution [3]. Knowing the uncertainty of the transformation might even be vital in image guided surgery when it comes to operate close to important anatomical structures.

Most existing methods for computing 3D rigid motion deal with sets of matched points and minimize the sum of square distances after registration.

This is called the *orthogonal Procrustes problem* in statistics, the *absolute orientation problem* in photogrammetry and the *pose estimation problem* in computer vision. Several closed form solutions have been developed, using unit quaternions [4], singular value decomposition (SVD) [9,11], Polar decomposition [5] or dual quaternions [12]. However, models of the real world often require more complex features like lines [2], planes, oriented points or frames. Traditional methods rely on the vector space structure of points and generalizing them directly to other types of features leads to paradoxes. For instance, depending on the representation used, the standard expectation could take an arbitrary value [7]. Moreover, if uncertainty handling is a central topic in several works, like [1], there are much fewer studies dealing with the accuracy of the estimated transformation.

We first review some notions of Riemannian geometry in order to introduce proper tools on geometric features. Then, we develop a pose estimation criterion based on the Riemannian least-squares and another based on the intrinsic Mahalanobis distance, and provide a way to compute an estimation of the result accuracy (generalizing the approach of [8] to any kind of features). In the last section, we investigate a practical case in Medical Image Analysis: the registration of MRI images of the head, where the availability of each image in two different echoes allows us to test for the uncertainty prediction.

2   Geometric Features

Geodesics Geometric features like lines, planes, oriented points, frames, etc. generally belong to a manifold and not to a vector space. In the geometric framework, one specifies the structure of a manifold $\mathcal{M}$ by a *Riemannian metric*. This is a continuous collection of dot products on the tangent space at each point x of the manifold. Thus, if we consider a curve on the manifold, we can compute at each point its instantaneous speed. The length of the curve is obtained as usual by integrating it along the curve. The distance between two points of a connected Riemannian manifold is the minimum length among the curves joining these points. The curves realizing this minimum for any two points of the manifold are called geodesics.

Exponential charts Let us develop the manifold in the tangent space at point x along the geodesics (think of rolling a sphere along its tangent plane). The geodesics going through that point are transformed into straight lines and the distance along these geodesics are conserved. This generates a chart called *the exponential chart*. It covers all the manifold except a set of null measure called the cut locus. Let $\overrightarrow{xy}$ be the representation of y in this chart. Then its distance to x is $\text{dist}(x,y) = \|\overrightarrow{xy}\|$. This means that the exponential chart is a linear representation of the manifold with respect to the development point.

Invariant distance Since we are working with a transformation group that models the possible image viewpoints, it is natural to choose an invariant Riemannian metric on the manifold. This way, all the measurements based on distance are independent of the image reference frame. Denoting by $f \star x$ the action of transformation f on feature x, the distance is invariant if $\text{dist}(x,y) = \text{dist}(f \star x, f \star y)$. Existence conditions for such a metric are detailes in [7].

Principal chart Let o be a point of the manifold that we call *the origin* and f_x be a "placement function" (a transformation such that $f_x \star o = x$). We call *principal chart* the exponential chart at the origin and we denote by $\vec{x}$ the representation of x in this chart. In this chart, the distance becomes: $\text{dist}(x,y) = \text{dist}(f_x^{(-1)} \star y, o) = \|f_{\vec{x}}^{(-1)} \star \vec{y}\|$. In fact, we can express all operations of interest for us from the following "*atomic operations*" and their Jacobians in the principal chart: **the action** $[\vec{f} \star \vec{x}]$ of a transformation and **the placement function** $[\vec{f}_{\vec{x}}]$.

The transformation group Since the group acts on itself, we just have to replace the action by **the composition** $[\vec{f} \circ \vec{g}]$ and add **the inversion** $[\vec{f}^{(-1)}]$ to the atomic operations. The placement function disappears (it is the identity). An important property of the invariant metric is that it relates the exponential chart at any point f with the principal chart. Using the non-orthogonal coordinate system induced by the principal chart, we have: $\vec{fg} = J_L(\vec{f})(\vec{f}^{(-1)} \circ \vec{g})$, where $J(\vec{f}) = \left.\frac{\partial(\vec{f} \circ \vec{e})}{\partial \vec{e}}\right|_{\vec{e}=Id}$ is the Jacobian of the left translation of the identity in the principal chart. From a practical point of view, this means that we can "translate" local calculations on points to the principal chart of our transformation group by replacing $g - f$ with $\vec{fg}$ and $f + \delta f$ with $\exp_{\vec{f}}(\vec{\delta f}) = \vec{f} \circ (J_L(\vec{f})^{(-1)} \vec{\delta f})$.

Example of features We have implemented this framework for 3D rigid transformations acting on frames, semi-oriented frames and points. Frames are composed of a point and an orthonormal trihedron and are equivalent to rigid transformations. The principal chart is made of the rotation vector representing the trihedron or the rotation and the translation of the point position vector. Semi-oriented frames model the differential properties of a point on a surface. In particular, they model the "extremal points" we will extract on medical images in Sec. 4. They are composed of a point and a trihedron (t_1, t_2, n) where $(t_1, t_2) \equiv (-t_1, -t_2)$ are the principal *directions* and n the normal of the surface.

3 Feature-Based Pose Estimation

3.1 Riemannian Least-Squares

Let $\{x_i\}$ and $\{y_i\}$ be two sets of matched features. The Least squares criterion is easily written using the invariant Riemannian distance:

$$C(f) = \frac{1}{2} \sum_i \text{dist}(y_i, f \star x_i)^2$$

Now, thanks to the good properties of the principal chart, it turns out that this criterion can be expressed as a classical sum of squares of vector norms. Let $\vec{z}_i = \vec{f}_{\vec{y}_i}^{(-1)} \circ (\vec{f} \star \vec{x}_i)$ be the *error vector* in the principal chart. The criterion becomes $2C(f) = \sum_i \text{dist}\left(f_{y_i}^{(-1)} \circ (f \star x_i), o\right)^2 = \sum_i \|\vec{z}_i\|^2$.

From the atomic operations, and using the composition rule for differentials, we can compute the error vector $\vec{z}_i$ and its Jacobians $\frac{\partial \vec{z}_i}{\partial x_i}$, $\frac{\partial \vec{z}_i}{\partial y_i}$, and $\frac{\partial \vec{z}_i}{\partial f}$. The first derivative of the criterion $C(f)$ is: $\Phi = \sum_i \frac{\partial \vec{z}_i}{\partial f}^T \vec{z}_i$. Neglecting the term in $\ddot{z}z$ with respect to the terms in $\dot{z}^2$ in the second derivatives, we obtain: $H = \frac{\partial \Phi}{\partial f} \simeq \sum_i \frac{\partial \vec{z}_i}{\partial f}^T \frac{\partial \vec{z}_i}{\partial f}$ and $\frac{\partial \Phi}{\partial \vec{z}_i} \simeq \frac{\partial \vec{z}_i}{\partial f}^T$.

A gradient descent algorithm Assume that f is a vector. The 2nd order Taylor expansion of the criterion is $C(f + \delta f) \simeq C(\hat{f}) + \Phi^T \delta f + \frac{1}{2} \delta f^T H \delta f$. The minimum of this approximation is obtained for $\delta f = -H^{(-1)} \Phi$. Now, since $\vec{f}$ is the expression of a transformation in the principal chart, we just have to replace $f + \delta f$ by $\exp_f(\overrightarrow{\delta f}) = \vec{f} \circ (J_L(\vec{f})^{(-1)} \overrightarrow{\delta f})$, and iterate the process:

$$\vec{f}_{t+1} = \vec{f}_t \circ \left(-J_L(\vec{f}_t)^{(-1)} H_t^{(-1)} \Phi_t \right) \quad (1)$$

As an initial estimate, we can choose the identity if nothing else is given. The process is stopped when the norm $\|\overrightarrow{\delta f}_t\|$ of the adjustment transformation becomes too small (we use $\varepsilon = 10^{-10}$) or when the number of iterations becomes too high (practically, it converges in about 10 iterations).

Estimation of the uncertainty at the minimum Let $\hat{\chi}$ be the vector of observed data and $\hat{f}$ the corresponding state vector. The minimum $f(\chi)$ of the criterion for a data vector χ is characterized by $\Phi(f(\chi), \chi) = 0$. A Taylor expansion around the actual values $(\hat{\chi}, \hat{f})$ gives a modification of the state $\delta f = -\hat{H}^{(-1)} \hat{J}_\Phi \delta \chi$ for a modification of the data vector $\delta \chi$, where $\hat{J}_\Phi = \frac{\partial^2 \Phi}{\partial \chi \partial f}$. Thus, the covariance of $\hat{f}$ is $\Sigma_{\hat{f}\hat{f}} = \mathbf{E}(\delta f \delta f^T) = \hat{H}^{(-1)} \hat{J}_\Phi \Sigma_{\hat{\chi}\hat{\chi}} \hat{J}_\Phi^T \hat{H}^{(-1)}$. Assuming that all our measurements are independent, we can simplify $\hat{J}_\Phi \Sigma_{\hat{\chi}\hat{\chi}} \hat{J}_\Phi^T$ to obtain:

$$\Sigma_{\hat{f}\hat{f}} = \hat{H}^{(-1)} \left(\sum_i \frac{\partial \hat{\Phi}}{\partial \vec{z}_i} \Sigma_{z_i z_i} \frac{\partial \hat{\Phi}}{\partial \vec{z}_i}^T \right) \hat{H}^{(-1)} \quad (2)$$

In our case, the data and the state are not vectors, but features and transformations in a Riemannian manifold. In fact, we can do the same derivation by replacing δf with $\overrightarrow{\delta f} = J(\hat{\vec{f}})(\hat{\vec{f}}^{(-1)} \circ \overrightarrow{\delta f})$ and $\delta \chi$ with a somehow similar expression. It turns out that the definition of the covariance is changed accordingly and that finally nothing is changed in equation (2).

3.2 Mahalanobis Distance Minimization

To allow different and non isotropic covariance matrices for different measures, we can minimize the sum of squared Mahalanobis distances after registration. It turns out that this Mahalanobis distance can be expressed with exactly the same error vector as before:

$$C(f) = \frac{1}{2} \sum_i \mu^2(\mathbf{y}_i, \mathbf{f} \star \mathbf{x}_i) = \frac{1}{2} \sum_i \vec{z}_i^T \Sigma_{z_i z_i}^{(-1)} \vec{z}_i$$

Thus, the algorithm is the same as for least squares, but the derivatives of the criterion are different: $\Phi = \left(\frac{\partial C}{\partial f}\right)^T = \sum_i \frac{\partial \vec{z}_i}{\partial f}^T \Sigma_{z_i z_i}^{(-1)} \vec{z}_i$, $H \simeq \sum_i \frac{\partial \vec{z}_i}{\partial f}^T \Sigma_{z_i z_i}^{(-1)} \frac{\partial \vec{z}_i}{\partial f}$ and $\frac{\partial \Phi}{\partial \vec{z}_i} \simeq \frac{\partial \vec{z}_i}{\partial f}^T \Sigma_{z_i z_i}^{(-1)}$. Now, with these new derivatives, the Taylor expansion for the criterion is the same, and the evolution for the gradient descent is still given by equation (1). We can use the same starting value and stopping criterion as before. Practically, we have observed a convergence in about 15 iterations when starting from identity and in 5 to 10 iterations when starting from the least-squares solution. For the uncertainty of the solution, we replace the values of H and $\frac{\partial \Phi}{\partial \vec{z}_i}$ into equation (2) and obtain: $\Sigma_{\hat{f}\hat{f}} = \hat{H}^{(-1)}$

3.3 Algorithm Comparison

We have performed test on synthetic data simulating the MRI data of Sect. (4) to evaluate these two algorithms (denoted by LSQ and MAHA). Since all our features can be simplified into points, we took as reference the unit quaternion technique (QUAT) [4]. Concerning accuracy, we found that QUAT and LSQ perform very similarly, but MAHA is 1.2 to 1.5 times more accurate. LSQ and MAHA computation times are much higher than QUAT (by a factor 10 to 40) but the times are still reasonable (we have applied these algorithms to more than 500 registrations of MR images in next section).

To verify the uncertainty prediction, we used the validation index developped in [8]: under the Gaussian hypothesis, the Mahalanobis distance between the estimated and the exact transformation (the validation index) should be χ_6^2 distributed. By repeating the registration experiment, we can verify that the empirical mean value $I = \bar{\mu}^2 = \frac{1}{N}\sum \mu_i^2$ and variance σ_I^2 correspond to the expected values (here 6 and 12 for a χ_6^2), and that the empirical distribution corresponds to the exact distribution using the Kolmogorov-Smirnov (K-S) test. As expected, the most accuracy estimation is given by MAHA ($I = 6.05$, $\sigma_I^2 = 11.90$), which proves that the uncertainty estimation is very accurate. For LSQ, the uncertainty on the transformation is still well predicted (but it is larger that the one of MAHA) and QUAT needs a minimum number of 15 matches tp pass the K-S test since we have to estimate the noise on features from mesurements.

As a conclusion, MAHA gives the most accurate transformation and a good uncertainty in all cases, even with very few matches, but it should be initialized with QUAT to keep the computation time low.

4 Registration of Real MRI Images

The experiment is performed using multiple 2D contiguous Magnetic Resonance images (MRI) which constitute a 3D representation of the head. The images are part of an extensive study of the evolution of the Multiple Sclerosis (MS) disease performed at the Brigham and Woman's Hospital (Harvard Medical School, Boston). Each patient underwent a complete head MR examination several times during one year (up to 24 different 3D acquisitions). Each acquisition provides a first echo image and a second echo image (256 x 256 x 54 voxels of size .9375 x .9375 x 3mm) representing the same T2 weighted signal imaged at different echo times. Thus, they are expected to be approximately in the same coordinate system. This protocol was designed to optimize the contrast in the two channels for an easier tissue segmentation. Considering two acquisitions A and B, the registration of echo-1 images (A_1 to B_1) and echo-2 images (A_2 to B_2) give two relatively independent estimates of the genuine transformation from A to B. The comparison of these two transformations gives a Real Validation Index which can be tested for the accuracy of the uncertainty estimation.

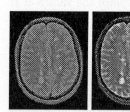 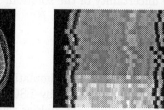

Fig. 1. Left: Example of MS images. The same slice of one acquisition in echo-1 (left) and echo-2 (right). **Right:** evolution of an image row going through a lesion across 24 time points over a year. Left: without registration; Right: after registration and intensity correction.

Our registration algorithm relies on the extraction of *Extremal Points* (see [10]) that we model as semi-oriented frames (see Sec. 2). Matches between extremal points of two images are determined using an iterative closest point algorithm adapted to such features. Typically, we match 1000 extremal points out of the about 3000 extracted with a residual mean square error (RMS) of about $1mm$. We initialize the registration with QUAT and then iterate a loop consisting of a noise estimation on features [8] followed by a MAHA registration.

In a first experiment, we compared directly the registrations between corresponding echo-1 and echo-2 images. This diagram represents three acquisitions A, B and C with the three echo-1 images (A_1, B_1, C_1) and the three echo-2 images (A_2, B_2, C_2). The echo-1 and echo-2 registrations are significantly different ($\mu^2(f_{AB_1}, f_{AB_2})$, $\mu^2(f_{AC_1}, f_{AC_2})$, $\mu^2(f_{BC_1}, f_{BC_2}) > 50$) but the intra-echo-1 and intra-echo2 registrations are compatible ($\mu^2(f_{BC_1} \circ f_{AB_1}, f_{AC_1}) \simeq 6$ and $\mu^2(f_{BC_2} \circ f_{AB_2}, f_{AC_2}) \simeq 6$). This led us to assume a global bias for each acquisition between echo-1 and echo-2 images, represented here by the transformations f_A, f_B, and f_C.

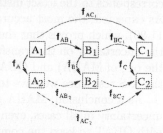

To estimate the biases, we observed first that the transformation from image A_1 to image B_2 can be written $f_{A_1 B_2} = f_B \circ f_{AB_1} = f_{AB_2} \circ f_A$. If measurements where perfect, the bias f_A could be expressed for any other image Z: $f_A = f_{AZ_2}^{(-1)} \circ f_Z \circ f_{AZ_1}$. Since measurements are noisy, we obtain an estimator of the bias f_A by taking the Fréchet mean value [7]. The biases we obtain are different for each acquisition and could be considered as translations of standard deviations $\sigma_x = 0.09$, $\sigma_y = 0.11$ and $\sigma_z = 0.13$ mm.

Although the biases appear very small, they are sufficient to explain the previous errors in the registration accuracy prediction: the mean value and standard deviation of this new index across all registrations are now very close to their theoretical value (see table 1). For the uncertainty of the transformations, we found a typical boundary precision around $\sigma_{corn} = 0.11$ mm and a typical object precision far below the voxel size: $\sigma_{obj} = 0.05$ mm for echo-1 registrations. Values are even a little smaller for echo-2 registrations: $\sigma_{corn} = 0.10$ and $\sigma_{obj} = 0.045$ mm.

	$\bar{I}$	σ_I	K-S test	num. im.	num. reg.
Theoretical values	6	$\sqrt{12} = 3.46$	0.01 − 1	$n \leq 24$	$n * (n - 1)/2$
patient 1	6.29	4.58	0.14	15	105
patient 2	5.42	3.49	0.12	18	153
patient 3	6.50	3.68	0.25	14	91
patient 4	6.21	3.67	0.78	21	210

Table 1. Real Validation Index with bias correction for different patients. The mean validation index is within 10% of its theoretical value and the K-S test exhibits impressively high values.

Most of the extremal points we match are situated on the surface of the brain and the ventricles. These surfaces appear differently in echo-1 and echo-2 images due to the difference in contrast. Other artifacts such as chemical shift or susceptibility effects may also account for the observed bias as they influence the detection of extremal points. Indeed, the two echoes are acquired with different receiver RF bandwidth to improve the signal/noise ratio [6]. Therefore, the chemical shift and the susceptibility effect are different in the two echoes. In a future work, we plan to correlate the biases with diverse quantities in the images in order to understand their origin. Ultimately, we would like to predict the biases in each acquisition before registration. This would allow the indubitable validation of the registration accuracy prediction.

5 Conclusion

We show in this article how to generalize the classical least squares and least Mahalanobis distance pose estimation algorithms to generic geometric features, and how to estimate the uncertainty of the result. The uncertainty prediction on the transformation is validated on synthetic data within a bound of 5% for all algorithms, decreasing to less than 1% of inaccuracy for the algorithm MAHA. We believe that these algorithms could be easily embedded in many applications and provide a thorough basis for computing many image statistics. Further improvements could include the generalization of this framework to non rigid transformations, the estimation of a multiple registration of n sets of matched features and the coupling with statistical matching algorithms to provide a complete registration system.

From the application point of view, we show an example in medical imaging where we reached a sub-voxel registration accuracy (0.05 mm) that allowd us to detect and estimate a systematic bias in each acquisition between features extracted from the echo-1 and the echo-2 images. After the correction of the biases, multiple experiments on several patients show that our prediction of the registration accuracy is validated within a bound of 10%. These experiments demonstrate that, using adapted and rigorous tools, we can detect very small modifications in medical images. In a future work, we plan to determine the origin of the bias in order to predict it. Other applications include the automatic detection and correction of the misalignment of the slices in contiguous slice images and the statistical study of deformations in MR images.

Acknowledgments

The authors would like to thank Pr. Eric Grimson and Pr. Ron Kikinis for making this collaboration possible. Part of this work was supported by a post-doctoral fellowship from INRIA at the A.I.Lab, in Pr. Grimson team. The serial MRI exams were obtained from studies of the natural course of multiple sclerosis support by the National Institute of Health (contract no. N01-NS-0-2397).

References

1. H.F. Durrant-Whyte. Uncertain geometry in robotics. *IEEE Journal of Robotics and Automation*, 4(1):23–31, February 1988.
2. W.E.L. Grimson. *Object Recognition by Computer - The role of Geometric Constraints*. MIT Press, 1990.
3. C.R.G. Guttmann, R. Kikinis, M.C. Anderson, M. Jakab, S.K. Warfield, R.J. Killiany, H.L. Weiner, and Jolesz F.A. Quantitative follow-up of patients with multiple sclerosis using mri: reproducibility. *JMRI*, 1998. To appear.
4. B.K.P. Horn. Closed form solutions of absolute orientation using unit quaternions. *Journal of Optical Society of America*, A-4(4):629–642, April 1987.
5. B.K.P. Horn, Hilden H.M., and S. Negahdaripour. Closed form solutions of absolute orientation using orthonormal matrices. *Journal of Optical Society of America*, A-5(7):1127–1135, 1988.
6. R. Kikinis, C.R.G. Guttmann, D. Metcalf, W.M. III Wells, G.J. Ettinger, H.L. Weiner, and F.A. Jolesz. Quantitative follow-up of patients with multiple sclerosis using mri: technical aspects. *JMRI*, 1998. to appear.
7. X. Pennec and N. Ayache. Uniform distribution, distance and expectation problems for geometric features processing. *Journal of Mathematical Imaging and Vision*, 9(1):49–67, July 1998.
8. X. Pennec and J.P. Thirion. A framework for uncertainty and validation of 3D registration methods based on points and frames. *Int. Journal of Computer Vision*, 25(3):203–229, 1997.
9. P.H. Schönemann. A generalized solution of the orthogonal Procrustes problem. *Psychometrika*, 31:1–10, 1966.
10. J-P Thirion. The extremal mesh and the understanding of 3D surfaces. *IJCV*, 19(2):115–128, 1996.
11. S. Umeyama. Least-squares estimation of transformation parameters between two point patterns. *IEEE Transactions on Pattern Analysis and Machine Intelligence*, 13(4):376–380, April 1991.
12. M.W. Walker and L. Shao. Estimating 3-D location paramters using dual number quaternions. *CVGIP: Image Understanding*, 54(3):358–367, Nov. 1991.

The Correlation Ratio as a New Similarity Measure for Multimodal Image Registration

Alexis Roche, Grégoire Malandain, Xavier Pennec, and Nicholas Ayache

INRIA Sophia Antipolis, EPIDAURE project, France
Alexis.Roche@sophia.inria.fr

Abstract. Over the last five years, new "voxel-based" approaches have allowed important progress in multimodal image registration, notably due to the increasing use of information-theoretic similarity measures. Their wide success has led to the progressive abandon of measures using standard image statistics (mean and variance). Until now, such measures have essentially been based on heuristics. In this paper, we address the determination of a new measure based on standard statistics from a theoretical point of view. We show that it naturally leads to a known concept of probability theory, the *correlation ratio*. In our derivation, we take as the hypothesis the functional dependence between the image intensities. Although such a hypothesis is not as general as possible, it enables us to model the image smoothness prior very easily. We also demonstrate results of multimodal rigid registration involving Magnetic Resonance (MR), Computed Tomography (CT), and Positron Emission Tomography (PET) images. These results suggest that the correlation ratio provides a good trade-off between accuracy and robustness.

1 Introduction

The general principle of voxel-based registration consists of quantifying the quality of matching with respect to a *similarity measure* of the images' overlapping voxels. As the measure is assumed to be maximal when the images are correctly aligned, these approaches are often implemented using an optimization scheme, or simulating a dynamic process [7].

Many similarity measures have been proposed in the literature (see [3, 15, 2, 6] for reviews). Considering the elementary problem of aligning two similar images, the first idea was to use a least squares criterion. Simple correlation measures were then proposed in order to cope with inter-image bias. Although these similarity measures have been used extensively in medical imaging, they basically assume a linear relationship between the image intensities. Such a hypothesis is generally too crude in multimodal registration.

More recently, Woods et al. [21, 20] have proposed an original criterion which proved itself to be efficient for matching PET with MR. Although the method needs some manual segmentation to work, Nikou et al. [9] have defined a robust version of the criterion that led to a fully automatic algorithm and extended its usage to several modality combinations.

But the currently most popular multimodal measure is probably mutual information [18, 17, 5, 13, 8] since it has been used with success for a large variety of combinations including MR, CT, PET, and SPECT[1]. Given two images X and Y, one can define their joint probability density function (joint pdf), $P(i,j)$, by simple normalization of their 2D-histogram (other approaches are possible, see section 2.3). Let $P_x(i)$ and $P_y(j)$ denote the corresponding marginal probability density functions (pdf's). Mutual information between X and Y is given by [1]:

$$I(X,Y) = \sum_{i,j} P(i,j) \log_2 \frac{P(i,j)}{P_x(i)P_y(j)}.$$

The mutual information measure is very general because it makes no assumptions regarding the nature of the relationship that exists between the image intensities (see [16] for an excellent discussion). It does not assume a linear, nor functional correlation but only a *predictable* relationship.

However, one pitfall of mutual information is to treat intensity values in a purely *qualitative* way, without considering any notion of proximity in the intensity space. As one tissue is never represented by a single intensity value, nearby intensities convey a lot of *spatial* information.

Let us illustrate this remark with a synthetic experiment (see figure 1). We consider two artificial images : a binary image A representing a "grey stripe" (40 × 30 pixels), and a gradation image B of the stripe (30 × 30 pixels) in which the intensity is uniform in any column but each column has a different intensity.

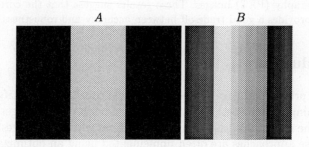

Fig. 1. *"Grey stripe" registration experiment.*

If we horizontally move B over A, we note that any translation corresponding to an integer number of pixels makes mutual information $I(A, B_T)$ maximal (provided that B_T totally falls into A). Then, $I(A, B_T)$ reaches 1, which is its theoretical upper bound in this case. This is to say that mutual information does not explain how to align the stripes.

Mutual information and the correlation ratio (later explained) have been computed for various horizontal translations of B, using bilinear interpolation for non-integer ones (see figure 2). Unlike mutual information, the correlation

---

[1] Single Photon-Emission Computed Tomography.

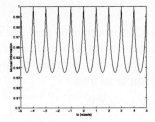 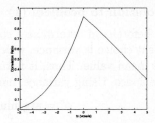

Fig. 2. *"Grey stripe" registration experiment. Left, plot of mutual information $I(A, B_T)$ vs. horizontal translation. Right, the correlation ratio. By convention, the null translation corresponds to the case where the stripes completely overlap. Notice that for any integer translation, $I(A, B_T)$ is maximal (for non-integer translations, smaller values are observed due to interpolation).*

ratio has an absolute maximum corresponding to the position where the stripes completely overlap.

This example suggests that mutual information may be under-constrained when reasonable assumptions can be made upon the existing relationship between the images. Practically, one often observes its tendency to handle many local maxima. In this paper, we address the case where a *functional* correlation can be assumed, but making minimal assumptions regarding the nature of the function itself. The similarity measure we propose is inherited from probability theory and is known as the *correlation ratio*.

2 Theory

We give an intuitive argument to introduce our approach. Suppose that we have two registered images, X and Y. If we randomly select voxels in their overlapping region, we will observe that the intensity couples we get are statistically consistent: all the voxels having a certain intensity i in X may also have clustered intensities in Y (possibly very different from i). Depending on the images type, any iso-set $X = i$ might project to one or several such clusters. In the case of a single cluster per iso-set, the intensity in Y could be approximately predicted from the intensity in X, by applying a simple function. This argument is valid only if the images are correctly registered. Thus, we could use the degree of *functional* dependence between X and Y as a matching criterion.

How now to measure the functional dependence? In the above thought experiment, images X and Y are considered as random variables. Evaluating the functional dependence between two variables comes down to an unconstrained regression problem. Suppose we want to determine how well X approximates Y. A natural approach is:

(1) find the function $\phi^*(X)$ that best fits Y among *all* possible functions of X,
(2) measure the quality of fitting.

2.1 A solution to problem (1)

One must beforehand determine a cost function in order to perform regression. A convenient choice is variance, which measures a variable's average dispersion around its mean value. Thus, it naturally imposes a constraint of proximity in the sample space. Using variance, our problem is to find

$$\phi^* = \arg\min_{\phi} Var\left[Y - \phi(X)\right]. \tag{1}$$

If no constraint is imposed on the functions ϕ (such as linearity), eq (1) is known to be minimized uniquely by the *conditional expectation* of Y in terms of X [10]. Recall that it is defined by,

$$E(Y|X) = \phi^*(X), \quad \text{with} \quad \phi^*(x) = \int y\, p(y|x)\, dy,$$

where $p(y|x)$ denotes the conditional pdf of Y assuming the event $X = x$. To a given event corresponds a given conditional pdf.

2.2 A solution to problem (2)

Now that we have optimally estimated Y in terms of X, we use a result known as the total variance theorem [12, 11], which relies on the orthogonality principle well-known in Kalman filtering:

$$Var(Y) = Var\left[E(Y|X)\right] + Var\left[Y - E(Y|X)\right]. \tag{2}$$

This may be seen as an energy conservation equation. The variance of Y is decomposed as a sum of two antagonist "energy" terms: while $Var\left[E(Y|X)\right]$ measures the part of Y which is predicted by X, $Var\left[Y - E(Y|X)\right]$ measures the part of Y which is functionally independent of X.

From eq (2), we remark that $Var\left[Y - E(Y|X)\right]$ can actually be low for two distinct reasons: either Y is well "explained" by X ($Var\left[E(Y|X)\right]$ is high), or Y gives little information ($Var(Y)$ is low). In a registration problem, $Var(Y)$ can only be computed in the overlapping region of the images. It may be arbitrarily low depending on the region size. Thus, minimizing $Var\left[Y - E(Y|X)\right]$ would tend to completely disconnect the images. Notice that for exactly the same reasons, mutual information is preferred to conditional entropy [16].

It seems more reasonable to compare the "explained" energy of Y with its total energy. This leads to the definition of the *correlation ratio*:

$$\eta(Y|X) = \frac{Var\left[E(Y|X)\right]}{Var(Y)} \iff \eta(Y|X) = 1 - \frac{Var\left[Y - E(Y|X)\right]}{Var(Y)}. \tag{3}$$

The correlation ratio measures the functional dependence between X and Y. It takes on values between 0 (no functional dependence) and 1 (purely deterministic dependence). Due to the use of a ratio instead of a subtraction, $\eta(Y|X)$ is invariant to multiplicative changes in Y, i.e. $\forall k$, $\eta(kY|X) = \eta(Y|X)$. Also note that the correlation ratio is asymmetrical by nature since the two variables fundamentally do not play the same role in the functional relationship; in general, $\eta(Y|X) \neq \eta(X|Y)$.

2.3 Application to registration

In order to compute the correlation ratio between two images, we must be able to define them as random variables, that is determine their marginal and joint pdf's. A common technique consists of normalizing the image pair 2D-histogram [4, 5, 2]. Then, the images may be seen as discrete random variables [11]. Viola [16] has proposed a continuous approach using Parzen density estimates.

If we choose the discrete approach, there is no need to manipulate explicitly the images 2D-histogram. Instead, the correlation ratio can be computed recursively by accumulating local computations. Let Ω denote the images overlapping region, and $N = \text{Card}(\Omega)$ the total number of voxels it contains. We consider the iso-sets of X, $\Omega_i = \{\omega \in \Omega, X(\omega) = i\}$ and their cardinals $N_i = \text{Card}(\Omega_i)$. The total and conditional moments (mean and variance) of Y are:

$$\sigma^2 = \frac{1}{N} \sum_{\omega \in \Omega} Y(\omega)^2 - m^2, \qquad m = \frac{1}{N} \sum_{\omega \in \Omega} Y(\omega).$$

$$\sigma_i^2 = \frac{1}{N_i} \sum_{\omega \in \Omega_i} Y(\omega)^2 - m_i^2, \qquad m_i = \frac{1}{N_i} \sum_{\omega \in \Omega_i} Y(\omega).$$

Starting from eq (3), we obtain a very simple expression for the correlation ratio (the complete proof can be found in [11]):

$$1 - \eta(Y|X) = \frac{1}{N \sigma^2} \sum_i N_i \sigma_i^2. \qquad (4)$$

The algorithm derived from these equations does not require the computation of the images 2D-histogram. This makes an important difference with mutual information. Classical algorithms for computing mutual information have an $\mathcal{O}(n_x n_y)$ complexity, n_x and n_y being the number of intensity levels in the X and Y images, respectively. Our computation of the correlation ratio has only an $\mathcal{O}(n_x)$ complexity, and is independent from n_y.

3 Related measures

The correlation ratio generalizes the correlation coefficient, which is a symmetrical measure of *linear* dependence between two random variables:

$$\rho(X,Y) = \frac{Cov(X,Y)^2}{Var(X)Var(Y)}.$$

The correlation coefficient is closely related to the various correlation measures that have been used in image registration. The linear dependence being a stronger constraint than the functional dependence, it can be shown that [12, 11],

$$\eta(Y|X) \geq \rho(X,Y), \qquad \eta(X|Y) \geq \rho(X,Y).$$

We now analyze two similarity measures which are based on standard statistics but not limited to the case of linear correlation.

3.1 Woods criterion

The heuristic criterion devised by Woods et al. [21] was originally intended for PET-MR registration, but it has also been used with other modalities [2]. This turns out to be very similar to the correlation ratio. According to the notations introduced in section 2.3, the Woods criterion can be written as follows:

$$W(Y|X) = \frac{1}{N} \sum_i N_i \frac{\sigma_i}{m_i}, \tag{5}$$

where the notation $W(Y|X)$ is used in order to emphasize that the criterion is asymmetrical, such as the correlation ratio. Notice that $W(Y|X)$ has to be *minimized*, just like $1 - \eta(Y|X)$.

Though different, eq (5) and eq (4) express the same basic idea. Even so, we can identify two differences. First, the correlation ratio sums variances, σ_i^2 whereas the Woods criterion sums normalized standard deviations, σ_i/m_i. Second, the multiplicative invariance property is achieved in the correlation ratio via a global division by σ^2; in the Woods criterion, every term of the sum is divided by a conditional mean, m_i.

3.2 Weighted neighbor likelihood

In [16], Viola already proposed performing registration by evaluating the degree of functional dependence between two images. This approach is very analogous to that we have proposed in section 2. First, a *weighted neighbor approximator* is used to estimate the Y image in terms of the X image. Second, a similarity measure is obtained by considering the estimation log-likelihood (under hypotheses we won't discuss here).

We have previously shown [11] that the approximator devised by Viola is nothing but the conditional expectation of Y in terms of a variable, $\tilde{X}$, whose pdf is the Parzen estimate of X. Furthermore, the weighted neighbor likelihood is negatively proportional to the estimation error:

$$L(Y|X) = -k \, Var\left[Y - E(Y|\tilde{X})\right], \qquad k > 0.$$

Maximizing the weighted neighbor likelihood is in fact equivalent to minimizing the *numerator* in eq (3) (up to the use of Parzen windowing). However, the correlation ratio involves a division by $Var(Y)$, which plays a critical role in registration problems since it prevents disconnecting the images (see section 2.2).

4 Results

We tested voxel-based 3D multimodal registration over ten patient brain datasets. For each patient, the following images were available :

- MR, T1 weighted ($256 \times 256 \times 20/26$ voxels of $1.25 \times 1.25 \times 4 \, mm^3$)

- MR, T2 weighted ($256 \times 256 \times 20/26$ voxels of $1.25 \times 1.25 \times 4\,mm^3$)
- CT ($512 \times 512 \times 28/34$ voxels of $0.65 \times 0.65 \times 4\,mm^3$)
- PET ($128 \times 128 \times 15$ voxels of $2.59 \times 2.59 \times 8\,mm^3$)

All images were stored with one byte per voxel. The gold standard transformations between each modality were known thanks to a prospective, marker-based registration method [19]. No preprocessing of the images was done.

We implemented an algorithm similar to that of Maes et al. [5], employing Powell's multidimensional direction set method as a maximization scheme. Four similarity measures were tested: the correlation ratio (CR), mutual information (MI), the correlation coefficient (CC), and the opposite of the Woods criterion (OW). The choice of the opposite is only for consistency: OW has to be maximized like MI, CR, and CC. In all registration experiments, the transformation was initialized as the identity.

We used two different interpolation techniques: trilinear interpolation (TRI) and trilinear partial volume interpolation [5] (PV). The results that are presented here were obtained using PV interpolation; on the whole, they are better than those obtained with TRI interpolation.

After each registration, a "typical" error ϵ was computed in the following way. We selected eight points in the transformed image, approximately situated on the skull surface. Registration errors corresponding to these points were computed according to the marker-based transformation, and then averaged to obtain ϵ.

Table 1. *Mean and median of the registration typical errors (based on positions of stereotaxic markers) obtained over ten intra-patient experiments.*

Experiment	Measure		Mean ϵ (mm)	Median ϵ (mm)
T1-to-T2	MI		4.30	1.48
	CR	(X:T2)	1.93	1.46
	OW	(X:T2)	2.65	2.00
	CC		2.42	2.37
CT-to-T1	MI		2.52	2.00
	CR	(X:T1)	3.27	3.24
PET-to-T1	MI		5.87	5.58
	CR	(X:T1)	4.60	3.65
	OW	(X:T1)	7.69	7.62

Statistics on typical errors over the ten patients are shown in table 1. We got non sensible results with CC in CT-to-T1 and PET-to-T1 registration, and with OW in CT-to-T1 registration. Conversely, MI and CR demonstrated suitable accuracy levels for every modality combination. MI gave the best results for CT-to-T1 registration, while CR was better for PET-to-T1 registration. In the case of T1-to-T2 registration, CR and MI generally provided the best results, but MI failed in two cases. Notice that for CT-to-T1 registration, the CT images were subsampled by factors $2 \times 2 \times 1$ in the x, y, and z direction, respectively; due to the large dimensions of the CT images, registration at full resolution was indeed too time consuming.

Several subsampling factors were also tested for every modality combination in order to speed up the registration process with minimal loss in terms of accuracy. A typical drawback of subsampling is to introduce local maxima in the similarity measure so that the global maximum becomes difficult to track.

Table 2. *The correlation ratio performances depending on resolution.*

Experiment	Subsampling	Mean ϵ (mm)	Median ϵ (mm)
T1-to-T2	$(2 \times 2 \times 1)$	1.90	1.48
	$(4 \times 4 \times 1)$	2.01	1.67
CT-to-T1	$(4 \times 4 \times 1)$	4.23	3.55
	$(8 \times 8 \times 1)$	6.65	5.96
PET-to-T1	$(2 \times 2 \times 1)$	6.82	6.20
	$(4 \times 4 \times 1)$	11.65	11.19

The influence of subsampling on the correlation ratio performances was remarkably moderate (see table 2). While CR allowed good registration at relatively low resolutions, other studies [11] (which could not be presented here) qualitatively demonstrated that CR was less sensitive to subsampling than MI and OW.

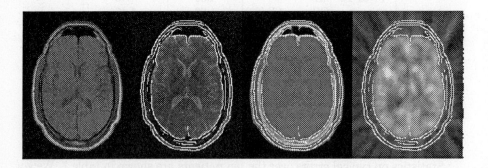

Fig. 3. *Multimodal registration by maximization of CR. Images from left to right : MR-T1, MR-T2, CT, and PET. The images are resampled in the same reference frame after registration. Contours extracted from the MR-T1 are superimposed to each other modality in order to visualize the quality of registration.*

5 Discussion and conclusion

Our experiments tend to show that assuming a functional correlation between certain multimodal images is not critical. Even if this is an approximation, notably in the CT-MR case (see [18] for a discussion), a preprocessing step might validate it. Van den Elsen et al. [14] have proposed a simple intensity mapping to the original CT image so that bone and air appear in the same intensity range as is the case in MR images. Then, low intensities in MR (air and bone) may project to nearby intensities in CT. Another possible strategy for CT-MR registration could be to use the correlation ratio for a quick guessing of the correct transformation (using subsampling), and then mutual information for probably more accurate alignment.

The case of PET images is particular because they are much more distorted than MR or CT. This might explain why mutual information is relatively inaccurate in PET-T1 registration. It is generally admitted that today Woods method is the best one for this specific problem. In some way, our results corroborate this observation, suggesting that taking into account nearby intensities in PET images might be crucial. Mutual information seems to be better adapted to low-noise images.

Finally, the discrepancies found experimentally between the correlation ratio and the Woods criterion are surprising since these two measures are formally based on similar considerations (see section 3.1). It seems that the correlation ratio gives not only a theoretical justification to the Woods criterion but also perceptible practical improvements.

Acknowledgments

The images and the standard transformations were provided as part of the project, "Evaluation of Retrospective Image Registration", National Institutes of Health, Project Number 1 R01 NS33926-01, Principal Investigator, J. Michael Fitzpatrick, Vanderbilt University, Nashville, TN.

Many thanks to Frederik Maes, Jean-Pierre Nadal, and Christophoros Nikou for fruitful discussion and to Janet Bertot for the proofreading of this article.

References

1. R. E. Blahut. *Principles and Practice of Information Theory*. Addison-Wesley Pub. Comp., 1987.
2. M. Bro-Nielsen. Rigid Registration of CT, MR and Cryosection Images Using a GLCM Framework. *CVRMed-MRCAS'97*, pages 171–180, March 1997.
3. L. G. Brown. A survey of image registration techniques. *ACM Computing Surveys*, 24(4):325–376, 1992.
4. D. L. G. Hill and D. J. Hawkes. Medical image registration using voxel similarity measures. *AAAI Sping Symposium Series: Applications of Comp. Vision in Med. Im. Proces.*, pages 34–37, 1994.

5. F. Maes, A. Collignon, D. Vandermeulen, G. Marchal, and P. Suetens. Multimodality Image Registration by Maximization of Mutual Information. *IEEE Transactions on Medical Imaging*, 16(2):187–198, 1997.
6. J. B. A. Maintz and M. A. Viergever. A survey of medical image registration. *MedIA*, 2(1):1–36, 1998.
7. G. Malandain, S. Fernández-Vidal, and J.C. Rocchisani. Improving registration of 3-D images using a mechanical based method . *ECCV'94*, pages 131–136, May 1994.
8. C. R. Meyer, J. L. Boes, B. Kim, P. H. Bland, K. R. Zasadny, P. V. Kison, K. Koral, K. A. Frey, and R. L. Wahl. Demonstration of accuracy and clinical versatility of mutual information for automatic multimodality image fusion using affine and thin-plate warped geometric deformations. *Medical Image Analysis*, 1(3):195–206, 1996/7.
9. C. Nikou, F. Heitz, J.-P. Armspach, and I.-J. Namer. Single and multimodal subvoxel registration of dissimilar medical images using robust similarity measures. *SPIE Conference on Medical Imaging*, February 1998.
10. A. Papoulis. *Probability, Random Variables, and Stochastic Processes*. McGraw-Hill, Inc., third edition, 1991.
11. A. Roche, G. Malandain, X. Pennec, and N.. Ayache. Multimodal Image Registration by Maximization of the Correlation Ratio. Technical Report 3378, INRIA, March 1998.
12. G. Saporta. *Probabilités, analyse des données et statistique*. Editions Technip, Paris, 1990.
13. C. Studholme, D. L. G. Hill, and D. J. Hawkes. Automated 3-D registration of MR and CT images of the head. *Medical Image Analysis*, 1(2):163–175, 1996.
14. P. A. van den Elsen, E.-J. D. Pol, T. S. Sumanaweera, P. F. Hemler, S. Napel, and J. R. Adler. Grey value correlation techniques for automatic matching of CT and MR brain and spine images. *Proc. Visualization in Biomed. Comp.*, 2359:227–237, October 1994.
15. P.A. van den Elsen, E.J.D. Pol, and M.A. Viergever. Medical image matching - a review with classification. *IEEE Engineering in Medicine and Biology*, 12(4):26–39, march 1993.
16. P. Viola. *Alignment by Maximization of Mutual Information*. PhD thesis, M.I.T. Artificial Intelligence Laboratory, 1995. also A.I.T.R. No. 1548, available at ftp://publications.ai.mit.edu.
17. P. Viola and W. M. Wells. Alignment by Maximization of Mutual Information. *Intern. J. of Comp. Vision*, 24(2):137–154, 1997.
18. W. M. Wells, P. Viola, H. Atsumi, and S. Nakajima. Multi-modal volume registration by maximization of mutual information. *Medical Image Analysis*, 1(1):35–51, 1996.
19. J. West and al. Comparison and evaluation of retrospective intermodality brain image registration techniques. *Journal of Comp. Assist. Tomography*, 21:554–566, 1997.
20. R. P. Woods, S. R. Cherry, and J. C. Mazziotta. Rapid Automated Algorithm for Aligning and Reslicing PET Images. *Journal of Comp. Assist. Tomography*, 16(4):620–633, 1992.
21. R. P. Woods, J. C. Mazziotta, and S. R. Cherry. MRI-PET Registration with Automated Algorithm. *Journal of Comp. Assist. Tomography*, 17(4):536–546, 1993.

Real-time Registration of 3D Cerebral Vessels to X-ray Angiograms

Yasuyo Kita[1] Dale L. Wilson[2] J. Alison Noble[2]

[1] Electrotechnical Laboratory, Ibaraki 305-8568, Japan
(terashi@robots.ox.ac.uk Tel:+44-1865-282185 Fax:+44-1865-273908)
[2] University of Oxford, Oxford OX1 3PJ, United Kingdom

Abstract. A quick method to obtain the 3D transformation of a 3D free-form shape model from its 2D projection data is proposed. This method has been developed for the real-time registration of a 3D model of a cerebral vessel tree, obtained from pre-operative data (eg. MR Angiogram), to a X-ray image of the vessel (eg. Digital Subtraction Angiogram) taken during an operation. First, the skeleton of the vessel in a 2D image is automatically extracted in a model-based way using a 2D projection of a 3D model skeleton at the initial state (up to ±20 degree difference in rotation). Corresponding pairs of points on the 3D skeleton and points on the 2D skeleton are determined based on the 2D Euclidean distance between the projection of the model skeleton and the observed skeleton. In the process, an adaptive search region for each model point, which is determined according to the projected shape, effectively removes incorrect correspondences. Based on a good ratio of correct pairs, linearization of a rotation matrix can be used to rapidly calculate the 3D transformation of the model which produces the 2D observed projection. Experiments using real data show the practical usefulness of the method.

Key words: 3D-2D registration, ICP (Iterative closest point) algorithm, multi-modal fusion and augmented reality visualizations.

1 Introduction

This work is being developed to aid the endovascular treatment of intracranial aneurysms by coil embolisation. In current practice, the neuroradiologist guides a catheter through a vessel while viewing its 2D projection (X-ray angiogram). It is hard for a neuroradiologist to visualize the complex 3D shapes of the vessels from one 2D projection, even with the 3D shape information from pre-operative data (eg. MR A(ngiography)). To help the neuroradiologist's understanding, Wilson and Noble[1] developed a method for reconstructing a 3D model of cerebral vessels from slices of MRA data. Fig. 1a shows a result of the reconstructed 3D model. If this 3D structure is superimposed on a 2D intra-operative X-ray image and the location of the catheter is displayed on the 3D reconstruction, it may aid the neuroradiologists in accurately deciding how they should manipulate the catheter. For this purpose, real-time determination of the posture and position of the 3D model from its 2D projection is required.

The determination of the position and posture of a 3D model from its 2D view is a fundamental and important problem in Computer Vision research. In the case that the object has some prominent features (points, edges etc) that can be robustly extracted and matched between the 3D model and its 2D view, the approach based on feature-matching can be taken. However, usually both robust feature extraction and robust feature matching are not easy, especially in the case of a free-form object. The iterative closest point (ICP) algorithm[2], originally developed for 3D-3D rigid registration, has appropriate characteristics for free-form shape registration. The basic idea of the method is to use iterative transformations of the 3D model towards the correct position and posture using the corresponding pairs between the observed and the model points, which are matched on the basis of the closeness at each state. If the initial position and posture is not far from the correct position and posture, so that the corresponding pairs include a high ratio of correct pairs, the model can converge to the correct state. For registration of a 3D model registration to its 2D view, that is, for obtaining the best 3D transformation of a model which produces a given 2D view, the difficulties of the extension of this approach are mainly two-fold:
I) The difficulty of finding correct pairs between the projection of the 3D model and the observed 2D view using only the 2D distance, and;
II) Even after finding the pairs, it is not easy to feedback the 2D difference to the 3D transformation of the model.

Concerning (I), in [3], the tangent of the projection of the 3D model and the observed 2D curve was used to decrease the number of bad correspondences. Although the effectiveness of using such additional attributes (curvatures, grey level etc) in addition to the geometrical distance has been shown in 3D-3D registration of free-form objects[4], it is not so effective in the 3D-2D case for two reasons: a) the tangent on the 2D image is not an invariant feature; and b) the projection of the complex 3D model often causes complicated self-overlapping, where the robust calculation of geometric features can be difficult.

Concerning (II), most proposed methods take similar approaches to a gradient descent method (eg. [5]) to find the best 3D transformation which minimizes the sum of 2D distances between corresponding pairs (or maximizes the similarity between the projection of the model and the observed data) over the six degrees of freedom. However, such approaches are time consuming and are not suitable for use in real-time applications. Fortunately, to address this problem, the Active Vision Research field has made advanced steps towards real-time object tracking from time-sequential 2D images. One solution that has been proposed is to linearize the 3D non-linear transformation[6]. The main difference between their application and ours is that, in their case, the feature correspondences are easier to find since special features (like corners) can be used. To use thier approach, we need to solve the problem (I) and robustly obtain a high ratio of correct pairs.

In this paper we propose a fast registration method which overcomes the two difficulties noted above as follows. Concerning (I), the model-based strategy plays an important role both in extracting the vessels from the X-ray image and

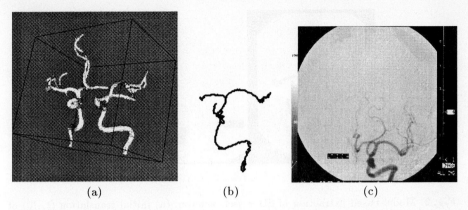

(a) (b) (c)

Fig. 1. The 3D model of the cerebral vessels and a digital subtraction angiography (DSA) image of the same vessels: (a) the 3D model of both carotid circulations; (b) a skeleton of the left internal carotid circulation; (c) a DSA image of the left internal carotid circulation.

in finding correct point matching pairs between the vessel and the 3D model. In particular, the search area for finding the corresponding observed points is effectively adjusted for each point in the 3D model depending on the shape of the model projection, so that most of the wrong pairs are excluded. Secondly, concerning (II), taking advantage of the high-ratio of correct pairs obtained by the first process, the 3D transformation of the model is calculated using separation of the translation effect and linearization of the rotation matrix. Although the correct position and posture of the model is not obtained at once, because of inaccurate matching pairs and linearization errors, the 3D model quickly converges to the correct state by iterating the point matching and model transformation processes.

2 Model-based 2D vessel extraction

2.1 Preprocessing

The input to our method is a skeleton of the 3D vessel model (eg. Fig.1b), obtained from the full 3D vessel reconstruction (Fig. 1a)[7], and a digital subtraction angiography (DSA) image of the vessels (eg. Fig. 1c). For full automation, the region of interest (which is almost a circle) is extracted from the X-ray image with simple image processing. The small black rectangle containing text is also removed from the region of interest.

2.2 Initial localization

Here we briefly explain our 3D coordinate frame, (X, Y, Z). The X-ray source of the X-ray machine is defined as the origin of the coordinate system. The image plane is on the $Z = f$ plane, where f is the distance between the source and the plane. The X and Y axes are defined as the same directions as I and J

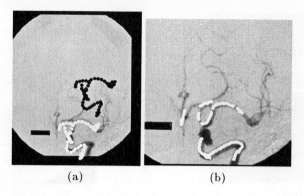

Fig. 2. Model-based extraction of 2D vessel skeleton: (a) initial translation (t_x, t_y) of 3D model (from black to white points); (b) resultant extraction (white lines).

of the image coordinates respectively. The 3D vessel model is placed between the source and the image plane and perspectively projected to the image. The model's initial position and posture is approximately known.

In the registration process we use n points which have been sampled at regular intervals from the 3D model skeleton. The 3D coordinates of these points are $\mathbf{X}_i = (X_i, Y_i, Z_i)^\top (i = 1, ...n)$. The 3D transformation of the model is represented by $\mathbf{R}$(the 3 × 3 rotation matrix) and $\mathbf{T} = (t_x, t_y, t_z)^\top$(the translation vector). The 2D projections of the 3D model points after the transformation of $\mathbf{R}$ and $\mathbf{T}$ have the 3D coordinates $(x_i, y_i, f)^\top$, where $x_i = fX'_i/Z'_i$, $y_i = fY'_i/Z'_i$ and $\mathbf{X}'_i = \mathbf{R}\mathbf{X}_i + \mathbf{T}$.

When real X-ray images are acquired, the patient's head is immobilized, and the X-ray source and the image plane are rotated together around the head. Here, inversely, we rotate the model (head) to give the same effect as the X-ray system rotation. Since the rotation angle of the system is known from the graduations, the position and posture of the 3D model can be estimated approximately. This includes about ± 20 degrees error in rotation and about (±100,±100,±200)(mm) in translation, since the position and posture of the head is not calibrated and is changed a little during the acquisition of the X-ray images. It is this calibration, or determination of the change in the patient position and orientation between MR and X-ray, that we wish to find.

In Fig. 2a black points represent the projection of the 3D model skeleton at its initial state. Using simple template matching between the projected shape of the 3D model skeleton at its initial state and the X-ray image, t_x, t_y is roughly estimated so that the projection optimally overlaps the dark regions (possible vessel regions) . In the case of Fig. 2a, the model is translated by (-14.8, 39.8, 0.0)(mm); the white points show the projection of the model after the translation.

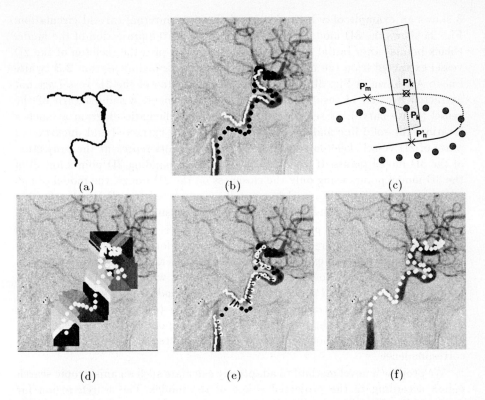

Fig. 3. Point matching search: (a) skeleton of the 3D model of the right internal carotid circulation; (b) initial position (black points) and extracted 2D skeleton (white lines); (c) anisotropy of the appropriate search regions(see text); (d) territory-based search regions; (e) result of point matching (only the large white dots made corresponding pairs); (f) the final registration result.

2.3 Skeleton extraction

After the initial localization, the projection of the model is classified into horizontal and vertical segments on the image. In the vicinity of each segment, a histogram of the grey levels of the image is calculated to decide an adaptive threshold of vessel brightness. Although the estimated thickness of the vessel from the 3D model can be also used to establish an adaptive threshold, we have not yet implemented this. Using the adaptive information of approximate vessel direction and brightness, the corresponding opposite edges of vessels are tracked more robustly than without a model. In Fig. 2b, the skeleton is well extracted despite the weak image contrast.

3 Territory-based correspondence search

Here our sub-goal is to find as many correct corresponding points on the 2D vessel skeleton for each point on the 3D model while avoiding wrong pairs. Fig.

3 shows an example of a X-ray image of the right internal carotid circulation: Fig. 3a shows the 3D model skeleton; Fig. 3b shows the projection of the model (black points) after initial localization (Section **2.2**) plus the skeleton of the 2D vessel extracted from the image by the method described at Section **2.3** (white lines). As shown in Fig. 3b, some parts of the skeleton of the 2D vessel are not extracted because of insufficient contrast enhancement, a sudden turn of the vessel (acute curve), or self-overlap. Fig. 3c is a schematic diagram at such a location: the solid line and the dotted line show the extracted and unextracted parts of 2D vessel skeleton respectively; the large dots represent the projection of the 3D model points. If we try to find the corresponding 2D points for all of the 3D model points using only the closeness on the 2D image, the model points whose corresponding 2D vessel has not been extracted (eg. P_k) will definitely have the wrong correspondences (eg. P'_m or P'_n) causing serious errors.

Removing such model points (matching outliers), is not an easy task since it is not known which parts are successfully extracted before the correct registration has been computed. For example, in [3], human interaction is required for this removal process. Note, however, that in many cases wrongly selected 2D vessel points, like P'_m or P'_n for P_k, are the correct corresponding points to other model points. If we can set an appropriate search region (eg. the shaded region in Fig. 3c) by considering the projected shape, model points whose corresponding 2D vessel part has not been extracted can be rejected as a point that has no correspondence.

We propose a novel method to adaptively calculate such an anisotropic search region according to the projected shape of the model. The search region for each model point is determined by segmenting the image into territories of the model points as follows. On the image, each projected point tries to extend its territory in the vicinity of the point at the same speed as the other points and to some width (the largest search width). Each pixel in the image belongs only to the search region of the point that first reaches the pixel. As a result, search regions become akin to Voronoi regions. Concretely, we implement this process by region growing using mask-processing. Fig. 3d shows the resultant search regions. We can see that points around more complicated projected shapes tend to have smaller search areas. As a result, the chance that model points find a wrong corresponding point (which actually corresponds to different parts of the model) are greatly decreased; while some points find the proper match at a far position as seen in Fig. 3e. This search mechanism is essential when we deal with complex 3D free-form models which cause complicated self-overlapping in the 2D projections.

4 3D-2D matching pairs → 3D transformation

Now we have m corresponding pairs of the observed position $\mathbf{x}_i^o, (x_i^o, y_i^o, f)^\top$ and a 3D model point $\mathbf{X}_i, (X_i, Y_i, Z_i)^\top$ whose projection is $\mathbf{x}_i, (x_i, y_i, f)^\top$. In many methods, the nonlinear minimization, $min(\sum_{i=1}^{m}((x_i^o - x_i)^2 + (y_i^o - y_i)^2))$ is solved iteratively to determine $\mathbf{R}$ and $\mathbf{T}$ at the same time. To speed up this calculation, we take the approach presented in [6]. We explain this method very briefly.

The minimization criteria is initially only based on rotation by separating out the translation effect using the following geometry. If we pick up two pairs from the m corresponding pairs, $\mathbf{X^o}_i - \mathbf{X^o}_j = \mathbf{R}(\mathbf{X}_i - \mathbf{X}_j)$ should be perpendicular to the vector $(\mathbf{x^o}_i \times \mathbf{x^o}_j)$. Therefore the optimal rotation is obtained by computing

$$\min_{\mathbf{R}} \sum_{i=1}^{m-1} \sum_{j=i+1}^{m} ((\mathbf{x}_i \times \mathbf{x}_j) \cdot \mathbf{R}(\mathbf{X}_i - \mathbf{X}_j))^2.$$

The rotation matrix can be represented by quaternions $\mathbf{q} = (q_0, q_1, q_2, q_3)^\top$ and linearized with some small error as follows.

$$\mathbf{R} = \begin{bmatrix} (q_0^2 + q_1^2 - q_2^2 - q_3^2) & 2(q_1 q_2 - q_0 q_3) & 2(q_1 q_3 + q_0 q_2) \\ 2(q_1 q_2 + q_0 q_3) & (q_0^2 - q_1^2 + q_2^2 - q_3^2) & 2(q_2 q_3 - q_0 q_1) \\ 2(q_1 q_3 - q_0 q_2) & 2(q_2 q_3 + q_0 q_1) & (q_0^2 - q_1^2 - q_2^2 + q_3^2) \end{bmatrix}$$

$$\approx \begin{bmatrix} q_0 & -2q_3 & 2q_2 \\ 2q_3 & q_0 & -2q_1 \\ -2q_2 & 2q_1 & q_0 \end{bmatrix}$$

Using this linearization, the equation of minimization on $\mathbf{R}$ becomes

$$\min_{\mathbf{q}} \sum_{i=1}^{n-1} \sum_{j=i+1}^{n} ((\mathbf{x}_i \times \mathbf{x}_j) \cdot (q_0 (\mathbf{X}_i - \mathbf{X}_j) + 2\mathbf{q}' \times (\mathbf{X}_i - \mathbf{X}_j)))^2,$$

where $\mathbf{q}' = (q_1, q_2, q_3)^\top$. The $\mathbf{q}$ which minimizes this function is obtained by solving the simultaneous equations of the partial differentials on $\mathbf{q}$.

Once the rotation is known, the translation can be calculated by solving $2m$ simultaneous equations on (t_x, t_y, t_z):

$$\frac{f(X_i^{o'} + t_x)}{Z_i^{o'} + t_z} = x_i' \quad \text{and} \quad \frac{f(Y_i^{o'} + t_y)}{Z_i^{o'} + t_z} = y_i',$$

where $\mathbf{X^{o'}} = \mathbf{R}\mathbf{X}$ using the calculated $\mathbf{R}$.

We tested this method using synthetic data. Although we omit the detail of the results, the experiments indicated that a high ratio of correct pairs (at least 50 %) is imperative for the success of this method.

5 Results

Fig. 3f shows a registration result on a real example. Although a lower part of the internal carotid artery is faded owing to insufficient contrast enhancement and many of the other arteries are self-overlapping, the 3D model is properly transformed so that the projection overlaps well with the 2D observed vessel. The final transformation is a 16.6 degree rotation around the axis (0.39, 0.67 , -0.64) and a (6.6, 6.5, -5.6)(mm) translation. Computational time for each step

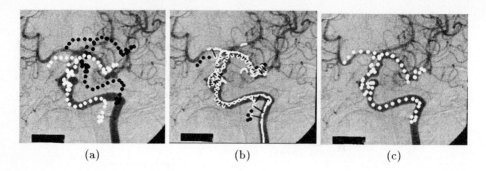

Fig. 4. Result: (a) initial localization (white points); (b) initial point correspondence; (c) final registration result.

was (1)preprocessing (0.2 sec), (2)initial localization (0.08 sec), (3)2D skeleton extraction (0.5 sec), (4)point correspondence (0.13sec) and (5)3D transformation (0.01 sec). Steps (4) and (5) were iterated 30 times for convergence and hence the total time was 5.5 sec (SUN IPX/ULTRA1).

Fig. 4 shows another result using a X-ray image of the vessels of the 3D model which is shown in Fig. 1b. Although the projected shape of the model at initial state is quite different from the observed vessel, the 3D transformation of the model is correctly obtained. The transformation is a 14.6 degree rotation around the axis (-0.77, -0.61, -0.18) and a translation of (-9.7, 4.8, -127.9)(mm). The large translation in the Z direction agrees with the fact that the height of the bed where the human subject lay was altered by approximately 10~15 cm during the acquisition of the images. Even though, at the middle of the internal carotid artery in the image, there is very complicated self-overlapping at which the topology of the initial projected shape is different from the actual one, territory-based search restriction helps to retain the high ratio of correct corresponding pairs. Computational time for each step was (1)preprocessing (0.2 sec), (2)initial localization (0.11 sec), (3)2D skeleton extraction (1.5 sec), (4)point correspondence (0.31 sec) and (5)3D transformation (0.01 sec). A total of 18 iterations were required for convergence and the total time was 5.7 sec (SUN IPX/ULTRA 1). We have applied the method to a total of 9 X-ray images for the two 3D models. All data have similar results except one which failed because of poor 2D skeleton extraction.

6 Conclusion

We have proposed a method for the real-time determination of the pose and position of a complicated 3D free-form shape with respect to its 2D projection. The method is fully automated. The robustness and speed of the method are supported by two characteristics:
1. Robust model-based 3D-2D point matching using territory-based search restriction.

2. Linear solution to obtain the 3D transformation from 3D-2D point correspondences.

Although the second part is not original, the first part enables the second part to work effectively even on complication data. The results using real data show that the proposed method is quite promising.

Our future work will focus on:
1. Assessment of the method by comparing it with 3D ground truth data. Unfortunately, we do not have the true value of the 3D transformation of the model in the experiments shown here. We will apply the method to real data where fiducial markers have been used to compute the transformation.
2. Improvement of the 2D skeleton extraction process. Since the model gradually becomes closer to the correct state, incremental extraction is more desirable.

Other aspects we will consider include:
1. Comprehensible display of the 3D model with the 2D view.
2. Fusion of two (or more) 2D views. The information about the distance in Z direction is fundamentally poor if we use just one view. Fusion of two different views is desirable to increase the accuracy of the localization of the model. It is especially important in the case where the 3D model has a simple linear shape.

Acknowledgments

We are thankful to Dr J. Byrne and Dr D. Royston for their clinical advice and the data used for the experiments. The first author thanks STA's middle-term researcher sending scheme. She is also thankful to Dr Tsukune, Dr Tsukiyama and the ETL administrators for their support of her research at the University of Oxford. She is grateful to Mr N. Kita for many useful discussions and encouragement.

References

1. D.L. Wilson and J.A. Noble: "Segmentation of cerebral vessels and aneurysms from MR angiography data", In *Proc. of Information Processing in Medical Imaging*, pp.423–428, 1997.
2. P. J. Besl and N. D.Mckay: "A method for registration of 3D shapes", *IEEE Trans. on Pattern Analysis and Machine Intelligence*, Vol.14, No.2, pp. 239–256, 1992.
3. J. Feldmar, G. Malandain, N. Ayache, S. Fernandez-Vidal, E. Maurincomme and Y. Trousset: "Matching 3D MR Angiography Data and 2D X-ray Angiograms", In *Proc. of CVRMed-MRCAS'97*, pp.129–138, 1997.
4. Y. Kita: "Force-based registration method using attribute values", In *Proc. of 14th International Conference on Pattern Recognition*, pp.34–39, 1996.
5. G.P. Penney, J.A. Little, D.L.G. Hill and D.J. Hawkes: "2D-3D registration for use in image guided interventions", In *Proc. of Medical Image Understanding and Analysis '97*, pp.49–52, 1997.
6. J.J. Heuring and D.W. Murray: "Visual head tracking and slaving for visual telepresence", In *Proc. of IEEE Int Conf. on Robotics and Automation*, pp.2908–2914, 1996.
7. D.L. Wilson, J.A. Noble and C. Pudney: "From MR Angiography to X-Ray Angiography", In *Proc. of Medical Image Understanding ans Analysis'97*, pp.161–164, 1997.

Multi-object Deformable Templates Dedicated to the Segmentation of Brain Deep Structures

F. Poupon[1,2,3], J.-F. Mangin[1], D. Hasboun[4], C. Poupon[1],
I. Magnin[2] and V. Frouin[1]

[1] Service Hospitalier Frédéric Joliot, DSV, DRM, CEA, 91406 Orsay Cedex, France
e-mail : poupon@shfj.cea.fr
[2] CREATIS-INSA Lyon, 69621 Villeurbanne, France
[3] IFSBM, 94805 Villejuif Cedex, France
[4] Service de Neuroradiologie H. Fischgold, CHU Pitié Salpêtrière, 75013 Paris, France

Abstract. We propose a new way of embedding shape distributions in a topological deformable template. These distributions rely on global shape descriptors corresponding to the 3D moment invariants. In opposition to usual Fourier-like descriptors, they can be updated during deformations at a relatively low cost. The moment-based distributions are included in a framework allowing the management of several simultaneously deforming objects. This framework is dedicated to the segmentation of brain deep nuclei in 3D MR images. The paper focuses on the learning of the shape distributions, on the initialization of the topological model and on the multi-resolution energy minimization process. Results are presented showing the segmentation of twelve brain deep structures.

1 Introduction

The wide diffusion of magnetic resonance imaging has given rise to numerous potential applications for 3D segmentation algorithms, ranging from morphometric or functional studies to neuro-surgical assistance. Unfortunately most methods proposed by the image processing community are still far from reaching the robustness required by clinical applications. With regard to the brain for instance, statistical analysis of gray levels is unsufficient to segment deep gray matter nuclei mainly because of partial volume effect [1]. A solution to overcome this kind of difficulties consists in embedding *a priori* knowledge in the segmentation algorithm, which is generally done using deformable models.

1.1 Deformable models

First active contours known as snakes [2] were introduced for regularization purpose. Since they include no *a priori* knowledge on global shape, they still required a precise initialization. The next generations of deformable models include global shape information. Hence they can be viewed as deformable templates. Two different directions have been investigated. The first one consists in using an elastic atlas which is mapped onto the image to be segmented, this atlas being generated by an expert manual delineation [3]. The second approach consists in restricting the class of admissible shapes to a family described by a few parameters using for instance superquadrics with global deformations [4]. This approach can be improved by allowing local deformations of the template using splines [5]. Other families of models have been proposed including a continuum of parameters from global to local shape information using modal analysis [6] or wavelet analysis [7].

The more recent efforts aim at including some knowledge on anatomical variability in the deformable template. This can be achieved by endowing the model parameters with some probability distribution. This distribution generally relies on the parameter expected values and variances which are inferred from a training set [8]. The segmentation goal is then defined using for instance a Maximum a Posteriori criterion which leads to an energy minimization. An alternative consists in using principal component analysis in order to restrict the space of admissible shapes according to the main modes of deformation of a mean model [9]. The 3D extension of this approach is rather difficult because of parametrization problems. A solution recently proposed in [10] allows the computation of a homogeneous parametrization of an arbitrarily shaped simply connected object. From this parametrization, 3D Fourier snakes including a restricted deformation space relying on eigenmodes are proposed. Because of the shape space restriction, a final minimization can be required to recover shape local details. A fairly complete bibliography on deformable models can be found in [11].

1.2 Paper overview

In this paper we propose a new way of embedding shape distributions in a framework allowing simultaneous deformation of several objects. The underlying model is simply a label image initially endowed with the *a priori* known topology which is preserved during the deformation process [12]. Performing simultaneous deformation of several templates increases the robustness of the segmentation. Indeed, each object is confined to a domain defined by surrounding objects. The segmentation is achieved through the coarse-to-fine minimization of a global energy including data-driven terms, regularization and shape distributions.

This paper focuses on the construction of the initial topological model from the training set and the way of embedding shape distributions in an energy-based multi-object segmentation framework.

The paper is organized as follows. First we present the 3D multi-object deformable topological template endowed with the *a priori* known information on shapes. Then we present what is inferred from the learning step on the training set. Next we present the way of constructing the initial topological model from the training set followed by the presentation of the particular energy minimization scheme. Finally we propose different results obtained by this 3D multi-object segmentation process.

2 The deformable model

The deformable model is based on deformable regions initially endowed with the *a priori* known topology. Then, segmentation amounts to applying topology preserving deformations in order to reach an energetic goal [12]. The deformations are performed by applying an homotopic transformation that is a sequence of addition or deletion of simple points in the objects. Those simple points are efficiently characterized by two numbers of connected components in the local neighborhood [13]. To respect Jordan's theorem an object and its background have to be taken with two different connectivity. Then the numbers are computed with the 26-connectivity for the objects of interest and with the 6-connectivity for the background defined by the surrounding of the set of objects. Knowledges on shapes are also embedded to constrain the deformations to an *a priori* known domain in the shape space during the segmentation process. These knowledges are shape distributions relying on descriptors corresponding to the 3D moment invariants [16, 14]. These descriptors are invariant relatively to location, orientation and scale.

The energy defining the segmentation goal has the form

$$E_g = \sum_M V_{l(M)}^{data}(i(M)) + \sum_{M_1,M_2} V^{Potts}(l(M_1), l(M_2)) + \sum_l V_l^{shape}, \quad (1)$$

where M is a point, $l(M)$ is a point label, $i(M)$ is the intensity of M, and M_1, M_2 are 6-neighbours. The $V_{l(M)}^{data}$ functions embed the data attraction on the deformable model. They are φ-functions roughly modeling for each region statistical knowledge on intensities

$$V_{l(M)}^{data}(i(M)) = \left(\frac{i(M) - m_{l(M)}}{\sigma_{l(M)}}\right)^4 / \left(1 + \left(\frac{i(M) - m_{l(M)}}{\sigma_{l(M)}}\right)\right)^4. \quad (2)$$

where $m_{l(M)}$ and $\sigma_{l(M)}$ are respectively the gray level mean and standard deviation of the object defined by the label $l(M)$.

V^{Potts} is a matrix of adjacency costs related to the Potts model used in Gibbs fields [15]. A set of potentials V_l^{shape} is added to the energy function to model the fact that the shape of each object is relatively stable between individuals. V_l^{shape} embeds the shape distributions related to the label l.

$$V_l^{shape} = V_l^v + V_l^g + V_l^o + \sum_{12} V_l^i(\tilde{I}_\beta^\alpha), \quad (3)$$

where V_l^v is related to the object volume, V^g is related to its gravity center position, V_l^o is related to its inertial frame orientation and $V_l^i(\tilde{I}_\beta^\alpha)$ is related to the moment invariants. The derivation of the $\tilde{I}_\beta^\alpha$ is described in [16, 14]. Those potentials are logarithm of Gaussians relying on statistical parameters inferred from a training set. Statistics on gravity center and orientation stem from an initial registration in the Talairach proportional reference frame like in [10].

3 The learning step

The various *a priori* knowledge embedded in the deformable template is learnt from a training set. This training set was generated by manual delineation of the 12 desired structures on 6 different brains (Fig. 2). During this step statistics on volume, gravity center position, moment invariants and orientation are computed to form the shape distributions.

3.1 Moment invariants

The influence of resolution on the invariants has been studied from a training set composed of 8 different lateral ventricles by resampling each ventricles with sixteen different resolutions. Fig. 1 shows the evolution curve of the invariant $\tilde{I}^2_{22}$ which is typical of other ones. It can be seen that the error on the values of the invariants becomes noticeable in low resolutions, which could be foreseeable since the object shape is perturbed. But by studying the inter-individual variability on this set of ventricles (Fig. 1) we have shown that the anatomical variability is greater than the variations induced by resolution. Therefore the coarse-to-fine implementation can be done with the same shape distribution at all resolution levels.

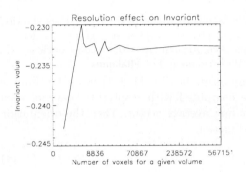

Invariants	R_LV m	R_LV σ	L_LV m	L_LV σ	P_LV
$\tilde{I}^2_{00}$	1.37	0.14	1.39	0.18	0.70
$\tilde{I}^3_{11}$	-0.79	0.13	-0.79	0.07	-0.35
$\tilde{I}^2_{22}$	0.97	0.10	0.99	0.14	0.41
$\tilde{I}^3_{33}$	-0.68	0.06	-0.68	0.06	-0.33
$\tilde{I}^2_{222}$	-1.07	0.11	-1.09	0.15	-0.44
$\tilde{I}^3_{3111}$	0.06	0.59	-0.15	0.57	0.23
$\tilde{I}^3_{3131}$	0.55	0.07	0.55	0.04	0.25
$\tilde{I}^3_{3331}$	-0.58	0.07	-0.58	0.05	-0.27
$\tilde{I}^3_{3333}$	0.66	0.06	0.66	0.07	0.32
$\tilde{I}^{2,3}_{112}$	-0.07	0.66	0.15	0.63	-0.25
$\tilde{I}^{2,3}_{312}$	-0.62	0.07	-0.63	0.05	-0.28
$\tilde{I}^{2,3}_{332}$	0.70	0.06	0.71	0.07	0.33

Fig. 1. Left: resolution curve of $\tilde{I}^2_{22}$ obtained for a lateral ventricle composed of 8836 voxels. Table: average (m) and standard deviation (σ) of the invariants evaluated for 8 right (R_LV) and left (L_LV) lateral ventricles and the invariants computed for a pathological one (P_LV).

It should be noted that most of the $\tilde{I}^\alpha_\beta$ show a relatively low variability between individuals. This result tends to prove that these $\tilde{I}^\alpha_\beta$ vary sufficiently slowly in the shape space to be efficiently used for constructing shape distributions. The results corresponding to a pathological ventricle show that it can be easily discriminated from the others due to its low values far from the distribution means. Nevertheless it means that in case of pathological structures some of the shape constraints have to be relaxed. This can be done either interactively or perhaps using a high level process driving the energy minimization.

3.2 Adjacencies

The adjacency cost matrix has also been constructed from the training set by looking for the different possible adjacencies in the manual segmentations. This can only be done if the manual delineations are performed in the same way to insure a reproductive topological arrangement of the brain structures. The twelve structure adjacency graph is given in Fig. 2.

3.3 Orientation

Since all the position and orientation parameters are computed in the Talairach reference frame we suppose that the orientations are relatively stable between individuals. Then each object average inertial frame is obtained by computing

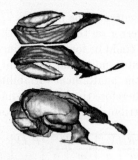 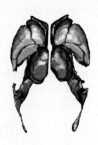 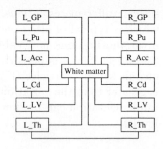

Fig. 2. Left: different views of a manually segmented brain of the training set showing the 12 structures of interest. Right: the 12 structures adjacency graph. L_ denotes Left and R_ denotes Right. Abbreviations: Acc, Accumbens; Cd, Caudate nucleus; GP, Globus Pallidus; LV, Lateral Ventricle; Pu, Putamen; Th, Thalamus.

the average vector of each frame components $\overrightarrow{m_i}$, $i \in \{1, 2, 3\}$ from the training set. The standard deviations σ_i are computed with respect to angle of each frame components with its corresponding average vector. Then the orientation potential is obtained by a specific φ-function

$$\Phi(x(\overrightarrow{v})) = x(\overrightarrow{v})^4/(1 + x(\overrightarrow{v})^4) \, , \qquad x(\overrightarrow{v}) = cos^{-1}(|\overrightarrow{m_i} . \overrightarrow{v}|)/\sigma_i \, . \qquad (4)$$

Only the first orientation vector corresponding to the maximum eigenvalue of the inertial matrix is taken into account. It avoids the possible misplacement of the other vectors due to the relative symmetry of the objects. Another better approach could be designed from third order moments like in [16].

3.4 Data attraction

The next statistics to be determined is related to the data attraction term. It relies on the gray-level of the different structures in the volume. Since the gray-level distributions are different between acquisitions we propose to estimate the gray-level statistic parameters of each nucleus from the histogram of the brain we want to segment. First, the gray and white matter modes are automatically detected by a scale-space analysis of the histogram [17]. Then we suppose that each nucleus gray-level average value can be defined as a weighted function of the gray and white matter average values stable between acquisitions. For a brain nucleus n, we define its gray-level average value μ_n as

$$\mu_n = \alpha_n m_W + (1 - \alpha_n) m_G \, , \qquad (5)$$

where m_W and m_G are respectively the white and gray matter gray-level average values and α_n the weighting coefficient for the nucleus n. The μ_n are inferred from the training set by computing the average gray-level value of the voxels belonging to a structure defined by a label. Then the α_n are estimated for each structure of each brain of the training set. These values are given in Tab. 1.

The α_n values are ranging from 0.0 for the gray matter to 1.0 for the white matter. Then the nuclei can be classified from the brightest to the darkest one as in Tab. 1.

Table 1. Average (m) and standard deviation (σ) of specific brain nuclei weighting coefficients α_n.

Nuclei	Globus Pallidus	Thalamus	Putamen	Caudate nucleus	Accumbens
$m(\alpha_n)$	0.911	0.618	0.458	0.287	0.244
$\sigma(\alpha_n)$	0.065	0.019	0.064	0.040	0.029

Anatomically, the nuclei we are interested in are made of neurons composing the gray matter. Each nucleus is connected to others or to the cortex by bright fibers composing the white matter. Some structures such as the thalamus are composed of a set of nuclei also connected to each other by white fibers. Then partial volume effects due to the MRI resolution results in a mixture of white and gray matter for some voxels where both neurons and fibers are present. That explains why some structures appear brighter than others. The definition proposed in eq. (5) was motivated by this assertion. Then α_n can be seen as an indicator that gives the proportion of gray and white matter gray-level that characterize a given nucleus. This α_n coefficients can not be computed for the Cerebro-Spinal Fluid (CSF) because its gray-level variations are too important between acquisitions. Anyway the CSF gray-level values are systematically lower than the gray matter ones. Therefore the ventricle attraction term is a simple linear potential function giving low values in the range $[0, m_G - 2\sigma_G[$, where σ_G is the standard deviation of the gray matter gray-level.

So the data attraction statistics of each nucleus of a new brain we want to segment except for the CSF is obtained by first extracting the gray and white matter gray-level average values from the brain histogram analysis [17] followed by the computation of their own average values according to eq. (5) using the α_n coefficients inferred from the training set in Tab. 1. Because nucleus standard deviations variability study is not yet achieved we chose them as the greatest values obtained during the learning step.

4 Energy minimization

The energy defined above stems from an extension of the usual Gibbs distribution form using additional global shape potentials. The global nature of these potentials and the topological constraints could lead to a failure of a simulated annealing algorithm. In fact, a good initialization can be provided to the minimization algorithm. Then, if the initial temperature is not to high, each objet will be confined to a restricted area leading to local potentials. In our case where a complex energy is involved with many parameters, applying simulated annealing in normal resolution results in a prohibitive computation time. To overcome this problem, the whole deformation process is performed with a coarse-to-fine strategy. In this multi-resolution scheme, simulated annealing is only applied on the coarsest resolution level. Then, the resampled solution from coarser level is entered as initialization to the next finer level where the energy minimization is refined by an ICM like algorithm [12].

The whole homotopic deformation process is implemented using a multi-front strategy. At high temperature threads can appear arround objects. They are difficult to delete during the following deformations because of the topological constraints. In order to prevent their apparition and to favour their deletion a sophisticated front scanning is used. The idea is to make the number of time a point is treated depend on its neighborhood configuration. The goal is the decrease of the growth potential of threads while increasing their potential of beeing removed. This is achieved by attaching to each local configuration a probability of beeing treated. We chose this not normalized probability to be

$$P_N(n) = \begin{cases} 0.02 & \text{if } n \leq N, \\ 0.5 & \text{if } N < n < 26 - N, \\ 5.0 & \text{if } n \geq 26 - N. \end{cases} \qquad (6)$$

where n is the number of identical labels in the 26-neighborhood and N is a parameter that specifies the two important transitions in the behaviour of the process (typically $N = 3$). The first condition forbids a point to be set to a specified label if there is not enough points of this label in its neighborhood so that the creation of threads is kept out. $P_N(n \leq N)$ is not set to 0.0 because if so, the relatively thin lines used for the initial topological model could not grow. $P_N(N \leq n \leq 26 - N)$ is set to 0.5 to randomize the treatment of points. Finally $P_N(n \geq 26 - N)$ is set to a high value to favour the deletion of threads. Practically this value is used to perform the Gibbs sampler probability test at most five times to have more chances to accept the transition of the label when we are in presence of threads.

5 The initial topological model

The initial topological model provides the first approximation of the organisation of the different structures to segment in the top-level pyramid volume. The major difficulty to generate this model is to assure the right topology with the good adjacencies.

Since all our objects are simply connected they can simply be defined as single points. This is the easier way to get the desired topology for the objects. The problem is the choice of such points because they must be relatively stable between individuals in the Talairach reference frame. Those points can not be the mean gravity center ones because since some of the structures are bended the gravity center can be located outside the object which could lead to energy minimization problems. So only points that are part of the objects should be used. We defined them as the one point reduction given by a homotopic skeletonization of the object. This skeleton is obtained from a front-based sequential deletion of simple points which assures a relatively stable localization of the final point between individuals. The statistics on the position of these points in the Talairach frame are computed during the learning step. Fig. 3.a shows the points obtained for the twelve structures of interest.

Next, we have to construct the adjacencies between these points. If the white matter is removed from the graph of Fig. 2, it simplifies to a simple chain of adjacent objects. So the skeleton points of the adjacent objects can simply be linked with lines to assure the right model adjacencies (Fig. 3.b).

Then we compute a Voronoï diagram associated to a simple chamfer distance conditionally to the connecting segments. This Voronoï diagram associates each line point to the closest seed (Fig. 3.c). Then this result is used as the initial topological model of the arrangement of the different structures at the top level of the pyramid according to the multi-resolution scheme.

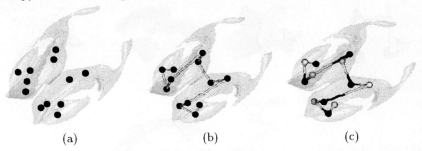

Fig. 3. Construction of the initial topological model. (a): the skeleton points in their surrounding structures. (b): the adjacent skeleton points linked by lines. (c): the initial topological model obtained after a Voronoï diagram.

6 Results

In the following the results are not presented using a triangulation-based rendering technique as in Fig. 2 but by representing each voxel by a cube to give a better insight of the topological nature of the process.

6.1 Without data attraction

The consistency of the shape information given by the moment invariants is studied at the top level of the multi-resolution segmentation scheme by minimizing the energy defined in eq. (1) without the data attraction term. Fig. 4 shows the results obtained for 4 of the structures with respect to their corresponding anatomical representations. They present a relatively good similarity with their anatomical corresponding structures. It should be noted that the purpose of the shape distributions is only to roughly characterize the shapes. Finer details have to be inferred from the data.

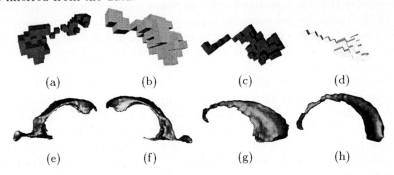

Fig. 4. Results obtained at the top level of the multi-resolution scheme only with shape information (top), with respect to their corresponding nuclei (bottom). (a), (e): right lateral ventricle. (b), (f): left lateral ventricle. (c), (g): right caudate nucleus. (d), (h): left caudate nucleus.

6.2 With data attraction

The whole multi-resolution scheme has been used to segment the twelve brain deep structures listed and represented in Fig. 2 in a given brain MR image.

The results obtained from the top level initial topological model to the normal resolution level of the pyramid are shown in Fig. 5.

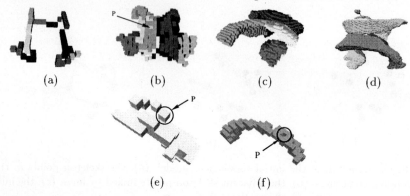

Fig. 5. Results obtained at the different level of the multi-resolution scheme. (a): initial topological model. (b): top level result. (c): intermediate level result. (d): normal resolution result. The arrow in (b) points out a particular configuration : in (e) P is 18-adjacent and the caudate nucleus is simply 26-connected and in (f) the ventricle is simply 26-connected. (e) and (f) have the expected topology, but P seems to create a hole in the ventricle (b).

The caudate nucleus point P in Fig. 5 can be seen as a hole for the ventricle but if we look at those structures separately (Fig. 5) both have the expected simple 26-connectivity. In fact, since each object topology is considered in 26-connectivity relatively to 6-connectivity for its complement, surprising configurations can arise when dealing with several objects. They are related to the usual paradoxes linked to Jordan theorem. Up to know, these strange configurations do not really perturb the segmentation process but further studies have to be done on the subject.

It appears that the structures well contrasted relatively to their surroundings such as the ventricles are correctly segmented. No problem is also encountered for the parts of the structures where the information is well defined in the model, i.e. where other structures are in competition with them. Their behavior leads to the desired result.

In return, areas where no competition occur can lead to errors. For instance the putamen can spread into the neighboring cortex; this result from the fact that both anatomical structures lead to similar gray levels. A solution to overcome these difficulties would consist in a better design of the attraction terms acting on background. Indeed in the current model the background is supposed to be made up from white matter which is far to be sufficient. We plan to devise a better attraction term for background by splitting it in three classes of tissues corresponding to CSF, gray and white matter. Each subclass would be regularized independently by the Potts model but the topological constraints would act on the union of the three sub-labels.

7 Conclusion

We have proposed a new method to embed global shape information in a framework allowing deformation of several objects. This information relies on shape distributions constructed from 3D moment invariants. Indeed these invariants have been shown to vary sufficiently slowly in the shape space to be relatively stable between individuals. The whole segmentation process has been tested for 12 brain deep structures. It shows a good behavior for the well defined parts of the model, i.e. the regions where competition occur. In return, a better management of the background class seems to be required to achieve acceptable results. The segmentation of these brain structures with a slow simulated annealing temperature decreasing at the coarsest resolution level (.995 geometric reason) takes 20 minutes on a SPARC-ULTRA 1 station.

References

1. T. Géraud, J.-F. Mangin, I. Bloch, and H. Maître. Segmenting internal structures in 3D MR images of the brain by Markovian relaxation on a watershed based adjacency graph. In *IEEE ICIP*, 1995, pp. 548–551.
2. M. Kass, A. Witkin, and D. Terzopoulos. Snakes : active contour models. *International Journal of Computer Vision*, vol. 1, 1988, pp. 321–331.
3. R. Bajcsy and R. Kovacic. Multiresolution elastic matching. *Computer Vision, Graphics and Image Processing*, vol. 46, 1989, pp. 1–21.
4. F. Solina and R. Bajcsy. Recovery of parametric models from range images: the case for superquadrics with global deformations. *PAMI*, vol. 12, 1990, pp. 131–147.
5. D. Terzopoulos and D. Metaxas. Dynamic 3D models with local and global deformations: deformable superquadrics. *IEEE PAMI*, vol. 13, 1991, pp. 703–714.
6. J. Martin, A. Pentland, and R. Kikinis. Shape analysis of brain structures using physical and experimental modes. In *IEEE CVPR, Seattle*, 1994, pp. 752–755.
7. B. C. Vemuri, A. Radisavljevic, and C. M. Leonard. Multi-resolution stochastic 3D shape models for image segmentation. In *13th IPMI, Flagstaff*, 1993, pp. 62–76.
8. L. H. Staib and J. S. Duncan. Model-based deformable surface finding for medical images. *IEEE Transactions on Medical Imaging*, vol. 15, no. 5, 1996, pp. 720–731.
9. T. F. Cootes, A. Hill, C. J. Taylor, and J. Haslam. Use of active shape models for locating structures in medical images. *Image and Vision Computing*, vol. 12, no. 6, 1994, pp. 355–365.
10. G. Székely, A. Kelemen, C. Brechbühler, and G. Gerig. Segmentation of 2D and 3D objects from MRI volume data using constrained elastic deformations of flexible Fourier contour and surface models. *MIA*, vol. 1, no. 1, 1996, pp. 19–34.
11. T. McInerney and D. Terzopoulos. Deformable models in medical image analysis: a survey. *Medical Image Analysis*, vol. 1, no. 2, 1996, pp. 91–108.
12. J.-F. Mangin, F. Tupin, V. Frouin, I. Bloch, R. Rougetet, J. Régis, and J. López-Krahe. Deformable topological models for segmentation of 3D medical images. In *14th IPMI, Brest, France*. Kluwer Academic Publishers, 1995, pp. 153–164.
13. G. Bertrand and G. Malandain. A new characterisation of three-dimensional simple points. *Pattern Recognition Letters*, vol. 15, 1994, pp. 169–175.
14. F. Poupon, J.-F. Mangin, V. Frouin, and I. Magnin. 3D multi-object deformable templates based on moment invariants. In *10th SCIA*, vol. I, 1997, pp. 149–155.
15. S. Geman and D. Geman. Stochastic relaxation, Gibbs distributions, and the bayesian restoration of images. *IEEE PAMI*, vol. 6, no. 6, 1984, pp. 721–741.
16. C.-H. Lo and H.-S. Don. 3D moment forms: their construction and application to object identification and positioning. *IEEE PAMI*, vol. 11, 1989, pp. 1053–1064.
17. J.-F. Mangin, O. Coulon, and V. Frouin. Robust brain segmentation using histogram scale-space analysis and mathematical morphology. In *1st MICCAI*, 1998.

Non-rigid Registration of Breast MR Images Using Mutual Information

D. Rueckert[1], C. Hayes[2], C. Studholme[1], P. Summers[1], M. Leach[2], and D. J. Hawkes[1]

[1] Computational Imaging Science Group
Division of Radiological Sciences
UMDS, Guy's Hospital, London SE1 9RT, UK
{email D.Rueckert@umds.ac.uk}
[2] Institute of Cancer Research
CRC Clinical Magnetic Resonance Research Group
Royal Marsden Hospital, Sutton SM2 5PT, UK

Abstract. We present a new approach for the non-rigid registration of contrast-enhanced breast MRI using normalised mutual information. A hierarchical transformation model of the motion of the breast has been developed: The global motion of the breast is modelled using affine transformation models while the local motion of the breast is modelled using spline-based free-form deformation (FFD) models. The algorithm has been applied to the fully automated registration of 3D breast MRI. In particular, we have compared the results of the proposed non-rigid registration algorithm to those obtained using rigid and affine registration techniques. The results clearly indicate that the non-rigid registration algorithm is much better able to recover the motion and deformation of the breast than rigid or affine registration algorithms.

1 Introduction

The application of voxel-based similarity measures for image registration has shown promising results over recent years. In particular, voxel-based similarity measures based on joint entropy [1], mutual information [2-5] and normalised mutual information [6-8] have been shown to align images acquired with different imaging modalities robustly. However, most of the approaches are either limited to rigid or affine transformations or global spline warps with a very limited number of degrees of freedom [9].

The registration of breast MRI is an important task which aids the detection of breast cancer. Currently, the detection and diagnosis of breast cancer primarily relies on X-ray mammography. Even though mammography is highly sensitive, there are a number of disadvantages such as the projective nature of the images and the exposure to radiation. This has led to the investigation of alternative imaging modalities like MRI for the detection of breast cancer. Typically, the detection of breast cancer in MRI requires the injection of a contrast agent whose uptake, it is proposed, will significantly increase the ability to differentiate between different types of malignant and healthy tissue. To quantify the rate of uptake, a 3D MRI scan is acquired prior to the injection of contrast media, followed by a dynamic sequence of 3D MRI scans. The rate of uptake can be estimated from the difference between pre- and post-contrast images. However, this assessment is complicated by misregistrations caused by patient motion, in particular respiratory motion.

To facilitate the analysis of pre- and post-contrast enhanced MRI, Zuo et al. [10] proposed a registration algorithm which minimises the ratio of variance between images. However, their algorithm is based on the assumption that the breast is only undergoing rigid motion. Kumar et al. [11] proposed a non-rigid registration technique which uses an optical-flow type algorithm and is based on the assumption that the intensities in the pre- and post-contrast enhanced images remain constant. To overcome the problems caused by non-uniform intensity change, Hayton et al. [12] developed a pharmacokinetic model which is used for an optical-flow registration algorithm.

In this paper we will present a new approach for the non-rigid registration of 3D breast MRI. We will use a hierarchical transformation model which captures the global and local motion of the breast. Normalised mutual information is used as a voxel-based similarity measure which is insensitive to changes of intensities between pre- and post-contrast enhanced images and independent of the amount of image overlap.

2 Image Registration

The goal of image registration in contrast-enhanced breast MRI is to relate any point in the post-contrast enhanced sequence to the pre-contrast enhanced reference image, i.e. to find the optimal transformation $\mathbf{T} : (x, y, z) \mapsto (x', y', z')$ which maps any point in the dynamic image sequence $I(x, y, z, t)$ at time t into its corresponding point in the reference image $I(x', y', z', t_0)$ taken at time t_0. In general, the motion of the breast is non-rigid so that rigid or affine transformations alone are not sufficient for the motion correction of breast MRI. Therefore, we develop a combined transformation $\mathbf{T}$ which consists of a global transformation and a local transformation:

$$\mathbf{T}(x, y, z) = \mathbf{T}_{global}(x, y, z) + \mathbf{T}_{local}(x, y, z) \qquad (1)$$

2.1 Global motion model

The global motion model describes the overall motion of the breast. The simplest choice is a rigid transformation which is parameterised by six degrees of freedom describing the rotations and translations of the breast. A more general class of transformations are affine transformations which have six additional degrees of freedom describing scaling and shearing. In 3D, an affine transformation can be written as

$$\mathbf{T}_{global}(x, y, z) = \begin{pmatrix} \alpha_{11} & \alpha_{12} & \alpha_{13} \\ \alpha_{21} & \alpha_{22} & \alpha_{23} \\ \alpha_{31} & \alpha_{32} & \alpha_{33} \end{pmatrix} \begin{pmatrix} x \\ y \\ z \end{pmatrix} + \begin{pmatrix} \alpha_{14} \\ \alpha_{24} \\ \alpha_{34} \end{pmatrix} \qquad (2)$$

where the coefficients α parameterise the twelve degrees of freedom of the transformation. In a similar fashion the global motion model can be extended to higher-order global transformations such as trilinear or quadratic transformations [13].

2.2 Local motion model

The affine transformation captures only the global motion of the breast. An additional transformation is required which models the local deformation of the breast. The nature of the local deformation of the breast can vary significantly across patients and with age. Therefore, it is difficult to describe the local deformation via parameterised transformations. Instead we have chosen a free-form deformation (FFD) model based on B-splines [14, 15] which is a powerful tool for modelling 3D deformable objects. The basic idea of FFDs is to deform an object by manipulating an underlying mesh of control points. The resulting deformation controls the shape of the 3D object and produces a smooth and C^2 continuous transformation.

To define a spline-based FFD we denote the domain of the image volume as $\Omega = \{(x, y, z) \mid 0 \leq x < X, 0 \leq y < Y, 0 \leq z < Z\}$. Let Φ denote a $n_x \times n_y \times n_z$ mesh of control points $\phi_{i,j,k}$ with uniform spacing. Then, the FFD can be written as the 3D tensor product of the familiar 1D cubic B-splines:

$$\mathbf{T}_{local}(x, y, z) = \sum_{l=0}^{3} \sum_{m=0}^{3} \sum_{n=0}^{3} B_l(u) B_m(v) B_n(w) \phi_{i+l, j+m, k+n} \quad (3)$$

where $i = \lfloor \frac{x}{n_x} \rfloor - 1, j = \lfloor \frac{y}{n_y} \rfloor - 1, k = \lfloor \frac{z}{n_z} \rfloor - 1, u = \frac{x}{n_x} - \lfloor \frac{x}{n_x} \rfloor, v = \frac{y}{n_y} - \lfloor \frac{y}{n_y} \rfloor, w = \frac{z}{n_z} - \lfloor \frac{z}{n_z} \rfloor$ and where B_l represents the l-th basis function of the B-spline [14, 15]

In general, the local deformation of the breast should be characterised by a smooth transformation. To constrain the spline-based FFD transformation to be smooth, one can introduce a penalty term which regularizes the transformation. The general form of such a penalty term has been described by Wahba [16]. In 3D, the penalty term takes the following form:

$$C_{smooth} = \iiint_{\Omega} \left(\frac{\partial^2 \mathbf{T}}{\partial x^2}\right)^2 + \left(\frac{\partial^2 \mathbf{T}}{\partial y^2}\right)^2 + \left(\frac{\partial^2 \mathbf{T}}{\partial z^2}\right)^2 + 2\left[\left(\frac{\partial^2 \mathbf{T}}{\partial xy}\right)^2 + \left(\frac{\partial^2 \mathbf{T}}{\partial xz}\right)^2 + \left(\frac{\partial^2 \mathbf{T}}{\partial yz}\right)^2\right] \quad (4)$$

This quantity is the 3D counterpart of the 2D bending energy of a thin-plate of metal and defines a cost function which is associated with the smoothness of the transformation. Note that the regularization term is zero for any affine transformations and therefore penalises only non-affine transformations.

The degree of local deformation which can be modelled by B-spline FFDs depends essentially on the resolution of the mesh of control points Φ. This enables a hierarchical multi-resolution approach in which the resolution of the control mesh is increased along with the image resolution in a coarse to fine fashion. Finally, B-splines are locally controlled splines which makes them computationally efficient even for a large number of control points compared to thin-plate splines [17] or elastic-body splines [18].

2.3 Normalised Mutual Information

To relate a post-contrast enhanced image to the pre-contrast enhanced reference image, we must define a similarity criterion which measures the degree of alignment between both images. Given that the image intensity might change after the injection of the contrast agent one cannot use a direct comparison of image intensities, i.e. sum of squared differences or correlation, as a similarity measure. Alternatively one can use mutual information (MI) which has been independently proposed by Collignon [2] and Viola [3, 4] as a voxel-based similarity measure. Mutual information is based on the concept of information theory and expresses the amount of information that one image A contains about a second image B,

$$\mathcal{C}_{similarity}(A, B) = H(A) + H(B) - H(A, B) \tag{5}$$

where $H(A), H(B)$ denote the marginal entropies of A, B and $H(A, B)$ denotes their joint entropy which are calculated from the joint histogram of A and B. If both images are aligned the mutual information is maximised. It has been shown by Studholme [6, 7] that mutual information itself is not independent of the overlap between two images. To avoid any dependency on the amount of image overlap, Studholme suggested the use of normalised mutual information (NMI) as a measure of image alignment:

$$\mathcal{C}_{similarity}(A, B) = \frac{H(A) + H(B)}{H(A, B)} \tag{6}$$

Similar forms of normalised mutual information have been proposed by Maes et al. [8].

To find the optimal transformation we minimise a cost function as a combination of the cost associated with the smoothness of the transformation C_{smooth} in eq. (4) and the cost associated with the image similarity $C_{similarity}$ in eq. (6):

$$\mathcal{C}(\mathbf{T}) = -\mathcal{C}_{similarity}(I(t_0), \mathbf{T}(I(t))) + \lambda \mathcal{C}_{smooth}(\mathbf{T}) \tag{7}$$

Here λ is the weighting parameter which defines the trade-off between the alignment of the two image volumes and the smoothness of the transformation. We have employed a simple gradient descent technique to minimise the cost function. For computational efficiency, the optimisation proceeds in a multi-resolution fashion: Initially, the affine transformation parameters are optimised at increasing levels of image resolution. During the subsequent refinement the non-affine transformation parameters are optimised at increasing levels of resolution of the control point mesh.

3 Results

We have applied the registration algorithm to volunteer as well as patient data. To test the ability of the algorithm to correct the non-rigid motion of the breast, two separate 3D MR scans of four volunteers were acquired (aged between 28 and 47 years). After the first scan each volunteer was asked to move inside the scanner. For the volunteer studies, a 3D FLASH sequence was used with TR = $12ms$, TE = $5ms$, flip angle = $35°$, FOV = $340mm$ and coronal slice orientation. The MR image were acquired on a 1.5 Tesla Siemens Vision MR system without contrast enhancement. The images have a size of $256 \times 256 \times 64$ voxels and spatial resolution of $1.33mm \times 1.33mm \times 2.5mm$.

Transformation	SSD (mean)	SSD (variance)	CC
–	38.52	53.90	0.8978
Rigid	23.09	33.38	0.9648
Affine	20.67	29.84	0.9736
Affine + FFD (20mm)	16.08	23.43	0.9845
Affine + FFD (15mm)	14.25	20.91	0.9878
Affine + FFD (10mm)	13.07	19.25	0.9899

Table 1. Comparison of the average registration error of the volunteer studies in terms of squared sum of intensity differences (SSD) and correlation coefficient (CC) for different types of transformation. The spline-based FFD has been evaluated at a control point spacing of $20mm$, $15mm$ and $10mm$.

An example of these images is shown in Figure 1. The effect of the misregistration due to the motion of the breast is clearly visible in the difference image. The corresponding registration results based on different transformation models are shown in Figure 2. To assess the quality of the registration in these images in more detail, we have calculated the mean and variance of the squared sum of intensity differences (SSD),

$$SSD = \frac{1}{n}\sqrt{\sum (I(x',y',z',t_0) - I(\mathbf{T}(x,y,z),t_1))^2} \qquad (8)$$

as well as the correlation coefficient (CC)

$$CC = \frac{\sum (I(x',y',z',t_0) - \overline{I}(t_0))(I(\mathbf{T}(x,y,z),t_1) - \overline{I}(t_1))}{\sqrt{\sum (I(x',y',z',t_0) - \overline{I}(t_0))^2 \sum (I(\mathbf{T}(x,y,z),t_1) - \overline{I}(t_1))^2}} \qquad (9)$$

Here $\overline{I}(t_0), \overline{I}(t_1)$ denote the average intensities of the images before and after motion and the summation includes all voxels within the overlap of both images. In these images, the squared sum of intensity differences and the correlation coefficient provides a reasonable metric for the assessment of misregistration as the position of the breast tissue changes but the tissue composition and hence image intensity does not. Since the motion of both breasts is normally uncorrelated, we have manually defined a region of interest (ROI) around each breast and then registered both ROIs independently.

Table 1 summarises the results of the registration quality of the volunteer datasets using different transformation models. We have compared three different types of transformations: Pure rigid and affine transformations as well as the proposed non-rigid transformation model which is a combination of an affine transformation and spline-based FFD. The results clearly show that the registrations which are based on rigid or affine transformations improve the correlation between the images before and after motion. However, both transformation models perform significantly worse than the proposed non-rigid transformation model. The results also show that the non-rigid registration performs better as the resolution of the control point mesh of the spline-based FFD increases. While a control point spacing of $20mm$ yields already improved correlation compared to affine transformations, a control point spacing of $15mm$ or less yields even higher correlation. The main reason for this is the increased flexibility of the spline-based FFD to describe local deformations of the breast as the number of control points increases.

Transformation	SSD (mean)	SSD (variance)	CC
–	149.64	205.13	0.8817
Rigid	72.78	91.75	0.9721
Affine	65.12	78.66	0.9784
Affine + FFD ($20mm$)	57.40	68.27	0.9836
Affine + FFD ($15mm$)	54.54	64.69	0.9852
Affine + FFD ($10mm$)	50.13	58.52	0.9877

Table 2. Comparison of the registration error in terms of squared sum of intensity differences (SSD) and correlation coefficient (CC) for the patient study in Figure 3. The region of increased uptake corresponding to the tumour has been excluded.

We have also applied the algorithm to a patient data set with contrast-enhanced MRI. An example of a pre- and post-contrast enhanced image of the patient data set without registration is shown in Figure 3. The difference image shows a substantial amount of motion artefacts. Again, we have used rigid, affine and the proposed non-rigid transformation model for the registration of these images. Figure 4 shows the post-contrast enhanced image and the corresponding difference images after registration. The results demonstrate that all three registrations techniques lead to a significantly improved localisation of the uptake of contrast agent. Again, we have calculated the quality of the registration in terms of squared sum of intensity differences (SSD) and correlation coefficient (CC). The region of increased uptake corresponding to the tumour has been excluded from the calculations. The results are summarised in Table 2 and show that the non-rigid transformation model is better able to correct the motion of the breast than the rigid and affine transformations.

4 Discussion

We have developed a fully automated algorithm for the non-rigid registration of 3D breast MRI based on normalised mutual information. The algorithm uses a non-rigid transformation model to describe the motion of the breast in dynamic MR images. The proposed combination of affine transformations and spline-based FFDs provides a high degree of flexibility to model the motion of the breast. In contrast to physics-based deformation models [19], the algorithm makes no assumptions about the elastic properties of the breast tissue. Even though physics-based deformation models might seem an attractive alternative, for example to model additional constraints such as incompressibility, they are usually difficult to evaluate and verify. Moreover, the elastic properties of the breast tissues can vary significantly across patients and with age which renders the application of such models problematic.

The experimental results have shown that the non-rigid registration of 3D breast MRI can significantly reduce motion artefacts between images. The results have also demonstrated that in many cases rigid or affine registration techniques are not sufficient to correct motion in 3D breast MRI. The registration of these images currently takes between

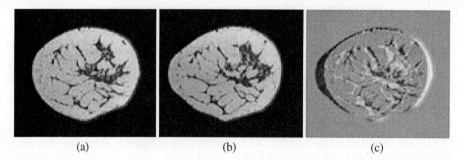

Fig. 1. Example of misregistration caused by motion of a volunteer: (a) before motion, (b) after motion and (c) after subtracting (b) from (a) without registration.

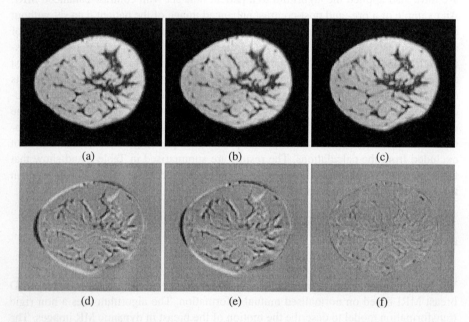

Fig. 2. Example of different transformations on the registration for the volunteer study in Figure 1: After (a) rigid, (b) affine and (c) non-rigid registration. The corresponding difference images are shown in (d) – (f).

15 and 30 $mins.$ of CPU time on a Sun Ultra 1 workstation which makes routine application in a clinical environment possible. We have also demonstrated the applicability of the algorithm to the motion correction in contrast-enhanced MRI. However, further work is needed to assess and evaluate the performance of the algorithm in these images. Future work will involve the application of the proposed registration algorithm to data from the MRC-supported UK study of MRI as a method of screening women at genetic risk of breast cancer.

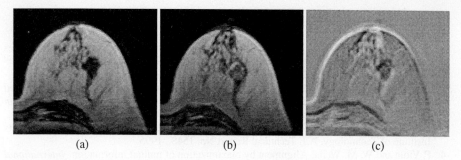

Fig. 3. Example of misregistration in a contrast-enhanced patient study: (a) before injection of the contrast media, (b) after injection of the contrast media and (c) after subtraction of (a) and (b) without registration.

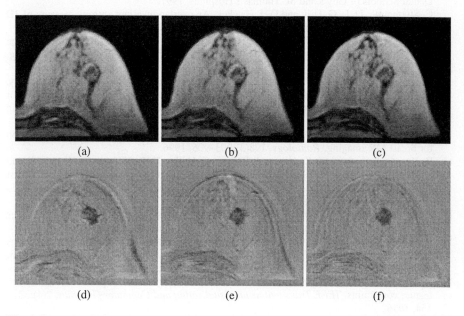

Fig. 4. Example of different transformations on the registration for the patient study in Figure 3: After (a) rigid, (b) affine and (c) non-rigid registration. The corresponding difference images are shown in (d) – (f).

Acknowledgements

We are grateful to EPSRC GR/L08519 for their financial support of this work. The support of the Medical Research Council G9600413 and the Cancer Research Campaign is gratefully acknowledged. We thank Dr. Hubertus Fischer, Siemens (Erlangen) for supplying acquisition sequences for the MRI measurements and the Advisory Group of the MR breast screening study for the measurement protocol.

References

1. C. Studholme, D. L. G. Hill, and D. J. Hawkes. Multiresolution voxel similarity measures for MR-PET registration. In *Information Processing in Medical Imaging: Proc. 14th International Conference (IPMI'95)*, pages 287–298, 1995.
2. A. Collignon, F. Maes, D. Delaere, D. Vandermeulen, P. Seutens, and G. Marchal. Automated multimodality image registration using information theory. In *Information Processing in Medical Imaging: Proc. 14th International Conference (IPMI'95)*, pages 263–274, 1995.
3. P. Viola. *Alignment By Maximization of Mutual Information*. PhD thesis, Massachusetts Institute of Technology. A.I. Technical Report No. 1548., 1995.
4. P. Viola and W. M. Wells. Alignment by maximization of mutual information. *International Journal of Computer Vision*, 24(2):137–154, 1997.
5. C. Studholme, D. L. G. Hill, and D. J. Hawkes. Automated 3-D registration of MR and CT images of the head. *Medical Image Analysis*, 1(2):163–175, 1996.
6. C. Studholme. *Measures of 3D Medical Image Alignment*. PhD thesis, United Medical and Dental Schools of Guy's and St. Thomas's Hospitals, 1997.
7. C. Studholme, D. L. G. Hill, and D. J. Hawkes. An overlap invariant entropy measure of 3D medical image alignment. *Pattern Recognition*, 1998. To appear.
8. F. Maes, A. Collignon, D. Vandermeulen, G. Marechal, and R. Suetens. Multimodality image registration by maximization of mutual information. *IEEE Transactions on Medical Imaging*, 16(2):187–198, 1997.
9. C. R. Meyer, J. L. Boes, B. Kim, P. H. Bland, K. R. Zasadny, P. V. Kison, K. Koral, K. A. Frey, and R. L. Wahl. Demonstration of accuracy and clinical versatility of mutual information for automatic multimodality image fusion using affine and thin-plate spline warped geometric deformations. *Medical Image Analysis*, 1(3):195–207, 1997.
10. C. S. Zuo, A. P. Jiang, B. L. Buff, T. G. Mahon, and T. Z. Wong. Automatic motion correction for breast MR imaging. *Radiology*, 198(3):903–906, 1996.
11. R. Kumar, J. C. Asmuth, K. Hanna, J. Bergen, C. Hulka, D. B. Kopans, R. Weisskoff, and R. Moore. Application of 3D registration for detecting lesions in magnetic resonance breast scans. In *Proc. SPIE Medical Imaging 1996: Image Processing*, volume 2710, pages 646–656, Newport Beach, USA, February 1996. SPIE.
12. P. Hayton, M. Brady, L. Tarassenko, and N. Moore. Analysis of dynamic MR breast images using a model of contrast enhancement. *Medical Image Analysis*, 1(3):207–224, 1997.
13. R. Szelski and S. Lavallee. Matching 3-D anatomical surfaces with non-rigid deformations using octree-splines. In *IEEE Workshop on Biomedical Image Analysis*, pages 144–153, 1994.
14. S. Lee, G. Wolberg, , K.-Y. Chwa, and S. Y. Shin. Image metamorphosis with scattered feature constraints. *IEEE Transactions on Visualization and Computer Graphics*, 2(4):337–354, 1996.
15. S. Lee, G. Wolberg, and S. Y. Shin. Scattered data interpolation with multilevel B-Splines. *IEEE Transactions on Visualization and Computer Graphics*, 3(3):228–244, 1997.
16. G. Wahba. *Spline Models for Observational Data*. Society for Industrial and Applied Mathematics, 1990.
17. F. L. Bookstein. Principal Warps: Thin-plate splines and the decomposition of deformations. *IEEE Transactions on Pattern Analysis and Machine Intelligence*, 11(6):567–585, 1989.
18. M. H. Davis, A. Khotanzad, D. P. Flamig, and S. E. Harms. A physics-based coordinate transformation for 3-D image matching. *IEEE Transactions on Medical Imaging*, 16(3):317–328, 1997.
19. P. J. Edwards, D. L. G. Hill, J. A. Little, and D. J. Hawkes. Deformation for image-guided interventions using a three-component tissue model. In *Information Processing in Medical Imaging: Proc. 15th International Conference (IPMI'97)*, pages 218–231, 1997.

A Comparison of Similarity Measures for Use in 2D-3D Medical Image Registration

Graeme P Penney[1], Jürgen Weese[2], John A Little, Paul Desmedt[3],
Derek LG Hill[1], and David J Hawkes[1]

[1] Division of Radiological Sciences, UMDS, Guy's & St Thomas' Hospitals, London SE1 9RT, UK. {email G.Penney@umds.ac.uk}
[2] Philips Research Hamburg, Rontgenstraße 24-26, 22335 Hamburg, Germany.
[3] EasyVision Advanced Development, Philips Medical Systems, Veenpluis 4-6, P.O. Box 10.000, 5680 DA Best, the Netherlands.

Abstract. A comparison of six similarity measures for use in intensity based 2D-3D image registration is presented. The accuracy of the similarity measures are compared to a "gold-standard" registration which has been accurately calculated using fiducial markers. The similarity measures are used to register a CT scan to a fluoroscopy image of a spine phantom. The registration is carried out within a region of interest in the fluoroscopy image which is user defined to contain a single vertebra. Many of the problems involved in this type of registration are caused by features which were not modelled by a phantom image alone. More realistic "gold standard" data sets were simulated using the phantom image with clinical image features overlaid. Results show that the introduction of soft tissue structures and interventional instruments into the phantom image can have a large effect on the performance of some similarity measures previously applied to 2D-3D image registration. Two measures were able to register accurately and robustly even when soft tissue structures and interventional instruments were present as differences between the images. These measures are called pattern intensity and gradient difference.

1 Introduction

Common modalities for guiding interventions are ultrasound or x-ray fluoroscopy. These modalities are "real-time" but only two dimensional, so they lack the spatial information contained in computed tomography (CT) and magnetic resonance (MR) images. There are also a number of important anatomical features which are not visualised well using these modalities, but can be observed using CT and/or MR. One method of allowing information from CT images to be used during interventional procedures is to register the CT scan to an intra-operative x-ray fluoroscopy image. A number of papers have described techniques to achieve this registration [1, 3, 4, 7, 8, 14]. Current techniques to achieve registration divide into those that match features, such as bony structures [1, 4, 7], and those that use image intensities directly [3, 8, 14]. The former relies on a pre-processing step to segment appropriate features and are therefore difficult to automate.

This paper compares six intensity based similarity measures to determine which is the most accurate and robust. Rigid body registrations are carried out between a CT scan and a fluoroscopy image of a spine phantom. The final registrations are compared to a "gold-standard" registration calculated using fiducial markers. More clinically realistic fluoroscopy images are simulated by overlaying structures segmented from clinical fluoroscopy images on to the fluoroscopy image of the spine phantom.

2 Comparing fluoroscopic images and DRRs

Digitally reconstructed radiographs (DRRs) are produced by casting rays through a CT volume and integrating the Hounsfield numbers along each ray. There are two main types of difference between DRRs and fluoroscopy images, those which are caused by changes in the imaged object and those due to differences in image formation.

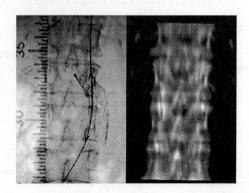

Fig. 1. Clinical fluoroscopy image (left) and digitally reconstructed radiograph (right) at registration.

2.1 Differences due to changes in imaged object

Overlying and underlying structures. We are assuming that the transformation between CT and fluoroscopy can be described by a perspective projection of rigid 3D motion. Soft tissue structures, however, can deform between the pre-operative CT image and interventional fluoroscopy. Because of this, we threshold the CT volume so no soft tissue structures are projected (see figure 1).

Interventional instruments in the field of view can create large differences between the images.

Spinal deformation can cause the vertebrae to be in different positions in the CT and fluoroscopy images.

2.2 Differences in image formation

Different x-ray energies between the modalities.
Heel effect and non-uniformity of the image intensifier response.
Different resolutions of fluoroscopy images and CT images.
Truncation when rays cut through the top or bottom of the CT scanned volume. Such rays are incomplete and so are not be compared to the fluoroscopy image.
Geometric distortion in the fluoroscopy image is corrected for using a suitable phantom and software [5].

3 Similarity measures

The following sections outline a number of similarity measures. Each similarity measure is used to compare a fluoroscopic image (intensity values I_{fl}) with a DRR (intensity values I_{DRR}). The position and orientation of the CT volume with respect to the fluoroscopy set are defined by ten parameters $\mathbf{P} = (X, Y, Z, \theta_x, \theta_y, \theta_z, c_s, l_s, k_1, k_2)$, see figure 2.

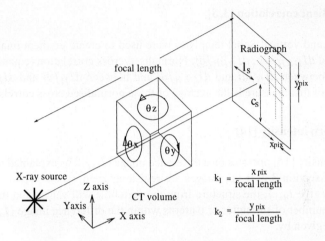

Fig. 2. Diagram showing the degrees of freedom in rigid body perspective projection. Six rigid body parameters, 3 translational X, Y and Z and 3 rotational θ_x, θ_y and θ_z. Four parameters c_s, l_s, k_1 and k_2 are associated with perspective projection: c_s and l_s are the coordinates on the film where the normal to the film goes through the x-ray source and k_1 and k_2 equal the pixel sizes x_{pix} and y_{pix} divided by the focal length.

3.1 Normalised Cross Correlation [8]

$$R = \frac{\sum_{(i,j)\in T}(I_{fl}(i,j) - \overline{I}_{fl})(I_{DRR}(i,j) - \overline{I}_{DRR})}{\sqrt{\sum_{(i,j)\in T}(I_{fl}(i,j) - \overline{I}_{fl})^2}\sqrt{\sum_{(i,j)\in T}(I_{DRR}(i,j) - \overline{I}_{DRR})^2}} \quad (1)$$

$\overline{I}_{fl}$ and $\overline{I}_{DRR}$ are the mean values of the images in the overlap region $(i,j) \in T$.

3.2 Entropy of the difference image [2]

$$I_{diff} = I_{fl} - s\, I_{DRR} \quad (2)$$

$$H(s) = -\sum_x p(x) \log p(x) \quad (3)$$

The entropy measure (H) described here operates on a single difference image (I_{diff}) which is created by subtracting the DRR from the fluoroscopy image using a suitable intensity scaling factor, s. A histogram is formed from the difference image and $p(x)$ denotes the probability of obtaining the pixel value x in I_{diff}.

3.3 Mutual information [9, 11–13]

$$S = \sum_{x,y} p(x,y) \log \frac{p(x,y)}{p(x)p(y)} \quad (4)$$

Where $p(x)$ and $p(y)$ are the probability distributions in individual images and $p(x,y)$ is the joint probability distribution.

3.4 Gradient correlation [3, 8]

Horizontal and vertical Sobel templates were used to create gradient images dI_{fl}/di, dI_{fl}/dj and dI_{DRR}/di, dI_{DRR}/dj. Normalised cross correlation (equation 1) is then calculated between dI_{fl}/di and dI_{DRR}/di and between dI_{fl}/dj and dI_{DRR}/dj. The final value of this measure is the average of these normalised cross correlations.

3.5 Pattern intensity [14]

Pattern intensity [14] operates on a difference image (I_{diff}) as explained in the entropy measure of section 3.2. If the images are registered then, when $s\, I_{DRR}$ is subtracted from I_{fl} to give I_{diff}, the structure from the vertebrae will vanish and there will be a minimum number of structures or patterns within the difference image (I_{diff}). Pattern intensity is given by,

$$P_{r,\sigma}(s) = \sum_{i,j} \sum_{d^2 \leq r^2} \frac{\sigma^2}{\sigma^2 + (I_{diff}(i,j) - I_{diff}(v,w))^2} \quad (5)$$

$$d^2 = (i-v)^2 + (j-w)^2 \quad (6)$$

where σ is a constant to reduce the effect of noise. The values chosen for the constants were $\sigma = 10$ and $r = 3$ pixels, as used in [14], although r was increased to 5 pixels when coarse images (see section 4.2) were used as this was found to increase the robustness of the measure.

3.6 Gradient difference

Gradient difference uses a difference image as explained in the entropy measure of section 3.2, though this time the difference image is calculated from gradient images (equation 8). It employs the same $1/(1+x^2)$ form as pattern intensity which should make the measure robust to thin line structures.

$$G(s) = \sum_{i,j} \frac{A_v}{A_v + (I_{diffV}(i,j))^2} + \sum_{i,j} \frac{A_h}{A_h + (I_{diffH}(i,j))^2} \quad (7)$$

$$I_{diffV}(i,j) = \frac{dI_{fl}}{di} - s\frac{dI_{DRR}}{di}, \quad I_{diffH}(i,j) = \frac{dI_{fl}}{dj} - s\frac{dI_{DRR}}{dj} \quad (8)$$

The gradients in equation 8 are described in the gradient correlation section 3.4, and A_v and A_h are constants, which for these experiments were the variance of the respective gradient fluoroscopy image.

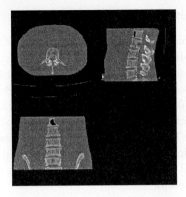 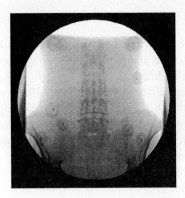

Fig. 3. Reformatted axial, sagittal and coronal slices from a CT image of a lumbar spine embedded in an acrylic matrix (left). Fluoroscopy image of the spine phantom (right).

4 Comparison using a gold standard

An experiment was carried out to investigate how accurately and robustly six similarity measures registered a CT scan of a spine phantom to a fluoroscopy image of the phantom. The phantom consisted of the five lumbar vertebrae and pelvis encased in acrylic which is approximately tissue equivalent at diagnostic x-ray energies. Registrations were compared to a "gold-standard" registration calculated using fiducial markers. Phantom images were used as it is an extremely difficult task to obtain an accurate "gold-standard" registration on clinical images. Many of the problems involved in our application are caused by image features which are not modelled by the phantom image alone. To assess how the similarity measures should perform on clinical images they were simulated by overlaying features segmented from clinical images onto the phantom image. Three clinical images were simulated by adding soft tissue, a stent (figure 4), and both soft tissue and a stent. No soft tissue structures were introduced to the CT volume as these would be removed during the thresholding stage (section 2.1).

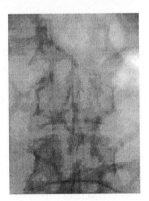 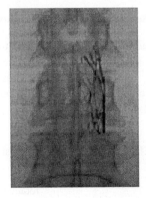

Fig. 4. Enlarged portion of the fluoroscopy image; (left) with soft tissue structures overlaid, (right) with interventional stent overlaid.

4.1 Calculation of the "gold-standard" registration

The "gold-standard" registration has been found using twelve fiducial markers (5mm diameter aluminium ball bearings cast in acrylic resin). A CT scan was acquired using a Philips TOMOSCAN SR 7000, which had voxel sizes 1.094x1.094x1.5mm and image dimensions 320x320x119 voxels. A fluoroscopy image was taken on a Philips multi DIAGNOST 3, which had image size 1024x1024 pixels. These images can be seen in figure 3. A distortion correction phantom and software were used to correct for pincushion distortion in the fluoroscopy image [5] and a cubic phantom of known dimensions was used to correct for any geometric scaling errors in the CT scan [6]. The "gold-standard" registration was calculated and its expected accuracy is given in table 1 (see [10] for a full description of the method used).

Table 1. Expected error in "gold-standard" parameters.

	rotation (degrees)			translation (mm)		
	θ_x	θ_y	θ_z	X	Y	Z
SD	0.09	0.09	0.09	1.34	0.15	0.15

4.2 The Registration Algorithm

The registration was carried out on the L3 vertebra. The search space for the algorithm was the six rigid body degrees of freedom. The parameters associated with perspective projection (c_s, l_s, k_1 and k_2) were held fixed at their "gold standard" values.

The search strategy alters each of the degrees of freedom in turn by $\pm\delta\mathbf{P}$ and calculates a new value of the similarity measure. When all the degrees of freedom have been checked a weighted movement is made in the directions which improve the similarity measure, with the parameter showing the greatest improvement being given the greatest weight. A multi-resolution approach is used. The algorithm starts at a coarse resolution (fluoroscopy image reduced, by blurring, to a 128x128 pixel image) and a large step size ($\delta\mathbf{P}$ set equal to 4 mm or 4°) and ends at a finer resolution (256x256) and small step size ($\delta\mathbf{P}$ = 0.5 mm or 0.5°).

4.3 Assessing accuracy and robustness

Each similarity measure was used to register a CT scan of the spine phantom to four different fluoroscopy images of the phantom. The starting estimates for registration were the "gold standard" value plus or minus ΔP (see table 2). There are sixty four possible combinations of "gold-standard" plus or minus ΔP which are at the corners of a six dimensional hyper-cuboid.

Table 2. The displacement (ΔP) of the starting positions from "gold-standard" for each of the six rigid body parameters.

	rotation (degrees)			translation (mm)		
	θ_x	θ_y	θ_z	X	Y	Z
$\Delta\mathbf{P}$	3.4	7.6	7.8	50.8	3.6	2.4

5 Results

Our results are presented in four tables, one for each of the different fluoroscopy images. They show the RMS error between "gold-standard" values and final registration positions (excluding failures) and the number of failed registrations. A failure was defined as when the final registration position, in any of the six degrees of freedom was further from "gold-standard" than ΔP as shown in table 2. The average registration took 74 seconds on a Sun Ultra 30 (300 MHz).

Table 3. RMS error values in rigid body parameters for registrations to fluoroscopy image of spine phantom with no added structures.

Similarity measure	rotation (degrees)			translation (mm)			No. fail, (%)
	θ_x	θ_y	θ_z	X	Y	Z	
Cross correlation	0.41	1.09	0.41	7.2	0.55	0.74	0
Entropy	0.32	0.72	0.36	10.4	0.64	0.46	0
Mutual Information	0.79	1.90	0.65	20.2	0.65	1.05	25
Gradient correlation	0.31	0.49	0.19	4.7	0.43	0.34	0
Pattern Intensity	0.28	0.49	0.26	4.1	0.45	0.34	0
Gradient difference	0.27	0.48	0.17	4.0	0.42	0.32	0

As can be seen from table 3 all six similarity measures, except for mutual information, performed well in registering to the fluoroscopy image of the spine phantom.

Table 4 shows how accurately the similarity measures registered when soft tissue structures were present. Soft tissue caused a large failure rate in mutual information (86%) and a fairly large failure rate in entropy (30%). The cross correlation measure failed relatively few times (8%), but the overall errors increased, particularly in X. Pattern intensity, gradient correlation and gradient difference were effected very little by the presence of soft tissue.

Table 4. RMS error values in rigid body parameters for registrations to fluoroscopy image of spine phantom with soft tissue structures overlayed.

Similarity measure	rotation (degrees)			translation (mm)			No. fail, (%)
	θ_x	θ_y	θ_z	X	Y	Z	
Cross correlation	1.64	1.63	0.41	13.2	0.86	1.06	8
Entropy	0.74	1.02	0.40	8.9	1.30	0.73	30
Mutual Information	2.00	2.43	0.57	21.0	0.97	1.42	86
Gradient correlation	0.51	0.49	0.27	6.9	0.39	0.39	0
Pattern Intensity	0.36	0.53	0.24	5.2	0.43	0.36	0
Gradient difference	0.37	0.36	0.21	6.5	0.40	0.39	0

When registrations to the fluoroscopy image with stent overlaid (table 5) were attempted two of the similarity measures, cross correlation and mutual information, failed to register a number of times and showed large errors when they did register (2.5° in θ_y and 22mm in X). Gradient correlation failed 3% of the time. Entropy was largely unaffected, with just a small general decrease in final accuracy. This result is expected, as the histogram used to compute entropy will be largely unaffected by a small number of pixels with a large difference in intensity. Pattern intensity and gradient difference performed best, with very little change in overall registration error.

Table 5. RMS error values in rigid body parameters for registrations to fluoroscopy image of spine phantom with stent overlayed.

Similarity measure	rotation (degrees)			translation (mm)			No. fail,
	θ_x	θ_y	θ_z	X	Y	Z	(%)
Cross correlation	1.40	2.34	1.11	23.7	0.48	1.46	33
Entropy	0.49	0.86	0.72	14.8	0.69	0.62	0
Mutual Information	0.98	2.37	1.93	21.0	0.55	1.58	48
Gradient correlation	0.23	0.75	0.23	8.5	0.27	0.59	3
Pattern Intensity	0.32	0.39	0.28	4.9	0.42	0.36	0
Gradient difference	0.27	0.49	0.22	3.5	0.43	0.33	0

On registering to the image which contained both soft tissue and a stent (table 6), cross correlation, entropy and mutual information all failed a large number of times and when registrations were deemed valid, they were not accurate. Gradient correlation failed to register 5% of the time, though successful registrations were accurate. Pattern intensity and gradient difference both achieved accurate registrations to this image with no failures. This investigation has only used one pair of CT and fluoroscopy images of a rigid phantom. Different sets of images, in particular different views, may yield different results.

Table 6. RMS error values in rigid body parameters for registrations to fluoroscopy image of spine phantom with soft tissue and stent overlayed.

Similarity measure	rotation (degrees)			translation (mm)			No. fail,
	θ_x	θ_y	θ_z	X	Y	Z	(%)
Cross correlation	2.33	2.25	0.89	27.2	0.29	1.39	45
Entropy	1.36	1.69	1.87	16.9	1.52	1.02	53
Mutual Information	2.67	3.94	2.94	30.3	1.34	5.07	95
Gradient correlation	0.48	0.49	0.42	12.1	0.25	0.50	5
Pattern Intensity	0.31	0.41	0.43	10.7	0.36	0.47	0
Gradient difference	0.28	0.45	0.26	6.7	0.37	0.47	0

6 Conclusions

This paper has compared the accuracy and robustness of six 2D-3D registration algorithms which used different intensity based similarity measures. Final registration positions were compared to an accurate "gold standard" registration found using fiducial markers. Clinical images were simulated by overlaying structures segmented from clinical fluoroscopy images onto a fluoroscopy image of a spine phantom. We have shown that the introduction of soft tissue structures and interventional instruments into the phantom image can have a large effect on the performance of some similarity measures previously applied to 2D-3D image registration. Correlation measures can be effected by thin line structures, such as an interventional stent, which introduces pixels which have a large difference in intensity. Entropy type measures are insensitive to thin line structures, but fail when soft tissue structures create slowly varying changes in background intensity. For a measure to work well with medical images it must be able to register accurately when soft tissue structures and thin line structures are present as differences between the images. Two of the measure described in this paper have achieved this: pattern intensity and gradient difference.

Acknowledgements

We would like to thank Philips Medical Systems, EasyVision Advanced Development for funding this work and providing software, particular thanks go to Alexander van Eeuwijk for his help with distortion correction and Frans Gerritsen for his encouragements and constructive criticisms. We would also like to thank Professor Andy Adam and Dr. Mark Cowling for their clinical input and to thank the radiographers at Guy's Hospital.

References

1. F. Betting and J. Feldmar. 3D-2D projective registration of anatomical surfaces with their projections. In *Proc. Information processing in medical imaging*, pages 275–286, 1995.
2. T.M. Buzug, J. Weese, C. Fassnacht, and C. Lorenz. Image registration: Convex weighting functions for histogram-based similarity measures. In J. Troccaz, E. Grimson, and R. Mösges, editors, *Proc. CVRMed/MRCAS*, pages 203–212. Berlin, Germany: Springer-Verlag, 1997.
3. L.M. Gottesfeld Brown and T.E. Boult. Registration of planar film radiographs with computed tomography. In *Proc. MMBIA*, pages 42–51, 1996.
4. A. Guéziec, P Kazanzides, B. Williamson, R.H. Taylor, and D. Lord. Anatomy based registration of CT-scan and X-ray fluoroscopy data for intra-operative guidance of a surgical robot. In *Proc. SPIE Medical Imaging*, 1998.
5. P. Haaker, E. Klotz, R. Koppe, and R. Linde. Real-time distortion correction of digital x-ray II/TV-systems: an application example for digital flashing tomosynthesis (DFTS). *International Journal of cardiac imaging*, 6:39–45, 1990.
6. D. L. G. Hill, C. R. Maurer, Jr., C. Studholme, J. M. Fitzpatrick, and D. J. Hawkes. Correcting scaling errors in tomographic images using a nine degree of freedom registration algorithm. *J. Comput. Assist. Tomogr.*, 22:317–323, 1998.
7. S. Lavallée, R. Szeliski, and L. Brunie. Matching 3-D smooth surfaces with their 2-D projections using 3-D distance maps. In *Proc. SPIE Geometric methods in computer vision.*, volume 1570, pages 322–336, 1991.
8. L. Lemieux, R. Jagoe, D.R. Fish, N.D. Kitchen, and D.G.T. Thomas. A patient-to-computed-tomography image registration method based on digitally reconstructed radiographs. *Med. Phys.*, 21(11):1749–1760, 1994.
9. F. Maes, A. Collignon, D. Vandermeulen, G. Marchal, and P. Seutens. Multimodality image registration by maximization of mutual, information. *IEEE Transactions on Medical Imaging*, 16(2):187–198, 1997.
10. G.P. Penney, J. Weese, J.L. Little, Desmedt P., D.L.G. Hill, and D.J. Hawkes. A comparison of similarity measures for use in 2D-3D medical image registration. *IEEE Transactions on Medical Imaging*, 1998 (Provisionally accepted).
11. C. Studholme, D.L.G. Hill, and D.J. Hawkes. Automated 3D registration of MR and CT images of the head. *Medical Image Analysis*, 1(2):163–175, 1996.
12. C. Studholme, D.L.G. Hill, and D.J. Hawkes. Automated 3D registration of MR and PET brain images by multi-resolution optimisation of voxel similarity measures. *Medical Physics*, 24:25–35, 1997.
13. P. Viola and W. M. Wells. Alignment by maximization of mutual information. In *Proc. 5th International Conference on Computer Vision (ICCV'95)*, pages 16–23, 1995.
14. J. Weese, T.M. Buzug, C. Lorenz, and C. Fassnacht. An approach to 2D/3D registration of a vertebra in 2D x-ray fluoroscopies with 3D CT images. In *Proc. CVRMed/MRCAS*, pages 119–128, 1997.

Elastic Model Based Non-rigid Registration Incorporating Statistical Shape Information

Yongmei Wang* and Lawrence H. Staib*+

Departments of Electrical Engineering* and Diagnostic Radiology+
Yale University, P.O. Box 208042, New Haven, CT 06520-8042
wang@noodle.med.yale.edu, lawrence.staib@yale.edu

Abstract. This paper describes a new method of non-rigid registration using the combined power of elastic and statistical shape models. The transformations are constrained to be consistent with a physical model of elasticity to maintain smoothness and continuity. A Bayesian formulation, based on this model, on an intensity similarity measure, and on statistical shape information embedded in corresponding boundary points, is employed to find a more accurate and robust non-rigid registration. A dense set of forces arises from the intensity similarity measure to accommodate complex anatomical details. A sparse set of forces constrains consistency with statistical shape models derived from a training set. A number of experiments were performed on both synthetic and real medical images of the brain and heart to evaluate the approach. It is shown that statistical boundary shape information significantly augments and improves elastic model based non-rigid registration. [1]

1 Introduction

Comparing function or morphology between individuals requires non-rigid registration, because the detailed anatomical structure differs, sometimes greatly, between individuals. The goal of our non-rigid registration is to remove structural variation between individuals by matching an atlas image to each individual, or study, image, in order to have a common coordinate system for comparison. Shape differences between the atlas and study's anatomy are contained in the non-rigid transformation.

There have been many approaches to non-rigid registration in recent years [2] [3] [4] [6] [8] [9] [10] [15]. Usually, the transformation is constrained in some way because of the ill-posedness (i.e. in this case, the existence of many possible solutions) of the problem. Physical models, for example, linear elastic models, are widely used to enforce topological properties on the deformation and then constrain the enormous solution space [2] [4] [8] [9] [10]. Here, we are particularly interested in intensity based deformation using elastic models. Our goal is to incorporate statistical shape information into this type of elastic model based registration and to develop a more accurate and robust algorithm.

Christensen et al. [4] present two physical models for non-rigid registration of the brain. The transformations are constrained to be consistent with the physical properties of deformable elastic solids in the first method and those of viscous

---
[1] This work was supported in part by a grant from the Whitaker Foundation.

fluids in the second. Viscous fluid models are less constraining than elastic models and allow long-distance, nonlinear deformations of small subregions. In these formulations, however, no matter what model is used, elastic solid [10], viscous fluid [5], or other physics model such as hyperelasticity [11], the deformed configuration of the atlas is always determined by driving the deformation using only pixel-by-pixel intensity difference between images. In many applications, however, this kind of warping is under-constrained and admits to unreasonable registration. Corresponding anatomical structure may shift or twist away from one position to another (Fig.1(a)(b)). Even if the driving force is very small, the transformation may not be accurate enough, or may even be completely wrong, *even though* the deformed atlas and study appear similar (Fig.1(b)(c)(d)). In these circumstances, if shape information had been included, the correct mapping or registration could have been found (Fig.1(g)(h)). In addition, due to the use of the gray-level gradient of the deformed atlas in the body force formulation [4], lower contrast objects deform much slower than high-contrast objects, independent of their importance. Sometimes objects do not deform well because their gradient is too low compared to high-gradient objects (Fig.2(c)(d)). With the incorporation of the shape information, the result is improved (Fig.2(h)).

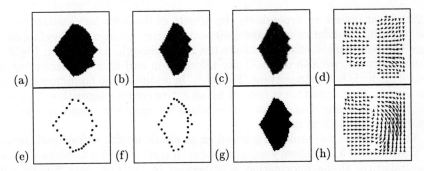

Fig. 1. Comparison of synthetic image (64 × 64) non-rigid registration methods. (a): atlas image; (b): study image; (c): deformed atlas image by Christensen&Miller's elastic method [4] [10] (based on our implementation, discussed in Section 5); (d): corresponding unreasonable vector map of (c) (The two bumps on the right side do not slide up to the corresponding bumps, as desired); (e): atlas image control points; (f): study image control points; (g): deformed atlas image by our method; (h): vector map of our elastic transformation showing correct tracking of features.

Davatzikos and Prince [8] propose a method where they first identify the boundaries of homologous brain regions in two images to be registered (e.g., cortex, ventricles, etc.), and establish a one-to-one mapping between them. Based on this mapping, they deform the boundaries in one image into those in the other image. The rest of the image is deformed by solving the equations describing the deformation of an elastic body using the boundary deformation as input. In this approach, although the mapping may be accurate on the boundary, the farther away the structure is from the boundary, the more error there is, because only information from object boundaries is used for registration. Also, the localization

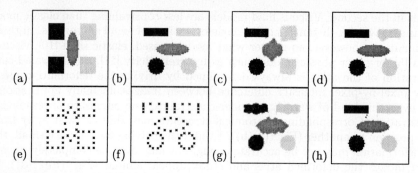

Fig. 2. Comparison of synthetic multi-gradient image (64 × 64) non-rigid registration methods. (a): atlas image; (b): study image; (c): deformed atlas at iteration 20 by Christensen&Miller's elastic method [4] [10] ; (d): deformed atlas at iteration 150 by Christensen&Miller's elastic method; (e): atlas image control points; (f): study image control points; (g): deformed atlas at iteration 150 by Davatzikos's elastic method [8], with body force solely determined by corresponding pairs of control points; (h): deformed atlas at iteration 150 by our elastic method showing good convergence without any boundary jiggling effect.

of the object boundary depends on the density of the boundary control points. The resulting boundaries can have quite severe errors producing a jiggling effect when the boundary control points are not dense enough, as shown in Fig.2(g). In our approach, we also use intensity information and thus the density of the control points is not as important (Fig.2(h)). In addition, the boundary information used in their approach is derived by an active contour algorithm [8], and it does not include any shape information which we believe is crucial in non-rigid registration for medical images.

The algorithm we employed is based on an elastic model, a gray level similarity measure and a consistency measure between corresponding boundary points. The statistical shape information is embedded in the boundary finding with correspondence process [16] applied to the study. This method uses statistical point models with shape, and shape variation, generated from sets of examples by principal component analysis of the covariance matrix. The power of elastic and statistical shape models are combined in our approach using a Bayesian framework.

2 Elastic Model

There is no true elastic model for deformation because, for example, one anatomical structure does not literally result from the deformation of another structure. We use an analogous linear elastic model to control the deformation. Without it, the results could be almost completely arbitrary.

An Eulerian reference is used in our elastic model formulation. In this frame, a particle is tracked with respect to its final coordinates. The non-rigid registration is defined by the transformation corresponding to a homeomorphic mapping of the coordinate system, defined in 2D by:

$$w = (x, y) \rightarrow (x - u_x(w), y - u_y(w)) \qquad (1)$$

where $u(w) = [u_x(w), u_y(w)]^T$ is the displacement at each pixel w whose coordinate is denoted as (x, y). This mapping allows for the detailed local transformation into the specific anatomy of the individual, or study.

We want to find this transformation that best matches the atlas with the study, constrained by the elastic model. The formulation of the elastic model is similar to that in [4]. For linear elastic solids, the force is proportional to the displacement. The spatial transformation satisfies the partial differential equation (PDE):

$$\mu \nabla^2 u + (\mu + \beta) \nabla (\nabla \cdot u) = F(u) \tag{2}$$

with certain boundary conditions such as that $u(w) = 0$ for w on the image boundary. In this equation, μ and β are Lamé constants. The body force, $F(u)$, is the driving function that deforms the atlas into the shape of the study, which will be formulated in detail in Section 4.

3 Statistical Shape Model Based Boundary Finding

Numerous deformable model based boundary finding methods have been proposed [7] [13] [14]. We have developed a statistical shape model based boundary finding with correspondence algorithm, which has been described in detail in [16]. Global shape parameters derived from the statistical variation of object boundary points in a training set are used to model the object [7]. A Bayesian formulation, based on this prior knowledge and the edge information of the input image, is employed to find the object boundary with its subset points in correspondence with the point sets of boundaries in the training set.

Given m aligned examples, and for each example, a set of N labeled points, $L_i = (x_i(1), y_i(1), x_i(2), y_i(2), \cdots, x_i(N), y_i(N))^T$, $(i = 1, 2, \cdots, m)$, we calculate the mean shape, $\bar{L}$, and the covariance about the mean, $C_{training}$. The t eigenvectors q_i of $C_{training}$ corresponding to the largest t eigenvalues, λ_i, give a set of uncorrelated basis vectors, or *modes of variation*, for a deformable model. A new example can be calculated using $L = \bar{L} + Qa$, where $Q = (q_1|q_2|\cdots|q_t)$ is the matrix of eigenvectors and $a = (a_1, a_2, \cdots, a_t)^T$ is the vector of weights, or shape parameters, to be determined. As a varies from zero, the corresponding shapes will be similar to those in the training set.

Given the statistical models, our aim is to match them to particular examples of structure in the individual images, and find the shape parameters, $a = (a_1, a_2, \cdots, a_t)^T$, and pose parameters: scale s, rotation θ, and translation T_x, T_y. The combined pose and shape parameter vector to be determined is $p = (s, \theta, T_x, T_y, a_1, a_2, ..., a_t)$.

A Bayesian formulation leads to ([16]):

$$M(p) = \sum_{j=1}^{t+4} \left[-\frac{(p_j - m_j)^2}{2\sigma_j^2} \right] + \frac{1}{\sigma_n^2} \sum_{n=1}^{N} E(x(p, n), y(p, n)) \tag{3}$$

where m_j is the mean of p_j; σ_j is the standard deviation for each of the parameters and σ_n is the standard deviation of the white zero mean Gaussian noise associated with the image noise model [16]. This equation is the maximum *a posteriori* objective incorporating a prior bias to likely shapes and poses (first term) and a match to edges in the image (second term). Additional features can easily be incorporated.

4 Elastic Model Incorporating Statistical Shape

While elastic models are useful in non-rigid registration, they are limited by themselves because they are too generic. With statistical information, we have a stronger bias to augment the elastic model. Statistical models can be powerful tools to directly capture the character of the variability of the individuals being modeled. Instead of relying on an elastic model to guide the deformation in a roughly plausible way, the statistics of a sample of images can be used to guide the deformation in a way governed by the measured variation of individuals. Thus, this paper proposes an algorithm which uses an elastic model, yet incorporates a statistical shape model to constrain solutions to more anatomically consistent deformations.

We pose the above displacement estimation problem in a maximum *a posteriori* framework. As input to the problem, we have both the intensity image of the study (individual), $I_s(w)$, and the boundary points of the study $b_s(\mathbf{p}, n) = (x_s(\mathbf{p}, n), y_s(\mathbf{p}, n))$, for $n = 1, 2, \cdots, N$, given the shape and pose parameters, $\mathbf{p}$, which are derived from the statistical shape model based boundary finding [16]. Thus, we want to maximize:

$$\Pr(u|I_s, b_s(\mathbf{p})) = \frac{\Pr(u, I_s, b_s(\mathbf{p}))}{\Pr(I_s, b_s(\mathbf{p}))} \qquad (4)$$

Ignoring the denominator, which does not change with u, and by using Bayes rule, our aim is to find:

$$\arg\max_{u} \Pr(u|I_s, b_s(\mathbf{p})) \equiv \arg\max_{u} \Pr(b_s(\mathbf{p})|u, I_s) \Pr(I_s|u) \Pr(u)$$
$$\propto \arg\max_{u} \Pr(b_s(\mathbf{p})|u) \Pr(I_s|u) \Pr(u) \qquad (5)$$
$$\equiv \arg\max_{u} [\ln \Pr(u) + \ln \Pr(I_s|u) + \ln \Pr(b_s(\mathbf{p})|u)] \quad (6)$$

where (5) is true if we ignore the dependence of $b_s(\mathbf{p})$ on I_s because $b_s(\mathbf{p})$ is obtained as a prior here and is not modified in this formulation. In the last equation, we have just taken the natural logarithm, which is a monotonically increasing function.

It is straightforward to directly connect the Bayesian posterior to the PDE in Eq.(2) [5]. This view is based on a variational principle from which the PDE can be derived. Such principles are well known in mechanics [12] and link the PDE formulation as the minimizer of some potential. The PDE for the linear elastic model, which is given in Eq.(2), is produced by setting the variation of the *generalized Lagrangian* energy density associated with constraints imposed by the linearized mechanics equal to zero [5]. The forcing function in the PDE (Eq. (2)) is then the variation of the likelihood function with respect to the vector displacement field [1] [10].

The first term in Eq.(6) corresponds to the transformation prior term, which is defined to give a high probability to transformations consistent with the elastic model and low probability to all other transformations. As mentioned above, it is a PDE of the deformation field, u, and is given by Eq.(2).

The second term in Eq.(6) is actually the likelihood term which depends on the study image. Let $I_a(w)$ be the intensity image of the atlas. We model the study image as a Gaussian process with mean given by the deformed atlas image, $I_a(w - u(w))$ [5] (since Eulerian reference frame is used here, a mass particle instantaneously located at w originated from point $w - u(w)$). That is,

$$\ln \Pr(I_s|u) = -\frac{1}{2\sigma_1^2} \int_\Omega [I_s(w) - I_a(w - u(w))]^2 \, dw \qquad (7)$$

where σ_1 is the standard deviation of the Gaussian process.

The first body force, F_1, is the gradient of this likelihood term with respect to u at each w [5] and is given by:

$$F_1(u) = -\frac{1}{\sigma_1^2} [I_s(w) - I_a(w - u(w))] \nabla I_a(w - u(w)) \qquad (8)$$

This force is a combination of $I_s(w) - I_a(w - u(w))$, the difference in intensity between the study and the deformed atlas, and $\nabla I_a(w - u(w))$, the gradient of the deformed atlas. The gradient term determines the directions of the local deformation forces applied to the atlas. As explained in the introduction, this kind of forcing by itself is often under-constrained.

The main contribution of this paper lies in the last term of Eq.(6), which incorporates statistical shape information into the non-rigid registration framework. The extra constraint of corresponding boundary points is used as an additional matching criterion. The boundary point positions are the result of the deformation of the model to fit the data in ways consistent with the statistical shape models derived from the training set, as described in Section 3. Let $b_a(n) = (x_a(n), y_a(n))$, for $n = 1, 2, \cdots, N$, denote the atlas boundary points positions, which are known since we have full information about the atlas. We now model $b_s(\mathbf{p})$ as a Gaussian process with mean given by the deformed atlas boundary position, expressed as $b_a(n) + u(w)$, for pixels w on the deformed atlas boundary points. Then,

$$\ln \Pr(b_s(\mathbf{p})|u) = -\frac{1}{2\sigma_2^2} \sum_{n=1}^{N} ||b_s(\mathbf{p}, n) - [b_a(n) + u(w)]||^2 \qquad (9)$$

where σ_2 is again the standard deviation of the Gaussian process.

The second body force, F_2, is then the gradient of Eq.(9) with respect to u for pixels w on the deformed atlas boundary points:

$$F_2(u) = \frac{1}{\sigma_2^2} ||b_s(\mathbf{p}, n) - [b_a(n) + u(w)]|| \qquad (10)$$

$F_2(u)$ is zero for pixels w not on the deformed atlas boundary points.

From Eq.(10), we can see that the calculated displacements at the sparse boundary points are constrained to match the vector difference of the corresponding atlas and study boundary point positions. This kind of forcing contains information from the statistical shape model. The result will match shape

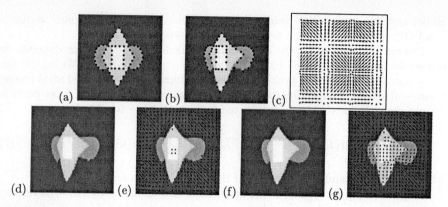

Fig. 3. Synthetic images (100 × 100) and displacement vectors. (a): atlas image with its control points; (b): study image with its control points; (c): true displacement vectors by Eq.(12); (d): our deformed atlas image; (e): errors in our estimated vectors on study image; (f): deformed atlas image by Christensen&Miller's elastic method; (g): errors in estimated vectors for (f) on study image.

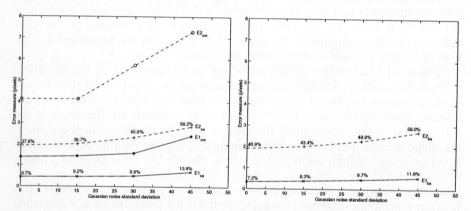

Fig. 4. Sensitivity to noise experiment for synthetic images. E_{om}: maximum displacement error over the deformed objects; E_{oa}: average displacement error over the deformed objects; E_{ba}: average displacement error on the sparse boundary points. Note: $E1$ and $E2$ are error measures by our method and Christensen&Miller's elastic method respectively; the percentages shown are the percentages of the average errors (E_{oa}, E_{ba}) relative to the true average displacements; the intensity range in the atlas and study images in Fig.3 is 50 to 250.

features of the atlas and the study, such as high curvature points and important anatomical landmarks, in addition to the intensity measure.

The total force term, $F(u)$, in Eq.(2) is then the weighted sum of $F_1(u)$ in Eq.(8) and $F_2(u)$ in Eq.(10), that is, for each w,

$$F(u) = c_1 F_1(u) + c_2 F_2(u) \qquad (11)$$

The two coefficients, c_1 and c_2, can be related to the image contrast and the deformation between the atlas and study image. If c_2 is too large, $F_2(u)$ will play a dominant role by matching only boundary points, which may cause discontinuity when the boundary points are not dense enough. On the other hand, if c_1 is too large, $F_2(u)$ will have almost no effect and the algorithm is then an elastic regularization method (as [10]) without statistical information. For the time being, they are fixed empirically so that $F_1(u)$ and $F_2(u)$ are of the same order and then have the best effect.

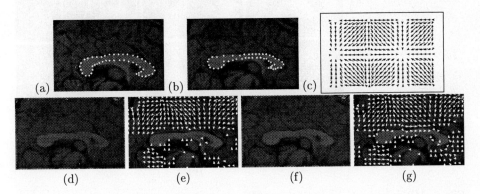

Fig. 5. MR sagittal corpus callosum images (100 × 64) and synthetic displacement vectors. (a): atlas image with control points; (b): study image with control points; (c): true displacement vectors; (d): our deformed atlas image; (e): errors in our estimated vectors on study image; (f): deformed atlas image by Christensen&Miller's elastic method; (g): errors in estimated vectors for (f) on study image.

We have presented an elastic model based non-rigid registration procedure that incorporates information obtained from statistical shape model based boundary finding. Our non-rigid registration method is then composed of Eq.(2) and Eq.(11). In order to solve the problem, we discretize the two equations and solve the resulting system iteratively by using successive over-relaxation (SOR). The value of the total body force is used as the stopping criterion for the iterations.

5 Experimental Results

For all of the experiments, we apply Christensen&Miller's elastic registration [10] [4] for a direct comparison based on our own implementation. We discretize and solve the resulting system iteratively by using SOR instead of stochastic gradient search, as in [10]. As to the computation time, while our method requires an extra force F_2 calculation at sparse boundary points, this leads to faster and accurate convergence. Also, since the boundary finding step takes negligible time, i.e. only several seconds, the total convergence time of our method is usually a little faster.

5.1 Evaluation Criterion

To evaluate the methodology, we quantify errors in the displacement field over the objects of interest, since warping of the background is irrelevant.

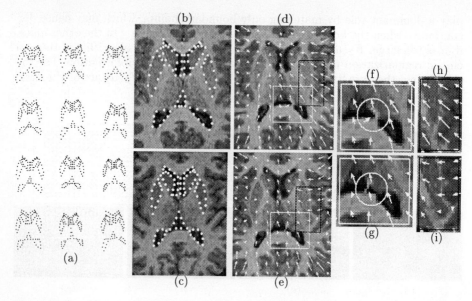

Fig. 6. MR axial brain images (80 × 100) and displacement vectors. (a): 12 examples of brain shapes from a training set with each example a 93 point model of basal ganglia and ventricle boundaries; (b): atlas image with its control points; (c): study image with its control points derived from our boundary finding algorithm [16]; (d): our estimated vectors over our deformed atlas; (e): estimated vectors by Christensen&Miller's elastic method over their deformed atlas; (f): enlargement of (d) showing correct mapping of the ventricle corners; (g): mis-matching due to Christensen&Miller's method; (h): well deformed putamen by our method (cropped); (i): poorly deformed putamen by Christensen&Miller's method.

Image (Fig.)	Error	Our method	Christensen&Miller's method
MR sagittal corpus callosum (Fig.5)	E_{oa} (%)	0.48 pixels (11.5%)	1.26 pixels (30.0%)
	E_{om}	1.33 pixels	3.56 pixels
	E_{ba} (%)	0.45 pixels (10.3%)	1.51 pixels (34.7%)
MR axial brain (Fig.6)	E_{ba}(%)	0.75 pixels (16.0%)	2.04 pixels (43.7%)
MR heart (Fig.7)	E_{ba}(%)	0.90 pixels (15.4%)	1.81 pixels (31.1%)

Table 1. Error measure for MR corpus callosum images with known warping, real axial brain and heart images. E_{oa}: average displacement error over corpus callosum; E_{om}: maximum displacement error over corpus callosum; E_{ba}: average displacement error on sparse boundary points. Note: the percentages shown with each average error are with respect to the true average displacement.

Given a known warp, we can measure detailed displacement errors throughout the object. For testing purposes, we can define a particular warp and apply it to an image generating a warped study image to which the algorithm can be applied. We use the following sinusoidal displacement field for transforming the atlas image to a study image (see Fig.3(c) or Fig.5(c)):

$$x_{new} = x_{old} + A_x sin(\pi x_{old}/32); \qquad y_{new} = y_{old} + A_y sin(\pi y_{old}/32) \quad (12)$$

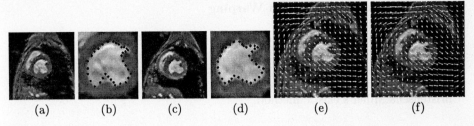

| (a) | (b) | (c) | (d) | (e) | (f) |

Fig. 7. MR heart images (150 × 150) and displacement vectors. (a): atlas image; (b): atlas image with its control points on the endocardium (cropped); (c): study image; (d): study image with control points derived from our boundary finding algorithm; (e): our estimated vectors over our deformed atlas image; (f): estimated vectors by Christensen&Miller's elastic method over their deformed atlas image.

where x_{old} and y_{old} are coordinates of a point in the atlas image and x_{new} and y_{new} are coordinates of the corresponding point in the transformed study image. A_x and A_y are the limits of the maximum displacement distances along the x and y directions.

For a known non-rigid warp, the average (E_{oa}) and maximum (E_{om}) differences between the estimated and actual displacement vectors over the objects are used to measure accuracy. We also use the average difference between the estimated and actual displacement vectors on the sparse boundary control points, E_{ba}. Since the control points are also derived from the known warp, all three measures only reflect the non-rigid registration, and do not include the boundary finding step. For true image pairs, we only use E_{ba} as an accuracy measure because we do not know the true warp, except at sparse boundary points determined by an expert. Since the study image boundary control points are derived by our statistical shape model based boundary finding, the error, E_{ba}, for true image pairs includes both the boundary finding step and the non-rigid registration step.

5.2 Synthetic Images with Known Warping

The synthetic study image, Figure 3(b), is obtained by resampling the synthetic atlas image, Fig.3(a), based on the predetermined displacement vectors (Eq.(12)). The study control points are also derived from the same predetermined displacement vectors. The atlas image is then registered to the synthetic study image using our image registration procedure. Although the resulting deformed atlases for our method and Christensen&Miller's method are similar, the estimated displacement vectors are not. From the errors in the estimated vectors (differences between the estimated and true displacement vectors), we can see that our method has almost zero error over the objects, while there is significant error in their approach.

The following experiment, shown in Fig.4, demonstrates the effect of noise on the two methods, by adding varying amounts of zero mean Gaussian noise to the synthetic images shown in Fig.3(a) and Fig.3(b). The error measures defined above are computed for our method ($E1_{oa}$, $E1_{om}$, $E1_{ba}$) and Christensen&Miller's elastic approach ($E2_{oa}$, $E2_{om}$, $E2_{ba}$).

5.3 Real Image with Known Warping

In this experiment (Fig.5), we apply a known warping (Eq.(12)) to a magnetic resonance (MR) sagittal brain image showing the corpus callosum. While the deformed atlases appear similar, the results (Fig.5 and Table 1) show that our method leads to a much better registration in the object of interest than Christensen&Miller's elastic method.

5.4 Real Atlas and Study Images

Results of the method applied to MR brain (axial) and heart image pairs are shown in Fig.6 and Fig.7. These are 2D slices roughly corresponding from different brains and hearts for demonstration purposes. The control points of the study image are derived from statistical shape model based boundary finding algorithm [16]. The shape model used for the brain examples incorporates multiple objects and thus also models the distance between the objects. From the error measures shown in Table 1, we see that even with the error in the boundary finding step, the final error of our method is still much better than Christensen&Miller's elastic method. Note particular in Fig.6, the corner of the third ventricle in the study was not registered to the atlas correctly by Christensen&Miller's method (Fig.6(g)). The structures of the study are shifted away from the corresponding ones in the atlas based on gray level information. Our method calculated the correct mapping (Fig.6(f)) by incorporating statistical shape information and using the corresponding boundary points as an extra constraint. Also note that the putamen did not deform well in Christensen&Miller's method (Fig.6(i)) because the contrast of the putamen is too low compared to the contrast of the ventricles. In our approach, the putamen deformed correctly (Fig.6(h)) since shape information of the putamen was included.

6 Conclusions

This work presents a systematic approach for non-rigid registration. Transformations are constrained to be consistent with physical deformations of elastic solids in order to maintain the topology, or integrity, of the anatomic structures while having high spatial dimension to accommodate complex anatomical details. Both intensity information and statistical shape information are used as matching criteria in a Bayesian formulation. The incorporation of statistical shape information into the framework is the main contribution of our work. From the experimental results, statistical boundary shape information has been shown to augment and improve an elastic model formulation for non-rigid registration.

Our current and future directions include exploring the use of fluid models to track long-distance, nonlinear deformations [17] and generalization to 3D. Although finding the landmark surface points and model construction in 3D will require new strategies, generalizing the purely elastic model deformation to 3D is straightforward and has been developed by Christensen *et al.* [4]. Of course, the computational cost increases with the number of voxels.

References

1. Y. Amit, U. Grenander and M. Piccioni, "Structural image restoration through deformable templates," *J. American Statistical Association*, Vol. 86, no. 414, pp. 376-387, June 1991.
2. R. Bajcsy and S. Kovacic, "Multiresolution elastic matching," *Computer Vision, Graphics and Image Processing*, Vol. 46, pp. 1-21, 1989.
3. F. L. Bookstein, "Shape and information in medical images: A decade of the morphometric synthesis," *Proc. Workshop Math. Meth. Biomed. Image Anal.*, pp. 2-12, June 1996.
4. G. E. Christensen, M. I. Miller and M. W. Vannier, "Individualizing neuroanatomical atlases using a massively parallel computer," *Computer*, pp. 32-38, January 1996.
5. G. E. Christensen, R. D. Rabbitt and M. I. Miller, "Deformable templates using large deformation kinematics," *IEEE Trans. on Image Processing*, Vol. 5, no. 10, pp. 1435-1447, October 1996.
6. D. L. Collins, A. C. Evans, C. Holmes and T. M. Peters, "Automatic 3D segmentation of neuro-anatomical structures from MRI," *Information Processing in Medical Imaging*, pp. 139-152, 1995.
7. T. F. Cootes, C. J. Taylor, D. H. Cooper and J. Graham, "Active shape models – their training and application," *Computer Vision and Image Understanding*, Vol. 61, no. 1, pp. 38-59, 1995.
8. C. Davatzikos and J. Prince, "Brain image registration based on curve mapping," *IEEE Workshop Biomedical Image Anal.*, pp. 245-254, 1994.
9. J. Gee, L. L. Briquer, C. Barillot and D. Haynor, "Probabilistic matching of brain images," *Information Processing in Medical Imaging*, pp. 113-125, 1995.
10. M. I. Miller, G. E. Christensen, Y. Amit and U. Grenander, "Mathematical textbook of deformable neuroanatomies," *Proc. National Academy of Science*, Vol. 90, no. 24, pp. 11944-11948, 1993.
11. R. D. Rabbitt, G. E. Christensen and M. I. Miller, "Mapping of hyperelastic deformable templates using finite element method," *Vision Geometry IV*, Vol. 2573, pp. 252-265, July 1995.
12. J. N. Reddy, *Energy and Variational Methods in Applied Mechanics*, New York: Wiley-Interscience, 1984.
13. L. H. Staib and J. S. Duncan, "Boundary finding with parametrically deformable models," *IEEE Trans. Pattern Analysis and Machine Intelligence*, Vol. 14, no. 11, pp. 1061-1075, 1992.
14. G. Székely, A. Keleman, C. Brechbuler and G. Gerig, "Segmentation of 2-D and 3-D objects from MRI volume data using constrained elastic deformations of flexible Fourier contours and surface models," *Medical Image Analysis*, Vol. 1, no. 1, pp. 19-34, 1996.
15. J. P. Thirion, "Non-rigid matching using demons," *Proc. Conf. Computer Vision and Pattern Recognition*, pp. 245-251, June 1996.
16. Y. Wang and L. H. Staib, "Boundary finding with correspondence using statistical shape models," *Proc. Conf. Computer Vision and Pattern Recognition*, pp. 338-345, Santa Barbara, California, June 1998.
17. Y. Wang and L. H. Staib, "Integrated approaches to non-rigid registration in medical images," *Fourth IEEE Workshop on Applications of Computer Vision*, in press, Princeton, New Jersey, October 1998.

Image Registration Based on Thin-Plate Splines and Local Estimates of Anisotropic Landmark Localization Uncertainties

Karl Rohr

Universität Hamburg, Fachbereich Informatik, AB Kognitive Systeme,
Vogt-Kölln-Str. 30, D-22527 Hamburg, Germany
rohr@informatik.uni-hamburg.de

Abstract. We present an approach to elastic registration of tomographic brain images which is based on thin-plate splines and takes into account landmark errors. The inclusion of error information is important in clinical applications since landmark extraction is always prone to error. In comparison to previous work, our approach can cope with anisotropic errors, which is significantly more realistic than dealing only with isotropic errors. In particular, it is now possible to include different types of landmarks, e.g., quasi-landmarks at the outer contour of the brain. Also, we introduce an approach to estimate landmark localization uncertainties directly from the image data. Experimental results are presented for the registration of 2D and 3D MR images.

1 Motivation

Image registration is fundamental to computer-assisted neurosurgery. Examples are the registration of tomographic images and the registration of images with digital atlases. In either case, the central aim is to increase the accuracy of localizing anatomical structures in 3D space. One principal approach to registration is based on thin-plate splines and anatomical point landmarks.

Previous work on thin-plate spline registration has concentrated on specifying the landmarks manually and on using an interpolating transformation model (e.g., [2],[6],[11]). The approach is efficient and well-suited for user-interaction which we consider important in clinical scenaria. However, with an interpolation scheme the corresponding landmarks are forced to match exactly. It is (implicitly) assumed that the landmark positions are known exactly, which, however, is generally not true in practical applications. Therefore, to take into account landmark localization errors, we have recently introduced an approximation scheme ([13]). This scheme is based on a minimizing functional, it uses scalar weights to represent landmark errors, and it has been described for images of arbitrary dimensions. The applicability of our approach has been demonstrated for 2D MR images. Bookstein [3] has proposed a different approach to relax the interpolation conditions. His approach, however, has not been related to a minimizing functional, but combines different metrics based on a technique called 'curve décolletage'. Also, the approach has only been described for 2D datasets, and experimental results have been reported for 2D synthetic data ('simulated PET images').

One problem with our approach in [13] is that scalar weights for the landmarks are only a coarse characterization of the localization errors. Generally, the errors are different in different directions and thus are anisotropic. Another problem is how to specify the landmark errors.

In this contribution, we describe an extension of our previous approach [13], which allows to incorporate full covariance matrices representing landmark position errors. Although the corresponding minimizing functional is more complicated than in the case of using only scalar weights, we still have an analytic solution the parameters of which can efficiently be computed by solving an analogous linear system of equations. Also, we introduce an approach to estimate the covariance matrices directly from the image data. In our case, these matrices represent the minimal localization uncertainty at landmark points (Cramér-Rao bound). An advantage of our approach is that we can now include different types of 3D point landmarks, e.g., 'normal' point landmarks as well as 'quasi-landmarks'. Quasi-landmarks are not uniquely definable in all directions (e.g., arbitrary edge points) and they are used, for example, in the reference system of Talairach [15] to define the 3D bounding box of the brain. The incorporation of such landmarks is important since 'normal' point landmarks are hard to define, for example, at the outer parts of the brain.

The remainder of this contribution is organized as follows. In the next section, we provide a statistical interpretation of our approach to landmark localization. This interpretation is also the basis for estimating landmark localization uncertainties directly from the image data as described in Section 3. Section 4 is then devoted to the thin-plate spline approach using weight matrices, and Section 5 demonstrates the applicability of our approach for 2D as well as 3D tomographic images of the human brain.

2 Statistical Interpretation of 3D Landmark Localization

3D anatomical point landmarks are usually localized manually. Generally, this procedure is difficult, time-consuming, and often lacks accuracy (e.g., [6],[9]). To improve on this, we use a semi-automatic procedure with the advantage that the user has the possibility to control the results (see also [13]). Semi-automatic means that landmark candidates are automatically detected within a specified region-of-interest (ROI) and then the user selects the most promising candidate. To simplify the selection, the landmark candidates are ordered based on the automatically computed operator responses. The anatomical landmarks we use are located on the skull base (e.g., tip of external protuberance, saddle point on zygomatic bone) as well as on the ventricular system (e.g., tips of frontal and occipital horns).

To extract anatomical point landmarks, we here consider a 3D extension of a 2D corner operator. In previous work ([13],[12]) this approach has been motivated by the criterion: 'Find points with high intensity variations'. This criterion, however, is rather unspecific. In this contribution, we show that a statistical interpretation is possible. We consider the 3D differential operator

$$det\mathbf{C}_g \rightarrow max, \qquad (1)$$

where $\mathbf{C}_g = \overline{\nabla g \, (\nabla g)^T}$ is a symmetric 3×3 matrix which represents the averaged dyadic product of the 3D intensity gradient $\nabla g = (g_x, g_y, g_z)^T$, $g(x,y,z)$ is the image function, and det denotes the determinant of a matrix. Note, that the operator in (1) requires to compute only first order partial derivatives of an image. Therefore, the operator is computationally efficient and does not suffer from instabilities of computing high order partial derivatives. In contrast to that, other 3D differential operators require partial derivatives up to order two or three (e.g., [17],[10]).

In the following, let σ_n^2 denote the variance of additive white Gaussian image noise and m the number of voxels in a local 3D window. Then, we can relate the matrix $\mathbf{C}_g$ to the minimal localization uncertainty of the center of the window $\mathbf{x} = (x,y,z)$. The minimal localization uncertainty is given by the Cramér-Rao bound (e.g., [18]) and is represented by the covariance matrix

$$\mathbf{\Sigma}_g = \frac{\sigma_n^2}{m} \mathbf{C}_g^{-1}. \qquad (2)$$

We see, that $\mathbf{\Sigma}_g$ is proportional to the inverse of $\mathbf{C}_g$. From (2) we can derive the 3D error ellipsoid of the position estimate with semi-axes σ_x, σ_y, and σ_z. A quantitative measure for the localization uncertainty of a landmark is the volume of the 3D error ellipsoid which is defined as

$$V = \frac{4}{3}\pi \sqrt{det\mathbf{\Sigma}_g}, \qquad (3)$$

where $det\mathbf{\Sigma}_g = \sigma_x^2 \sigma_y^2 \sigma_z^2$. The smaller $det\mathbf{\Sigma}_g$ the smaller is the localization uncertainty. Thus, we can formulate the following criterion for localizing 3D point landmarks: 'Find points with minimal localization uncertainty', i.e., minimal volume of the 3D error ellipsoid. This requirement can be stated as

$$det\mathbf{\Sigma}_g \rightarrow min. \qquad (4)$$

Since $det\mathbf{\Sigma}_g = 1/det\mathbf{\Sigma}_g^{-1}$ and with (2) we see that (4) is equivalent to the operator in (1). Thus, this operator extracts 3D points with minimal localization uncertainty. Note, that in the case we have no Gaussian image noise, we consider (2) as an approximation. Note also, that $\mathbf{C}_g$ and thus $\mathbf{\Sigma}_g$ can directly be computed from the image data, and that $det\mathbf{C}_g$ is invariant w.r.t. translations and rotations.

3 Estimation of Landmark Localization Uncertainties

Our aim is to integrate landmark errors in elastic registration of 3D images, and in the general case we have to deal with anisotropic errors. But how should we specify these errors ? One possibility is to exploit error information from anatomical studies concerning the variability of brain structures. However, currently we are not aware that such anatomical knowledge is available. Alternatively, a user in a certain registration application may provide confidence levels of how well localization of single landmarks is possible (e.g., high, middle, low confidence) as well as may specify certain directions where the uncertainty is extremal. A disadvantage of this procedure is, however, that it is time-consuming.

Instead, we here propose a different approach which allows to estimate landmark localization uncertainties directly from the image data. With this approach we exploit the minimal stochastic error due to the intensity variations in the neighborhood of a landmark. The minimal error is determined by the Cramér-Rao bound stated in (2). This bound depends on the local variation of the image gradient as well as on the image noise. Note, that since we use a lower bound this procedure is applicable to any point within an image, independently of how this point has been localized (manually or automatically). The required first order image derivatives in (2) in our case are computed by applying Gaussian derivative filters or Beaudet filters. Averaging is generally performed in a $5 \times 5 \times 5$ neighborhood.

Based on (2) we can distinguish different types of 3D landmark points. Landmarks with locally high intensity variations in all directions have low localization uncertainties in all directions and we refer to them as 'normal' point landmarks. Arbitrary points on image edges have low localization uncertainties perpendicular to the edge but high localization uncertainties along the edge. Such landmarks will be denoted as 'quasi-landmarks' since they are not uniquely definable in all directions (e.g., the 3D bounding box landmarks of Talairach [15]). Finally, normal landmarks and quasi-landmarks can be distinguished from points in homogeneous regions where we have high localization uncertainties in all directions (see [7] for an analogous classification in the case of 2D aerial images).

Note, that our error characterization is based on the minimal errors, which are generally different from the errors obtained by an anatomical study or specified by a user. However, in either case we suspect that the localization errors depend on the geometry of the landmark, e.g., for an edge point we have large uncertainties along the edge but low uncertainties perpendicular to the edge. Also, all approaches should share the property that increasing the image noise generally leads to larger localization errors, which is the case with our scheme.

As an example, we show in Fig. 1 the estimated error ellipses (68.3% probability corresponding to 1σ regions) for the tip of the frontal horn of the ventricular system as well as for an arbitrary edge point at the outer contour of the head within a 2D MR dataset. The selected points are examples for normal landmarks and quasi-landmarks. Note, that the error ellipses have been enlarged by a factor of 30 for visualization purposes. It can be seen that the error ellipse of the tip is small and close to a circle which means that the localization uncertainty for this

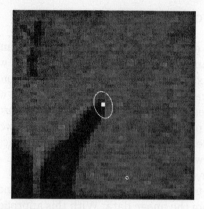 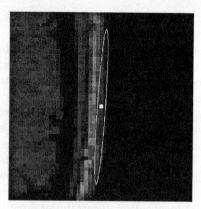

Fig. 1. Estimated 2D error ellipses (enlarged by a factor of 30) for a 2D MR dataset: tip of ventricular system (left) and edge point at the outer contour of the head (right).

point is low in arbitrary directions. For the edge point, however, the error ellipse is largely elongated and indicates a large localization uncertainty along the contour and a low localization uncertainty perpendicular to the contour. This is what we expect from the local intensity structure at the considered points.

4 Thin-Plate Splines with Anisotropic Errors

In [13] we have introduced an approach for nonrigid matching of medical images using approximating thin-plate splines. This approach is based on the mathematical work in [19] and is an extension of the original interpolating thin-plate spline approach [2]. For related approaches in the context of surface approximation and modification of facial expressions, see, e.g., [8],[5],[16],[1].

To find the transformation $\mathbf{u}$ between two images of dimension d we assume to have two sets of n landmarks $\mathbf{p}_i$ and $\mathbf{q}_i$, $i = 1\ldots n$, in the first and second image, resp., as well as information about the landmark localization errors in terms of scalar weights σ_i^2. Then, $\mathbf{u}$ results as the solution of a minimizing functional which measures the distance between the two landmark sets and the smoothness of the transformation:

$$J_\lambda(\mathbf{u}) = \frac{1}{n}\sum_{i=1}^n \frac{|\mathbf{q}_i - \mathbf{u}(\mathbf{p}_i)|^2}{\sigma_i^2} + \lambda J_m^d(\mathbf{u}), \qquad (5)$$

where m is the order of the involved derivatives of $\mathbf{u}$, and the parameter $\lambda > 0$ weights the two terms. This functional can be separated into a sum of functionals which only depend on one component of $\mathbf{u}$. The solution to the single functionals can be stated analytically as

$$u(\mathbf{x}) = \sum_{\nu=1}^M a_\nu \phi_\nu(\mathbf{x}) + \sum_{i=1}^n w_i U(\mathbf{x}, \mathbf{p}_i), \qquad (6)$$

with polynomials ϕ up to order $m-1$ and suitable radial basis functions U as defined in [19]. For example, in the case $m = d = 2$ we have the well-known function $U(\mathbf{x}, \mathbf{p}) = 1/(8\pi)|\mathbf{x} - \mathbf{p}|^2 \ln |\mathbf{x} - \mathbf{p}|$.

The coefficients $\mathbf{a} = (a_1, \ldots, a_M)^T$ and $\mathbf{w} = (w_1, \ldots, w_n)^T$ of the transformation can be computed through the following system of linear equations:

$$(\mathbf{K} + n\lambda \mathbf{W}^{-1})\mathbf{w} + \mathbf{P}\mathbf{a} = \mathbf{v} \qquad (7)$$
$$\mathbf{P}^T \mathbf{w} = 0,$$

where $\mathbf{v}$ is a vector of one component of the coordinates of the landmarks $\mathbf{q}_i$, $K_{ij} = U(\mathbf{p}_i, \mathbf{p}_j)$, and $P_{ij} = \phi_j(\mathbf{p}_i)$. The matrix

$$\mathbf{W}^{-1} = \text{diag}\{\sigma_1^2, \ldots, \sigma_n^2\} \qquad (8)$$

contains the scalar weights representing isotropic landmark localization errors.

This approach can further be extended when replacing the scalar weights σ_i^2 by covariance matrices $\mathbf{\Sigma}_i$ representing anisotropic landmark errors. With $\epsilon_i = \mathbf{q}_i - \mathbf{u}(\mathbf{p}_i)$ now our functional reads as

$$J_\lambda(\mathbf{u}) = \frac{1}{n} \sum_{i=1}^{n} \epsilon_i^T \mathbf{\Sigma}_i^{-1} \epsilon_i + \lambda J_m^d(\mathbf{u}). \qquad (9)$$

Although this generalized functional can no longer be separated into the components of $\mathbf{u}$, the solution can still be stated in analytic form with the same basis functions and the same structure of the computational scheme as in (7), see also [20],[14]. In our case, the weight matrix in (7) is given by

$$\mathbf{W}^{-1} = \text{diag}\{\mathbf{\Sigma}_1, \ldots, \mathbf{\Sigma}_n\} \qquad (10)$$

and is a block-diagonal matrix. Note, that the $\mathbf{\Sigma}_i$ represent the localization errors of two corresponding landmarks. Thus, to end up with one matrix we have to combine the covariance matrices of corresponding landmarks. If we assume that the two covariance matrices depend only slightly on the elastic part of the transformation, then we can combine these matrices by applying a linear transformation (rotation, scaling) to one of the matrices before adding them. The other matrices in (7) are given by $\mathbf{K} = (K_{ij}\mathbf{I}_d)$, where $K_{ij} = U(\mathbf{p}_i, \mathbf{p}_j)$ and $\mathbf{I}_d$ is the $d \times d$ unity matrix, and $\mathbf{P} = (P_{ij}\mathbf{I}_d)$, where $P_{ij} = \phi_j(\mathbf{p}_i)$.

With the extended registration scheme it is now possible to include 'quasi-landmarks'. Note, that our approximation scheme using weight matrices is also a generalization of the work in [4], where the interpolation problem is solved while the landmarks are allowed to slip along straight lines within a 2D image. Actually, this is a special case of our approximation scheme since for straight lines the variance in one direction is zero whereas in the perpendicular direction it is infinity.

5 Experimental Results

5.1 2D Data

We have applied our approach to the registration of 2D MR brain images of different patients shown in Fig. 2. In this 2D example we have manually selected normal landmarks and quasi-landmarks and have automatically estimated the error ellipses at these points (note, that the ellipses drawn in Fig. 2 have been enlarged by a factor of 7 for visualization purposes). Fig. 3 on the left shows the registration result when applying interpolating thin-plate splines while using all landmarks. The edges of the second image have been overlayed onto the transformed first image. We see that an unrealistic deformation towards the top left is obtained since corresponding landmarks are forced to match exactly although they are generally not homologous points. Using instead approximating thin-plate splines and equal scalar weights ($m = d = 2$ in (5)) the registration result is improved but it is still not satisfactory (Fig. 3 on the right). A further improvement is obtained if we apply this procedure only to the normal landmarks (numbers 1-6 and 8) in the inner parts of the brain (Fig. 4 on the left). However, the best result is achieved if we use both the normal landmarks and the quasi-landmarks together with the estimated ellipses, and apply approximating thin-plate splines with anisotropic errors (Fig. 4 on the right). It can be seen that the combination of both types of landmarks significantly improves the registration accuracy, particularly at the outer contour of the brain.

5.2 3D Data

We also demonstrate the applicability of our approach for the registration of 3D MR images of different patients. The datasets consist of $179 \times 236 \times 165$ and $177 \times 245 \times 114$ voxels, resp. (see Fig. 5). We have used normal landmarks as well as quasi-landmarks while setting $m = 2$ and $d = 3$ in (9). The normal point landmarks have semi-automatically been localized using the 3D differential operator in (1). As quasi-landmarks we have used the 3D bounding box landmarks of the brain (Talairach [15]) as well as two landmarks at the top of the ventricular system. The quasi-landmarks have been localized manually. For all landmarks the weight matrices have automatically been estimated from the image data according to (2). Fig. 6 shows that we generally obtain a good registration result (see slices 29, 41, and 67), while some deviations can be observed at the bottom left of the slices 41 and 67.

6 Conclusion

We have introduced a thin-plate spline approach to elastic image registration which can cope with anisotropic landmark errors. The covariance matrices of landmark errors are directly estimated from the image data and represent the

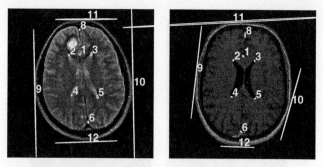

Fig. 2. 2D MR datasets of different patients: normal landmarks, quasi-landmarks, and estimated error ellipses (enlarged by a factor of 7).

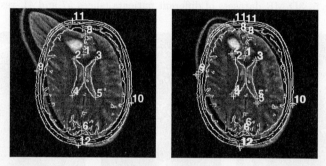

Fig. 3. Registration result: Thin-plate spline interpolation (left), and approximation with equal scalar weights (right) using normal landmarks and quasi-landmarks.

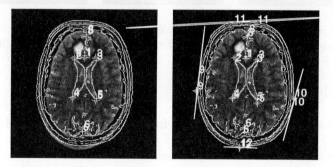

Fig. 4. Registration result: Thin-plate spline approximation using normal landmarks and equal scalar weights (left), and normal landmarks, quasi-landmarks and estimated error ellipses (right).

minimal stochastic localization uncertainties. Besides the handling of error information an additional advantage is that we can include different types of landmarks, e.g., quasi-landmarks. Our experiments for 2D and 3D tomographic images of the human brain have shown that the incorporation of quasi-landmarks significantly improves the registration result.

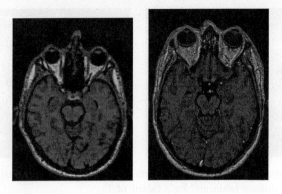

Fig. 5. 3D MR datasets of different patients (slices 57 and 41, resp.).

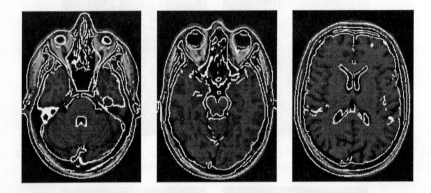

Fig. 6. 3D registration result using approximating thin-plate splines, normal landmarks, quasi-landmarks and estimated 3D weight matrices (slices 29, 41, and 67).

Acknowledgement

This work has been supported by Philips Research Hamburg, project IMAGINE. For discussions I thank S. Frantz, R. Sprengel, and H.S. Stiehl. The tomographic images have kindly been provided by Philips Research Hamburg, the AIM project COVIRA as well as W.P.Th.M. Mali, L. Ramos, and C.W.M. van Veelen (Utrecht University Hospital) via ICS-AD of Philips Medical Systems Best.

References

1. N. Arad, N. Dyn, D. Reisfeld, and Y. Yeshurun, "Image warping by radial basis functions: Application to facial expressions", *Computer Vision, Graphics, and Image Processing* 56:2 (1994) 161-172
2. F.L. Bookstein, "Principal Warps: Thin-Plate Splines and the Decomposition of Deformations", *IEEE Trans. on Pattern Anal. and Machine Intell.* 11:6 (1989) 567-585

3. F.L. Bookstein, "Four metrics for image variation", *Proc. IPMI'89*, In *Progress in Clinical and Biological Research*, Vol. 363, D. Ortendahl and J. Llacer (Eds.), Wiley-Liss New York, 1991, 227-240
4. F.L. Bookstein, "Landmark methods for forms without landmarks: morphometrics of group differences in outline shape", *Medical Image Analysis* 1:3 (1996/7) 225-243
5. T.E. Boult and J.R. Kender, "Visual surface reconstruction using sparse depth data", *Proc. CVPR'86*, June 22-26, Miami Beach, FL, 1986, 68-76
6. A.C. Evans, W. Dai, L. Collins, P. Neelin, and S. Marrett, "Warping of a computerized 3-D atlas to match brain image volumes for quantitative neuroanatomical and functional analysis", *Medical Imaging V: Image Processing*, 1991, San Jose, CA, Proc. SPIE 1445, M.H. Loew (Ed.), 236-246
7. W. Förstner, "A Feature Based Correspondence Algorithm for Image Matching", *Intern. Arch. of Photogrammetry and Remote Sensing* 26-3/3 (1986) 150-166
8. W.E.L. Grimson, "An Implementation of a Computational Theory of Visual Surface Interpolation", *Computer Vision, Graphics, and Image Processing* 22 (1983) 39-69
9. D.L.G. Hill, D.J. Hawkes, J.E. Crossman, M.J. Gleeson, T.C.S. Cox, E.E.C.M. Bracey, A.J. Strong, and P. Graves, "Registration of MR and CT images for skull base surgery using point-like anatomical features", *The British J. of Radiology* 64:767 (1991) 1030-1035
10. J.B.A. Maintz, P.A. van den Elsen, and M.A. Viergever, "Evaluation of ridge seeking operators for multimodality medical image matching", *IEEE Trans. on Pattern Anal. and Machine Intell.* 18:4 (1996) 353-365
11. K. Mardia and J. Little, "Image warping using derivative information", In *Mathematical Methods in Medical Imaging III*, 25-26 July 1994, San Diego, CA, Proc. SPIE 2299, F.L. Bookstein, J. Duncan, N. Lange, and D. Wilson (Eds.), 16-31
12. K. Rohr, "On 3D Differential Operators for Detecting Point Landmarks", *Image and Vision Computing* 15:3 (1997) 219-233
13. K. Rohr, H.S. Stiehl, R. Sprengel, W. Beil, T.M. Buzug, J. Weese, and M.H. Kuhn, "Point-Based Elastic Registration of Medical Image Data Using Approximating Thin-Plate Splines", *Proc. VBC'96*, Hamburg, Germany, Sept. 22-25, 1996, *Lecture Notes in Computer Science* 1131, K.H. Höhne and R. Kikinis (Eds.), Springer Berlin Heidelberg 1996, 297-306
14. K. Rohr, R. Sprengel, and H.S. Stiehl, "Incorporation of Landmark Error Ellipsoids for Image Registration based on Approximating Thin-Plate Splines", *Proc. CAR'97*, Berlin, Germany, June 25-28, 1997, H.U. Lemke, M.W. Vannier, and K. Inamura (Eds.), Elsevier Amsterdam Lausanne 1997, 234-239
15. J. Talairach and P. Tornoux, *Co-planar Stereotactic Atlas of the Human Brain*, Georg Thieme Verlag Stuttgart New York 1988
16. D. Terzopoulos, "Regularization of Inverse Visual Problems Involving Discontinuities", *IEEE Trans. on Pattern Anal. and Machine Intell.* 8:4 (1986) 413-424
17. J.-P. Thirion, "New Feature Points based on Geometric Invariants for 3D Image Registration", *Intern. J. of Computer Vision* 18:2 (1996) 121-137
18. H.L. van Trees, *Detection, Estimation, and Modulation Theory*, Part I, John Wiley and Sons, New York London 1968
19. G. Wahba, *Spline Models for Observational Data*, Society for Industrial and Applied Mathematics, Philadelphia, Pennsylvania, 1990
20. G. Wahba, "Multivariate function and operator estimation, based on smoothing splines and reproducing kernels", in *Nonlinear Modeling and Forecasting, SFI Studies in the Sciences of Complexity*, Vol. XII, M. Casdagli and S. Eubank (Eds.), Addison-Wesley 1992, 95-112

Segmentation of Carpal Bones from 3D CT Images Using Skeletally Coupled Deformable Models

T. B. Sebastian[1], H. Tek[1], J. J. Crisco[2], S. W. Wolfe[3], and B. B. Kimia[1]

[1] LEMS, Division of Engineering, Brown University, Providence RI 02912
{tbs,tek,kimia}@lems.brown.edu, http://www.lems.brown.edu
[2] Department of Orthopaedics, Rhode Island Hospital, Providence, RI 02903
Joseph_Crisco_III@Brown.edu
[3] Department of Orthopaedics, Yale University School of Medicine
Scott.Wolfe@yale.edu

Abstract. The in vivo investigation of joint kinematics in normal and injured wrist requires the segmentation of carpal bones from 3D (CT) images and their registration over time. The non-uniformity of bone tissue, ranging from dense cortical bone to textured spongy bone, the irregular, small shape of closely packed carpal bones which move with respect to one another, and with respect to CT resolution. augmented with the presence of blood vessels, and the inherent blurring of CT imaging renders the segmentation of carpal bones a challenging task. Specifically, four characteristic difficulties are prominent: (i) gaps or weak edges in the carpal bone surfaces, (ii) diffused edges, (iii) textured regions, and, (iv) extremely narrow inter-bone regions. We review the performance of statistical classification, deformable models, region growing, and morphological operations for this application. We then propose a model which combines several of these approaches in a single framework. Specifically, initialized seeds grow in a curve evolution implementation of active contours, but where growth is modulated by a skeletally-mediated competition between neighboring regions, thus combining the advantages of local and global region growing methods, region competition and active contours. This approach effectively deals with many of the difficulties presented above as illustrated by numerous examples.

Acknowledgements: We gratefully acknowledge the support of the Whitaker Foundation, and NIH grant AR44005.

1 Introduction

Segmentation is an important pre-processing step in medical imaging for visualization, registration, kinematic analysis, *etc.* For our application, namely, the segmentation and registration of carpal bones in the wrist from CT images, which is used primarily to investigate joint loading and joint kinematics, the task has proved to be rather challenging. A key fact is that bone tissue cannot

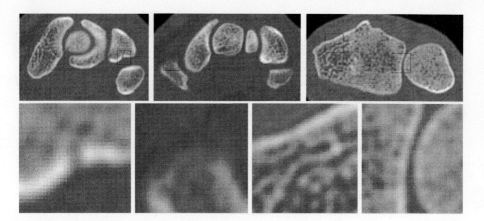

Fig. 1. Three slices from a three-dimensional CT image of carpal bones (top row) demonstrate typical cases of gaps or weak edges, diffused edges, textured areas, and extremely narrow inter-bone regions that make automatic segmentation difficult. Each window is zoomed in the bottom row detailing the above features, respectively.

be characterized uniformly: the outer layer of the bone tissue, or *cortical bone*, is denser than the *spongy bone* it encases. Thus, under CT imaging cortical bone appears brighter and smooth, while spongy bone appears darker and textured. In addition, due to the close spacing of some carpal bones with respect to CT resolution and inherent blurring in CT imaging, the inter-bone space often appears brighter than the background (soft tissue), drastically reducing boundary contrast in these regions. Finally, blood vessels resemble the background, creating gaps in the surface of bone images. In the image domain, challenging areas can be categorized into four predominant groups, Figure 1: *(i)* gaps in the cortical shell; *(ii)* weak or diffused bone boundaries due to partial volume effect in CT imaging; *(iii)* textured areas corresponding to the spongy bone; *(iv)* the narrow inter-bone regions which tend to be diffused.

While is possible for medical experts to segment these images by using thresholding or manual seeding, *e.g.* using the ANALYZE package, this process considering the time required for manual correction is labor intensive. Thus the development and use of segmentation techniques that minimize user interaction is highly desirable. We have implemented and evaluated a large number of techniques for the segmentation of carpal bones from 3D CT images, including global thresholding, statistical methods, seeded region growing [1], deformable models like snakes [7], balloons [4], and bubbles [18], morphological watersheds [20], and region competition [21]. The experience with the use of these techniques in our domain has prompted us to combine three of these approaches in a single framework. Specifically, this framework evolves from the approach taken by Tek *et al.* [18], numerous seeds are initialized which then grow by image-dependent forces and in the process merge and slow down near boundaries, thus trapping the boundary between the inner and outer regions. The success of this technique is dependent on the existence of boundaries with sufficient contrast or symmetric initialization in the case of weak boundaries. This is due to the monotonic nature of growth: once a region has evolved beyond object boundaries it can no longer return to capture it. Region competition [21], on the other hand, also relies on the growth of seeds, but implements a non-monotonic adjustment based on *local* competition between regions, once they become adjacent. The back and forth movements of adjacent regions is dependent on a statistical decision on which of these regions a point is more likely to belong to. The central assumption underlying this scheme is that the growth of seeds leads to regions that characterize distinct areas. This assumption fails, *e.g.* in asymmetrically initialized seeds, where the growing seeds in "waiting" for other regions to arrive, acquire and encompass two statistically distinct domains, thus disabling a reversal. Seeded region growing [1] avoids this difficulty by implementing a *global* competition among growing regions, but does not implement the "back and forth" competition between them, thus not allowing for recovery from errors.

The approach presented in this paper combines these ideas, namely, deformable models implemented in the curve evolution framework, probabilistic growth, local back and forth competition, and global competition under one framework. The main idea is to rely on the *inter-region skeleton* as a predictor of boundaries resulting from the current seeds, assuming current growth conditions, and to feed back this information into the growth process by modulating the deformation speed. In other words, if points on the skeleton are more likely to belong to one region as compared to another, then the former region should grow faster to capture it. Region competition then becomes a special case, *i.e.*, when the two regions become adjacent. The idea of global competition in seeded region growing is implemented by the long-distance competition among neighboring seeds, mediated by the inter-region skeleton.

2 Medical Application: Segmentation of Carpal Bones

Degenerative joint disease is commonly attributed to alterations in joint loading and joint kinematics due to traumatic injury. In the wrist, despite widespread clinical awareness of dynamic and static wrist instability, little is known about the pathoanatomy and kinematics of these conditions. Patients may continue to be incapacitated by pain following stressful activities months after injury, even though radiographs and other static imaging studies appear normal. Attempts to treat these conditions surgically usually involve limiting abnormal carpal bone motion by restricting normal carpal motion through arthrodesis or ligamentous reinforcement. Characterizing the true 3D kinematics of the carpal bones following these ligament injuries would provide better insight for development of diagnostic techniques and more appropriate treatment strategies. Clarifying the relationship of partial and complete tears of the scapholunate interosseous ligament, for example, to alterations in carpal kinematics would help guide clinicians in decisions regarding surgical or conservative management of this common injury.

The significance of accurately measuring 3D in vivo carpal kinematics in normal wrists and in those with specific ligament injuries is the understanding

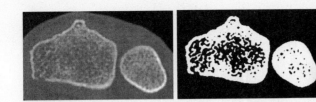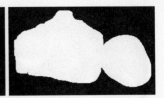

Fig. 2. An example of a 2D slice where global thresholding fails. Observe that there are holes in the bones and also a gap in the bone contour. While morphological filtering can close the holes and gaps, the inter-bone region will also be closed and the shape of the boundary will be slightly altered.

gained from these studies can benefit diagnosis, surgical treatment, rehabilitation, and the design of prosthetic devices. Our long-term research is aimed at studying degenerative changes, surgical reconstructions, and rehabilitation in joints. More broadly, these methods can noninvasively measure 3D motion of any joint using any 3D imaging modality.

Studying 3D skeletal joint motion is most often accomplished using marker systems implanted in the bones of cadaveric specimens. Similar methods have also been used to study joint motion in vivo in the knee and hip [6, 10, 11], but these studies are not widely performed due to their invasive nature. More recently, researchers have measured the 3D kinematics of the knee joint in vivo using non-invasive techniques based on single-plane fluoroscopy and three dimensional models [2]. However, given the small size, narrow articular spaces and complex joint surfaces, such methods are not applicable to the wrist. We now review an application of some of the currently available techniques to this domain, and then proceed by an approach that combines some of the current techniques.

3 Segmentation of Carpal Bones: Current Approaches

We have investigated the use of several segmentation techniques for the recovery of carpal bone surfaces from CT images. These methods include global thresholding, statistical classification, seeded region growing [1], region competition [21], deformable models like snakes [7], balloons [4], their curve evolution counterparts [12, 3, 17], and watershed segmentation [20]. See also [16] for a similar application. This section briefly reviews our experience with the application of these techniques to carpal bone segmentation and motivates the approach present in Section 4.

Global thresholding is the simplest statistical segmentation technique, where pixels are classified based on their intensity values. However, choosing the right intensity threshold is difficult and typically varies from one dataset to another. Interactive manual selection of the threshold is tedious and operator-sensitive. Even with the optimal threshold, final segmentation based on thresholding has holes and in some images, two adjacent bones merge. The choice of the intensity threshold can be automated by using the expectation maximization (EM) algorithm [5] to fit a mixture of Gaussian distributions to the intensity values and using classical Bayes Decision theory to find the decision boundaries.

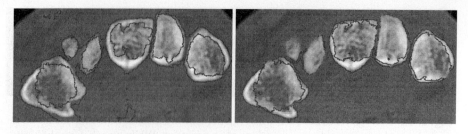

Fig. 3. This figure illustrates a shortcoming of the bubbles [17] approach. (Left) Randomly initialized seeds have grown to near bone boundaries; note the convergence of bubbles in the small bone on the top left. (Right) Further iterations, which are necessary for convergence in other places, *e.g.*, inter-bone regions will push out the bubble inside the small bone.

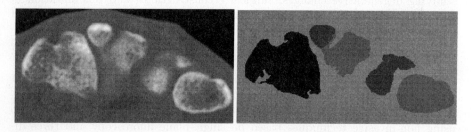

Fig. 4. This figure illustrates a shortcoming of seeded region growing [1]. Seeded region growing can leak through gaps in the bones.

Deformable models (snakes or active contours [7]) need to be initialized close to the boundaries for proper convergence, one snake per boundary. *Balloons* overcome the first restriction by transporting the initialized model close to the edges by adding a constant inflation force to the snake [4]. However, this inflation term also often pushes the evolving contour over weak/diffused edges. Curve evolution snake models [12, 3, 17] address the second restriction since they have the ability to change their topology during the deformation process. However, for carpal bone segmentation, the deformable models encounter similar problems, as in using statistical classification: *(i)* not all models converge at weak/diffused boundaries; *(ii)* the contour smoothing terms does not allow entry into the narrow inter-bone region; *(iii)* as these models rely only on the local information along the boundary, the texture inside the bone slows snakes down, resulting in poor convergence on the bone boundary.

Another class of techniques for segmentation is *region growing* and *merging*, where initialized seeds grow by annexing "similar" (as defined by a statistical test) pixels. Region growing methods are sensitive to seed initialization, and result in jagged boundaries and poorly localized edges. *Seeded region growing* [1] improves traditional region growing by introducing a "competition" between growing regions by ordering all candidate "growth" pixels according to some suitability criteria. However, seeded region growing, like traditional region growing doesn't incorporate any geometrical information and hence can "leak" through

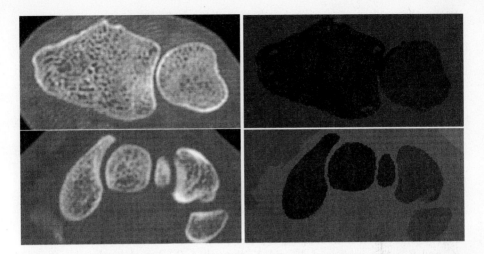

Fig. 5. While region competition [21] frequently captures the correct bone boundaries, in some cases it does not, as illustrated here. In the first case, region competition merges the bones and there are some holes in the captured regions. In the second case region competition fails to segment the bone on the extreme left of the image. Here the seeds that were initialized lost statistical character, resulting in the wrong segmentation, a mislabelling of some bones. The main flaw is that seeds compete only after they have fully grown and become adjacent.

narrow gaps (like the ones seen in the cortical shell, Figure 1). It also tends to merge bones that are very close to each other. *Region competition* [21] combines the geometrical features of the deformable models and the statistical features of region growing, by using a combination of statistical and smoothing forces for seed growth. It also introduces a local competition between regions when they contact each other, thus allowing recovery from errors. This is a powerful technique that works even when seeds are initialized across boundaries. However, for carpal bone segmentation it was observed that occasionally, initialized regions which have grown to a great extent beyond object boundaries, lose their "character" and hence are unable to be pushed back. Also, the discrete nature of region competition allows the boundaries to move by one pixel or not at all, resulting in jagged boundaries.

Finally, *watershed segmentation* [20] can be viewed as a region-growing technique [18] which often results in over-segmentation, unless specialized marker methods [20] are used. See [13] for details.

4 Skeletally Coupled Deformable Models

Our proposed approach is an iterative one where initialized seeds grow by a local statistical force, modulated by the desirability of a simulated segmentation, assuming current conditions prevail. The main idea is *(i)* at each step a local growth force is computed, *(ii)* the skeleton of the inter-seed region is used as a predictor of the final segmentation, *(iii)* each skeleton point is viewed as the

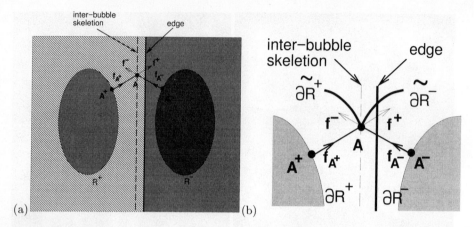

Fig. 6. (a) A sketch of the coupling of forces between nearby regions, (seeds of bubbles) R^+ and R^-, e.g., coupling of A^+ and A^- through A. (b) Actual coupling in a cropped portion; the thin solid lines are the boundaries of each each deformable model, R^+ and R^-, the thick solid line is the deformable true boundary (edge), and the dashed line is the inter-bubble skeleton. The skeleton is a preview of the final segmentation should the current growth conditions prevail. The relative desirability of growth from A^+ to A as compared to that of A^- to A modulates the growth of A^+ and A^- in each iteration, in this case inhibiting the growth of A^- and encouraging the speedier growth of A^+. Hence the skeleton, recomputed in each iteration converges onto the edge.

front of competition for a pair of points, each from a different seed, (iv) the desirability of growth of each seed point, along its respective paths to form the skeleton, is statistically measured and compared, and (v) the relative merit of each path is used to modulate the local growth force at each seed point to improve the segmentation results. This approach, namely, *skeletally coupled deformable models* (SCDM) thus implements a "long range coupling" that allows for the competition at a distance and prevents the seeds from losing their statistical characterization when seeds are initialized close to or over the boundary.

To see how long range coupling is mediated by the inter-region skeleton, consider Figure 6, which illustrates two seeds R^+ and R^- and the background R_B. Let S denote the *shocks*[1] of R_B as defined in [8, 9, 14, 19]. Each shock point A couples two[2] seed points $A^+ \in \partial R^+$ and $A^- \in \partial R^-$, where ∂R is the boundary of R. This coupling of the deformable models' boundary points, A^+ and A^-, allows for competition for their growth with respect to capturing A. Let the local statistical growth force at a point P be denoted by f_P, typically $f_P = \log(\frac{1}{\sqrt{2\pi\sigma^2}} e^{-\frac{(I(x,y)-\mu)^2}{2\sigma^2}})$, where $I(x,y)$ is the intensity at P and μ and σ are the mean and standard deviation of the region. This defines local forces f_A-

---

[1] Shocks are the skeleton points augmented with the notions of speed, direction, type, label, grouping, and a hierarchy of these groups [9].
[2] Generically, each shock point couple two or three boundary (characteristic) points. The discussion for shocks with three characteristic points is similar.

and f_{A^+}, at A^- and A^+, respectively,

$$f_{A^-} = \log(\frac{1}{\sqrt{2\pi\sigma^{-2}}}e^{-\frac{(I(x,y)-\mu^-)^2}{2\sigma^{-2}}}), \qquad f_{A^+} = \log(\frac{1}{\sqrt{2\pi\sigma^{+2}}}e^{-\frac{(I(x,y)-\mu^+)^2}{2\sigma^{+2}}}). \tag{1}$$

These forces are adjusted to produce net forces, F_{A^-} and F_+, respectively by using feedback indicating the desirability of a predicted segmentation at A, assuming A^- and A^+ evolve in a simulated growth up to collision at A. Since only infinitesimal adjustments are needed, we consider whether it is more appropriate for the skeleton to move left or right, and by what amount. This is accomplished by comparing the predicted statistical forces f^+ and f^- at A.

$$f^+ = \log P(A \in R^+), \qquad f^- = \log P(A \in R^-). \tag{2}$$

Thus, the net force at each skeletal point A, $f^+ - f^-$, is propagated to each boundary point to modulate the growth force there. This force is only needed when boundaries are at a distance. Second, in addition to the local skeleton force, we feed back a measure of growth at A^+ to A^- (and vice-versa) via coupling at the skeleton, as adjusted by a monotonically decreasing function of the distance $\lambda(d) = \frac{1}{\sqrt{2\pi\sigma_d^2}}e^{-\frac{d^2}{2\sigma_d^2}}$. Thus, the net force is

$$F_{A^-} = f_{A^-} - \lambda_0 f_{A^-} + (1-\lambda_0)(f^- - f^+) \tag{3}$$
$$F_{A^+} = f_{A^+} - \lambda_0 f_{A^+} + (1-\lambda_0)(f^+ - f^-) \tag{4}$$

where $\lambda_0 = \lambda(2d(A^-, A))$. When two regions are close to each other, or adjacent, $\lambda_0 \approx 1$, $F_{A^-} = f_{A^-} - f_{A^+}$, effectively implementing the region competition approach. However, when the two regions are not close, the approach implements a *long range, predicted competition*. In Figure 6, this long range force has the effect of slowing A^- down and speeding up A^+, allowing A^+ to "catch up" before A^- has grown beyond the edge, thus symmetrizing the regions R^+ and R^- with respect to the edge.

5 Implementation: Curve Evolution and ENO Interpolation

This approach is implemented in the curve evolution framework by embedding the curve as the zero level-set of an evolving surface. This allows for partial movement of the curve on a discrete grid. Partial movements are essential to avoid jagged boundaries and to allow regions to move at different speeds. However, a subpixel implementation of region competition requires regions to be adjacent, thus constantly operating in a mode where more than one curve is present within a pixel, a situation not easily represented by an embedding surface. Specifically, the reliable identification of the subpixel boundary and the computation of forces at subcell points are especially challenging.

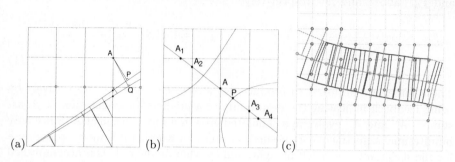

Fig. 7. The subpixel deformation of a curve via updating its embedding surface by the movement of the closest point to each grid point. (a) The subpixel computation of force at P requires a two stage ENO interpolation; one along the line normal to the curve $\{A_i\}$ and one for each A_i along either the horizontal or vertical directions (solid dot). (c) The coupling between two contours ∂R^+ and ∂R^- when they are roughly two pixels apart. Details are omitted here due to space constraints.

As a solution, we use a piecewise circular (PC) approximation [15], of the subpixel boundary *within each pixel*. This representation can be extracted accurately from its distance transform using an approach based on Essentially Non Oscillatory (ENO) interpolation [15]. The accuracy of the PC curve reconstruction from its embedding surface, implies that the surface can be transformed in such a way that the modified surface is the distance transform of the modified curve. Hence, the surface point at A in Figure 7(a) should be updated by the change from AP to AQ, which for small movements can be approximated by PQ. This requires computing the force at subcell point point P, which requires the accurate computation of the image intensity and image derivatives along the normal to the curve at P. This is done using an ENO interpolation along the line orthogonal to the curve, along the subpixel grid samples $\{A_i\}$ in Figure 7(b), which in turn is found using an ENO interpolation along grid lines. The details of the implementation are involved and beyond the scope of this paper [13].

6 Results and Discussion

In this section we present the results of applying the SCDM method to carpal bone segmentation, especially to illustrate the performance of SCDM in the problem areas listed in Section 1, namely, gaps and weak edges, diffused edges, bone texture, and narrow inter-bone spaces. Seeds were initialized manually, one seed per bone (this can be automated at a later stage by relying on statistical classification). Figure 8 illustrates the effectiveness of this approach in images with gaps (a), low contrast edges (b) and (c), narrow regions (d), and diffused edges (e). These are typical results and the application of this method to carpal bone images has led to reliable and robust segmentation. For further examples, animation of growth, and comparison to other techniques, we refer the reader to *http://www.lems.brown.edu/vision/researchAreas/SCDM/bone-segmentation/bone-segmentation.html*.

References

1. R. Adams and L. Bischof. Seeded region growing. *PAMI*, 16(6):641–647, 1994.
2. S. A. Banks and W. A. Hodge. Accurate measurement of three-dimensional knee replacement kinematics using single-plane fluorscopy. *IT Biomed Eng*, 43(6):638–649, 1996.
3. V. Caselles, F. Catte, T. Coll, and F. Dibos. A geometric model for active contours in image processing. *Numerische Mathematik*, 66, 1993.
4. L. D. Cohen and I. Cohen. Finite element methods for active contour models and balloons for 2D and 3D images. *PAMI*, 15:1131–1147, 1993.
5. A. Dempster, N. Laird, and D. Rubin. Maximum likelihood from incomplete data via the EM algorithm. *J. of Royal Stat. Soc.*, Series B, 39:1–38, 1977.
6. J. Karrholm, L. Elmqvist, G. Selvik, and L. Hansson. Chronic antrolateral instability of the knee: a Roentgen stereophotogrammetric evaluation. *Am. J. Sports Medicine*, 17(4):555–563, 1989.
7. M. Kass, A. Witkin, and D. Terzopoulos. Snakes: Active contour models. *IJCV*, 1:321–331, 1988.
8. B. B. Kimia, A. R. Tannenbaum, and S. W. Zucker. Toward a computational theory of shape: An overview. In *ECCV '90*, pages 402–407, 1990.
9. B. B. Kimia, A. R. Tannenbaum, and S. W. Zucker. Shapes, shocks, and deformations, I: The components of shape and the reaction-diffusion space. *IJCV*, 15:189–224, 1995.
10. T. J. Koh, M. Grabiner, and R. DeSwart. In vivo tracking of the human patella. *J. Biomech.*, 25(6):637–644, 1992.
11. M. Lafortune, P. Cavanagh, H. Sommer, and A. Kalenak. Three-dimensional kinematics of the human knee during walking. *J. Biomech.*, 25(4):347–358, 1992.
12. R. Malladi, J. A. Sethian, and B. C. Vemuri. Evolutionary fronts for topology-independent shape modelling and recovery. In *ECCV '94*, pages 3–13, 1994.
13. T. B. Sebastian, H. Tek, J. J. Crisco, and B. B. Kimia. Skeletally coupled deformable models. Tech. Rep. LEMS 169, LEMS, Brown University, January 1998.
14. K. Siddiqi and B. B. Kimia. A shock grammar for recognition. In *CVPR '96*:507–513, 1996.
15. K. Siddiqi, B. B. Kimia, and C. Shu. Geometric shock-capturing ENO schemes for subpixel interpolation, computation and curve evolution. *GMIP*, 59(5):278–301, 1997.
16. H. D. Tagare and K. W. Elder. Location and geometric descriptions of carpal bones in CT images. *Annals of Biomedical Engineering*, 21:715–726, 1993.
17. H. Tek and B. B. Kimia. Image segmentation by reaction-diffusion bubbles. In *ICCV*, pages 156–162, Boston, June 1995.
18. H. Tek and B. B. Kimia. Volumetric segmentation of medical images by three-dimensional bubbles. *CVIU*, 64(2):246–258, 1997.
19. H. Tek, F. Leymarie, and B. B. Kimia. Multiple generation shock detection and labeling using CEDT. In *IWVF '97*, Italy, May 1997.
20. L. Vincent and P. Souille. Watersheds in digital spaces: an efficient algoritm based on immersion simulations. *PAMI*, 13(6):583–598, 1991.
21. S. C. Zhu and A. L. Yuille. Region competition: Unifying Snakes, Region growing, and Bayes/MDL for multiband Image Segmentation. *PAMI*, 18(9):884–900, 1996.

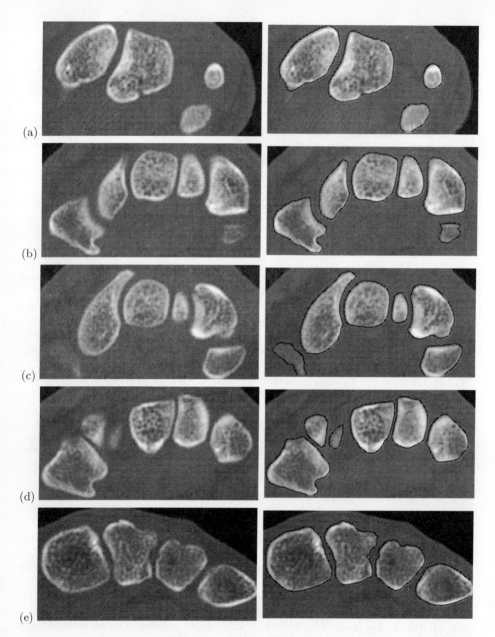

Fig. 8. Examples of carpal bone segmentation using skeletally coupled deformable models. Observe that SCDM works well in images having a gap in the bone contour, (a). It captures low contrast contours, *e.g.*, the bone on the bottom right in (b) and the bone on the extreme left in (c). Observe how it allows growth into the narrow inter-bone spaces, (d). It also does well in case of diffused edges, *e.g.*, second bone in (e). Also note that the region-based statistical force allows growth in textured areas, as evidenced by all these examples.

Segmentation of Bone in Clinical Knee MRI Using Texture-Based Geodesic Active Contours*

Liana M. Lorigo[1], Olivier Faugeras[1,2], W.E.L. Grimson[1], Renaud Keriven[2,3], and Ron Kikinis[4,5]

[1] MIT AI Laboratory, Cambridge MA, USA
liana@ai.mit.edu
[2] INRIA, Sophia Antipolis, France
[3] Cermics, ENPC, France
[4] Dept. Of Radiology, Brigham and Womens Hospital, Boston MA, USA
[5] Harvard Medical School, Boston MA, USA

Abstract. This paper presents a method for automatic segmentation of the tibia and femur in clinical magnetic resonance images of knees. Texture information is incorporated into an active contours framework through the use of vector-valued geodesic snakes with local variance as a second value at each pixel, in addition to intensity. This additional information enables the system to better handle noise and the non-uniform intensities found within the structures to be segmented. It currently operates independently on 2D images (slices of a volumetric image) where the initial contour must be within the structure but not necessarily near the boundary. These separate segmentations are stacked to display the performance on the entire 3D structure.

1 Introduction

We address the problem of automatically segmenting clinical MRI of knees. There are many applications of this capability, including diagnosis, change-detection, as a pre-cursor to registration with a model, and in the building of an initial model for surgical simulation. Moreover, the segmentation system can be used as a tool to replace or expedite the tedious process of manual segmentation.

There are two primary strategies for detecting image boundaries. Region growing uses local properties of the region of interest along with techniques for splitting and merging regions [2, 1]. Deformable or "active" contour models ("snakes") use only the boundary of the object which deforms over the image to minimize some energy function based on properties of the curve (such as smoothness) and of the image (such as gradients) [12, 6, 18]. Several methods explicitly combine both the region and contour approaches [23, 16]. Active boundary methods are commonly applied to medical images because they can capture the irregular shapes and shape deformations found in anatomical structures [14]. Several

---

* This report describes research supported in part by NSF under contract 1R1-9610249 and in part by MERL, A Mitsubishi Electric Research Laboratory.

approaches to knee segmentation have been explored, including a model based approach to segmenting both bone and cartilage using region-growing, snakes, and spatial information [11], and a knowledge-based approach which uses information about the shape and the imaging process to localize the femur [19]. While such approaches are important for utilizing anatomical knowledge in guiding segmentation, we believe that new measurements of similarity can improve basic segmentation methods and provide a stronger basis for knowledge-rich segmentation. We use a deformable boundary model to capture the shape, but we extend it to include texture information for better performance.

In particular, trabecular bone has an apparent visual texture in MRI data which is approximately constant; it is this texture pattern that we wish to exploit. This implies that the method is best-suited to handle the portions of the bones near joints, since these portions contain much trabecular structure. The shafts of the bones contain much less of this structure and may not be as readily segmented by our method, depending on their appearance in the MR images. For this work, we address the problem of segmenting the trabecular bone in the portions of the femur and tibia near their respective joints. The method has not been applied to other areas of the bones. It should be further noted that we do not find cortical bone directly in this work. Should that segmentation be desired, our method may be useful as a pre-processing step, since it can be viewed as providing a rough segmentation of the interior boundary of cortical bone.

Segmenting the trabecular region of the bone can also be viewed as classifying the pixels in that region, since the boundary is initialized to contain intensity and texture corresponding to trabecular bone, then grows outward to find the true boundary of that bone region. However, no classification is performed on the rest of the image, and the classification of trabecular bone is performed locally only.

For the deformable model, we use geodesic active contours ("geodesic snakes") which are described below [4, 3, 13]. The advantage of geodesic snakes over classical snakes [12] is that the former are independent of the parameterization of the curve and can handle topological changes automatically. Moreover, implementation by level-set methods provides accuracy and stability [15]. This segmentation method has been applied to various medical imaging domains in [20].

The energy function used by either active contour method is normally based on the intensity gradients in the image so the snake will lock onto strong edges. MRI images, however, are often too complex for gradient information alone to be reliable. Intensities often vary non-uniformly throughout a single structure and the boundary between neighboring structures may be noisy. This is where a less local approach, moving toward region-growing, is of benefit. Specifically, texture information can be incorporated to model these image attributes.

Many different distributions can be used to represent or learn texture classes [21, 22]. Additionally, filters at different scales can be used to decompose an image into low-level texture features [7]. Texture modeling is used for denoising, texture synthesis, classification, and segmentation. We have chosen to incorporate texture information directly into the weighting function of the geodesic snakes. We add only variance at this time, but more statistics such as directional filters or multiscale filters could be incorporated easily if needed. Specifically, we define the snake to be attracted to intensity gradients as well as variance gradients, where variance is computed in a small neighborhood around each pixel. We use the vector-valued snakes approach to combine these measures in a manner formally consistent with the original snakes formulation [17].

This paper presents a system which automatically detects closed boundaries in 2D magnetic resonance images of knees. Both the femur and the tibia are segmented separately from each image of a volumetric set. Also input must be a small patch that is known to be within the desired structure but does not need to be anywhere near the true boundary; the snake flows outward from this patch until convergence. This is an improvement over many similar optimization approaches where the initial contour must be near the boundary, and the user may need to guide the contour. Each 2D image is segmented independently at this time, with the results stacked to give the volumetric segmentation. Future work will generalize the method to 3D. No user-interaction is required.

2 Geodesic Snakes

This work uses the framework of geodesic active contours as in [4, 3, 13, 17].

2.1 ... Basic Formulation

The task of finding the curve that best fits the boundary of the object is posed as a minimization problem over all closed planar curves $C(q) : [0, 1] \to R^2$. The objective function is

$$\int_0^1 g(|\nabla I(C(q))|)|C'(q)|dq$$

where $I : [0, a] \times [0, b] \to R^+$ is the image and $g : [0, \infty) \to R^+$ is a strictly decreasing function such that $g(r) \to 0$ as $r \to \infty$. That is, we are looking for the minimal distance curve where distance is weighted by the function g which acts on intensity gradients, so that the curve is attracted to intensity edges in the image. For example, one common choice is $g(|\nabla I|) = \frac{1}{1+|\nabla I|^2}$.

To minimize this objective function by steepest descent, consider C to be a function of time t as well as parameter q. Then one can compute the Euler-Lagrange equation of the objective function to determine the evolution of the curve, i.e., its derivative with respect to time. This yields the curve evolution equation

$$\frac{\partial C(t)}{\partial t} = g\kappa \boldsymbol{N} - (\nabla g \cdot \boldsymbol{N})\boldsymbol{N}$$

where κ is the Euclidean curvature and $\boldsymbol{N}$ is the unit inward normal.

In order to make this flow intrinsic to the curve (independent of its parameterization), a surface $u : [0, a] \times [0, b] \to R$ can be defined to give the distance from any image point to the curve $C(\cdot)$. Then u is evolved instead of C, which is identically the zero level-set of u. The evolution equation is

$$u_t = g\kappa|\nabla u| + \nabla g \cdot \nabla u.$$

An additional term c can be used either to increase the speed of the flow or to force the contour to flow outward, similar to the balloon force in [6], to yield

$$u_t = g(c+\kappa)|\nabla u| + \nabla g \cdot \nabla u.$$

2.2 ... on Vector-Valued Images

As described above, I is assumed to have one value at each pixel. The same minimization can be achieved on multi-valued images [17]. Let $\Phi(u_1, u_2) : R^2 \to R^m$ be an m-valued image, so the value of the image at any point is a vector in R^m. The quadratic form $d\Phi^2(v)$ gives the rate of change of the image in the v direction:

$$d\Phi^2 = \begin{bmatrix} du_1 \\ du_2 \end{bmatrix}^T \begin{bmatrix} g_{11} & g_{12} \\ g_{21} & g_{22} \end{bmatrix} \begin{bmatrix} du_1 \\ du_2 \end{bmatrix}$$

where $g_{ij} := \frac{\partial \Phi}{\partial u_i} \cdot \frac{\partial \Phi}{\partial u_j}$. The extrema of $d\Phi^2$ are obtained in the directions of the eigenvectors of $[g_{ij}]$, the attained values are the corresponding eigenvalues $\lambda_\pm$.

We then want to define our function g to be used in the evolution equations according to the steepest-descent method. One approach is to make g be a function of either λ_+ or $(\lambda_+ - \lambda_-)$, still requiring that $g(r) \to 0$ as $r \to \infty$.

3 Segmentation Algorithm

Our segmentation algorithm uses these evolution equations in conjunction with local variance [10]. The algorithm also uses an image-dependent balloon force [9], requires an initial contour, and detects convergence automatically. Finally, a post-processing step is added to counteract the effects of smoothing and windowing on the energy function g.

3.1 Incorporating Texture

Although the trabecular bone regions of the MR images vary in intensity, there is a fairly uniform texture throughout those regions. This led us to use variance along with intensity for segmentation. In particular, local variance $S : [0,a] \times [0,b] \to R^+$ is computed over a fixed-sized window. We now treat the original image as a two-valued image with intensity and local variance as the values at each pixel. We choose $g = \frac{1}{1+\sqrt{\lambda_+}}$, computed at each pixel in the image, and use the geodesic snakes formulation. An example of g on an image is shown in Figure 1.

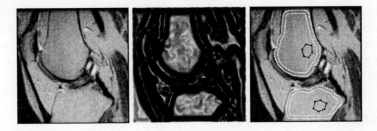

Fig. 1. Intermediate steps in algorithm. (1) An example image slice. (2) The weighting function g used in minimization, operating on that slice. (3) The output of the segmentation algorithm: the inner boundary is the true boundary based on g, the outer boundary is the result after compensation for windowing and smoothing, the starting contour is shown in black.

3.2 Image-Dependent Balloon Force

Our system performs outward flow with the balloon force proportional to g at each point on the curve. This means that the curve will push outward quickly when g is high (far from the boundary) and slowly when g is near zero. Note that this is an important deviation from the definition of geodesic active contours which may change the behavior of the partial differential equation, affecting the existence and uniqueness of the solution.

3.3 Initial Contour

The algorithm requires an initial closed curve which must be within the structure to be segmented. Our system does not require it to be anywhere near the actual boundary as shown in Figure 1. The initial contour does not need to be connected but could be a set of "bubbles" within the object or objects to be segmented.

3.4 Convergence

Convergence is detected automatically when the curve has not moved with respect to the image resolution over a fixed number of iterations. For the parameter settings used in our experiments, this number could be set between 10 and 20 with good results.

3.5 Windowing Effect

Because g is computed over a window of the image, the final contour more closely matches the centers of the respective windows which is a fixed distance (the radius of the window) inside of the true boundary. Additionally, the smoothing used in the computation of the gradients of the intensity and variance images shrinks the apparent boundary of the structure related to the amount of smoothing and to the structure's curvature. For these reasons the final contour is expanded by a constant k at each point as shown in Figure 1, where k depends on the window size used in the variance computation and the amount of smoothing. This is only an approximation, as k should also vary locally depending on the curvature of the boundary and on the appearance of neighboring structures. These factors are not currently incorporated, and k is constant over the curve.

4 Experimental Results

This algorithm has been run on one clinical volumetric knee image. This image consists of 45 2D slices (greyscale images), each with resolution 256x256. The slices on the ends were not used in the experiments since the femur and tibia were not prominent in them, leaving 37 slices used. The program is run on each slice independently. The same initial contours were used in each image, except for slices early in the sequence and late in the sequence where separate initial curves had to be defined so that the initial curve was within the structure. The femur and tibia were segmented separately, and are overlaid on the same image for display purposes only. The window-size for variance computation was 7x7, sigma of 4 was used in the gradient computations, the compensation factor k was 8, and convergence was defined to be movement less than image resolution over 12 iterations. Most segmentations required approximately 200 iterations for convergence, dependent primarily on the size of the structure in the image, and took approximately 30 seconds on a 250MHz UltraSparc.

4.1 Performance

Segmentations of the 35 central slices are pictured in Figure 2. The segmentation was performed separately for the femur and tibia, although this is not a requirement of the algorithm. Notice that the boundary is well approximated by most segmentations, and the starting contours are not near the boundaries. These segmentations were fully automatic, with fixed initial contours used for the early, middle, and late slices respectively, and all other parameters constant on all images. The exact settings were not crucial; many settings yield qualitatively equivalent results. The convergence criteria can be tightened to allow more outward flow, and this change would fix the error in the femur segmentation in one image in Figure 2 where a dark region within the femur causes the flow to stop. If the criteria is made too strict, however, the contours would leak into neighboring structures. The segmentations are rendered together to show the total segmentation of the bones in Figure 3.

4.2 Comparison to Intensity Only

This algorithm was run using only the intensity gradients, as in the traditional active contour definition. In this case, the energy function was defined as $g(|\nabla I|) = \frac{1}{1+|\nabla I|^2}$. This method worked for some images and settings but was much less stable than the two-valued method. Areas of low gradients (high

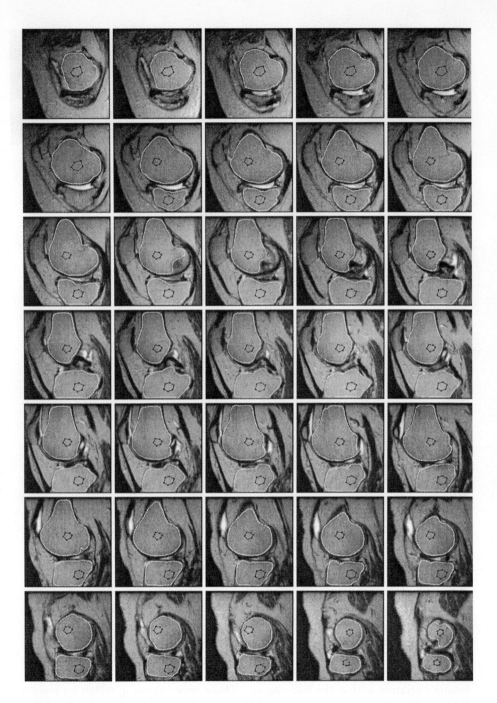

Fig. 2. 35 image slices shown with segmentations overlaid in white. Initial contour is shown in black.

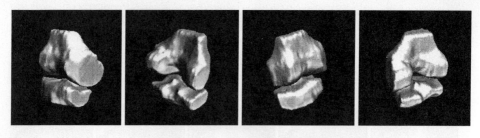

Fig. 3. Segmentations from 37 slices rendered together to show volumetric information.

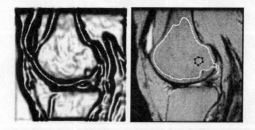

Fig. 4. Segmentation using only intensity gradients. (1) The energy function $g(|\nabla I|) = \frac{1}{1+|\nabla I|^2}$. (2) Curve flow showing leaking into neighboring structures, convergence not yet detected.

values of g) near the boundary often caused the contour to leak into other areas of the image. Figure 4 shows an example run using this energy function. The snake was stopped after a fixed number of iterations; it did not yet detect convergence. However, it had already leaked beyond the boundary of the femur, and subsequent iterations would cause it to leak much more. No compensation for smoothing was applied, but there is less of a need than in the two-valued case. Note again that the use of a balloon force that depends on g has changed the partial differential equations from the derivation of geodesic snakes, so the existence and uniqueness of a solution may not be assured as in the original formulation [4].

4.3 Comparison to Variance Only

Variance was also tested alone using the energy function $g(|\nabla S|) = \frac{1}{1+|\nabla S|^2}$, where S is the variance image. It attained much better results than intensity alone, rivaling the two-valued approach. It almost always converged to a reasonable boundary. Compared to the two-valued approach, it appeared slightly more likely to leak through a region boundary but was better able to handle large intensity variation within the bone region. Three experiments in which its results differed from those of the two-valued algorithm are shown in Figure 5. Again, the inner boundary is the result before compensation for windowing. The first experiment was stopped after some number of iterations: convergence was not detected. The second segmentation is better than that achieved in the two-valued

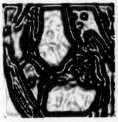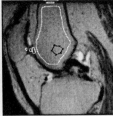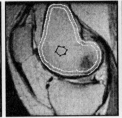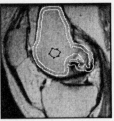

Fig. 5. Segmentation using only variance component of image. (1) The energy function $g(|\nabla S|) = \frac{1}{1+|\nabla S|^2}$, where S is the variance image. (2) Curve flow showing leaking into neighboring structures, convergence not yet detected (and stretching by k not applied). (3) A difficult segmentation. (4) A third segmentation where the result differs from the two-valued segmentation.

case for the same image and initial contour (Figure 2). Whether or not the third segmentation is better than the corresponding two-valued segmentation depends on what a radiologist would consider ground truth for that particular image, as the boundary is not clear. Overall the results for variance alone were good, and one could use this approach for segmentation but may need to be more careful when choosing parameters settings.

5 Future Work

One direction for future work is to extend the system to operate on 3D images directly, so that a surface is evolved instead of curves on individual slices. The geodesic snakes method was generalized to volumetric data in [5], and the vector-valued extension will hold in 3D as well. In that case, the data would be a vector-valued volume where one would consider mappings from R^3 to R^m where m is the number of (3D) texture features used.

A second direction is the incorporation of other texture measures which may be necessary for other applications or may improve the results for this application. Such measures include orientational filters and gray-level co-occurrence [8]. We also plan to consider textures across multiple scales to be able to handle a wide variety of textures and scenarios.

Acknowledgments

The authors thank Polina Golland for the program used to render the 2D slices as a volume. Also, thanks to Tina Kapur for discussions on this project.

References

1. R. Adams and L. Bischof. Seeded region growing. *IEEE Trans. Patt. Analysis and Mach. Intell.*, 16(6):641–647, 1994.

2. J. R. Beveridge, J. Griffith, R. R. Kohler, A. R. Hanson, and E. M. Riseman. Segmenting images using localized histograms and region merging. *Int'l Journal Comp. Vision*, 2:311–347, 1989.
3. V. Caselles, F. Catte, T. Coll, and F. Dibos. A geometric model for active contours. *Numerische Mathematik*, 66:1–31, 1993.
4. V. Caselles, R. Kimmel, and G. Sapiro. Geodesic active contours. *Int'l Journal Comp. Vision*, 22(1):61–79, 1997.
5. V. Caselles, R. Kimmel, G. Sapiro, and C. Sbert. Minimal surfaces: A three dimensional segmentation approach. Technical Report 973, Technion, Dept. EE, June 1995.
6. L. D. Cohen. On active contour models and balloons. *CVGIP: Image Understanding*, 53(2):211–218, 1991.
7. J. De Bonet and P. Viola. Structure driven image database retrieval. In *Neural Information Processing Systems*, 1997.
8. R. M. Haralick and L. G. Shapiro. *Computer and Robot Vision*. Addison-Wesley Publishing Company, Inc., 1992.
9. T. Kapur. Segmentation of brain tissue from magnetic resonance images. Technical Report 1566, MIT Artificial Intelligence Laboratory, Jan. 1995.
10. T. Kapur, P. Beardsley, and S. Gibson. Segmentation of bone in clinical mri. Technical report, MERL, A Mitsubishi Electric Research Company, Aug. 1997.
11. T. Kapur, P. Beardsley, S. Gibson, W. Grimson, and W. Wells. Model-based segmentation of clinical knee MRI. In *Proc. IEEE Int'l Workshop on Model-Based 3D Image Analysis*, pages 97–106, 1998.
12. M. Kass, A. Witkin, and D. Terzopoulos. Snakes: Active contour models. *Int'l Journal Comp. Vision*, 1(4):321–331, 1988.
13. A. Kichenassamy, A. Kumar, P. Olver, A. Tannenbaum, and A. Yezzi. Gradient flows and geometric active contour models. In *Proc. IEEE Int'l Conf. Comp. Vision*, pages 810–815, 1995.
14. T. McInerney and D. Terzopoulos. Deformable models in medical image analysis: a survey. *Medical Image Analysis*, 1(2):91–108, 1996.
15. S. Osher and J. Sethian. Gradient flows and geometric active contour models. *Journal of Computational Physics*, 79:12–49, 1988.
16. R. Ronfard. Region-based strategies for active contour models. *Int'l Journal Comp. Vision*, 13(2):229–251, 1994.
17. G. Sapiro. Vector-valued active contours. In *Proc. IEEE Conf. Comp. Vision and Patt. Recog.*, pages 680–685, 1996.
18. L. Staib and J. Duncan. Boundary finding with parametrically deformable contour models. *IEEE Trans. Patt. Analysis and Mach. Intell.*, 14(11), 1992.
19. M. Wolf, P. Weierich, and H. Niemann. Automatic segmentation and 3d-registration of the femoral bone in mr-images of the knee. *Pattern Recognition and Image Analysis: Advances in Mathematical Theory and Application, Russian Academy of Sciences*, 7, 1997.
20. A. Yezzi, S. Kichenassamy, A. Kumar, P. Olver, and A. Tannenbaum. A geometric snake model for segmentation of medical imagery. *IEEE Trans. Medical Imaging*, 16(2):199–209, 1997.
21. S. C. Zhu and D. Mumford. Prior learning and gibbs reaction-diffusion. *IEEE Trans. Patt. Analysis and Mach. Intell.*, 19(11), Nov. 1997.
22. S. C. Zhu, Y. Wu, and D. Mumford. Frame: Filters, random fields, and minimax entropy. In *Proc. IEEE Conf. Comp. Vision and Patt. Recog.*, pages 686–693, 1996.
23. S. C. Zhu and A. Yuille. Region competition. *IEEE Trans. Patt. Analysis and Mach. Intell.*, 18(9), 1996.

Tensor Controlled Local Structure Enhancement of CT Images for Bone Segmentation

C-F. Westin, S. Warfield, A. Bhalerao, L. Mui, J. Richolt, and R. Kikinis

Surgical Planning Lab, Radiology, Brigham and Women's Hospital,
westin@bwh.harvard.edu, Harvard Medical School, Boston

Abstract. This paper addresses the problem of segmenting bone from Computed Tomography (CT) data. In clinical practice, identification of bone is done by thresholding, a method which is simple and fast. Unfortunately, thresholding alone has significant limitations. In particular, segmentation of thin bone structures and of joint spaces is problematic. This problem is particularly severe for thin bones such as in the skull (the paranasal sinus and around the orbit). Another area where current techniques often fail is automatic, reliable and robust identification of individual bones, which requires precise separation of the joint spaces. This paper presents a novel solution to these problems based on three-dimensional filtering techniques. Improvement of the segmentation results in more accurate 3D models for the purpose of surgical planning and intraoperative navigation.

1 Introduction

Three-dimensional renderings of bone that are based on thresholding are currently available on most state-of-the-art CT consoles. Unfortunately, using only thresholding to segment the CT data leads to suboptimal and unsatisfying results in the vast majority of the cases. It is seldom possible to automatically separate the different bones adjacent to a given joint (e.g. femur and pelvis) or different fracture fragments. Problems also exist in areas with very thin bone, such as the paranasal sinuses and around the orbits. So far bone and joint disorders are primarily visualized by plain radiographs or cross sectional CT and MR images. Neither of them are intuitive tools for displaying the patient's anatomy, especially if the spatial relationships of different structures are more complex. 3D visualization can be very helpful for example in cases of pelvic, hip and shoulder disorders. Also pathoanatomic findings in areas with small joints (such as the wrist, hindfoot and spine) are much easier to understand when displayed in 3D.

The adaptive filtering algorithm presented in [1] has been implemented for the specific needs of CT segmentation. The major change presented here is adding the ability to create filters on grids which have different spatial resolutions in different directions to cope with the large out-of-plane/in-plane voxel ratio. Additionally, filters that have a well tuned frequency characteristic in all directions of the data is important as many of the structures of interest have a size close to the signal spacing.

In this paper an adaptive filtering algorithm is designed to emphasize structures of interest in CT data to make segmentation of bone easier. This is an extension of our work presented in [2] where information of locally planar structures were used in an adaptive thresholding algorithm.

Most image enhancement algorithms presented in the literature have design criteria based on characteristics of the perceived quality, such as that the human eye is more sensitive to noise in dark regions and less sensitive to noise in bright and structured ones. Since our goal is not to improve the human visual perception of the data but to perform filtering to improve segmentation, our constraints are slightly different. This paper is based on an adaptive filtering algorithm proposed by Knutsson, Wilson and Granlund [3, 4, 1]. The reason for choosing this particular image enhancement algorithm is that extra edge sharpening can be obtained while smoothing along structures in a very controlled way. Algorithms that are based on anisotropic diffusion information [5, 6] or level set theory (so called "geometric diffusion") [7, 8] also perform smoothing along structures which to some extent sharpen edges. However, how best to incorporate a stable and controllable sharpening into schemes based on anisotropic diffusion is an open question. Some sharpening can be obtained by running the diffusion equation "backwards", but causes instability and may give unpredictable results. In the literature several methods have been reported to obtain more robust and accurate bone segmentation based on for example region growing and deformable contours. In principle, any of these methods can be used in conjunction with the method proposed in this paper.

2 Algorithmic description

The approach we have taken is to filter the CT data using adaptive filters for the purpose of enhancing the local image structure. The organization of this section is that we begin with presenting a list of the main steps involved in the segmentation scheme. A detailed description of each of the items in the list then follows.

1. Design filters for the data grid which is not equally spaced in all directions.
2. Resample the data in the slice direction to obtain dense enough sampling to describe a classification result as a binary label map.
3. Estimate local image structure and represent it by tensors, and use the local structure tensors to locally control the adaptation of the filters.
4. Segment the adaptively filtered result.

Step 1: Filter design on non-cubic grids

In CT data, the voxels are in general non-cubic, i.e. the distance between the samples are not the same in all direction. The in-plane resolution in CT image volumes is often more than a factor of 5-10 higher than the through-plane resolution, e.g. $0.5 \times 0.5 \times 3$ mm^3. Data sampled like this has a frequency content that varies with the direction of the data. In order to get invariance of a filter response, i.e. to get the same sensitivity of structures independent of the orientation of the structure, the frequency characteristic of the filters used must be altered to compensate for the differences in the data. Spatially designed kernels can be compressed in the slice direction before being sampled. However, when designing filters in the frequency domain there is, in most cases, no closed spatial form of the filter available. This is particularly true when other additional constraints, such as locality of the filters, are introduced during the optimization procedure when creating the filters. This means that there is not a spatial filter function that can be resampled, and any compensation of the non-isotropic sampling grid must first be applied in the frequency domain. The relation of a filter, $f(\mathbf{x})$, and linearly transformed version, $g(\mathbf{x}) = f(\mathbf{A}\mathbf{x})$, in the Fourier domain is

$$G(\mathbf{u}) = \frac{1}{|\det \mathbf{A}|} F(|\mathbf{A}^T|^{-1}\mathbf{u}) \qquad (1)$$

A scaling of the spatial grid along the coordinate axes can be written,

$$\mathbf{A} = \begin{pmatrix} a & 0 & 0 \\ 0 & b & 0 \\ 0 & 0 & c \end{pmatrix} \qquad (2)$$

where a, b and c are the scaling factors. According to Equation 1, this implies the following relation of the two Fourier transforms F and G.

$$G(u_1, u_2, u_3) = \frac{1}{abc} F(\frac{u_1}{a}, \frac{u_2}{b}, \frac{u_3}{c}) \qquad (3)$$

Step 2: Resampling

The output from segmenting gray-level data is in general a label map, with label values of low order. In the case of a two class problem as in this paper; bone and no bone, this label map is binary. From an information preserving point of view, the description of a sampled gray-level signal with samples of lower dimensionality, requires a higher sample density. For example, describing an 8-bit signal with binary values would require 8 times the samples to be able to describe the same amount of information. For images, where the signal spectrum is highly biased towards low spatial frequencies, the actual required sample density is lower. However, in CT data, where the size of the structures of interest are comparable to the voxel dimensions (in the slice direction) a higher sampling rate is preferable.

In the CT data used in this paper the voxel dimensions are $0.82 \times 0.82 \times 3$ mm^3. We found it necessary to resample the data by a factor of two in the slice direction to adequately be able to describe the segmentation result, i.e. double the number of slices. This was done by upsampling by factor of two in the slice direction followed by smoothing with a $3 \times 3 \times 3$ Gaussian filter kernel, which gives the new voxel dimensions $0.82 \times 0.82 \times 1.5$ mm^3. Note that the voxels still are non cubic. A reason for not expanding the original data more than necessary is that interpolation to higher resolution is a difficult problem in itself [9, 10].

CT data used for the experiments in this paper has voxel dimensions $(a, b, c) = (0.82, 0.82, 3)$, and after resampling $(a', b', c') = (0.82, 0.82, 1.5)$. The ratio between the in-plane and the out-of-plane distance is then, $r = \frac{c'}{a'} = 1.83$

Step 3: Tensor controlled adaptive filtering

The adaptive filtering scheme consists of two main parts: 1) filtering the data with a filter set consisting of six directed quadrature filters producing a description of local structure, and 2) filtering the data with a basis filter set consisting of one low-pass filter and six directed high-pass filters. The final filter result is a combination of the basis filter outputs controlled by the information of the local structure. The affine frequency model discussed in the previous section is applied to all the filters involved.

A tensor $\mathbf{T}$, describing local structure, can be obtained by a linear summation of lognormal quadrature filter output magnitudes, $|q_k|$, weighted by predefined tensors $\mathbf{M}_k$ associated with each filter [11]. For the CT data presented in this paper we have experimentally found that a lognormal filter with centre frequency, $\rho_0 = \pi/4$, and relative bandwidth, $B = 2$, was appropriate for structures in-plane, which gives the out-of-plane filter center frequency $r\frac{\pi}{4}$, $((r = 1.83)$, from above). For details see [11]. It is desirable that the model describing the local neigbourhood varies slower than the signal it is describing. To ensure a slowly varying adaptive filter and to reduce the impact of noise the estimated tensor field, $\mathbf{T}$, is relaxed by applying a $7 \times 7 \times 5$ Gaussian filter. The output from this relaxation is denoted $\mathbf{T}_r$.

The filter set used in the adaptive scheme consists of a low-pass filter and six directed high-pass filters. This basis set can construct filters of a variety of shapes; filters that can smooth along lines, along planes, high-pass filtering across lines or across planes. The basic idea is to compose a filter that fits the local structure of the data,

$$F = F_{lp} + h(\|\hat{\mathbf{T}}_r\|) \sum_k \langle \mathbf{M}_k, \mathbf{C} \rangle F_{hp}^k \tag{4}$$

where $\hat{\mathbf{T}}_r = \frac{\mathbf{T}_r}{\|\mathbf{T}_r\|_{max}}$ and $\mathbf{C}$ is the tensor $\mathbf{T}_r$ normalized with the corresponding largest eigenvalue, $\mathbf{C} = \frac{\mathbf{T}_r}{\lambda_1}$. $\mathbf{C}$ defines the angular behaviour of the adaptive filter. The function, $h(\|\hat{\mathbf{T}}_r\|)$ in Equation 4, controls how much over-all high pass information is allowed through the adaptive filter F. In noisy regions without well defined structures the norm of the tensor $\|\hat{\mathbf{T}}_r\|$ will generally be small compared to areas with well defined structures such as edges. A desired behaviour of the adaptive filter is that when no structures are present, lowpass filtering should be performed in all direction in order to smooth out the noise (isotropic lowpass filtering). Therefore, the function h is designed to be zero for small arguments. The consequence of this will be that the highpass term in Equation

4 is cancelled in regions not having well defined structures and that lowpass filtering is performed instead. The function used is not critical as long as it can be tuned to the described behaviour. The following function was used

$$h(|\hat{\mathbf{T}}_r|) = \frac{|\hat{\mathbf{T}}_r|^\beta}{|\hat{\mathbf{T}}_r|^{\beta+\alpha} + \sigma^\beta} \tag{5}$$

with $\alpha = 1$, $\beta = 2$, and $\sigma = 0.05$.

Step 4: Segmentation

This step has been implemented in a very straight forward way. However, despite its simplicity, it was shown to work satisfactorily. The procedure is as follows.

First the adaptively filtered data was thresholded. An example of this step is shown in Figure 2, where the lower left image shows the adaptively filters result, and the lower middle image shows the result of thresholding. Then the thresholded data was labelled into connected components. Isolated islands of voxels inside larger structures were merged into the largest one. The result of this can be seen in the lower right image in Figure 2.

3 Results

Figure 1 displays the results of thresholding a CT data set of a hip joint before and after adaptive filtering. Although the filter was applied in 3D, a single slice is displayed and compared to thresholding at different signal intensity levels. The size of the 6 filters used for the local structure estimation was $9 \times 9 \times 7$, and $15 \times 15 \times 9$ for the 7 basis filters used in adaptive filtering scheme (1 lowpass and 6 directed highpass filters).

The top left image shows the CT scan. This slice shows the hip joint. The top middle image shows the segmentation using a high enough threshold to separate the joint space. Unfortunately important parts of the bone are missing, e.g. the hole in the femoral head (false negatives). The top left image shows segmentation using a low enough threshold to capture most of the important bone. Unfortunately, the result is very noisy and now the femur and the pelvis are connected (false positives). These are the same reasons that make it difficult to capture thin bone structures. Thin bright structures disappear [2] and dark thin structures get filled and this artificially connects different bones (Figure 1 top right). A threshold that separates the joint space inevitably introduces severe artifacts and removes large parts of real bone (false negatives).

The bottom left image shows the result of 3D adaptive filtering of the CT data. The lower right image shows segmentation of the filtered data. The same threshold as in the top right image was used. Note the reduction of the noise level and that the joint space is free from falsely segmented bone structures. Note also that the boundaries of the segmented structures have not moved. This is because smoothing of the data has been performed along the structures and not across them, at the same time extra sharpening is obtained across the structures.

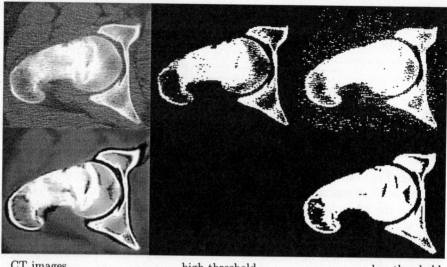

CT images   high threshold   low threshold

Fig. 1. *Adaptive filtering of CT data through the hip joint* **Top:** *Original gray-scale image (left). The middle image shows the segmentation using a threshold high enough to separate the joint space. The rightmost image shows segmentation using a threshold low enough that is captures all of the important bone.* **Bottom:** *The left image shows a gray-scale image as the result after 3D adaptive filtering of the CT data. The lower right image shows segmentation of the filtered data. The same threshold as in the top right image was used.*

Figure 2 shows adaptive filtering of a second data set. This data set is displayed differently than in Figure 1. The images presented are slices from the volume orthogonal to the slice direction of the data acquisition. The top left image clearly shows that the voxels dimension are non-cubic. The ratio of the vertical and horizontal resolution is $3/0.82 = 3.7$. The top middle image shows the effect of thresholding the original data. It is impossible to find a threshold that separates the femur and the pelvis without removing most of the data. The top right image shows the result of manual segmentation by an orthopaedic surgeon. The lower left image shows the result after resampling the original data by a factor of two in the slice acquisition direction followed by adaptive filtering. The result of thresholding this data is shown by the lower middle image. The two bone parts are now separated and well defined. A connected component labeling and filling of interior regions gives the final segmentation result presented in lower right image.

In Figure 3 the manually segmented femur and the automatically segmented femur are visualized side by side using surface models. The voxel overlap between the two data sets is 98%. In the voxel overlap calculation, the automatically obtained segmentation result was subsampled by a factor of two in the slice direction in order to get the same resolution as the manually segmented data.

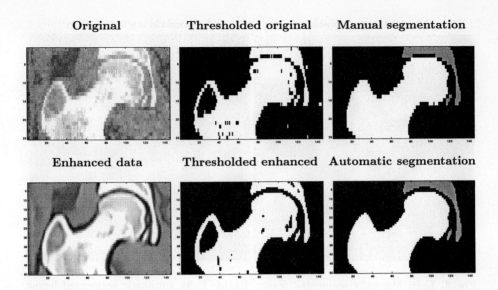

Fig. 2. Top: An image from the original CT volume of a hip joint perpendicular to the slice direction (the pelvis is seen in the top part of the images and the femur in the lower part). The middle image shows the result from thresholding the original CT data. The right image shows the result from careful manual segmentation by an orthopaedic surgeon. **Bottom**: Automatic segmentation using resampling and adaptive filtering to enhance local structure (left image), thresholding of the filtered result (middle), final segmentation by connected component labeling (right).

4 Summary and future work

A three-dimensional adaptive filtering scheme has been implemented for the particular needs of enhancing CT data to improve bone segmentation. It was shown how the frequency characteristic of the filters can be designed to fit the data geometry and compensate for the non-isotropic voxel dimensions normally present in CT data. This also gives well tuned frequency characteristics in all directions of the volume, which is of importance since many of the structures of interest have a size close to the signal spacing. By using adaptive filtering, structures of interest can be emphasized and thus more easily segmented. We have shown that the presented method can automatically segment and separate bones that are close spatially, such as femur and pelvis in the hip joint. For the few cases we have segmented so far, we have obtained around 98% agreement in terms of voxel overlap between automatic and manual segmentation of the data. Future work will be focused on extending our implementation of the linear model in Equation 1, i.e. not only perform scaling of the Fourier domain along the axes when designing filters to get the desired frequency behaviour, but to incorporate shift and shear as well. By introducing subvoxel shifts by modulation in the frequency domain, a resampling to a new grid can be done inside the adaptive filtering scheme.

Manual segmentation   Automatic segmentation

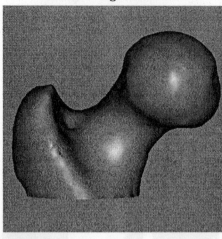 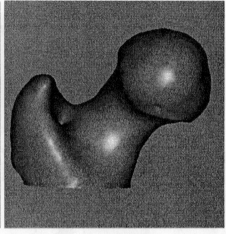

Fig. 3. Left: Manually segmented femur. **Right**: Fully automatic segmented femur using adaptive filtering to enhance local structure followed by thresholding and connected component labeling. The voxel overlap between the manually segmented and the automatic segmentation result is 98 %.

References

1. G. H. Granlund and H. Knutsson. *Signal Processing for Computer Vision*. Kluwer Academic Publishers, 1995. ISBN 0-7923-9530-1.
2. C-F Westin, A. Bhalerao, H. Knutsson, and R. Kikinis. Using local 3D structure for segmentation of bone from computer tomography images. In *Proceedings of IEEE Computer Society Conference on Computer Vision and Pattern Recognition*, pages 794–800, Puerto Rico, June 1997.
3. H. Knutsson, R. Wilson, and G. H. Granlund. Anisotropic non-stationary image estimation and its applications — part I: Restoration of noisy images. *IEEE Trans on Communications*, COM-31(3):388–397, March 1983.
4. R. Wilson, H. Knutsson, and G. H. Granlund. Anisotropic non-stationary image estimation and its applications — part II: Predictive image coding. *IEEE Trans on Communications*, COM-31(3), March 1983.
5. P. Perona and J. Malik. Scale space and edge diffusion using anisotropic diffusion. *IEEE Transactions on Pattern Analysis and Machine Intelligence*, 12(7):629–639, July 1990.
6. G. Gerig, O. Kübler, R. Kikinis, and F. Jolesz. Non-linear anisotropic filtering of MRI data. *IEEE Transaction on Medical Imaging*, 11(2):221–232, June 1992.
7. A. Kumar, A. Tannenbaum, and G. Balas. Optical flow: A curve evolution approach. *IEEE Trans. on Image Processing*, 5(4):598–610, April 1996.
8. J.A. Sethian. Curvature and the evolution of fronts. *Commun. Math. Phys.*, 1985.
9. J. A. Parker, R. V. Kenyon, and D. E. Troxel. Comparison of interpolation methods for image resampling. *IEEE Transactions on Medical Imaging*, 2(1), 1983.
10. C-H Lee. Restoring spline interpolation of CT images. *IEEE Transactions on Medical Imaging*, 2(3), 1983.
11. H. Knutsson. Representing local structure using tensors. In *The 6th Scandinavian Conference on Image Analysis*, pages 244–251, Oulu, Finland, June 1989.

Segmentation of Magnetic Resonance Images Using 3D Deformable Models

Jyrki Lötjönen[1,2,3], Isabelle E. Magnin[1], Pierre-Jean Reissman[1,2], Jukka Nenonen[2,3], and Toivo Katila[2,3]

[1] Creatis, INSA 502, 69621 Villeurbanne Cedex, France
Isabelle.Magnin@creatis.insa-lyon.fr
[2] Laboratory of Biomedical Engineering, Helsinki University of Technology, P.O.B. 2200, FIN-02015 HUT, Finland
{Jyrki.Lotjonen, Jukka.Nenonen, Toivo.Katila}@hut.fi
[3] BioMag Laboratory, Helsinki University Central Hospital, P.O.B. 503, FIN-00029 HYKS, Finland

Abstract. A new method to segment MR volumes has been developed. The method matches elastically a 3D deformable prior model, describing the structures of interest, to the MR volume of a patient. The deformation is done using a deformation grid. Oriented distance maps are utilized to guide the deformation process. Two alternative restrictions are used to preserve the geometrical prior knowledge of the model. The method is applied to extract the body, the lungs and the heart. The segmentation is needed to build individualized boundary element models for bioelectromagnetic inverse problem. The method is fast, automatic and accurate. Good results have been achieved for four MR volumes tested so far.

1 Introduction

Multichannel magneto- and electrocardiographic (MCG and ECG) recordings have been proved useful in non-invasive localization of bioelectromagnetic sources such as cardiac excitation sources [1]. In the bioelectromagnetic forward and inverse problems, the anatomy of the patient has to be modeled as a volume conductor. Usually the modeling is done using magnetic resonance (MR) images of the patient [2]. However, the segmentation of the structures of interest remains in practice the most time consuming part in the modeling process, thus drastically limiting the use of the individualized models.

In medical imaging field, accurate delineation of anatomic structures from image data sequences is still an open problem. In practice, manual extraction of the objects of interest is often considered as the most reliable technique. However, such methods remain time consuming and are affected by intra- and interobserver variability. Various computer methods have been recently proposed for segmentation of medical images [3, 4]. They can be divided into region-based and boundary based approaches [5]. In region based methods, some features based on the intensity of the images are used to merge voxels. One of the limitations of these approaches is the difficulty to automatically choose seed points. To overcome the problem, higher control can be used with graph theory approaches and prior knowledge of the image content [6, 7]. The boundary based methods [8, 9] rely on an intensity gradient detection. Unfortunately, they are sensitive to impulsive noise, which cause spurious and partial edge maps. Deformable methods [9, 10] allow to group partial edges with a chosen parametrization [11]. Their main drawback is the lack of control on the resulting shape [12]. This is especially true when the images contain several nested structures of interest [13]. To deal with the problem, we propose an automatic segmentation technique, based on the deformable pyramidal model [14] that highly relies on the prior geometrical knowledge [15, 16] of the anatomic structures to be segmented. The theory of the method is represented more detailed in a recent doctorate thesis [17].

2 Methods

The aim of this work is to extract the body surface, lungs and heart from the MR-images as automatically and fast as possible starting from a 3D prior geometrical deformable model. The model used is a triangulation representing the surfaces of the structures of interest (Fig. 1).

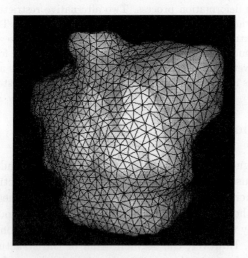

Fig. 1. *The prior geometrical model used in the 3D deformation process. It has been built from MR-images of a female patient.*

2.1 The energy function

1. Isotropic distance maps. The model is elastically deformed in 3D to match to edges in MR images. The edges can be extracted from MR-images using a classical edge detection algorithm [18]. In practice, thresholding separates body surface and lungs from MR-images well enough and the edges can be easily found from the binarized volume.

Once the edges have been extracted from the volume, the energy function is defined by calculating a distance map $f = f(x,y,z)$ for the edges (Fig. 2) [19]. Each voxel in the distance map gives the shortest chamfer distance to the nearest edge in the 3D MR volume. This leads to so called isotropic distance map. The mismatch energy E_{data} between the edges in the MR volume and the triangulated prior model is calculated as follows:

$$E_{data} = \frac{1}{N_{nd}} \sum_{l=1}^{N_{nd}} f(x_{nd,l}, y_{nd,l}, z_{nd,l}), \quad (1)$$

where N_{nd} is the total number of nodes in the model and $x_{nd,l}, y_{nd,l}, z_{nd,l}$ are the coordinates of the node l.

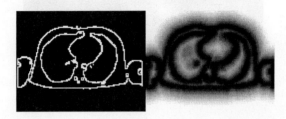

Fig. 2. *Calculation of the distance map: a) the edges and b) the corresponding distance map.*

2. Oriented distance maps. The prior knowledge about the objects to be segmented can be utilized in the creation of the distance maps; so called oriented distance maps are defined. The idea is that the boundaries of given orientation in the model have to match with similarly oriented edges extracted from the MR-data. In other words, if the surface normal of the model is locally oriented towards the positive y-axis, this part of the surface is allowed to deform only towards the edges in MR data with the same normal directions. To accomplish this, oriented edges are searched from the MR data (Fig. 3). In the middle of Fig. 3, all edges found from a MR-slice are represented. The arrows on the surrounding subimages give the average normal direction of the edges, $\mathbf{n}_{mr,i}$ on each subimage. The normals of the edges within a subimage differ less than $90°$ from the vector $\mathbf{n}_{mr,i}$. The number of different orientations is 8 in 2D (9 neighborhood) and 26 in 3D (27 neighborhood). The normal directions of the edges are estimated from the thresholded MR volume as follows: 1) Calculate the center of mass for each edge point using 27 voxel neighborhood. 2) The normal of the voxel is the vector from the center of mass to the edge point.

Actually all 26 oriented distance maps are not calculated on the highest resolution level for two reasons: 1) The size of the distance maps would be tens of megabytes. 2) The execution time would be about 2-3 minutes longer. The problem is solved by calculating only 6 oriented distance maps. The vectors $\mathbf{n}_{mr,i}$ are along x-, y- and z-axis. Since the angle between $\mathbf{n}_{mr,i}$ and the normal of each edge point in an oriented distance map is less than $90°$, Eq. 3 gives a good distance map for any $\mathbf{n}_{nd,l}$. If the angle is 90 degrees, in practice, 6 distance maps can be used instead of 26 in each resolution level.

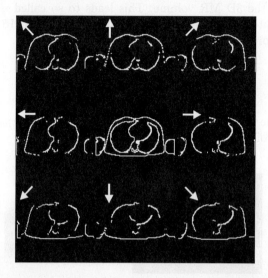

Fig. 3. *Oriented edges. The middle image shows all edges extracted from one MR slice. The edges oriented to 8 directions are presented in the surrounding subimages.*

The oriented distance maps are created by calculating distance maps separately for these 26 volumes including the oriented edges. The energy of the model can be calculated as follows

$$E_{data} = \frac{1}{N_{nd}} \sum_{l=1}^{N_{nd}} f_i(x_{nd,l}, y_{nd,l}, z_{nd,l}), \qquad (2)$$

where

$$f_i, i \in \{1, .., 26\} : \mathbf{n}_{mr,i} \cdot \mathbf{n}_{nd,l} \geq \mathbf{n}_{mr,k} \cdot \mathbf{n}_{nd,l}, \forall k \in \{1, .., 26\}. \qquad (3)$$

Here, the vector $\mathbf{n}_{mr,i}$ is the mean orientation of the edges in the distance map f_i, the vector $\mathbf{n}_{nd,l}$ is the normal of the surface of the model at the node l and $\cdot$ is for dot product. The matching process is now performed in two steps.

2.2 Coarse matching

The model is coarsely registered with the MR volume. Surface registration methods, such as [21], can be used to registrate the model with the edges extracted from the MR volume. If the rotation component is small, the bounding box, set around the model, can be scaled in such a way that it coincides with the bounding box set around the thresholded volume.

2.3 Detailed matching

The final registration step is done by placing the model inside a 3D deformation grid G (Fig. 4). When a grid point is moved, the model is deformed correspondingly. The benefit in using a deformation grid is, that the topology of the model can be easily preserved during the deformation process. The grid points are not moved more than half the distance between two neighboring grid points. The Bernstein polynomials or trilinear interpolation can be used to calculate the new positions for the nodes of the model [22]. In this paper trilinear interpolation is used. The grid divides space into box shaped subvolumes and each node of the triangulated model belongs to one of these boxes. The new position of a node in the model can be calculated as follows

$$\mathbf{p}_{nd} = \mathbf{p}_{nd}^{*} + \sum_{k=n}^{n+1}\sum_{j=m}^{m+1}\sum_{i=l}^{l+1} a_{G_{ijk}} \mathbf{v}_{G_{ijk}}, \qquad (4)$$

where $\mathbf{p}_{nd}^{*}$ is the original position of the node represented in the vector form, the summing is through the grid points, which define the box around the node, $\mathbf{v}_{G_{ijk}}$ is the displacement vector of the grid point G_{ijk} from its original position and $a_{G_{ijk}}$ is a weighting factor. The factor is calculated using trilinear interpolation.

All grid points G_{ijk} are sequentially moved towards a new position, which minimizes the energy of the model. This energy is computed from the distance map as defined in Eq. 2. within a $3 \times 3 \times 3$ or $5 \times 5 \times 5$ voxel neighborhood. Each grid point G_{ijk} is moved within the neighborhood and displacement is done sequentially for every point in the grid G. The process is iterated until the energy does not decrease anymore.

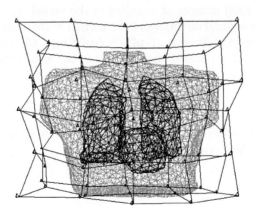

Fig. 4. *The 5x3x5 deformation grid G and the model placed inside.*

The deformation can be started for example by a $3 \times 3 \times 3$ grid, so providing a global match between the model and the MR volume. When the minimum is found for a given grid size, the number of grid points can be increased to $5 \times 5 \times 5$,

$7 \times 7 \times 7$ etc. Initial positions of the points in the new grid are regularly placed and not interpolated from the earlier, deformed grid.

To ensure a theoretical convergence towards the global minimum, methods such as simulated annealing should be used [20]. Since these methods are very time consuming, we chose the pyramid approach [21]. It does not guarantee the global minimum but works better than the method using local gradient alone.

In the case where the extraction of the edges from MR data does not succeed, some false edges may appear or some true edges may remain undetected. If the minimum of energy is defined using only gradient information, the deformation can lead to unacceptable results. In that case restrictions for deformation strength should be set. Reissman [17] proposed to limit the displacements of the grid points (LGD=Limit Grid Displacements) and proposed the deformation component of the energy to be calculated as follows,

$$E_{model} = \frac{1}{N_G} \sum_{l=1}^{N_G} \|\mathbf{p}_{G,l} - \mathbf{p}_{G,l}^*\|, \qquad (5)$$

where N_G is the number of grid points, $\mathbf{p}_{G,l}$ is the deformed position of the grid point l and $\mathbf{p}_{G,l}^*$ its original position.

Another way to preserve the prior knowledge of the model during deformation is to directly control the changes in the shape of the model. If the directions of the surface normals are used (LCN = Limit Change of Normals), the deformation energy E_{model} can be calculated as follows

$$E_{model} = \frac{1}{N_{tr}} \sum_{l=1}^{N_{tr}} (1.0 - \mathbf{n}_{tr,l} \cdot \mathbf{n}_{tr,l}^*), \qquad (6)$$

where N_{tr} is the total number of triangles in the model, $\mathbf{n}_{tr,l}$ and $\mathbf{n}_{tr,l}^*$ are the deformed and the original directions of the normal of the triangle l, respectively, and $\cdot$ is the dot product. Since $\mathbf{n}_{tr,l} \cdot \mathbf{n}_{tr,l}^* = cos(\angle(\mathbf{n}_{tr,l}, \mathbf{n}_{tr,l}^*))$, the large changes in the normal direction penalize more deeply to the energy than small changes.

Using deformation component in the energy, the total energy is defined by

$$E_{total} = E_{data} + \gamma E_{model}, \qquad (7)$$

where γ is a user defined parameter to control the balance between the data feature and the deformation components.

3 Results

The method was tested to segment the thorax, lungs and heart of four patients from their MR volumes using an IBM RS6000 workstation. In each case the algorithm produced a good result, with few interactive corrections of small magnitude. Next, the results for one thorax MR are represented. The size of the MR volume is 128x128x100. Fig. 5 shows the result of prior model deformation, when

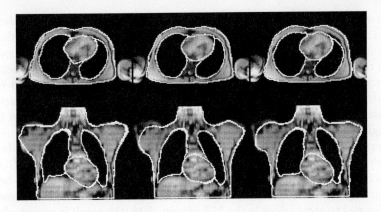

Fig. 5. *Segmentation result with $\gamma = 0.0$, with the LGD-method ($\gamma = 0.01$) and with the LCN-method ($\gamma = 5.0$)*

$\gamma = 0.0$, when the LGD-method was used with $\gamma = 0.01$ and when the LCN-method was applied with $\gamma = 5$. The results are not very sensitive to γ-values in the LGD- and LCN-methods: increase by factor 10 produces fairly similar results. The numbers of grid points on each pyramid level are represented in Table 1a. The iteration with each grid size was stopped, when the change in the energy was less than user defined parameter $\epsilon = 0.02$. The computing time to segment MR images and the energies at convergence related to the Fig. 5 are represented in Table 1b. The star '*' indicates that the oriented distance maps are not used at the highest resolution level, other parameters being equal. E_{data} corresponds to the average distance (in mm) between the nodes of the model and the edges in the MR volume. Since the voxel size at the highest resolution is 3.52 mm, the average distance of the nodes from edges is 0.17 voxel.

4 Discussion

A. General discussion. The segmentation error with the automatic method is low: about 87% of the nodes of the model are located on the edges of the MR data and the average error is about 0.17 voxel for the case presented in the

Level	Resolution	Grid	Model
2	32x32x25	3x3x3, 5x5x5	983
1	64x64x50	5x5x5, 5x5x5	2713
0	128x128x100	7x7x7, 9x9x9 11x11x11	9811

Method	Time	Edata	Emodel	Etotal
$\gamma = 0.0$	156	0.56	0.00	0.56
LGD	155	0.58	0.11	0.69
LCN	211	0.61	0.10	0.71
$\gamma = 0.0$*	94	0.61	0.00	0.61
LGD*	95	0.59	0.11	0.80
LCN*	150	0.62	0.11	0.73

Table 1. *a) The sizes of the grid and the number of nodes in the model at the different pyramid levels. b) Computing time (seconds) and matching energy for each method.*

results section. This error can be still reduced by increasing the size of the deformation grid. It is remarkable that, when only the E_{data} component is minimized ($\gamma = 0.0$), the energy value is higher than in the case of the LGD-method. This means the algorithm does not find the global minimum. However, in most cases the results are 'good' local minima. The segmentation results are also visually accurate, which is even more important than the absolute value of the error. The absolute value should not be emphasized too much, since the error can be low, although the model has deformed to wrong edges.

The model may also include edges, which can not be found from the data. For example, for the thorax three areas exist: 1) The model used in our MCG/ECG studies does not include arms (Fig. 1). 2) The edges of the heart can not be easily found in regions where the heart is not in contact with the lungs. If these areas are deformed to some edges in the MR volume data, the result is wrong, although the E_{total} can be minimum. 3) The quality of the MR images is poor nearby the shoulders, and the edges extracted from the volume does not describe well the real anatomy. In these cases, it is almost compulsory to use E_{model} component, which preserves the geometrical prior knowledge.

The balance between the E_{data} and E_{model} components can be set locally to improve the handling of the mismatch problem of the model and real data. This can be accomplished, for example, by attaching a weight $t_{nd,l}$ to each node of the model and multiplying the E_{data} term of the corresponding node by this weight.

In this paper two different methods to define E_{model} were described: the LGD- and the LCN-methods. The biggest benefit of the LGD-method is its speed. The quality of the results did not differ a lot for the cases we tested. However, the LCN-method preserves better the geometrical prior knowledge.

B. Implementation. Several factors affect to the execution time. If the oriented distance maps are used, the running time is higher (Table 1) but the robustness of the program is better. However, the results are fairly similar to the results with the oriented distance maps. The optimization time is directly dependent on the number of the nodes in the model. However, the number of the nodes can not be reduced too much. Otherwise, the probability that the model attaches to noise increases considerably. The average distance between the nodes was about two voxels at each resolution level. The size of the deformation grid does not affect much the execution time. If the size is higher, the number of the nodes connected to each grid point is correspondingly lower. Each grid size affects the run time cumulatively. For example, if a 11 × 11 × 11-grid had not been used in Table 1, the time would have been 10 s lower. The average error of the deformation would have been 0.81 mm, not 0.56 mm.

In summary, a new method to segment MR volumes has been developed. Since the method is fast and the results have been good for all tested data, it can be regarded useful in practice.

References

1. Nenonen, J.: Solving the inverse problem in magnetocardiography. *IEEE Eng. Med. Biol.* **13** (1994) 487-496
2. Lötjönen, J., Reissman, P.-J., Magnin, I.E., Nenonen, J. and Katila, T.: A Triangulation Method of an Arbitrary Point Set for Biomagnetic Problems. *IEEE Trans. Magn.* in press
3. Amit, Y., Kong, A.: Graphical templates for model registration. *IEEE Trans. PAMI* **18** (1996) 225-236
4. Philip, K.P., Dove, E.L., McPherson, D., Gotteiner, N.L., Vonesh, M.J., Stanford, W., Reed, J.E., Rumberger, J.A., Chanbran, K.B.: Automatic detection of myocardial contours in cine computed tomographic images. *IEEE Trans. Med. Imag.* **13** (1994) 241-253
5. Worring, M.W., Smeulders, A.W.M., Staib, L.H., Duncan, J.S.: Parameterized feasible boundaries in gradient vector fields. *Comput. Vision Imag. Under.* **63** (1996) 135-144
6. Fwu, J.K., Djurie, P.M.: Unsupervised vector image segmentation by a tree structure-ICM algorithm. *IEEE Trans. Med. Imag.* **15** (1996) 871-880
7. Sonka, M., Tadikonda, S.K., Collins, S.M.: Knowledge-based interpretation of MR brain images. *IEEE Trans. Med. Imaging* **44** (1996) 443-452
8. Goshtasby, A., Turner, D.A.: Segmentation of cardiac cine MR images for extraction of right and left ventricular chambers. *IEEE Trans. Med. Imag.* **14** (1995) 56-64
9. Chakrabotry, A., Staib, L.H., Duncan, J.S.: Deformable boundary finding in medical images by integrating gradient and region information. *IEEE Trans. Med. Imag.* **15** (1996) 859-870
10. Davatzikos, C.A., Bryan, R.N.: Using a deformable surface model to obtain a shape representation of the cortex. *IEEE Trans. Med. Imag.* **15** (1996) 785-795
11. Cohen, L.D., Cohen, I.: Finite-element methods for active contour models and balloons for 2-D and 3-D images. *IEEE Trans. PAMI* **15** (1993) 1131-1147
12. Kass, M., Witkin, A., Terzopoulos, D.: Snakes: active contour models. *Inter. Journ. Comp. Vision* **1** (1988) 321-331
13. Davatzikos, C.A., Prince, J.L.: An active contour model for mapping the cortex. *IEEE Trans. Med. Imag.* **14** (1995) 65-80
14. Reissman, P-J., Magnin, I.E.: Modeling 3D deformable object with the active pyramid. *Int. J. Patt. Rec. & Art. Int.* **11** (1997) 1129-1139
15. Jain, A.K., Zhong, Y., Lakshmannan, S.: Object matching using deformable templates. *IEEE Trans. PAMI* **14** (1996) 267-278
16. Terzopoulos, D., Waters, K.: Analysis and synthesis of facial image sequences using physical and anatomical models. *IEEE Trans. Med. Imag.* **15** (1993) 569-579
17. Reissman, P-J.: Modélisation et mise en correspondance par pyramides actives: Application à l'imagerie cardique par résonance magnétique, *Doctorate thesis, L'Institut National Des Sciences Appliquees de Lyon* France (1997)
18. Canny, J.: A computational approach to edge detection. *IEEE Trans. PAMI* **8** (1986) 679-698
19. Borgefors, G.: Distance transformation in digital images. *Computer Vision Graphics and Image Processing* **48** (1986) 344-371
20. Geman, S., Geman, D.: Stochastic relaxation, Gibbs distributions, and the Bayesian restoration of image. *IEEE PAMI* **6** (1984) 721-741
21. Borgefors, G.: Hierarchical chamfer matching: A parametric edge matching algorithm. *IEEE Trans. PAMI* **10** (1988) 849-865
22. Sederberg, T., Parry, S.: Free-form deformation of solid geometrical models. *SIGGRAPH* **20** (1986) 151–160

Automatic Segmentation of Brain Tissues and MR Bias Field Correction Using a Digital Brain Atlas

Koen Van Leemput, Frederik Maes, Dirk Vandermeulen, and Paul Suetens

Katholieke Universiteit Leuven, Medical Image Computing, Radiology-ESAT,
UZ Gasthuisberg, Herestraat 49, B-3000 Leuven, Belgium
Koen.VanLeemput@uz.kuleuven.ac.be

Abstract. This paper [1] proposes a method for fully automatic segmentation of brain tissues and MR bias field correction using a digital brain atlas. We have extended the EM segmentation algorithm, including an explicit parametric model of the bias field. The algorithm interleaves classification with parameter estimation, yielding better results at every iteration. The method can handle multi-channel data and slice-per-slice constant offsets, and is fully automatic due to the use of a digital brain atlas.

1 Introduction

Accurate segmentation of magnetic resonance (MR) images of the brain is of increasing interest in the study of many brain disorders such as schizophrenia and epilepsia. For instance, it is important to precisely quantify the total amounts of grey matter, white matter and cerebro-spinal fluid, as well as to measure abnormalities of brain structures. In multiple sclerosis, accurate segmentation of white matter lesions is necessary for drug treatment assessment. Since such studies typically involve vast amounts of data, manual segmentation is too time consuming. Furthermore, such manual segmentations show large inter- and intra-observer variability. Therefore, there is an increasing need for automated segmentation tools.

A major problem when segmenting MR images is the corruption with a smooth inhomogeneity bias field. Although not always visible for a human observer, such a bias field can cause serious misclassifications when intensity-based segmentation techniques are used.

Early methods for estimating and correcting bias fields used phantoms [1]. However, this approach assumes that the bias field is patient independent, which it is not. Homomorphic filtering [2] assumes that the frequency spectrum of the bias field and the image structures are well separated. This assumption, however, fails in the case of MR images. Other approaches use an intermediate classification or require that the user manually selects some reference points [3] [4].

---

[1] This paper is a short version of a technical report KUL/ESAT/PSI/9806 which can be obtained from the first author (Koen.VanLeemput@uz.kuleuven.ac.be)

Wells et al. [5] introduced the idea that estimation of the bias field is helped by classification and vice versa. This leads to an iterative method, interleaving classification with bias correction. In the Expectation-Maximization (EM) algorithm [6], which interleaves classification with class-conditional parameter estimation, Wells et al. substituted the step for estimating the class parameters by a bias estimation step. This requires that the user manually selects representative points for each of the classes considered. But such user interaction is time consuming, yields subjective and unreproducible segmentation results, and should thus be avoided if possible.

This paper describes a new method, based on the same idea of interleaving classification with bias correction. Rather than substituting the class-conditional parameter estimation step, as Wells et al. do, we propose an extension of the EM algorithm by including a bias field parameter estimation step. Furthermore, we use a digital brain atlas in the form of *a priori* probability maps for the location of the tissue classes. This method yields fully automatic classifications of brain tissues and MR bias field correction.

2 Method

2.1 The Expectation-Maximization (EM) algorithm

The EM algorithm [6] applied to segmentation interleaves a statistical classification of image voxels into K classes with estimation of the class-conditional distribution parameters. If each class is modeled by a normal distribution, then the probability that class j has generated the voxel value y_i at position i is $p(y_i \mid \Gamma_i{=}j, \theta_j) = G_{\sigma_j}(y_i - \mu_j)$ with $\Gamma_j \in \{j\}$ the tissue class at position i and $\theta_j = \{\mu_j, \sigma_j\}$ the distribution parameters for class j. Defining $\theta = \{\theta_j\}$ as the model parameters, the overall probability for y_i is

$$p(y_i \mid \theta) = \sum_j p(y_i \mid \Gamma_i{=}j, \theta_j) p(\Gamma_i{=}j)$$

The Maximum Likelihood estimates for the parameters μ_j and σ_j can be found by maximization of the likelihood $\prod_i p(y_i \mid \theta)$, equivalent to minimization of $\sum_i -\log(p(y_i \mid \theta))$. The expression for μ_j is given by the condition that

$$\frac{\partial}{\partial \mu_j}\left(\sum_i -\log\left(\sum_j p(y_i \mid \Gamma_i{=}j, \theta_j) p(\Gamma_i{=}j) \right) \right) = 0$$

Differentiating and using Bayes' rule

$$p(\Gamma_i{=}j \mid y_i, \theta) = \frac{p(y_i \mid \Gamma_i{=}j, \theta_j) p(\Gamma_i{=}j)}{\sum_j p(y_i \mid \Gamma_i{=}j, \theta_j) p(\Gamma_i{=}j)} \quad (1)$$

yields

$$\mu_j = \frac{\sum_i y_i \, p(\Gamma_i{=}j \mid y_i, \theta)}{\sum_i p(\Gamma_i{=}j \mid y_i, \theta)} \quad (2)$$

The same approach can be followed to find the expression for σ_j:

$$\sigma_j^2 = \frac{\sum_i p(\Gamma_i{=}j \mid y_i, \theta)(y_i - \mu_j)^2}{\sum_i p(\Gamma_i{=}j \mid y_i, \theta)} \quad (3)$$

Note that equation 1 performs a classification, whereas equation 2 and 3 are parameter estimates. Together they form a set of coupled equations, which can be solved by alternately iterating between classification and parameter estimation.

2.2 Extension of the EM algorithm

In order to estimate the bias field, we propose to make an extension of the EM algorithm. As in the original algorithm, each class j is modeled by a normal distribution, but now we also add a parametric model for the field inhomogeneity: the bias is modeled by a polynomial $\sum_k C_k \phi_k(x)$. Field inhomogeneities are known to be multiplicative; we first compute the logarithmic transformation on the intensities so that the bias becomes additive. Our model is then

$$p(y_i \mid \Gamma_i{=}j, \theta_j, C) = G_{\sigma_j}(y_i - \mu_j - \sum_k C_k \phi_k(x_i))$$

and

$$p(y_i \mid \theta, C) = \sum_j p(y_i \mid \Gamma_i{=}j, \theta_j, C) p(\Gamma_i{=}j)$$

with $C = \{C_k\}$ the bias field parameters. In order to find the bias field, the parameters μ_j, σ_j and C_k maximizing the likelihood $\prod_i p(y_i \mid \theta, C)$ must be searched. The C_k then allow calculating the estimated bias field.

Following the same approach as for equations 2 and 3, the expressions for the distribution parameters μ_j and σ_j are

$$\mu_j = \frac{\sum_i p(\Gamma_i{=}j \mid y_i, \theta, C)(y_i - \sum_k C_k \phi_k(x_i))}{\sum_i p(\Gamma_i{=}j \mid y_i, \theta, C)} \quad (4)$$

and

$$\sigma_j^2 = \frac{\sum_i p(\Gamma_i{=}j \mid y_i, \theta, C)(y_i - \mu_j - \sum_k C_k \phi_k(x_i))^2}{\sum_i p(\Gamma_i{=}j \mid y_i, \theta, C)} \quad (5)$$

Equations 4 and 5 are no surprise, as they are in fact the same equations which arise in the original EM algorithm (equations 2 and 3). The only difference is that the data is corrected for a bias field before the distribution parameters are calculated.

Setting the partial derivate for C_k to zero yields

$$\begin{bmatrix} C_1 \\ C_2 \\ \vdots \end{bmatrix} = (A^T W A)^{-1} A^T W r \quad \text{with} \quad A = \begin{bmatrix} 1 & \phi_1(x_1) & \phi_2(x_1) & \ldots \\ 1 & \phi_1(x_2) & \phi_2(x_2) & \ldots \\ \vdots & \vdots & \vdots & \ddots \end{bmatrix} \quad (6)$$

and with weights W and residue r

$$W_{mn} = \begin{cases} \sum_j \frac{p(\Gamma_m=j|y_m,\theta,C)}{\sigma_j^2} & \text{if } m = n \\ 0 & \text{otherwise} \end{cases} \qquad r = \begin{bmatrix} y_1 - \frac{\sum_j p(\Gamma_1=j|y_1,\theta,C)\mu_j/\sigma_j^2}{\sum_j p(\Gamma_1=j|y_1,\theta,C)/\sigma_j^2} \\ y_2 - \frac{\sum_j p(\Gamma_2=j|y_2,\theta,C)\mu_j/\sigma_j^2}{\sum_j p(\Gamma_2=j|y_2,\theta,C)/\sigma_j^2} \\ \vdots \end{bmatrix}$$

Equation 6 is a weighted least-squares fit. From the intermediate classification and Gaussian distribution estimates, a prediction of the signal without bias is constructed and subtracted from the original data. A weight is assigned to each voxel of the resulting residue image, inversely proportional to a weighted variance. The bias is then the weighted least-squares fit to that residue. In the special case in which each voxel is exclusively assigned to one single class, the predicted signal contains the mean of the class each voxel belongs to. The weights are then inversely proportional to the variance of that class.

Iterating between equations 1, 4, 5 and 6 interleaves classification (step 1), distribution parameter estimation (step 2) and bias estimation (step 3). This has to be compared to the original EM algorithm, where only steps 1 and 2 were used. Wells *et al.* [5], on the contrary, only use steps 1 and 3.

2.3 Further extensions

We have further extended the algorithm to handle multi-channel data input. Furthermore, we have included a model for the background noise as well as for slice-per-slice constant offsets. We just summarize the results here; more details can be found in [7].

Multi-channel data The algorithm is easily extended to multi-channel data by substituting the Gaussian distributions by multivariate normals with mean μ and covariance matrix Σ.

Background noise Since the background signal only contains noise and is not affected by the bias field, we have included an explicit model for the background noise. Pixels assigned to the background automatically get a zero weight for the bias estimation.

Slice-per-slice constant offsets In addition to a smoothly varying field inhomogeneity, 2D multi-slice sequence MR images, which are acquired in an interleaved way, are typically corrupted with additional slice-per-slice intensity offsets. We model these variations by assigning a 2D polynomial to each slice separately.

2.4 Digital brain atlas

In order to make the algorithm more robust and fully-automatic, a priori information is used in the form of an atlas. This atlas [8] contains a priori probability maps for white matter, grey matter and csf, as shown in figure 1.

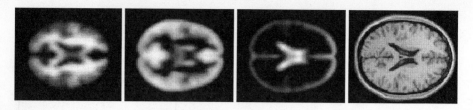

Fig. 1. The atlas consists of a priori probability maps for white matter, grey matter and csf, and a T1 template needed for registration of the subject to the space of the atlas

As a preprocessing step, we normalize the study images to the space of the atlas using the affine multi-modality registration technique described in [9]. At initialization, the atlas is used to sample the image for calculating the tissue-specific distribution parameters μ_j and σ_j. This approach frees us from interactively indicating representative pixels for each class. During subsequent iterations, the atlas is further used to spatially constrain the classification by using the spatially varying priors for $p(\Gamma_i=j)$ in equation 1. Thus, the voxels are not only classified based on their intensity, but also based on their spatial position. This makes the algorithm more robust, especially when the images are corrupted with a heavy bias field.

3 Results

We have implemented the algorithm as a modification of the SPM96 [10] segmentation tool, which originally used the EM algorithm without bias correction. We have performed experiments on various artificial and real MR data sets. In all the tests, a fourth order polynomial model for the bias was used. We here only shortly present some examples on real MR images of the head. A more detailed description can be found in [7], as well as some quantitative results on simulated MR data.

Single-channel data In figure 2, the classification of a high-resolution T1-weighted MR image is shown obtained with the EM algorithm without bias correction and with our extended EM algorithm using a 3D polynomial. For visualization purposes, we have made a hard segmentation from the probability maps by assigning each pixel exclusively to the class where it most probably belongs to. Because of a relatively strong bias field reducing the intensities in the slices at the top of the head, white matter is wrongly classified as the darker grey matter in those slices when the EM algorithm without bias correction is used. Our extended EM algorithm succeeds in compensating for this and provides better segmentations.

Multi-channel data The segmentation on a two-channel (PD and T2-weighted) MR image of the head is shown in figure 3. Although the effect of the bias field is hardly visible, it has a big impact on the resulting segmentation when the

EM algorithm without bias correction is used. With the extended algorithm, the segmentation is clearly improved.

MS lesion segmentation It is possible to assign multiple classes to the same a priori probability map. As an example, consider the problem of segmenting MS lesions. Since by far most of these lesions are located inside white matter, we have used the a priori white matter probability map for both the white matter and MS lesion class. The result for three-channel data of an MS patient, including T1, T2 and PD-weighted images, is shown in figure 4.

Slice-per-slice constant offsets As an example of bias correction for images with slice-per-slice constant offsets, we have processed the image shown in figure 5. The slice-per-slice offsets can clearly be seen as an interleaved bright-dark intensity pattern in a cross-section orthogonal to the slices. The estimated bias is also shown; it can be seen that the algorithm has found the slice-per-slice offsets.

4 Discussion

The algorithm that is proposed is based on Maximum-Likelihood parameter estimation using the EM algorithm. The method interleaves classification with parameter estimation, increasing likelihood at each iteration step.

The bias is estimated as a weighted least-squares fit, with the weights inversely proportional to the variance of the class each pixel belongs to. Since white matter and, in a lesser extend, grey matter have a narrow histogram, voxels belonging to the brain automatically get a large weight compared to non-brain tissues. We use a polynomial model for the bias field, which is a well-suited way for estimating bias fields in regions where the bias cannot be confidently estimated, i.e. regions with a low weight. The bias field is estimated from brain tissues and extrapolated to such regions.

At every iteration, the normal distribution parameters μ_j and σ_j for each class are updated. In combination with the atlas which provides a good initialization, this allows the algorithm to run fully automatic, avoiding manual selection of pixels representative for each of the classes considered. This yields objective and reproducible results. Furthermore, tissues surrounding the brain are hard to train for manually since they consist of a combination of different tissues types. Since our algorithm re-estimates the class distributions at each iteration, non-brain tissues automatically get a large variance and thus a low weight for the bias estimation.

We use an atlas which provides a priori information about the expected location of white matter, grey matter and csf. This information is used for initialization, avoiding user interaction which can give unreproducible results. Furthermore, the atlas makes the algorithm significantly more robust, since voxels are forced to be classified correctly even if the intensities largely differ due to a heavy bias field.

5 Summary and conclusions

In this paper, we have proposed a method for fully automatic segmentation of brain tissues and MR bias field correction using a digital brain atlas. We have extended the EM segmentation algorithm, including an explicit parametric model of the bias field. Results were presented on MR data with important field inhomogeneities and slice-per-slice offsets. The algorithm is fully automatic, avoids tedious and time-consuming user interaction and yields objective and reproducible results.

6 Acknowledgments

This research was performed within the context of the BIOMORPH project "Development and Validation of techniques for Brain Morphometry" supported by the European Commission under contract BMH4-CT96-0845 in the BIOMED2 programme and the research grant KV/E/197 (Elastische Registratie voor Medische Toepassingen) of the FWO-Vlaanderen to Dirk Vandermeulen.

References

1. M. Tincher, C.R. Meyer, R. Gupta, and D.M. Williams. Polynomial modeling and reduction of RF body coil spatial inhomogeneity in MRI. *IEEE transactions on medical imaging*, 12(2):361–365, june 1993.
2. R.C. Gonzalez and R.E. Woods. *Digital Image Processing*. Addison-Wesley, 1993.
3. Benoit M. Dawant, Alex P. Zijdenbos, and Richard A. Margolin. Correction of intensity variations in MR images for computer-aided tissue classification. *IEEE transactions on medical imaging*, 12(4):770–781, december 1993.
4. C.R. Meyer, P.H. Bland, and J. Pipe. Retrospective correction of MRI amplitude inhomogeneities. In N. Ayache, editor, *Proc. CVRMed '96, Computer Vision, Virtual Reality, and Robotics in Medicine; Lecture Notes in Computer Science*, pages 513–522. Berlin, Germany: Springer–Verlag, 1995.
5. W.M. Wells, III, W.E.L. Grimson, R. Kikinis, and F.A. Jolesz. Adaptive segmentation of MRI data. *IEEE transactions on medical imaging*, 15(4):429–442, august 1996.
6. A. P. Dempster, N. M. Laird, and D. B. Rubin. Maximum likelihood from incomplete data via the EM algorithm. *J. Roy. Stat. Soc.*, 39:1–38, 1977.
7. K. Van Leemput, D. Vandermeulen, and P. Suetens. Automatic segmentation of brain tissues and MR bias field correction using a digital brain atlas. Technical Report KUL/ESAT/PSI/9806, ESAT/PSI, june 1998.
8. Evans A.C., Collins D.L., Mills S.R., Brown E.D., Kelly R.L., and Peters T.M. 3d statistical neuroanatomical models from 305 MRI volumes. In *Proc. IEEE Nuclear Science Symposium and Medical Imaging Conference*, pages 1813–1817, 1993.
9. F. Maes, A. Collignon, D. Vandermeulen, G. Marchal, and P. Suetens. Multimodality image registration by maximization of mutual information. *IEEE transactions on medical imaging*, 16(2):187–198, april 1997.
10. John Ashburner, Karl Friston, Andrew Holmes, and Jean-Baptiste Poline. *Statistical Parametric Mapping*. The Wellcome Department of Cognitive Neurology, University College London.

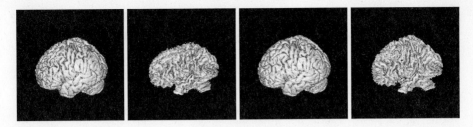

Fig. 2. 3D rendering of grey matter and white matter segmentations of a T1-weighted MR image of the head. From left to right: grey matter and white matter segmentation obtained with the EM algorithm without bias correction; grey matter and white matter segmentation obtained with the extended EM algorithm

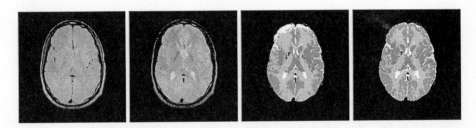

Fig. 3. Segmentation of multi-channel data. From left to right: PD and T2-weighted images, segmentation with the EM algorithm without bias correction and with the extended EM algorithm.

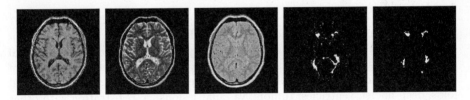

Fig. 4. MS lesion segmentation. From left to right: T1, T2, PD-weighted image, automatic lesion segmentation, manual segmentation

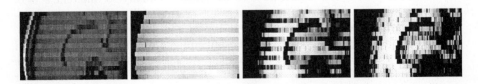

Fig. 5. An example of slice-per-slice offsets. From left to right: original data, estimated bias, white matter classification with the EM algorithm without bias correction and with the extended EM algorithm

Robust Brain Segmentation Using Histogram Scale-Space Analysis and Mathematical Morphology

J.-F. Mangin[1], O. Coulon[1,2], and V. Frouin[1]

[1] Service Hospitalier Frédéric Joliot, Département de Recherche Médicale, Direction des Sciences du Vivant, Commissariat à l'Énergie Atomique
E-mail: mangin@shfj.cea.fr, P-mail: place du Général Leclerc, 91406 Orsay, France
[2] Département Signal et Image, ENST Paris

Abstract. In this paper, we propose a robust fully non-supervised method dedicated to the segmentation of the brain in T1-weighted MR images. The first step consists in the analysis of the scale-space of the histogram first and second derivative. We show first that the crossings in scale-space of trajectories of extrema of different derivative orders follow regular topological properties. These properties allow us to design a new structural representation of a 1D signal. Then we propose an heuristics using this representation to infer statistics on grey and white matter grey level values from the histogram. These statistics are used by an improved morphological process combining two opening sizes to segment the brain. The method has been validated with 70 images coming from 3 different scanners and acquired with various MR sequences.

1 Introduction

Brain segmentation in magnetic resonance (MR) T1-weighted images has been one of the most addressed applications of image analysis in the field of medical imaging. Indeed, brain segmentation is usually a first step before detection of embedded anatomical or pathological structures (hemispheres, tissues, cortical folds, deep nuclei, ventricles, tumors, vascular lesions...), registration with other modalities or atlases, and 3D visualisation (neurosurgical planning, brain mapping...). A lot of methods have been proposed, but none of them has reached a level of robustness sufficient to be used routinely by clinicians. Usual methods rely on a few parameters which have to be tuned manually to different sets of acquisition parameters. In this paper we propose a new fully non supervised approach designed to assure a high quality result for a large range of MR sequences.

In the following, we assume that the only image which has been acquired is a 3D T1-weighted MR image covering most of the head. Situations where T2-weighted or proton-density images can also be used could lead to further developments integrating their additional discriminative power. We do not address such developments, first because such images are not always acquired due to timing considerations, second because slice thickness of T1-weighted images is usually much lower, finally because T1-weighted images are sufficient for our brain segmentation purpose.

The wide variety of methods proposed in literature to segment the brain in T1-weighted images can be browse according to the few recurrent schemes involved. It should be noted that a simple classification scheme based for instance on texture analysis is a priori not sufficient to solve the problem. Therefore, the more frequent approach consists in using mathematical morphology or region growing algorithms to discriminate the brain from the surrounding structures in a preclassified binary image [9,6]. Multi-resolution or scale-space analysis appears to be an interesting alternative to the previous scheme [11]. Other approaches relying on the deformable model paradigm seem to be more difficult to master mainly because of initialisation difficulties [10].

Our paper proposes several improvements of the mathematical morphology based scheme, which has been the most successful one. These improvements lead to a segmentation method robust for a large range of images. This method has been validated on a set of 70 images acquired on three different scanners using gradient-echo and inversion-recovery sequences with various parameters. In the next section, a rapid survey of the mathematical morphology based scheme will help us to catch some of its intrinsic weaknesses which will be overcome throughout the paper.

2 The classical scheme

2.1 Histogram analysis

The first step consists in binarizing the initial grey level image. All voxels which could belong to the brain are selected according to a range [Tlow,Thigh] of grey level values supposed to include grey matter and white matter tissues (cf. Fig. 1). This binarization aims at disconnecting as much as possible the brain from surrounding structures. The low threshold eliminates the cerebrospinal fluid (CSF) and the skull while the high threshold eliminates the fat and the vascular system. Since the MR signal do not correspond to an absolute measure of some physical property, both thresholds have to be tuned for each image. This adaptation is difficult to perform automatically because of large variations of the image contrast according to the MR sequence parameters (spin-echo, gradient-echo, inversion-recovery, echo time, repetition time, excitation number, slice thickness...) and according to the subjects (anatomy, pathologies...) (cf. Fig. 2).

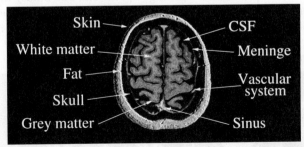

Fig. 1. *A simple description of the various head tissues observed in T1-weighted MR images.*

The only a priori knowledge on the MR signal nature which seems to be invariant across T1-weighted sequences is the relative positions of tissues along

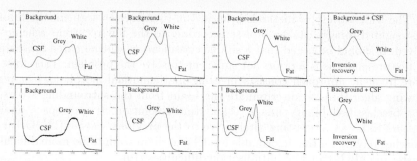

Fig. 2. *The histograms of 3D T1-weighted MR images turn out to be especially variable.*

the grey level scale. The first part of this paper proposes a fully non supervised process using this structural information to analyse the scale-space of the image histogram. This analysis gives statistical parameters on brain tissue grey levels from which is computed the binarization. Because the classical "finger print" analysis based on first derivative extrema fails for some configurations where grey and white matter are especially mixed, we have designed a new histogram mode detection method using the structure of the two first derivative extrema in the scale-space. Some crossings of extremum trajectories follow simple topological properties which help to analyse the scale-space structure according to a priori knowledge.

2.2 Morphological processing

Unfortunately, a reasonable estimation of the two thresholds is not always sufficient to assure a good behaviour of the segmentation process. Indeed, the quality of the result can be significantly lowered by a slight modification of the thresholds, especially the lowest one. Moreover, for some images, which can appear visually very good, not a pair of thresholds give acceptable segmentation. This instability is easy to understand from a description of the process (cf. Fig. 3).

In order to achieve a whole disconnection between the brain and the surrounding structures preserved by the binarization (with "good" thresholds: scalp, meninges, eyes, sinuses), different methods have been proposed. They all rely on the effect of the morphological "opening" operation. The binary image is eroded to cut the remaining connections. Then the largest or the more central 3D connected component is selected as a seed of the brain. Finally the brain shape is recovered by a geodesic dilation of the seed conditionally to the initial binary image (which is often related to region growing).

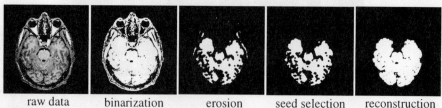

Fig. 3. *The classical morphological scheme to segment the brain in T1-weighted MR images.*

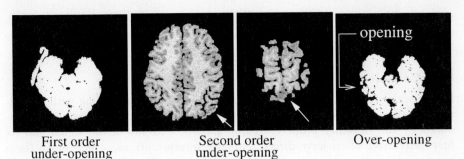

Fig. 4. *The classical morphological scheme (cf. Fig. 3) presents intrinsic weaknesses which can lead to three kinds of problems.*

The erosion and dilation structuring element diameters, like the two thresholds, influence largely the quality of the final result. Three kinds of failures can occur, sometimes simultaneously and with various amplitudes (cf. Fig. 4). First, the eyes or a large part of the scalp can be included in the brain segmentation which means that the erosion has not done its job, either because the binarization was too permissive or because the erosion diameter was too low. These situations will be called first order under-opening problems. Second, a part of the brain like a gyrus can be removed because of the opening effect of the erosion-dilation sequence. This can happen when the binarization is too selective or when the erosion diameter is too large. We will talk about over-opening problems. The unstability of the process stems from the two conflictual constraints imposed to the parameter choice by these two opposite kinds of problems. The domain of acceptable parameters can be especially narrow or even empty. Finally, the last kind of errors called second order under-opening problems correspond to connections with some small pieces of sinus or meninges. These problems are the more difficult to get completely rid of because they often occur when previous problems have been solved.

In this paper, the classical morphological process is modified in order to obtain a correct behaviour for a large parameter domain. A first modification relies on a simple regularization of the binarization. Then a two step geodesic reconstruction process restricts the opening effect potentially removing gyri to the smallest one. It should be noted that because of frequent non stationarities in MR images, simple thresholding operations are not always sufficient to get good binarizations for the whole brain. In the following, we assume that the amplitude of these non stationarities is slight, otherwise a preprocessing could be required which is beyond the scope of the paper [15].

3 1D scale-space analysis

In this section, we described the automatic analysis of the histogram scale-space which leads to an estimation of mean and standard deviations of grey and white matter grey levels. Each tissue class is represented by a specific histogram mode. The more important ones, which are related to background, CSF, grey matter, white matter, fat and vascular system, always appear with the same order along the grey scale (cf. Fig. 2). Various approaches have been proposed to deal with the detection of these modes, including K-means [6] and fit with a sum of Gaussians or with other a priori models [13]. Our own unsuccessful experiments with such methods when dealing with a wide set of sequence parameters led us to search for a more robust approach.

3.1 Cascades of singularities

Linear scale-space analysis is an appealing approach when dealing with 1D signals because of the surprisingly simple geometry of extremum trajectories induced by the causality property [16, 5]. Indeed, extrema of the signal and its first derivatives often have direct semantic interpretations, which make them good candidates for deriving structural descriptions. Usual approaches rely only on extrema of one single derivative. For instance, finger prints stem from first derivative extrema [16] while blob based primal sketches stem from signal (or Laplacian) extrema [7, 2]. Finger print based analysis has been proposed to initialise the decomposition of 1D signals in mixtures of Gaussians [1, 4]. In the case of MR image histograms, the Gaussian hypothesis may appear justified at first glance. In fact such an hypothesis does not take into account partial volume effect, signal non stationarities, Gibbs artefacts, subject motions and other MRI specific artefacts. Therefore, to get a more robust approach, we make the histogram mode detection rely directly on histogram scale-space.

The goal of our analysis is the detection of grey and white matter modes. Because these two neighboring modes can be especially mixed, histogram and first derivative extrema are not sufficient in all cases to detect them (cf. Fig. 5). Simple experiments with sums of Gaussians will show that higher derivatives have a better detection power in such situations.

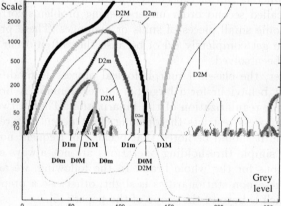

Fig. 5. *The derivative extrema of a histogram (D0) and its two first derivatives (D1 and D2) in the scale-space. DiM denotes a maximum while Dim denotes a minimum. Grey and white matter modes are too mixed to be detected from D0 and D1 extrema. In return, D2 extrema reveal the mixture.*

Straightforward considerations on 1D functions with zero values on their domain bounds lead to the recursive property that N extrema in the ith derivative implies at least $(N+1)$ nested extrema in the $(i+1)^{th}$ derivative. Thus one single Gaussian leads to one signal extremum, two first derivative extrema, three second derivative extrema, etc (cf. Fig. 6). These extrema can be tracked

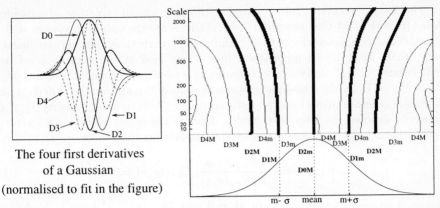

Fig. 6. *The derivative extrema of a binarized Gaussian in the scale-space computed from heat equation. DiM denotes a maximum while Dim denotes a minimum of the ith derivative. Extrema which do not reach scale 100 have not been tracked.*

throughout the scale-space (cf. Fig. 6). The sum of two Gaussians lead to different extremum patterns according to their relative localizations, amplitudes, means and standard deviations. Intuitively, when the two Gaussians are sufficiently distant from each other, the pattern of the sum extrema corresponds to the juxtaposition of two single Gaussian extrema patterns. When the Gaussians are brought closer to each other, some extrema disappear. For very closed Gaussians, the sum extrema pattern differs from the single Gaussian extrema pattern only for high derivative extrema.

Because of the nature of the linear scale-space, which amounts to convolutions with Gaussians (the Gaussian is the Green function of the heat equation), a sum of two Gaussians remains a sum of two Gaussians throughout the whole scale-space. Therefore, since smoothing the sum is similar to bringing the two Gaussians "closer" to each other (while increasing their standard deviations), the structure of the sum extrema trajectories in the scale-space corresponds to a sequence of extremum extinction (cf. Fig. 7). These extinctions, which are the well known singularities related to scale-space bifurcations [7], follow a simple rule giving rise to what we will call singularity cascades.

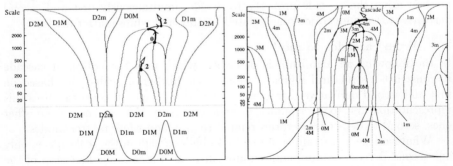

Fig. 7. *The derivative extrema of the sum of two Gaussians in the scale-space giving rise to cascades of singularities (left: two cascades of order 0 and 2 are shown, right: the cascade of order 0 is followed until the singularity of order 4).*

The simple syntactic rule leading to the nice nested structure of cascades stems from the fact that the order i singularities are the only locations in scale-space where the trajectories of the ith and $(i+1)^{th}$ derivative extrema can "meet" each other. This can be understood first if one look at the expression of the drift velocity of a ith derivative extremum under scale-space smoothing. Let D_i : $\mathbb{R}_+ \times \mathbb{R}_+ \to \mathbb{R}$ be the scale-space representation of the histogram i^{th} derivative. In non-degenerate situations, an estimate of a D_i extremum velocity $v_i(g, s)$ (where g denotes the grey level and s denotes the scale) along its trajectory defined by $D_{i+1}(g, s) = 0$, is given by the implicit function theorem [7]:

$$v_i(g, s) = -\frac{1}{2} \frac{D_{i+3}(g, s)}{D_{i+2}(g, s)}, D_{i+1}(g, s) = 0. \tag{1}$$

Hence, a crossing between $D_{i+1}(g, s) = 0$ and $D_{i+2}(g, s) = 0$ would lead to a degenerate situation where the drift velocity tends to infinity. Therefore singularities of order i are the only locations where such trajectories can meet.

Second, since at least one extremum of the $(i + 1)^{th}$ derivative has to exist between a pair of minimum and maximum of the ith derivative at every scale where this pair exists, one $(i + 1)^{th}$ derivative extremum trajectory is bound to cross a pair extinction. Then, the structure of extinctions of Fig. 7 is invariant whatever the two Gaussian parameters are, namely one cascade of order 0 linking singularities of order 0, 1, 2 and more (cf. Fig. 7), one cascade of order 2 linking singularities of order 2 and more, and higher order cascades which do not appear in the figures.

Previous observations on singularity cascades lead to the conclusion that the mixture of two histogram modes can be untangled if high derivative extrema are used. Indeed, the mixture of very close modes will simply lead to cascades of higher order than usual. With MRI histograms, second derivative extrema turn out to be sufficient to deal with the grey and white matter mode detection for all the configurations in our database.

If we assume now that a MRI histogram mode is relatively symmetric, a good estimation of its mean value is provided by the related second derivative minima. Then, an estimation of standard deviation can be derived from the neighboring first derivative extrema (cf. Fig. 6). Therefore, we have devised a method using the cascade property to detect simultaneously first and second derivative extremum trajectories related to grey and white matter modes.

3.2 From cascades to modes

In the following an algorithm is described which uses the notion of cascade to construct a structural representation of the histogram scale-space based on first and second derivative extremum trajectories. Then, an heuristics uses this representation first to discriminate inversion-recovery MR sequences from other ones, second to detect trajectories related to grey and white matter modes.

Whatever the histogram is, if one looks high enough in the scale-space, only one second derivative minimum remains alive (cf. Fig. 6). The first step of the process consists in computing the scale-space of the histogram first and second derivatives until the first scale where only one second derivative minimum exists. This is done using the usual discretization of heat equation [7]. Then all extrema reaching a minimum scale (in practice 5) are tracked from their extinction scale until scale zero. The different trajectories are gathered in families corresponding to the cascade notion. "Maximum/minimum" couples of trajectories of the same order mating in a singularity are detected first. Then each order 1 singularity leads to a link between one order 1 couple and one order 2 couple. Two kinds of families are obtained: "full ones" include two couples and "childless ones" include only one order 2 couple. Finally the few trajectories reaching the maximum scale are gathered in the "infinity family" (cf. Fig. 8).

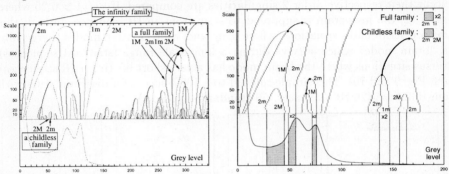

Fig. 8. *First and second derivative extremum trajectories are gathered in three kinds of families (left). Each family is endowed with a volume (right).*

We assume now that a histogram mode can have different signatures in the scale-space according to its surrounding. A dominant mode will lead in the lowest scales to a signature similar to the Gaussian signature of Fig. 6, namely a hand-shaped 5-uplet of trajectories $SG = (D2M, D1M, D2m, D1m, D2M)$. In case of competition between modes, only partial signatures appear which simply means that the initial scale was to high to unravel the full signatures. Since we can not compute the missing part of the scale-space because of the well-known unstability of the inversed heat equation, we have to cope with these partial signatures [12].

Full or partial signatures of the modes of interest will be reconstituted step by step. First, the few families supposed to include the central $D2m$ trajectories of these signatures will be selected, all other families being removed. Then all remaining trajectories are ordered according to their location at scale 0. This operation leads to a sequence in which full and partial signatures are detected by a simple pattern matching method using the signature SG as model. The $D2m$ trajectories represent seeds to which are added other trajectories if the SG sequence is respected.

The crucial part of the process is the initial family selection, which includes an automatic discrimination between inversion-recovery (IR) sequences and other ones because of the very different nature of both kinds of histograms (cf. Fig. 2).

All families apart from the infinity one are sorted according to what will be called the "family volume", which is a rough measure of importance (cf. Fig. 8). It should be noted that the highest scale reached by a family is not a good selection criterion because it depends only on mode surrounding. Therefore, extrema stemming from grey level highest values can survive a very long time in the scale-space (cf. Fig. 8).

We assume that two types of families exist, which are related to the two cascades of Fig. 7. Those which are related to the order 0 cascade include the $D2m$ trajectory of one specific histogram mode. They can be full or childless. The other families, related to order 2 cascade of Fig. 7 are just bringing the $D2M$ trajectories required to complete the signatures. They are necessarily childless. A family volume corresponds to the integral of the histogram over a specific range which is illustrated in Fig. 8.

The two biggest families are selected. Then the two scales $s1$ and $s2$ where occur their respective order 2 singularities are compared. If $s2/s1 > 0.25$ where $s1 > s2$, the histogram is supposed to stem from an IR sequence. Indeed, this ratio discriminates situations where grey and white matter modes merge into a "brain mode" which survive during a long scale range (standard sequences) versus situations where the brain mode has a very short life time (IR sequences) (cf. Fig. 9 and 10). This simple rule led to a 100% successful discrimination with our database (20 IR sequences, 50 standard sequences).

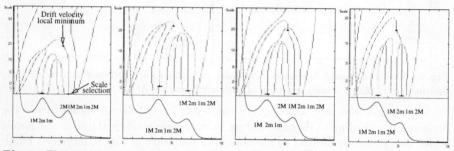

Fig. 9. *The signatures and scale selections of grey and white matter modes in four different histograms stemming from Inversion Recovery MR sequences.*

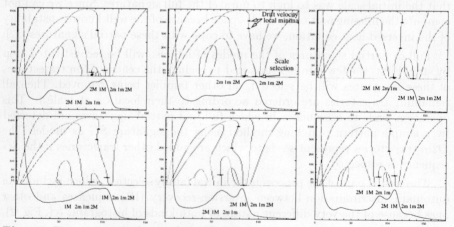

Fig. 10. *The signatures and scale selections of grey and white matter modes in six different histograms stemming from standard T1-weighted MR sequences.*

Then, in the IR situation, the pattern matching algorithm previously described is applied to the trajectory set made up by the infinity family and the two biggest families. This analysis provides the grey and white matter signatures (cf. Fig. 9).

In the other situations, a first signature analysis is applied to the trajectory set made up by the infinity family and the family endowed with the highest order 2 singularity in scale-space. This first analysis provides the "brain mode" signature. Then two new families are added to the trajectory set. The first one is selected as the highest family (once again highest means highest order 2 singularity in scale-space) which $loc_0(D2m)$ is located in the range $[loc_0(D1M_{brain}), loc_0(D1m_{brain})]$, where $D1i_{brain}$ denotes order 1 trajectories belonging to the brain mode signature and loc_0 denotes location at 0 scale. The second one is selected as the highest family which $loc_0(D2m)$ is located in the range $[loc_0(D1m_{background}), loc_0(D1M_{brain})]$. Finally a second analysis is applied with this four family set which provides the grey and white matter signatures (cf. Fig. 10).

3.3 Scale selection

In this section, we describe how mean and standard deviation of a mode are estimated from its signature. Scale selection is one major problem of linear scale-space analysis, mainly because the hypothesis that an extremum trajectory in scale-space arises from a single event is rarely true. Therefore, the simple "select at high scale and track until lowest scale" strategy is far from being sufficient. Intuitively, at highest scales extrema are related to a mixture of modes (like the brain) while at lowest scales they are related to noise or minor histogram modes. We propose an heuristics based on local minima of the second derivative minimum drift absolute velocity. This particular points turn out to be especially similar from histogram to histogram which make them good candidates to develop a new kind of primal sketch (cf. Fig. 9 and 10), but such an approach is beyond the scope of this paper. Our heuristics stems from the idea that extremum trajectories alternate periods of high drift velocity with periods of stability which could be related to scale ranges where they are catched by some underlying event. It should be noted that drift velocity minima are also strongly related to crossings between order i and order $(i+2)$ trajectories, which can be understood from Eq. 1 (cf. Fig. 7).

Using Eq. 1 to detect velocity minima leads to bad results induced by trajectory discretization effect. Therefore we have developed a more robust approach which inferred drift velocity estimations with discrete computations. The trajectory is considered has a sequence of segments of constant abcisse. Then each segment is endowed with a velocity inversely proportional to its length. Finally, using also velocity sign, all absolute velocity minima are detected.

This method provides the points pointed out in Fig. 9 and 10. Then, the scale s_{mode} from which is estimated a mode mean value is given by the first local minimum of the drift velocity appearing along the $D2m_{mode}$ trajectory under the lowest order 2 singularity of the whole family set. Finally, the two "standard deviations" are estimated from the $D1M_{grey}$ and $D1m_{white}$ trajectories, which always exist.

The whole histogram analysis algorithm has been applied with success on the 70 histograms of our database. The analysis takes less than one second on a standard sparc station.

4 Morphological process

Now, we propose briefly an improved morphological process qualitatively robust to small variations of the values extracted from the histogram.

4.1 Regularized binarization

The first step of the process consists in a regularized binarization. The regularizing effect is classically obtained from the classical Markovian approach relying on Ising model [3,9]. The closing effect on the binarization allows us to use a relatively selective low threshold $m_G - 2\sigma_G$. This improves the effect of the following erosion and reduces the risk of first order under opening (cf. Fig. 4). It should be noted that the regularization is restricted to a range of grey levels which limits the risk of creating thick connections between the brain and the surrounding tissues (meninges, sinus, skull marrow).

4.2 Brain segmentation

In order to reduce over-opening effects often induced by the standard morphological process (cf. Fig. 3, 4), we propose to combine two morphological openings related to two different structuring element diameters. The largest opening $\mathcal{O}_l$ will have to fully disconnect the brain from surrounding tissues, leading to the brain seed. The smallest opening $\mathcal{O}_s$ will have to define the final brain shape, which means mainly removing meninges and noise. The whole process can be summarized as follows:

- Apply $\mathcal{O}_s$ opening to binarization B to get object $\mathcal{O}_s(B)$ (structuring element: 26-neighbourhood);
- Apply 3mm erosion to $\mathcal{O}_s(B)$ (structuring element: 3mm radius ball) [8];
- Select largest 26-connected component as brain seed S;
- Compute geodesic chamfer distance to S conditionally to $\mathcal{O}_s(B)$ (denoted $d(S)$)n;
- Threshold the previous distance to get brain complement $T_{>8mm}(d(S))$;
- Dilate brain complement conditionally to $T_{>4mm}(d(S))$ until convergence;
- Removes the dilation result from $T_{<=8mm}(d(S))$ to get the final brain segmentation.

The largest opening $\mathcal{O}_l$ is related to the 3mm radius ball structuring element, which is defined from a chamfer distance adapted to the voxel anisotropy [8]. This choice makes the opening effect of $\mathcal{O}_l$ independent of the voxel geometry. The 26-neighborhood has been chosen for $\mathcal{O}_s$ to assure a minimum opening effect in all directions whatever the voxel geometry is. Geodesic chamfer distances are efficiently implemented using a thick front propagation [14].

The whole segmentation has been applied to the 70 images of our database (40 healthy subjects/30 epileptic subjects involved in a neurosurgery protocol). The process takes about one minute on standard sparc stations. In 68 cases, the process was globally successfull apart from some second order under-opening errors in a few cases and slight over-opening errors in temporal lobes for one specific MR sequence with non-homogeneities (see. Fig. 4). For one of the remaining cases, the $\mathcal{O}_l$ structuring element radius had to be increased to 4mm to get a good result. The last case was presenting large non-homogeneities which call for a preprocessing step [15].

5 Conclusion

We have proposed a robust fully non-supervised method to segment the brain in T1-weighted MR images. Hence, this method can now be considered as a reliable preprocessing before more sophisticated image analysis approaches. The statistics inferred from the histogram can be used for other segmentation purposes when the contrast between grey and white matter is of interest. The scale-space based approach proposed in this paper could be used to analyse other kinds of histograms. Finally, the extension of the cascade notion to higher dimension signals would be very interested but the question appears rather involved at first glance.

References

1. M. J. Carlotto. Histogram analysis using a scale-space approach. *IEEE PAMI*, 9(1):121–129, 1987.
2. O. Coulon, I. Bloch, V. Frouin, and J.-F. Mangin. Multiscale measures in linear scale-space for characterizing cerebral functional activations. In *Scale-Space'97, Utrecht*, number 1252 in LNCS, Springer, pp. 188–199, 1997.
3. S. Geman and D. Geman. Stochastic relaxation, Gibbs distributions and the Bayesian restoration of images. *IEEE PAMI*, 6(6):721–741, 1984.
4. A. Goshtasby and W. D. O'Neil. Curve fitting by a sum of Gaussians. *CVGIP: Graphical Models and Image Processing*, 56(4):281–288, 1994.
5. J.J. Koenderink. The structure of images. *Biol. Cybernetics*, 50:363–370, 1984.
6. F. Kruggel and G. Lohmann. Automatical adaption of the stereotactical coordinate system in brain MRI datasets. In *XVth IPMI, Poultney, USA*, pages 470–476, 1997.
7. T. Lindeberg. *Scale-space theory in computer vision*. Kluwer, 1994.
8. J.-F. Mangin, I. Bloch, J. Lopez-Krahe, and V. Frouin. Chamfer distances in anisotropic 3D images. In *VII Europ. Signal Proces. Conf.*, pp 975–978, 1994.
9. J.-F. Mangin, V. Frouin, I. Bloch, J. Regis, and J. López-Krahe. From 3D magnetic resonance images to structural representations of the cortex topography using topology preserving deformations. *J. Math. Imag. Vision*, 5(4):297–318, 1995.
10. T. McInerney and D. Terzopoulos. Deformable models in medical image analysis: a survey. *Medical Image Analysis*, 1(2):91–108, 1996.
11. W. J. Niessen, K. L. Vincken, and M. A. Viergever. Comparison of multiscale representations for a linking-based image segmentation model. In *IEEE/SIAM MMBIA, San Francisco*, pp. 263–272, 1996.
12. I. Pollak, A. S. Willsky, and H. Krim. Scale space analysis by stabilized inverse diffusion equation. In *Scale-Space'97*, LNCS-1252, Springer, pp. 200–211, 1997.
13. L. Vérard, P. Allain, J.-M. Travère, J. C. Baron, and D. Bloyet. Fully automatic identification of AC and PC landmarks on brain MRI using scene analysis. *IEEE TMI*, pages 610–616, 1997.
14. B. J. H. Verwer, P. W. Verbeek, and S. T. Dekker. An efficient uniform cost algorithm applied to distance transforms. *IEEE PAMI*, 11(4):425–428, 1989.
15. W. M. Wells III, W. E. L. Grimson, R. Kikinis, and F. A. Jolesz. Adaptive segmentation of MRI data. *IEEE TMI*, 15(4):429–442, 1996.
16. A.P. Witkin. Scale-space filtering. In *International Joint Conference on Artificial Intelligence*, pages 1019–1023, 1983.

Vascular Shape Segmentation and Structure Extraction Using a Shape-Based Region-Growing Model

Yoshitaka Masutani, Thomas Schiemann and Karl-Heinz Höhne

Institute of Mathematics and Computer Science in Medicine (IMDM),
University Hospital Hamburg - Eppendorf
Martinistr. 52, 20246 Hamburg, Germany
Tel. +49-40-4717-3652, Fax. +49-40-4717-4882
masutani@uke.uni-hamburg.de

Abstract. A new, practical, and efficient approach is proposed for 3D vascular segmentation and bifurcation structure extraction. The method uses a combination of mathematical morphology, region-growing schemes, and shape features in addition to greyscale information. By an extension of math-morphological operations within bounded space of vascular shape, smooth and natural region-growing and sensitivity-controllable bifurcation detection were realized. The algorithm was implemented in the interactive segmentation and visualization software package VOXEL-MAN and validated with clinical data of X-ray CT angiography and MRA.

Introduction

Segmentation is one of the most important and difficult procedures in medical image analysis and in its clinical application, and blood vessels are especially difficult to segment. Except for large structures like the abdominal aorta, even visualization is not as easy as for other organs. Additional structural information is often required for special purposes beyond visualization and segmentation, for example construction of a structured vascular atlas [Pommert94], functional analysis of blood supply [Hoehne95], or navigation of catheters for endovascular treatment [Masutani97]. These procedures need information like bifurcation structure or radii of blood vessels. As seen in several reports, common methods for obtaining such information are usually based on three-dimensional thinning algorithms [Tsao81][Malandain93][Szekely94]. However, these thinning-based approaches fail to manage abnormal vessel structures like aneurysms which are important in clinical routine. Preliminary separation of such objects from vessels [Masutani95] is suitable to measure their volumes, however the relationship between them (e.g. neck shape of aneurysm) is spoiled.

The most serious problem in thinning is that such algorithms try to keep topology of original objects. Therefore, segmentation procedures must be carefully carried out to get topologically correct vascular shapes. However, practically, this is too hard to achieve without any manual correction or compilation. The main reason for such difficulties is low resolution of current medical imaging modalities regarding the size of blood vessels. This causes partial volume effects which connect vascular structures to other organs like bones in X-ray CT. In case of MRA (Magnetic Resonance Angiography), flow-void, which is lack of signals in vessels, often causes disconnection of extracted vascular objects. Therefore, it is almost impossible to solve these problems without any a priori knowledge. For such reasons, recent methods using deformable models are promising for relatively larger structures like brains or livers. Because these methods originally assume and utilize global smoothness of the target objects. However, blood vessels are not globally smooth and have bifurcation structures. Recent reports by McInerney [McInerny97] showed an improvement for such drawback by a more flexible deformable model.

Our goal is to obtain structured vascular shape with minimum interaction for constructing a digital atlas, image-guided surgery, and so on. For these purposes, vascular structures must be separated in groups of vessel branches and abnormal structures. Therefore, we developed a region (voxel)-based approach for the convenience of bifurcation analysis. In this paper, we propose a new model based on region-growing controlled by math-morphological information of local shape, which has the ability of topological correction.

Materials and Methods

1. Overview

Our method for vascular shape segmentation and structure extraction consists of two parts. First, the initial shape is acquired by thresholding. Then, region-growing is processed basically in the space limited by the initial shape. Structural information of the shape is simultaneously obtained. The region grows while avoiding non-vessel regions and keeps its local smoothness based on math-morphological information and local shape processing. In the next two sections, details of math-morphological information and local math-morphological shape processing are described.

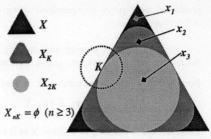

$X_{nK} = \phi \ (n \geq 3)$

$x_1 \in X, x_1 \notin X_K, x_1 \notin X_{2K} \Leftrightarrow S_m(x_1, X, K) = 1$
$x_2 \in X, x_2 \in X_K, x_2 \notin X_{2K} \Leftrightarrow S_m(x_2, X, K) = 2$
$x_3 \in X, x_3 \in X_K, x_3 \in X_{2K} \Leftrightarrow S_m(x_3, X, K) = 3$

Fig. 1. Computation example of morphological size

2. Mathematical morphology

Mathematical morphology is a well-known theory for structure analysis and processing of binary shapes [Robert87]. Most math-morphological operations and analysis methods can be defined in terms of the basic operations erosion, dilation, closing and opening. One of the most important characteristics of them is controllability of their results by size and shape of a filter kernel (structuring element). A math-morphological quantity, called morphological size, is used in our region-growing model. It is an attribute of voxels which belong to an object. Distribution of morphological size in a shape is called pattern spectrum [Maragos89] to represent the characteristics of the whole shape.

Let x denote a voxel in a shape X, K a kernel for opening and nK, the n-scaled kernel of K. Morphological size of a voxel x, $S_m(x, X, K)$ is defined as:

$$S_m(x, X, K) = \min\{n \mid x \in X, x \notin X_{nK}\} \quad (n \geq 1) \tag{1}$$

where X_K reperesent the shape of X opened by K. That is, morphological size of a voxel in an object means the minimum size of kernels which can remove the voxel from the shape by opening operation (Fig.1). It represents local thickness of the object at the position of voxel x.

3. Mathematical morphology in bounded space

Math-morphological operations are usually performed in unlimited space. In this paper, an extension of these operations in bounded space is introduced to generalize region growth and to process the shape of its growth-front. Beside X and K, give a constant boundary shape B which is never changed by any operations and let B^C be its complement. The two most fundamental operations, dilation and erosion are defined as follows:

Bounded space dilation of a shape X in B by K:

$$X \bullet_B K = X_N = (X_{N-1} \bullet \tilde{K}) \cap B = \ldots \quad \bullet : \textit{original dilation} \tag{2}$$

$$X_i = (X_{i-1} \bullet \tilde{K}) \cap B, \quad X_0 = X, \quad \tilde{K} = \frac{1}{N} K$$

Bounded space erosion of a shape X in B by K:

$$X \circ_B K = ((X^c \cap B) \bullet_B K)^c \cap B \tag{3}$$

N must be large enough to avoid jump and diffraction of growing as shown in Fig.2. In discrete space, the radius of $\tilde{K}$ is 1.

Most properties of original dilation and erosion, such as translation invariability, distributivity, local knowledge, and increasing are kept in bounded space extension while iterativity is not. Regarding the definition of bounded space dilation, our previous approach [Masutani96] prohibited only jump of operations using a connectivity filter. This new method also restricts diffraction of growing.

Like original closing and opening, bounded space versions of closing and opening are defined by combinations of the above operations:

Bounded space closing of a shape X in B by K:

$$^{B}X^{K} = (X \bullet_{B} K) \circ_{B} K \tag{4}$$

Bounded space opening of a shape X in B by K:

$$^{B}X_{K} = (X \circ_{B} K) \bullet_{B} K \tag{5}$$

They also have smoothing effects on shapes. Two interesting properties for smoothing are convex-filling (closing only) and growth-front smoothing as shown in Fig.3. Zahlten proposed a method [Zahlten95] similar to our model and reported that a growth-front sometimes becomes oblique to its growing direction after going through narrow and curved parts of bounded space. Bounded space closing or opening with a kernel of relatively large size tries to modify such an oblique front perpendicular to the growing direction. As shown in Fig.3(a), the kernel radius must be larger than the width of the narrow structure to get obvious smoothing effect. The convex-filling property shown in Fig.3(b) is important to control the sensitivity of the bifurcation detection. This property is explained in the next section with a simplified example.

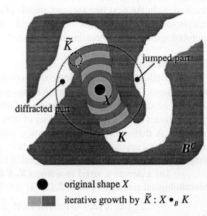

Fig. 2. Bounded space dilation (N=6)

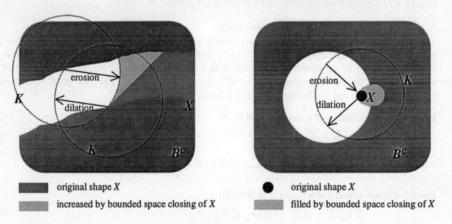

Fig. 3. Properties of bounded space closing. Growth-front smoothing (left) and convex filling (right)

4. Description of the algorithm

(a) Initial shape acquisition

A thresholding operation is performed to get an initial binary shape. Except for blood vessels, it may include other structures like bone, and some vessels may be connected to other vessels, or may be partially disconnected (Fig.4). Threshold values (minimum and maximum) should be interactively adjusted to minimize the need for correction by the following processing.

(b) Seed definition

A seed is positioned, which defines the starting shape for iterative dilation in bounded space.

(c) Shape-based region-growing model

The model iterates basically two processes, simple growing and growth-front smoothing. The former is bounded space dilation and the latter is bounded space closing, both with different kernels. Other optional processes and growing conditions for certain purposes are defined in section (d).

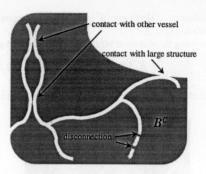

Fig. 4. Example of initial shape

A compact set of voxels, which belong to the same growth generation, is defined as a cluster, which is an unit of iterative growth (Fig.5). C_0 denotes a seed voxel (or region), and C_1 is a differential regions after the first growth step. If voxels after bounded space dilation are disconnected, these regions must be distinguished as individual clusters. This situation defines bifurcation. Therefore, for an initial boundary shape B, clusters grow as:

$$\bigcup_{i=0}^{m} C_{n+i} = \left\{ (\bigcup_{i=0}^{n-1} C_i) \bullet_B K_G \right\}^{K_S} \quad (n \geq 1, m \geq 0) \tag{6}$$

where m is summation of bifurcation, K_G and K_S are kernels for simple-growing and growth-front smoothing respectively.

During iterative cluster generation, attributes of clusters are measured (e.g. volume, growing direction, center of gravity, morphological size and connectivity to other clusters).

(d) Optional growing configuration

-morphological size upper limitation

We used the morphological size computed with a spherical kernel radius 1 as an attribute similar to greyscale values. Similar to conventional region-growing, morphological size is used for limitation of the growing process. Note that this condition is not applied in growth-front smoothing. This operation prevents clusters from explosive growing into connected large structures.

-object boundary opening of clusters

This operation is used to neglect thin contacts of a cluster with other structures (Fig.6). It is realized by conventional opening. However, erosion and dilation must be from/to object boundary not from/to cluster boundary. Therefore, a cluster C processed by object boundary opening C_K is:

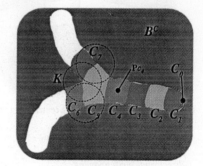

C_i : i-th cluster

P_c: cluster's center of gravity

Fig. 5. Shape-based region-growing model

$$C_K = C \cap B_K \tag{7}$$

where B is a boundary shape and K is a kernel.

-directional growing

The kernel shape for simple growing K should be spherical so that it can grow in any direction

uniformly. However, if a kernel is directional and its direction is controlled by the growing direction,
growing skips several bifurcation structures (Fig.7). A directional version of K in a direction v, K_v is:

$$K_v(t) = \{y \mid y \in K, \frac{y}{|y|} \cdot \frac{v}{|v|} \geq t\} \quad (-1 \leq t \leq 1) \tag{8}$$

where t is a threshold value for the dot product and therefore $K_v(-1.0)=K$.

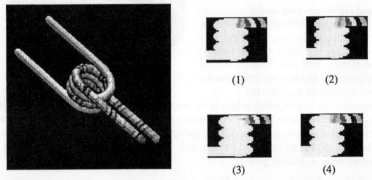

Fig. 6. Neglecting thin contact by cluster opening (synthetic data). The whole shape and final result are shown (left). Clusters are painted in repeated 12 gray tones. The procedure of cluster opening is shown (right). From a cluster (1), the region grows over thin contact (2). By erosion of the cluster and the region, the contact is removed and the disconnected region is removed (3). Dilation recovers the thickness of the clusters (4).

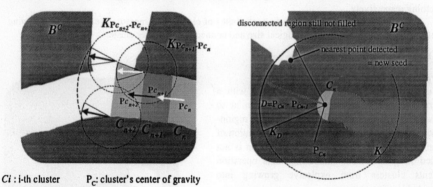

Ci : i-th cluster P_c: cluster's center of gravity

Fig. 7. Directional growing   Fig. 8. Directional jump growing from an end cluster

-directional jump growing
If no region grows after several iterations, clusters with connectivity number 1 try to grow out of the initial shape. This means that local ends try to establish connections to other regions (Fig.8), which have not been filled before. These ends search disconnected regions with a directional kernel. If such regions are detected, a new seed is thrown to continue further growing. This process is iterated until no disconnected region is detected.

(e) Control of kernel sizes and shapes
Basically, kernel shapes are spherical both for simple growing and growth-front smoothing. Since the size of the growing kernel K_G controls the length of the clusters in their growth directions, the kernel radius should be 1. Otherwise, in the final process described in section (f), certain quantization effects of branch grouping are observed. However, for the kernels with radius 1 of digital spherical shape, directional control is difficult. Therefore, directional kernels should have relatively

larger radius (about 5 voxels). The radius of the growth-front smoothing kernel controls the sensitivity of the bifurcation detection. With smaller kernels, smaller convex shapes are detected as bifurcation. As shown in Fig.8(a), a convex part of a vascular shape is detected as bifurcation, if a growth-front smoothing kernel does not completely fill the convex structure in the bounded space dilation process when the growth-front reached the boundary to separate the rest of the shape into two parts. While this bifurcation detection property depends on the width W and the length L of the convex shape, it is obvious and interesting that it is independent of the local width D of the main branch, if the kernel size is constant.

In our model, the radius of the kernel is adaptively set as the width of the previous cluster in order to smooth the growth-front. The cluster width is defined as double of its morphological size. Therefore, convex shapes with width 1 and length smaller than D are not detected as bifurcations. Fig.8(b) shows examples of neglected convex shapes.

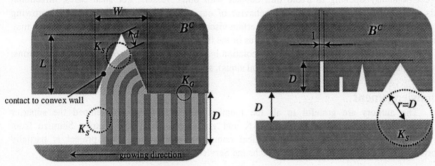

If d > radius of Ks, bifurcation is detected.

Fig. 8. Bifurcation detection control. (a) an example of bifurcation detection (left) (b) examples of neglected convex shapes in the case of r = D (right)

(f) Cluster grouping (Constructing branches)

Finally, a set of clusters with their connection graph is obtained as an extracted shape. To make anatomically relevant information, i.e. sets of branches or other structures, clusters are grouped based on their attributes. Making branches is realized by grouping of clusters according to their connectivity number. A branch is defined as a set of connected clusters, which have connectivity numbers smaller than 3. Those branches can be further divided into several groups according to their growing directions. Other connected clusters with irregularly larger volumes are also grouped, e.g. abnormal structures like aneurysms.

Results

This algorithm was implemented within the segmentation section [Schiemann92] of the software VOXEL-MAN [Hoehne95]. Except for initial shape acquisition and seed definition, users select one of the modes for optional processing described above. The growth termination condition is also variable. For example, if bifurcation detection is set as condition, it functions as a single branch grabber tool. Other conditions are limitation of total volume, cluster volume or generation of growth.

Interactive segmentation of cerebral blood vessel structures was performed on clinical data from phase contrast MRA (matrix size:256x256x240) and X-ray CT angiography (256x256x90). In Fig.10, an initial shape was obtained from MRA, and clusters were grouped into branches in different colors (12 colors repeated). For X-ray CT data, a vessel, which contacted with the skull bone was extracted using limitation of morphological size between 1 and 3 (Fig.11).

Discussion and Summary

Based on the extension of mathematical morphology to bounded space, a new model for segmentation and structure extraction of vascular shapes was proposed. By theoretical investigation and clinical application, new features of the model, like quantitative bifurcation detection, its sensitivity control and topological correction of vascular shapes were shown.

As it is often discussed, conventional thinning algorithms yield noisy branches due to high sensitivity to convex shape. One of the important properties of our model is controllability of the bifurcation detection by the size of the growth-front smoothing kernel. The definition of sensitivity for bifurcation gave reasonable results for cerebral vascular shapes.

In our results, any line structure enhancement filters were not employed. Such filters may contribute to a reduction of disconnection in the initial shape. As shown in detail by Sato [Sato98], however, false responses like connection between adjacent vessels spoil small structures. We also investigated response properties for other situations like contact with bone and non-vessel like structures (e.g. aneurysms) to conclude that more improvement is needed for our purpose.

In cerebral arteries, some vessels are less than three voxels in diameter. This is critical for use of object boundary opening to avoid thin contact with other vessels. For such cases, directional kernels showed better performance. The behavior of our model, especially with optional growing conditions can be compared to a fluid with a certain viscosity. Use of parameters in such analogy may give a better user-interface than the kernel radius or the threshold for dot products.

Future work will address shape interpolation between end clusters and disconnected regions. For non-circular sections of vessels (e.g. sagittal sinus), shapes of end clusters should be utilized.

Acknowledgement

The authors are grateful to all the members in IMDM, who developed the superior visualization software package VOXEL-MAN and guest researcher Dr. Akinobu Shimizu from Nagoya University, Japan for giving practical comments and advice. This project is partially supported by DAAD (German Academic Exchange Service).

References

[Pommert94] A. Pommert, et al. Symbolic Modeling of Human Anatomy for Visualization and Simulation, SPIE Vol. 2359, Proc. of Visualization on Biomedical Computing (VBC) '94, pp412-423, 1994

[Hoehne95] K. H. Höhne, et al. A new representation of knowledge concerning human anatomy and function, Nature Medicine, Vol.1, No. 6, 1995

[Masutani97] Y. Masutani, et al. Interactive Virtualized Display System for Intravascular Neurosurgery, LNCS Vol. 1205, Proc. of CVRMed (Computer Vision Virtual Reality and Robotics in Medicine) '97, pp427-434, 1997

[McInerney97] T. McInerney, et al. Medical image segmentation using topologically adaptable surfaces, LNCS Vol. 1205, Proc. of CVRMed'97, pp23-32, 1997

[Szekely94] G. Szekely, et al. Structural description and combined 3-D display for superior analysis of cerebral vascularity from MRA, SPIE Vol. 2359, Proc. VBC'94, pp272-281, 1994

[Tsao81] Y. F. Tsao, et al. A Parallel Thinning Algorithm for 3-D Pictures, Computer Graphics and Image Processing Vol.17, 1981 pp315-331

[Malandain93] G. Malandain, et al. Topological segmentation of discrete surfaces, International Journal of Computer Vision, Vol.10, No.2, pp183-197, 1993

[Masutani95] Y. Masutani, et al. Quantitative Vascular Shape Analysis for 3D MR-Angiography Using Mathematical Morphology, LNCS Vol. 905, Proc. CVRMed '95, pp449-454, 1995

[Robert87] M. Robert, et al. Image Analysis Using Mathematical Morphology, IEEE trans. Pattern Analysis and Machine Intelligence, Vol. PAMI-9, No. 4, pp532-550, 1987

[Maragos89] P. Maragos, et al. Pattern Spectrum and Multiscale Shape Representation, IEEE trans. Pattern Analysis and Machine Intelligence, Vol. PAMI-11, No. 9, pp701-716, 1989

[Masutani96] Y. Masutani, et al. Region-Growing Based Feature Extraction Algorithm for Tree-like Objects, LNCS Vol. 1131, Proc. VBC '96, pp161-171, 1996

[Zahlten95] C. Zahlten, et al. Reconstruction of branching blood vessels from CT-data, Proc. 5th Eurographics Workshop on Visualization in Scientific Computing, pp41-52, 1995

[Schiemann92] T. Schiemann, et al. Interactive 3D-segmentation, SPIE Vol. 1808, Proc. VBC '92, pp376-383, 1992

[Sato98] Y. Sato, et al. Three-dimensional multi-scale line filter for segmentation and visualization of curvilinear structures in medical images, Medical Image Analysis vol.2, No.2, pp143-168, 1998

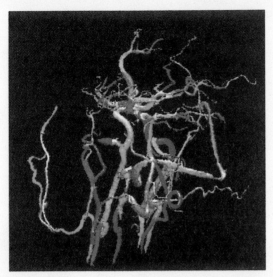
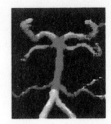

Segmented basilar arteries

Fig. 10. Clinical application results (1), Structures of cerebral arteries (MRA). After defining a seed, the whole object was structured as clusters and these were grouped into branches using the connectivity number (left: Branches are colored in repeated 12 colors). A part of the whole structure, basilar arteries are shown (right).

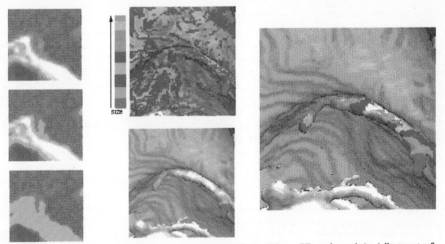

Fig. 11. Clinical application results (2), Bone structure avoidance (X-ray CT angiography). Adjustment of threshold values can not separate bone and vessels because of the partial volume effects (left). Using the threshold range shown in the bottom image (left), the morphological size was computed (middle upper). A seed area is given on the vessel (middle lower), the vessel was extracted (right, Clusters are shown in repeated 12 colors).

Author Index

Adachi, Y., 397
Adler, J., 241
Amini, A.A., 110, 167
Anderson, J.H., 404
Andresen, P.R., 710
Anno, H., 870
Aoyama, H., 926
Arnold, A.S., 539
Asano, T., 926
Atalar, E., 189
Ateshian, G.A., 9
Atsumi, H., 63, 74
Auberger, T., 352
Auer, T., 352
Avis, D., 650
Axel, L., 177
Ayache, N., 1115

Baguet, J.-P., 1049
Bakker, C.J.G., 317
Bale, R.J., 352
Bani-Hashemi, A., 119
Bansal, R., 1075
Barbe, C., 1041
Barillot, C., 509
Barnes, A., 197
Barth, K., 119
Barwise, J.A., 51
Bashein, G., 102
Bauer, J., 285
Bell, W., 899
Belliveau, J.W., 670
Bello, F., 964
Bender, H.-J., 679
Berger, M., 832
Bergmann, H., 343
Berman, L., 1016
Bettega, G., 21, 688
Bhalerao, A., 1205
Birkfellner, W., 343
Black, P., 63, 74
Blackwell, M., 232, 421
Blanchet, E., 269
Bland, P., 944
Blank, W., 899

Bloch, I., 489
Boes, J., 944
Bolson, E.L., 102
Bookstein, F.L., 788
Borup, D.T., 606
Bos, C., 317
Bosson, J.L., 1032
Brady, M., 499
Brammer, M.F., 842
Brechbuehler, C., 550
Bricault, I., 261
Brinkmann, B.H., 1087
Brucq, D. de, 562
Brunner, T., 119
Buatois, H., 269
Buchanan, T.S., 539
Bullitt, E., 952
Byrne, J., 814
Bzostek, A., 1041

Calmon, G., 761
Carrat, L., 84, 1041
Carroll, J.D., 377
Castellano Smith, A.D., 842
Chabrerie, A., 63, 74
Champleboux, G., 269
Chan, C., 1007
Chassat, F., 277
Chauhan, S., 386
Chavanon, O., 1041
Chen, S.-Y.J., 377
Chen, Y., 167
Chen, Z., 1075
Cheung, J., 822
Chirossel, J.-P., 84
Cinquin, P., 261, 1049
Cobb, J., 996
Cohen, Z.A., 9
Colchester, A.C.F., 469, 964
Colgan, B., 421
Collins, D.L., 509, 974
Colot, O., 562
Colucci, D., 934
Cornelius, N., 899
Coudert, J.L., 269

Coulon, O., 1230
Cox, T.C.S., 842
Crawford, J.R., 934
Crisco, J.J., 696, 1184

Dale, A.M., 670
Davatzikos, C., 531
Davies, B.L., 386, 996
DeJong, S.C., 146
Delaere, P., 918
Delp, S.L., 539
Desmedt, P., 1153
Devillers, S., 822
Devinoy, R., 562
Diaz, F., 253
DiGioia, A.M., 232, 421, 700
Dohi, T., 207, 215, 1067
Drake, S.H., 934
Duffy, F., 74
Duncan, J.S., 519, 641, 1075
Duncker, H.-R., 798
Durbhakula, M.M., 539
Duret, F., 732
Durlak, P., 119
Dutt, V., 606

Eberhardt, K.E.W., 660
Eguchi, K., 449
Ehman, R.L., 598, 606
Eichberger, P., 352
Ekatodramis, D., 578
Elayyadi, M., 110
Eldridge, P., 761
Ellis, R.E., 39
Elwes, R., 842
Emrich, R.J., 335
Enislidis, G., 343
Epitaux, M., 241
Ertl, T., 660
Etemad, M.E., 481
Ettinger, G., 63
Evans, A.C., 439, 509, 650, 974
Everett, P., 1
Ewers, R., 343

Faugeras, O., 1195
Felmlee, J.P., 598
Ferretti, G., 261
Fitzpatrick, J.M., 51
Fleute, M., 879

Forghani, R., 439
Fortin, T., 269
Frangi, A.F., 130
Freysinger, W., 352
Frouin, V., 489, 1134, 1230
Fuchs, H., 934
Furst, J.D., 780

Gaber, O., 352
Gaens, T., 1099
Garza-Jinich, M., 325
Gee, A., 1016
Gerig, G., 469, 578, 832
Gerritsen, F.A., 822
Gibson, S.F.F., 679, 888
Gieser, J., 910
Girod, B., 1
Golland, P., 720
González Ballester, M.Á., 499
Graumann, R., 119
Greenleaf, J.F., 606
Grimson, W.E.L., 63, 74, 457, 1057, 1195
Grzeszczuk, R., 241
Guan, C.G., 1007
Guimond, A., 631
Gunkel, A.R., 352
Guttmann, C.R.G., 469, 1107

Haber, E., 177
Hadley, S.W., 223
Halle, M., 720
Halperin, H., 189
Hansen, K.V., 305
Harris, S.J., 996
Harrison, M.M., 39
Hartov, A., 743
Hasboun, D., 1134
Hasegawa, J.-i., 870
Hashimoto, D., 207
Hastreiter, P., 660
Hata, N., 1067
Hattori, A., 397
Hawkes, D.J., 842, 1144, 1153
Hayes, C., 1144
Heinze, P., 1024
Helmers, S., 74
Henry, D., 1032
Henry, J.H., 9
Hensler, E., 352
Hern, N., 1007

Hibberd, R.D., 996
Hill, D.L.G., 51, 842, 1153
Hodgson, A.J., 335
Höhne, K.-H., 853, 1242
Holmes, G., 74
Hoogenboom, T., 317
Hoopes, J., 743
Horwitz, B., 623
Hutter, R., 550

Ikemoto, A., 397
Ikuta, K., 293, 411
Inkpen, K.B., 335
Ionescu, G., 1041
Iseki, H., 215

Jakopec, M., 996
Jan, U. von, 1024
Jaramaz, B., 421, 700
Ji, L.H., 215
Jiang, Z., 253
Johnson, L.S., 223
Jolesz, F., 74
Jolesz, F.A., 431, 926, 1067
Jones, T.N., 156
Joskowicz, L., 29, 325
Jumrussirikul, P., 189

Kainuma, O., 926
Kakinuma, R., 449
Kanade, T., 232
Kanazawa, K., 449
Kaneko, M., 449
Kaplan, C., 285
Kapur, T., 457
Katada, K., 870
Katila, T., 1213
Kato, T., 411
Kaus, M., 431
Kavoussi, L.R., 404
Kawata, Y., 449
Keeve, E., 74
Keller, K., 934
Kenmochi, T., 926
Kennedy, F., 743
Keriven, R., 1195
Kikinis, R., 1, 63, 74, 431, 457, 720, 861, 926, 1067, 1195, 1205
Kim, B., 944
Kimia, B.B., 1184

Kita, Y., 1125
Knisely, J., 1075
Kobayashi, E., 207
Kockro, R.A., 1007
Kreiborg, S., 710
Kriete, A., 798
Krummel, T., 899
Künzel, K.H., 352
Kumano, T., 397
Kutka, M., 197
Kyriacou, S.K., 531

Lardo, A.C., 189
Larsen, O.V., 305
Lavallée, S., 21, 84, 277, 879
Lazovic, D., 1024
Le Bihan, D., 489
Le Goualher, G., 509, 974
Leach, M., 1144
Lee, E.C.K., 1007
Lee, Y.H., 1007
Leventon, M.E., 63, 74, 1057
Li, D., 110
Li, Q., 253
Little, J.A., 1153
Liu, A.K., 670, 952
Livingston, M.A., 934
Lötjönen, J., 1213
Lorensen, W.E., 926
Lorigo, L.M., 1195
Lowe, M.J.S., 386
Lukas, P.H., 352

MacDonald, D., 650
Maciunas, R.J., 51
Männer, R., 679
Maes, F., 1099, 1222
Magnin, I.E., 1134, 1213
Makram-Ebeid, S., 822
Malandin, G., 1115
Mandal, C., 753
Manduca, A., 598, 606
Mangin, J.-F., 489, 1134, 1230
Mani, V., 167
Marchal, G., 918, 985
Martin, A., 352
Martin, R.W., 102
Masamune, K., 207, 215
Masutani, Y., 1242
Maurer, C.R., 51, 842

McCarthy, D.M., 9
McDonald, J., 102
McGee, K.P, 598
McGovern, R.D., 696
McInerney, T., 861
McVeigh, E., 189
Medioni, G., 732
Meijering, E.H.W., 590
Mendoza-Sagaon, M., 197
Merloz, P., 84
Metaxas, D.N., 156, 177
Meunier, J., 631
Meyer, A.A., 934
Meyer, C., 944
Miga, M., 743
Milgrom, C., 29, 325
Millis, M.B., 1
Mollard, B., 21
Moody Jr., J.E., 421
Moreau-Gaudry, A., 1049
Mori, K., 870
Moriyama, N., 449
Moul, J.W., 285, 358
Mow, V.C., 9
Mui, L., 1205
Mulet-Parada, M., 806
Mullan, B.P., 1087
Mun, S.K., 285, 358
Murray, W.M., 539
Muthupillai, R., 606

Nadar, M.S., 119
Nagata, S., 411
Nakagohri, T., 926
Nakajima, S., 63, 74
Namiki, T., 293
Nath, R., 1075
Navab, N., 119
Nenonen, J., 1213
Neumann, P.F., 910
Nielsen, M., 710
Niessen, W.J., 130, 138
Nijlunsing, P., 822
Niki, N., 449
Nikou, C., 232, 421, 700
Noble, J.A., 806, 814, 1125
Nowinski, W.L., 1007

O'Brien, T.J., 1087
O'Connor, M.K., 1087

O'Toole, R., 899
Ohmatsu, H., 449
Okuda, S., 926
Ottensmeyer, M.P., 368
Overhoff, H.M., 1024
Ozlen, F., 63, 74

Pachot-Clouard, M., 489
Paulsen, K., 743
Pavel, D.G., 623
Payan, Y., 688
Pelizzari, C.A., 223
Pennec, X., 1107, 1115
Penney, G.P., 1153
Pflesser B., 853
Pham, D.L., 481
Pichot, O., 1032
Pike, G.B., 614
Pittet, L., 84
Pizer, S.M., 780, 952
Playter, R., 899
Polkey, C.E., 842
Poorten, V.V., 918
Poulouse, B., 197
Poupon, C., 489, 1134
Poupon, F., 489, 1134
Prager, R., 1016
Prause, G.P.M., 146
Prima, S., 770
Prince, J.L., 481

Qin, H., 753
Quintana, J.C., 623

Rademacher, P., 934
Radeva, P., 110
Raibert, M., 899
Rangarajan, A., 1075
Raphaël, B., 688
Raskar, R., 934
Rau, W., 798
Régis, J., 489
Reissman, P.-J., 1213
Rezk-Salama, Ch., 660
Rhomberg, A., 550
Richolt, J.A., 1, 720, 1205
Riviello Jr., J., 74
Robb, R.A., 1087
Roberts, D., 743
Roberts, N., 761, 770

Roberts, W., 899
Roche, A., 1115
Rodkey, W.G., 9
Roglic, H., 9
Rohr, K., 1174
Royston, D., 814
Rudan, J., 39
Rueckert, D., 1144

Sadler, L.L., 910
Salinas, S., 539
Satoh, H., 449
Saxena, P., 623
Schiemann, T., 1242
Schill, M.A., 679
Schmid, P., 550
Schultz, R.T., 519
Schutyser, F., 918
Sebastian, T.B., 1184
Serra, L., 1007
Sesterhenn, I.A., 285, 358
Shahidi, R., 241
Sheehan, F.H., 102
Shenton, M.E., 720
Sheridan, T.B., 368
Simkin, A., 29, 325
Simmons, A., 842
Škrinjar, O., 641
Sled, J.J., 614
Smits, H.F.M., 317
Sombo, A., 562
Sonka, M., 146
Spencer, D., 641
Staib, L.H., 519, 1075, 1162
State, A., 934
Steadman, J.R., 9
Steenberghe, D. van, 985
Stoianovici, D., 404
Studholme, C., 1144
Subsol, G., 770
Suenaga, Y., 870
Suetens, P., 918, 985, 1099, 1222
Summers, P., 1144
Sun, J., 167
Suzuki, M., 215
Suzuki, N., 397
Szankay, A., 352
Székely, G., 469, 550, 578

Takakura, K., 215

Takatsu, A., 397
Takeichi, M., 293
Talamini, M., 197
Tang, C.-K., 732
Taylor, C.J., 570
Taylor, R.H., 197, 404
Tek, H., 1184
Teschner, M., 1
Thirion, J.-P., 631, 761, 770, 1107
Thompson, J.M., 368
Thumfart, W.F., 352
Tiede, U., 853
Tockus, L., 29
Tokoro, Y., 926
Tomandl, B., 660
Tonetti, J., 84
Toriwaki, J.-i., 870
Troccaz, J., 1032, 1041
Truppe, M., 343
Tso, C.Y., 39

Umans, C., 720

Vaals, J.J. van, 317
Van Cleynenbreugel, J., 918, 985
Van Leemput, K., 1222
Vandermeulen, D., 1099, 1222
Veldhuizen, A., 822
Vemuri, B.C., 753
Verdonck, B., 822
Verstreken, K., 985
Viergever, M.A., 130, 138, 317, 590
Vinas, F., 253
Vincken, K.L., 130
Vogele, M., 352

Wahle, A., 146
Wang, B., 241
Wang, M.Y., 51
Wang, Y., 358, 1162
Wanschitz, F., 343
Warfield, S.K., 431, 1067, 1205
Watz, H., 798
Watzinger, F., 343
Weese, J., 1153
Weide, R. van der, 317
Welch, E.B., 598
Wells, W.M., 457, 1067
Welti, D., 469
Westin, C.-F., 1205

Wever, D.J., 822
Whitcomb, L.L., 404
Wiesent, K., 119
Wilson, D.L., 814, 1125
Wink, O., 138
Wolfe, S.W., 696, 1184

Xu, C., 481
Xuan, J., 358

Yang, C., 197
Yaniv, Z., 325

Yeung, C., 189
Young, A.A., 92
Yu, D.N., 481

Zamorano, L., 253
Zeng, J., 285
Zeng, X., 519
Zijdenbos, A., 439
Zisserman, A., 499
Zuiderveld, K.J., 317, 590
Zwiggelaar, R., 570

Lecture Notes in Computer Science

For information about Vols. 1–1428

please contact your bookseller or Springer-Verlag

Vol. 1429: F. van der Linden (Ed.), Development and Evolution of Software Architectures for Product Families. Proceedings, 1998. IX, 258 pages. 1998.

Vol. 1430: S. Trigila, A. Mullery, M. Campolargo, H. Vanderstraeten, M. Mampaey (Eds.), Intelligence in Services and Networks: Technology for Ubiquitous Telecom Services. Proceedings, 1998. XII, 550 pages. 1998.

Vol. 1431: H. Imai, Y. Zheng (Eds.), Public Key Cryptography. Proceedings, 1998. XI, 263 pages. 1998.

Vol. 1432: S. Arnborg, L. Ivansson (Eds.), Algorithm Theory – SWAT '98. Proceedings, 1998. IX, 347 pages. 1998.

Vol. 1433: V. Honavar, G. Slutzki (Eds.), Grammatical Inference. Proceedings, 1998. X, 271 pages. 1998. (Subseries LNAI).

Vol. 1434: J.-C. Heudin (Ed.), Virtual Worlds. Proceedings, 1998. XII, 412 pages. 1998. (Subseries LNAI).

Vol. 1435: M. Klusch, G. Weiß (Eds.), Cooperative Information Agents II. Proceedings, 1998. IX, 307 pages. 1998. (Subseries LNAI).

Vol. 1436: D. Wood, S. Yu (Eds.), Automata Implementation. Proceedings, 1997. VIII, 253 pages. 1998.

Vol. 1437: S. Albayrak, F.J. Garijo (Eds.), Intelligent Agents for Telecommunication Applications. Proceedings, 1998. XII, 251 pages. 1998. (Subseries LNAI).

Vol. 1438: C. Boyd, E. Dawson (Eds.), Information Security and Privacy. Proceedings, 1998. XI, 423 pages. 1998.

Vol. 1439: B. Magnusson (Ed.), System Configuration Management. Proceedings, 1998. X, 207 pages. 1998.

Vol. 1440: K.S. McCurley, C.D. Ziegler (Eds.), Advances in Cryptology 1981 – 1997. Proceedings. Approx. XII, 260 pages. 1998.

Vol. 1441: W. Wobcke, M. Pagnucco, C. Zhang (Eds.), Agents and Multi-Agent Systems. Proceedings, 1997. XII, 241 pages. 1998. (Subseries LNAI).

Vol. 1442: A. Fiat. G.J. Woeginger (Eds.), Online Algorithms. XVIII, 436 pages. 1998.

Vol. 1443: K.G. Larsen, S. Skyum, G. Winskel (Eds.), Automata, Languages and Programming. Proceedings, 1998. XVI, 932 pages. 1998.

Vol. 1444: K. Jansen, J. Rolim (Eds.), Approximation Algorithms for Combinatorial Optimization. Proceedings, 1998. VIII, 201 pages. 1998.

Vol. 1445: E. Jul (Ed.), ECOOP'98 – Object-Oriented Programming. Proceedings, 1998. XII, 635 pages. 1998.

Vol. 1446: D. Page (Ed.), Inductive Logic Programming. Proceedings, 1998. VIII, 301 pages. 1998. (Subseries LNAI).

Vol. 1447: V.W. Porto, N. Saravanan, D. Waagen, A.E. Eiben (Eds.), Evolutionary Programming VII. Proceedings, 1998. XVI, 840 pages. 1998.

Vol. 1448: M. Farach-Colton (Ed.), Combinatorial Pattern Matching. Proceedings, 1998. VIII, 251 pages. 1998.

Vol. 1449: W.-L. Hsu, M.-Y. Kao (Eds.), Computing and Combinatorics. Proceedings, 1998. XII, 372 pages. 1998.

Vol. 1450: L. Brim, F. Gruska, J. Zlatuška (Eds.), Mathematical Foundations of Computer Science 1998. Proceedings, 1998. XVII, 846 pages. 1998.

Vol. 1451: A. Amin, D. Dori, P. Pudil, H. Freeman (Eds.), Advances in Pattern Recognition. Proceedings, 1998. XXI, 1048 pages. 1998.

Vol. 1452: B.P. Goettl, H.M. Halff, C.L. Redfield, V.J. Shute (Eds.), Intelligent Tutoring Systems. Proceedings, 1998. XIX, 629 pages. 1998.

Vol. 1453: M.-L. Mugnier, M. Chein (Eds.), Conceptual Structures: Theory, Tools and Applications. Proceedings, 1998. XIII, 439 pages. (Subseries LNAI).

Vol. 1454: I. Smith (Ed.), Artificial Intelligence in Structural Engineering. XI, 497 pages. 1998. (Subseries LNAI).

Vol. 1456: A. Drogoul, M. Tambe, T. Fukuda (Eds.), Collective Robotics. Proceedings, 1998. VII, 161 pages. 1998. (Subseries LNAI).

Vol. 1457: A. Ferreira, J. Rolim, H. Simon, S.-H. Teng (Eds.), Solving Irregularly Structured Problems in Prallel. Proceedings, 1998. X, 408 pages. 1998.

Vol. 1458: V.O. Mittal, H.A. Yanco, J. Aronis, R-. Simpson (Eds.), Assistive Technology in Artificial Intelligence. X, 273 pages. 1998. (Subseries LNAI).

Vol. 1459: D.G. Feitelson, L. Rudolph (Eds.), Job Scheduling Strategies for Parallel Processing. Proceedings, 1998. VII, 257 pages. 1998.

Vol. 1460: G. Quirchmayr, E. Schweighofer, T.J.M. Bench-Capon (Eds.), Database and Expert Systems Applications. Proceedings, 1998. XVI, 905 pages. 1998.

Vol. 1461: G. Bilardi, G.F. Italiano, A. Pietracaprina, G. Pucci (Eds.), Algorithms – ESA'98. Proceedings, 1998. XII, 516 pages. 1998.

Vol. 1462: H. Krawczyk (Ed.), Advances in Cryptology - CRYPTO '98. Proceedings, 1998. XII, 519 pages. 1998.

Vol. 1463: N.E. Fuchs (Ed.), Logic Program Synthesis and Transformation. Proceedings, 1997. X, 343 pages. 1998.

Vol. 1464: H.H.S. Ip, A.W.M. Smeulders (Eds.), Multimedia Information Analysis and Retrieval. Proceedings, 1998. VIII, 264 pages. 1998.

Vol. 1465: R. Hirschfeld (Ed.), Financial Cryptography. Proceedings, 1998. VIII, 311 pages. 1998.

Vol. 1466: D. Sangiorgi, R. de Simone (Eds.), CONCUR'98: Concurrency Theory. Proceedings, 1998. XI, 657 pages. 1998.

Vol. 1467: C. Clack, K. Hammond, T. Davie (Eds.), Implementation of Functional Languages. Proceedings, 1997. X, 375 pages. 1998.

Vol. 1468: P. Husbands, J.-A. Meyer (Eds.), Evolutionary Robotics. Proceedings, 1998. VIII, 247 pages. 1998.

Vol. 1469: R. Puigjaner, N.N. Savino, B. Serra (Eds.), Computer Performance Evaluation. Proceedings, 1998. XIII, 376 pages. 1998.

Vol. 1470: D. Pritchard, J. Reeve (Eds.), Euro-Par'98: Parallel Processing. Proceedings, 1998. XXII, 1157 pages. 1998.

Vol. 1471: J. Dix, L. Moniz Pereira, T.C. Przymusinski (Eds.), Logic Programming and Knowledge Representation. Proceedings, 1997. IX, 246 pages. 1998. (Subseries LNAI).

Vol. 1473: X. Leroy, A. Ohori (Eds.), Types in Compilation. Proceedings, 1998. VIII, 299 pages. 1998.

Vol. 1474: F. Mueller, A. Bestavros (Eds.), Languages, Compilers, and Tools for Embedded Systems. Proceedings, 1998. XIV, 261 pages. 1998.

Vol. 1475: W. Litwin, T. Morzy, G. Vossen (Eds.), Advances in Databases and Information Systems. Proceedings, 1998. XIV, 369 pages. 1998.

Vol. 1476: J. Calmet, J. Plaza (Eds.), Artificial Intelligence and Symbolic Computation. Proceedings, 1998. XI, 309 pages. 1998. (Subseries LNAI).

Vol. 1477: K. Rothermel, F. Hohl (Eds.), Mobile Agents. Proceedings, 1998. VIII, 285 pages. 1998.

Vol. 1478: M. Sipper, D. Mange, A. Pérez-Uribe (Eds.), Evolvable Systems: From Biology to Hardware. Proceedings, 1998. IX, 382 pages. 1998.

Vol. 1479: J. Grundy, M. Newey (Eds.), Theorem Proving in Higher Order Logics. Proceedings, 1998. VIII, 497 pages. 1998.

Vol. 1480: F. Giunchiglia (Ed.), Artificial Intelligence: Methodology, Systems, and Applications. Proceedings, 1998. IX, 502 pages. 1998. (Subseries LNAI).

Vol. 1481: E.V. Munson, C. Nicholas, D. Wood (Eds.), Principles of Digital Document Processing. Proceedings, 1998. VII, 152 pages. 1998.

Vol. 1482: R.W. Hartenstein, A. Keevallik (Eds.), Field-Programmable Logic and Applications. Proceedings, 1998. XI, 533 pages. 1998.

Vol. 1483: T. Plagemann, V. Goebel (Eds.), Interactive Distributed Multimedia Systems and Telecommunication Services. Proceedings, 1998. XV, 326 pages. 1998.

Vol. 1484: H. Coelho (Ed.), Progress in Artificial Intelligence – IBERAMIA 98. Proceedings, 1998. XIII, 421 pages. 1998. (Subseries LNAI).

Vol. 1485: J.-J. Quisquater, Y. Deswarte, C. Meadows, D. Gollmann (Eds.), Computer Security – ESORICS 98. Proceedings, 1998. X, 377 pages. 1998.

Vol. 1486: A.P. Ravn, H. Rischel (Eds.), Formal Techniques in Real-Time and Fault-Tolerant Systems. Proceedings, 1998. VIII, 339 pages. 1998.

Vol. 1487: V. Gruhn (Ed.), Software Process Technology. Proceedings, 1998. VIII, 157 pages. 1998.

Vol. 1488: B. Smyth, P. Cunningham (Eds.), Advances in Case-Based Reasoning. Proceedings, 1998. XI, 482 pages. 1998. (Subseries LNAI).

Vol. 1489: J. Dix, L. Fariñas del Cerro, U. Furbach (Eds.), Logics in Artificial Intelligence. Proceedings, 1998. X, 391 pages. 1998. (Subseries LNAI).

Vol. 1490: C. Palamidessi, H. Glaser, K. Meinke (Eds.), Principles of Declarative Programming. Proceedings, 1998. XI, 497 pages. 1998.

Vol. 1493: J.P. Bowen, A. Fett, M.G. Hinchey (Eds.), ZUM '98: The Z Formal Specification Notation. Proceedings, 1998. XV, 417 pages. 1998.

Vol. 1495: T. Andreasen, H. Christiansen, H.L. Larsen (Eds.), Flexible Query Answering Systems. IX, 393 pages. 1998. (Subseries LNAI).

Vol. 1496: W.M. Wells, A. Colchester, S. Delp (Eds.), Medical Image Computing and Computer-Assisted Intervention – MICCAI'98. Proceedings, 1998. XXII, 1256 pages. 1998.

Vol. 1497: V. Alexandrov, J. Dongarra (Eds.), Recent Advances in Parallel Virtual Machine and Message Passing Interface. Proceedings, 1998. XII, 412 pages. 1998.

Vol. 1498: A.E. Eiben, T. Bäck, M. Schoenauer, H.-P. Schwefel (Eds.), Parallel Problem Solving from Nature – PPSN V. Proceedings, 1998. XXIII, 1041 pages. 1998.

Vol. 1499: S. Kutten (Ed.), Distributed Computing. Proceedings, 1998. XII, 419 pages. 1998.

Vol. 1501: M.M. Richter, C.H. Smith, R. Wiehagen, T. Zeugmann (Eds.), Algorithmic Learning Theory. Proceedings, 1998. XI, 439 pages. 1998. (Subseries LNAI).

Vol. 1502: G. Antoniou, J. Slaney (Eds.), Advanced Topics in Artificial Intelligence. Proceedings, 1998. XI, 333 pages. 1998. (Subseries LNAI).

Vol. 1503: G. Levi (Ed.), Static Analysis. Proceedings, 1998. IX, 383 pages. 1998.

Vol. 1504: O. Herzog, A. Günter (Eds.), KI-98: Advances in Artificial Intelligence. Proceedings, 1998. XI, 355 pages. 1998. (Subseries LNAI).

Vol. 1508: S. Jajodia, M.T. Özsu, A. Dogac (Eds.), Advances in Multimedia Information Systems. Proceedings, 1998. VIII, 207 pages. 1998.

Vol. 1510: J.M. Zytkow, M. Quafafou (Eds.), Principles of Data Mining and Knowledge Discovery. Proceedings, 1998. XI, 482 pages. 1998. (Subseries LNAI).

Vol. 1511: D. O'Hallaron (Ed.), Languages, Compilers, and Run-Time Systems for Scalable Computers.

Vol. 1512: E. Giménez, C. Paulin-Mohring (Eds.), Types for Proofs and Programs. Proceedings, 1996. VIII, 373 pages. 1998.

Vol. 1513: C. Nikolaou, C. Stephanidis (Eds.), Research and Advanced Technology for Digital Libraries. Proceedings, 1998. XV, 912 pages. 1998.

Vol. 1514: K. Ohta,, D. Pei (Eds.), Advances in Cryptology – ASIACRYPT'98. Proceedings, 1998. XII, 436 pages. 1998.

Vol. 1516: W. Ehrenberger (Ed.), Computer Safety, Reliability and Security. Proceedings, 1998. XVI, 392 pages. 1998.

Vol. 1518: M. Luby, J. Rolim, M. Serna (Eds.), Randomization and Approximation Techniques in Computer Science. Proceedings, 1998. IX, 385 pages. 1998.